Primer of
Diagnostic
Imaging
Third Edition

Ralph Weissleder, M.D., Ph.D.

Professor
Harvard Medical School;
Radiologist
Massachusetts General Hospital
Boston, Massachusetts

Jack Wittenberg, M.D.

Professor
Harvard Medical School;
Radiologist
Massachusetts General Hospital
Boston, Massachusetts

Mukesh G. Harisinghani, M.D.

Assistant Professor
Harvard Medical School;
Assistant Radiologist
Massachusetts General Hospital
Boston, Massachusetts

with 1,815 illustrations

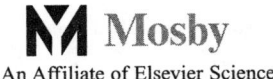 Mosby

An Affiliate of Elsevier Science

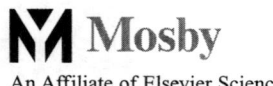

An Affiliate of Elsevier Science

The Curtis Center
Independence Square West
Philadelphia, Pennsylvania 19106

PRIMER OF DIAGNOSTIC IMAGING   ISBN 0-323-02328-2
Third Edition

Editor: Janice M. Gaillard
Senior Developmental Editor: Hazel Hacker
Editorial Assistant: Danielle Burke

TG/QWV

Printed in the United States of America

Last digit is the print number: 9 8 7 6 5 4 3 2 1

Primer of
Diagnostic
Imaging

*To all the radiologists whose
knowledge, research, and wisdom contributed to this book.*

Reviewers

A number of present and former (*) staff members of the Department of Radiology, Massachusetts General Hospital, have reviewed and contributed to the different editions of *Primer of Diagnostic Imaging*. Our special thanks goes to Mark Rieumont, who was Associate Editor of the second edition of the *Primer*.

Chest Imaging

Meenakshi P. Bhalla, M.D.*
Theresa C. McLoud, M.D.
Jo-Anne O. Shepard, M.D.

Cardiac Imaging

Farouc Jaffer, M.D.
Stephen W. Miller, M.D.*

Gastrointestinal Imaging

Peter R. Mueller, M.D.

Genitourinary Imaging

Debra A. Gervais, M.D.
Michael J. Lee, M.D.*
Nicholas Papanicolaou, M.D.*

Musculoskeletal Imaging

Felix S. Chew, M.D.*
Damian E. Dupuy, M.D.*
James T. Rhea, M.D.

Obstetric-Gynecologic Imaging

Genevieve L. Bennett, M.D.*
Deborah A. Hall, M.D.

Mammography

Debra A. Gervais, M.D.
Daniel B. Kopans, M.D.

Neuroradiology

Bradley R. Buchbinder, M.D.
Kenneth R. Davis, M.D.
R. Gilberto Gonzalez, M.D., Ph.D.
Michel H. Lev, M.D.
Pamela W. Schaefer, M.D.
David Schellingerhout, M.D.

Head and Neck Imaging

P. Pearse Morris, M.D.*
David Schellingerhout, M.D.
Daniel Silverstone, M.D.*
Alfred L. Weber, M.D.*

Vascular Imaging

Stuart C. Geller, M.D.
John A. Kaufman, M.D.*

Pediatric Imaging

Johan G. Blickman, M.D., Ph.D.*
Robert T. Bramson, M.D.*
Susan Connolly, M.D.

Nuclear Medicine

Edward E. Webster, Ph.D.*
Edwin L. Palmer, M.D.

Physics

Ronald J. Callahan, Ph.D.
Edward E. Webster, Ph.D.*
Umar Mahmood, Ph.D., M.D.

General Comments

Jerry Glowniak, M.D.
Ross Titon, M.D.
Arastoo Vossough, M.D., Ph.D.

Preface

Current, comprehensive, and *clinically revelant.* With these "C" words in mind, we offer our newest edition. Staying current is the major impetus, mindful that magnetic resonance imaging (MRI) is now nudging its way into many subspecialties other than neuroradiological and musculoskeletal imaging. We have made every effort to update information in these latter subspecialties and indicate where MRI is staking its toehold in the remainder. Since newer computed tomographic (CT) techniques have also affected our practice, additional information on the impact of multislice helical technology has been added. We recognize that the book is approaching the upper limits of portability but have deleted little in an effort to comply with our intention of the other "C" words.

We welcome Dr. Mukesh Harisinghani as our new co-author. Dr. Harisinghani brings additional knowledge, careful review of content, and enthusiasm with him. He has an authoritative background in MRI and CT imaging. As before, many other colleagues in our and other departments have added comments and peer reviews. Their acknowledgments in the list of contributors always seems to fall short of the thanks we owe them.

We hope this new edition fulfills your every expectation.

Ralph Weissleder
Jack Wittenberg
Mukesh G. Harisinghani

Preface to the First Edition

The idea for this work began when one of us (RW) contemplated the enormity of material one needed to master during the radiology residency. A strategy was called for that would enhance retention of facts, techniques, and images and simplify their recall when, inevitably, they were forgotten. Thus was born the discipline at the end of each workday of computer processing important material, along with an accompanying sketch or two if sleep didn't intervene. At the very least it would be there in the computer for review those last 6 months before "Armageddon"; at the least it might help future Massachusetts General Hospital (MGH) residents. Five years later it all seems justified.

The MGH curriculum provides for rotations through all subspecialty divisions, 4 weeks at a time. A minimum of three staff and often several fellows comprise a subspecialty division, providing a wealth of educational resources. The information you find here is basically a distillation of teaching from these radiologists supplemented by reading. Already you can recognize the potential for bias. Aside from the fellows who have trained elsewhere, much of what you will read in this book has the threat of being overly inbred. We have worked hard to avoid this pitfall. The decision as to what to include, emphasize, illustrate with a drawing, append as a pearl or two, is largely from a resident's point of view, although certainly influenced by the senior author. It's an eye on the average working day spent at a viewbox or passing needles and catheters, practical and functional. The emphasis is on the fundamentals, trying to give "low tech" its rightful place alongside the "high tech" of CT and MR. The more lengthy differential diagnostic lists and occasional appended esoteria come mostly from night and weekend refinements. By the third rotation in the fourth year, an organization of the assembled facts began to take place; the lean, bullet-type textual format served for a quick and efficient review. The leanness of the format was also gratefully received by divisional staff, who agreed to sacrifice precious summer hours to reassure us they had not been misquoted. The oft-repeated comment was, "It's like a record of my daily words being played back to me."

One of the unique strengths of this offering is the anatomic drawings, which one of us (JW) had nothing to contribute to other than sharpening pencils for the other (RW). Visuals are the critical other language of radiologic education. Unquestioned reliance on the specificity of an image suffers from the perils of an Aunt Minnie approach, but it's a good starting point to be able to recognize the variations in all her siblings. Furthermore, a drawing will never substitute for the hard copy. We hope that sort of companion tool will soon follow, perhaps in a suitable handy electronic form.

The format and size of the book are specifically designed to be a handy, readily available refresher of important signs, anatomic landmarks, common radiopathologic alterations, and practical differential diagnoses. It is not intended as a long-range substitute for the kind of sophisticated pathophysiologic, clinical information one needs to be the most effective radiologist. As the title indicates, we intend to prime the pump of intellectual curiosity. That quality of information comes from reading the more in-depth radiologic and other medical literature. Our judgment is that having mastered the information herein, you should certainly have enough information to intelligently and wisely discuss radiologic interpretation. However, a rich exchange with the internist, surgeon, neurologist, or obstetrician demands a mastering of much more material than you will find in this book.

It is critical that the authors be scrupulous in their acknowledgment of their sources of information. If we fail to do so with any of our resources, it is not out of immodesty or unintended claims of original material. The proffered information, while largely accumulated over 5 years, certainly represents a body of work (and therefore workers) that spans almost a century now. We have tried to filter out folklore and myths, but you know very well that much of what we all say, repeat, defend is experiential and not always defensible on the basis of sensitivity, specificity, and accuracy of data. We have intended to describe information that we feel there are reasonable facts to support. If true data go unreferenced, however, we hope those authorities who recognize a little of their personal experience accept the unintended oversight as a mandate of the leanness and intent of our style.

It would be imprudent and graceless for us not to acknowledge some of the more local sources of major information. We are pretty sure that much of what we describe began with Drs. George Holmes and Aubrey Hampton; we recognize with clear certainty the leadership role in radiology of Drs. Laurence Robbins, Juan Taveras, and James Thrall. The most identifiable contributors are the present, often quoted, staff of our department. We are eternally grateful for their tireless daily educational tours de force and, in particular, thank those acknowledged contributors who took the time to review in detail the text we took from their lips. The many textbooks that served us particularly well in providing a bounty of useful information are listed in the Suggested Readings sections at the end of each chapter. These books were consulted, and information contained therein has been amalgamated with MGH teaching to provide a more seamless, complete, and less biased description of radiologic features. Lecture notes have been particularly helpful in distilling more complex information into readable text. After 5 years of compilation it is impossible to accurately trace each individual source of information.

Ralph Weissleder
Jack Wittenberg

Preface to the Second Edition

The second edition of the *Primer of Diagnostic Imaging* follows closely on the heels of the first to make up for our original gaps, omissions, and inconsistencies. In an attempt to provide as many fundamentals as possible the first time around, we emphasized certain modalities over others, but this time we have expanded on the newer modalities such as MRI and CT. We have also added new and updated graphics based on the positive feedback from the first edition. We hope these changes improve on our intent to provide a comprehensive review of radiology for residents, fellows, and possibly board certified radiologists. The differential diagnosis sections now follow after each chapter rather than being aggregated at the end of the book. Finally, we have recruited a co-editor. Dr. Mark Rieumont, a recent ABR-minted radiologist and colleague, provides the balance of currency, perspective, focus, and feedback that sometimes eludes grizzly veterans.

What has fortunately not changed is the dedication of our MGH colleagues to peer review our material. We are extremely grateful to all of them for keeping us from making serious gaffes. Our lean style of bulletlike factual presentation persists to fill our perceived need for a comprehensive yet digestible source of information. While style of curricula certainly vary among institutions, the basic fund of knowledge composing a curriculum should remain reasonably constant. A reminder of caution: this work should be viewed as a necessary infrastructure upon which we all must build a sophisticated superstructure of medical information.

Ralph Weissleder
Mark Rieumont
Jack Wittenberg

Contents

Abbreviations

5-HIAA = 5-hydroxyindoleacetric acid
AA = aortic arch
Aa = alveolar-arterial PO_2 difference
AAA = abdominal aortic aneurysm
ABC = aneurysmal bone cyst
ABPA = allergic bronchopulmonary aspergillosis
ABS = amniotic band syndrome
AC = acromioclavicular
ACA = anterior cerebral artery
ACC = agenesis of corpus callosum
ACL = anterior cruciate ligament
ACTH = adrenocorticotropic hormone
AD = abdominal diameter; autosomal dominant; average distance
ADEM = acute disseminated encephalomyelitis
ADH = antidiuretic hormone
AFL = air fluid level
AFP = alpha-fetoprotein
AFV = amniotic fluid volume
AHD = acquired heart disease
AICA = anterior inferior cerebellar artery
AICD = automatic intracardial defibrillation
AIDS = acquired immunodeficiency syndrome
AMI = acute myocardial infarction
AML = angiomyolipoma; anterior mitral leaflet
ANCA = antineutrophil cytoplasmic antibody
AP = anterior-posterior
APKD = adult polycystic kidney disease
APUD = amine precursor uptake and decarboxylation
AR = autosomal recessive
ARDS = acquired respiratory distress syndrome
AS = ankylosing spondylitis; aortic stenosis
ASA = anterior spinal artery
ASD = air space disease; atrial septal defect
ATN = acute tubular necrosis
AV = arteriovenous; atrioventricular
AVM = arteriovenous malformation

AVN = avascular necrosis
BBBD = blood-brain barrier disruption
BCP = basic calcium phosphate
BCS = Budd-Chiari syndrome
BE = barium enema
BFM = bronchopulmonary foregut malformation
BHCG = beta–human chorionic gonadotropin
BIP = bronchiolitis obliterans interstitial
BOOP = bronchiolitis obliterans and organizing pneumonia
BPD = bronchopulmonary dysplasia; biparietal diameter
BPF = bronchopleural fistula
BPH = benign prostatic hyperplasia
BRBPR = bright red blood per rectum
C-section = cesarean section
CA = carcinoma
CABG = coronary artery bypass graft
CAD = coronary artery disease
CAH = chronic active hepatitis
CBD = common bile duct
CC = craniocaudad
CCA = common carotid artery
CCAM = congenital cystic adenoid malformation of the lung
CCF = carotid cavernous sinus fistula
CCK = cholecystokinin
CCU = coronary care unit
CD4 = cluster designation 4 antigen
CDH = congenital dislocation of the hip
CECT = contrast enhanced CT
CFA = cryptogenic fibrosing alveolitis
CHA = calcium hydroxyapatite; common hepatic artery
CHD = congenital heart disease
CHF = congestive heart failure
CI = cardiothoracic index
CLC = corpus luteum cyst

CMC = carpometacarpal joint
CMD = corticomedullary differentiation
CMV = cytomegalovirus
CNS = central nervous system
COPD = chronic obstructive pulmonary disease
CP = cerebellopontine
CPA = cerebellopontine angle
CPPD = calcium pyrophosphate dihydrate
CREST = calcinosis, Raynaud's esophageal dysmotility, sclerodactyly, telangiectasia
CRL = crown-rump length
CSF = cerebrospinal fluid
CT = computed tomography
CTAP = CT arterial portography
CVA = cerebrovascular accident
CVS = chorionic villous sampling
CWP = coal worker's pneumoconiosis
CXR = chest radiograph
D-TGA = complete transposition of great arteries
DA = double arch
DAI = diffuse axonal injury
DCIS = ductal carcinoma in situ
DDX = differential diagnosis
DES = diffuse esophageal spasm
DIC = disseminated intravascular coagulation
DIP = distal interphalangeal joint
DISH = diffuse idiopathic skeletal hyperostosis
DJD = degenerative joint disease
DM = diabetes mellitus
DNA = deoxyribonucleic acid
DORV = double outlet right ventricle
DSA = digital subtraction angiography
DTPA = diethylenetriaminepentaacetic acid
DVT = deep vein thrombosis
DW = Dandy Walker
EA = esophageal atresia
EAC = external auditory canal
EBV = Epstein-Barr virus
ECA = external carotid artery
ECD = endocardial cushion defect
ECG = electrocardiogram
ECMO = extracorporeal membrane oxygenation
EDV = end-diastolic volume
EF = ejection fraction
EFW = estimated fetal weight
EG = eosinophilic granuloma
ERCP = endoscopic retrograde cholangiopancreatography
ERPF = effective renal plasma flow
ESR = erythrocyte sedimentation rate
ESV = end-systolic volume

ET = endotracheal tube
EVR = expiratory reserve volume
FCD = fibrous cortical defect
FL = femur length
FMC = focal myometrial contraction
FMD = fibromuscular dysplasia
FNH = focal nodular hypoplasia
FSE = fast spin echo
FTA-ABS = fluorescent treponemal antibody absorption (test)
GB = gallbladder
GBM = glio-blastoma multiforme
GBPS = gated blood pool study
GCT = giant cell tumor
Gd = gadolinium
GDA = gastroduodenal artery
GE = gastroesophageal
GEJ = gastroesophageal junction
GFR = glomerular filtration rate
GI = gastrointestinal
GIP = giant cell interstitial pneumonia
GM = gray matter
GSD = genetically significant dose
GTD = gestational trophoblastic disease
GU = genitourinary
GvH = graft versus host
GWM = gray-white matter
HA = hepatic artery
HbAS = sickle cell trait
HbSS = sickle cell disease
HC = head circumference
HCC = hepatocellular carcinoma
HCG = human chorionic gonadotropin
HD = Hunter and Driffield
HGH = human growth hormone
HIDA = hepatic iminodiacetic acid derivative
HIV = human immunodeficiency virus
HLA = human leukocyte antigen
HMD = hyaline membrane disease
HPO = hypertrophic pulmonary osteoarthropathy
HPS = hypertrophic pyloric stenosis
HPT = hyperparathyroidism
HR = heart rate
HRCT = high-resolution CT
HSV = herpes simplex virus
HU = Houndsfield unit
HVL = half-value layer
IAA = interruption of aortic arch
IABP = intraaortic balloon pump
IAC = internal auditory canal

IBD =	inflammatory bowel disease
ICA =	internal carotid artery
ICU =	intensive care unit
ICV =	internal cerebral vein
ID =	internal diameter
IDA =	iminodiacetic acid
IG =	immunoglobulin
IgG =	immunoglobulin G
IHF =	immune hydrops fetalis
IHSS =	idiopathic hypertrophic subaortic stenosis
IJV =	internal jugular vein
IL-2 =	interlukin-2
IMA =	inferior mesenteric artery
IMV =	internal mammary vein
INF =	inferior
INH =	isoniazid
IPKD =	infantile polycystic kidney disease
IRV =	inspiratory reserve volume
IUGR =	intrauterine growth retardation
IV =	intravenous
IVC =	inferior vena cava
IVDA =	intravenous drug abuse(r)
IVP =	intravenous pyelogram
IVS =	interventricular septum
JRA =	juvenile rheumatoid arthritis
KS =	Kaposi sarcoma
kVp =	kilovolt (peak)
L =	left
L-TGA =	corrected transposition of great arteries
LA =	left atrium
LAD =	left anterior descending
LAM =	lymphangioleiomyomatosis
LAO =	left anterior oblique
LBBB =	left bundle branch block
LBWC =	limb body wall complex
LCA =	left carotid artery; left coronary artery
LCIS =	lobular cancer in situ
LCP =	Legg-Calvé-Perthes disease
LCX =	left circumflex artery
LDH =	lactate dehydrogenase
LES =	lower esophageal sphincter
LET =	linear energy transfer
LFT =	liver function test
LGA =	large for gestational age; left gastric artery
LHA =	left hepatic artery
LIMA =	left internal mammary artery
LIP =	lymphocytic interstitial pneumonia
LL =	lower lobe
LLL =	left lower lobe
LMB =	left mainstem bronchus
LMP =	last menstrual period
LN =	lymph node
LOCA =	low osmolar contrast agents
LPO =	left posterior oblique
LPV =	left portal vein
L-R shunt =	left-to-right shunt
LSA =	left subclavian artery
LUL =	left upper lobe
LUQ =	left upper quadrant
LUS =	lower uterine segment
LV =	left ventricle
LVH =	left ventricular hypertrophy
mA =	milliampere
MA =	meconium aspiration; milliampere seconds
MAA =	macroaggregated albumin
MAG =	methyl-acetyl-gly
MAG$_3$ =	methyl-acetyl-gly-gly-gly
MAI =	*Mycobacterium avium intracellulare*
MALT =	mucosa-associated lymphoid tissue
MAO =	monoamine oxidase inhibitor
mAs =	milliampere second
MCA =	middle cerebral artery
MCD =	medullary cystic disease
MCDK =	multicystic dysplastic kidney
MCTD =	mixed connective tissue disease
MCV =	middle cerebral vein
MDP =	methylene diphosphonate
MEN =	multiple endocrine neoplasia
MFH =	malignant fibrous histiocytoma
MGH =	Massachusetts General Hospital
MI =	myocardial infarction
MIBI =	methoxyisobutylisonitrile
MIBG =	meta-iodobenzyl guanidine
MLD =	maximum transverse diameter to left from midline
MLO =	mediolateral oblique
MNG =	multinodular goiter
MOCE =	multiple osteocartilaginous exostoses
MOM =	multiples of median
MRA =	magnetic resonance angiography
MRI =	magnetic resonance imaging
MRSA =	methicillin-resistant *Staphylococcus aureus*
MRV =	magnetic resonance venography
MS =	multiple sclerosis
MSAFP =	maternal serum alpha-fetoprotein
MSD =	mean sac diameter
MT =	magnetization transfer
MTP =	metatarsal phalangeal joint

MVA =	motor vehicle accident		**PIE** =	pulmonary interstitial emphysema
MW =	molecular weight		**PIOPED** =	prospective investigation of pulmonary embolus detection
N =	nerve (cranial)			
NEMD =	nonspecific esophageal motility disorders		**PIP** =	postinflammatory polyps; proximal interphalangeal joint
NEC =	necrotizing enterocolitis		**PMC** =	pseudomembranous colitis
NF1 =	neurofibromatosis, type 1		**PMF** =	progressive massive fibrosis
NF2 =	neurofibromatosis, type 2		**PMHR** =	predicted maximal heart rate
NG =	nasogastric		**PML** =	posterior mitral leaflet; progressive multifocal leukoencephalopathy
NH =	nonhereditary			
NHL =	non-Hodgkins lymphoma		**PMT** =	photomultiplier tube
NIHF =	nonimmune hydrops fetalis		**PNET** =	primitive neuroectodermal tumor
NOF =	nonossifying fibroma		**PO$_2$** =	oxygen tension
NP =	neonatal pneumonia		**PRL** =	prolactin
NPO =	fasting		**PROM** =	premature rupture of membranes
NSAIDs =	nonsteroidal antiinflammatory drugs		**PSS** =	progressive systemic sclerosis
NTBM =	nontuberculous mycobacteria		**PT** =	prothrombin time
OA =	osteoarthritis		**PTA** =	percutaneous transluminal angioplasty
OEIS =	omphalocele, exstrophy, imperforate anus, special anomaly		**PTH** =	parathormone
			PTT =	partial thromboplastin time
OFD =	occipitofrontal diameter		**PTU** =	propylthiouracil
OIC =	osteogenesis imperfecta congenita		**PUD** =	peptic ulcer disease
OIT =	osteogenesis imperfecta tarda		**PUL** =	percutaneous uretero lithotomy
OMC =	osteomeatal complex		**PUV** =	posterior urethral valves
ORIF =	open reduction and internal fixation		**PV** =	portal vein
OSA =	osteosarcoma		**PVH** =	pulmonary venous hypertension
PA =	posterior-anterior; pulmonary artery		**PVNS** =	pigmented villonodular synovitis
PAH =	pulmonary arterial hypertension		**PWMA** =	periventricular white matter abnormality
PAN =	polyarteritis nodosa			
PAPVC =	partial anomalous pulmonary venous connection		**R** =	right
			RA =	right atrium; rheumatoid arthritis
PAVM =	pulmonary arteriovenous malformation		**RAO** =	right anterior oblique
PC =	phase contrast		**RBBB** =	right bundle branch block
PCA =	posterior cerebral artery		**RBC** =	red blood cell(s)
PCL =	posterior cruciate ligament		**RBE** =	relative biologic effectiveness
PCN =	percutaneous nephrostomy		**RCA** =	right carotid artery; right coronary artery
PCO =	polycystic ovary			
PCP =	*Pneumocystis carinii* pneumonia		**RCC** =	renal cell carcinoma
PDA =	persistent patent ductus arteriosus		**RDS** =	respiratory distress syndrome
PDW =	proton density weighted		**RES** =	reticuloendothelial system
PE =	pulmonary embolism		**RF** =	rheumatoid factor
PEEP =	positive end-expiratory pressure		**RGA** =	right gastric artery
PET =	positron emission tomography		**Rh** =	rhesus factor
PFA =	profunda femoral artery		**RHA** =	right hepatic artery
PFC =	persistent fetal circulation		**RIMA** =	right internal mammary artery
PGE$_1$ =	prostaglandin E-1		**R-L shunt** =	right-to-left shunt
PHA =	pulse height analyzer		**RLQ** =	right lower quadrant
PHS =	pulse height selector		**RMB** =	right mainstem bronchus
PICA =	posterior inferior cerebellar artery		**RML** =	right middle lobe
PID =	pelvic inflammatory disease		**RNA** =	ribonucleic acid
			RPN =	renal papillary necrosis

RPO =	right posterior oblique
RPV =	right portal vein
RSA =	right subclavian artery
RSV =	respiratory syncytial virus
RT =	radiotherapy
RTA =	renal tubular acidosis
RTPA =	recombinant tissue plasminogen activator
RUL =	right upper lobe
RUQ =	right upper quadrant
RV =	right ventricle
RVA =	right vertebral artery
RVT =	renal vein thrombosis
S/P =	status post
SA =	sinoatrial
SAH =	subarachnoid hemorrhage
SB =	small bowel
SBFT =	small bowel follow-through
SBO =	small bowel obstruction
SC =	subcutaneous
SCA =	superior cerebellar artery
SCC =	squamous cell carcinoma
SCFE =	slipped capital femoral epiphysis
SCG =	small for gestational age
SD =	standard deviation
SDAT =	senile dementia Alzheimer's type
SDH =	subdural hematoma
SE =	spin echo
SFA =	superior femoral artery
SGOT =	serum glutamic-oxaloacetic transaminase
SI =	sacroiliac; signal intensity
SK =	streptokinase
SL =	sublingual
SLE =	systemic lupus erythematosus
SMA =	superior mesenteric artery
SNR =	signal-to-noise ratio
SPECT =	single photon emission computed tomography
ST =	ST complex on EKG
SUP =	superior
SVC =	superior vena cava
T1W =	T1 weighted (images)
T2W =	T2 weighted (images)
T_3 =	triiodothyronine
T_4 =	thyroxine
TA =	truncus arteriosus
TAPVC =	total anomalous pulmonary venous connection
TAS =	transabdominal ultrasound
TB =	tuberculosis
TBI =	traumatic brain injury

TCC =	transitional cell cancer
TDLU =	terminal duct lobular unit
TEE =	transesophageal echocardiography
TEF =	tracheoesophageal fistula
TFCC =	traingular fibrocartilage complex
TGA =	transposition of great arteries
THR =	total hip replacement
TIPS =	transjugular intrahepatic portal shunt
TKR =	total knee replacement
TLA =	translumbar approach
TMC =	toxic megacolon
TNM =	tumor node metastases
TOA =	tuboovarian abscess
TOF =	time of flight
TORCH =	toxoplasma, rubella, cytomegalovirus, herpes simplex virus
TPO =	tracheopathia osteoplastica
TSH =	thyroid-stimulating hormone
TTN =	transient tachypnea of the newborn
TURP =	transurethral resection of prostate
TV =	transvaginal
UA =	umbilical artery
UBC =	unicameral bone cyst
UC =	ulcerative colitis
UCD =	uremic cystic disease
UGI =	upper gastrointestinal
UIP =	usual interstitial pneumonia
UK =	urokinase
UL =	upper lobe
UPJ =	ureteropelvic junction
US =	ultrasound
UTI =	urinary tract infection
UV =	umbilical vein
UVJ =	ureterovesical junction
V/Q =	ventilation-perfusion ratio
VA =	vertebral artery
VACTERL =	vertebral body, anal, cardiovascular, tracheoesophageal, renal, limb anomalies
VCUG =	voiding cystourethrogram
VHL =	von Hippel-Lindau syndrome
VMA =	vanillylmandelic acid
VP =	ventriculoperitoneal
VR =	Virchow-Robin (spaces)
VSD =	ventricular septal defect
VUR =	vesicoureteral reflux
VZ =	varicella zoster
WBC =	white blood cell(s)
WM =	white matter
WPW =	Wolf Parkinson White
yr =	year

Symbols

$<$	less (common) than
$<<$	much less (common) than
$\leq$	less than or equal to
$>$	more (common) than
$>>$	much more (common) than
$\geq$	greater than or equal to
$\rightarrow$	leads to
$\varnothing$	normal, unchanged
$\uparrow$	increased
$\downarrow$	decreased

Chapter 1

1

Chest Imaging

Chapter Outline

Imaging Anatomy
   Gross lung anatomy
   Parenchymal anatomy
   Pulmonary function
   Mediastinum
   Imaging protocols
Infection
   General
   Bacterial Infections
   Viral pneumonia
   Fungal infections
AIDS
   General
   Chest
Neoplasm
   General
   Bronchogenic carcinoma
   Tumor staging
   Specific lung tumors
   Lung metastases from other primaries
Chronic Lung Disease
   Idiopathic diseases
   Lymphoproliferative disorders
   Collagen vascular diseases
   Vasculitis and granulomatoses
   Other chronic disorders
Inhalational Lung Disease
   Pneumoconiosis
   Antigen-antibody mediated lung disease
   Toxin-induced interstitial pneumonitis/fibrosis

Airway Disease
   Trachea
   Chronic bronchial disease
Lung Injury
   Postoperative chest
Pulmonary Vasculature
   Pulmonary artery hypertension
   Pulmonary edema
   Pulmonary embolism
   Vasculitis
   Venous abnormalities
Pleura
   General
   Fluid collections
   Pleural tumors
   Other
Mediastinum
   General
   Anterior mediastinal tumors
   Middle mediastinal tumors
   Posterior mediastinal tumors
   Other mediastinal disorders
Differential Diagnosis
   General
   Atelectasis
   Consolidation
   Pulmonary masses
   Cystic and cavitary lesions
   Interstitial lung disease
   Abnormal density
   Tracheobronchial lesions
   Pleural disease
   Mediastinum

Imaging Anatomy

Gross Lung Anatomy

ANATOMICAL SEGMENTAL ANATOMY

Right lung

Upper lobe	Apical	B1
	Anterior	B2
	Posterior	B3
Middle lobe	Lateral	B4
	Medial	B5
Lower lobe	Superior	B6
	Medial basal	B7
	Anterior basal	B8
	Lateral basal	B9
	Posterior basal	B10

Left lung

Upper lobe		
Upper	Apicoposterior	B1, 3
	Anterior	B2
Lingula	Superior	B4
	Inferior	B5
Lower lobe	Superior	B6
	Medial basal	B7
	Anterior basal	B8
	Lateral basal	B9
	Posterior basal	B10

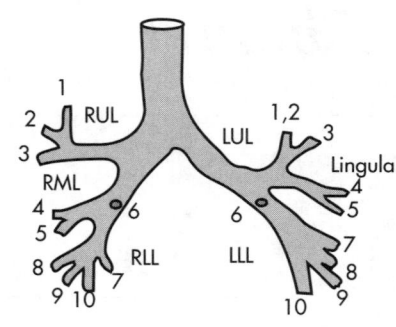

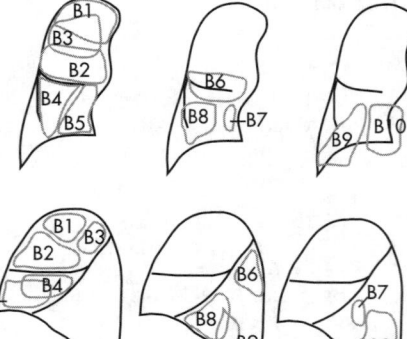

SEGMENTAL CT ANATOMY

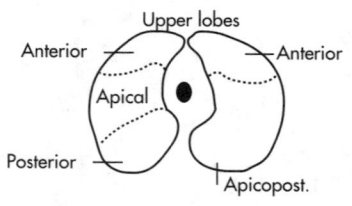
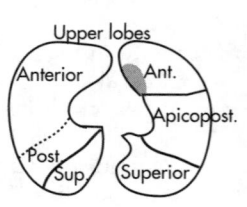
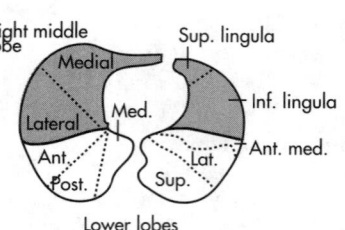
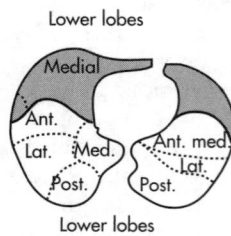

BRONCHIAL CT ANATOMY

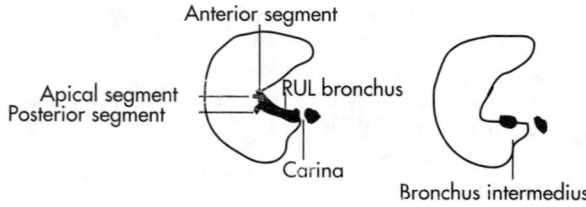
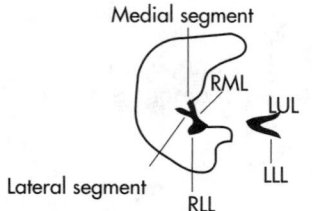
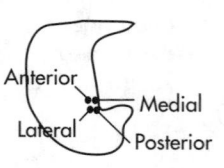

PLAIN FILM ANATOMICAL LANDMARKS

Lines

- Anterior junction line: 2 mm linear line that projects over the trachea. Represents the anterior right and left pleura.
- Posterior junction line: extends above clavicles
- Azygoesophageal line: interface between RLL air and mediastinum
- Left paraspinal line: extends from aortic arch to diaphragm
- Right paraspinal line

Paratracheal stripe

- Abnormal if > 4 mm
- Never extends below right bronchus

Fissures

- Minor (horizontal) fissure
- Major (oblique) fissures
- Azygos fissure
- Other fissures
    - Superior accessory lobe
    - Inferior accessory lobe

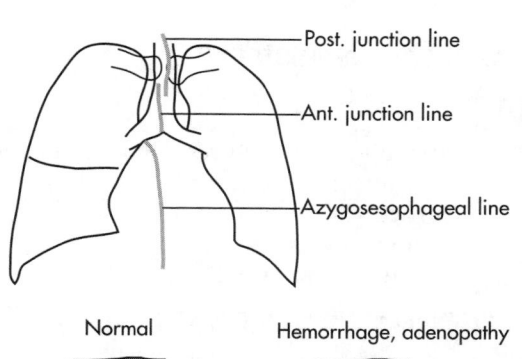

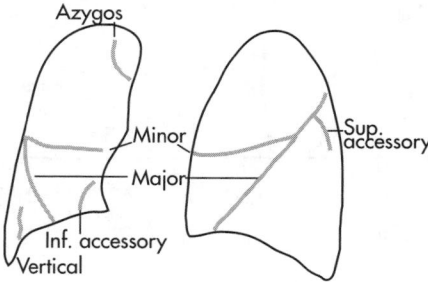

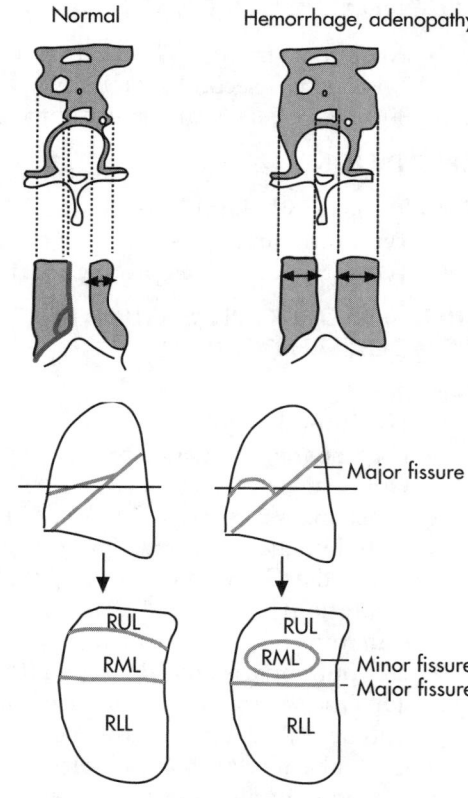

Upper lobe bronchi

- RUL bronchus is always higher than the LUL on lateral view
- Posterior wall of bronchus intermedius (right) is normally < 2 mm

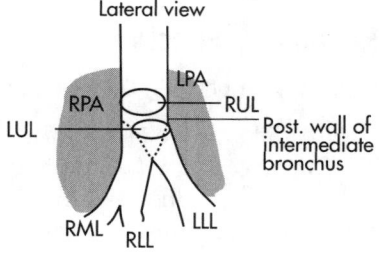

Parenchymal Anatomy

ACINUS

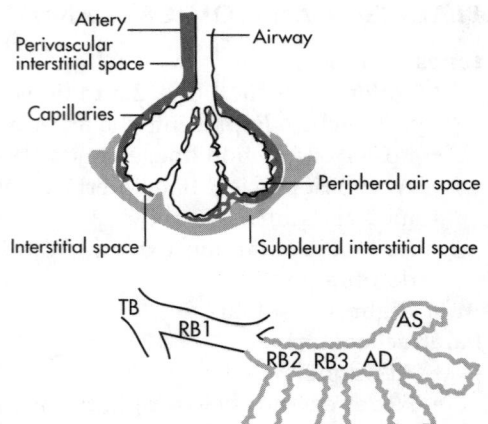

- Includes all structures distal to one terminal bronchiole. The terminal bronchiole is the last purely air-conducting structure
- Acinus measures 7 mm
- Acinus contains ~400 alveoli

SECONDARY PULMONARY LOBULE

- Polygonal structure, 1.5-2 cm in diameter
- 3-5 acini per secondary lobule
- Supplied by several terminal bronchioles

EPITHELIUM

The alveolas epithelium is made up of two cell types:
- Type 1 pneumocytes
- Type 2 pneumocytes produce surfactant, have phagocytic ability and regenerate

HIGH-RESOLUTION COMPUTED TOMOGRAPHY (HRCT)

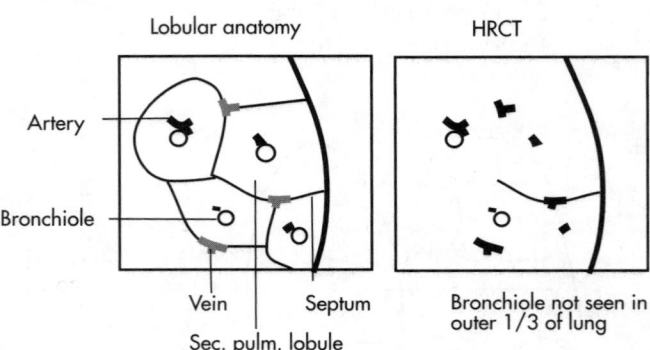

Technique
- 1-1.5 mm thin collimation
- High spatial frequency reconstruction
- Optional
Increase in kVp or mA (140 kVp, 170 mA)
Targeted image reconstruction (one lung rather than both to improve spatial resolution)

HRCT anatomy
The basic pulmonary unit visble by HRCT represents the secondary pulmonary lobule:
- Polyhedral 1.5 cm structure surrounded by connective tissue (interlobular septa)
- Central artery and bronchiole
- Peripheral pulmonary veins and lymphatics in septum

Pulmonary Function

LUNG VOLUMES, CAPACITIES, AND FLOW RATES

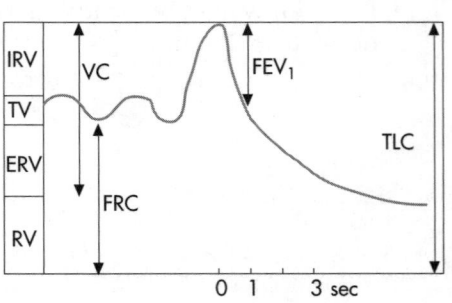

- Tidal volume (TV): normal respiratory cycle
- Vital capacity (VC): amount of gas that can be expired after maximum inspiration without force
- Functional residual capacity (FRC): volume remaining in lung after quiet expiration
- Total lung capacity (TLC): volume contained in lung at maximum inspiration
- Forced expiratory volume (FEV): amount of air expired during one second (FEV_1)

Mediastinum

- Superior mediastinum, plane above aortic arch; thoracic inlet structures
- Anterior mediastinum; contains thymus, lymph nodes, mesenchymal tissue; some classifications include the heart
- Middle mediastinum; contains heart, major vessels, bronchi, lymph nodes, and phrenic nerve
- Posterior mediastinum; starts at anterior margin of vertebral bodies; contains descending aorta, esophagus, thoracic duct, lymph nodes, nerves, and paravertebral areas

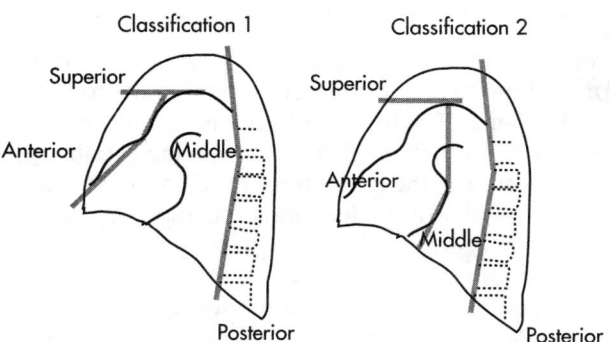

Imaging Protocols

STANDARD CHEST CT PROTOCOL

Supine position. Scan in suspended inspiration at total lung capacity. Scan set up:

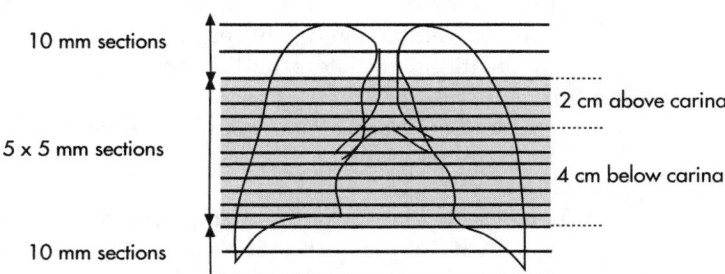

- 5 × 5 mm sections from 2 cm above carina to 4 cm below carina
- 10 × 10 mm sections through remainder of lung
- Six 1.5 mm high resolution cuts throughout lung at 3.5-cm intervals.
  In interstitial lung disease, the six cuts are repeated in prone position.
  Reconstruction with high resolution bone algorithm

Use of IV contrast

- Evaluation of vascular structures, AVM, aortic dissection
- Evaluation of mediastinal tumors, enlarged lymph nodes
- Hilar masses
- Neck masses

HELICAL CHEST CT PROTOCOL

- Scan in detail algorithm
- 1 mm reconstructions through pulmonary nodules
- Number of different combinations of pitch and section thickness. Set thickness to 7-10 mm.

PUMONARY EMBOLISM CT PROTOCOL

- Patient in supine position
- Scan range: adrenals to lung apex
- Injection of 140 mL of nonionic iodinated contrast at 3 mL/second, 25-30 seconds delay. Scanning is performed with suspended respiration.
- Scans are retrospectively reconstructed from the dome of the diaphragm as 2.5 mm thick slices with 1 mm spacing.

DIAGNOSTIC RADIOLOGY REPORT (ACR)

An authenticated written interpretation should be performed on all radiological procedures. The report should include the following items.

1. Name of patient and other identifier, such as birth date, Social Security number, or hospital or office identification number
2. Name of the referring physician to provide more accurate routing of the report to one or more locations specified by the referring physician (hospital, office, clinic, etc.)
3. History
4. Name or type of examination
5. Dates of the examination and transcription
6. Time of the examination (for ICU/CCU patients), to identify multiple examinations (e.g., chest) that may be performed on a single day
7. Body of the report.
   - Procedures and Materials

     Include in the report a description of the procedures performed and any contrast media (agent, concentration, volume and reaction, if any), medications, catheters, and devices.
   - Findings

     Use precise anatomical and radiological terminology to describe the findings accurately
   - Limitations

     Where appropriate, identify factors that can limit the sensitivity and specificity of the examination. Such factors might include technical factors, patient anatomy, limitations of the technique, incomplete bowel preparation, wrist examination for carpal scaphoid.
   - Clinical Issues

     The report should address or answer any pertinent clinical issues raised in the request for the imaging examination. For example, to rule out pneumothorax state "There is no evidence of pneumothorax"; or to rule out fracture, "There is no evidence of fracture." It is not advisable to use such universal disclaimers as "The mammography examination does not exclude the possibility of cancer."
   - Comparative Data

     Comparisons with previous examinations and reports when possible are a part of the radiological consultation and report and optionally may be part of the "impression" section.
8. Impression (conclusion or diagnosis)
   - Each examination should contain an "impression" section
   - Give a precise diagnosis whenever possible
   - Give a differential diagnosis when appropriate
   - Recommend, only when appropriate, follow-up and additional diagnostic radiological studies to clarify or confirm the impression

Infection

General

PATHOGENS

Bacterial pneumonia
- *Streptococcus pneumoniae (pneumococcus)*
- *Staphylococcus*
- *Pseudomonas*
- *Klebsiella*
- *Nocardia*
- *Chlaymidia*
- *Neisseria meningitides*
- *Haemophilus influenzae*
- *Anaerobes*
- *Legionella*
- *Mycoplasma pneumoniae*
- Actinomyces israeli
- Tuberculosis

Viral pneumonia (25% of community-acquired pneumonias)
- Influenza
- Varicella, herpes zoster
- Rubeola
- CMV
- Coxsackie, parainfluenza, adenovirus, RSV

Fungal pneumonia
- Histoplasmosis
- Coccidioidomycosis
- Blastomycosis
- Aspergillosis
- Cryptococcosis
- Candidiasis
- Zyogomyocoses

Parasitic pneumonias
- *Pneumocystis carinii*
- *Toxoplasma gondii*

ACQUISITION OF PNEUMONIA

Community-acquired pneumonia
- *S. pneumoniae, Haemophilus*
- *Mycoplasma*

Hospital-acquired pneumonia (incidence 1%, mortality 35%): nosocomial infection
- Gram negatives: *Pseudomonas, Proteus, E. coli, Enterobacter, Klebsiella*
- Methicillin-resistant *Staphylococcus aureus* (MRSA)
- Vancomycin-resistant Enterococcus (VRE)

Pneumonia in immunosuppressed patients
- Bacterial pneumonia (gram negative) still most common
- TB
- Fungal
- PCP

Endemic pneumonias
- Fungal: histoplasmosis, coccidioidomycosis, blastomycosis
- Viral

Aspiration-associated pneumonia (important)

RISK FACTORS

The radiographic appearance of pulmonary infections is variable depending on pathogen, underlying lung disease, risk factors, and prior or partial treatment. Common pathogens associated in community-acquired infections are:

COMMUNITY-ACQUIRED INFECTIONS	
Risk Factor	**Pathogens**
Alcoholism	Gram negatives, *Strep. pneumoniae*, TB, aspiration (mouth flora)
Old age	*Strep. pneumoniae*, *S. aureus*, aspiration
Aspiration	Mouth flora (anaerobes)
Cystic fibrosis	*Pseudomonas*, *S. aureus*, *Aspergillus*
Chronic bronchitis	*Strep. pneumoniae*, *H. influenzae*

Other risk factors for developing pneumonia
- Bronchiectasis
- Coma, anesthesia, seizures (aspiration)
- Tracheotomy
- Antibiotic treatment
- Immunosuppression (renal failure, diabetes, cancer, steroids, AIDS)
- Chronic furunculosis (*Staphylococcus*)

RADIOGRAPHIC SPECTRUM OF PULMONARY INFECTIONS

SUMMARY		
Type	Pathogen	Imaging

LOBAR PNEUMONIA
 	
Infection primarily involves alveolus
Spread through pores of Kohn and canals of Lambert throughout a segment and ultimately an entire lobe
Bronchi are not primarily affected and remain air-filled; therefore:
    Air bronchograms
    No volume loss because airways are open
Nowadays uncommon due to early treatment
Round pneumonia (children): *S. pneumoniae*
	S. pneumoniae
	K. pneumoniae
	Others:
	  S. aureus
	  H. influenzae
	  Fungal	

BRONCHOPNEUMONIA
 	
Primarily affects the bronchi and adjacent alveoli
Volume loss may be present as bronchi fill with exudate
Bronchial spread results in multifocal patchy opacities
	S. aureus
	Gram negatives
	Other:
	  H. influenzae
	  Mycoplasma	

NODULES
 	
Variable in size
Indistinct margins
	Fungal
	  Histoplasma
	  Aspergillus
	  Cryptococcus
	  Coccidioides
	Bacterial
	  Legionella
	  Nocardia
	Septic emboli
	  S. aureus	

CAVITARY LESIONS Abscess: necrosis of lung parenchyma ± bronchial communication Fungus ball (air crescent sign) Pneumatoceles due to air leak into pulmonary interstitium (*S. aureus*)	Anaerobes Fungal TB	
DIFFUSE OPACITIES Reticulonodular pattern: interstitial peribronchial areas of inflammation (viral) Alveolar location (PCP) Miliary pattern: hematogenous spread (TB)	Viral *Mycoplasma* PCP	

Complications of Pneumonia
- Parapneumonic effusion
    - Stage 1: exudation: free flowing
    - Stage 2: fibropurulent: loculated
    - Stage 3: organization, erosion into lung or chest wall
- Empyema
- Bronchopleural fistula (fistula between bronchus and pleural space) with eroding pleural-based fluid collections
- Bronchiectasis
- Pulmonary fibrosis, especially after necrotizing pneumonia or ARDS
- Adenopathy

RESOLUTION OF PNEUMONIA

- 80% to 90% resolve within 4 weeks
- 5% to 10% resolve within 4 to 8 weeks (usually in older or diabetic patients). Subsequent films should always show interval improvement compared to the prior films.
- Nonclearance
    - Antibiotic resistance
    - Consider other pathogen, (e.g., TB)
    - Recurrent infection
    - Obstruction pneumonitis due to tumor

Bacterial Infections

GENERAL

Common pathogens
- *S. pneumoniae*, 50% (40-60 years)
- *Mycoplasma*, 30%
- Anaerobes, 10%
- Gram negatives, 5%
- *Staphylococcus*, 5%
- *Haemophilus*, 3% (especially in infants and patients with COPD)

Clinical findings

Pneumonic syndrome
- Fever
- Cough
- Pleuritic pain
- Sputum

Ancillary findings
- Headache, arthralgia, myalgia
- Diarrhea
- Hemoptysis

STREPTOCOCCAL PNEUMONIA

Radiographic features
- Lobar or segmental pneumonia pattern
- Bronchopneumonia pattern
- Round pneumonia (in children)

STAPHYLOCOCCAL PNEUMONIA

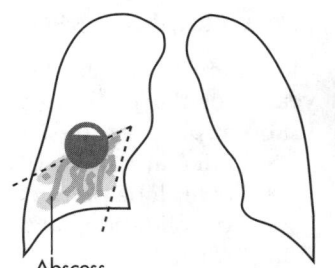

Abscess

Radiographic features
- Bronchopneumonia pattern
- Bilateral in > 60%
- Abscess cavities in 25%-75%
- Pleural effusion, empyema, 50%
- Pneumatoceles, 50% (check valve obstruction), particularly in children
- Central lines
- Sign of endocarditis

PSEUDOMONAS PNEUMONIA

Typical clinical setting
- Hospital-acquired infection
- Ventilated patient
- Reduced host resistance
- Patients with cystic fibrosis

Radiographic features

Three presentations:
- Extensive bilateral parenchymal consolidation (predilection for both lower lobes)
- Abscess formation
- Diffuse nodular disease (bacteremia with hematogenous spread; rare)

LEGIONNAIRES' DISEASE

Severe pulmonary infection caused by *Legionella pneumophila*; 35% require ventilation, 20% mortality. Most infections are community acquired. Patients have hyponatremia. Seroconversion for diagnosis takes 2 weeks.

Radiographic features

Common features
- Initial presentation starts as peripheral patchy consolidation
- Bilateral severe disease
- Rapidly progressive
- Pleural effusions < 50%
- Lower lobe predilection

Uncommon features
- Abscess formation
- Lymph node enlargement

HAEMOPHILUS PNEUMONIA

Caused by *Haemophilus influenzae*. Occurs most commonly in children, immuno-compromised adults or patients with COPD. Often there is concomitant meningitis, epiglottitis, bronchitis.

Radiographic features
- Bronchopneumonia pattern
- Lower lobe predilection, often diffuse
- Empyema

MYCOPLASMA PNEUMONIA

Most common nonbacterial pneumonia (atypical pneumonia). Mild course. Age 5-20 years. Positive cold agglutinins, 60%.
Radiographic features
- Reticular pattern
- Lower lobe predominance, often diffuse
- Consolidation, 50%

Complications
- Autoimmune hemolytic anemia
- Erythema nodosum, erythema multiforme
- Stevens-Johnson syndrome
- Meningoencephalitis

KLEBSIELLA (FRIEDLÄNDER'S) PNEUMONIA

Gram-negative organism. Often in debilitated patients and/or alcoholics.
Radiographic features
- Consolidation appears similar to S. Pneumonia
- Lobar expansion
- Cavitation in 30-50%, typically multiple
- Massive necrosis (pulmonary gangrene)
- Pleural effusion is uncommon

TUBERCULOSIS (TB)

Transmitted by inhalation of infected droplets *Mycobacterium tuberculosis* or *M. bovis*. TB usually requires constant or repeated contact with sputum-positive patients as the tubercle does not easily grow in the immunocompetent human host. Target population:
- Patients of low socioeconomic scale (homeless)
- Alcoholics
- Immigrants: Mexico, Philippines, Indochina, Haiti
- Elderly patients
- AIDS patients
- Prisoners

Primary infection
Usually heals without complications. Sequence of events:
- Pulmonary consolidation (1-7 cm); cavitation is rare; lower lobe (60%) > upper lobes
- Caseous necrosis 2-10 weeks after infection

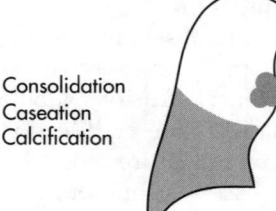

Primary TB

1. Consolidation
2. Caseation
3. Calcification

Nodes

- Lymphadenopathy (hilar and paratracheal), 95%
- Pleural effusion, 10%
- Spread of a primary focus occurs primarily in children or immunosuppressed patients

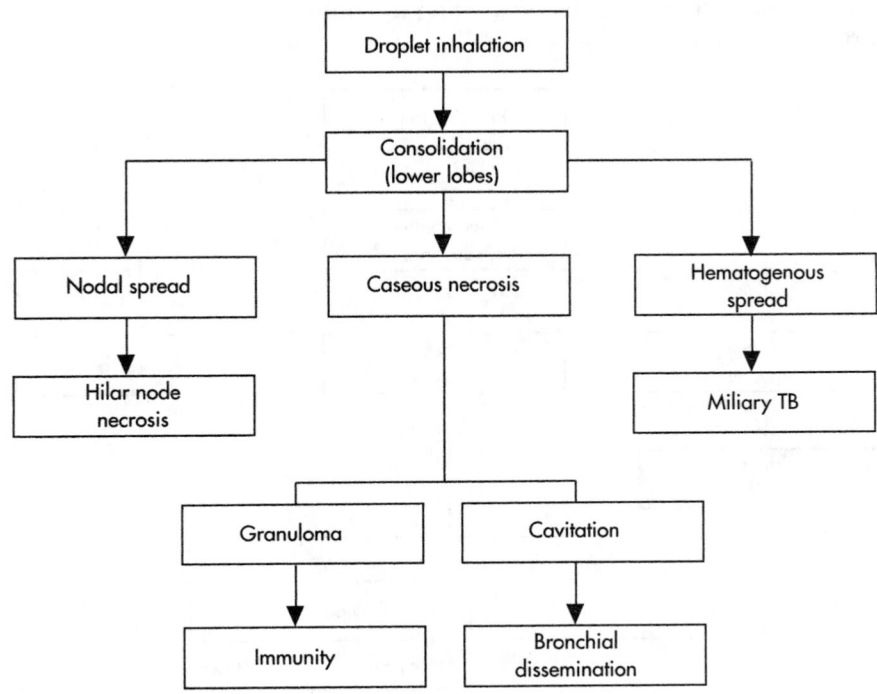

Secondary infection

Active disease in adults most commonly represents reactivation of a primary focus. However, primary disease is now also common in adults in developed countries scince there is no exposure in childhood. Distribution is as follows:

- Typically limited to apical and posterior segments of upper lobes or superior segments of lower lobes (because high P_{O_2}?)
- Rarely in anterior segments of upper lobes (in contradistinction to histoplasmosis)

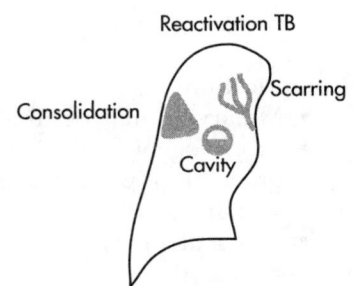

Radiographic features

- Exudative tuberculosis
    Patchy or confluent airspace disease
    Adenopathy is uncommon
- Fibrocalcific tuberculosis
    Sharply circumscribed linear densities radiating to hilum
- Cavitation, 40%

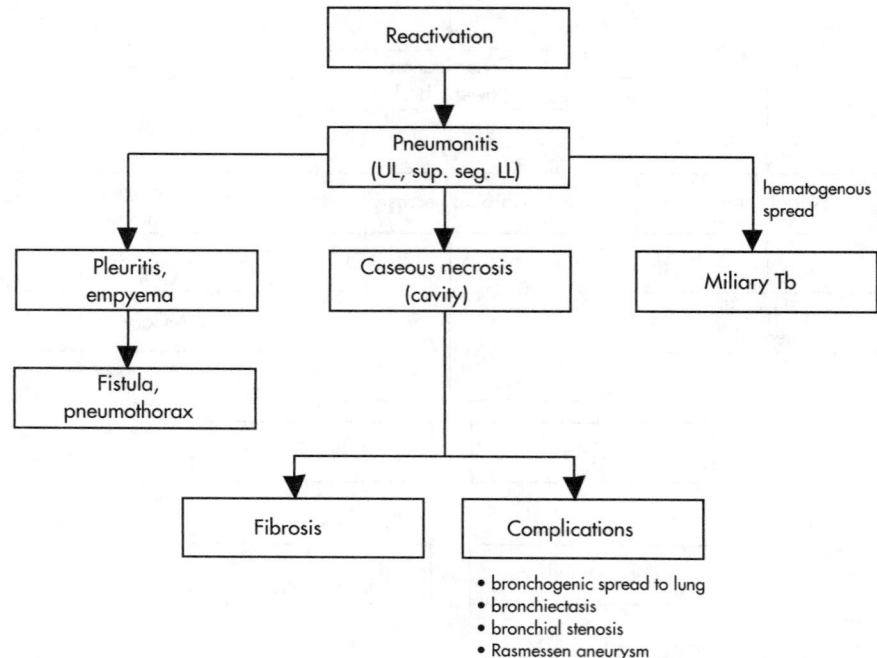

Complications

- Miliary TB may occur after primary or secondary hematogenous spread
- Bronchogenic spread occurs after communication of the necrotic area with a bronchus; it produces an acinar pattern (irregular nodules approximately 5 mm in diameter)
- Tuberculoma (1-7 cm): nodule during primary or secondary TB; may contain calcification
- Effusions are often loculated
- Bronchopleural fistula
- Pneumothorax

COMPARISON		
	Primary TB	**Reinfection TB**
Location	Usually bases	Upper lobes, sup. segment LL
Appearance	Focal	Patchy
Cavitation	No	Frequent
Adenopathy as only finding	Common	No
Effusion	Common	Uncommon
Miliary pattern	Yes	Yes

NONTUBERCULOUS MYCOBACTERIAL (NTBM) INFECTIONS

The two most common NTBM pathogens are *M. avium-intracellulare* and *M. kansasii* (less common: *M. xenopi, M. chelonei, M. gordoniae, M. fortuitum* = "fast grower"). Unlike TB, NTBM infections are not acquired by human-human transmission, but are a direct infection from soil or water. There is also no pattern of primary disease or reactivation: the infection is primary, although some may become chronic. Often occurs in elderly patients with COPD, older women in good health, and AIDS patients.

Radiographic features
- NTBM may be indistinguishable from classic TB
- Atypical features such as bronchiectasis and bronchial wall thickening are common
- Nodules are common in older women

CT FINDINGS		
Findings	TB (%)	MAI (%)
Nodules < 1 cm	80	95
Nodules 1-3 cm	40	30
Mass > 3 cm	10	10
Consolidation	50	50
Cavity	30	30
Bronchiectasis	30	95
Bronchial wall thickening	40	95
Septal thickening	50	15
Emphysema	20	20
Calcified granuloma	15	5

NOCARDIA PNEUMONIA

Caused by *Nocardia asteroides,* worldwide distribution. Common opportunistic invader in:
- Lymphoma
- Steroid therapy; especially transplant patients
- Pulmonary alveolar proteinosis (common)

Radiographic features
- Focal consolidation (more common)
- Cavitation
- Irregular nodules

ACTINOMYCOSIS

Actinomycosis is caused by *Actinomyces israelii,* a gram-positive normal saprophytes in oral cavity, Pulmonary disease develops from aspiration of organism (poor dentition) or from direct penetration into the thorax.

Radiographic features
- Focal consolidation > cavitating mass
- Lymphadenopathy is uncommon
- Extension into the chest wall and pleural thickening is less common today but still occurs and represents an important differential feature

PULMONARY ABSCESS

The spectrum of anaerobic pulmonary infections includes:
- Abscess: single or multiple cavities > 2 cm, usually with air-fluid level
- Necrotizing pneumonia: analogous to abscess but more diffuse and cavities < 2 cm
- Empyema: suppurative infection of the pleural space, most commonly as a result of pneumonia

Predisposing conditions
- Aspiration (alcoholism, neurologic disease, coma, etc.)
- Intubation
- Bronchiectasis, bronchial obstruction

Treatment:
- Antibiotics, postural drainage
- Percutaneous drainage of empyema
- Drainage/resection of lung abscess only if medical therapy fails

SICKLE CELL ANEMIA

- Patients with sickle cell disease are at increased risk of pneumonia and infarction. These entities are difficult to differentiate, hence called *acute chest syndrome.*
- Pneumonias were originally due to pneumococci but now are due viruses, mycoplasma. Differential: atelectasis; infarct
- Infarcts more frequent in adults than in children. Rare in children under 12 years of age.
- Consolidation is seen on chest films; resolves slower than in general population and tends to recur.

Viral Pneumonia

GENERAL

Classification
DNA viruses
    Unenveloped
- Parvoviruses
- Papavoviruses
- Adenoviruses
- Hepatitis viruses (hepatitis B)

    Enveloped
- Herpesviruses (herpes simplex, Epstein-Barr, varicella zoster, CMV)
- Poxviruses (variola, molluscum contagiosum)

RNA viruses
    Unenveloped
- Picornaviruses (hepatitis A, coxsackievirus)
- Caliciviruses
- Reoviruses

    Enveloped
- Retroviruses (HIV)
- Arenaviruses
- Coronaviruses
- Togaviruses

- Bunyaviruses
- Orthomyxoviruses (influenza)
- Paramyxoviruses (mumps, measles, respiratory syncytial virus, parainfluenza)

Spectrum of disease
- Acute interstitial pneumonia: diffuse or patchy interstitial pattern, thickening of bronchi, thickened interlobar septae
- Lobular inflammatory reaction: multiple nodular opacities 5-6 mm (varicella; late calcification)
- Hemorrhagic pulmonary edema: mimics bacterial lobar pneumonia
- Pleural effusion: usually absent or small
- Chronic interstitial fibrosis (broncholitis obliterans)

INFLUENZA PNEUMONIA

Influenza is very contagious and thus occurs in epidemics. Pneumonia, however, is uncommon.

Radiographic features
- Acute phase: multiple acinar densities
- Coalescence of acinar densities to diffuse patchy air space disease (bronchopneumonia type)

VARICELLA ZOSTER PNEUMONIA

15% of infected patients have pneumonias; 90% are older than 20 years.

Radiographic features
- Acute phase: multiple acinar opacities
- Coalescence of acinar opacities to diffuse patchy air space disease
- 1-2 mm calcifications throughout lungs after healing

CMV PNEUMONIA

Occurs most commonly in neonates or immunosuppressed patients.

Radiographic features
- Predominantly interstitial infection, multiple small nodules (common)
- Adenopathy may be present

Fungal Infections

GENERAL

Two broad categories:

Endemic human mycoses (prevalent only in certain geographic areas):
- Histoplasmosis (Ohio, Mississippi, St. Lawrence river valleys)
- Coccidioidomycosis (San Joaquin Valley)
- Blastomycosis

Opportunistic mycoses (worldwide in distribution) occur primarily in immuno-compromised patients (aspergillosis and cryptococcosis may also occur in immunocompetent hosts)
- Aspergillosis
- Candidiasis
- Cryptococcosis
- Mucormycosis

Radiographic features
- Acute phase: pneumonic type of opacity (may be segmental, nonsegmental, or patchy); miliary (hematogenous) distribution in immunosuppressed patients
- Reparative phase: nodular lesions with or without cavitations and crescent sign
- Chronic phase: calcified lymph nodes or pulmonary focus with fungus (e.g., histoplasmosis)
- Disseminated disease (spread to other organs) occurs primarily in immunocompromised patients

HISTOPLASMOSIS

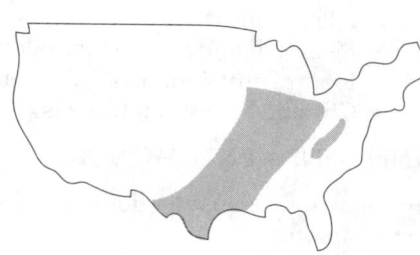

Histoplasma capsulatum is particularly prevalent in the Ohio, Missisippi, St. Lawrence river valleys although the agent is worldwide in distribution. The organism is most prevalent in soil that contains excrement of bats and birds (bat caves, chicken houses, old attics or buildings). Clinical: most patients are asymptomatic or have nonspecific respiratory symptoms, increased complement fixation titer, positive *H. capsulatum* antigen.

Radiographic features

Consolidation (primary histoplasmosis)
- Parenchymal consolidation
- Adenopathy is very common and may calcify heavily later on

Nodular form (chronic histoplasmosis, reinfection)
- Histoplasmoma: usually solitary, sharply circumscribed nodule, most commonly in lower lobes
- Fibrocavitary disease in upper lobes indistinguishable from post-primary TB
- Cavitary nodules

Disseminated form (immunocompromised patients)
- Miliary nodules
- Calcifications in liver and spleen

Mediastinal histoplasmosis

Mediastinal histoplasmosis may follow pulmonary histoplasmosis. Two distinct entities (which may not always be separable from each other):

Mediastinal granuloma
- Results from spread of *H. capsulatum* to lymph nodes
- Granulomas are usually calcified

Mediastinal fibrosis (fibrosing mediastinitis)
- May cause superior vena cava syndrome, airway compression, PA occlusion, pericarditis
- Diffuse infiltration of mediastinum
- Multiple densely calcified nodes

COCCIDIOIDOMYCOSIS

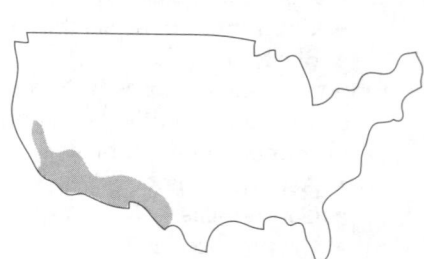

Coccidioides immitis is endemic in the southwest United States (San Joaquin valley, "valley fever"), and in Central and South America. Infection occurs due to inhalation of spores in soil. Human-to-human infection does not occur. Clinical: cutaneous manifestations common, 70% are asymptomatic.

Radiographic features

Consolidation (primary form)
- "Fleeting" parenchymal consolidation, most commonly lower lobes
- Adenopathy in 20%

Nodular form (chronic form, 5%)
- 15% cavitate
  - 50% have thin-walled cavity (suggestive of diagnosis)
  - 50% have thick-walled cavity (i.e., nonspecific)
  - May present with pneumothorax
- Nodules rarely calcify
- Hilar or paratracheal adenopathy

Disseminated form (immunocompromised patients; rare: 0.5% of all forms)
- Miliary nodules
- Extrapulmonary spread

NORTH AMERICAN BLASTOMYCOSIS

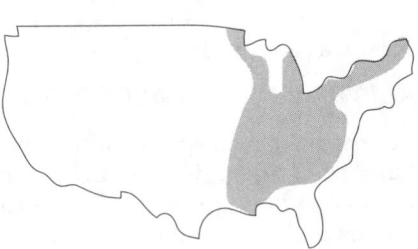

- Caused by *Blastomyces dermatitidis;* uncommon infection. Most infections are self-limited.
- CXR is nonspecific: airspace disease > nodule (15% cavitate) or solitary mass > miliary spread
- Focal blastomycosis typically occurs in paramediastinal location and has an air bronchogram, findings that may suggest the diagnosis
- Satellite nodules around primary focus are common
- Adenopathy, pleural effusions and calcifications are very uncommon
- Bone lesions, 25%
- Skin lesions are common

ASPERGILLOSIS

Aspergillus is a ubiquitous fungus that, when inhaled, leads to significant lung damage. The fungus grows in soil, water, decaying vegetation, hospital air vents. *Aspergillus fumigatus* > *A. flavus*, *A. niger*, *A. glaucus*. There are 4 unique forms of pulmonary aspergillosis, each associated with a specific immune status.

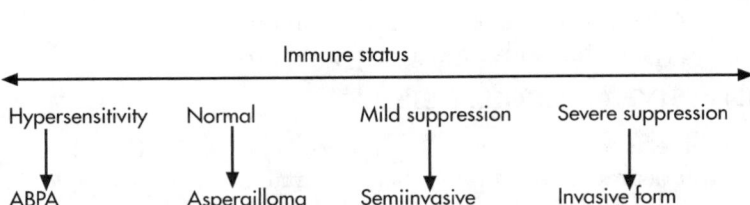

TYPES OF ASPERGILLOSIS			
Type	**Lung Structure**	**Immune Status**	**Pathology**
Allergic (ABPA)	Normal	Hypersensitivity	Hypersensitivity → bronchiectasis, mucus plugging
Aspergilloma	Preexisting cavity	Normal	Saprophytic growth in preexisting cavity
Invasive	Normal	Severely impaired	Vascular invasion, parenchymal necrosis
Semiinvasive	Normal	Normal or impaired	Chronic local growth, local cavity formation

ALLERGIC BRONCHOPULMONARY ASPERGILLOSIS (ABPA)

ABPA represents a complex hypersensitivity reaction (type 1) to *Aspergillus*, occuring almost exclusively in patients with asthma and occasionally cystic fibrosis. The hypersensitivity initially causes bronchospasm and bronchial wall edema (IgE mediated); ultimately there is bronchial wall damage, bronchiectasis and pulmonary fibrosis. Clinical: elevated *Aspergillus*-specific IgE, elevated precipitating IgG against *Aspergillus*, peripheral eosinophilia, pos. skin test. Treatment: oral prednisone.

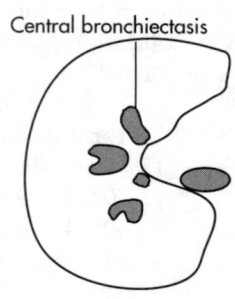

Central bronchiectasis

Radiographic features

- Fleeting pulmonary alveolar opacities (common manifestation)
- Central, upper lobe saccular bronchiectasis (hallmark)
- Mucus plugging ("finger in glove appearance ") and bronchial wall thickening (common)
- Chronic disease may progress to pulmonary fibrosis predominately in upper lobe (endstage)
- Cavitation, 10%

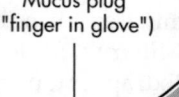

Mucus plug ("finger in glove")

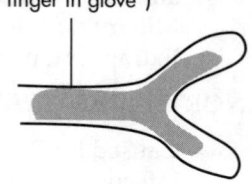

ASPERGILLOMA (MYCETOMA, FUNGUS BALL)

Represents a saprophytic infection in preexisting structural lung disease (cavitary or bulla from TB, endstage sarcoid, emphysema). Commonly in upper lobes, solitary lesions. The fungus grows in the cavity creating a "fungus ball" consisting of fungus, mucus and inflammatory cells. Treatment: surgical resection, intracavitary administration of amphotericin.

Radiographic features

- Focal intracavitary mass (3-6 cm), typically in upper lobes
- Air may surround the aspergilloma (Monod sign), mimicking the appearance of cavitation seen with invasive aspergillosis
- Small area of consolidation around cavity is typical
- Adjacent pleural thickening common
- Fungus ball moves with changing position

INVASIVE ASPERGILLOSIS

Invasive aspergillosis has a high mortality (70%-90%) and occurs mainly in severely immunocompromised patients (bone marrow transplants, leukemia). The infection starts with endobronchial fungal proliferation and then leads to vascular invasion with thrombosis and infarction of lung ("angioinvasive infection"). Additional sites of infection (in 30%) are: brain, liver, kidney, GI tract. Treatment: systemic and/or intracavitary administration of amphotericin.

Radiographic features

- Multiple pulmonary nodules, 40%
- Nodules have a characteristic halo of ground glass appearance (represents pulmonary hemorrhage)
- Within 2 weeks, 50% of nodules undergo cavitation which results in the air crescent sign. The appearance of the cresent signs indicates the recovery phase (increased granulocytic response). Note that the air crescent sign may also be seen in TB, actinomycosis, mucormycosis, septic emboli, tumors. Do not confuse the air crescent sign with the Monod sign (clinical history helps to differentiate).
- Other manifestations:
    Peribronchial opacities
    Focal areas of consolidation

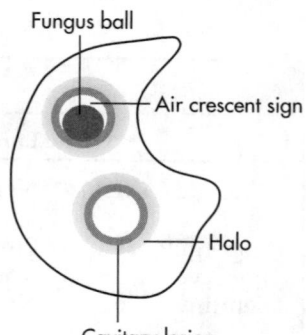

Fungus ball

Air crescent sign

Halo

Cavitary lesion

1

SEMI-INVASIVE ASPERGILLOSIS

This form of aspergillosis occurs in mildly immunocompromised patients and has a similar pathophysiology as invasive aspergillosis except that the disease progresses more chronically over months (mortality 30%). Risk factors: diabetes, alcoholism, pneumoconioses, malnutrition, COPD. Treatment: systemic and/or intracavitary administration of amphotericin.

Radiographic features
- Similar appearance as invasive aspergillosis
- Cavitation occurs at 6 months after infection

CRYPTOCOCCOSIS

Caused by *Cryptococcus neoformans* which is worldwide in distribution and ubiquotous in soil and pigeon excreta. Infection occurs through inhalation of contaminated dust. Clinical: common in patients with lymphoma, steroid therapy, diabetes, AIDS.

Radiographic features
- Most common findings in lung are: pulmonary mass, multiple nodules or segmental or lobar consolidation
- Cavitation, adenopathy, effusions are rare
- Disseminated form: CNS, other organs

CANDIDIASIS

Caused by *Candida albicans* > other *Candida* species. Clinical: typically in patients with lymphoreticular malignancy, suspect pulmonary disease if associated with oral disease. Often there is disseminated fungemia.

Radiographic features:
- Plain film is nonspecific: opacities (lower lobe) > nodules
- Nodular disease in disseminated form
- Pleural effusion, 25%
- Cavitation and adenopathy are rare

ZYOGOMYCOSES

Group of severe opportunistic mycoses caused by fungi of the zygomycetes class:
- Mucormycosis (*Mucor*)
- *Rhizopus*
- *Absidia*

Zygomycoses usually have two major clinical manifestations:
- Pulmonary mucormycosis
- Rhinocerebral mucormycosis

Zygomycoses are uncommon infections and occur primarily in immunocompormised patients (leukemia, AIDS, chronic steroid use, diabetics).

Radiographic features
- Similar radiographic features as invasive aspergillosis because of angioinvasive behavior of fungi

AIDS

General

Acquired immunodeficiency syndrome is caused by HTLV type III (human T-cell lymphotrophic virus = HIV: human immunodeficiency virus). HIV-1 and HIV-2 are single-stranded RNA viruses that bind to CD4 present on T-lymphocytes (other cells: glial cells, lung monocytes, dendritic cells in lymph nodes). The viral RNA genome is copied into DNA with the help of reverse transcriptase and integrated into the host cellular DNA.

EPIDEMIOLOGY

To date (2001) AIDS has been reported in > 750,000 individuals with > 450,000 deaths in the United States. Groups at highest risk:
- Homosexual males, bisexual males, 60%
- IV drug abusers (IVDA), 25%
- Recipients of blood products, 3%
- Congenital from AIDS-positive mothers
- Heterosexual females: most rapidly growing group due to partners who are IVDA

Known routes of HIV transmission:
- Blood and blood products
- Sexual activity
- In utero transmission
- During delivery

CLINICAL

The disease is characterized by:
- Lymphadenopathy
- Opportunistic infections
- Tumors: lymphoma, Kaposi's sarcoma
- Other manifestations:
  > Lymphocytic interstitial pneumonia (LIP)
  > Spontaneous pneumothorax (development of cystic spaces, interstitial
  >   fibrosis related to PCP)
  > Septic emboli

Clinical findings supportive of AIDS:
- CD4 count < 200/mm³; the dysfunction of the immune system is inversely related to the CD4 count; PCP: CD4 < 200 cells/mm³, MAI: CD4 < 50 cells/mm³
- > 1 case of bacterial pneumonia per year

Opportunistic infections
- *Pneumocystis carinii*, 70%
- Mycobacterial infection, 20%; CD4 counts often < 50 cells/mm³
- Bacterial infection, 10% (*S. pneumoniae, Haemophilus*)
- Fungal infection (< 5% of AIDS patients)
- *Nocardia*, < 5%: cavitating pneumonia
- CMV pneumonia (common at autopsy)

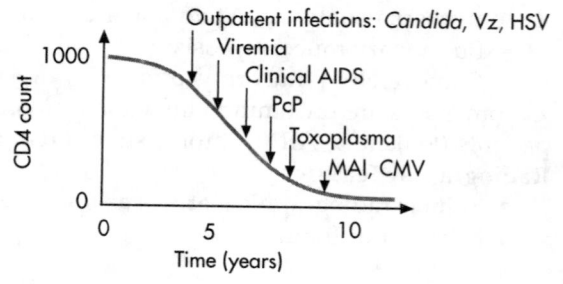

Chest

GENERAL

- 50% of all AIDS patients have pulmonary manifestations of infection or tumor
- A normal CXR does not exclude the diagnosis of PCP
- CMV is common at autopsy but does not cause significant morbidity or mortality; CMV antibody titers are present in virtually all patients with AIDS
- Use of chest CT in AIDS patients:
    Symptomatic patient with normal CXR; however, patients will commonly first undergo induced sputum, bronchoscopy or be put on empirical treatment for PCP
    Clarify confusing CXR
    Work-up of focal opacities, adenopathy, nodules

SPECTRUM OF CHEST MANIFESTATIONS

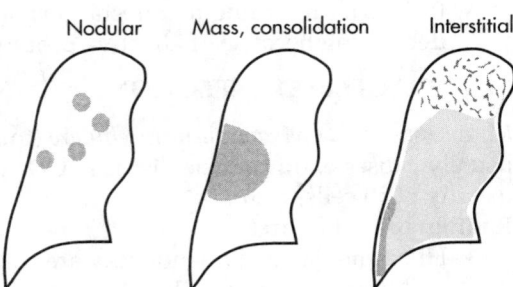

Nodular   Mass, consolidation   Interstitial

Nodules
- Kaposi sarcoma (usually associated with skin lesions)
- Septic infarcts (rapid size increase)
- Fungal: *Cryptococcus, Aspergillus*

Large opacity: consolidation, mass
- Hemorrhage
- NHL
- Pneumonia

Linear or interstitial opacities
- PCP
- Atypical mycobacteria
- Kaposi sarcoma

Lymphadenopathy
- Mycobacterial infections
- Kaposi sarcoma
- Lymphoma
- Reactive hyperplasia, rare in thorax

Pleural effusion
- Kaposi's sarcoma
- Mycobacterial, fungal infection
- Pyogenic empyema

PCP INFECTION

Radiographic features
- Interstitial pattern, 80%
    CXR: bilateral perihilar or diffuse
    HRCT: ground glass appearance predominately in upper lobe with cysts
- Progression to diffuse consolidation within days

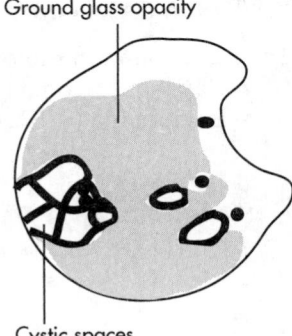

Ground glass opacity

Cystic spaces

- Normal CXR in the presence of pulmonary PCP infection, 10%
- Multiple upper lobe air-filled cysts or pneumatoceles (10%) causing
    Pneumothorax
    Bronchopleural fistulas

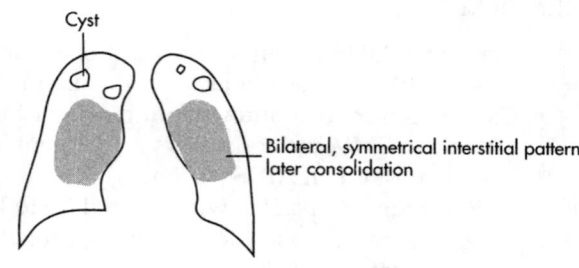

- Upper lobe PCP involvement is common because aerosolized pentamidine may not get to upper lobes; upper lobe disease may mimic TB but the latter may have pleural effusions or lymphadenopathy, both of which are uncommon in PCP
- Atypical patterns, 5%
    Unilateral disease
    Focal lesions, cavitary nodules
- PCP as a presenting manifestations of AIDS is decreasing because of effective prophylaxis

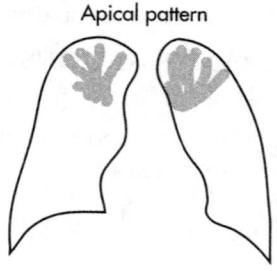

MYCOBACTERIAL INFECTION

M. tuberculosis > *M. avium-intracellulare* (this pathogen usually causes extrathoracic disease). CD4 cell count usually < 50 cells/mm^3.

Radiographic features

- Hilar, mediastinal adenopathy are common.
    Necrotic lymph nodes (TB) have a low attenuation center and only rim-enhance with contrast.
    MTB is more commonly associated with necrosis from MAI.
    Adenopathy in Kaposi's sarcoma or lymphoma enhances uniformly.
- Pleural effusion
- Other findings are similar to non-AIDS TB (upper lobe consolidations, cavitations)

FUNGAL INFECTIONS

Fungal infections in AIDS are uncommon (< 5% of patients).

- Cryptococcosis (most common); 90% have CNS involvement
- Histoplasmosis: nodular or miliary pattern most common; 35% have normal CXR
- Coccidioidomycosis: diffuse interstitial pattern, thin-walled cavities

KAPOSI'S SARCOMA

The most common tumors in AIDS are:

- Kaposi's sarcoma (15% of patients); incidence declining; M:F = 50:1
- Lymphoma (< 5% of patients)

Pulmonary manifestations of Kaposi's sarcoma (almost always preceded by cutaneous/visceral involvement):

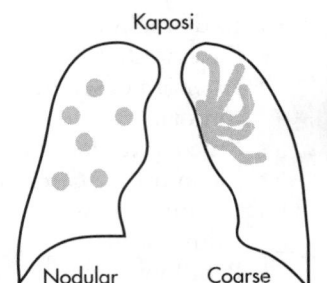

- Nodules
    1-3 cm
    Single or multiple
    Virtually always associated with skin lesions
- Coarse linear opacities emanating from hilum
- Pleural effusions (serosanguinous), 40%
- Adenopathy
- Lymphangitic tumor spread

AIDS-RELATED LYMPHOMA

Non-Hodgkin's lymphoma (usually aggressive B-cell type) > Hodgkin's lymphoma. Poor prognosis. Spectrum:
- Solitary or multiple pulmonary masses ± air bronchogram, 25%
- AIDS-related lymphoma is typically an extranodal disease (CNS, GI tract, liver, bone marrow): adenopathy not very prominent
- Pleural effusions are common

LYMPHOID INTERSTITIAL PNEUMONIA

Diffuse interstitial infiltrate composed of lymphocytes, plasma cells, histiocytes. Radiographic features: diffuse reticulonodular pattern, basilar in distribution, late honeycombing. Diagnosis is established by biopsy. Occurs with:

Non-AIDS
- Sjögren
- SLE
- CAH

AIDS
- Common in pediatric AIDS patients

Neoplasm

General

LOCATION

Chest neoplasms are best categorized by their primary location:
- Lung tumors
- Pleural tumors
- Mediastinal tumors
- Tumors of the airway
- Chest wall tumors

CLASSIFICATION OF PULMONARY NEOPLASM

Malignant tumors
- Bronchogenic carcinoma
- Lymphoma
- Metastases
- Sarcomas, rare

Low-grade malignancies (previously bronchial adenoma)
- Carcinoid, 90%
- Adenoid cystic carcinoma (previously cylindroma, resembles salivary gland tumor), 6%
- Mucoepidermoid carcinoma, 3%
- Pleomorphic carcinoma, 1%

Benign tumors, rare
- Hamartoma
- Papilloma
- Leiomyoma
- Hemangioma
- Chemodectoma
- Pulmonary blastoma
- Chondroma
- Multiple pulmonary fibroleiomyomas
- Pseudolymphoma

PERCUTANEOUS BIOPSY

True positive rate of percutaneous lung biopsy is 90%-95%. False negative results are usually due to poor needle placement, necrotic tissue, etc. Tumor seeding is extremely uncommon (1:20,000). Contraindications to biopsy are usually relative:
- Severe COPD
- Pulmonary hypertension
- Coagulopathy
- Contralateral pneumonectomy
- Suspected echinococcal cysts

Technique
- Fluoroscopic or CT localization of nodule
- Pass needle over superior border of rib to avoid intercostal vessels
- Avoid passing through fissures
- Coaxial needle system
    20-gauge outer needle
    22-gauge inner needle
- Cytopathologist should be present in room to determine if sample is adequate and diagnostic
- Chest film after procedure to determine presence of pneumothorax

Complications
- Pneumothorax, 25%; 5%-10% require a chest tube (i.e., pneumothorax > 25% or if patient is symptomatic)
- Hemoptysis, 3%

Bronchogenic Carcinoma

Bronchogenic carcinoma refers broadly to any carcinoma of the bronchus. However, the use of the term is usually restricted to the following entities:

CLASSIFICATION

Adenocarcinoma (most common), 40%
- Bronchoalveolar carcinoma
- Papillary adenocarcinoma
- Acinar adenocarcinoma
- Solid adenocarcinoma with mucus formation

Squamous cell carcinoma, 30%
- Spindle cell carcinoma

Small cell carcinoma, 15%
- Oat cell
- Intermediate cell type
- Combined oat cell carcinoma

Large cell carcinoma, 1%
- Giant cell carcinoma
- Clear cell carcinoma

Adenosquamous tumor

RISK FACTORS FOR BRONCHOGENIC CARCINOMA

- Smoking: 98% of male patients and 87% of female patients with lung cancer smoke. 10% of heavy smokers will develop lung cancer. The strongest relationship between smoking and cancer has been established for SCC followed by adenocarcinoma; the least common association is for bronchoalveolar carcinoma
- Radiation, uranium miners
- Asbestos exposure
- Genetic predisposition (HLA-Bw44 associated?)

RADIOGRAPHIC SPECTRUM

Primary signs of malignancy
- Mass (> 6 cm) or nodule (< 6 cm) with spiculated, irregular borders
- Unilateral enlargement of hilum: mediastinal widening, hilar prominence
- Cavitation
    Most common in upper lobes or superior segments of lower lobes
    Wall thickness is indicative of malignancy
    < 4 mm: 95% of cavitated lesions are benign
    > 15 mm: 85% of cavitated lesions are malignant
    Cavitation is most commonly seen in squamous cell carcinoma

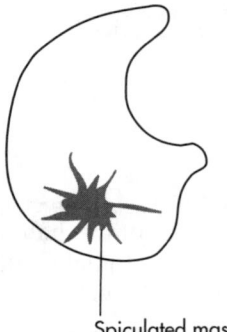

Spiculated mass

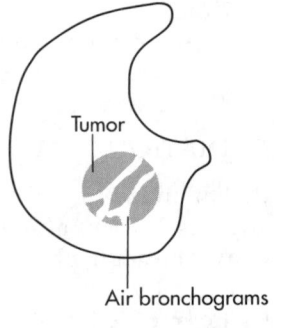

Tumor

Air bronchograms

- Certain tumors may present as chronic air space disease: bronchoalveolar carcinoma, lymphoma
- Some air bronchograms are commonly seen by HRCT in adenocarcinoma

Secondary signs of malignancy
- Atelectasis (Golden's inverted "S" sign in RUL, LUL collapse)
- Obstructive pneumonia
- Pleural effusion
- Interstitial patterns: lymphangitic tumor spread
- Hilar and mediastinal adenopathy
- Metastases to ipsilateral, contralateral lung

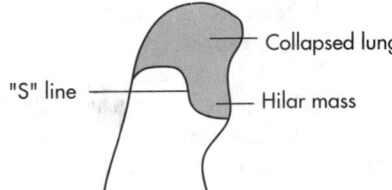

Collapsed lung

"S" line

Hilar mass

LOCATION OF TUMORS			
Tumor	Frequency	Location	Comments
Adenocarcinoma	40%	Peripheral	Scar carcinoma
Squamous cell carcinoma	30%	Central, peripheral*	Cavitation
Small cell carcinoma	15%	Central, peripheral*	Endocrine activity
Large cell carcinoma	1%	Central, peripheral	Large mass

*Rarely present as a resectable T1 lesion.

PARANEOPLASTIC SYNDROMES OF LUNG CANCER

Incidence: 2% of bronchogenic carcinoma.
Metabolic
  - Cushing's syndrome (ACTH)
  - Inappropriate antidiuresis (ADH)
  - Carcinoid syndrome (serotonin, other vasoactive substances)
  - Hypercalcemia (PTH, bone mets)
  - Hypoglycemia (insulin-like factor)
Musculoskeletal
  - Neuromyopathies
  - Clubbing of fingers (HPO)
Other
  - Acanthosis nigricans
  - Thrombophlebitis
  - Anemia

RADIATION PNEUMONITIS

Radiation pneumonitis represents the acute phase of radiation damage and usually appears 3 weeks after treatment. Minimum radiation to induce pneumonitis is 30 Gray. The acute phase is typically asymptomatic but may be associated with fever and cough. Fibrosis usually occurs after 6-12 months.

Radiographic features
  - Diffuse opacities in radiation port
  - HRCT allows better assessment of extent than plain film

Tumor Staging

TNM STAGING SYSTEM

Primary tumor (T)
  - T0 No evidence of a primary tumor
  - T1 < 3 cm, limited to lung
  - T2 > 3 cm; > 2 cm distal to carina
  - T3 Tumor of any size with direct extension to:
        Chest wall, superior sulcus, diaphragm
        Pleura, pericardium
        Within 2 cm of carina
  - T4 Mediastinal organs, carinal, vertebral body invasion or malignant pleural effusion; unresectable. Malignant pleural effusion even if not associated with any other findings suggests unresectable status

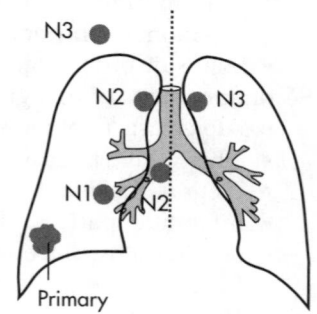

Nodes (N)
- N0 No lymph node involvement
- N1 Ipsilateral hilar nodes
- N2 Ipsilateral mediastinal or subcarinal nodes
- N3 Contralateral hilar or mediastinal nodes; supraclavicular nodes

Metastases (M)
- M0 no metastases
- M1 distant metastases

Unresectable stages
- Tumors are unresectable if T4, N3, or M1
- Stage 3b: N3, M0, any T
    T4, M0, any T
- Stage 4: M1, any T, any N

5-year survival
- Stage 1: 60%
- Stage 2: 40%
- Stage 3a (limited disease): 20%
- Stage 3b, 4: 0%

LYMPH NODE IMAGING

Anatomy
Anterior mediastinal nodes
- Parietal node group
    Internal mammary nodes
    Superior diaphragmatic nodes
- Prevascular node group (anterior to the great vessels)

Middle mediastinal nodes
- Paratracheal*; the lowest node is the azygos node
- Subcarinal*: below bifurcation; drainage to right paratracheal nodes
- Subaortic; AP window node
- Tracheobronchial (pulmonary root, hilar)

Posterior mediastinal nodes
- Paraaortic
- Prevertebral
- Paraspinous: lateral to vertebral body

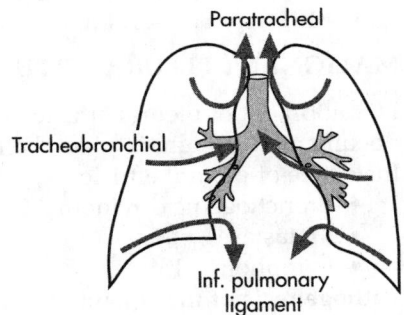

American Thoracic Society classification
This classification system assigns numbers to regional lymph nodes:
- 2R, 2L: paratracheal
- 4R, 4L: superior tracheobronchial
- 5, 6: ant. mediastinal
- 7: subcarinal
- 8, 9: posterior mediastinal
- 10R, 10L: bronchopulmonary
- 11R, 11L: pulmonary
- 14: diaphragmatic

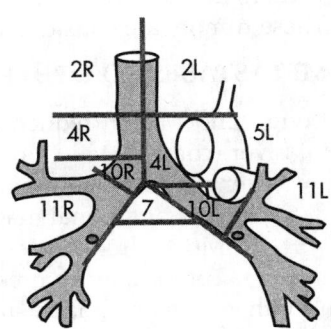

CT Criterion for abnormal nodes
Short axis lymph node diameter > 1 cm (approximately 60%-70% accuracy for differentiating between malignant and benign adenopathy).

*These nodes are best assessed by mediastinoscopy; the remainder of nodes are best assessed by CT.

CHEST WALL INVASION

Accuracy for detection of chest wall invasion by CT is 40%-60%.

Radiographic features

Reliable signs
- Soft tissue mass in chest wall
- Bone destruction

Unreliable signs
- Obtuse angles at contact between tumor and pleura
- > 3 cm of contact between tumor and pleura
- Pleural thickening
- Increased density of extrapleural fat

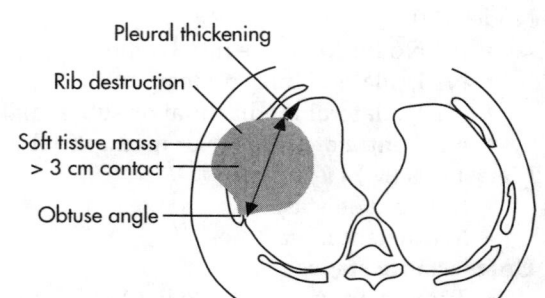

MEDIASTINAL INVASION

Contiguous invasion of mediastinal organs, heart, great vessels, aerodylative tract and vertebra indicates nonresectability.

Radiographic features
- Diaphragmatic paralysis (phrenic nerve involvement)
- Mediastinal mass with encasement of mediastinal structures
- MRI may be useful to detect vascular invasion

MALIGNANT PLEURAL EFFUSION

Development of pleural effusions usually indicates a poor prognosis. Presence of a documented malignant pleural effusion makes a tumor unresectable (T4 tumor).

Incidence of pleural effusion:
- Bronchogenic carcinoma, 50%
- Metastases, 50%
- Lymphoma, 15%

Pathogenesis of malignant effusions
- Pleural invasion increases capillary permeability
- Lymphatic or venous obstruction decreases clearance of pleural fluid
- Bronchial obstruction → atelectasis → decrease in intrapleural pressure

CENTRAL BRONCHIAL INVOLVEMENT

Tumors that involve a central bronchus usually cause lung collapse or consolidation. These tumors are considered unresectable (T4 tumors) only if they involve the carina.

METASTASES TO OTHER ORGANS

Lung tumors most frequently metastasize to:

Liver (common)

Adrenal glands (common)
- 30% of adrenal masses in patients with adenocarcinoma are adenomas
- Most adrenal masses in patients with small cell carcinomas are metastases
- Tumor may be present in a morphologically normal appearing gland

Other sites (especially small and large cell tumors)
- Brain (common)
- Bones
- Kidney

Specific Lung Tumors

ADENOCARCINOMA

Now the most frequent primary lung cancer. Typically presents as a multilobulated, peripheral mass. May arise in scar tissue: scar carcinoma.

BRONCHIOLOALVEOLAR CARCINOMA

Subtype of adenocarcinoma. Slow growth. The characteristic radiographic presentations are:
- Morphologic type
    Small peripheral nodule (solitary form), 25% (most common)
    Multiple nodules
    Chronic air space disease
- Air bronchogram
- Absent adenopathy
- Cavitation may be seen by HRCT (cheerio sign)

SQUAMOUS CELL CARCINOMA (SCC)

SCC is most directly linked with smoking. SCC carries the most favorable prognosis. The most characteristic radiographic appearances are:
- Cavitating lung mass, 30%
- Peripheral nodule, 30%
- Central obstructing lesion causing lobar collapse
- Chest wall invasion

PANCOAST TUMOR (SUPERIOR SULCUS TUMOR)

Tumor located in the lung apex that has extended into the adjacent chest wall. Histologically, Pancoast tumors are often squamous cell carcinoma. Clinical: Horner syndrome, pain radiating into arm (invasion of pleura, bone, brachial plexus, or subclavian vessels).

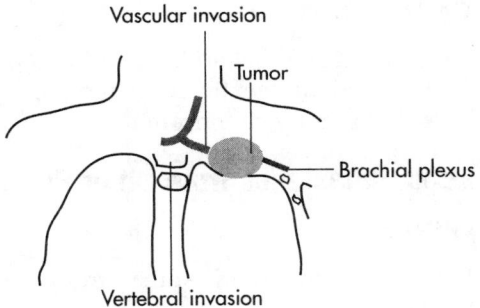

Radiographic features:
- Apical mass
- Chest wall invasion
- Involvement of subclavian vessels
- Brachial plexus involvement
- Bone involvement: rib, vertebral body

SMALL CELL CARCINOMA (NEUROENDOCRINE TUMOR, TYPE 3)

Most aggressive lung tumor with poor prognosis. At diagnosis, 80% of patients already have extrathoracic spread:
- Typical initial presentation: massive bilateral lymphadenopathy
- With or without lobar collapse
- Brain metastases

LARGE CELL CARCINOMA

Usually presents as large (> 70% are > 4 cm at initial diagnosis) peripheral mass lesions. Overall uncommon tumor.

CARCINOID (NEUROENDOCRINE TUMOR, TYPES 1 AND 2)

Represent 90% of low-grade malignancy tumors of the lung. The 10-year survival with surgical treatment is 85%. Types:
- Typical carcinoid: local tumor (Type 1)
- Atypical carcinoid (10%-20%): metastasizes to regional lymph nodes (Type II); liver metastases are very rare and therefore the carcinoid syndrome rarely develops.

Radiographic features:

Centrally located carcinoid, 80%
- Segmental or lobar collapse (most common finding)
- Periodic exacerbation of atelectasis
- Endobronchial mass

Peripherally located carcinoid, 20%
- Pulmonary nodule
- May enhance with contrast

HAMARTOMA

Hamartomas are benign tumors and are composed of cartilage (predominant component), connective tissue, muscle, fat, and bone. 90% are peripheral, 10% are endobronchial.

Radiographic features
- Well-circumscribed solitary nodules
- Chondroid "popcorn" calcification is diagnostic, but uncommon (< 20%)
- Fat attenuation within a lesion by HRCT is pathognomonic

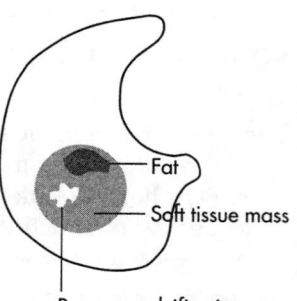

Fat

Soft tissue mass

Popcorn calcification

CARNEY'S TRIAD

- Gastric epitheloid leiomyosarcoma
- Functioning extra adrenal paraganglioma
- Pulmonary chondroma

Lung Metastases from Other Primaries

GENERAL

Pathways of metastatic spread from a primary extrathoracic site to lungs (in order of frequency):
- Spread via pulmonary arteries
- Lymphatic spread (celiac nodes → posterior mediastinal nodes + paraesophageal nodes) and in lung parenchyma
- Direct extension
- Endobronchial spread

Neoplasms with rich vascular supply draining into systemic venous system
- Renal cell carcinoma
- Sarcomas
- Trophoblastic tumors
- Testicle
- Thyroid

Neoplasms with lymphatic dissemination
- Breast (usually unilateral)
- Stomach (usually bilateral)
- Pancreas
- Larynx
- Cervix

Other neoplasms with high propensity to localize in lung
- Colon
- Melanoma
- Sarcoma

Radiographic features
- Multiple lesions, 95% > solitary lesion 5%
- Lung bases > apices (related to blood flow)
- Peripheral, 90% > central, 10%
- Metastases typically have sharp margins
- Fuzzy margins can result from peritumoral hemorrhage (choriocarcinoma, chemotherapy)
- Cavitations are common in squamous cell carcinomas from head and neck primaries

CALCIFIED METASTASES

Calcifications in lung metastases are observed in:

Bone tumor metastases
- Osteosarcoma
- Chondrosarcoma

Mucinous tumors
- Ovarian
- Thyroid
- Pancreas
- Colon
- Stomach

Metastases after chemotherapy

GIANT METASTASES ("CANNON BALL" METASTASES) IN ASYMPTOMATIC PATIENT

- Head and neck tumors cancer
- Testicular and ovarian tumors camcer
- Soft tissue tumors cancer
- Breast cancer
- Renal cancer
- Colon cancer

STERILE METASTASES

This term refers to pulmonary metastases under treatment that contain no viable tumor. Nodules typically consist of necrotic and/or fibrous tissue.

Chronic Lung Disease

Idiopathic Diseases

OVERVIEW OF IDIOPATHIC INTERSTITIAL PENUMONIAS		
Diagnosis	Clinical Features	HRCT Features
IPF	40-70 years, M > F, > 6 month history of dyspnea, cough, crackles, clubbing	Peripheral, basal, subpleural reticulation and honey-combing ± ground glass opacity
NSIP	40-50 years, M = F, dyspnea, cough, fatigue, crackles	Bilateral, patchy, subpleural ground glass opacity, ± reticulation
RB-ILD	30-50 years, M > F, dyspnea, cough	Ground glass, centrilobular nodules, ± centrilobular emphysema
AIP	Any age, M = F, acute onset dyspnea, diffuse crackles and consolidation	Ground glass consolidation, traction bronchiectasis and architectural distortion
COP	Mean 55 years, M = F, < 3 month history of cough, dyspnea, fever	Subpleural and peribronchial consolidation ± nodules in lower zones
DIP	30-54 years, M > F, Insidious onset weeks to months of dyspnea and cough	Ground glass, lower zone, peripheral
LIP	Any age, F > M	Ground glass opacity, ± poorly defined centrilobular nodules, thin walled cysts and air trapping may be found

NSIP, Nonspecific interstitial pneumonia; *RB-ILD*, respiratory bronchiolitis associated interstitial lung diseas; *AIP*, acute interstitial pneumonia; *COP*, cryptogenic organizing pneumonia; *DIP*, desquamative interstitial pneumonia; *LIP*, lymphoid interstitial pneumonia; *DAD*, diffuse alveolar damage.

IDIOPATHIC PULMONARY FIBROSIS (IPF)

Progressive inflammation, fibrosis, and destruction of lung (end-stage lung) of unknown cause. Synonyms: usual interstitial pneumonia (UIP, pathology term), cryptogenic fibrosing alveolitis (CFA, British term). Hamman-Rich syndrome is an acute, rapidly fatal form of IPF (IPF has also been termed "chronic" Hamman-Rich syndrome). Prognosis: mean survival 4 years (range 0.4 to 20 years). Lung biopsy is necessary for diagnosis. Treatment: steroids useful in 50%. Cytotoxic agents

Clinical findings
- Clubbing, 60%
- Nonproductive cough, 50%
- Dyspnea
- Weight loss, 40%

Pathology
Pathological changes are nonspecific and also occur in a variety of secondary disorders such as collagen vascular disease, drug reactions, pneumoconiosis. Liebow classification:
- UIP: alveolar fibrosis with inflammatory cells
- Desquamative interstitial pneumonitis (DIP): alveolar spaces are filled with macrophages

- Giant cell interstitial pneumonia (GIP); also found in cobalt and tungsten exposure, measles
- Bronchiolitis obliterans interstitial pneumonitis (BIP)
- Lymphoid interstitial pneumonia (LIP); may progess to lymphoma in < 20%: AIDS, viral pneumonia, Sjögren, RA, lupus. A localized form of LIP has been called "pseudolymphoma" because of histologic resemblance to lymphoma. Uncommonly progresses.

Radiographic features

Distribution

- Primarily in lower lung zones
- Peripheral subpleural involvement,

HRCT pattern

- Early: ground glass appearance
- Later: reticular pattern predominantly in lower lobes
- Endstage: honeycombing
- Traction bronchiectasis indicates fibrosis

Other

- Low lung volumes (fibrosis)
- Pulmonary hypertension with cardiomegaly (fibrosis), 30%
- Uncommon findings
  - Pleural thickening, 5%
  - Pneumothorax, 5%
  - Effusion, 5%

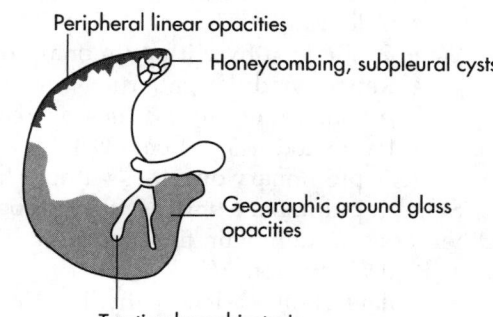

Peripheral linear opacities
Honeycombing, subpleural cysts
Geographic ground glass opacities
Traction bronchiectasis

SARCOID

Systemic granulomatous disease of unknown etiology (lung, 90% > skin, 25%> eye, 20% > hepato-splenomegaly, 15% > CNS, 5% > salivary glands > joints > heart). Clinical: 10-20 times more common in blacks than in whites, 30% are asymptomatic. Treatment: steroids. Prognosis:

Adenopathy only: more benign course
- 75% regress to normal within 3 years
- 10% remain enlarged
- 15% progress to stages 2 and 3

Parenchymal abnormalities: 20% develop progressive pulmonary fibrosis

Diagnosis

Biopsy

- Bronchial and transbronchial biopsy (sensitivity 90%)
- Open lung biopsy (sensitivity 100%)
- Lymph node, parotid gland or nasal mucosa biopsy (sensitivity 95%)
- Mediastinoscopy (sensitivity 95%)

Kveim test (sensitivity 70%-90%). Problems:

- Unavailability of validated tissue suspension (made from splenic tissue of infected patients)
- Lack of reactivity late in the disease
- Delay of 4-6 weeks before reactivity occurs

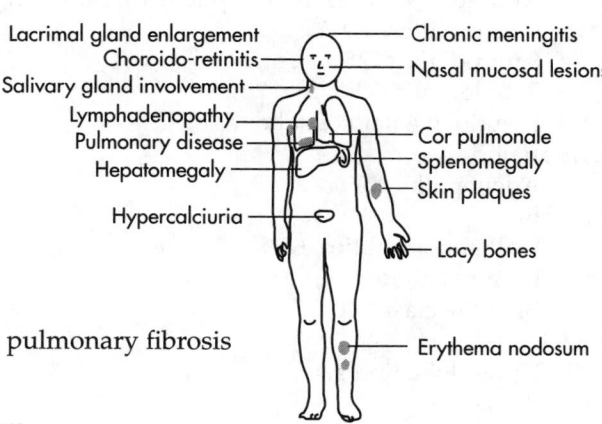

Lacrimal gland enlargement
Choroido-retinitis
Salivary gland involvement
Lymphadenopathy
Pulmonary disease
Hepatomegaly
Hypercalciuria
Chronic meningitis
Nasal mucosal lesions
Cor pulmonale
Splenomegaly
Skin plaques
Lacy bones
Erythema nodosum

Radiographic features
Stages (Silzbach classification, plain film)
  Stage 0: initial normal film, 10%
  Stage 1: adenopathy, 50%
  • Symmetric hilar adenopathy
  • Paratracheal, tracheobronchial, and azygos adenopathy is commonly associated with hilar adenopathy (Garland's triad)
  • Calcification, 5%
  Stage 2: adenopathy with pulmonary opacities, 30%
  • Reticulonodular pattern
  • Acinar pattern may coalesce to consolidation
  • Large nodules > 1 cm (2%)
  Stage 3: pulmonary opacities without hilar adenopathy, 10%
  Stage 4: pulmonary fibrosis, upper lobes with bullae
Other less common plain film findings:
  • Pleural effusion, 10%
  • Unilateral hilar adenopathy, 1%-3%
  • Eggshell calcification of lymph nodes
  • Complications of stage 3:
    Pneumothorax (blebs, bullae)
    Aspergillus with fungus ball
  • Bronchostenosis with lobar/segmental collapse

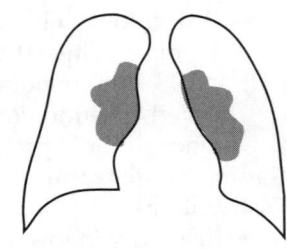

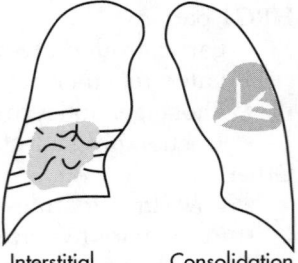

Interstitial   Consolidation

CT Features
Lung parenchyma
  • Nodules, (90%), along lymphatic distribution, i.e. central or axial and subpleural
  • Linear pattern, 50%
  • Ground glass, 25%
  • Subpleural thickening, 25%
  • Pseudoalveolar consolidation, 15%
Lymph nodes
  • Adenopathy, 80%
Bronchi
  • Wall abnormalities, 65%
  • Luminal abnormalities, 25%
  • Bronchiectasis, 10%
Endstage
  • Upper lobe fibrosis
  • Bullae
  • Traction bronchiectasis

Lymphoproliferative Disorders

Spectrum of lymphoid abnormalities in the chest characterized by accumulation of lymphocytes and plasma cells in the pulmonary interstitium or mediastinal/hilar lymph nodes. Believed to be due to stimulation of bronchus associated lymphoid tissue by antigens. Types:

Nodal disorders
- Castleman's disease (see medistinal masses)
- Infectious mononucleosis
- Angioimmunoblastic lymphadenopathy: drug hypersensitivity

Pulmonary parenchymal disorders
- Plasma cell granuloma (inflammatory pseudotumor, histiocytoma)
- Pseudolymphoma
- Lymphoid interstitial pneumonia (LIP)
- Lymphomatoid granulomatosis

OVERVIEW OF LYMPHOPROLIFERATIVE DISEASES				
Diagnosis	Lung	Nodes	Effusion	Malignancy
NODES				
Castleman's disease	Unaffected	Yes	No	No
Infectious mononucleosis	Mediastinal adenopathy	Yes	No	No
Angioimmunoblastic lymphadenopathy	Interstitial and alveolar opacity	Yes	10%	30%
PARENCHYMAL				
Plasma cell granuloma	Solitary pulmonary mass	No	No	No
Pseudolymphoma	Single or multiple parenchymal masses, air bronchograms	No	No	20%
LIP	Bilateral interstitial disease	No	No	< 20%
Lymphomatoid granulomatosis	Multiple pulmonary nodules, frequent cavitation	Rare	35%	30%

DIFFERENTIATION OF LYMPHOMA AND LYMPHOPROLIFERATIVE DISEASE		
Parameter	Lymphoproliferative Disorder	Lymphoma
Location	Parenchyma *or* lymph nodes but not both	Parenchyma *and* lymph nodes
Lymphoid population	Polyclonal	Monoclonal
Onset	Young patients (< 30 years)	Old patients (> 50 years)
Prognosis	Usually benign or low grade malignancy	Malignant

PLASMA CELL GRANULOMA

Local cellular proliferation of spindle cells, plasma cells, lymphocytes and histicytes in lung. Most common tumor-like pulmonary abnormality in children < 15 years.
Treatment: resection.
Radiographic features
- Solitary lung mass 1-12 cm
- No or very slow growth
- Cavitation and calcification are uncommon

LYMPHANGIOLEIOMYOMATOSIS (LAM)

Proliferation of smooth muscle cells along lymphatics in lung, thorax and abdomen. Unknown etiology. Rare. Clinical: young women presenting with spontaneous pneumothorax, chylothorax, hemoptysis, slowly progressive dyspnea. 10-year survival 75%. Similar lesions may be seen in tuberous sclerosis (LAM has been dubbed a *forme frust* of tuberous sclerosis). Extrapulmonary LAM is rare.

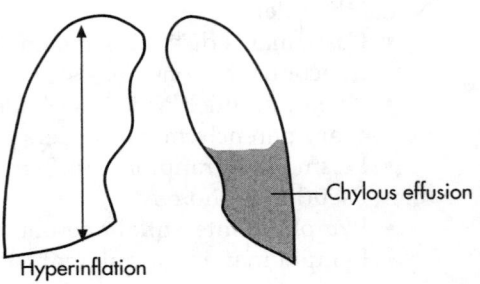

Hyperinflation — Chylous effusion

Radiographic features

Plain film/HRCT

- Numerous cystic spaces, 90%
    Size of cysts usually < 5-10 mm
    Thin walled
    Surrounded by normal lung
- Recurrent pneumothorax, 70%
- Chylous pleural effusions, 25%
- Plain film: overinflation, irregular opacities, cysts

Lymphangiography

- Obstruction of lymphatic flow at multiple levels
- Dilated lymphatics
- Increased number of lymphatics

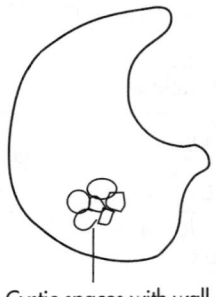

Cystic spaces with wall

TUBEROUS SCLEROSIS

Identical lesions as in LAM

Collagen Vascular Diseases

Collagen vascular diseases have a common pathogenesis in the lung: immune response → inflammation (interstitial pattern, granuloma) → vasculitis → obstruction (respiratory insufficiency, PA hypertension, etc.).

Pearls

- Lower lungs are more frequently affected (higher blood flow)
- Vasculitides of large arteries (e.g., periarteritis nodosa) cause pulmonary hypertension
- Most common complication is infection (secondary to immunosuppressive medications)

RHEUMATOID ARTHRITIS (RA)

There are seven forms of pleuropulmonary disease associated with RA:

Rheumatoid lung nodules, 20% (necrobiotic)

- Usually multiple
- Nodules may change rapidly in size, or disappear completely
- Association between cutaneous and pulmonary nodules

Pleural effusion and pleuritis

- Clinically, pleuritis is the most common pulmonary feature of RA
- Effusions are bilateral in the majority of patients
- Proportionately more common in men

- Fluid has low pH and low glucose
- Effusions are usually unilateral

Caplan's syndrome
- Nodular rheumatoid lung disease associated with pneumoconiosis

Fibrosing alveolitis
Constrictive bronchiolitis
Lymphoid hyperplasia
Pulmonary hypertension

Radiographic findings
- Bibasilar patchy alveolar opacities are early findings
- Dense reticulo (nodular) pattern is most frequent
- Pleural involvement, 20%
- Endstage: honeycombing, PAH

ANKYLOSING SPONDYLITIS (AS)

- Pulmonary fibrocystic changes in 1%-10%
- Upper lobe fibrotic scarring, infiltration, cystic air spaces
- Complications: tuberculosis and aspergillosis, 40%
- Ancillary findings:
  - Ossification of spinal ligaments, sacroileitis
  - Cardiomyopathy

SYSTEMIC LUPUS ERYTHEMATOSUS (SLE)

Pleural abnormalities are the most common findings
- Pleural thickening
- Recurrent pleural effusions
- Pleuritis is thought to be pathogenetically similar to polyserositis affecting joints
- Glucose level of pleural effusion is normal (decreased in RA)

Pulmonary disease: wide spectrum of findings but the usual presentation is as acute lupus pneumonitis
- Acute lupus pneumonitis: vasculitis and hemorrhage resulting in focal opacities at the lung bases
- Alveolar opacities, which may progress to ARDS
- Fibrosing alveolitis, rare
- Elevating diaphragm, atelectasis at bases (shown to be due to diaphragmatic dysfunction)
- Lupus-like disease can also be seen with drugs like hydralazine and procainamide

OTHER COLLAGEN VASCULAR DISEASES WITH PULMONARY MANIFESTATIONS

- Progressive systemic sclerosis (PSS) exists in two forms:
  - PSS with scleroderma
    - After esophagus, lung is the second most common site.
    - Interstitial fibrosis is the most commonpulmonary manifestation.
    - Pulmonary vascular and pleural changes are less common.
  - PSS with CREST (**c**alcinosis, **R**aynaud's, **e**sophageal dysmotility, **s**clerodactyly, **t**elangiectasia)
    - Usually in older women
    - Long history of PSS with swollen fingers
    - Mild disease, slowly progressive, greater life expectancy

- Polymyositis, dermatomyositis
- Mixed connective tissue disease (MCTD)

Vasculitis and Granulomatoses

WEGENER'S GRANULOMATOSIS

Systemic granulomatous process with destructive angiitis involving lung, upper respiratory tract, and kidney (necrotizing glomerulonephritis). Type IV immune mechanism.

Radiographic features

- Multiple nodules with cavitation (common)
- Interstitial, reticulonodular opacities at lung bases (earliest finding)
- Diffuse opacities (common) are due to:
    Atelectasis: bronchoconstriction
    Confluent nodules and masses
    Pulmonary hemorrhage
    Superimposed infection
- Other findings:
    Pleural effusions, 25%
    Adenopathy (rare)

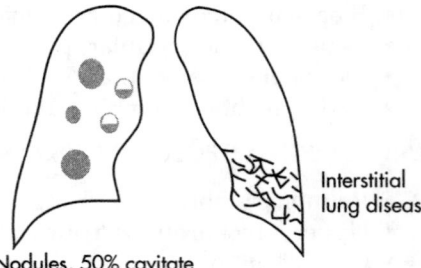

Nodules, 50% cavitate

Interstitial lung disease

LYMPHOMATOID GRANULOMATOSIS

Now considered a B cell lymphoma. Men > women. The multiple nodules are smaller than those in Wegner's. Nodules are not numerous and tend to cavitate.

CHURG-STRAUSS—ALLERGIC ANGITIS AND GRANULOMATOSIS

- Similar to polyarteritis nodosa, but patients have pulmonary diseases and asthma. Affects skin, kidneys, lung, heart and CNS, eosinophilia.

Radiographic features

- Patchy peripheral areas of consolidation
- Fleeting opacities
- Multiple nodules

Other Chronic Disorders

EOSINOPHILIC GRANULOMA (LANGERHANS CELL HISTIOCYTOSIS)

Langerhans cell histiocytosis consists of 3 clinical syndromes:
    Letterer-Siwe: acute disseminated form
    Hand-Schüller-Christian: chronic disseminated form
    Eosinophilic granuloma:

- Solitary bone lesion
- Small cystic spaces in lung parenchyma
- 3-10 mm pulmonary nodules
- Apical reticulonodular pattern
- Pneumothorax, 30%

IDIOPATHIC PULMONARY HEMORRHAGE (IPH)

Recurrent pulmonary hemorrhage which may result in interstitial fibrosis.
Age: usually < 10 years.

Radiographic features
- Diffuse air space pattern (radiographic appearance similar to Goodpasture's syndrome)
- Hilar adenopathy

AMYLOID

Extracellular deposition of protein derived from light chains of monoclonal Ig. Classification:
- Primary amyloid: heart, lung (70%), skin, tongue, nerves
- Amyloid associated with multiple myeloma (carpal tunnel syndrome, common)
- Secondary amyloid: (liver, spleen, kidney) in:
    - Chronic infections
    - Chronic inflammations
    - Neoplasm
- Hereditofamilial amyloidosis (Mediterranean fever; other syndromes)
- Local amyloidosis in isolated organs
- Amyloid associated with aging

Radiographic features
- Adenopathy and calcifications are common
- Plain film findings are nonspecific; multiple nodules or diffuse linear patterns
- Pulmonary involvement can be either diffuse or focal
- Diagnosis requires biopsy

NEUROFIBROMATOSIS

20% of patients with neurofibromatosis have pulmonary involvement:
- Progressive pulmonary fibrosis
- Bullae in upper lobes and chest wall
- Chest wall and mediastinal neurofibromas
- Intrathoracic meningoceles
- Ribbon deformities of the ribs

PULMONARY ALVEOLAR MICROLITHIASIS

Tiny calculi within alveoli. Unknown cause (hereditary). Rare.
Radiographic features
- Sandlike microcalcifications
- Bilateral, symmetrical involvement
- Pulmonary activity on bone scan

ALVEOLAR PROTEINOSIS

Proteinaceous, lipid-rich surfactant from type II pneumocytes accumulates in alveoli. Unknown etiology (may be associated with lymphoma or acute silicosis). Clinical: extensive sputum production (liters/day). Diagnosis: biopsy, sputum electron microscopy for alveolar phospholipids. Prognosis: 35% full recovery, 35% stable disease, 35% fatal. Complications: nocardiosis, aspergillosis, cryptococcosis, lymphoma. Treatment: aerosolized proteolytic agents, bronchoscopic lung lavage with 10-20 L saline (therapy of choice).

Radiographic features
- Bilateral, symmetric air space disease (butterfly, batwing pattern)
- Acinar pattern may become confluent (consolidation)
- CT: multifocal, panlobular, ground glass and air space opacities with septal thickening "crazy paving"
- Other findings from superimposed opportunistic infection

DRUG-INDUCED LUNG DISEASE

A large number of therapeutic drugs can cause lung toxicity. Because the findings are often nonspecific, a high index of suspicion is required. The most common abnormalities are:

Diffuse interstitial opacities
- Cytotoxic agents: bleomycin, methotrexate, carmustine, cyclosphosphamide
- Gold salts

Pulmonary nodules (uncommon)
- Cyclosporine
- Oil aspiration

Focal ASD
- Amiodarone accumulates in lysomes of phagocytes; high iodine content results in increased CT density of affected lung and liver

Diffuse ASD (pulmonary edema, hemorrhage)
- Cytotoxic agents: cytosine arabinoside, IL-2, OKT3
- Tricyclic antidepressants
- Salicylate
- Penicillamine
- Anticoagulants

Adenopathy
- Phenytoin (Dilantin)
- Cytotoxic agents: cyclosporine, methotrexate

Pleural effusions
- Drug-induced SLE
- Bromocryptine
- Methysergide, ergotamine tartrate

Inhalational Lung Disease

Pneumoconiosis

Pneumoconioses are caused by inhalation of inorganic dust particles that overwhelm the normal clearance mechanism of the respiratory tract. Types:

Benign pneumoconiosis: radiographic abnormalities are present while there are no symptoms or only minimal symptoms (not fibrogenic):
- Tin = stannosis
- Barium = baritosis
- Iron = siderosis

Fibrogenic pneumoconiosis (symptomatic)
- Silica = silicosis
- Asbestos = asbestosis
- Coal worker's pneumoconiosis (CWP)

INTERNATIONAL LABOR CLASSIFICATION (ILO)

The ILO classification can be used to classify or follow pneumoconioses. All pneumoconioses have similar radiographic features which range from few tiny nodules to end-stage lung disease. Classification:

Small opacities

Size:

- Nodules: p = < 1.5 mm, q = < 3 mm, r = > 3-10 mm
- Reticular: s = fine, t = medium, u = coarse
- Reticulonodular: x = fine, y = medium, z = coarse (This is not part of KO classification)

Location ("zone"): upper middle and lower zone of each lung field

How many (profusion = concentration): category 1 = few nodules, category 2 = lung markings still visible, category 3 = lung markings obscured

Large opacities

Size: A = < 5 cm, B = half of upper lung zone affected, C = > half of upper lung zone affected

Other features

Pleural thickening, plaques

Pleural calcification, diffuse

Small rounded opacities: size
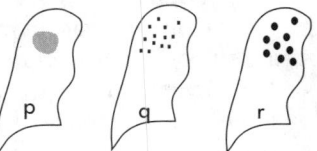

Small linear opacities: size
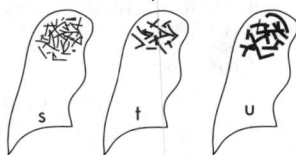

Small reticulonodular opacities: size
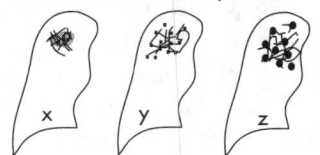

Small opacities: profusion
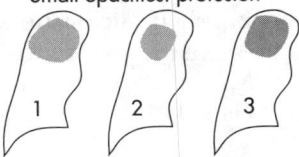

Large opacities
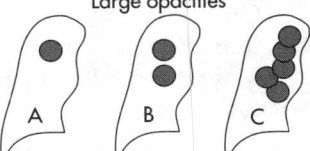

SILICOSIS

Causative agent is silicone dioxide (SiO_2) in quartz, cristobalite, tridy-mite. The severity of disease is related to the total amount of inhaled dust. Inhaled particles need to be < 5 μm in diameter since larger particles are removed by upper airways. Treatment: stop exposure; however, in contrast to CWP, silicosis may be progressive despite removal from dust environment. Isoniazid (INH) chemoprophylaxis. Occupations most at risk (only 5% of patients with > 20 years exposure will develop complicated form of pneumoconiosis) are:

- Mining (gold, tin, copper, mica)
- Quarrying (quartz)
- Sandblasting

Pathology

- Silica is phagocytosed by pulmonary macrophages
- Cytotoxic reaction causes formation of noncaseating granuloma
- Granulomas develop into silicotic nodules (2-3 mm in diameter)
- Pulmonary fibrosis develops as nodules coalesce

Clinical presentations

Chronic silicosis

- 20-40 years of exposure
- Predominantly affects upper lobes
- Rarely develops into massive fibrosis

Accelerated silicosis

- 5-15 years of heavy exposure
- Middle and lower lobes are also affected
- Radiographic appearance is similar to alveolar proteinosis

- Concomitant diseases:
    - TB, 25% (silicotuberculosis)
    - Collagen vascular disease, 10% (scleroderma, RA, SLE, Caplan's syndrome)

Acute silicosis (silicoproteinosis)

- < 3 years of exposure
- Fulminant course: diffuse multifocal ground glass or air space consolidations
- TB, 25%

Caplan syndrome

- RA
- Lung disease:
    - Silicosis (less common) or CWP (more common)
    - Rheumatoid nodules

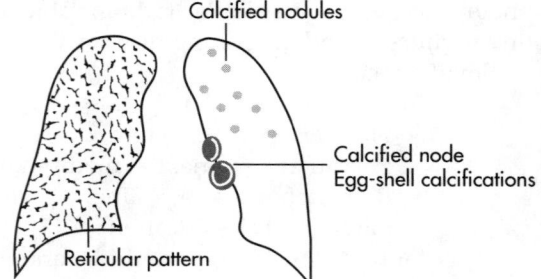

Radiographic features

Nodular pattern (common)

- Nodules 1-10 mm
- Calcific nodules, 20%
- Upper lobe > lower lobe
- Coalescent nodules cause areas of conglomerate opacities

Reticular pattern may precede or be associated with the nodular pattern

Hilar adenopathy

- Common
- Eggshell calcification, 5%

Progressive massive fibrosis (PMF)

- Masses (> 1 cm) formed by coalescent nodules
- Usually in posterior segment of upper lobes
- Vertical orientation
- Cavitation due to ischemia or superinfection from TB
- Often bilateral
- Retracts hila superiorly
- Main differential diagnosis: neoplasm, TB, fungus

Concomitant TB

COAL WORKERS' PNEUMOCONIOSIS (CWP)

Development of pneumoconiosis depends on the kind of inhaled coal: anthracite (50% incidence of pneumoconiosis) > bituminous > lignite (10% incidence). Pathology: coal macule around respiratory bronchioli with associated focal dust (centrilobular emphysema).

Radiographic features

Radiographically indistinguishable from silicosis

- Simple (reticulonodular) pneumoconiosis
    - Upper and middle lobe predominance
    - Nodules 1-5 mm
    - Centriacinar emphysema surrounds nodules
- Complicated pneumoconiosis with progressive massive fibrosis
    - Usually evolves from simple CWP
    - Mass lesions > 1 cm in diameter

ASBESTOS

Asbestos exposure causes a variety of manifestations:

Pleura
- Pleural plaques (hyalinized collagen)
- Diffuse thickening
- Benign pleural effusion
- Pleural calcification

Lung
- Interstitial fibrosis (asbestosis)
- Rounded atelectasis with Comet tail sign of vessel leading to atelactatic lung
- Fibrous masses

Malignancy
- Malignant mesothelioma
- Bronchogenic carcinoma
- Carcinoma of the larynx
- GI malignancies

Pathogenicity of fibers: crocidolite (South Africa) > amosite > chrysolite (Canada).

Risk professions:
- Construction, demolition workers
- Insulation workers
- Pipe-fitters and shipbuilders
- Asbestos miners

ASBESTOS-RELATED PLEURAL DISEASE

Focal pleural plaques

Hyalinized collagen in submesothelial layer of parietal pleura. Focal interrupted areas of pleural thickening.
- Pleural plaques have no functional significance
- Most common manifestation of asbestos exposure
- Preferred location: bilateral, posterolateral mid and lower chest
- Only 15% of pleural plaques are visible by CXR

Diffuse pleural thickening

- Less frequent than focal plaques
- Unlike focal plaques, diffuse thickening may cause respiratory symptoms (abnormal pulmonary function tests)
- Thickening of interlobar fissures
- May be associated with round atelectasis

Pleural calcifications

Pleural calcification in absence of other histories (hemothorax, empyema, TB, previous surgery) is pathognomonic of asbestos exposure.
- Calcium may form in center of plaques
- Contains uncoated asbestos fibers but no asbestos bodies
- Usually requires > 20 years to develop

Benign pleural effusions

Early sign of asbestos-related disease. Usually sterile, serous exudate. The diagnosis is one of exclusion: rule out other causes of pleural effusion:
- Malignant mesothelioma
- Bronchogenic carcinoma
- TB

Round atelectasis

Round-appearing peripheral atelectasis associated with pleural thickening. Although not unique to asbestos exposure, round atelectasis is common in patients with asbestos exposure and pleural thickening. Most commonly in posterior part of lower lobe.

Radiographic features

- Round mass in lung periphery
- Thickened pleura (due to asbestos-related disease)
- Mass is most dense at its periphery
- Mass is never completely surrounded by lung
- Atelectasis forms an acute angle with pleura
- Comet sign: bronchi and vessels curve toward the mass
- Signs of volume loss: displaced fissure

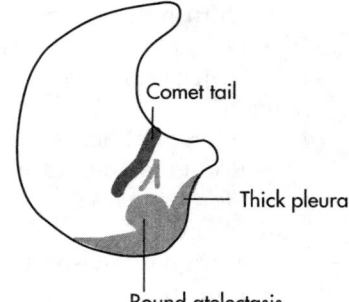

Comet tail

Thick pleura

Round atelectasis

ASBESTOSIS

Refers exclusively to asbestos related interstitial pulmonary fibrosis. Radiographically, features are similar to IPF:

- Reticular, linear patterns
- Initial subpleural location
- Progression from bases to apices
- Honeycombing occurs later in the disease
- No hilar adenopathy

MALIGNANCY IN ASBESTOS-RELATED DISEASE

- 7000-fold increase of mesothelioma (10% risk during lifetime; latency > 30 years after exposure)
- 7-fold increase of bronchogenic carcinoma
- 3-fold increase of GI neoplasm

Antigen-Antibody Mediated Lung Disease

Allergic reactions in lung can cause one of four patterns of disease:

- Granulomatous alveolitis
    Hypersensitivity alveolitis
    Chronic beryllium disease
- Pulmonary eosinophilia (pulmonary infiltrations with eosinophilae, PIE)
- Asthma
- Goodpasture's syndrome

HYPERSENSITIVITY PNEUMONITIS (EXTRINSIC ALLERGIC ALVEOLITIS)

Granulomatous inflammation of bronchioles and alveoli caused by immunologic response to inhaled organic material. Type III (Ag-Ab complex mediated) and type IV (cell mediated) hypersensitivity reactions. Antigens are often fungal spores or avian-related antigens.

HYPERSENSITIVITY ALVEOLITIS		
Disease	Antigen Source	Antigen
Farmer's lung	Moldy hay	*Micropolyspora faeni*
Bird fancier's lung (pigeons, parakeets)	Avian excreta	Avian serum proteins
Humidifier lung	Contaminated air conditioners	Thermophilic actinomyces
Bagassosis	Moldy bagasse dust	*Thermoactinomyces sacchari*
Malt worker's lung	Moldy malt	*Aspergillus clavatus*
Maple bark stripper's lung	Moldy maple bark	*Crystostroma corticale*
Mushroom worker's lung	Spores from mushrooms	Thermophilic actinomyces

Radiographic features
Acute, reversible changes
- Diffuse ground glass pattern
- Reticulonodular interstitial pattern
- Patchy areas of consolidation (rare)

Chronic, irreversible changes
- Progressive interstitial fibrosis (often upper lobe predominance) with honeycombing
- Pulmonary hypertension

CHRONIC BERYLLIUM DISEASE

T-lymphocyte dependent granulomatous response to inhaled beryllium (beryllium copper alloy, fluorescent strip lighting). Now a rare disease.

Radiographic features
Many similarities to sarcoidosis:
- Reticulonodular pattern → fibrosis
- Bilateral hilar lymph node enlargement

Distinction between berylliosis and sarcoidosis:
- History of exposure to beryllium
- Positive beryllium transformation test
- Increased concentration of beryllium in lung or lymph nodes
- Negative Kveim test

PULMONARY INFILTRATIONS WITH EOSINOPHILIA (PIE)

Group of diseases characterized by transient pulmonary opacities and eosinophilia ($> 500/mm^3$).

Types
Loeffler's syndrome (idiopathic origin)
- Benign transient pulmonary opacities
- Minimally symptomatic, self-limited
- Rare

Chronic eosinophilic pneumonia (idiopathic origin)
- Severe, chronic pneumonia
- Predominantly peripheral opacities

Pneumonias of known origin:
- Allergic bronchopulmonary mycoses (type 1 + 2 hypersensitivity)
    Aspergillus (ABPA is the most important one)
    Rare: *Candida, Curcularia lunata, Dreschlera hawaiiensis,* helminosporium,
        Stemphylium lanuginosum
- Helminth infection (nodular opacities, very high eosinophilia count, high IgE):
    Ascaris
    Schistosomiasis, 50% have pulmonary involvement
    Toxocara canis
    Microfilariasis
- Drugs
    Penicillin, tetracycline, sulfonamides
    Salicylates
    Chlorpropamide, imipramine
    Nitrofurantoin (causes chronic interstitial eosinophilic alveolitis with
        progression to fibrosis)

GOODPASTURE'S SYNDROME

Three main features: pulmonary hemorrhage, iron deficiency anemia, and
glomerulonephritis. Binding of circulating antibodies to glomerular and alveolar
basement membranes. Symptoms: hemoptysis, renal failure. Diagnosis:
antiglomerular basement membrane antibody, immunofluorescence of antibody, renal
biopsy.

Radiographic features
- Pulmonary hemorrhage: consolidation with air bronchogram
- Clearing of pulmonary hemorrhage in 1-2 weeks
- Repeated hemorrhage leads to hemosiderosis and pulmonary fibrosis →
  interstitial reticular pattern
- Renal findings

Toxin-Induced Interstitial Pneumonitis/Fibrosis

DRUG-INDUCED PULMONARY TOXICITY

Chemotherapeutic drugs
- Bleomycin
- BCNU
- Cyclophosphamide
- Methotrexate
- Procarbazine

Other drugs
- Amiodarone
- Nitrofurantoin
- Gold
- Carbamazepine

SILO FILLER'S DISEASE

- Due to NO_2 production (yellow gas) in silos
- NO_2 forms nitric acid (HNO) in lungs causing pulmonary edema and later to
  BOOP
- Silo fillers disease only occurs in September and October, when silos are being
  filled
- Safe NO_2 levels below 5 ppm

Airway Disease

Trachea

MALIGNANT TRACHEAL NEOPLASM

90% of all tracheobronchial tumors are malignant.

Types:

Primary malignancies
- Squamous cell carcinoma (most common)
- Adenoid cystic carcinoma (second most common)
- Mucoepidermoid (less common)
- Carcinoid (less common; strong contrast enhancement, octreotide uptake)

Metastases
- Local extension (common)
  Thyroid cancer
  Esophagal cancer
  Lung cancer
- Hematogenous metastases (rare)
  Melanoma
  Breast cancer

BENIGN NEOPLASM

Only 10% of tracheobronchial tumors are benign. Benign tumors are typically < 2 cm.

Types

Papilloma
- Common laryngeal tumors in children, rare in adults, often multiple
- May cause lung nodules
- Malignant potential (these lesions are caused by the papilloma virus and are benign, but may degenerate into malignancies)

Hamartoma
- Fat density is diagnostic
- Often calcified (popcorn pattern)

Adenoma
- Rare

SABER-SHEATH TRACHEA

Reduced coronal diameter (< 50% of sagittal diameter). Only affects the intrathoracic trachea; the extrathoracic trachea appears normal.
- 95% of patients have COPD
- More common in male patients
- Tracheal ring calcification is common

TRACHEOPATHIA OSTEOPLASTICA (TPO)

Foci of cartilage and bone develop in the submucosa of the tracheobronchial tree. Benign, rare condition. Most cases are discovered incidentally at autopsy.

Symptoms
- Dyspnea, hoarseness, expiratory wheeze/stridor (airway obstruction)
- Hemoptysis (mucosal ulceration)
- Cough and sputum production
- Rarely: atelectasis, pneumonia

Radiographic features
- Calcified tracheobronchial tree, nodules, osteocartilaginous growth
- Thickening of tracheal cartilage
- Sparing of the posterior membranous portion
- Narrowed lumen
- Distal ¾ of the trachea and the proximal bronchi are most commonly involved

RELAPSING POLYCHONDRITIS

Collagen vascular disease characterized by inflammation and progressive destruction of cartilage throughout the body (ribs, trachea, earlobes, nose, joints). Rare.

Diagnostic criteria (> 3 needed)
- Recurrent chondritis of auricles (painful ear)
- Inflammation of ocular structures (conjunctivitis, scleritis, keratitis, etc.)
- Chondritis (painful) of laryngeal/tracheal cartilage
- Cochlear or vestibular damage

Radiographic features
Trachea
- Diffuse narrowing (slitlike lumen)
- Thickening of tracheal wall

Location
- Ear, 90%
- Joints, 80%
- Nose, 70%
- Eye, 65%
- Respiratory tract, 55%
- Inner ear, 45%
- Other: cardiovascular, 25%, skin, 15%

TRACHEOBRONCHOMALACIA

Refers to weakening of tracheal and bronchial walls. Causes:
Primary (uncommon)
- Occurs in children
- May be associated with laryngomalacia

Secondary (more common)
- Intubation
- COPD
- Less common causes: recurrent infections, trauma, relapsing polychondritis
- Compression of trachea by vessels or mediastinal mass

Radiographic features
- Collapsed walls of trachea and bronchi
- Recurrent pneumonia

TRACHEOBRONCHOMEGALY (MOUNIER-KUHN DISEASE)

Atrophy and dysplasia of trachea and proximal bronchi. Associated with Ehlers-Danlos syndrome. The trachea measures > 3 cm and/or bronchi measure > 2.4 cm.

Chronic Bronchial Disease

Group of diseases characterized by increased airway resistance and reduction in expiratory flow. Entities include: chronic bronchitis, emphysema, asthma, bronchiectasis, and cystic fibrosis. The most common combination is chronic bronchitis and emphysema, often referred to as chronic obstructive pulmonary disease (COPD).

CHRONIC OBSTRUCTIVE PULMONARY DISEASE (COPD)

COPD is characterized by progressive obstruction to airflow. Two components:
- Chronic bronchitis is a clinical diagnosis: excessive mucus formation and cough for > 3 months during 2 consecutive years; all other causes of expectoration have to be ruled out. The diagnosis of chronic bronchitis is based on clinical history; chest films add little information except to exclude other underlying abnormalities.
- Emphysema is a pathological diagnosis: abnormal enlargement of air space distal to the terminal nonrespiratory bronchiole.

The exact etiology of COPD is unknown:
- Tobacco smoke
- Industrial air pollution
- Alpha$_1$-antitrypsin deficiency (autodigestion)

Clinical syndromes

Blue-bloaters
- Bronchitis, tussive type of COPD
- Episodic dyspnea due to exacerbation of bronchitis
- Young patients

Pink-puffers
- Emphysematous type of COPD
- Progressive exertional dyspnea due to the emphysema
- Old patients

Radiographic features

Features are nonspecific:

Tubular shadows (thickened bronchial walls)
- Parallel shadows if bronchiole is imaged in longitudinal section
- Thickening of bronchi imaged in axial section

Increased lung markings (dirty chest)
- Accentuation of linear opacities throughout the lung
- Very subjective finding

EMPHYSEMA

Abnormal enlargement of distal air spaces with destruction of alveolar walls with or without fibrosis. Underlying cause: imbalance of proteases and antiproteases. Clinical: chronic airflow obstruction, decreased FEV_1.

TYPES OF EMPHYSEMA*			
	Panacinar	Centroacinar	Paraseptal
Predominant location	Lower lobes	Upper lobes	Along septal lines (periphery of lung and branch points of vessels)
Distribution	Homogenous	Patchy	Peripheral
Associations	Alpha$_1$-antitrypsin deficiency, smoking	Chronic bronchitis, smoking	Smoking
Involvement	All components of acinus homogenously involved	Center of pulmonary acinus involved	Usually entire secondary pulmonary lobule
Imaging	Panlobular emphysema	Normal pulmonary lobule — central artery and bronchiole / Centrilobular emphysema	

*The designations "lobular" and "acinar" refer to the number of acini affected (few acini make up a lobule).

Radiographic features

Overinflation
- Flattening of hemidiaphragms (reliable sign): highest level of the dome is < 1.5 cm above a straight line drawn between the costophrenic and the vertebrophrenic junctions
- Tenting of diaphragm (invagination of thickened visceral pleura attached to septa between basal bullae)
- Saber sheath trachea
- Other less reliable signs:
    - Increase of retrosternal air space > 3 cm measured at level 3 cm below the sternomanubrial junction
    - Craniocaudal diameter of lung > 27 cm
    - Anterior bowing of sternum
    - Accentuated kyphosis
    - Widely spaced ribs

Vascular abnormalities
- Decreased number of vessels in areas of abnormal lung
- Absence of peripheral pulmonary vessels
- Fewer arterial branches
- Central pulmonary artery increased in size

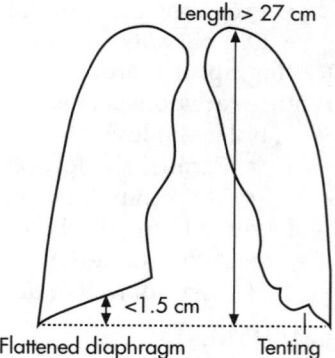

Length > 27 cm

<1.5 cm

Flattened diaphragm   Tenting

Emphysema
- Decreased attenuation of abnormal lung
- An air-fluid level indicates infection of a bulla

HRCT
- Centriacinar (centriacinar): the central portion of the pulmonary lobule is involved
- Panlacinar (panolobular): the whole acinus is involved, and central arteries and bronchioles can be seen (usually at apices)
- Paraseptal: emphysematous changes adjacent to septal lines in periphery and along fissures

Pearls
- As emphysema becomes more severe with time, the CT differentiation of the three types of emphysema becomes more difficult
- Different types of emphysema may co-exist
- Moderate to severe emphysema can be detected on CXR; for the detection of mild forms an HRCT is usually required
- HRCT is currently the most sensitive method to detect emphysema; however, a normal HRCT does not rule out the diagnosis of emphysema
- Always look at CXR before interpreting an HRCT; occasionally, CXR changes of emphysema are more evident than on HRCT changes (e.g., hyperinflation)
- 20% of patients with emphysema have normal HRCT
- 40% of patients with abnormal HRCT have normal pulmonary function tests
- Bullous lung disease is a severe form of emphysema that is highly localized and > 1 cm in size

ASTHMA

Hyperirritability of airways causes reversible airway obstruction (bronchial smooth muscle contraction, mucosal edema, hypersecretion of bronchial secretory cells: bronchospasm). The etiology is unknown (lgE participation).

Types
Extrinsic, allergic form
- Childhood asthma
- Immunologically mediated hypersensitivity to inhaled antigens

Intrinsic asthma
- Adults
- No immediate hypersensitivity

Radiographic features
Normal CXR in majority of patients
Severe or chronic asthma:
- Air trapping, hyperinflation: flattened diaphragm, increased retrosternal air space
- Limited diaphragmatic excursion

Bronchial wall thickening (tramlines), a nonspecific finding, is also seen in chronic bronchitis, cystic fibrosis, bronchiectasis, pulmonary edema
Complications:
- Acute pulmonary infection
- Mucous plugs
- Allergic bronchopulmonary aspergillosis (ABPA)
- Tracheal or bronchial obstruction
- Pneumomediastinum/pneumothorax

BRONCHIECTASIS

Irreversible dilatation of bronchi (reversible bronchial dilatation may be seen in viral and bacterial pneumonia). Clinical: recurrent pneumonias and/or hemoptysis. HRCT is now the method of choice for workup of bronchiectasis.

Types

Congenital (rare)
- Abnormal secretions: cystic fibrosis
- Bronchial cartilage deficiency: Williams-Campbell syndrome
- Abnormal mucociliary transport: Kartagener's syndrome
- Pulmonary sequestration

Postinfectious (common)
- Childhood infection
- Chronic granulomatous infection
- ABPA
- Measles

Bronchial obstruction
- Neoplasm
- Inflammatory nodes
- Foreign body
- Aspiration

MORPHOLOGIC CLASSIFICATION OF BRONCHIECTASIS			
	Cylindrical	**Varicose**	**Cystic**
Terminal divisions* Pathology CXR, HRCT	20 Not end-stage Fusiform dilatation, tramlines, signet signs	18 Destroyed lung Tortuous dilatation rare	4 Destroyed lung Saccular dilatation, "string of cysts," AFL common

*Normal tracheobronchial tree has 23-24 divisions.

Radiographic features

Plain film
- Tramline: horizontal, parallel lines corresponding to thickened, dilated bronchi
- Bronchial wall thickening (best seen end-on)
- Indistinctness of central vessels due to peribronchovascular inflammation
- Atelectasis

HRCT
- Conspicuous bronchi
    - Bronchi can be seen in outer third of lung
    - Bronchi appear larger than accompanying vessels
- Bronchial walls
    - Thickened wall
    - Signet ring sign: focally thickened bronchial wall adjacent to pulmonary artery branch

Signet ring sign

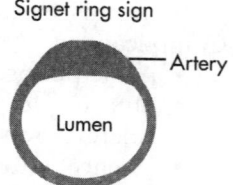

Pearls
- Bronchography may be indicated if clinical suspicion of bronchiectasis is high and CT is negative; CT has a low positive predictive value for mild forms of bronchiectasis. Bronchography is rarely performed alone
- Differentiation of cystic bronchiectasis and cystics spaces in IPF (honeycombing) is difficult; bronciectasis usually involves lower lobes; honeycombing is not associated with air-fluid levels
- To distinguish emphysema from bronchiectasis expiratory scans will show air trapping in bullae, cystic bronchiectasis will collapse

CYSTIC FIBROSIS

Caused by an abnormality in the cystic fibrosis transmembrane conductance regulator protein, which regulates the passage of ions through membranes of mucus-producing cells. Autosomal recessive disease (incidence 1:2000). Pathophysiology:
- Dysfunction of exocrine glands causing thick, tenacious mucus that accumulates and causes bronchitis and pneumonia
- Reduced mucociliary transport: airway obstruction with massive mucous plugging

Spectrum of disease

Pulmonary, 100%
- Chronic cough
- Recurrent pulmonary infections: colonization of plugged airways by *Staphylococcus* and *Pseudomonas*
- Progressive respiratory failure
- Finger clubbing: hypertrophic osteoarthropathy from hypoxemia

GI tract
- Pancreatic insufficiency 85%: steatorrhea, malabsorption
- Liver cirrhosis
- Rectal prolapse
- Neonates: meconium ileus, meconium peritonitis, intussusception

Other
- Sinusitis: hypoplastic frontal sinus, opacification of other sinuses
- Infertility in males

Radiographic features

Severity of bronchiectasis
- Mild: lumen equal to adjacent blood vessels
- Moderate: lumen 2-3 times the size of adjacent blood vessels
- Severe: lumen > 3 times the size of adjacent blood vessels

Peribronchial thickening
- Wall thickness ≥ than the diameter of adjacent blood vessels

Mucous plugging
- Determine number of pulmonary segments involved
- Air trapping → increased lung volumes
- Collapse, consolidation
- Bullae

Location: predominantly upper lobes and superior segments of lower lobes

Other
- Reticular, cystic pattern of lung fibrosis
- Prominent hila:
    Adenopathy
    Large pulmonary arteries (PAH)
- Recurrent pneumonias

Complications

Early

- Lobar atelectasis (especially RUL)
- Pneumonia

Late

- Respiratory insufficiency, hypertrophic osteoarthropathy
- Recurrent pneumothorax (rupture of bullae or blebs)
- Cor pulmonale and pulmonary arterial hypertension
- Hemoptysis
- *Aspergillus* superinfection

BRONCHIOLITIS OBLITERANS

Bronchiolitis obliterans (Swyer-James syndrome, unilateral emphysema) refers to unilateral air trapping caused by obstruction of distal bronchioles. Etiology of adult bronchiolitis:

Obliterative

- Exposure to toxic fumes
- Bone marrow transplant
- Viral infections
- Drugs

Proliferative

- Acute infectious
- Respiratory bronchiolitis
- BOOP
- COPD
  - Asthma
  - Chronic bronchitis

Radiographic features (CT)

- Nodules with branching opacities: tree-in-bud appearance
- Ground glass attenuation and consolidation
- Moasiac pattern
  - Seen with obliterative bronchiolitis
  - Moasiac pattern due to hypoxic vasoconstriction in ares of bronchiolar obstruction with redistribution to normal areas
  - Decreased size and number of vessels in affected lung with air trapping on inspiration/expiration CT, thus the apparent ground glass appearing lung is normal
- Other nonspecific findings
  - Bronchiectasis
  - Bronchial wall thickening

Lung Injury

TRAUMA

Four major mechanisms of injury:

- Direct impact
- Sudden deceleration (motor vehicle accident): sudden torsion at interfaces of fixed (e.g., paraspinal) and mobile (e.g., lung) components
- Spallation: broad kinetic shock wave, which is partially reflected at a liquid-gas interface, leading to local disruption of alveoli and supporting structures
- Implosion: low-pressure afterwave that causes rebound overexpansion of gas bubbles

Other mechanisms of chest trauma include:
- Posttraumatic aspiration
- Inhalation injury
- Increased capillary permeability: fat emboli, oligemic shock, neurogenic pulmonary edema

Pearls
- Radiographic and clinical evidence of lung trauma is often absent in the first 2-3 hours after trauma
- There is no consistent relationship between external chest wall injury and underlying lung injury, especially in children
- Radiographic studies usually underestimate the true extent of pulmonary trauma

PNEUMOTHORAX

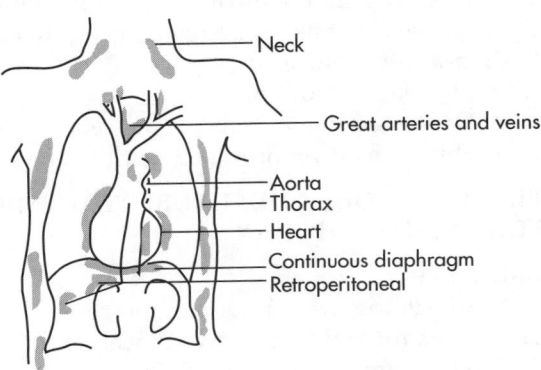

Common causes:
Iatrogenic
- Percutaneous biopsy, 20%
- Barotrauma, ventilator, 20%

Trauma
- Lung laceration
- Tracheobronchial rupture

Cystic lung disease
- Bulla, bleb: often in healthy young men; 30% recurrence
- Emphysema, asthma
- PCP
- Honeycombing: end-stage interstitial lung disease
- Lymphangioleiomyomatosis (pneumothorax in 75% of cases)
- Eosinophilic granuloma (pneumothorax in 20% of cases)

Parenchymal necrosis
- Lung abscess, necrotic pneumonia, septic emboli, fungal disease, TB
- Cavitating neoplasm, osteogenic sarcoma
- Radiation necrosis

Other
- Catamenial: recurrent spontaneous pneumothorax during menstruation, associated with endometriosis of pleura

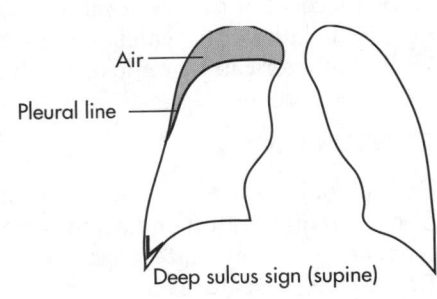

Deep sulcus sign (supine)

Radiographic features
Appearance
- Upright position
  Air in pleural space is radiolucent
  White line of the visceral pleura is distinctly visible
  Volume loss of underlying lung
- Supine position
  Deep sulcus sign: anterior costophrenic angle sharply delineated

Detection
- Lateral decubitus (suspected side should be up, whereas it should be down for fluid); 5 mL of air detectable
- Upright expiration film
- CT most sensitive

Size of pneumothorax can be estimated but is rarely of practical use
- Average distance (AD in cm) = (A + B + C)/3
- % pneumothorax ≈ AD (in cm) × 10, e.g.,:
  - AD of 1 cm corresponds to a 10% pneumothorax
  - AD of 4 cm corresponds to a 40% pneumothorax

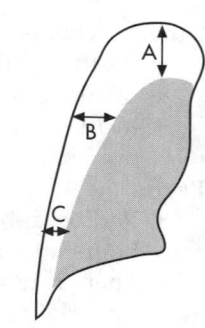

Pneumothorax

Effusion

TENSION PNEUMOTHORAX

Valve effect during inspiration/expiration leads to progressive air accumulation in thoracic cavity. The increased pressure causes shift of mediastinum and ultimately vascular compromise. Treatment: emergency chest tube placement.

Radiographic features
- Overexpanded lung
- Depressed diaphragm
- Shift of mediastinum and heart to contralateral side

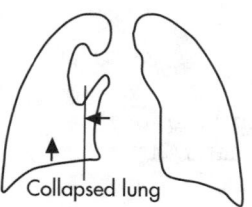

Pneumothorax

Collapsed lung

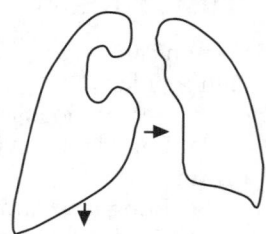

Tension pneumothorax

PERCUTANEOUS CHEST TUBE PLACEMENT FOR PNEUMOTHORAX

Indication
- All symptomatic pneumothoraces

Technique for Heimlich valve placement (for biopsy induced pneumothorax)
1. Entry: mid-clavicular line 2nd-4th anterior intercostal space
2. Aspirate air with 50-mL syringe
3. Use small drainage kits that includes a Heimlich valve (one-way airflow system). During expiration, positive intrapleural pressure causes air to escape through the valve

Technique for chest tube placement (any pneumothorax)
1. Entry: posterior or lateral or region of largest pneumothorax
2. Local anesthesia
3. Place 12 Fr drainage catheter using trocar technique
4. Put catheter to wall suction
5. Catheter can be removed if there is no pneumothorax 24 hours after clamping of the catheter

CONTUSION

Endothelial damage causes extravasation of blood into interstitium and alveoli. Occurs mainly in lung adjacent to solid structures (ribs, vertebra, heart, liver, etc). Appears 6-24 hours after injury. Clinical: hemoptysis, 50%. Mortality rate: 15%-40%.

Radiographic features
- Pulmonary opacities are due to hemorrhage and edema
- Air bronchograms are commonly seen by CT, but are not always present if there is associated bronchial obstruction
- Contusions usually appear 6-24 hours after trauma and resolves by 7-10 days
- Opacities that do not resolve by 7-10 days may represent:
  - Postlaceration hematoma
  - Aspiration
  - Hospital-acquired pneumonia
  - Atelectasis
  - ARDS

LUNG LACERATION

Produced by sharp trauma (rib fractures), deceleration, shearing, or implosion. Pathogenetically, there is a linear tear (may be radiographically visible) that becomes round or ovoid (pneumatocele) with time. Usually accompanied by hemoptysis and pleural and parenchymal hemorrhage. Bronchopleural fistulas are a common complication. Detection of a laceration is clinically important as lacerations can become secondarily infected and also lead to bronchopleural fistula requiring prolonged chest tube drainage.

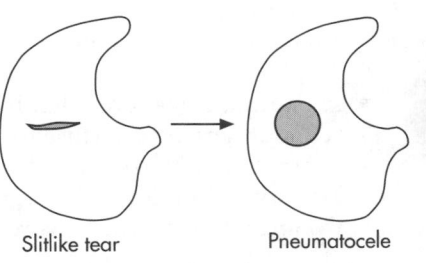

Slitlike tear   Pneumatocele

TYPES OF PULMONARY LACERATIONS			
Type	Location	Penumothorax	Mechanism
1	Mid lung	Variable	Shear between parenchyma and tracheobronchial tree
2	Paraspinal	Uncommon	Shear due to sudden herniation of lower lobe parenchyma in front of vertebral column
3	Subpleural	Usual	Puncture by displaced rib fracture
4	Subpleural	Usual	Shear at site of transpleural adhesion

FAT EMBOLISM

Lipid emboli from bone marow enter pulmonary and systemic circulation. When complicated by ARDS fat embolism has high mortality. Frequently CNS is also affected.

Radiographic features

- Suspect in patients with initially clear lungs, sudden onset of dyspnea, and multiple fractures
- Interstitial and alveolar hemorrhagic edema produces a varied radiographic appearance
- Radiographic opcaities induced by fat embolism become evident only 48 hrs after the incidenct ("delayed onset")
- Opacities clear in 3-7 days

TRACHEOBRONCHIAL TEAR

High mortality (30%). Requires early bronchoscopy for early detection to avoid later bronchostenosis. Two presentations:

- Tear of right mainstem and distal left bronchus: pneumothorax not relieved by chest tube placement. Most common locations are main bronchi (R > L); 75% occur within 2 cm of tracheal carina.
- Tear of trachea and left mainstem bronchus: air leaks are usually confined to mediastinum and subcutaneous tissues

DIAPHRAGMATIC TEAR

90% of tears occur on the left side. 90% of clinically significant hemidiaphragm ruptures are overlooked initially and 90% of strangulated diaphragmatic hernias are of traumatic etiology

Radiographic features
- Air-fluid levels or abnormal air collection above diaphragm
- Abnormal elevation of left hemidiaphragm with or without herniated gastric fundus, or colon
- Contralateral tension displacement of mediastinum
- Abnormal location of NG tube
- Confirmation of tear by coronal MRI

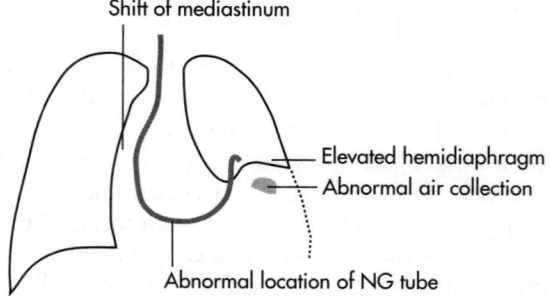

Shift of mediastinum

Elevated hemidiaphragm
Abnormal air collection

Abnormal location of NG tube

ESOPHAGEAL TEAR

- Esophageal tear (thoracic inlet, gastroesophageal junction)
- Blunt injuries usually seen in phrenic ampulla and cervical esophagus, while penetrating injuries can occur anywhere
- Chest radiographs are nonspecific and usually show wide mediastinum, left pleural effusion, or hydropneumothorax
- Pneumomediastinum is common but is a nonspecific finding
- Pleural effusion has low pH and high amylase levels

OTHER INJURIES

- Aortic injury
- Hemothorax
- Chylothorax
- Cardiac injury
- Fractures: rib, spine

Postoperative Chest

COMPLICATIONS OF SURGICAL PROCEDURES

Mediastinoscopy
Complication rate: < 2%:
- Mediastinal bleeding
- Pneumothorax
- Vocal cord paralysis (recurrent nerve injury)

Bronchoscopy
- Injury to teeth, aspiration
- Transient pulmonary opacities, 5%
- Fever, 15%
- Transbronchial biopsy:
    Pneumothorax, 15%
    Hemorrhage (> 50 ml), 1%

Wedge resection
- Air leaks (common)
- Contusion
- Recurrence of tumor

Median sternotomy complications
Complication rate 1%-5%:
- Mediastinal hemorrhage
- Mediastinitis (focal fluid collection)
- Sternal dehiscence
- False aneurysm
- Phrenic nerve paralysis
- Osteomyelitis of sternum

Chest tube placement
- Horner syndrome (pressure on sympathetic ganglion)
- False aortic aneurysm

PNEUMONECTOMY

Radiographic features
- ⅔ of the hemithorax fills with fluid in 4-7 days; it is important that successive films demonstrate gradual fill-in and that the residual air bubble does not get bigger; an air bubble increasing in size suggests the presence of a bronchopleural fistula
- Gradual shift of the mediastinum and heart toward the pneumonectomy side
- Contralateral lung may normally be herniated toward the pneumonectomy side at the apex and mimic the presence of residual lung

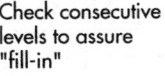

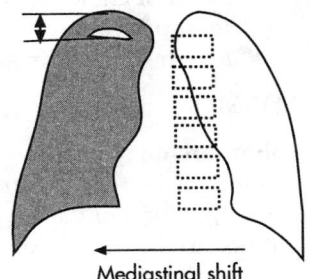

Check consecutive levels to assure "fill-in"

Opacification (fluid)

Mediastinal shift

Lobectomy
- Remaining lobes expand to fill the void; splaying of vessels
- Slight shift of mediastinum, elevation of hemidiaphragm

(Sub)segmental resection
- Little or no parenchymal rearrangement
- Postoperative opacities (hemorrhage, contusion, edema) are common

Postpneumonectomy syndrome
This rare syndrome refers to airway obstruction that occurs after pulmonary resections and is due to an extreme shift of the mediastinum or rotation of hilar structures. Occurs most commonly after right pneumonectomy, or after a left pneumonectomy when a right arch is present. Radiographic features

Airway obstruction
- Air trapping: hyperinflated lung
- Recurrent pneumonia, bronchiectasis

Narrowing of bronchi or trachea, bronchomalacia
Postsurgical changes
- Hyperinflation of contralateral lung
- Marked shift of mediastinum

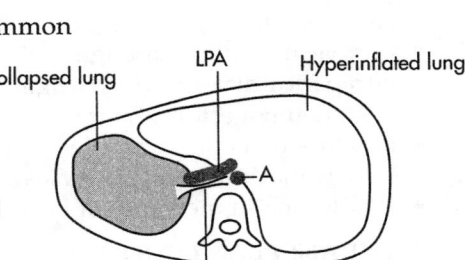

Collapsed lung   LPA   Hyperinflated lung

A

Collapsed L main bronchus

BRONCHOPLEURAL FISTULA (BPF)

A fistula between bronchus and pleural space develops in 2%-4% of pneumonectomy patients; with large fistulas the fluid in the pneumonectomy cavity may drown the opposite healthy lung. Factors that predispose to BPF:
- Active inflammation (TB), necrotizing infection
- Tumor in bronchial margin
- Devascularized bronchial stump, poor vascular supply
- Preoperative irradiation
- Contamination of the pleural space

Radiographic features
Plain film
- Persistent or progressive pneumothorax
- Sudden shift of mediastinum to the normal side

Nuclear medicine
- Xenon leak

Sinography with non-ionic contrast material
- Exam of choice to define the size of a pleural cavity and bronchial communication
- Alternatively thin section CT may show communication

TORSION

Lobar torsion

A prerequisite for torsion is the presence of complete fissures. Predisposing factors: masses, pleural effusion, pneumothorax, pneumonia, surgical resection of inferior pulmonary ligament. Rare.
- Most commonly the right middle lobe (RML) rotates on its bronchovascular pedicle
- Causes obstruction of venous flow, ischemia, necrosis
- Plain film: mobile opacity at different locations on different views

Cardiac herniation

Rare. 50%-100% mortality. Most often occurs following a right pneumonectomy requiring intrapericardial dissection.

Radiographic features
- Heart is rotated to the right
- Cardiac herniation through pericardial sac results in intrapericardial air, which originates from the postpneumonectomy space
- Presence of a notch
- Intracardiac catheters are kinked
- "Snowcone" appearance of heart border

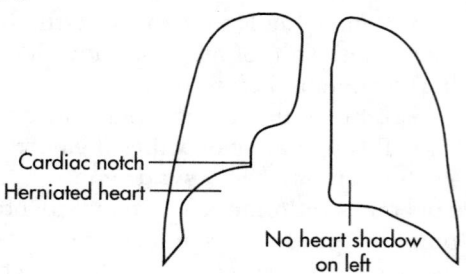

Cardiac notch
Herniated heart
No heart shadow on left

LUNG TRANSPLANTATION

Transplantation of the left lung is technically easier because of the longer left bronchus.

Radiographic features

Reimplantation response
- Diffuse alveolar pattern of noncardiogenic pulmonary edema develops within 4-5 days in the transplanted lung due to capillary leak. It never develops later
- The alveolar pattern lasts one to several weeks

Rejection
- Acute rejection is most commonly detected by biopsy when there are no associated radiographic findings; when radiographic findings are present, they are:

    Diffuse interstitial pattern in peribronchovascular distribution
    Septal thickening
    Pleural effusion
    Alveolar edema
- Chronic rejection

    Bronchiolitis obliterans (air-trapping on expiratory scans)
    Bronchiectasis

Infections, 50% of patients
- Infections usually involve the transplanted, not the native lung, due to poor mucociliary clearance, and/or lymphatic interruption
- Pathogens: *Pseudomonas*, *Staphylococcus* > other bacterial, viral, fungal infections

Airways
- Leaks at bronchial anastomosis site are the most common abnormality and usually present as pneumomediastinum and/or pneumothorax in perioperative period
- Operations to prevent leaks
  Omental flap around anastomosis
  Telescope type anastomosis
- Bronchial strictures may require stenting

Pulmonary Vasculature

Pulmonary Artery Hypertension

GENERAL

PAH is defined as $P_{sys} > 30$ mm Hg or $P_{mean} > 25$ mm Hg. Normal pulmonary arterial pressures in adult:
- P_{sys}: 20 mm Hg
- P_{dias}: 10 mm Hg
- P_{mean}: 14 mm Hg
- Capillary wedge pressure: 5 mm Hg

Causes of PAH
Primary PAH (females 10-40 years; rare)
Secondary PAH (more common)
- Eisenmenger
- Chronic PE
- Emphysema, pulmonary fibrosis

Classification
Precapillary hypertension
  Vascular
- Increased flow: L-R shunts
- Chronic PE
- Vasculitis
- Drugs
- Idiopathic
  Pulmonary
- Emphysema
- Interstitial fibrosis
- Fibrothorax, chest wall deformities
- Alveolar hypoventilation
Postcapillary hypertension
  Cardiac
- LV failure
- Mitral stenosis
- Atrial tumor

Pulmonary venous
- Idiopathic venoocclusive disease
- Thrombosis

Radiographic features
- Enlarged main PA (diameter correlates with pressure): > 29 mm is indicative of PAH
- Rapid tapering of PA towards the periphery
- Decreased velocity of pulmonary flow by MRA
- Calcification of the pulmonary arteries is pathognomonic but occurs late in the disease
- Cardiomegaly (cor pulmonale)
- If the ratio of pulmonary artery diameter to aortic diameter is greater than one (rPA > 1) by CT, there is a strong correlation with elevated mean pulmonary artery pressure, particularly in patients less than 50 years of age.
- By HRCT scans, both primary and secondary forms of pulmonary hypertension may produce a mosaic pattern of lung attenuation, a finding suggestive of regional variations in parenchymal perfusion. A vascular cause for the mosaic pattern is suggested when areas of high attenuation contain larger caliber vessels and areas of low attenuation contain vessels of diminished size.

Pulmonary Edema

TYPES OF PULMONARY EDEMA

Signs	Cardiac	Renal	Lung Injury
Heart size	Enlarged	Normal	Normal
Blood flow	Inverted	Balanced	Normal
Kerley lines	Common	Common	Absent
Edema	Basilar	Central: butterfly	Difuse
Air bronchograms	Not common	Not common	Very common
Pleural effusions	Very common	Common	Not common

Causes of pulmonary edema
Cardiogenic
    Adults
- LV failure from CAD (most common)
- Mitral regurgitation (common)
- Ruptured chordae
- Endocarditis

    Neonates
- TAPVC below diaphragm
- Hypoplastic left heart
- Cor triatriatum

Renal
- Renal failure
- Volume overload

Lung injury (Increased permeability: capillary leak)
- Septic shock, neurogenic shock
- Fat embolism
- Inhalation: SO_2, O_2, Cl_2, NO_2
- Aspiration, drowning

GRADING OF CARDIOGENIC PULMONARY EDEMA

Fluid accumulation in the lung due to cardiogenic causes (CHF; pulmonary venous hypertension) follows a defined pattern:

Grade 1: vascular redistribution (10-17 mm Hg)
- Diameter of upper lobe vessels equal or increased over diameter of lower lobe vessels at comparable distance from hilum
- Pulmonary veins in 1st intercostal space > 3 mm in diameter

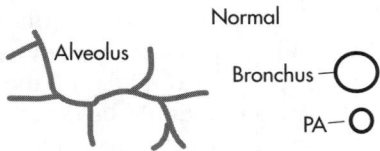

Grade 2: interstitial edema (18-25 mm Hg)
- Peribronchiovascular cuffing, perihilar haziness
- Kerley lines (differential diagnosis: chronic fibrosis from edema, hemosiderin, tumor, etc.)
- Unsharp central pulmonary vessels (perivascular edema)
- Pleural effusion

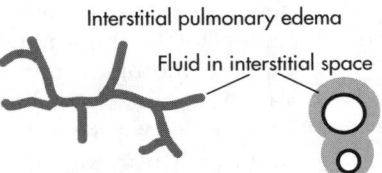

Grade 3: alveolar edema (> 25 mm Hg)
- Air space disease: patchy consolidation, air bronchograms

ASYMMETRICAL PULMONARY EDEMA

- Gravitational (most common)
- Underlying COPD (common)
- Unilateral obstruction of pulmonary artery: PE
- Unilateral obstruction of lobar pulmonary vein: tumor

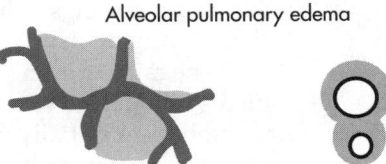

Pulmonary Embolism

Acute pulmonary embolism is associated with significant morbidity and mortality causing 120,000 deaths/year in United States. Types:
- Incomplete infarct: hemorrhagic pulmonary edema without tissue necrosis; resolution within days
- Complete infarct: tissue necrosis; healing by scar formation

Risk factors
- Immobilization > 72 hours (55% of patients with proven PE have this risk factor)
- Recent hip surgery, 40%
- Cardiac disease, 30%
- Malignancy, 20%
- Estrogen use (prostate cancer, contraceptives), 6%
- Prior deep vein thrombosis (DVT), 20%; risk factors:
    - Myocardial infarction
    - Thoracoabdominal surgery
    - Permanent pacemaker
    - Venous catheters

Clinical findings
Chest pain 90%, tachypnea (>16 resp/min) 90%, dyspnea 85%, rales 60%, cough 55%, tachycardia 40%, hemoptysis 30%, fever 45%, diaphoresis 25%, cardiac gallop 30%, syncope 15%, phlebitis 35%

Radiographic features
Radiographic signs are nonspecific and are present only if a significant infarction occurs.

Imaging algorithm
- Patients with normal CXR are evaluated by V/Q scans. Patients with normal or very low probability scintigraphic findings are presumed not to have pulmonary emboli. Patients with a high-probability scan usually undergo anticoagulation therapy. All other patients should be evaluated with helical CT pulmonary angiography, conventional pulmonary angiography, or lower-extremity ultrasound (US), depending on the clinical situation.

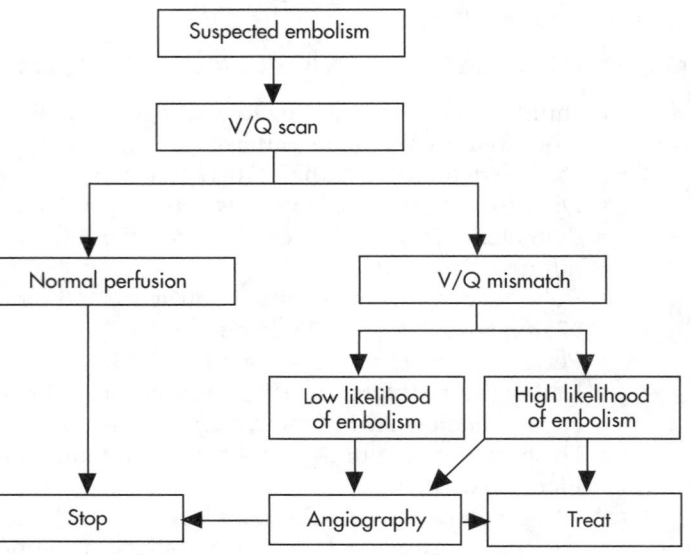

- Patients with abnormal chest radiographic findings, especially chronic obstructive pulmonary disease, are unlikely to have definitive scintigraphic findings. These patients undergo helical CT pulmonary angiography as well as axial CT of the inferior vena cava and the iliac, femoral, and popliteal veins. If the findings at helical CT pulmonary angiography are equivocal or technically inadequate (5%-10% of cases) or clinical suspicion remains high despite negative findings, additional imaging is required.
- Patients who have symptoms of deep venous thrombosis but not of pulmonary embolism initially undergo US, which is a less expensive alternative. If the findings are negative, imaging is usually discontinued; if they are positive, the patient is evaluated for pulmonary embolism at the discretion of the referring physician.
- Specific indications for CTA
  Clinically suspected PE in patients with a reduced likelihood of a diagnostic-quality nuclear medicine ventilation/perfusion (V/Q) study
  Equivocal lung ventilation/perfusion study
  Rapid diagnosis of pulmonary embolism is essential
  Candidates for pulmonary thromboendarterectomy, with chronic pulmonary hypertension
  Contraindication to conventional catheter pulmonary arteriography

Plain film
- Westermark sign: localized pulmonary oligemia (rare)
- Hampton's hump: triangular peripheral cone of infarct = blood in secondary pulmonary lobules (rare)
- Fleischner sign: increased diameter of pulmonary artery (> 16 mm) seen in acute PE. It usually disappears within a few days.
- Cor pulmonale: sudden increase in size of RV, RA
- Pulmonary edema, atelectasis, pleural effusion (50%)

CT findings in PE
- Adequately performed CT studies are essentially > 90% sensitive and specific for large central emboli
- Intraluminal filling defect surrounded by contrast
- Expanded un opacified vessel
- Eccentric filling defect
- Peripheral wedge shaped consolidation
- Pleural effusion
- Allows evaluation of the inferior vena cava and the lower-extremity veins to the knee

Scintigraphy
- Ventilation-perfusion mismatch (see Chapter 6)

Angiography
- Constant intraluminal filling defects in PA
- Complete cutoff of PA or its branches
- Prolongation of the arterial phase; delayed filling and emptying of venous phase

Vasculitis

OVERVIEW OF PULMONARY VASCULITIDES		
Syndrome	Pathology	Other Affected Vessels
Polyarteritis nodosa	Necrotizing vasculitis	Renal, hepatic, and visceral aneurysm
Allergic granulomatous angiitis (Churg-Strauss syndrome)	Granulomatous vasculitis	Allergic history, eosinophilia
Hypersensitivity vasculitis	Leukocytoclastic vasculitis	Skin (common)
Henoch-Schönlein purpura	Leukocytoclastic vasculitis	Skin, gastrointestinal, renal involvement usual
Takayasu's arteritis	Giant cell arteritis	Aortic arch
Temporal arteritis	Giant cell arteritis	Carotid branches
Wegener's granulomatosis	Necrotizing granulomatous vasculitis	Upper and lower respiratory tracts, glomerulonephritis

Venous Abnormalities

PULMONARY ARTERIOVENOUS MALFORMATION (AVM)

Abnormal communication between pulmonary artery and veins. A communication between systemic arteries and pulmonary veins is much less common (< 5%).

Types

Congenital, 60%
- Osler-Weber-Rendu disease (hereditary hemorrhagic telangiectasia)

Acquired, 40%
- Iatrogenic
- Infection
- Tumor

Radiographic features
- Location: lower lobes, 70% > middle lobe > upper lobes
- Feeding artery, draining veins
- Sharply defined mass

- Strong enhancement
- Change in size with Valsalva/Mueller procedure

Complications

- Stroke, 20%
- Abscess, 10% (AVM acts as a systemic shunt)
- Rupture: hemothorax, hemoptysis, 10%

PULMONARY VARICES

Uncommon lesions that are typically asymptomatic and do not require treatment. Usually discovered incidentally.

Radiographic features

- Dilated vein
- Usually near left atrium

AORTIC NIPPLE

Normal variant (10% of population) caused by the left superior intercostal vein seen adjacent to the aortic arch. Maximum diameter of vein: 4 mm

PULMONARY VENOOCCLUSIVE DISEASE (PVOD)

In the typical form there is occlusion of small pulmonary veins. The proposed initial insult in PVOD is venous thrombosis, possibly initiated by infection, toxic exposure, or immune complex deposition. The unique histologic hallmarks of

Radiographic features

- Edema without cephalization
- Pleural effusions
- Cardiomegaly
- CT findings
    Secondary pulmonary arterial hypertension
    Markedly small central pulmonary veins
    Central and gravity-dependent ground-glass lung attenuation
    Smoothly thickened interlobular septa
    Normal-sized left atrium
    Centrilobular nodules

Pleura

GENERAL

NORMAL PLEURAL ANATOMY

- Visceral pleura: covers lung
- Parietal pleura: covers rib (costal pleura), diaphragm (diaphragmatic pleura), mediastinum (mediastinal pleura)

Visceral amd parietal pleura are continued at the pulmonary hilum and continue inferiorly as the inferior pulmonary ligament. Normal pleura (0.2-0.4 mm) is not visible by CT. Plerual thickening is present when a stripe of soft tissue is seen internal to a rib.

DIAGNOSTIC THORACENTESIS

Success rate 97%. Pneumothorax: 1-3% (less than with blind thoracentesis).
Indication
- Suspected malignancy
- Suspected infection

Technique
1. Use US to determine skin entry site
2. Anesthetize skin, subcutaneous, and deep tissues
3. Advance 18-22 G spinal needle into collection going over the superior border of the rib to avoid the neurovascular bundle
4. Aspirate 20-30 mL

THERAPEUTIC THORACENTESIS

Success rate 95%. Pneumothorax 7%.
Indication
- Respiratory compromise from large pleural effusions

Technique
1. Perform diagnostic thoracentesis
2. Skin nick
3. Place 8-12 Fr catheters or Turkell needle system for therapeutic thoracentesis. Remove catheter
4. Obtain CXR to check for pneumothorax

Expansion pulmonary edema
Pulmonary edema may occur as a result of rapid evacuation of large amounts of pleural effusion. We routinely evacuate 2-3 L without complications. Do not aspirate both lungs in the same sitting because of the risk of expansion pulmonary edema and/or bilateral pneumothoraces

Vacuthorax
If the lung parenchyma is abnormally stiff (fibrosis) it can not reexpand and fill the pleural space resulting in a "vacuthorax". The patient is unlikely to benefit from thoracentesis in this circumstance.

PNEUMOTHORAX MANAGEMENT

Success rate > 90%.
Indication for intervention
- Symptomatic pneumothorax
- Pneumothorax > 20%
- Enlarging pneumothorax on subsequent CXR
- Tension pneumothorax
- Poor lung function or contralateral lung disease

Technique
1. Two approaches
   - 2nd-4th anterior intercostal space, midclavicular line
   - 6th-8th intercostal space, midaxilary line or posterior
2. Local anesthesia, skin nick
3. Place 8-12 Fr catheters using a trocar technique. For the anterior approach small Heimlich valve sets may be used.
4. After the lung is fully re-expanded for 24 hrs, the catheter is placed on water seal for 6 hrs and then removed if there is no pneumothorax

Persistent pneumothorax in patient with chest catheter
- Persistent leak from airways (bronchial injury, lung laceration)
- Loculated pneumothorax
- Anterior pneumothorax
- Obstructed catheter

EMPYEMA DRAINAGE

Success rate 80%. Complications (hemorrhage, lung injury), 2%.
Indication:
- Pus on diagnostic thoracentesis
- Positive Gram stain
- Positive culture

Technique
1. Choose entry site adjacent to largest collection using US or CT
2. Local anesthesia
3. Diagnostic tap with 18 G needle. Sent specimen for bacteriologic testing
4. Choice of drainage catheters
   - 10-16 Fr pigtail catheter for liquid effusions (usually placed by trocar technique)
   - 24 Fr catheter for thick collections (usually placed by Seldinger technique); dilators, 8, 10, 12, 14, 16, 20, etc.
5. Put catheter to suction
6. Intrapleural urokinase may be necessary for loculated effusions. 80,000 units of urokinase are administered in 150 mL of saline 3 times per day for 30 minutes for 3 days

Complications
- Technical catheter problems (clogging: change for larger catheter)
- Nonclearance of collection: surgical removal

Fluid Collections

PLEURAL EFFUSIONS

Excess fluid in the pleural space. There are two generic types: transudates and exudates:
  Transudate: ultrafiltrate of plasma; highly fluid, low in protein, devoid of inflammatory cells
  Exudate: increased permeability of microcirculation; rich in protrein, cells and debris

DIFFERENTIATION OF TRANSUDATE AND EXUDATE		
	Transudate	**Exudate**
Protein	< 3 g/dL	> 3g/dL
Protein (plasma/fluid)	< 0.5	> 0.5
LDH	< 200 IU	> 200 IU
	< 70% of serum level	> 70% of serum level
Common causes	CHF, renal failure cirrhosis	Infection (parapneumonic) tumor, embolism

Causes of pleural effusions

Tumor
- Bronchogenic carcinoma
- Pleural metastases
- Malignant mesothelioma
- Lymphoma

Inflammation
- Pneumonia, TB, empyema
- Collagen vascular disease
- Abdominal disease
    - Pancreatitis
    - Subphrenic abscess
    - Boerhaave's syndrome
    - Meigs' syndrome (benign ovarian fibroma)

Cardiovascular
- Congestive heart failure
- Pulmonary embolism
- Renal failure

Congenital
- Hydrops (neonate)

Metabolic
- Hypoproteinemia

Trauma

RADIOGRAPHIC FEATURES OF PLEURAL EFFUSIONS

Lateral decubitus films
- Most sensitive: may detect as little as 25 mL

PA, lateral films: blunting of costophrenic angles
- Posterior costophrenic angle (> 75 mL required)
- Lateral costophrenic angles (> 175 mL required)

Large effusions
- All cardiophrenic angles obliterated
- Mediastinal shift
- Elevated diaphragm

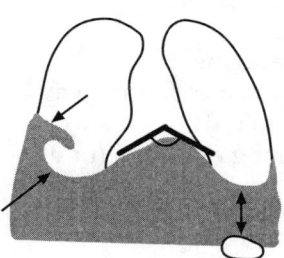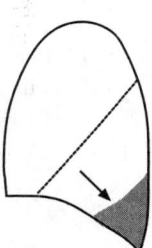

Split pleura sign (CT, MRI): loculated fluid between visceral and parietal pleura with thickening of pleura. Thickened pleura may enhance with IV contrast.

EMPYEMA

Empyema refers to either pus in the pleural space or an exudate that contains organism on a Gram stain (polymicrobial anaerobe 35%, mixed aerobe/anaerobe 40%, culture negative 20%). There are three stages in the development of an empyema.

OVERVIEW			
Parameter	Stage 1	Stage 2	Stage 3
Pathology	Exudative	Fibrinopurulent	Fibrinous
WBC	Normal	> 15,000/cm^3	15,000/cm^3
pH	Normal	< 7	< 7
Glucose	ormal	< 40 mg%	< 40 mg%
LDH	> 200 IU/L	> 200 IU/L	> 200 IU/L
Protein	> 3 g/L	> 3 g/L	> 3 g/L
Treatment	Antibiotics	Percutaneous drainage	Surgery

Causes
- Postinfection (parapneumonic), 60%
- Postsurgical, 20%
- Posttrauma, 20%

Radiographic features
- Pleural fluid collection
- Thick pleura
- Pleural enhancement
- Gas in empyema collection may be due to:
    BPF (common)
    Gas-forming organism (rare)

DIFFERENTIATION OF EMPYEMA VS ABSCESS		
	Abscess	Empyema
Cause	Necrotizing pneumonia (anaerobes, fungus)	Abscess extends to pleura; trauma, surgery
Shape	Round	Elliptical along chest wall
Air fluid level	A = B	A ≠ B
Margins	Sharp or irregular	Sharp
Wall	Thick	Thin
Lung	Normal position	Displaced
Pleura	Not seen	Split
Vessel/bronchi	Within	Displaced
Treatment	Antibiotics, postural drainage, percutaneous drainage in non-responders	Percutaneous drainage

CHYLOTHORAX

Chylothorax is caused by disruption of the thoracic duct. Daily chyle production: 1.5-2.5 L. Chyle contains chylomicrons from intestinal lymphatics and appears milky. Causes:

Tumor, 55% (especially lymphoma)
Trauma, 25%
  • Iatrogenic duct laceration
  • Sharp, blunt trauma
Idiopathic, 15%
Rare causes
  • Lymphangioleiomyomatosis
  • Filiariasis

Pleural Tumors

FIBROUS TUMOR OF THE PLEURA

Unifocal tumor of the pleura. No relationship to asbestos exposure. Fibrous tumors originate from visceral (70%) or parietal (30%) pleura usually on a pedicle. Clinical: respiratory symptoms, HPO, 15%; hypoglycemia, 5%. Types:
  • Benign, 80% (previously classified as benign mesothelioma)
  • Invasive, 20% (unlike malignant mesothelioma, this tumor grows only locally)

Radiographic features
- Well-delineated, solitary pleural-based mass; often lobulated
- Pedunculated 30%; mass may flop into different locations from film to film
- Chest wall invasion may be seen in the invasive form, absent in benign form
- Tumor may grow in fissure and simulate the appearance of a solitary pulmonary nodule
- Recurrence rate after surgical resection, 10%
- May have associated pleural effusion, necrosis

MALIGNANT MESOTHELIOMA

Incidence: 500 new cases/year in United States. Risk is 300 times larger in asbestos workers than in general population. Highest rates in Seattle (shipyard industry) and St. Louis. 20-40 years between asbestos exposure and tumor development. Three histological variants (diagnosis usually requires an open pleural biopsy):
- Epithelial: difficult to differentiate from adenocarcinoma
- Mesenchymal
- Mixed

Radiographic features
- Pleural thickening together with effusion, 60%
    Isolated pleural thickening, 25%
    Isolated pleural effusion, 15%
- Hemithoracic contraction, 25%
- Pleural calcification, 5%
- CT best shows full extent of disease:
    Contralateral involvement
    Chest wall and mediastinal involvement, 10%, diaphragm and
        abdominal extension
    Pericardial involvement
    Pulmonary metastases
- MRI useful to show chest wall or diaphragmatic extent

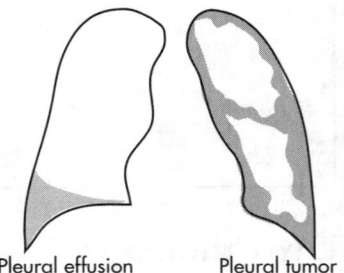

Pleural effusion   Pleural tumor

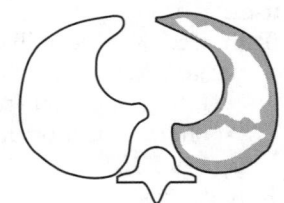

Other

DIAPHRAGMATIC PARALYSIS

Paralysis of the diaphragm can be unilateral or bilateral. Clinical: unilateral paralysis is usually asymptomatic, bilateral paralysis results in respiratory symptoms. Causes:

Phrenic nerve paralysis
- Bronchogenic carcinoma
- Neuropathies, postinfectious, nutritional
- Spinal cord injury, myelitis
- CNS injury: stroke
- Cardiac surgery
- Erb's palsy (birth trauma)

Muscular disorders
- Myasthenia
- Polymyositis
- Muscular dystrophy

Idiopathic, 70%

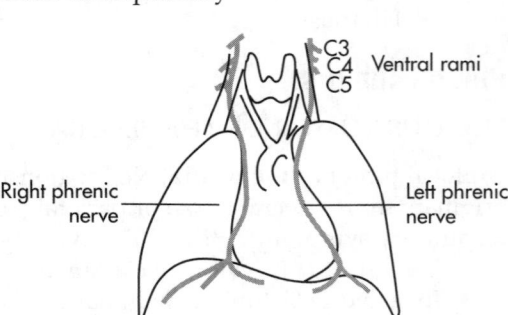

C3
C4   Ventral rami
C5

Right phrenic   Left phrenic
   nerve   nerve

Radiographic features
- Elevated hemidiaphragm
- No motion of hemidiaphragm by fluoroscopy
- Paradoxical motion of hemidiaphragm using "sniff test"
- Reduced lung volume

Mediastinum

General

APPROACH TO MEDIASTINAL MASSES

- Location
    - Anterior mediastinum
    - Superior mediastinum
    - Middle mediastinum
    - Posterior mediastinum
- Invasive or noninvasive mass
- Content: fat, cystic, solid, enhancement

DIFFERENTIATION OF MEDIASTINAL AND PULMONARY MASSES	
Mediastinal Mass	**Pulmonary Mass**
Epicenter in mediastinum	Epicenter in lung
Obtuse angles with the lung	Acute angles
No air bronchograms	Air bronchograms possible
Smooth and sharp margins	Irregular margins
Movement with swallowing	Movement with respiration
Bilateral	Unilateral

NORMAL VARIANTS CAUSING A WIDE MEDIASTINUM

- Anteroposterior (AP) projection instead of posteroanterior (PA) projection
- Mediastinal fat: obesity, steroid therapy
- Vascular tortuosity: elderly patients
- Low inspiratory supine position

Anterior Mediastinal Tumors

THYMOMA

Thymoma is the most common anterior mediastinal tumor in the adult (very rare in children). 30% are invasive (malignant thymoma). Parathymic syndromes are present in 40% of patients:
- 35% of thymoma patients have myasthenia gravis (15% of myasthenia gravis patients have thymoma)
- Aplastic anemia (50% have thymoma)
- Hypogammaglobulinemia (15% have thymoma)
- Red cell aplasia

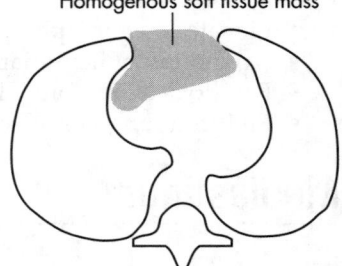

Homogenous soft tissue mass

Pathology

Benign thymoma, 75%
- Common in patients with myasthenia

Malignant thymoma, 25%
- Local spread into pleura but no hematogenous metastases
- More common in patients without myasthenia

Radiographic features

- Anterior mediastinal soft tissue mass
    - Asymmetrical location on one side
    - Homogenous density and signal intensity
    - Some have cystic components
    - Contrast enhancement
- Invasive thymomas show growth through capsule into adjacent tissue. Drop metastases into pleural space are common.
- Calcifications, 20%

THYMOLIPOMA

Thymolipomas are benign, encapsulated mediastinal tumors that contain both thymic and adipose tissue. The tumor occurs most frequently in children and young adults. Tumors usually grow to large sizes (75% are > 500 g) with little or no symptoms. Associations:
- Myasthenia gravis (in 3% of thymolipomas)
- Aplastic anemia
- Graves' disease
- Hypogammaglobulinemia
- Lipomas in thyroid, pharynx

Radiographic features

- Anterior mediastinal mass contains fatty and soft tissue elements
- The mass is usually large and displaces mediastinal structures and/or lungs
- Small tumors may be difficult to detect
- Large tumors mimic liposarcoma

BENIGN THYMIC HYPERPLASIA

Causes

- Myasthenia
- Thyrotoxicosis
- Collagen vascular diseases:
    - SLE
    - Scleroderma
    - Rheumatoid arthritis
- Rebound thymic hyperplasia:
    - Chemotherapy (hyperplasia is often a good prognostic indicator)
    - Addison's disease
    - Acromegaly

Radiographic features

- Enlarged thymus without focal masses; fat interspersed in parenchyma
- Size and morphology of normal thymus:
    - > 20 years of age: < 13 mm
    - > 30 years of age: convex margins are abnormal
- No increase in size over time
- If clinical suspicion for malignancy is high, a biopsy should be performed

THYROID MASSES

Thyroid masses that extend into the mediastinum: goiter >> adenoma, carcinoma, lymphoma. Location of goiters within mediastinum:
- Anterior to brachiocephalic vessels, 80%
- Posterior to brachiocephalic vessels, 20%

Radiographic features

Goiters
- Thoracic inlet masses (thymomas are lower in the anterior mediastinum)
- Mass is contiguous with cervical thyroid and is well defined
- Heterogenous density by CT: calcium, iodine (70-120 HU), colloid cysts
- Tracheal displacement is the most common finding by CXR
- CT: marked and prolonged contrast enhancement
- Nuclear scan with ^{99m}Tc, ^{131}I confirms the diagnosis

Other
- Thyroid carcinoma has irregular borders
- Thyroid lymphomas generally show little enhancement

GERM CELL TUMORS

Tumors arise from rests of primitive cells and are of variable malignant potential (mnemonic "SECTE"):
- **S**eminoma
- **E**mbryonal cell carcinoma
- **C**horiocarcinoma
- **T**eratoma (70% of germ cell tumors), teratocarcinoma
- **E**ndodermal sinus tumors (yolk sac tumors)

Teratoma
- 20% are malignant; therefore all mediastinal teratomas should be surgically removed
- Teratomas typically present as large mass lesions
- Variable tissue contents:
    Calcification, 30%
    Fat, fat-fluid levels
    Cystic areas
    Soft tissue

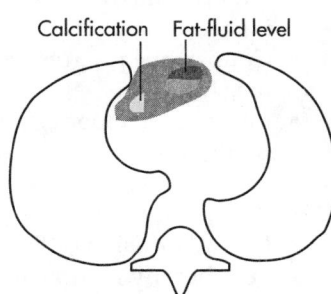
Calcification   Fat-fluid level

Seminoma
- Rarely infiltrative
- Large, unencapsulated lesions
- Occasionally associated with testicular atrophy

Embryonal cell carcinoma
- Mediastinal invasion is the rule: bad prognosis (mean survival time < 10 months)
- Elevated AFP and human chorionic gonadotropin (HCG)

HODGKIN'S LYMPHOMA

The pathologic diagnosis is based on the presence of Reed-Sternberg cells. The cell of origin is the antigen-presenting interdigitating cells in the paracortical regions of the lymph node (not B or T cells). 90% originate in the lymph nodes, 10% originate in extranodal lymphoid tissues of parenchymal organs (lung, GI tract, skin). Incidence: 1:50,000. Bimodal age distribution with peaks at 30 and 70 years.

TYPES OF HODGKIN'S LYMPHOMA		
Type	Frequency	Prognosis
Lymphocyte predominant (LP)	< 5% (young patients)	Most favorable
Nodular sclerosing (NS)	70%	Less favorable than LP
Mixed cellularity (MC)	25% (old patients)	Less favorable than NS
Lymphocyte depleted (LD)	< 5%	Worst prognosis

STAGING (ANN ARBOR)	
Stage*	Involvement
I	Single node group or region
IE	Single extranodal site
II	Two or more nodes on same side of diaphragm
IIE	Localized disease in an organ and node on same side of diaphragm
III	Node groups on both sides of diaphragm
IIIE	Above diaphragm + localized extralymphatic
IIIS	Above diaphragm + spleen
IV	Extension beyond above limit

*Constitutional symptoms (classification B) are present in 25%: fever, night sweats, weight loss.

Radiographic features

- Superior mediastinal nodal (prevascular, paratracheal) involvement, 95%
- Contiguous progression from one lymph node group to the next
- Lung involvement, 15%
    Pulmonary mass lesion, air bronchograms
    Direct extension into lung from involved nodes (most common)
- Pleural effusions, 15%
- Posttherapy mediastinal changes are common
    Thymic cysts
    Thymic hyperplasia
    Persistent mediastinal masses may be present without representing active disease: ^{67}Ga, PET scanning may be helpful for differentiation

Pearls

- Recurrence of lymphoma
    Radiation treatment: recurrence usually occurs outside the treatment field, (commonly paracardiac region)
    No radiation: recurrence usually in sites of previous involvement
- 5% of treated Hodgkin's patients will develop aggressive leukemias
- Radiation pneumonitis occurs 6-8 weeks after completion of the radiation and evolves to mature fibrosis by 1 year

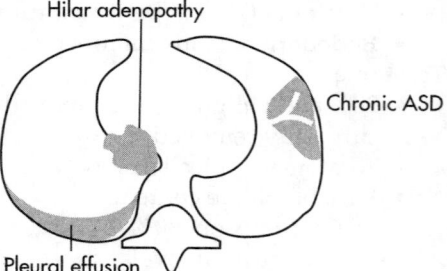

Hilar adenopathy

Chronic ASD

Pleural effusion

NON-HODGKIN'S LYMPHOMA

60% originate in lymph nodes, 40% in extranodal sites. 85% arise from B cells, 15% from T cells. Occurs in all age groups (mean age 50 years). Increased incidence in patients with altered immune status:
- Transplant patients
- AIDS
- Congenital imunodeficiency
- Collagen vascular diseases: RA, SLE

CLASSIFICATIONS OF NON-HODGKIN'S LYMPHOMA*		
Working Formulation	Rappaport	Comment
LOW GRADE		
Small, lymphocytic	Lymphocytic, well-differentiated	Uncommon
Follicular, small cleaved	Nodular, poorly differentiated	Most frequent type
Follicular, mixed cells	Nodular, mixed	
INTERMEDIATE GRADE		
Follicular, large cells	Nodular, histiocytic	
Diffuse, small cleaved	Diffuse, lymphocytic	
Diffuse, mixed cell	Diffuse, mixed	
Diffuse, large cell	Diffuse, histiocytic	GI involvement 25%
HIGH GRADE		
Immunoblastic	Diffuse, histiocytic	GI involvement 25%
Lymphoblastic	Lymphoblastic	Mediastinal mass, young patient
Small, noncleaved	Diffuse undifferentiated (Burkitt and non-Burkitt	Abdominal form (North America), craniofacial (Africa)

*Constitutional symptoms are more common than in HD.

Radiographic features
Mediastinal and hilar adenopathy
- Often generalized at presentation
- Adenopathy may be noncontiguous

Lung involvement
- May occur without adenopathy
- Patterns: mass, chronic ASD

Extrathoracic spread
- Nasooropharynx
- GI tract
- Spread to unusual sites common

Middle Mediastinal Tumors

BRONCHOPULMONARY FOREGUT MALFORMATIONS

Abnormalities in budding and differentiation of the primitive foregut. Depending on type, duplication cysts are also classified as posterior mediastinal masses. The lining of the cyst wall determines the cyst type:
- Bronchogenic cysts: ventral defects containing respiratory epithelium
- Enteric cysts: posterior defects containing gastrointestinal epithelium (gastric mucosa > esophageal mucosa > small bowel mucosa > pancreatic tissue)

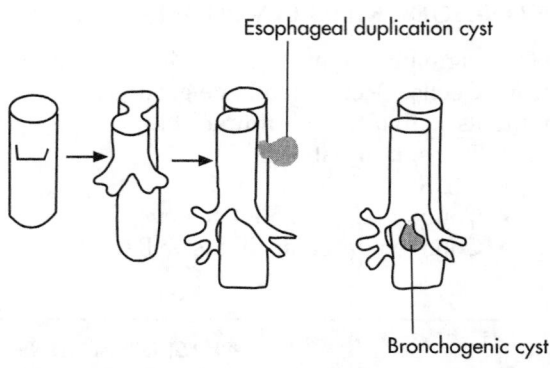

Esophageal duplication cyst

Bronchogenic cyst

DIFFERENTIATION OF BRONCHOGENIC VS. ENTERIC CYSTS		
	Bronchogenic Cyst	Enteric Cyst
Location	Ventral	Dorsal
Level	Subcarinal	Supracarinal
Cyst wall	Imperceptible	Thick wall
Symptoms	Asymptomatic unless there is mass effect; usually as an incidental finding	Symptomatic: peptic ulceration, distention
Other imaging findings	May contain calcification Associated rib anomalies CT: no contrast enhancement T2 hypointense	Vertebral body anomalies Hemivertebra Scoliosis Spina bifida

Radiographic features
- Round mass of water/protein density
- Location

    Bronchogenic cysts are mediastinal (75%) or pulmonary (25%). Mediastinal locations: subcarinal, 50%; paratracheal, 20%; hilar, paracardiac, 30%. Esophageal duplication cysts are located along the course of the esophagus.
- High CT density (40%) may be due to debris, hemorrhage, infection
- Calcifications in wall (rare finding)

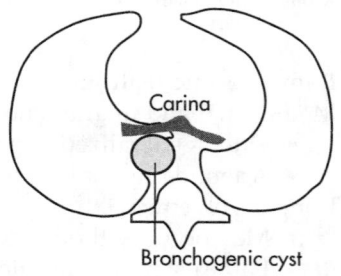

Carina

Bronchogenic cyst

CASTLEMAN'S DISEASE (GIANT BENIGN LYMPH NODE HYPERPLASIA)

Large, benign mediastinal lymph node masses. Rare. Etiology is is unknown (nodal hyperplasia vs. benign tumor). Two histological types: hyaline vascular 90%, plasma cell 10% (associated with general symptoms: night sweats, fever, etc.). Age: < 30 years (70%). Treatment: surgical excision. Two types:
- Hyaline vascular type
- Plasma cell type

Radiographic features
- Bulky mediastinal mass lesion (3-12 cm): anterior > middle > posterior mediastinum
- Dense homogenous contrast enhancement is the key feature ("vascular lesions")
- Nodal calcification may be present
- Involvement of lymph nodes in neck, axilla, pelvis is rare
- Slow growth

FIBROSING MEDIASTINITIS

Causes: mediastinal histoplasmosis, idiopathic. May result in obstruction of pulmonary artery, veins, bronchi. Calcified lymph nodes.

Posterior Mediastinal Tumors

NEURAL TUMORS

Posterior mediastinal neural tumors arise from:
Peripheral nerves, 45% = benign
- Schwannoma (arise from nerve sheath)
- Neurofibroma (contain all elements of nerve)

Sympathetic ganglia (varying malignant potential)
- Ganglioneuroma (benign)
- Ganglioneuroblastoma
- Neuroblastoma (malignant)

Paraganglion cells, 2%
- Paraganglioma (= chemodectoma, histologically similar to pheochromocytoma): functional tumors, may secrete catecholamines. Intense contrast enhancement. Found in AP window

Radiographic features
Schwannoma, neurofibroma
- Arise posteriorly, frequently in neural foramina
- May cause widening and erosion of neural foramina
- Usually round or oval and < 2 vertebral bodies long
- Enhancement with contrast
- T2-weighted (T2W) very hyperintense

Sympathetic ganglia tumors
- Arise anterolateral (more conspicuous on plain film)
- Usually elongated and fusiform (resembling sympathetic chain) and > 2 vertebral bodies long

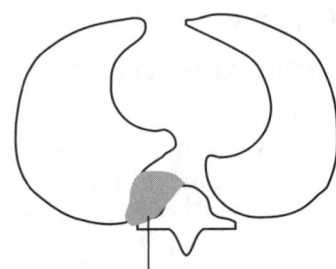

Vascular, T2 bright, bone erosion

EXTRAMEDULLARY HEMATOPOIESIS

Paravertebral masses represent bone marrow extruded through cortical defects of vertebral bodies. Seen in congenital anemias (thalassemia, etc.). Suspect diagnosis if:
- Multiple bilateral posterior mediastinal masses
- Cortical bone changes by CT
- Clinical history of anemia
- Marked contrast enhancement

Other Mediastinal Disorders

PNEUMOMEDIASTINUM

Sources of mediastinal air
Intrathoracic
- Trachea and major bronchi
- Esophagus
- Lung
- Pleural space
Extrathoracic
- Head and neck
- Intraperitoneum and retroperitoneum

Radiographic features
- Subcutaneous emphysema
- Elevated thymus: Thymic sail sign
- Air anterior to pericardium: Pneumoprecordium
- Air around pulmonary artery and main branches: ring around artery sign
- Air outlining major aortic branches: tubular artery sign
- Air outlining bronchial wall: double bronchial wall sign
- Continous diaphragm sign: due to air trapped posterior to pericardium
- Air between parietal pleura and diaphragm:extrapleural sign
- Air in pulmonary ligament

Differential Diagnosis

General

APPROACH TO CXR

1. Lungs
   - Focal or diffuse abnormalities
   - Lung volumes
      Increased or decreased
      Right/left difference in density
   - Hypolucent areas
2. Trachea and bronchi
3. Mediastinal lines
   - Paratracheal stripe
   - AP window
   - Azygoesophageal recess
   - Paraspinal lines
   - Other lines
      Anterior and posterior junction line
      Posterior wall of intermediate bronchus
4. Hila and cardiac contour
5. Pleura, fissures
6. Bones
   - Focal metastases
   - Rib notching
   - Clavicles

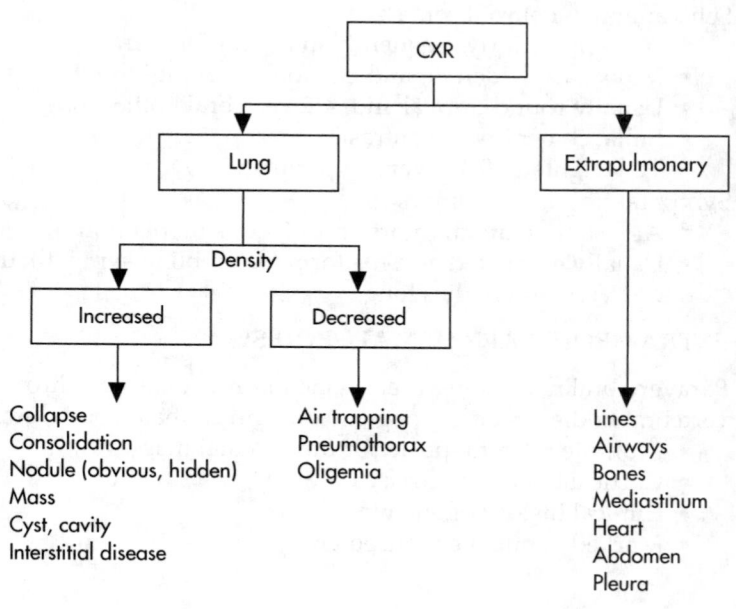

APPROACH TO ICU FILMS

1. Lines (check position)
2. Pneumothorax, pneumomediastinum
3. Focal parenchymal opacities
   - Atelectasis
   - Pneumonia
   - Aspiration
   - Hemorrhage
   - Contusion
4. Diffuse parenchymal opacities
   - ARDS
   - Pneumonia
   - Edema
   - Less common:
     Aspiration
     Hemorrhage

DIRECTED SEARCH IN APPARENTLY NORMAL CHEST FILMS

Lungs
   - Hidden nodules
   - Subtle interstitial disease
   - Differences in lung density
   - Retrocardiac disease
   - Bronchiectasis
   - Pulmonary embolism

Mediastinum
   - Posterior mediastinal mass
   - Tracheal lesions, deviation
   - Subtle hilar mass lesions

Bones
   - Lytic, sclerotic lesions
   - Rib notching

GENERIC APPROACHES TO FILM INTERPRETATION

The 4 Ds
   - **D**etection
   - **D**escription
   - **D**ifferential diagnosis
   - **D**ecision about management

Lesion description
   - Location
   - Extent
   - Characteristics
     Signal intensity, density, echogenicity, etc.
     Behavior after administration of contrast material
   - Differential diagnosis

UNIVERSAL DIFFERENTIAL DIAGNOSIS (MNEMONIC "TIC MTV")

- **Tumor**
- **Inflammation**
    Infectious
    Noninfectious causes
- **Congenital**
- **Metabolic**
- **Trauma, iatrogenic**
- **Vascular**

Atelectasis

LOBAR, SEGMENTAL ATELECTASIS

Endobronchial lesion
Extrinsic bronchial compression
- Tumor
- Lymphadenopathy
    Malignant
    Benign adenopathy (rarely causes lobar collapse), i.e. sarcoid
Rare causes
- Bronchial torsion

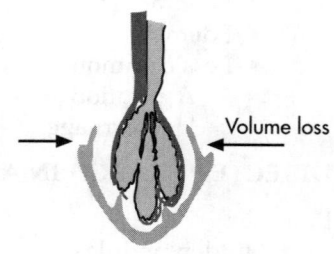

SIGNS OF LOBAR ATELECTASIS

Direct signs
- Displacement of interlobar fissures (lobar collapse)
- Increase in opacity of the involved segment or lobe
Indirect signs
- Displacement of hila
- Mediastinal displacement
- Elevation of hemidiaphragm
- Overinflation of remaining normal lung
- Approximation of ribs

RUL collapse
- Elevation of minor fissure
- Shift of trachea to right
- Elevation of hilum
- Thickening of right paratracheal in complete collapse

RML collapse
- Best seen on lordotic views
- RML syndrome: recurrent atelectasis despite an open orifice:
    Absent collateral ventilation
    Bronchus is surrounded by enlarged lymph nodes (TB)
    May have coexistent bronchiectasis

RLL collapse
- Triangular opacity in right retrocardiac region on PA film with obliteration of diaphragm
- Posterior displacement of right margin.
- Opacity over the spine

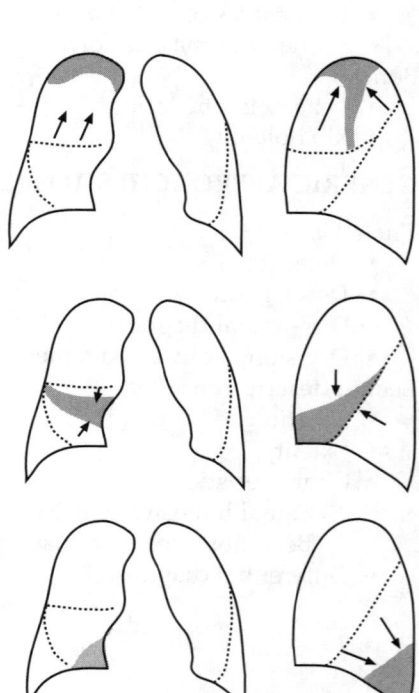

LUL collapse
- May be difficult to see: hazy density can be easily confused with loculated pleural effusion on PA film
- "Luftsichel": radiolucency in upper lung zone that results from upward migration of superior segment of the left lower lobe (LLL)
- Anterior displacement of major fissure on lateral view

LLL collapse
- Left retrocardiac triangular opacity on PA film
- Posterior displacement of left major fissure on lateral film

CT findings of lobar collapse
- Increased density of collapsed lobe
- See figure for patterns

TYPES OF PERIPHERAL ATELECTASIS

Relaxation
- Pleural effusion
- Pneumothorax
- Bullous disease

Atelectasis associated with fibrosis
- Granulomatous infections
- Pneumoconiosis
- Sarcoid

Resorptive atelectasis secondary to obstruction
- Platelike, discoid atelectasis

Depletion of surfactant (adhesive atelectasis; airways patent)
- ARDS of the newborn
- Radiation injury

Rounded atelectasis
- Due to pleural disease

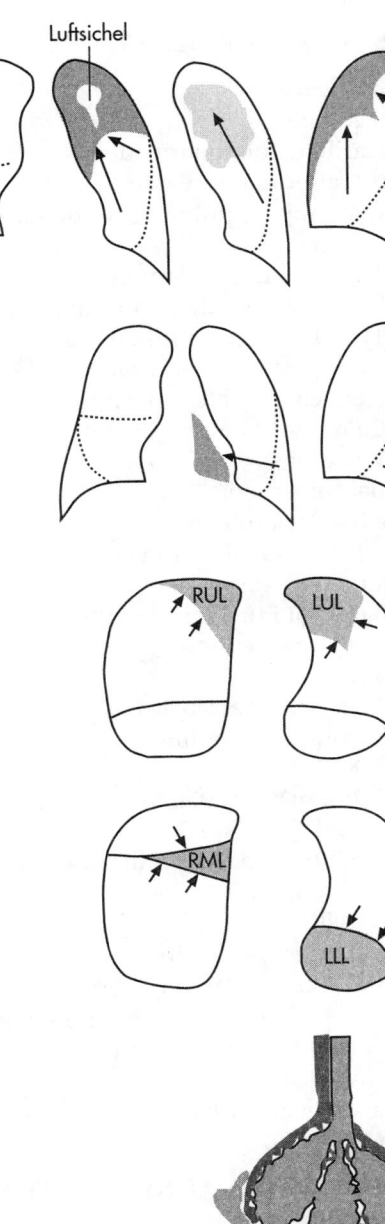

Consolidation

Radiographic features

Acinar shadow
- Air in acini (7 mm in diameter) is replaced by fluid or tissue
- May be confluence to form patchy densities

Air bronchogram
- Represents aerated airways in consolidated lung
- Air bronchogram may also be seen in some forms of collapse

Absence of volume loss
- No displaced fissures
- No elevation of diaphragm

Nonsegmental distribution
- Intersegmental spread is common because channels of interalveolar communication (channels of collateral drift) allow passage of air and fluid
- Channels of collateral drift include:
    Pores of Kohn (interalveolar openings)
    Channels of Lambert (bronchioalveolar communications)
    Direct airway anastomosis, 120 μm in diameter

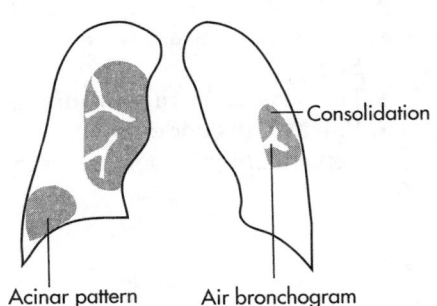

Acinar pattern   Air bronchogram

CAUSES OF CONSOLIDATION

Fluid in acini

Water (edema)
- Cardiac pulmonary edema
- Renal pulmonary edema
- Lung injury, pulmonary edema

Blood
- Trauma (most common)
- Bleeding disorder: anticoagulation, etc.
- Type II antigen-antibody reaction
- Goodpasture's syndrome
- Henoch-Schönlein purpura
- Pulmonary infarct (Hampton hump)
- Vasculitis

Proteinaceous fluid
- Alveolar proteinosis

Inflammatory exudate in acini

Infection
- Bacterial infections (pus)
- Nocardia, actinomycosis, TB

Noninfectious
- Allergic hypersensitivity alveolitis
- Chronic eosinophilic pneumonia
- BOOP
- Pulmonary infiltration with eosinophilia
      Loeffler's syndrome
      Chronic eosinophilic pneumonia
      Pneumonitis
      ABPA
      Drugs: penicillin
- Aspiration of lipid material
- Sarcoid (resides only in interstitial space but encroacheson airspace to produce a pattern that mimics ASD)

Tumor in acini

Bronchioalveolar carcinoma
Lymphoma

PULMONARY RENAL SYNDROMES

These syndromes are characterized by pulmonary hemorrhage and nephritis. Pulmonary findings usually present as consolidation on CXR.
- Goodpasture's syndrome (anti-GBM positive)
- Wegener's disease (ANCA positive; nodules are more common than ASD)
- SLE
- Henoch-Schönlein purpura
- Polyarteritis nodosa
- Penicillamine hypersensitivity

ACUTE RESPIRATORY DISTRESS SYNDROME (ARDS)

Clinical syndrome characterized by sudden onset of triad:
- Respiratory distress
- Hypoxemia
- Opaque, stiff lungs

After an incipient catastrophic event mediators of injury are activated → inflammatory response → endothelial damage → injury, pulmonary edema (ARDS): ARDS runs independent course from initiating disease. Radiograph: diffuse alveolar consolidation, commonly indistinguishable from pneumonia or pulmonary edema; end stage: interstitial fibrosis and scarring.

Causes
- Massive pneumonia
- Trauma
- Shock
- Sepsis
- Pancreatitis
- Drug overdose
- Near drowning
- Aspiration

CHRONIC AIR SPACE DISEASE

Tumors
- Bronchioalveolar carcinoma
- Lymphoma

Inflammation
- Tuberculosis, fungus
- Eosinophilic pneumonia
- Pneumonitis, BOOP
- Alveolar sarcoid (mimics ASD)

Other causes
- Alveolar proteinosis
- Pulmonary hemorrhage
- Lipoid pneumonia, chronic aspiration

Pulmonary Masses

APPROACH TO SOLITARY PULMONARY NODULE

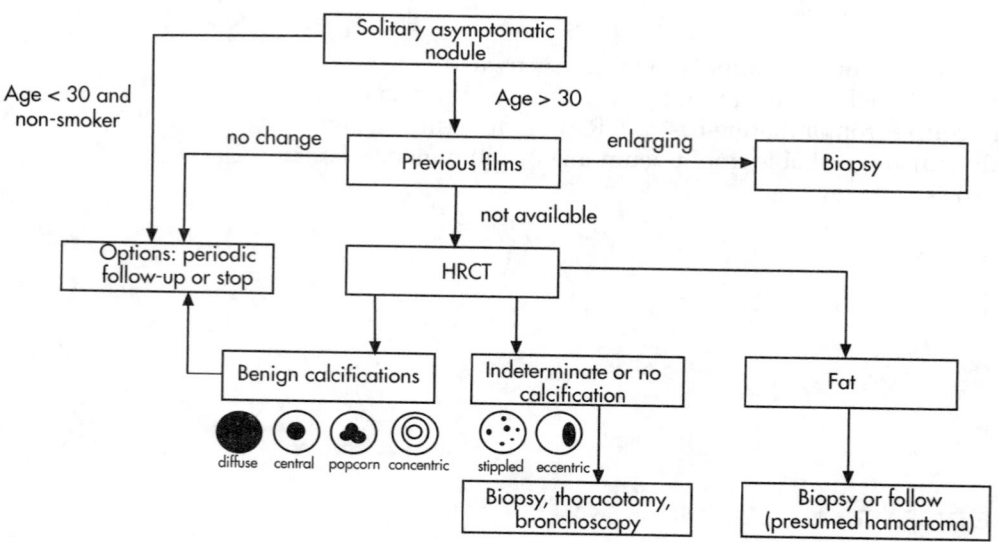

DIFFERENTIATION OF BENIGN AND MALIGNANT NODULES		
	Benign	**Malignant**
Shape	Round	Irregular
Size	< 3 cm	> 3 cm
Spiculations	No	Yes
Edge	Well-defined	Ill-defined
Satellite lesions	Yes	No
Cavitation	No	Yes
Doubling time (in volume)	< 1 month or > 2 years	> 1 month or < 2 years

The above-listed criteria *do not* allow reliable differentiation of a solitary pulmonary nodule. There are only *three* criteria by which a solitary pulmonary nodule can be judged benign:
- If there is fat density
- If there are specific types of benign calcifications (diffuse, central, popcorn, concentric):
    > 10% of a nodule consists of calcium with HU > 200
    Large or homogenous calcification throughout nodule (exceptions: multiple metastases from osteosarcoma, thyroid carcinoma, etc.)
- If old films show no interval growth within a 2-year period

Pearls
- Always get a second imaging modality (CT >> MR >> angio) before biopsying a solitary pulmonary nodule to exclude AV malformations. However, remember that 97% of all solitary nodules are either granulomas or primary carcinomas

- Extrapulmonary densities may mimic pulmonary lesions
    Artifact (nipple, skin, electrodes)
    Pseudotumor (fluid in fissure)
    Pleural mass or plaque
    Rib fracture
- Solitary pulmonary metastases seen on CXR will be truly solitary in only 50% of the cases
- Any solitary pulmonary nodule in cancer patients requires further workup:
    Comparison to old films
    Percutaneous biopsy if large enough
    Close follow-up (usually 3 month intervals)
- HRCT for nodule densitometry
    Perform only in nodules < 3.0 cm in diameter
    Densities of > 200 HU indicate presence of calcification

HIDDEN ZONES

Subtle pulmonary nodules are often missed if < 3 cm and located in:

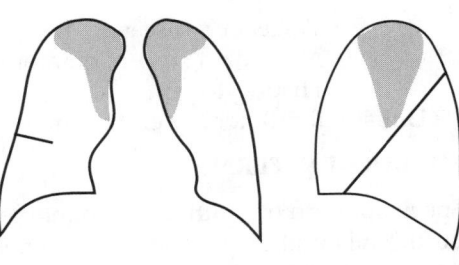

- Upper lobes (apices)
- Central, paramediastinal
- Superimposed onto ribs and clavicle

An effort should be made to perform a directed search in these regions to detect subtle lung cancer. This zone has also been called the lawyer zone. The threshold of lesion detection by plain film is approximately 9 mm.

SOLITARY NODULE

Criteria: < 6 cm. May be smooth, lobulated, discrete, circumscribed, calcified, cavitated, or have satellite lesions.

Tumor (45%)
- Primary carcinoma, 70%
- Hamartoma, 15%
- Solitary metastasis, 10%

Inflammation (53%); regional variations
- Histoplasmoma
- Tuberculoma
- Coccidioidomycosis

Other (2%)
- Vascular, 15%
    AV fistula
    Pulmonary varix (dilated pulmonary vein)
    Infarct, embolism
- Congenital, 30%
    Sequestration
    Bronchial cyst
- Miscellaneous, 45%
    Round pneumonia
    Loculated effusion in fissure
    Mucous plug
    Enlarged subpleural lymph node
    Silicosis (usually multiple nodules)

MULTIPLE NODULES

Multiplicity of pulmonary nodules often indicates hematogenous dissemination.
Causes:
- Metastases
- Abscess
    - Pyogenic: *Staphylococcus* > *Klebsiella* > *Streptococcus*
    - Immunocompromised patient: *Nocardia, Legionella*
- Granulomatous lung diseases
    - Infectious
        - TB
        - Fungus: *Aspergillus, Histoplasma*
    - Noninfectious
        - Sarcoid
        - Rheumatoid nodules
        - Silicosis
        - Wegener's disease
        - Necrotizing granulomatous vasculitis
        - Histiocytosis
- Unilateral pulmonary embolism

MILIARY PATTERN

Special pattern of multiple pulmonary nodules characterized by small size and diffuse bilateral distribution (too numerous to count). If the nodules are small enough, also consider the differential diagnosis for nodular interstitial disease.
Causes:
Soft tissue opacities
- Hematogenous, miliary infection: TB, histoplasmosis
- Hematogenous tumor seeding:
    - Metastases: thyroid, melanoma, breast, choriocarcinoma
    - Eosinophilic granuloma
    - Bronchioalveolar cancer
- Silicosis
- Sarcoid
High Density opacities

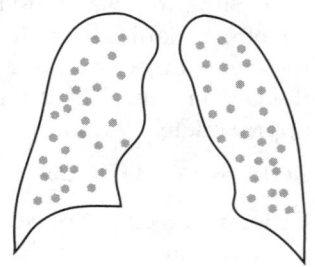

CALCIFIED LUNG NODULES

Larger (>1 mm)
- Tumor
    - Metastases from medullary thyroid cancer
    - Mucinous or osteogenic metastases
- Infection
    - Previous varicella pneumonia
    - Histoplasmosis, coccidiodomycosis TB
    - Parasites: schistosomiasis
- Other
    - Silicosis
Very small (0.1-1 mm; sandlike)
- Alveolar microlithiasis
- Chronic pulmonary venous hypertension
- "Metastatic" calcification from severe renal disease

LARGE (> 6 CM) THORACIC MASS

Pulmonary
- Tumor
    Bronchogenic carcinoma
    Metastases (SCC from head and neck)
- Abscess
- Round atelectasis
- Intrapulmonary sequestration
- Hydatid disease

Extrapulmonary
- Fibrous tumor of the pleura
- Loculated pleural effusion
- Torsed pulmonary lobe
- Chest wall tumors (Askin tumor)
- AAA
- Mediastinal masses

Cystic and Cavitary Lesions

APPROACH

The wall thickness and morphology arehelpful (but not definitive) to determine if a cavitary lesion is benign or malignant.

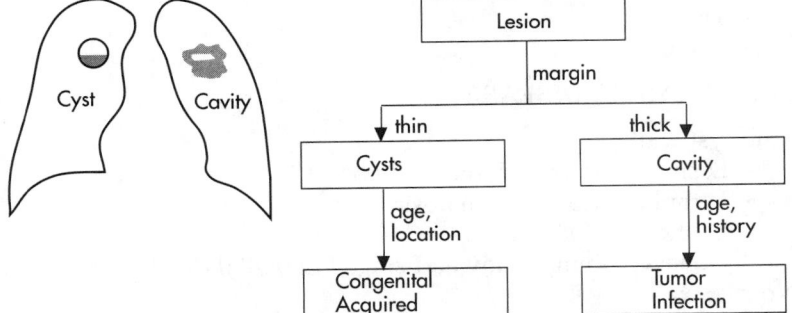

Thickness (not always reliable)
- < 2 mm, benign in 95%
- 2-15 mm, malignant in 50%
- > 15 mm, malignant in > 95%

Morphology, (not reliable)
- Eccentric cavity: suggests malignancy
- Shaggy internal margins: suggests malignancy

CYSTS

Parenchyma-lined space, filled with air or fluid.
- Pneumatocele (posttraumatic, postinfectious): common
- Bulla (located within lung parenchyma), bleb (located within the 9 histologic layers of the visceral pleura)
- Cystic bronchiectasis
- Congenital cysts
    Intrapulmonary bronchogenic cysts (rib and vertebral body anomalies common)
    Cystic adenomatoid malformation (multiple lesions)
    Sequestration
- Hydatid cyst (onion skin appearance)

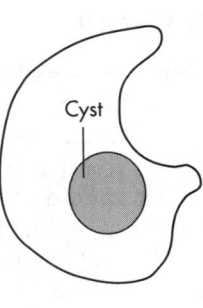

CAVITY

Parenchymal necrosis due to inflammation (benign) or tumor (malignant).

Abscess
- Pyogenic: *Staphylococcus > Klebsiella > Streptococcus*
- Immunocompromised patient: *Nocardia, Legionella*

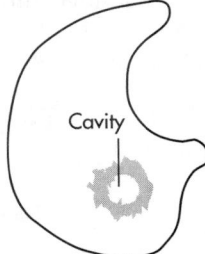

Cavitated tumor
- Squamous cell carcinoma (primary SCC > head and neck SCC > sarcoma metastases)
- Sarcoma
- Lymphoma
- TCC of the bladder

Cavitated granulomatous mass (often multiple)
- Fungus: *Aspergillus,* Coccidiodimycosis (thin wall)
- TB
- Sarcoid, Wegener's disease, rheumatoid nodules
- Necrotizing granulomatous vasculitis

Cavitated posttraumatic hematoma

AIR CRESCENT SIGN IN CAVITY

This sign was originally described in aspergillosis and is most commonly seen there. More recently, the sign has also been described with other entities:
- Mucormycois
- Actinomycosis
- Septic emboli
- *Klebsiella pneumoniae*
- TB
- Tumors

SMALL CYSTIC DISEASE

True cyst wall
- Eosinophilic granuloma
- Lymphangioleiomyomatosis
- Cystic form of PCP
- Honeycombing in any end-stage interstitial disease

No cyst wall
- Emphysema

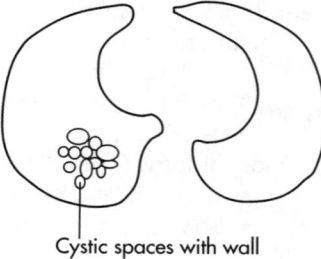

Cystic spaces with wall

Interstitial Lung Disease

RADIOGRAPHIC PATTERNS OF INTERSTITIAL DISEASE

Types of densities
- Linear or reticular densities: thickened interlobular septa, fibrosis
- Reticulonodular densities: inflammation in peribronchovascular interstitium
- Nodular densities: granulomas
- Ground glass opacity: usually represents acute interstitial disease (occasionally seen with chronic fibrosis)
   Hazy increase in lung density
   Vessels can be clearly seen through haze
- Honeycombing: ring shadows 2-10 mm; end-stage lung disease

Kerley lines (linear densities)

Kerley B lines, peripherally located in interlobular septa:
- < 2 cm long
- Peripheral
- Perpendicular to pleura

Kerley A lines:
- 2-6 cm long
- Central
- No relationship to bronchioarterial bundles

Kerley C lines
- Fine network caused by superimposition of Kerley B lines

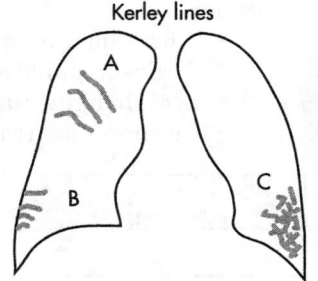

Kerley lines

APPROACH

Define the following parameters:
- Type of pattern
- Distribution
- Lung volumes
- Evolution
- Pleural disease
- Lymph nodes

Generic approach

Interstitial disease is due to thickening of interlobular septa (lymphatics, veins, or infiltration by cells), alveolar walls, and interstitium. Causes of thickening:

Fluid
- Water
    Pulmonary edema
    Venous obstruction (thrombosis)
- Proteinaceous material
    Congenital pulmonary lymphangiectasia (very rare)

Inflammation
- Infectious (interstitial pneumonias)
    Viral
    Granulomatous (TB, fungal)
    PCP
- Idiopathic
    IPF
    Sarcoid
- Collagen vascular disease
    RA
    Scleroderma
    Ankylosing spondylitis
- Extrinsic agents
    Pneumoconiosis, (asbestos, silicosis, CWP)
    Drugs

Tumor
- Interstitial tumors
    Eosinophilic granuloma
- Lymphangitic tumor spread
- Desmoplastic reaction to tumor

MNEMONIC APPROACH TO DDX	
Examples of Common Entities	
DISTRIBUTION	
Upper lobes ("CASSET P")	Cystic fibrosis (not an interstitial disease)
	Ankylosing spondylitis
	Silicosis
	Sarcoid
	Eosinophilic granuloma (sparing of costophrenic angles)
	Tuberculosis
	Pneumocystis carinii
Lower lobes ("BADAS")	Bronchiectasis (not an interstitial disease)
	Aspiration
	Drugs, DIP
	Asbestosis
	Scleroderma, other collagen vascular diseases
EVOLUTION	
Acute ("HELP")	Hypersensitivity (allergic alveolitis)
	Edema
	Lymphoproliferative
	Pneumonitis, viral
Chronic ("LIFE")	Lymphangitic spread
	Inflammation, infection
	Fibrosis
	Edema
LUNG VOLUMES	
Increased	Cystic fibrosis (associated with this pattern but not an interstitial disease)
	Eosinophilic granuloma (pneumothorax, 20%)
	Lymphangioleiomyomatosis (pneumothorax)
Decreased	Idiopathic pulmonary fibrosis
	Scleroderma
PLEURAL DISEASE	
Pleural plaques	Asbestosis
Pleural effusion	CHF
	Lymphangitic carcinomatosis
	Rheumatoid disease
LYMPH NODES	
Enlarged	Malignant adenopathy
	TB, fungus
	Sarcoid
Calcified	Silicosis

HRCT PATTERNS OF INTERSTITIAL LUNG DISEASE		
	Imaging	Causes

GROUND GLASS OPACITY

Increased haze
All acute interstitial diseases

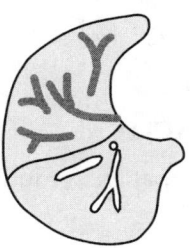

Allergic hypersensitivity
All acute interstitial disease
    DIP
    Active IPF
    Viral
PCP
BOOP
Eosinophilic pneumonia
Pulmonary edema

RETICULONODULAR OPACITIES

Peribronchovascular thickening
    (peribronchial cuffing on CXR)

Thickening of interlobular septae
    (Kerley lines)

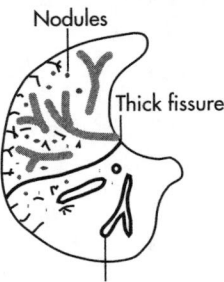

Pulmonary edema
Viral, mycoplasmal pneumonia,
    and PCP
Lymphangitic tumor spread
Pulmonary fibrosis
    IPF
    Secondary fibrosis
        Drugs
        Radiation
        Collagen vascular disease
        Hemosiderosis
Asbestosis

NODULAR OPACITIES

1-2 mm interstitial nodules:

Often associated with reticular
    opacities

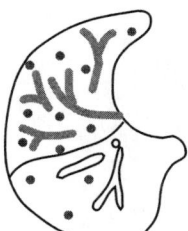

Hematogenous infection
Hematogenous metastases
Sarcoid
Pneumoconiosis
    Silicosis
    CWP
Histiocytosis (EG, also cysts)

CYSTIC SPACES

With or without walls

Lymphangioleiomyomatosis
Cystic PCP
Histiocytosis
Honeycombing
    IPF
        Any end-stage interstitial disease

CRAZY PAVING APPEARANCE ON HRCT

Ground glass opacity with overlying geometric structures
- Pulmonary alveolar proteinosis
- ARDS
- PCP
- Lipoid pneumonia

HALO PATTERN OF GROUND GLASS OPACITY

- Early invasive aspergillosis in a leukemic patient: ground glass around a nodule of consolidation
- Hemorrhage around a neoplasm
- Post biopsy pseudonodule

PERIPHERAL GROUND GLASS OPACITY AND CONSOLIDATION

- BOOP
- Infarcts
- Septic Emboli
- Collagen vascular disease
- Contusion
- DIP
- Drug toxicity
- Eosinophilic pneumonia
- Fibrosis
- Sarcoidosis

HONEY COMBING PATTERN ON HRCT

- UIP (idiopathic pulmonary fibrosis)
- Scleroderma/RA
- Asbestosis
- Chronic hypersensitivity pneumonitis
- Sarcoidosis
- Silicosis
- EG
- Drug toxicity: bleomycin

DISEASES SPREADING ALONG BRONCHOVASCULAR BUNDLE

- Sarcoidosis
- Lymphoma
- Lymphangitic spread of tumor
- TB
- Kaposi's sarcoma

TREE IN BUD APPEARANCE:

Infection
- TB
- Bronchopneumonia
- Fungal
- Asian panbronchiolitis
- Viral pneumonias

Bronchial disease
- Bronchiolitis

Congential disoders
- Cystic fibrosis
- Dyskinetic cilia syndrome

Other
- Allergic bronchopulmonary aspergillosis
- Lymphangitis carcinomatosis
- EG

Abnormal Density

HYPERLUCENT LUNG

Criteria: hyperlucency may be lobar, segmental, subsegmental, or generalized.
Hyperlucency may or may not be associated with overexpansion of lungs. Causes:

Airways
- Obstruction of airways (air trapping); inspiratory/expiratory films may be of use to accentuate the hyperlucency

    Emphysema, bullae
    Large airway obstruction: asthma, mucous plug
    Small airway obstruction (bronchioli): Swyer-James syndrome
        (bronchiolitis obliterans)
    Compensatory hyperexpansion of residual lung after: Surgical lobectomy,
        chronic lobar collapse

- Cysts
- Congenital

    Hypogenetic lung syndrome
    Congenital lobar emphysema

Vascular (hyperlucency caused by oligemia)
- PE
- Pulmonary artery stenosis

Chest wall abnormalities
- Mastectomy
- Poland's syndrome (congenital absence of pectoralis muscle)

Pleural
- Pneumothorax

SMALL LUNG

May be associated with either decreased or increased density.
- Hypogenetic lung syndrome
- Agenesis of pulmonary artery
- Chronic atelectasis
- Bronchiolitis obliterans (Swyer-James syndrome)

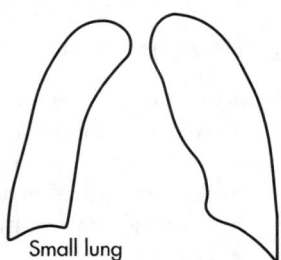

Small lung

Tracheobronchial Lesions

ENDOBRONCHIAL LESIONS

Criteria: focal bronchial abnormality. Causes:
  Tumors, 80%
  - Malignancy, 70%:
    Squamous cell carcinoma (most common)
    Low-grade malignancies
      Adenoidcystic carcinoma
      Mucoepidermoid carcinoma
    Small cell carcinoma
    Carcinoid
  - Metastases, 5%: RCC, melanoma, colon, breast, thyroid
  - Other: hamartoma, mucoepidermoid carcinoma, hemangioma
  Inflammatory disease, 20%
  - Tuberculosis
  Other
  - Mucous plug
  - Foreign body (fishbone, dental)
  - Trauma
  - Broncholith

DIFFUSE TRACHEAL LUMINAL ABNORMALITIES

Increased diameter
  - Tracheobronchomegaly (Mounier-Kuhn disease)
  - Pulmonary fibrosis
  - Tracheomalacia
Decreased diameter
  - Saber-sheath trachea (most common cause)
  - Tracheopathia osteochondroplastica
  - Tracheomalacia (decreased diameter on expiration)
  - Relapsing polychondritis
  - Amyloidosis
  - Sarcoidosis
  - Wegener's disease
  - Tuberculous and fungal stenosis

BRONCHIECTASIS

Postinfectious (most common)
  - Any childhood infection
  - Recurrent aspiration
  - ABPA: central bronchiectasis
  - Chronic granulomatous infection
  - Pertussis
Bronchial obstruction
  - Neoplasm
  - Foreign body

Congenital
- Cystic fibrosis (abnormal secretions)
- Bronchial cartilage deficiency: Williams-Campbell syndrome
- Abnormal mucociliary transport: Kartagener's syndrome

UPPER LOBE BRONCHIECTASIS

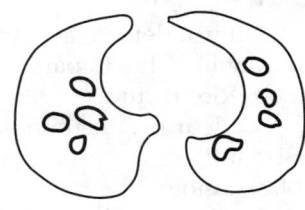

- Cystic fibrosis
- TB
- Radiation
- ABPA (most commonly central)

MUCOID (BRONCHIAL) IMPACTION

Criteria: bronchus filled with soft tissue density (inspissated mucus); bronchi may be enlarged (bronchocele) or be of normal size. No contrast enhancement. Causes:
- Asthma
- Cystic fibrosis
- ABPA
- Congenital bronchial atresia

Pleural Disease

PLEURAL-BASED MASS

Criteria: soft tissue mass along the chest wall; obtuse angles with chest wall.

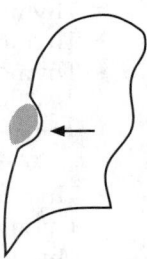

   Tumor
- Mesothelioma (malignant): multifocal, diffuse
- Fibrous tumor of the pleura (benign); unifocal may be locally invasive
- Malignant thymoma, lymphoma often have similar appearance as mesothelioma
- Metastases: breast, lung, prostate, thyroid, renal
- Lipoma (most common benign tumor)
- Extrapleural tumors
     Rib tumors
     Children: EG, ABC, Ewing's sarcoma, neuroblastoma
     Adults: metastases > multiple myeloma > Paget's disease, fibrous dysplasia
     Plexiform neurofibromas in neurofibromatosis (bilateral)

   Inflammatory
- Infectious: TB
- Asbestos related
- Actinomycosis (rib destruction)

   Trauma, surgery, chest tubes

CALCIFIED PLEURAL PLAQUES

The most common causes of calcified pleural plaques (mnemonic "TAFT") are:
- **T**uberculosis (usually diffuse plaques)
- **A**sbestos-related plaques (usually focal plaques)
- **F**luid (empyema, hematoma)
- **T**alc

ELEVATED HEMIDIAPHRAGM

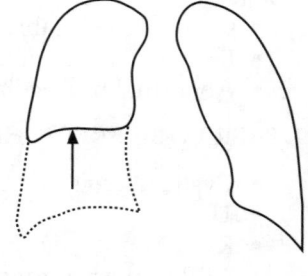

Phrenic nerve paralysis
- Tumor
- Surgery
- Birth defect: Erb's paralysis

Immobility due to pain
- Rib fractures
- Pleuritis, pneumonia
- PE

Mass lesions
- Abdominal masses, subphrenic collection, abscess
- Diaphragmatic hernia
- Pleural tumors
- Subpulmonic effusion (apparent elevation of hemidiaphragm)

Mediastinum

ANTERIOR MEDIASTINAL MASSES

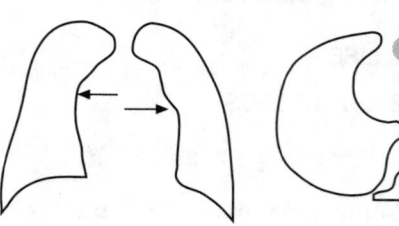

Thymic masses
- Thymic cyst
- Thymolipoma
- Thymoma
    Cystic
    Benign (noninvasive) thymoma
    Malignant (invasive) thymoma
- Thymic carcinoma
- Thymic carcinoid
- Thymic lymphoma

Germ cell tumors (male >> female)
- Seminoma
- Embryonal cell carcinoma
- Choriocarcinoma
- Teratoma

Lymphadenopathy: lymphoma, sarcoid, TB, etc.

Aneurysm and vascular abnormalities (involve both the anterior and superior mediastinal compartments)

Mnemonic for anterior mediastinal masses ("4 Ts")
- **T**hymoma (most common anterior mediastinal mass) + other thymic lesions
- **T**hyroid lesions
- **T** cell lymphoma (Hodgkin and NHL)
- **T**eratoma and other germ cell tumors (seminoma, choriocarcinoma), 10%

Cystic anterior mediastinal mass
- Thymic cyst (3rd pharyngeal pouch remnant)
- Cystic thymoma (contains solid components besides cysts)
- Teratoma
- Bronchogenic cysts (usually located in middle mediastinum)
- Pericardial cyst

SUPERIOR MEDIASTINAL MASS

Descending through thoracic inlet
- Thyroid masses
- Adenopathy (primary head and neck tumors)
- Lymphatic cysts, cystic hygroma

Ascending through thoracic inlet
- Small cell carcinoma of the lung

Lymphoma

Aneurysm and vascular anomalies may involve both the anterior and superior mediastinal compartments

MIDDLE MEDIASTINAL MASS

Adenopathy (often bilateral)
- Benign: sarcoid, TB, fungal infection, chronic beryllium exposure
- Malignant: metastases, lymphoma, leukemia

Congenital cysts
- Bronchogenic cysts (subcarinal, anterior trachea)
- Pericardial cysts

Aneurysm
- Aorta, aortic branches
- Pulmonary artery

Esophagus
- Hiatal hernia (common)
- Neoplasm
- Diverticula
- Megaesophagus: achalasia, hiatal hernia, colonic interposition

Other
- Mediastinal hemorrhage
- Mediastinal lipomatosis
- Bronchogenic cancer arising adjacent to mediastinum
- Aberrant RSA with diverticulum
- Varices
- Neurinoma from recurrent laryngeal nerve
- Malignancy of trachea
- Pancreatic pseudocyst

ADENOPATHY

Low-attenuation lymph nodes
- TB and fungal infections in AIDS (ring enhancement)
- Necrotic metastases (aggressive neoplasm)
- Lymphoma (occasionally)

Vascularized lymph nodes
- Castleman's disease (giant benign nodal hyperplasia)
- Vascular metastases: renal cell, thyroid, small cell, melanoma

Calcified lymph nodes
- TB
- Histoplasmosis, other fungus
- Sarcoidosis
- Silicosis
- Radiation therapy

POSTERIOR MEDIASTINAL MASS

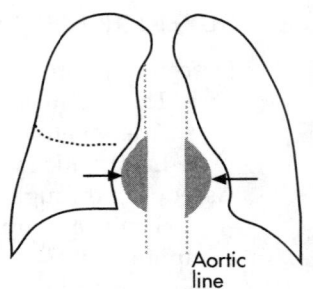

Neurogenic, 90%
- Peripheral nerves (20-40 years; < 2 vertebral bodies long): schwannoma and neurofibroma, 45%
- Sympathetic ganglia (< 20 years; > 2 vertebral bodies long): ganglioneuroma, neuroblastoma, sympathicoblastoma
- Paraganglionic cells: pheochromocytoma, paraganglioma (least common)
- Lateral meningomyelocele

Thoracic spine
- Neoplasm
- Hematoma
- Extramedullary hematopoiesis (bilateral)
- Discitis

Vascular
- Aneurysm
- Azygos continuation (congenital absence of IVC with dilated azygos and hemiazygos veins)

CARDIOPHRENIC ANGLE MASS

- Fat pad (most common cause)
- Diaphragmatic hernia (second most common)
    Morgagni (anterior; 90% on right side)
    Bochdalek (posterior; more common on left; not a true cardiophrenic mass)
- Pericardial cyst
- Cardiophrenic angle nodes (lymphoma usually recurrent. s/p radiation)
- Aneurysm
- Dilated right atrium
- Anterior mediastinal mass
- Primary lung or pleural mass

FATTY MEDIASTINAL LESIONS

Purely fatty lesions
- Mediastinal lipomatosis
- Morgagni hernia (omentum)
- Bochdalek hernia (omentum)
- Periesophageal fat herniation

Tumors with fatty components
- Lipoma
- Liposarcoma
- Thymolipoma (children and young adults, lesions are usually very large)
- Germ cell tumors (also contain calcifications, cystic and solid region)

HIGH-DENSITY MEDIASTINAL LESIONS (NONCONTRAST CT)

Calcified lymph nodes
Calcified primary mass
- Tumor
- Goiter
- Aneurysm

Hemorrhage

DENSELY ENHANCING MEDIASTINAL MASS

Vascular
- Aneurysm
- Vascular abnormalities
- Esophageal varices

Hypervascular tumors: paraganglioma, metastasis from thyroid cancer, RCC
Goiter
Castleman's disease

PROMINENT HILA

Tumors
- Central bronchogenic carcinoma
- Lymphoma

Adenopathy
- Infectious: TB, fungi, histoplasmosis
- Inflammatory: sarcoid, silicosis
- Tumor: commonly oat cell, lymphoma, metastases

Pulmonary artery enlargement

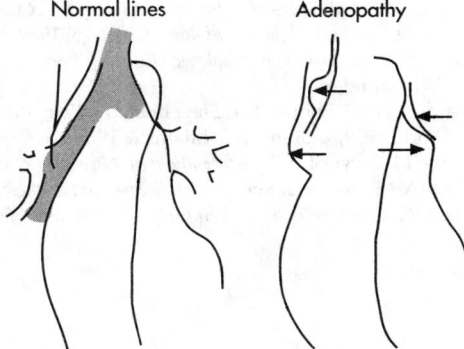

Normal lines   Adenopathy

EGGSHELL CALCIFICATION IN HILAR NODES

- Silicosis, CWP
- Treated lymphoma
- Granulomatous disease such as histoplasmosis rarely contains eggshell calcification; diffuse calcifications are more common
- Sarcoid (rare and late in disease)

PNEUMOMEDIASTINUM

Pulmonary
- Asthma (common)
- Barotrauma (intubation, diver)
- Childbirth
- Pneumothorax

Mediastinum
- Tracheobronchial laceration
- Esophageal perforation
- Mediastinal surgery
- Boerhaave's syndrome

Abdomen
- Intraperitoneal or retroperitoneal bowel perforation
- Retroperitoneal surgery

Head and neck
- Esophageal rupture
- Facial fractures
- Dental or retropharyngeal infection, mediastinitis

Primer of Diagnostic Imaging

SUGGESTED READINGS

Eisenberg RL: *Clinical imaging: an atlas of differential diagnosis*, Rockville, Md, 1988, Aspen Publishers.

Felson B: *Chest roentgenology*, Philadelphia, 1973, WB Saunders.

Fraser RG, Paré JAP, Paré PD, et al: *Diagnosis of disease of the chest*, ed 3, Philadelphia, 1991, WB Saunders.

Fraser RG et al: *Diagnosis of diseases of the chest*, ed 3, Philadelphia, 1991, WB Saunders.

Freundlich IM, Bragg D: *A radiologic approach to diseases of the chest*, Baltimore, 1996, Williams & Wilkins.

Gale M, Karlinsky J: *Computed tomography of the chest: a teaching file*, St Louis, 1988, Mosby.

Goodman LR, Putnam CE: *Critical care imaging*, ed 3, Philadelphia, 1992, WB Saunders.

Green R, Muhm J, editors: *Syllabus: a categorical course in diagnostic chest radiology*, Oak Brook, Ill, 1992, Radiological Society of North America.

Holleb AI, Fink DJ, Murphy GP: American Cancer Society textbook of clinical oncology, Atlanta, 1991, American Cancer Society

Kassner E, et al: *Atlas of radiologic imaging*, St Louis, 1989, Mosby.

Mann H, Bragg D: *Chest radiology*, Chicago, 1989, Yearbook Medical Publishers.

Muller NL, editor: *The radiologic clinics of North America: imaging of diffuse lung disease*, Philadelphia, 1991, WB Saunders.

Naidich DP, Zerhouni EA, Siegelman SS: *Computed tomography and magnetic resonance of the thorax*, New York, 1999, Lippincott Williams & Wilkins.

Newell J, Tarver R: *Thoracic radiology*, New York, 1993 Lippincott Williams & Wilkins.

Pare JAP, Fraser RG: *Synopsis of diseases of the chest*, Philadelphia, 1993, WB Saunders.

Reed JC: *Chest radiology: plain film patterns and differential diagnosis*, St Louis, 1997, Mosby.

Chapter 2

Cardiac Imaging

2

Chapter Outline

Cardiac Imaging Techniques

Plain Film Interpretation

NORMAL PLAIN FILM ANATOMY

Posteroanterior (PA) view

Right cardiac margin has three segments
- Superior vena cava (SVC)
- Right atrium (RA)
- Inferior vena cava (IVC)

Left cardiac margin has four segments
- Aortic arch (AA) (more prominent with age)
- Main pulmonary artery (PA) at level of left main stem bronchus
- Left atrial appendage (may not be visible in normal hearts)
- Left ventricle (LV)
- RV is usually not seen in frontal projection

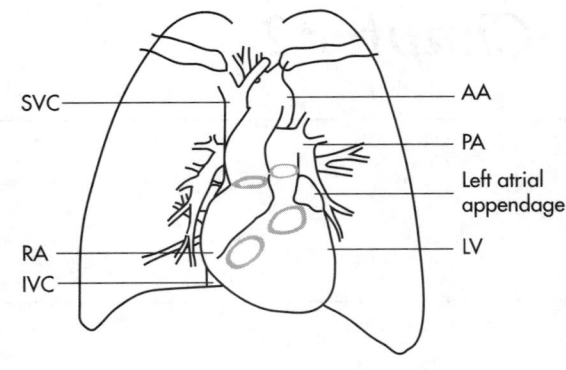

Lateral view

Anterior cardiac margin has three segments
- Right ventricle (RV) is in apparent contact with sternum
- Main PA
- Ascending aorta

Posterior cardiac margin has two segments
- LV
- Left atrium (LA)

Other anatomical landmarks
- Trachea, bronchi
- Right PA en face anterior to carina
- Aortopulmonary window (triangle between aorta and PA)

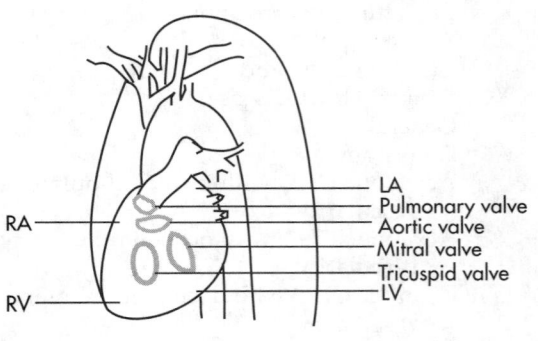

Oblique views

Right anterior oblique (RAO) and left anterior oblique (LAO) views are mainly used in coronary angiography and ventriculography. These views rarely add any diagnostic information in routine clinical practice. RAO view does not show calcified mitral or tricuspid valve.

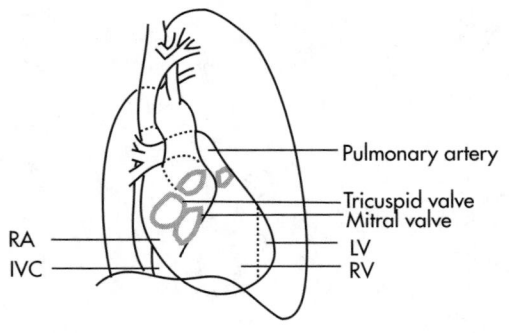

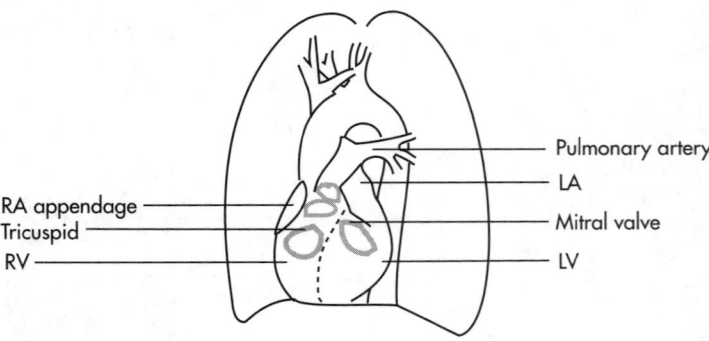

RADIOGRAPHIC APPROACH TO INTENSIVE CARE UNIT (ICU) FILMS

1. Patient data present
2. Date and time of exam are essential to report
3. Postsurgical? If so, what type of surgery?
4. Appliances: intravascular, catheters, endotracheal tube, tubes, drains, etc. New appliances? Any catheters removed or repositioned?
5. Cardiac, mediastinal size and shape
6. Pneumothorax present?
7. Lung disease: progression/regression?
8. Most important: any change from previous film?

Pearls

- Always obtain end-inspiratory films; varying lung volumes in inspiratory films will change the apparent extent and distribution of alveolar fluid
- Positive end-expiratory pressure (PEEP) ventilation may underestimate air space consolidation
- PEEP decreases vascular mediastinal width
- Quality of portable film is often suboptimal because:
    Exposure time is longer than with routine films; this, along with the inability to often suspend respiration, causes indistinct vascular margins, which should not be mistaken as interstitial edema
    Patient positioning suboptimal
    Anteroposterior (AP) not PA position
    Patient semierect not readily detectable
        Small pleural effusions not readily detectable
        Pulmonary vascularity may be "cephalized"
        Varying tube-film distance
        Varying cardiac/mediastinal silhouette
- Technique
    Lower (80-90) peak kilivolt (kVp) than normal (120-140)
    Variable daily density (exposure occurs at toe of HD curve): inadequate display of retrocardiac and mediastinal structures

ENDOTRACHEAL TUBE (ET)

Inflated cuff should not bulge tracheal wall. Tip of ET should be above the carina and below thoracic inlet:
- Neutral neck: 4-6 cm above carina
- Flexed neck: moves tip inferiorly by 2 cm
- Extended neck: moves tip superiorly by 2 cm

Complications of ET placement:
- Misplacement: atelectasis secondary to bronchial obstruction
- Tracheomalacia occurs above cuff pressures of 25 cm H_2O
- Tracheal rupture; radiographic findings include:
    Pneumothorax
    Pneumomediastinum
    Subcutaneous emphysema
- Tracheal stenosis
- Dislodged teeth
- Laceration of nasooropharynx

NASOGASTRIC TUBE

Tip with end-holes should be located in stomach. Complications:
- Placement in airway
- Gastric and/or duodenal erosion

SWAN-GANZ CATHETER

Tip should be located in left or right PA, within 1 cm from hilum. There should be no loops in RA, RV (may cause arrhythmias). Types:
- Swan-Ganz catheter for measurement of wedge pressure
- Swan-Ganz catheter with integrated pacemaker (metallic bands visible)

Complications:
- Pulmonary infarct
- Pulmonary hemorrhage
- Pulmonary artery pseudoaneurysm
- Infection

INTRAAORTIC BALLOON PUMP (IABP)

Tip should be located just distal to the takeoff of the left subclavian artery (LSA) and be 2-4 cm below aortic knob. Inflation may be seen during diastole. Complications:
- CVA (position too high)
- Renal or mesenteric ischemia (position too low)
- Aortic dissection
- Limb ischemia
- Infection
- Note initial position of electrodes as may migrate

EPICARDIAL PACING WIRE

Wires are typically anchored in the anterior myocardium; some slack may be left in pericardium. Multiple wires may be present. Wires exit through anterior chest wall.

AUTOMATIC INTRACARDIAC DEFIBRILLATION DEVICE

Rectangular or ovoid antenna around RV and LV. Types:
- New models have pin sensors
- Old models have spring sensors

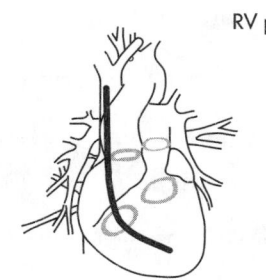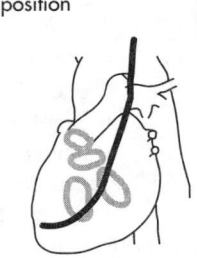

RV position

CENTRAL VENOUS LINES

Tip should end in the SVC below the anterior first rib. Always rule out pneumothorax. Signs of impending catheter perforation (hemothorax, pneumothorax):
- Position of the tip against the vessel wall
- Sharply curved catheter tip
- Infection, thrombosis

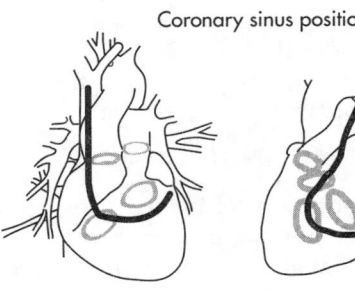

Coronary sinus position

PACEMAKER

Typical location is in apex of RV. May be located in atrial appendage for atrial pacing and in coronary sinus for atrial left ventricular pacing. Complications:
- Displacement of electrodes
- Broken wires (rare with modern pacemakers)
- Twiddlers syndrome: rotation of pulse generator due to manipulation in a large pacemaker pocket
- Perforation
- Infection
- Venous thrombosis, vascular obstruction

CHEST TUBES

Sideport (interruption of radiodense band) has to be within thoracic cavity, otherwise there may be a leak. The tip of tube should not abut the mediastinum. Complications:
- Residual pneumothorax
- Sideport outside the thoracic wall

PROSTHETIC CARDIAC VALVES

Tissue valves (no anticoagulation necessary; early breakdown)
  Heterografts
    Porcine valves
      - Edwards-Carpentier valve
      - Hancock valve
    Bovine valves
      - Ionescu-Shiley valve (presently not used)

Mechanical valves (more durable than tissue valves but require anticoagulation)
  Homografts
    Aortic in setting of endocarditis
  Autografts
    Native pulmonary valve, aortic valve
  Caged ball
    • Starr-Edwards valve (presently not used)
    • McGovern-Cromie (presently not used)
    • Smellof-Cutter valve (presently not used)
  Caged disk
    • Beal valve (presently not used)
  Tilting disk
    • Bileaflet—St. Judes valve
    • Single leaflet—Bjork-Shiley valve (presently not used)
    • Hall-Medtronics

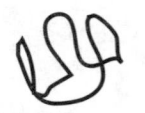 Edwards-Carpentier   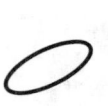 Hancock   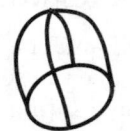 Starr-Edwards   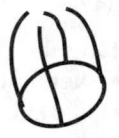 McGovern-Cromie

 St. Judes    Lillehei-Kaster   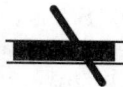 Bjork-Shiley   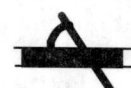 Hall-Medtronics

Angiography

CARDIAC ANGIOGRAPHY

Technique for left ventriculography
  • Femoral approach
  • Pigtail for ventricular injections
  • Straight endhole cathethercatheter for pressure measurements
  • 36-45 mL (3-4 sec injection) at 15 mL/sec

Evaluation
  1. Cardiac chamber size
  2. Wall motion
  3. Ejection fraction
  4. Valvular stenosis, regurgitation, or shunts

Ejection fraction

$$EF = \frac{(EDV - ESV)}{EDV} = \frac{\text{stroke volume}}{EDV}$$

Where EDV = end-diastolic volume, ESV = end-systolic volume

Wall motion abnormalities
  • Hypokinesis
  • Akinesis
  • Dyskinesis

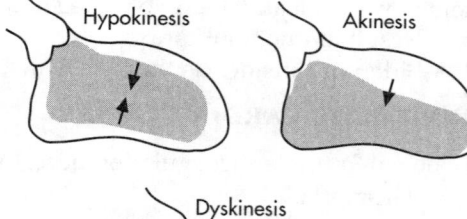

CORONARY ANGIOGRAPHY

Judkins catheters (6 Fr, groin) are the most commonly used catheters. Right and left Judkins catheters have different shapes:

Contrast medium
  • Hand injection: 7-9 mL for left coronary artery (LCA), 4-6 mL for right coronary artery (RCA)

- Low osmolar contrast agents are usually used
- Hyperosmolarity leads to electrocardiogram (ECG) changes
- Citrate in contrast medium may cause hypocalcemia
- 3000 U heparin IV; reversed by 350 mg of protamine

Complications
- Hematoma
- Arrhythmia
- Vasovagal reaction
- Contrast reaction/renal failure
- Acute myocardial infarction (AMI) < 1%
- Stroke < 1%
- Coronary air embolus

Interpretation
Steps in evaluation of coronary angiograms:
1. Which artery is being opacified?
2. Which projection (LAO or RAO)?
3. Stenosis present? If yes, grading of stenosis
4. Ventriculogram; analyze:
   Wall motion
   Ejection fraction
   Presence of mitral regurgitation?

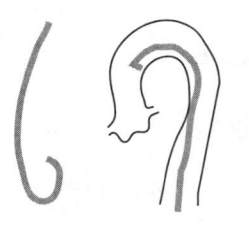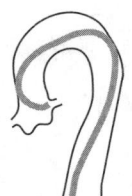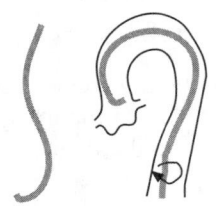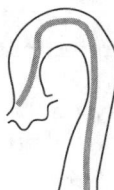

CORONARY ANGIOGRAM

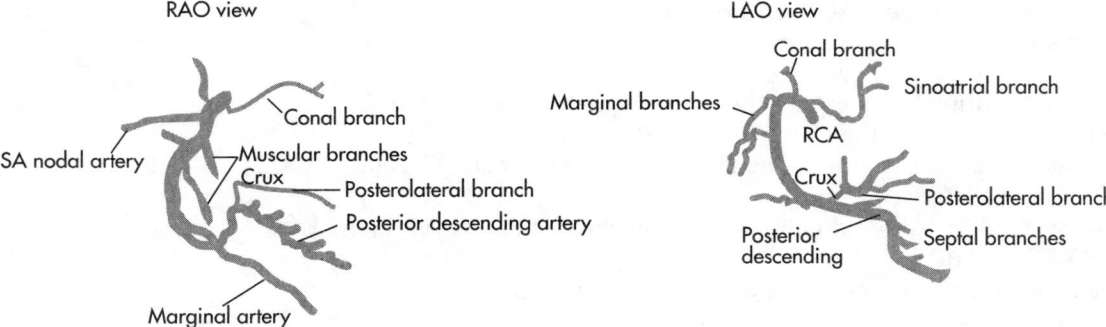

RCA
- Conus artery
    First branch of RCA
    Runs anteriorly
- Sinoatrial (SA) nodal artery
    Branch of RCA in 40%-55%
- Muscular branches
- Acute marginal branch
- Posterior descending artery
- Arterioventicular (AV) nodal artery
    Branch of RCA in 90%
- Posterolateral ventricular branches

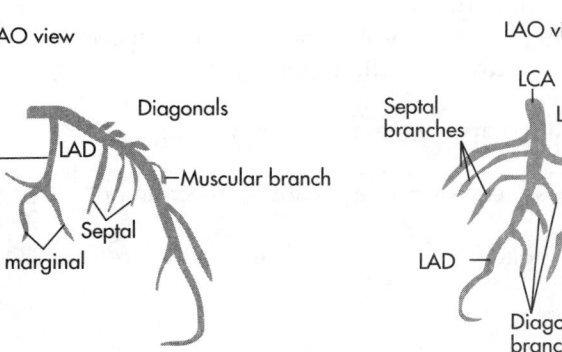

LCA
- Left anterior descending (LAD)
  Longest vessel
  Only vessel that extends to apex
  Septal branches
  Diagonal branches
- Left circumflex artery (LCX)
  Left atrial circumflex
  Marginal branches

Projections

LAO view projects the spine to the *left* (relative to the heart, i.e., on the right side of the image). RAO projects the spine to the *right* (relative to the heart, i.e., to the left side of the image).

Different projections (LAO, RAO) and angulations (caudad, cranial) are required to visualize all portions of the coronary arteries. Most commonly, the following injections are obtained:
- LAO with cranial angulation
- AP cranial or caudal angulation
- RAO cranial or caudal angulation
- Lateral (rarely used)

Although AP views are good for visualizing left main, they are not as useful as RAO and LAO views because arteries overlie the spine.

Dominance

Refers to the artery that ultimately supplies the diaphragmatic aspect of the interventricular septum (IVS) and the LV
- 85% of patients have right-sided dominance: RCA is larger than LCA and gives rise to the AV nodal artery
- 10% of patients have left-sided dominance: LCA is larger than RCA and gives rise to the AV nodal artery
- 5% of patients have balanced coronary artery tree (codominant): two posterior descending arteries are present, one from the left cirumflex and one from the RCA

Pitfalls

- Intramyocardial bridge: LAD enters deep into the myocardium and may be compressed during systole; appears normal in diastole
- Spasm of coronary arteries may be catheter induced (spasm can be provoked with ergot derivatives during angiography)
- Totally occluded arteries/bypasses may escape detection
- Orifice stenoses can be missed if aortic injection not performed
- In adequate opacification—need to see contrast reflux into aorta

Veins

- Epicardial veins accompany arteries and drain into coronary sinus
- Thebesian venous system drains directly into atria

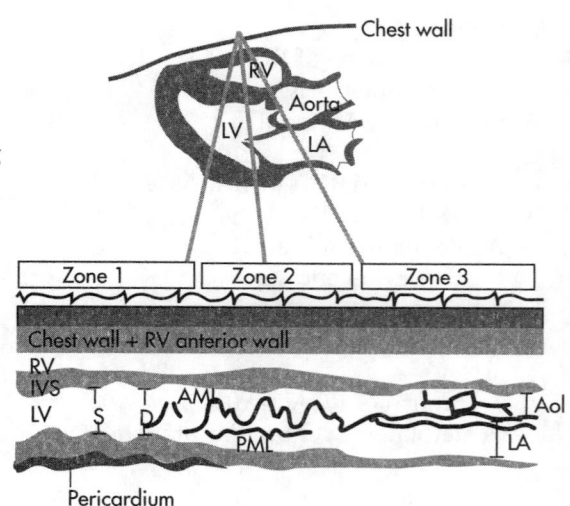

MR CORONARY ANGIOGRAPHY

Tremendous advances in magnetic resonance (MR) coronary angiography during the past decade have demonstrated promising potential for noninvasive diagnosis of coronary artery disease (CAD). The in-plane image resolution of current coronary artery MR imaging techniques is about 1 mm, which is sufficient for detection of stenoses in large coronary arteries but inadequate for accurate detection of disease in smaller branches of the coronary vasculature.

- Fast gradient-echo sequence are commonly used (TR < 10 msec, TE < 3 msec)
- Multislice 2D sequences are commonly used for breathhold sequences. 3D sequences are commonly used for non-breathhold sequences (using navigator correction for respiratory motion).
- Fat saturation is used to suppress epicardial coronary fat.
- Newer phased array coils have increased signal to noise ratio (SNR).
- ECG-gating minimizes motion artifacts.
- Gated, segmented k-space acquisition is commonly used.
- Spiral imaging is an alternative imaging modality that samples k space along trajectories that start at the center of k space and spiral outward. This scheme is a more natural sampling pattern that has high sampling densities near the center of k space, where the power spectrum of the image is generally highest.
- Low-dose nitrate (coronary vasodilatation) or beta blocker pretreatment (to slow down heart rate) has been used.

CT ANGIOGRAPHY OF CORONARY ARTERIES

Computed tomography (CT) is very sensitive in (1) detecting and quantitating coronary artery calcifications, (2) surveying the entire coronary tree noninvasively and (3) determining the luminal diameter. For the purposes of coronary calcium evaluation, CT examinations are performed without contrast agent administration and therefore display only calcified components of plaque. Usually, tissue densities ≥ 130 Hounsfield units are set as the attenuation level corresponding to calcified plaque. A calcium scoring system has been devised that is based on the maximum x-ray attenuation coefficient, or CT number measured in Hounsfield units, and the area of calcium deposits (traditional Agatston calcium score). Callister et al evaluated an alternative method of determining the calcium score by quantifying the actual volume of plaque analogous to that possible in prior histological studies (total calcium volume score, CVS). Both calcium scoring algorithms can be applied to fast multidetector CT images and provide a measure of total coronary plaque burden.

Cardiac Ultrasound

M-MODE ULTRASOUND

M-mode = motion mode = one-dimensional echocardiography; infrequently done today but included here for historical purposes. Structures with broad surfaces perpendicular to the beam reflect well. The transducer is swept through 3 zones:
Zone 1
- Ventricular measurement area permits estimation of stroke volume and ejection fraction
- Measurement of LV wall and IVS wall thickness
- Pericardial effusion may be detected

Zone 2
- Anterior (AML) and posterior mitral leaflets (PML) are identified

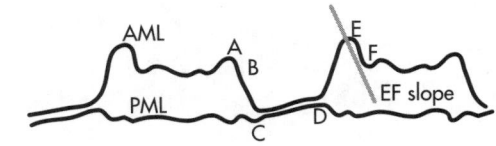

- Mitral valve (MV) excursion (measured from D to E) is an index of MV mobility and inflow volume
- EF slope: represents the rate of middiastolic posterior excursion of the AML; the EF slope is an index of mitral valve inflow

Zone 3
- Aorta and aortic valve (rhomboid structure) are seen
- Measurement of LA

TWO-DIMENSIONAL CARDIAC ULTRASOUND

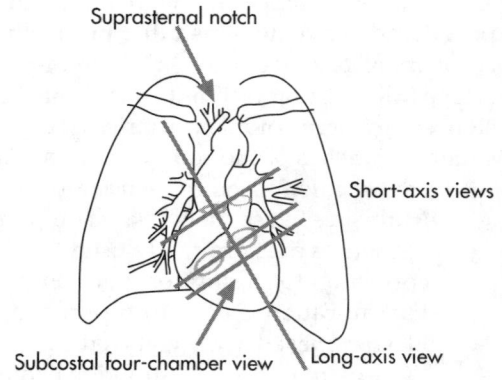

There are four common views:
- Long-axis view
- Short-axis view
- Apical views
- Suprasternal notch view

LONG-AXIS VIEW

Location: transducer in 3rd or 4th intercostal space so that the beam is parallel to a line from the right shoulder to the left flank. Image is oriented so that LA and LV are posterior and LA and aorta are left.

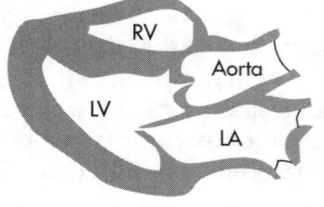

SHORT-AXIS VIEWS

Location: transducer in 3rd or 4th intercostal space but the beam is perpendicular to the long-axis view. Several levels are usually scanned, from cephalad to caudad: great arteries, plane of MV, and plane of papillary muscles (MPM = posteromedial papillary muscle; LPM = anterolateral papillary muscle). Image is oriented so that MPM is at 8 o'clock and LPM is at 4 o'clock.

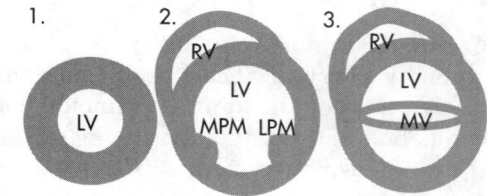

APICAL VIEWS

Apical four-chamber view
Location: patient in left lateral decubitus. Transducer at maximum point of impulse. Image is oriented so that RV and LV are anterior and LV and LA are on the right.

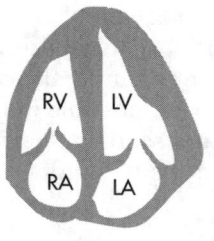

Apical two-chamber view (RAO view of the LV)
Location: transducer at maximum point of impulse and directed in a plane parallel to the IVS. Image is oriented so that LV is anterior.

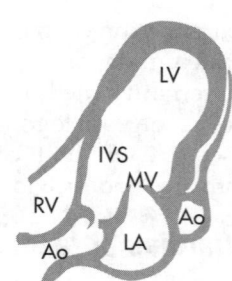

SUPRASTERNAL NOTCH VIEW

Location: transducer in the suprasternal notch with inferior and posterior beam angulation. Image is oriented so that the ascending aorta is on the left and the descending aorta is on the right.

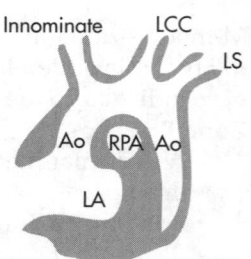

Congenital Heart Disease

General

INCIDENCE OF CONGENITAL HEART DISEASE

Overall incidence of all anomalies is approximately 1% of newborns. The most common structural defects are bicuspid aortic valve and mitral valve prolapse (MVP), most of which are asymptomatic. Incidence of symptomatic congenital heart diseases (CHD) are listed in the table.

INCIDENCE OF SYMPTOMATIC CHD	
	Frequency
MOST COMMON CONGENITAL ANOMALIES (ALL AGE GROUPS; BICUSPID AORTIC VALVE AND MVP EXCLUDED)	
Ventricular septal defect (VSD)	30%
Atrial septal defect (ASD)	10%
Tetralogy of Fallot	10%
Patent ductus arteriosus (PDA)	10%
Coarctation of aorta	7%
Transposition of great arteries (TGA)	5%
FIRST MONTH OF LIFE (SERIOUS CLINICAL PROBLEMS, HIGH MORTALITY)	
Hypoplastic left heart	35%
TGA	25%
Coarctation	20%
Multiple serious defects	15%
Pulmonary atresia/stenosis	10%
Severe tetralogy of Fallot	10%

APPROACH

Evaluate 5 structures on the chest x-ray:
- Pulmonary vascularity
- Chamber enlargement
- Situs
- Side of AA
- Bone and soft tissue changes

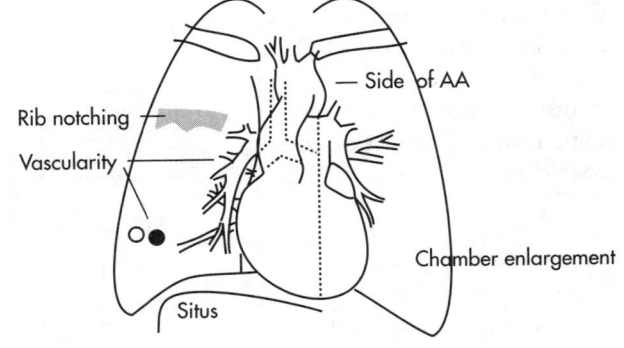

Pulmonary vascularity

Normal vascularity
- Right main PA = same size as trachea at level of AA
- Peripheral arteries (seen on-end) = same size as adjacent bronchus

Pulmonary arterial overcirculation (shunt vascularity): common in CHD, less common in acquired heart disease (AHD)

Pulmonary venous hypertension (PVH) (edema) grades:
- Grade 1: vascular redistribution (10-17 mm Hg)
- Grade 2: interstitial edema (18-25 mm Hg)
- Grade 3: alveolar edema (> 25 mm Hg)

Pulmonary arterial hypertension (PAH)
- Large main PA
- Usually normal hilar arteries

Eisenmenger pulmonary vasculature
- Combination of shunt and PAH
- Aneurysmal hilar arteries
- Calcified vessels (rare)

Cyanosis: there are no definitive signs to predict cyanosis by plain film; however, as a rule of thumb, cyanotic patients (right-to-left shunt) have small pulmonary arteries and the main PA segment may not be visible or is concave.

Chamber enlargement
Lateral view is more helpful in young children:
- LA enlargement
  - Posterior displacement of esophagus during barium swallow
  - Posterior displacement of left mainstem bronchus (LMB)
- LV enlargement: posterior displacement behind IVC
- RV enlargement: filling of retrosternal clear space

PA view; criteria for cardiomegaly:
- Cardiothoracic index > 0.55

Situs
- Liver or IVC determines on which side the RA is located
- Tracheobronchial tree: right mainstem bronchus (RMB) has a more acute angle than LMB
- Incidence of CHD in situs inversus: 5%

Algorithm

CLASSIFICATION

The radiographic classification of CHD relies mainly on clinical information (cyanosis) and plain film information (pulmonary vasculature).

Acyanotic CHD with increased pulmonary vascularity
Common: L-R shunt where pulmonary flow is greater than aortic flow; the shunt can be located in:

IVS
- Ventricular septal defect (VSD)

Atrium
- Atrial septum defect (ASD)

Large vessels
- Patent ductus arteriosus (PDA)
- Aorticopulmonary window (uncommon)

Other
- Endocardial cushion defect (ECD)
- Partial anomalous pulmonary venous connection (PAPVC)

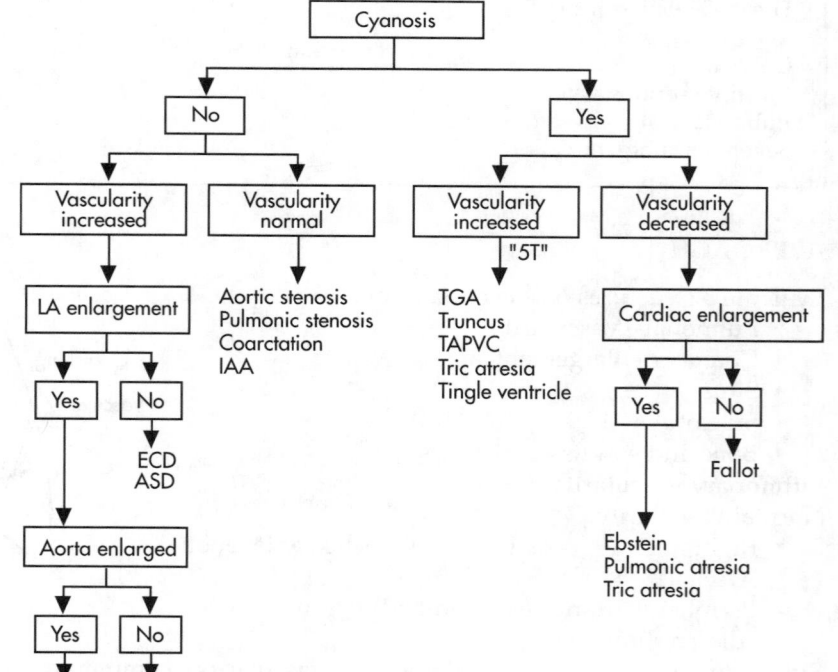

Acyanotic CHD with normal pulmonary vascularity
Normal pulmonary vascularity is associated with either outflow obstruction or valvular insufficiency prior to onset of congestive heart failure (CHF):
    Outflow obstruction
- Coarctation of aorta
- Interruption of aortic arch (IAA)
- Aortic stenosis
- Pulmonic stenosis

    Valvular insufficiency (rarely congenital)
    Corrected transposition of great arteries (L-TGA) (isolated)

Cyanotic CHD with decreased pulmonary vascularity
Decreased pulmonary vascularity due to obstruction of pulmonary flow. In addition, there is a R-L shunt due to an intracardiac defect.
    Normal heart size
- Tetralogy of Fallot
- Fallot variants
- Tricuspid atresia

    Increased heart size
- Ebstein's anomaly
- Pulmonary stenosis with ASD
- Pulmonary atresia

Cyanotic CHD with increased pulmonary vascularity (admixture lesions)
Common denominator of these lesions is that there is an "admixture" of systemic and pulmonary venous blood (bidirectional shunting). The mixing of venous and systemic blood may occur at the level of:
    Large veins
- Total anomalous pulmonary venous connection (TAPVC) (ASD is also present)

    Large arteries
- Truncus arteriosus (TA) (VSD is also present)

    Multiple
- Transposition of great arteries (TGA) (VSD, ASD, or PDA is also present)

    Ventricle
- Single ventricle (VSD is present)
- Double outlet right ventricle (DORV) (VSD is present)

CHD with PVH/CHF
- Cor triatriatum
- Mitral stenosis
- Hypoplastic left heart syndrome
- Coarctation of the aorta
- Cardiomyopathy
- Primary endocardial fibroelastosis
- Anomalous ICA
- Obstructed TAPVC

Increased incidence in females: ASD, PDA, and Ebstein's anomaly
Increased incidence in males: AS, coarctation, pulmonary/tricuspid atresia, hypoplastic left heart, TGA

USE OF IMAGING MODALITIES FOR EVALUATION OF CHD

Chest film
- Determine to which of the 4 categories a CHD belongs (based on pulmonary vascularity and cardiac contour abnormalities)

- Abdomen: determination of situs
- Bones: certain CHD are associated with osseous abnormalities such as 11 ribs, hypersegmented sternum (Down syndrome)

Ultrasound
- Often allows diagnosis of a specific disease entity

Angiography
- Confirmation of diagnosis
- Pressure measurements
- Oxygenation
- Intervention

Magnetic resonance imaging (MRI)
- Diagnostic test for anomalies in pulmonary arteries, aorta, and vena cava

Acyanotic CHD with Increased Pulmonary Vascularity

VENTRICULAR SEPTAL DEFECT (VSD)

Second most common congenital cardiac anomaly.

Types
- Membranous, 80%
- Muscular, 10%
- AV, 5%
- Conal, 5% (mostly supracristal)

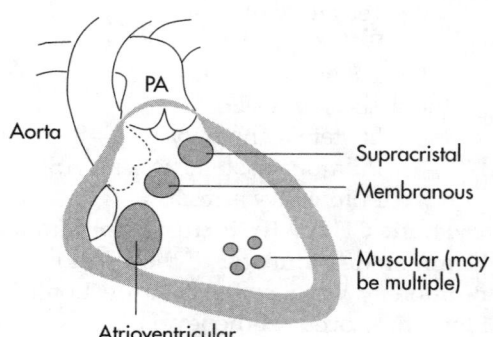

Clinical findings
- Small to moderate defects are initially asymptomatic
- Large defects lead to CHF at 2-3 months of age
- 75% close spontaneously by age 10
- 3% of patients develop infundibular stenosis
- Eisenmenger's syndrome (elevated pulmonary resistance leads to increased right-sided pressures) may develop in long-standing large defects; the end result is a R-L shunt with cyanosis

Hemodynamics
- Blood flow from LV through IVS into RV
- Redundant flow: LV → VSD → RV → PA → LA → LV

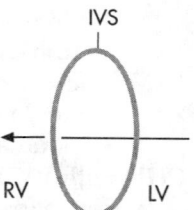

Radiographic features
Because of the variation in size of VSD, the radiographic features are variable and may range from normal cardiac size and pulmonary vessels to large RV, LV, LA.

Chest film findings
- Small VSD: normal CXR
- Significant shunt ($Q_{pulm}/Q_{aorta} > 2$): enlargement of heart, pulmonary arteries and LA
- Eisenmenger physiology
   Enlarged pulmonary arteries
   Cardiac and LA enlargement may decrease
   RVH
   Peripheral pulmonary arteries become constricted ("pruning")
   Calcified PA (rare)

Ultrasound is the diagnostic method of choice

Angiography: commonly performed preoperatively (pressure measurement, oxygenation)

Therapy

Expectant in small asymptomatic VSD because there is spontaneous closure in
infancy, 30%

Surgical therapy (patch) in patients with CHF, pulmonary hypertension, or
progressive worsening

ATRIAL SEPTAL DEFECT (ASD)

Most common congenital cardiac
anomaly.

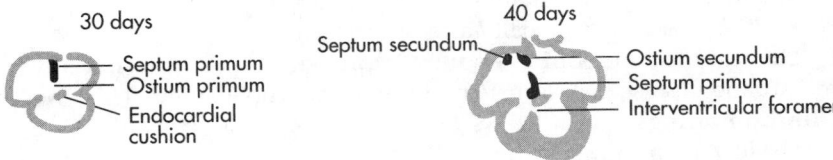

Types

- Ostium secundum type: most
  common, 60%
- Ostium primum ASD: part of
  the ECD syndromes, 35%
- Sinus venosus defect (at
  entrance of SVC): always
  associated with PAPVC
  anomalous venous return, 5%

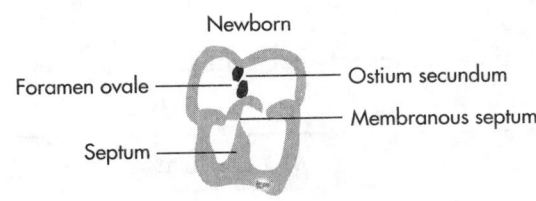

Associations

- Holt-Oram syndrome: ostium secundum defect
- Lutembacher syndrome: ASD and mitral stenosis
- Down syndrome: ostium primum defect

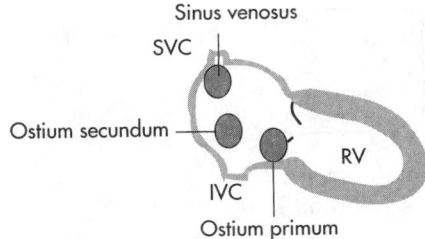

Clinical findings

- May be asymptomatic for decades because of the low atrial
  pressure even large defects are much better tolerated than
  VSD or PDA.
- Female preponderance
- May present with pulmonary hypertension

Hemodynamics

Blood flows from LA to RA

HEMODYNAMICS OF ASD		
	Right Side	Left Side
Atrium	Enlarged	No change
Ventricle	Enlarged	No change
Vasculature	Increased	Aorta no change

Radiographic features

Plain film

- RA, RV, and PA enlargement; no LA enlargement (different from VSD)
- The AA appears small (but in reality is normal) because of the prominent
  pulmonary trunk and clockwise rotation of heart (RV enlargement)

Ultrasound

- Imaging modality of choice for diagnosis

Angiography

- Useful for identifying associated anomalous pulmonary veins

PATENT DUCTUS ARTERIOSUS (PDA)

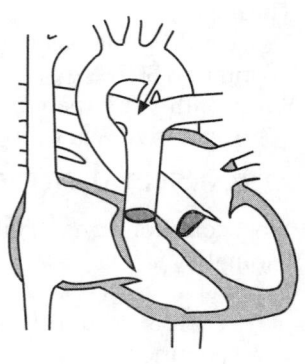

In the fetus, a PDA represents a normal pathway of blood flow.
- Fetal circulation: flow from PA to aorta as intrauterine bypass of non-aerated lungs
- PDA closes functionally 48 hours by delivery
- PDA closes anatomically after 4 weeks

Highest incidence of PDA occurs in premature infants (especially if hyaline membrane disease is present) and in maternal rubella; females > males.

Clinical findings
- Most are asymptomatic
- Large defects lead to CHF at 2-3 months of age

Hemodynamics
There is a L-R shunt because the pressure in the aorta is higher than in the pulmonary circulation.

HEMODYNAMICS OF PDA		
	Right Side	**Left Side**
Atrium	No change	Enlarged
Ventricle	No change	Enlarged
Vasculature	Enlarged	Aorta enlarged

Radiographic features
- Small PDA: normal CXR
- Increased pulmonary vascularity
- Enlargement of LA, LV
- Eisenmenger physiology may develop in long-standing, severe disease

All the above features are identical to those seen in VSD; specific features to suggest PDA are:
- Unequal distribution of pulmonary arterial blood flow, especially sparing of left upper lobe
- Enlargement of aorta and AA
- PDA may be seen as faint linear density through the PA (occasionally calcifies)

Therapy
- Indomethacin (inhibits PGE_1, which is a potent dilator of the duct); successful in 60% of infants
- Ligation of ductus through left thoracotomy
- Catheter closure with umbrella device

ENDOCARDIAL CUSHION DEFECT (ECD)

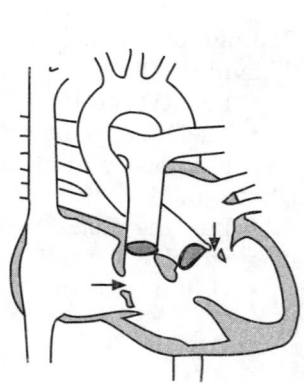

40% of ECD patients have trisomy 21 (Down syndrome).

Types
- Partial AV canal (ostium primum defect ± cleft in anterior mitral or septal tricuspid leaflets)
- Transitional AV canal (ostium primum defect, cleft in both AV valves, defect in superior IVS)
- Complete AV canal (ostium primum defect, cleft in both AV valves, large defect in IVS: either common AV valve or separate mitral and tricuspid valves)

Clinical findings
- Partial canals may be asymptomatic; both the degree of mitral insufficiency and the shunt through the ASD determine the clinical picture.
- Complete AV canal consist of large L-R shunts (ASD, VSD), mitral insufficiency, and CHF.

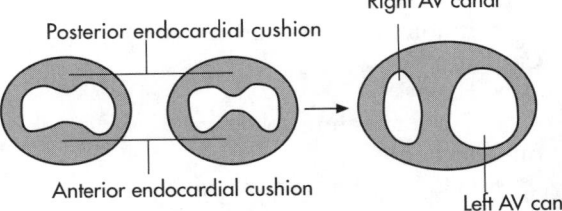

Embryology
Endocardial cushion tissue contributes to the formation of the ventricular septum, the lower atrial septum, and the septal leaflets of the MV and tricuspid valves. If the anterior and posterior endocardial cushions do not fuse, the AV valves (MV and tricuspid valves) do not develop properly.

Hemodynamics

HEMODYNAMICS OF ECD		
	Right Side	**Left Side**
Atrium	Enlarged	Enlarged
Ventricle	Enlarged	Enlarged
Vasculature	Enlarged	Aorta no change

Radiographic features
Plain film
- Cardiomegaly
- Increased pulmonary vascularity
- Screen for other trisomy 21 findings: 11 ribs, multiple manubrial ossification centers

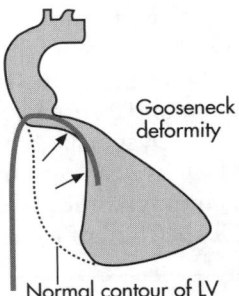

Angiography
- Gooseneck deformity of left ventricular outflow tract on RAO view
- Abnormal prolapse of anterior MV leaflet in diastole

Therapy
- Primary surgical repair before age 2

AORTOPULMONARY WINDOW

Synonym: aortopulmonary septal defect, partial truncus arteriosus.
- Defect between ascending aorta and main or right PA
- L-R shunt
- Plain film findings are identical to those seen in PDA
- Differentiation from truncus arteriosus:
    Two semilunar valves are present
    No VSD
- Associated with PDA 10%-15%
- Also associated with VSD and coarctation

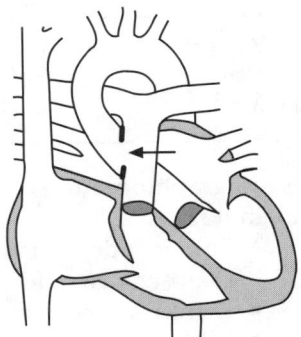

PARTIAL ANOMALOUS PULMONARY VENOUS CONNECTION (PAPVC)

Some but not all pulmonary veins drain to the systemic circulation rather than in to the LA. Anomalous pulmonary venous connection is a L-R shunt. Pulmonary veins connect to RA or systemic veins. Cyanosis occurs because of Eisenmenger's syndrome. PAPVC is not always cyanotic. Common connections of pulmonary veins:
Supracardiac
- Right SVC (most common)
- Left SVC

- Azygos vein
- Innominate (via vertical vein)

Cardiac

- RA
- Coronary sinus

Infracardiac

- IVC (scimitar syndrome)
- Portal vein

Associations

ASD, 15% (especially the sinus venosus defect)

Radiographic features

- Supracardiac and cardiac types resemble ASD findings
- The anomalous vein of the infracardiac type looks like a Turkish scimitar (= sword): scimitar sign
- Infracardiac PAPVC is part of hypogenetic lung syndrome (see chest section)

Acyanotic CHD with Normal Pulmonary Vascularity

VALVULAR PULMONARY STENOSIS (PS)

Clinical findings

- Most patients are asymptomatic
- Dysplastic type may show familial inheritance; also associated with Noonan's syndrome (short stature, webbed neck, hypogonadism)

Normal   Dome-shaped   Dysplastic

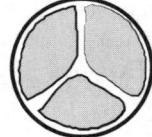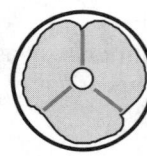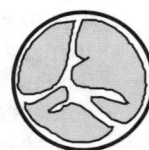

Types

- Dome-shaped type (95%); valve with a small orifice and 3 fused commissural raphes
- Dysplastic type (5%); thickened, redundant, immobile leaflets; commissures are not fused

Hemodynamics

Obstruction of right ventricular outflow.

HEMODYNAMICS OF PS		
	Right Side	**Left Side**
Atrium	No change	No change
Ventricle	Enlarged	No change
Vasculature	Poststenotic dilatation (only MPA & LPA)	Aorta no change

Radiographic features

Plain film

- Poststenotic dilatation of main and/or left PA (jet through stenosed valve dilates PA)
- Right PA is normal in size
- RV (hypertrophy)

Ultrasound

- Systolic doming of leaflets
- Thickened leaflets
- Doppler measurements

Treatment

- Most stenosis are amenable to balloon valvuloplasty
- Surgical reconstruction may be necessary for dysplastic types

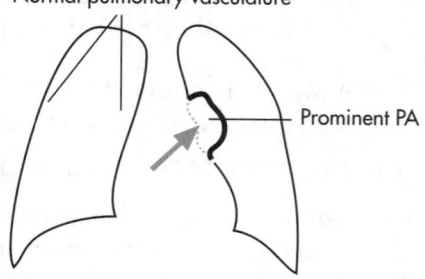

Normal pulmonary vasculature

Prominent PA

CONGENITAL PERIPHERAL PULMONARY ARTERY STENOSIS

Causes
- Maternal rubella (common)
- Williams syndrome

Types
- Type 1: single, main PA stenosis
- Type 2: stenosis at bifurcation of right and left PA
- Type 3: multiple peripheral stenosis
- Type 4: central and peripheral stenosis

Radiographic features
- PA enlargement if associated valvular stenosis
- RV hypertrophy

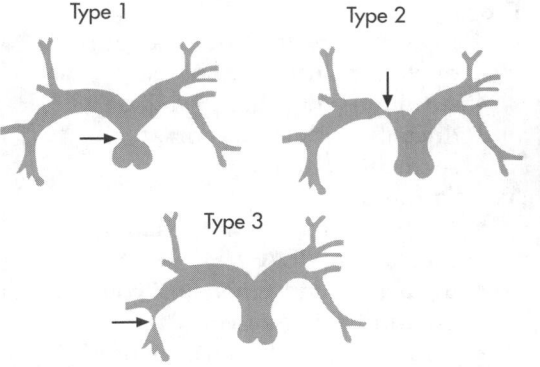

CONGENITAL AORTIC STENOSIS

Clinical findings
- Most are asymptomatic
- Severe AS leads to CHF in infancy
- Supravalvular type associated with Williams syndrome:
    Mental retardation
    Peripheral pulmonary stenoses
    Diffuse aortic stenoses

Types
Subvalvular aortic stenosis
- Membranous subaortic stenosis
- Hypertrophic subaortic stenosis (fibromuscular tunnel)

Valvular aortic stenosis (most common)
- Bicuspid aortic valve (most common congenital heart anomaly)
- Unicommissural valve (single horseshoe-shaped valve)

Supravalvular aortic stenosis
- Localized
- Diffuse

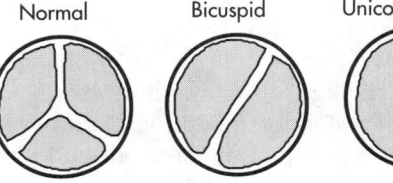

Radiographic features
Plain film
- Cardiomegaly: LV hypertrophy
- Poststenotic dilatation of aorta is present only in valvular AS
- CHF

Ultrasound and angiography
- Domed valve
- Jet through valve
- Hourglass deformity of ascending aorta (supravalvular AS)

COARCTATION OF AORTA

Types
- Infantile type (diffuse type, pre-ductal): tubular hypoplasia
- Adult type (localized type, post-ductal, periductal): short segment; common

Associations
- Coarctation syndrome: triad of coarctation, PDA, VSD
- In Turner syndrome, most common cardiac abnormality
- Bicuspid aortic valve, 50%
- Hypoplasia of the aortic isthmus (small arch)
- Circle of Willis aneurysms
- PDA aneurysm
- Intracardiac defects; occur in 50% with infantile type

Clinical findings
- Blood pressure difference between arms and legs
- Diffuse type presents as neonatal CHF
- Adult type is frequently asymptomatic; presents in young adult

Hemodynamics
- Preductal type has concomitant R-L shunting via PDA or VSD
- Postductal coarctation has L-R flow through PDA
- Collaterals to descending aorta
    Internal mammary-intercostals
    Periscapular arteries-intercostals

Radiographic features
Plain film
- Aortic figure-3 configuration 50%
    Prestenotic dilatation of aorta proximal to coarctation
    Indentation of aorta caused by the coarctation
    Poststenotic dilatation
- Inferior rib notching:
    Secondary to dilated intercostal arteries
    Only ribs 3-8 involved
    Only in children > 8 years
- Reverse 3 sign of barium-filled esophagus
- Prominent left cardiac border from left ventricular hypertrophy (LVH)
- Normal pulmonary vascularity

MRI
- Diagnostic study of choice
- Adequately shows site and length of coarctation
- Has replaced angiography (however, angiography allows pressure measurements)
- Allow evaluation of collaterals

Therapy
- Resection of coarctation and end-to-end anastomosis
- Patch angioplasty: longitudinal incision with placement of a synthetic patch
- Subclavian patch: longitudinal incision of coarctation; division of subclavian artery and longitudinal opening to be used as a flap
- Percutaneous balloon angioplasty

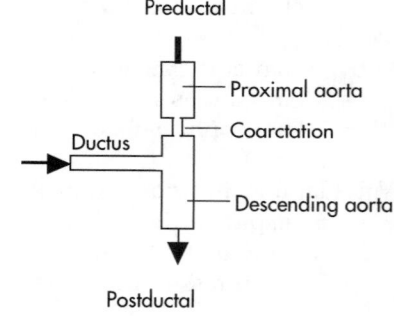

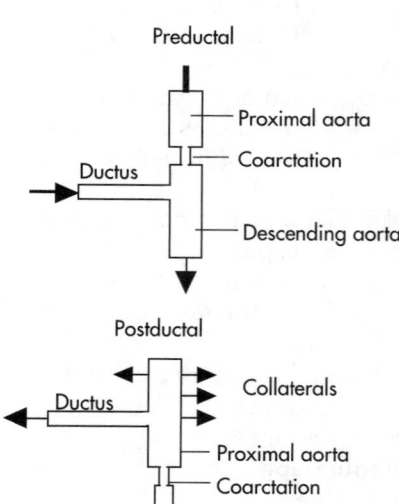

Cyanotic CHD with Decreased Pulmonary Vascularity

TETRALOGY OF FALLOT

The most common cyanotic CHD of childhood.

Tetrad
- Obstructed RV outflow tract
- Right ventricular hypertrophy (RVH)
- VSD
- Aorta overriding the interventricular septum

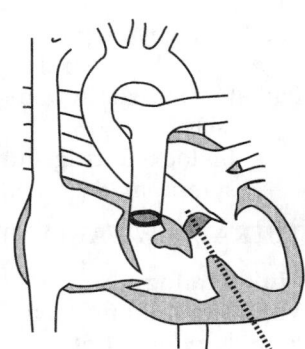

Clinical findings
- Squatting when fatigued (to increase pulmonary flow and thus O_2 saturation)
- Episodic loss of consciousness
- Cyanosis by 3-4 months; time of presentation depends on degree of RV outflow obstruction

Associations
- Pulmonary infundibular or valve stenosis in most cases
- Right AA anomalies with aberrant vessels and vascular sling or rings, 25%
- Anomalies of coronary arteries, 5% (LAD from RCA, single RCA)
- Rare
  Tracheoesophageal fistula
  Rib anomalies, scoliosis

Hemodynamics

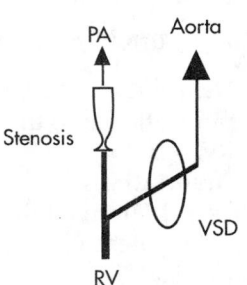

HEMODYNAMICS OF FALLOT		
	Right Side	**Left Side**
Atrium	No change	No change
Ventricle	Enlarged	No change
Vasculature	Decreased	Aorta normal

Radiographic features

Plain film
- Boot-shaped heart (enlarged RV): coeur en sabot
- Right AA, 25%
- Small or concave PA

MRI
- Used to determine extent of systemic collateral vessels coming off the aorta

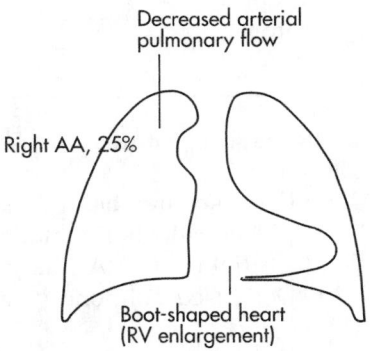

Therapy

Total corrective repair

- VSD closure and reconstruction of RV outflow tract

Palliative shunts: systemic to PA shunt allows growth of pulmonary
  vessels

- Blalock-Taussig shunt (subclavian artery → PA) indicated in
  symptomatic patients who are poor surgical candidates

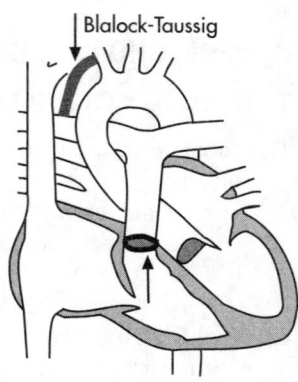

TETRALOGY VARIANTS

Pink tetralogy

VSD with mild pulmonic stenosis.

Pentalogy of Fallot

Tetralogy + ASD.

Trilogy of Fallot

PA stenosis, RVH with patent foramen ovale.

EBSTEIN'S ANOMALY

Deformity of the triscupid valve with distal displacement of the tricuspid leaflets into the RV inflow tract; results in atrialization of superior
RV.

Associations

- Maternal lithium intake
- Patent foramen ovale or ASD nearly always present, 80%

Clinical

- Tricuspid regurgitation and/or obstruction
- Arrhythmias (RBBB, WPW)
- 50% mortality in first year

Hemodynamics

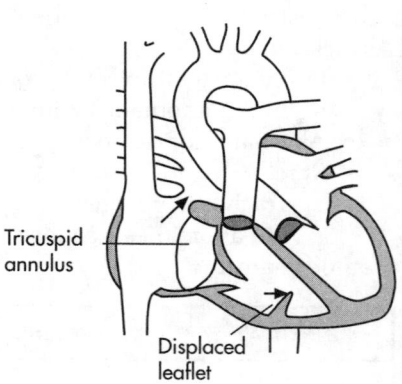

HEMODYNAMICS OF EBSTEIN'S ANOMALY		
	Right Side	**Left Side**
Atrium	Enlarged	No change
Ventricle	Enlarged	No change
Vasculature	No change	Aorta no change

Radiographic features

Plain film

- Large squared heart (box-shaped heart) due to:
      Left side: horizontal position of RV outflow tract
      Right side: RA enlargement
- Decreased pulmonary vascularity

Ultrasound

- Displacement of tricuspid leaflets

Therapy

- Extracorporeal membrane oxygenation (ECMO) for
  temporization
- Tricuspid valve reconstruction
- Cardiac pacemaker for arrhythmias
- Bidirectional Glenn shunt (SVC-PA to increase pulmonary blood flow)

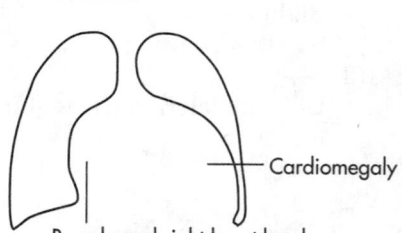

TRICUSPID ATRESIA

Complete agenesis of the tricuspid valve with no direct communication of the RA and RV.

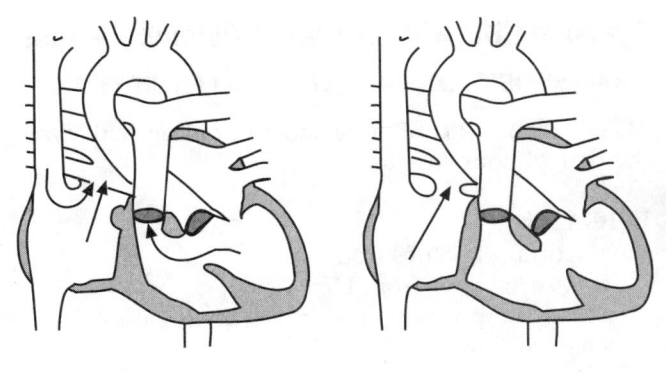

Associations
- Patent foramen ovale or ASD are always present
- Complete transposition of great arteries (D-TGA), 35%
- VSD is common
- Pulmonary atresia
- Hypoplastic right heart
- Extracardiac anomalies (GI, bone)

Hemodynamics
All blood crosses through a large ASD into the LA.

HEMODYNAMICS OF TRICUSPID ATRESIA		
	Right Side	**Left Side**
Atrium	Enlarged	Enlarged
Ventricle	Decreased	Enlarged
Vasculature	Decreased	Aorta no change

Radiographic features
Plain film
- May be normal
- No TGA: similar appearance as Fallot
- If TGA is present there is:
    Increased pulmonary flow
    Cardiomegaly
    Narrow vascular pedicle

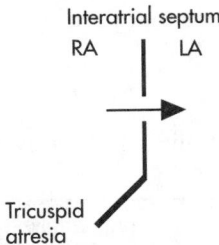

Therapy
Palliative
- Maintain patent PDA with prostaglandins
- Blalock-Taussig
- Glenn anastamosis (SVC → PA)

Definitive (older patients)
- Fontan procedure: RA is connected to main PA

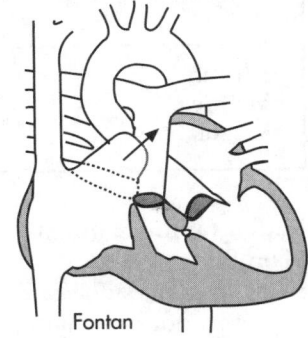

Fontan

Cyanotic CHD with Increased Pulmonary Vascularity

TRANSPOSITION OF GREAT ARTERIES (TGA)

TGA is the most common CHD presenting with cyanosis in the first 24 hours of life.

Types

D-TGA

- Aorta originates from RV
- PA originates from LV
- Normal position of atria and ventricles: AV concordance

L-TGA

- Transposition of great arteries
- Inversion of ventricles: AV discordance

Relative position of aorta and PA can be derived from the diagram in the right.

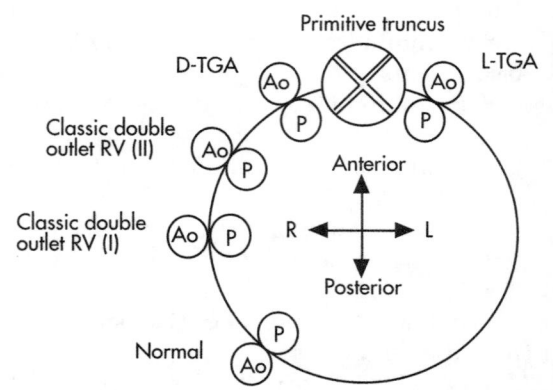

COMPLETE TRANSPOSITION OF GREAT ARTERIES (D-TGA)

Two independent circulations exist:

- Blood returning from body → RV → blood delivered to body
- Blood returning from lung → LV → blood delivered to lung

This circulatory pattern is incompatible with life unless there are associated anomalies that permit mixing of the two circulations, e.g., ASD, VSD, or PDA.

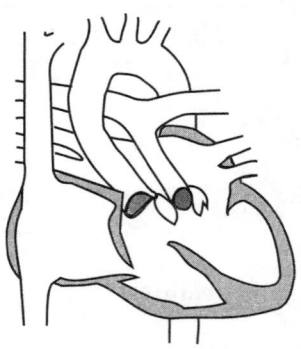

Hemodynamics

Depend on the type of mixing of the two circulations.

HEMODYNAMICS OF D-TGA		
	Right Side	**Left Side**
Atrium	Normal, enlarged	No change
Ventricle	Normal, enlarged	No change
Vasculature	No change, enlarged	Aorta no change

Radiographic features

Plain film

- "Egg-on-side" cardiac contour: narrow superior mediastinum secondary to hypoplastic thymus (unknown cause) and abnormal relationship of great vessels
- As pulmonary resistance decreases, pulmonary vascularity increases
- Right heart enlargement
- Pulmonary trunk not visible because of its posterior position

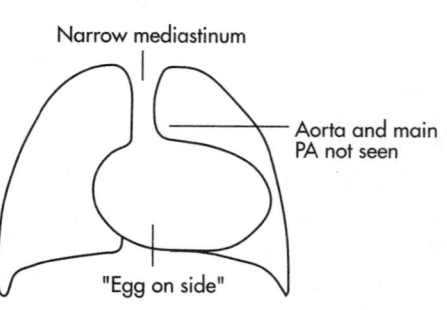

Ultrasound

- Aorta lies anterior, PA posterior
- Transposition of arteries is obvious

Therapy

PGE_1 is administered to prevent closure of PDA. Palliative: temporization methods before definitive repair. Corrective operation during first year of life:

- Correct reattachment of large vessels (Jatene Arterial Switch procedure)
- Creation of an atrial baffle (Mustard, Senning, or Schumaker procedure)
- Rashkind procedure: atrial septostomy with balloon catheter
- Blalock-Hanlon: surgical creation of atrial defect

TAUSSIG-BING COMPLEX (DORV II)

Represents a partial transposition. Aorta connected to RV, PA arises from both LV and RV, and supracristal VSD. Radiographic appearance similar to D-TGA.

CORRECTED TRANSPOSITION OF GREAT ARTERIES (L-TGA)

Large vessels and ventricles are transposed (AV discordance and ventricular-arterial discordance). Poor prognosis because of associated cardiac anomalies. If isolated, this is an acyanotic lesion.

Associations

- Perimembranous VSD, > 50%
- Pulmonic stenosis, 50%
- Anomaly of tricuspid valve
- Dextrocardia

Radiographic features

Plain film

- Pulmonary trunk and aorta are not apparent because of their posterior position
- LA enlargement
- Abnormal AA contour because of the leftward position of the arch
- Right pulmonary hilus elevated over left pulmonary hilus

Ultrasound

- Anatomical LV on right side
- Anatomical RV on left side

TRUNCUS ARTERIOSUS

Results from failure of formation of the spiral septum within the truncus arteriosus. As a result, a single vessel (truncus) leaves the heart and gives rise to systemic, pulmonary, and coronary circulation. The truncus has 2-6 cusps and sits over a high VSD.

Associations

- All patients have an associated high VSD
- Right AA, 35%

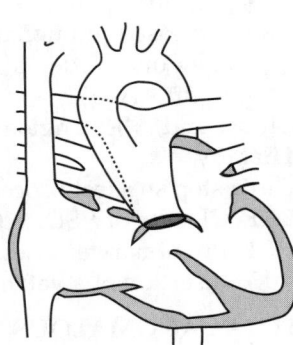

Types

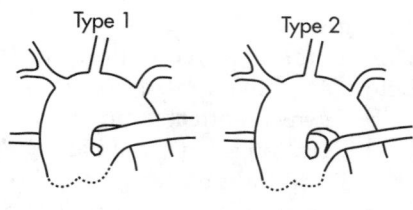

- Type 1: (most common): short main PA from truncus
- Type 2: two separate PA from truncus (posterior origin)
- Type 3: (least common): two separate PA from truncus (lateral origin)
- Type 4: (pseudotruncus) PA from descending aorta = pulmonary atresia with VSD; findings of a tetralogy of Fallot combined with pulmonary atresia

Hemodynamics

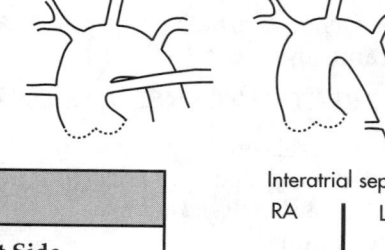

Admixture lesion with both L-R (truncus → PA) shunt and R-L (RV → VSD → overriding aorta) shunt.

HEMODYNAMICS OF TA		
	Right Side	**Left Side**
Atrium	No change	No change
Ventricle	Enlarged	Enlarged
Vasculature	Enlarged	Aorta enlarged

Radiographic features

Plain film

- Enlargement of aortic shadow (which actually represents the truncus)
- Cardiomegaly due to increased LV volume
- Increased pulmonary vascularity
- Pulmonary edema, occasionally present
- Right AA, 35%

Ultrasound, MRI, angiography to determine type

Therapy

Three-step surgical procedure:

1. Closure of VSD so that LV alone empties into truncus
2. Pulmonary arteries removed from truncus and RV-PA conduit placed
3. Insertion of a valve between the RV and PA.

TOTAL ANOMALOUS PULMONARY VENOUS CONNECTION (TAPVC)

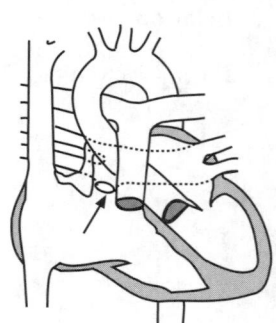

Pulmonary veins connect to systemic veins or the RA rather than to the LA. TAPVC exists when all pulmonary veins connect anomalously. The anomalous venous return may be obstructed or nonobstructed.

Types

Supracardiac connection (50%)

Supracardiac TAPVC is the most common type; infrequently associated with obstruction.

- Left vertical vein
- SVC
- Azygos vein

Cardiac connection (30%)
- RA
- Coronary sinus
- Persistent sinus venosus

Infracardiac connection (15%); majority are obstructed
- Portal vein
- Persistent ductus venosus
- IVC (caudal to hepatic veins)
- Gastric veins
- Hepatic veins

Mixed types (5%)

Associations
- Patent foramen ovale, ASD (necessary to sustain life)
- Heterotaxy syndrome (asplenia more common)
- Cat's eye syndrome

Clinical
- Symptomatology depends on presence or absence of obstruction
- Obstructed: pulmonary edema within several days after birth
- Nonobstructed: asymptomatic at birth. CHF develops during first month
- 80% mortality by first year

Hemodynamics

Unobstructed pulmonary vein

TAPVC causes a complete L-R shunt at the atrial level; therefore to sustain life, an obligatory R-L shunt must be present. Pulmonary flow is greatly increased, leading to dilatation of RA, RV, and PA.

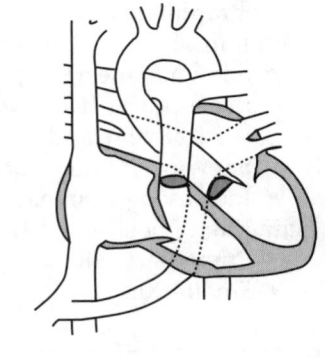

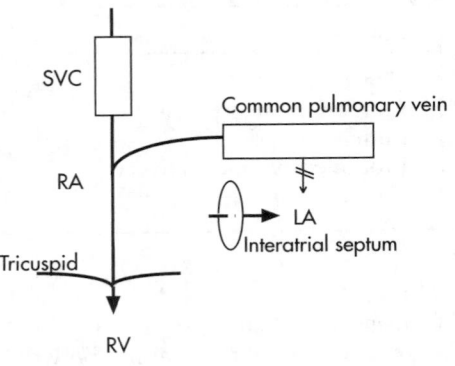

HEMODYNAMICS OF UNOBSTRUCTED TAPVC		
	Right Side	**Left Side**
Atrium	Enlarged	No change, decreased
Ventricle	Enlarged	No change, decreased
Vasculature	Enlarged	Aorta no change

Obstructed pulmonary vein

Obstruction has 3 consequences:
1. Pulmonary venous hypertension (PVH) and pulmonary arterial hypertension (PAH)
2. Pulmonary edema
3. Diminished pulmonary return to the heart, which results in low cardiac output

HEMODYNAMICS OF OBSTRUCTED TAPVC		
	Right Side	**Left Side**
Atrium	No change	Decreased
Ventricle	No change, increased	Decreased
Vasculature	No change	Aorta decrease

Radiographic features

Plain film of nonobstructed TAPVC
- Snowman heart (figure-of-eight heart) in supracardiac type; the supracardiac shadow results from dilated right SVC, vertical vein, and innominate vein
- Snowman configuration not seen with other types
- Increased pulmonary vascularity

Plain film of obstructed TAPVC
- Pulmonary edema
- Small heart

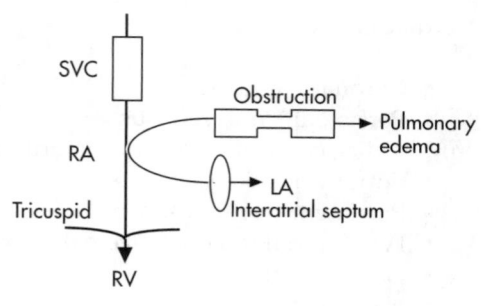

RADIOGRAPHIC FEATURES OF TAPVC		
Feature	Obstructed TAPVC	Nonobstructed TAPVC
Heart size	Normal	Enlarged
Pulmonary artery size	Normal	Enlarged
Pulmonary edema	Present early	Absent
Prominent venous density (snowman)	Rare (only in obstructed supracardiac TAPVC)	Frequent (especially in supracardiac forms of TAPVC)

Therapy

Consists of a 3-step procedure:
- Creation of an opening between the confluence of pulmonary veins and the LA
- Closure of the ASD
- Ligation of veins connecting to the systemic venous system.

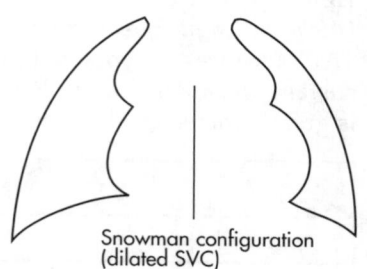

Snowman configuration (dilated SVC)

SINGLE VENTRICLE

Most commonly, the single ventricle has LV morphology and there is a rudimentary RV. The great arteries may originate both from the dominant ventricle or one may originate from the small ventricle. Rare anomaly with high morbidity. Common ventricle: absence of the interventricular septum.

Associations
- Malposition of the great vessels is usually present

Radiographic features
- Variable appearance: depends on associated lesions
- Pulmonary circulation may be normal depending on the degree of associated pulmonic stenosis

DOUBLE OUTLET RIGHT VENTRICLE (DORV)

The great vessels originate from the RV. A VSD is always present; other malformations are common. Rare anomaly. Radiographic features are similar to those of other admixture lesions and depends on concomitant anomalies.

Aorta

PSEUDOCOARCTATION

Asymptomatic variant of coarctation: no pressure gradient across lesion (aortic kinking)

Associations
- Bicuspid aortic valve (common)
- Many other CHD

Radiographic features
- Figure-3 sign
- No rib notching
- Usually worked up because of superior mediastinal widening (especially on left) on CXR

INTERRUPTION OF AORTIC ARCH

Types
- Type A: occluded after LSA similar to coarctation
- Type B: occluded between LCA and LSA
- Type C: occluded between brachiocephalic artery and LCA

Associations
- Usually associated with VSD and PDA
- DORV and subpulmonic VSD (Taussig-Bing malformation)
- Subaortic stenosis

Radiographic features
- Neonatal pulmonary edema
- No aortic knob; large PA

AORTIC ARCH ANOMALIES

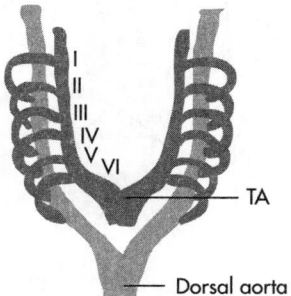

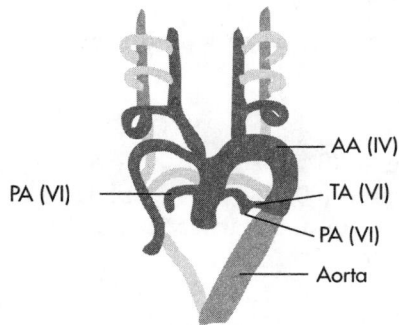

Normal development
- Right subclavian: arch IV (proximal) and 7th intersegmental artery
- Left subclavian: 7th intersegmental artery
- AA: arch IV (in part)
- Pulmonary arteries: arch VI
- Distal internal carotid artery ICA: primitive dorsal aorta
- Proximal ICA: arch III
- Common carotid: arch III

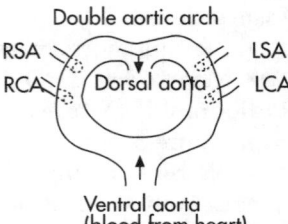

Double aortic arch

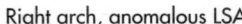

Pearls
- A large number of AA anomalies exist; however, only 3 are common:
     L arch with an aberrant right subclavian artery (RSA) (asymptomatic)
     R arch with an aberrant retroesophageal LSA (asymptomatic)
     Double arch (symptomatic)
- Most significant abnormalities occur in tetralogy of Fallot
- Normal lateral esophagram excludes significant arch anomalies and sling
- Fluoroscopy of trachea may be helpful for classification
- AP esophagram distinguishes double arch (bilateral esophageal indentations) from right arch
- MRI helpful to delineate vascular anatomy

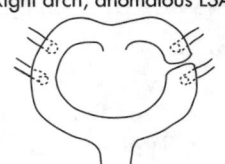

Right arch, anomalous LSA

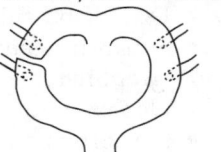

Left arch, anomalous RSA

LEFT AORTIC ARCH WITH ABERRANT RIGHT SUBCLAVIAN ARTERY

Most common congenital AA anomaly (interruption #4 on diagram). Asymptomatic.

Radiographic features
- Left arch
- Abnormal course of RSA
     Behind esophagus (80%) = retroesophageal indentation
     Between esophagus and trachea 15%
     Anterior to trachea 5%

Associations
- Absent recurrent right laryngeal nerve

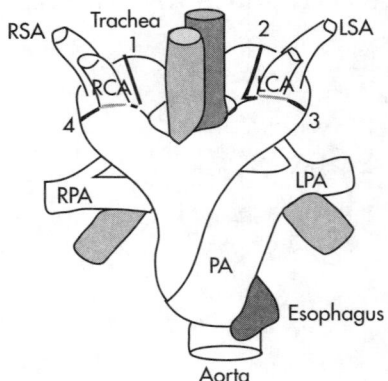

RIGHT AORTIC ARCH WITH ABERRANT LEFT SUBCLAVIAN ARTERY

Interruption #3 on above diagram. Only 5% have symptoms secondary to airway or esophageal compression.

Radiographic findings
- Right arch
- Retroesophageal indentation
- Diverticulum of Kommerell: aortic diverticulum at origin of aberrant subclavian artery

Associated with CHD in 10%
- Tetralogy of Fallot (70%)
- ASD, VSD
- Coarctation

RIGHT AORTIC ARCH WITH MIRROR IMAGE BRANCHING

Interruption #2 on diagram. No vascular ring symptoms.
Radiographic features
- Right AA
- No posterior indentation of esophagus

Associated with cyanotic heart disease in 98%
- Tetrology of Fallot (90%)
- TA (30%)
- Multiple defects

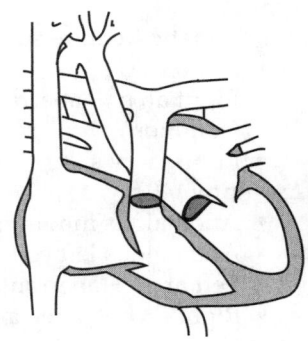

RIGHT ARCH WITH ISOLATED LEFT SUBCLAVIAN ARTERY

LSA attached to left PA via ductus arteriosus. The LSA is isolated from aorta and obtains blood supply from left vertebral artery; produces congenital subclavian steal. Interruptions near #2 and at #3.
Radiographic features
- Right arch
- No posterior esophageal indentation

Associations
- Almost all are associated with tetralogy of Fallot

DOUBLE AORTIC ARCH

Persistence of both fetal arches; concomitant CHD is rare. Most common type of vascular ring. Most symptomatic of vascular rings.
Radiographic features
- Right arch is higher and larger than the left arch
- Widening of the superior mediastinum
- Posterior indentation of the esophagus on lateral view
- Bilateral indentations of the esophagus on AP view

Pulmonary Artery

PULMONARY SLING

Aberrant left PA arises from the right PA and passes between the trachea (T) and esophagus (E). Compresses both trachea and esophagus. Tracheobronchiomalacia and/or stenosis occurs in 50%.

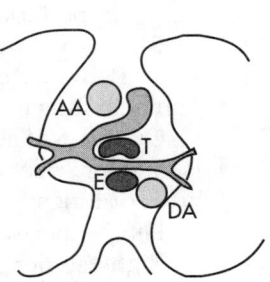

VASCULAR RINGS AND SLINGS

Vascular rings and slings are anomalies in which there is complete encirclement of the trachea and esophagus by the AA and its branches or PA. Symptoms are usually due to tracheal compression (stridor, respiratory distress, tachypnea); esophageal symptomatology is less common.

Types

Symptomatic (require surgery)
- Double AA
- Right arch + aberrant LSA + PDA (common)
- Pulmonary sling

Asymptomatic
- Anomalous innominate artery
- Anomalous left common carotid
- Left arch + aberrant RSA
- Right arch + aberrant LSA (mirror image to above)

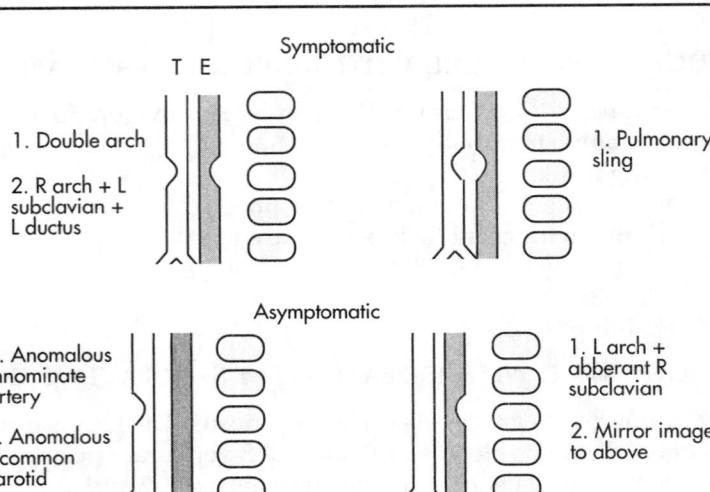

Symptomatic

T E

1. Double arch

2. R arch + L subclavian + L ductus

1. Pulmonary sling

Asymptomatic

1. Anomalous innominate artery

2. Anomalous L common carotid

1. L arch + abberant R subclavian

2. Mirror image to above

Situs Anomalies

GENERAL

Abdominal situ

Refers to position of liver and stomach:
- Abdominal situs solitus: liver on right, stomach on left (normal)
- Abdominal situs inversus: liver on left, stomach on right
- Abdominal situs ambiguous: symmetrical liver, midline stomach

Thoracic situ

Refers to position of the tracheobronchial tree:
- Thoracic situs solitus (normal)
    LMB longer than RMB
    Left upper lobe bronchus inferior to left PA (hyparterial bronchus)
    Right upper lobe bronchus superior to right PA (epiarterial bronchus)
- Thoracic situs inversus:
    Opposite of above
- Isomerism: refers to symmetric development of heart or lungs
    Left isomerism: 2 left lungs or 2 LA
    Right isomerism: 2 right lungs or 2 RA
- AV connections: refers to relation of atria to ventricles
    Concordant: correct atrium with its ventricle, (e.g., RA → RV)
    Discordant: mismatch of atrium and ventricle, (e.g., RA → LV)
- Version: refers to position of an asymmetric anatomic structure
    Dextroversion: dextrocardia and situs solitus
    Levoversion: levocardia and situs inversus
- Position of bronchi
    Epiarterial: bronchus above PA (normally on right)
    Hyparterial: bronchus below PA (normally on left)
- Cardia: refers to position of heart on chest film. May have nothing to do with situs or cardiac structure
    Levocardia (normal): heart on left side of chest
    Dextrocardia: heart on right side of chest (e.g., shift of mediastinum)

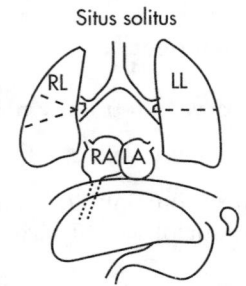

Situs solitus

RL   LL

RA LA

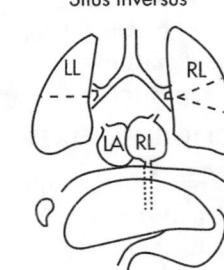

Situs inversus

LL   RL

LA RL

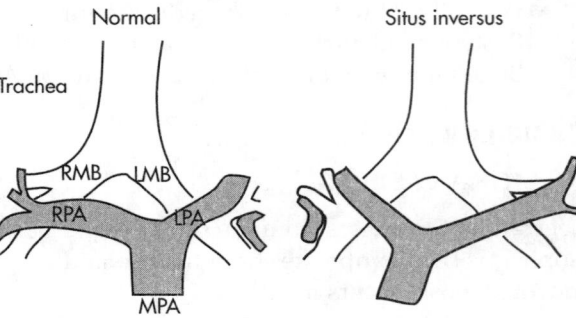

Normal

Trachea

RMB   LMB

RPA   LPA

MPA

Situs inversus

FREQUENCY OF CHD IN SITUS ANOMALIES	
Situs	**Frequency**
Situs solitus 1 levocardia (normal)	1%
Situs solitus 1 dextrocardia	98% (corrected TGA 5 L-TGA)
Situs inversus 1 dextrocardia	4% (L-TGA)
Situs inversus 1 levocardia	100%

2

CARDIOSPLENIC SYNDROMES

Abnormal relationship between heart and abdominal organs and isomerism. Always consider polysplenia/asplenia when the cardiac apex and situs are discordant. The tracheobronchial anatomy is the best indicator of situs.

CARDIOSPLENIC SYNDROMES		
	Asplenia (Right Isomerism)	Polysplenia (Left Isomerism)
RADIOGRAPHIC FINDINGS		
Pulmonary vascularity	Decreased (obstructed flow)	Increased (overcirculation)
Bronchi	Epiarterial	Hyparterial
Minor fissure	Bilateral	None, normal
Heart	Cardiomegaly/complex CHD	Cardiomegaly/moderate CHD
Atrium	Common atrium	ASD
Single ventricle	50%	DORV
Pulm veins	TAPVC	PAPVC
Great vessels	TGA 70%	Normal
SVC	Bilateral 50%	Bilateral 30%
Bowel	Malrotation	Malrotation
Spleen	Absent	Multiple
Abdominal situs	Ambiguous/inversus	Ambiguous/inversus
IVC/azygous	Normal	Azygous continuation

CLNICAL FINDINGS	**SEVERE DISEASE**	**MILDER DISEASE**
Age	Neonates	Infant
Cyanosis	Yes	No
Common problem	Infections (asplenia)	No infections
Prognosis	Poor	Good
CHD	L-TGA, pulmonary stenosis, single ventricle	PAPVC, ASD, VSD
Blood smear	Heinz and Howell-Jolly bodies	

Other

HYPOPLASTIC LEFT HEART (SHONE SYNDROME)

Spectrum of cardiac anomalies characterized by underdevelopment of LA, LV, MV, aortic valve, and aorta. Survival requires a large ASD and PDA with R-L and L-R shunting.

Clinical features
- Neonatal CHF within several days after birth
- Most infants die within first week as PDA closes
- Cardiogenic shock; metabolic acidosis

Radiographic features
- Increased pulmonary vascularity
- Severe pulmonary edema
- Prominent right heart, especially RA

Therapy
- Norwood procedure: PA-descending aorta conduit, followed by PA banding; palliative
- Heart transplant: curative attempt

COR TRIATRIATUM

Incomplete incorporation of pulmonary veins into LA causing obstruction to pulmonary venous return; very rare.

Radiographic features
- Mimics congenital mitral stenosis
- LA size usually normal
- Associated lesions:
    Parachute mitral valve
    Mitral web
- PVH and CHF

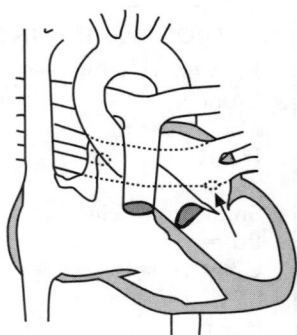

PERSISTENT FETAL CIRCULATION

Refers to persistent severe pulmonary hypertension in the neonate and consequent R-L shunting via a patent PDA. Treatment: ECMO.

Causes of neonatal pulmonary hypertension
- Idiopathic
- Meconium aspiration
- Neonatal pneumonia
- Diaphragmatic hernia
- Hypoxemia

AZYGOS CONTINUATION OF THE IVC

Developmental failure of the hepatic and/or infrahepatic IVC. Associated with polysplenia.

Radiographic features
- Enlarged azygos vein
- Enlarged hemiazygos vein
- Absent IVC

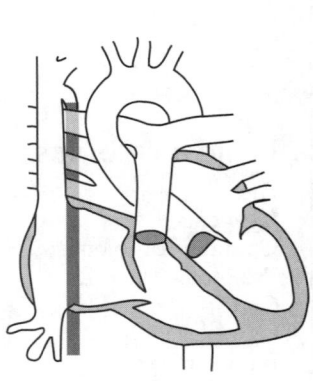

DOWN SYNDROME

- ECD, 25%
- ASD
- VSD
- PDA
- Cleft MV
- AV communis
- 11 rib pairs, 25%
- Hypersegmented manubrium, 90%

MARFAN SYNDROME

Autosomal dominant connective tissue disease (arachnodactyly) with cardiac abnormalities in 60%:

- Ascending aorta
    - Aneurysm
    - Aortic regurgitation (common)
    - Dissection
- Mitral valve
    - Prolapse (myxomatous degeneration)
    - Mitral regurgitation
- Coarctation
- Chest deformity, kyphosis
- Arachnodactyly,
- Excessive limb length

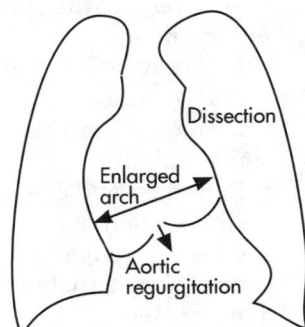

TURNER SYNDROME

- Coarctation, 15%
- Bicuspid aortic valve

Acquired Heart Disease

CARDIOMEGALY

Global cardiomegaly

$$CI = \frac{MRD + MLD}{ID}$$

MRD = maximum transverse diameter to the right from midline
MLD = maximum transverse diameter to the left from midline
ID = internal diameter of the thorax drawn through the tip of the dome of the right diaphragm

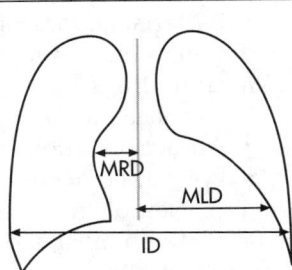

Causes

- Valvular disease
- Cardiomyopathy
- CHD
- Pericardial effusion
- Mass lesions

CHAMBER ENLARGEMENT

LA enlargement
- LA measurement (right LA border to LMB > 7 cm)
- Barium-filled esophagus is displaced posteriorly (lateral view)
- Double density along right cardiac border; a similar appearance may also be found in:
     Patients with normal-sized LA
     Confluence of pulmonary veins
- Bulging of LA appendage
- Widening of the angle of the carina (> 60°)

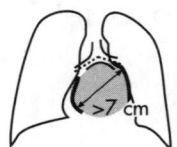 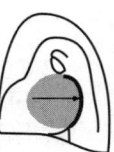

LV enlargement
- Left downward displacement of the apex (elongation of ventricular outflow tract)
- Round left cardiac border

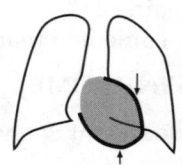 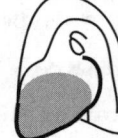

RV enlargement
- Rounding and elevation of cardiac apex
- Obliteration of retrosternal space on lateral view; normally, > ⅓ distance from anterior costophrenic angle to the angle of Louis (manubrosternal junction)

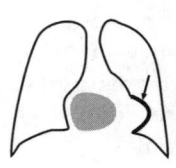 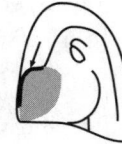

RA enlargement
- Difficult to assess by plain film
- Increased convexity of lower right heart border on PA view

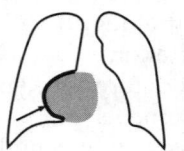 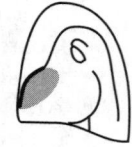

Valvular Heart Disease

Mitral and aortic valves are the most commonly affected valves. Rheumatic fever is the leading cause of acquired valve disease.

MITRAL STENOSIS

Causes
- Rheumatic fever (most common)
- Bacterial endocarditis and thrombi
- Prolapse of LA myxoma

Clinical findings
- Dyspnea on exertion and later at rest
- Atrial fibrillation and mural thrombus
- Episodes of recurrent arterial embolization
     Neurological deficit
     Abdominal and flank pain (renal, splanchnic emboli)

Hemodynamics

MITRAL VALVE		
Condition	Valve Area	LA Pressure
Normal	4-6 cm²	< 10 mm Hg
Symptomatic during exercise	1-4 cm²	> 20 mm Hg
Symptomatic at rest	< 1 cm²	> 35 mm Hg

Radiographic features
Plain film
- PVH in nearly all patients
- Normal overall heart size (pressure overload) but enlargement of LA
- Severe stenosis
    - Increase in pulmonary arterial pressure leads to RVH
    - Pulmonary hemosiderosis (ossified densities in lower lung fields)
    - Calcification of LA wall (laminated clot)

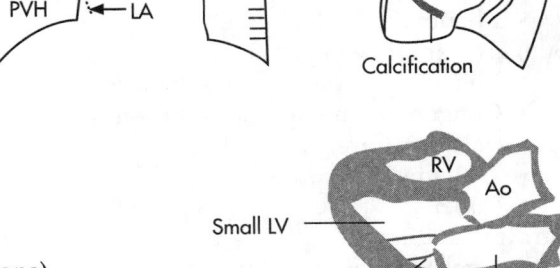

Ultrasound
- Increased LA dimensions (normal LV)
- RV enlargement if pulmonary hypertension is present
- Multiple echoes on MV leaflets (calcifications, vegetations)
- Doming of leaflets
- Doppler: velocity measurements

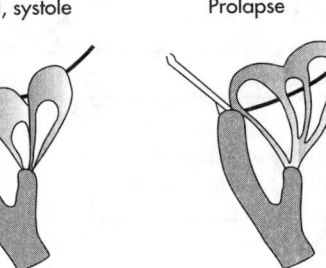

MITRAL REGURGITATION

Causes
- Rheumatic fever
- MVP (Barlow's syndrome)
- Rupture of papillary muscle (secondary to MI, bacterial endocarditis)
- Marfan syndrome
- Bacterial endocarditis
- Rupture of chordae

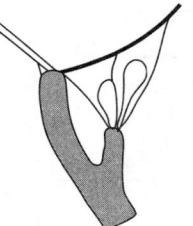

Clinical findings
- Often well tolerated for many years
- Decompensation by sudden onset of hypertension
- Acute presentation: MI, endocarditis

Hemodynamics
- MVP: movement of leaflet of MV into LA during systole

Radiographic features
Plain film
- "Big heart disease" (volume overload, cardiomegaly)
- Enlarged chambers: LA + LV
- PVH (usually less severe than in mitral stenosis)
- Calcification of mitral annulus
- Often coexistent with mitral stenosis

Ultrasound
- MVP
- Enlarged LA, LV

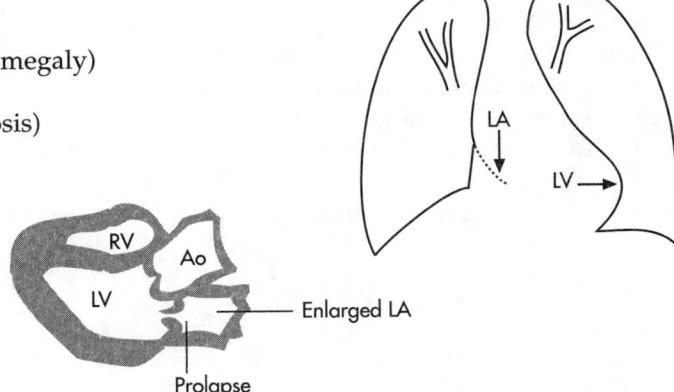

AORTIC STENOSIS

Types
Valvular (60%-70%, most common form)
- Degenerative leaflets in patients > 70 years
- Bicuspid
- Rheumatic

Subvalvular (15%-30%)
- Idiopathic hypertrophic subaortic stenosis (IHSS); 50% are autosomal dominant
- Congenital (membranous, fibromuscular tunnel)

Supravalvular (rare)
- Williams syndrome
- Rubella

Clinical findings
- Symptoms of LV failure (common)
- Angina, 50%; many patients also have underlying CAD
- Syncope (in severe stenosis)
- Sudden death in children, 5%

AORTIC VALVE	
Condition	**Valve Area**
Normal	2.0-4.0 cm^2
Symptomatic at exercise	< 1.0 cm^2
Symptomatic at rest	< 0.75 cm^2

Radiographic features
Plain film
- Often difficult to detect abnormalities by plain film (usually no chamber enlargement)
- Enlargement of ascending aorta (does not occur with supravalvular AS)
- Calcification of aortic valve: rare before age 40

Ultrasound
- Multiple aortic valve echoes
- Poststenotic dilatation of aorta
- Doming of the aortic valve
- LVH
- Doppler: velocity measurements

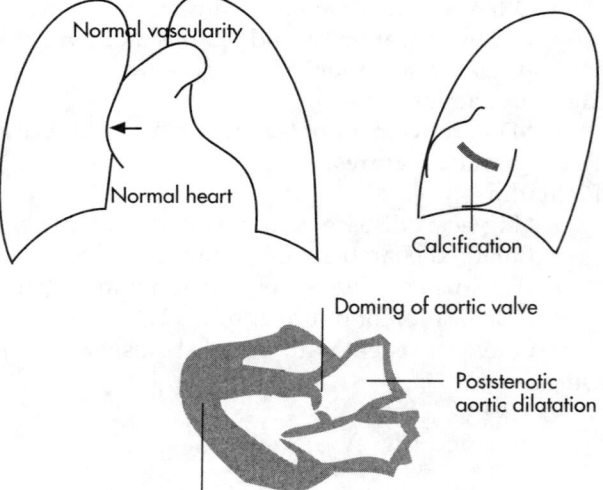

Normal vascularity
Normal heart
Calcification
Doming of aortic valve
Poststenotic aortic dilatation
LVH

AORTIC REGURGITATION

Causes
- Rheumatic fever
- Systemic hypertension (may lead to dilatation of the aortic root)
- Aortic dissection
- Endocarditis
- Rare causes: Marfan syndrome, syphilitic aortitis, trauma, collagen vascular diseases (ankylosing spondylitis)

Radiographic features
Plain film
- Cardiomegaly
- Dilated structures: LV, aorta

Ultrasound
- Dilatation of LV and aorta
- Atypical valve leaflets
- High-frequency vibrations of the anterior mitral leaflet

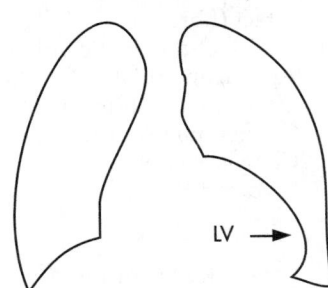
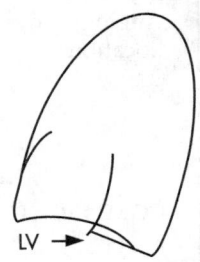

Normal vascularity

Myocardium

ACUTE MYOCARDIAL INFARCTION (AMI)

Diagnosis of AMI is made by clinical history, ECG, and serum enzymes; role of imaging studies is ancillary:

Angiography
- Evaluate CAD
- Therapeutic angioplasty

Plain film
- Monitoring of pulmonary edema

Thallium
- Evaluate for segmental ischemia and scar tissue

Gated blood pool study
- Wall motion kinetics
- Determination of ejection fraction

Ultrasound, MRI
- Imaging of complications (false, true aneurysm, thrombus)

Complications of AMI
- Papillary muscle rupture: acute mitral regurgitation
- Septum perforation: volume overload
- Pericardial tamponade from free wall rupture (death)
- Aneurysm formation (true, false)
- LV thrombus
- Arrhythmia

ANEURYSM

TYPES OF ANEURYSM		
Parameter	True Aneurysm	False Aneurysm
Myocardial wall	Intact (fibrous)	Ruptured wall
Angiography	Dyskinetic/akinetic bulge in wall	Neck, delayed emptying
Location	Apical, anterolateral	Posterior, diaphragmatic
Cause	Transmural MI (most common)	MI
	Congenital (Ravitch syndrome)	Trauma
	Chagas' disease	
	Myocarditis	
COMPLICATIONS		
	Low risk of rupture	High risk of rupture
	Mural thrombus; embolization	
	CHF	
	Arrhythmias	

CARDIOMYOPATHIES

Causes

Hypertrophic cardiomyopathy (obstructed LV outflow segment)
- Familial: autosomal dominant (50%)
- Sporadic

Dilated cardiomyopathy (congested; unable to contract effectively during systole)
- Infectious
- Metabolic
- Toxic: alcohol, Adriamycin
- Collagen vascular disease

Restrictive cardiomyopathy (unable to dilate effectively during diastole: impaired distensibility)
- Amyloid
- Sarcoidosis
- Loeffler's eosinophilic endocarditis
- Hemochromatosis

Pearls
- Restrictive cardiomyopathy and constrictive pericarditis have similar physiologic features
- CT and MRI may be helpful
    - 50% of patients with constrictive pericarditis have calcified pericardium easily detected by CT
    - Thickened pericardium can be easily detected by MRI

Coronary Arteries

VARIANTS/ANOMALIES OF CORONARY ARTERIES

- Anomalous origin of LCA from PA
    Venous blood flows through LCA resulting in myocardial ischemia
    15% of patients survive into adulthood because of collaterals
- Anomalous origin of both coronary arteries from right sinus of Valsalva
    Ectopic LCA takes an acute angle behind PA
    30% sudden death (infarction)
- Anomalous origin of both coronary arteries from left sinus of Valsalva
    RCA is ectopic
- Congenital coronary AV fistula
    Both arteries are orthotopic
    Venous side of fistula originates in RA, coronary sinus, or RV
- RCA terminates at crux: 10%
- SA nodal artery is a branch of the proximal RCA in > 50%; less commonly, the SA nodal artery arises from the proximal left circumflex
- Kugel's artery: collateral that connects the SA nodal artery and the AV nodal artery (anastomotic artery magnum)
- Vieussens' ring: collateral branches from right conus artery to LAD

CORONARY ARTERY DISEASE (CAD)

Three stages of atherosclerotic disease:
- Intimal fatty streaks in childhood (nonobstructive, clinically silent)
- Development of fibrous plaques during adulthood (narrowing of lumen: angina)
- Late occlusive disease: calcifications, plaques, hemorrhage (angina, AMI)

Risk factors

Strong correlation
- Family members with atherosclerotic disease
- Smoking
- Hypertension
- Hyperlipidemia
- Diabetes
- Male

Weaker correlation
- Obesity
- Stress
- Sedentary life

Treatment
- Avoidance of risk factors
- Reversal of risk factors
- Medication
- Transluminal coronary angioplasty
- Surgery
    Saphenous vein aortocoronary bypass
    Left internal mammary coronary bypass

Annual mortality
- 1 vessel disease: 2%-3%
- 2 vessel disease: 3%-7%

- 3 vessel disease: 6%-11%
- Low ejection fraction, doubles mortality
- Abnormal wall motion, doubles mortality

Radiographic features

Plain films

- Calcification of coronary arteries are the most reliable plain film sign of CAD (90% specificity in symptomatic patients), but calcified coronary arteries are not necessarily stenotic.
- LV aneurysm is the second most reliable plain film sign of CAD. It develops in 20% MI.
- Location
  - Anteroapical wall: 70%
  - Inferior wall: 20%
  - Posterior wall: 10%
- CHF causing:
  - Pulmonary edema
  - Least reliable sign of CAD

Coronary angiography

Stenosis occurs primarily in:

- Proximal portions of major arteries
- LAD > RCA > LCX

Collaterals develop if > 90% of the coronary diameter is obstructed; two types of anastomosis:

- Connections between branches of the same coronary artery (homocoronary)
- Connections between the branches of the three major coronary arteries (intercoronary)

Common pathways of intercoronary anastomoses in descending order of frequency are:

1. Surface of apex
2. Surface of pulmonary conus
3. Between anterior and posterior septal branches
4. In the AV groove: LCX and distal RCA
5. On the surface of the RV wall
6. On the atrial wall around SA node

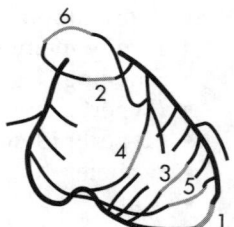

Left ventriculography

- RAO view most helpful
- Evaluate LV function, valvular insufficiency, shunts, mural thrombus

Other techniques employed at cardiac catheterization

- Transvalvular pressure measurements
- Cardiac output measurement
- O_2 saturation measurements: shunt detection
- Right heart catheterization

GRADING OF STENOSIS	
Type	**Diameter**
Not significant	< 50% decrease
Significant	50%-75% decrease
Severe	> 75% decrease

KAWASAKI DISEASE (MUCOCUTANEOUS LYMPH NODE SYNDROME)

Idiopathic acute febrile multisystem disease in children. Most cases are self-limited and without complications. Mortality from AMI: 3%. Treatment: aspirin, gamma globulin.

Clinical features
- Fever and cervical lymphadenopathy
- Desquamating rash on palms/soles
- Vasculitis of coronary arteries

Radiographic features
- Spectrum of coronary disease
    - Aneurysm: present in 25% (most are multiple when present)
    - Stenoses
    - Occlusion
    - Rupture
- Coronary artery aneurysms: usually is proximal segments and detectable by US
- Transient gallbladder hydrops

Pericardium

NORMAL ANATOMY

Pericardium consists of two layers:
- External fibrous pericardium
- Internal serous epicardium

The normal pericardial cavity has 10-50 mL of clear serous fluid. Normal structures:
- Fat stripe: fat on surface of heart beneath pericardium seen on lateral chest film
- Superior pericardial recess (commonly seen by CT or MRI)

CONGENITAL ABSENCE OF THE PERICARDIUM

May be total or partial. Partial absence is more common, occurs mainly on the left, and is usually asymptomatic. Large defects may cause cardiac strangulation. Small defects are usually asymptomatic.

Radiographic features

Total absence of the pericardium
- Mimics the appearance of the large silhouette seen in pericardial effusions

Partial absence of the pericardium
- Heart is shifted and rotated into left pleural cavity
- PA view looks like an RAO view
- Heart separated from sternum on cross-table lateral view
- Left hilar mass: herniated left atrial appendage and pulmonary trunk

PERICARDIAL CYSTS

Pericardial cysts represent congenital malformations (persistent coelom).
- 90% unilocular, 10% multilocular
- 75% are asymptomatic; occur at all ages
- If there is communication with pericardial cavity, the entity is termed *pericardial diverticulum.*

Radiographic features
- Well-defined, rounded soft tissue density on plain film
- Most common location: cardiophrenic angles
- Other locations: anterior and middle mediastinum
- CT is helpful in establishing diagnosis.

PERICARDIAL EFFUSION

Causes
Tumor
- Metastases (melanoma, breast, lung)

Inflammatory/idiopathic
- Rheumatic heart disease
- Collagen vascular disease
- Dressler syndrome
- Postpericardiotomy syndrome
- Drug hypersensitivity

Infectious
- Viral
- Pyogenic
- Tuberculosis (TB)

Metabolic
- Uremia
- Myxedema

Trauma
- Hemopericardium
- Postoperative

Vascular
- Acute MI
- Aortic dissection
- Ventricular rupture

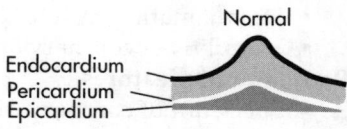

Normal

Endocardium
Pericardium
Epicardium

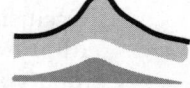

Pericardial effusion

Radiographic features
Plain film
- > 250 mL are necessary to be detectable
- Subpericardial fat stripe measures > 10 mm (a stripe 1-5 mm can be normal)
- Symmetrical enlargement of cardiac silhouette (water-bottle sign)
- Postsurgical loculated pericardial effusion may mimic an LV aneurysm

Ultrasound
- Study of choice
- Echo-free space between epicardium and pericardium

CONSTRICTIVE PERICARDITIS

Causes
- TB (most common cause)
- Other infections (viral, pyogenic)
- Cardiac surgery
- Radiation injury

Radiographic features

- Calcifications are common
  - 50% of patients with calcification have constrictive pericarditis.
  - 90% of patients with constrictive pericarditis have pericardial calcification.
  - Pericardial calcification is more common in the atrioventricular grooves.
- Pleural effusion, 60%
- PVH, 40%
- Elevated RV pressure: dilated SVC and azygos, 80%

Differential Diagnosis

Congenital Heart Disease

ACYANOTIC HEART DISEASE

Increased pulmonary vascularity (L-R shunt)
With LA enlargement (indicates that shunt is not in LA)
- VSD (normal AA)
- PDA (prominent AA)

With normal LA
- ASD
- ECD
- PAPVC and sinus venosus ASD

Normal pulmonary vascularity
- Aortic stenosis
- Coarctation
- Pulmonic stenosis

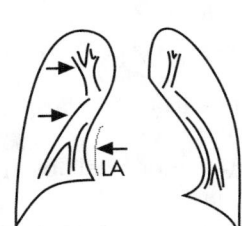
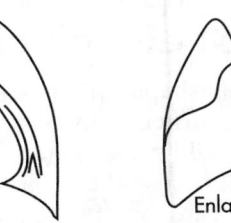

Enlarged LA

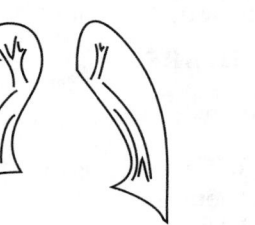
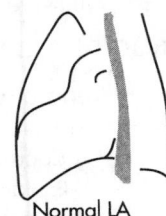

Normal LA

CYANOTIC HEART DISEASE

Normal or decreased pulmonary vascularity
Normal heart size
- Tetralogy of Fallot (common)
- Fallot variants

Cardiomegaly (RA enlarged)
- Ebstein's malformation
- Tricuspid atresia
- Pulmonic atresia

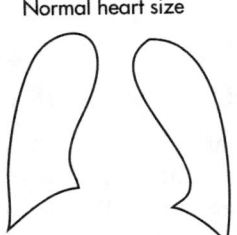

Normal heart size

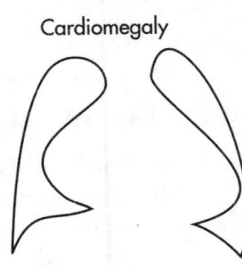

Cardiomegaly

Pearls
Increased pulmonary vascularity (5 "Ts")
- **T**GA (most common)
- **T**A
- **T**APVC
- **T**ricuspid atresia
- **T**ingle = single ventricle

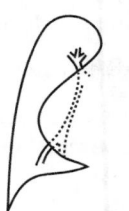
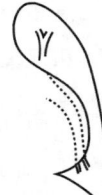

PULMONARY EDEMA IN NEWBORNS

- Cardiac
    Edema + large heart: hypoplastic RV or LV
    Edema + normal heart: TAPVC below diaphragm
- Transient tachypnea of the newborn (TTN)
- Pulmonary lymphangiectasia
- Other rare CHD causing obstruction to pulmonary venous return:
    Pulmonary vein atresia
    Cor triatriatum
    Supravalvular mitral ring
    Parachute mitral valve

MASSIVE CARDIOMEGALY IN THE NEWBORN

- Box-shaped right heart (RA enlargement)
    Ebstein's anomaly
    Uhl's disease (focal or total absence of RV myocardium; very rare)
    Tricuspid atresia
- Herniation of liver into pericardial sac
- Massive pericardial effusion

BOOT-SHAPED HEART

- Tetralogy of Fallot
- Adults
    Loculated pleural effusion
    Cardiac aneurysm
    Pericardial cyst

CHD WITH NORMAL HEART SIZE AND NORMAL LUNGS

- Coarctation
- Tetralogy of Fallot

SKELETAL ABNORMALITIES AND HEART DISEASE

- Rib notching: coarctation
- Hypersegmented manubrium, 11 pairs of ribs: Down syndrome
- Pectus excavatum: prolapse MV, Marfan syndrome
- Multiple sternal ossification centers: cyanotic CHD
- Bulging sternum: large L-R shunt
- Scoliosis: Marfan syndrome, tetralogy of Fallot

INFERIOR RIB NOTCHING

- Aortic obstruction
    Coarctation
    IAA
- Subclavian artery obstruction
    Blalock-Taussig shunt (upper 2 ribs)
    Takayasu's disease (unilateral)
- Severely reduced pulmonary blood flow (very rare)
    Tetralogy of Fallot
    Pulmonary atresia
    Ebstein's anomaly

- SVC obstruction
- Vascular shunts
    Arteriovenous malformation (AVM) of intercostals
- Intercostal neuroma
- Osseous abnormality (hyperparathyroidism)

SUPERIOR RIB NOTCHING

Abnormal osteoclastic activity
- Hyperparathyroidism (most common)
- Idiopathic

Abnormal osteoblastic activity
- Poliomyelitis
- Collagen vascular disease such as rheumatoid arthritis, systemic lupus erythematosus
- Local pressure
- Osteogenesis imperfecta
- Marfan syndrome

DIFFERENTIAL DIAGNOSIS OF CHD BY AGE OF PRESENTATION

- 0-2 days: hypoplastic left heart, aortic atresia, TAPVC, 5 "Ts"
- 7-14 days: coarctation, aortic stenosis, AVM, endocardial fibroelastosis
- Infants: VSD, PDA
- Adults: ASD

Aorta

RIGHT AORTIC ARCH AND CHD

Right aortic arches are associated with CHD in 5%
- TA, 35%
- Tetralogy of Fallot, 30%
- Less common associations, 35%
    TGA, 5%
    Tricuspid atresia, 5%
    Pulmonary atresia with VSD, 20%
    DORV
    Pseudotruncus
    Asplenia
    Pink tetralogy

Acquired Heart Disease

APPROACH

- Pressure overload (stenosis, hypertension) causes hypertrophy: normal heart size
- Volume overload (regurgitation, shunt) causes dilatation: large heart size
- Wall abnormalities

ABNORMAL LEFT HEART CONTOUR

Pressure overload (normal heart size)
- Aortic or mitral stenosis
- Systemic hypertension
- Coarctation

Volume overload (large heart disease)
- Mitral or aortic regurgitation
- Shunts: ASD, VSD
- High output states

Wall abnormalities
- Aneurysm, infarct
- Cardiomyopathy

ABNORMAL RIGHT HEART CONTOUR

Pressure overload (normal heart size)
- PA hypertension
- Pulmonic stenosis (rarely isolated except in CHD)

Volume overload (large heart disease)
- Pulmonic or tricuspid regurgitation
- Shunts: ASD, VSD
- High output states

Wall abnormalities
- Aneurysm, infarct
- Cardiomyopathy
- Uhl's anomaly

SMALL HEART

- Normal variant (deep inspiration)
- Addison's disease
- Anorexia nervosa/bulimia
- Dehydration
- Severe COPD

Film analysis

- Cardiac size, chamber enlargement
- Calcifications
- Pulmonary vascularity: CHF
- Catheters (CCU films), prostheses
- Bones

↓

Categorize lesion

- Pressure overload
- Volume overload (large heart)
- Wall abnormality

OVERVIEW OF PLAIN FILM FINDINGS				
Lesion	Calcification	CHF	LAE	LVE
Mitral stenosis	+	+	+	−
Mitral regurgitation	−	−	++	+
Aortic stenosis	++	−	−	−
Aortic regurgitation	−	−	−	+

LAE, LA enlargement; *LVE*, LV enlargement; − usually absent; + present; ++ marked.

CARDIAC MASSES

- Thrombus
- Infectious vegetation
- Neoplasm
    Metastases
    Atrial myxoma (left > right)
    Rhabdomyoma in infants (tuberous sclerosis)
    Pericardial cyst
    Angiosarcoma

PERICARDIAL EFFUSION

Transudate
- CHF
- AMI
- Postsurgical
- Autoimmune
- Renal failure

Infectious
- Viral

Tumor
- Pericardial metastases

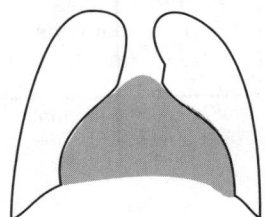

HIGH CARDIAC OUTPUT STATES

- Severe anemia
- Peripheral AVM
- Thyrotoxicosis
- Pregnancy

CARDIOVASCULAR CALCIFICATIONS

OVERVIEW	
Type	Comments
PERICARDIAL	
Pericarditis*	TB, uremia, AIDS, coxsackie, pyogenic
Pericardial cysts	In AMI
MYOCARDIAL	
Coronary arteries	Always significant in patients < 40 years
Calcified infarct	Curvilinear calcification (necrosis)
Aneurysm	
Postmyocarditis	
INTRACARDIAC	
Calcified valves	Indicates stenosis; most common: rheumatic fever
Calcified thrombus	In infarcts and aneurysm; 10% calcify
Tumors	Atrial myxoma is the most common calcified tumor
AORTA	
Atherosclerosis	In > 25% of patients > 60 years
Syphilitic aortitis	In 20% of syphilis patients
Aneurysm	Predominantly in ascending aorta

AIDS, Acquired immunodeficiency syndrome.
*Follows fat distribution.

PNEUMOPERICARDIUM

- Iatrogenic (aspiration, puncture)
- Cardiac surgery
- Barotrauma
- Fistula from bronchogenic or esophageal carcinoma

CORONARY ANEURYSM

- Atherosclerotic
- Congenital
- Periarteritis nodosa
- Kawasaki disease
- Mycotic
- Syphilis
- Trauma

Pulmonary Artery

PULMONARY ARTERY ENLARGEMENT

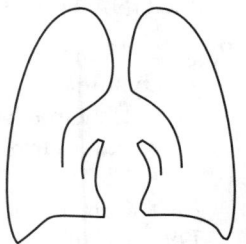

PAH
- Primary PAH (young females, rare)
- Secondary PAH

PA stenosis
- Williams syndrome (infantile hypercalcemia)
- Rubella syndrome
- Takayasu's disease
- Associated with CHD (especially tetralogy of Fallot)

PA dilatation
- Poststenotic jet
- AVM: Osler-Weber-Rendu disease

Aneurysm cystic medial necrosis
- Behçet's syndrome
- Takayasu's disease

PULMONARY ARTERIAL HYPERTENSION (PAH)

$P_{sys} > 30$ mm Hg

Classification

Precapillary hypertension
- Vascular
  - Increased flow: L-R shunts
  - Chronic PE
  - Vasculitis
  - Drugs
  - Idiopathic
- Pulmonary
  - Emphysema
  - Interstitial fibrosis
  - Fibrothorax, chest wall deformities
  - Alveolar hypoventilation

Postcapillary hypertension
- Cardiac
  - LV failure
  - Mitral stenosis
  - LA myxoma
- Pulmonary venous
  - Idiopathic venoocclusive disease
  - Thrombosis
  - Tumor

PULMONARY VENOUS HYPERTENSION (PVH)

$P_{wedge} > 12$ mm Hg

LV dysfunction
- Ischemic heart disease: CAD
- Valvular heart disease
- CHD
- Cardiomyopathy

Left atrium
- Cor triatriatum: stenosis of pulmonary veins at entrance to LA
- LA myxoma

EISENMENGER'S PHYSIOLOGY

Chronic L-R shunt causes high pulmonary vascular resistance, which ultimately reverses the shunt (R-L shunt with cyanosis). Causes:
- VSD
- ASD
- PDA
- ECD

SUGGESTED READINGS

Burton WF: *Congenital heart disease,* St Louis, 1985, Mosby.

Chen JT: *Essentials of cardiac roentgenology,* Philadelphia, 1998, Lippincott Williams & Wilkins.

Fink BW: *Congenital heart disease: a deductive approach to its diagnosis,* St Louis, 1991, Mosby.

Higgins CB: *Essentials of cardiac radiology and imaging,* Philadelphia, 1992, Lippincott Williams & Wilkins.

Hugo SF: *Radiology of the heart: cardiac imaging in infants, children, and adults,* New York, 1985, Springer-Verlag.

Miller SW: *Cardiac angiography,* Boston, 1984, Little, Brown.

Miller SW: *Cardiac radiology: the requisites,* St Louis, 1996, Mosby.

Mullins CE, Mayer DC: *Congenital heart disease: a diagramatic atlas,* New York, 1988, Alan R. Liss.

Chapter 3

Gastrointestinal Imaging

Chapter Outline

Esophagus

General

ANATOMY

Normal esophageal contour deformities:
- Cricopharyngeus
- Postcricoid impressions (mucosal fold over vein)
- Aortic impression
- Left mainstem bronchus (LMB)
- Left atrium (LA)
- Diaphragm
- Peristaltic waves

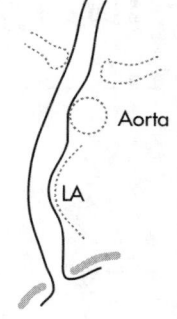

Gastroesophageal junction (GEJ) anatomy
- Phrenic ampulla: normal expansion of the distal esophagus; does not contain gastric mucosa
- A-line (for **a**bove; Wolf ring): indentation at upper boundary of the phrenic ampulla
- B-line (for **b**elow): indentation at lower boundary of the phrenic ampulla; normally not seen radiologically unless there is a hiatal hernia
- Z-line (**z**igzag line): squamocolumnar mucosal junction between esophagus and stomach; not visible radiologically
- The esophagus lacks a serosa. Upper one-third has striated muscle; lower two-thirds has smooth muscle

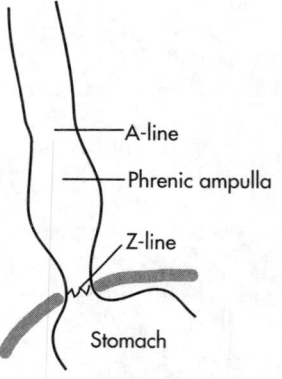

Peristaltic waves
- Primary contractions: initiated by swallowing; distally progressive contraction waves strip the esophagus of its contents; propulsive wave
- Secondary contractions: anything not cleared from the esophagus by a primary wave may be cleared by a locally initiated wave; propulsive wave
- Tertiary contractions: nonpropulsive, uncoordinated contractions; incidence of these random contractions increase with age and are rarely of clinical significance in absence of symptoms of dysphagia; nonpropulsive wave; only peristaltic activity in achalasia

Peristalsis should always be evaluated fluoroscopically with the patient in horizontal position. In the erect position the esophagus empties by gravity.

SWALLOWING

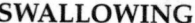

NORMAL SWALLOW				
Swallowing Phase	**Tongue**	**Palate**	**Larynx**	**Pharyngeal Constrictors**
1. Oral	Dorsum controls bolus; base assumes vertical position	Resting	Resting	Resting
2. Early pharyngeal	Strips palate and moves dorsally	Velopharynx closure	Epiglottis deflects, larynx moves anterosuperiorly	Middle constrictors
3. Late pharyngeal	Meets relaxing palate	Begins descent	Vocal folds close, epiglottis retroflects	Inferior constrictors
4. Esophageal	Returns to resting	Resting	Returns to resting	Completion of constriction, resting

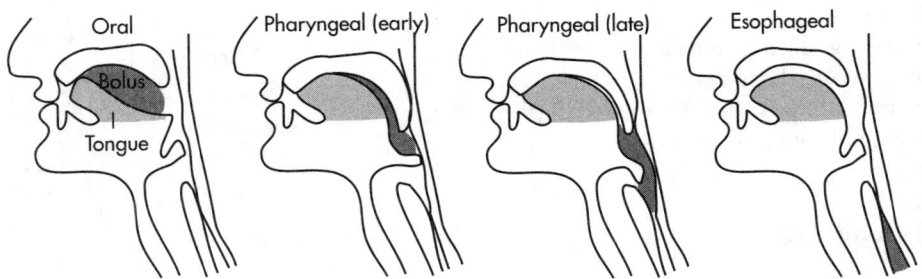

ESOPHAGEAL ULTRASOUND

Endoscopic esophageal transabdominal or gastric ultrasound (US) is performed mainly for staging of cancer or detection of early cancer. Most mass lesions and lymph nodes appear as hypoechoic structures disrupting the normal US "gut signature," consisting of different layers of hyper and hypoechogenic lines.

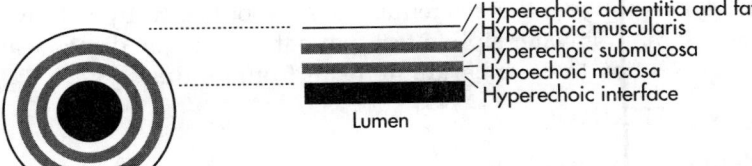

Esophageal Disease

SCHATZKI'S RING

Thin annular narrowing at junction of esophageus with stomach (B-line level). Present in 10% of population, 30% of which are symptomatic. Symptoms (dysphagia, heartburn) usually occur if rings cause esophageal narrowing of ≤ 12 mm.

ESOPHAGEAL WEBS AND RINGS

Mucosal structures (web = asymmetrical, ring = symmetrical) that may occur anywhere in the esophagus. Associations:
- Iron-deficiency anemia (cervical webs)
- Hypopharyngeal carcinoma

HIATAL HERNIA

There are 2 types:

Sliding hernia (axial type), 95%
- GEJ is above the diaphragm.
- Reflux is more likely with larger hernias.
- May be reducible in erect position.

Paraesophageal hernia, 5%
- GEJ is in its normal position (i.e., below diaphragm).
- Part of the fundus is herniated above the diaphragm through esophageal hiatus and lies to the side of the esophagus.
- Reflux is not necessarily associated.
- More prone to mechanical complications.
- Usually nonreducible.

Radiographic features

Criteria for diagnosing sliding hernia
- Gastric folds above diaphragm
- Concentric indentation (B-line) above diaphragm
- Schatzki's ring above diaphragm

Associated findings
- Esophagitis, 25%
- Duodenal ulcers, 20%

Approach
- Maximally distend distal esophagus in horizontal position; distention can be achieved by sustained inspiratory effort
- Determine the type of hernia
- Determine if there is reflux and/or esophagitis by Valsalva's maneuver or Grammy water siphon test (patient continually drinks water while in RPO position to see if barium refluxes from fundus)

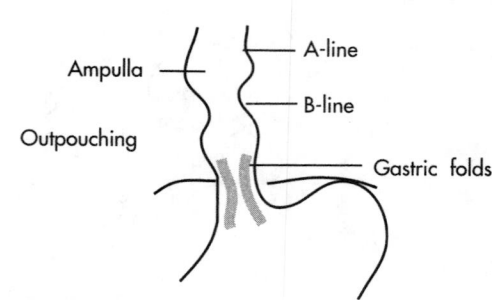

DIVERTICULA

Zenker's diverticulum

Pulsion diverticulum originates in the midline of the posterior wall of the hypopharynx at an anatomical weak point known as Killian's dehiscence (above cricopharyngeus at fiber divergence with inferior pharyngeal constrictor). During swallowing, increased intraluminal pressure forces mucosa to herniate through the wall. The etiology of Zenker's diverticulum is not firmly established, but premature contraction and/or motor incoordination of the cricopharyngeus muscle are thought to play a major role. Complications:
- Aspiration
- Ulceration
- Carcinoma

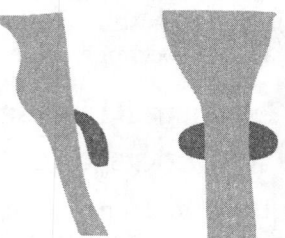

Killian Jamieson diverticulum
- Below cricopharyngeus
- Off midline
- Lateral to cervical esophagus

Epiphrenic diverticulum
- May occasionally be recognized on chest radiographs by presence of soft tissue mass (often with air fluid level) that mimics a hiatal hernia.
- Large diverticulum can compress the true esophageal lumen, causing dysphagia.

Pseudodiverticulosis

Numerous small esophageal outpouchings representing dilated glands interior to the muscularis. usually after 50 years. Clinical: dysphagia. Underlying diseases: candidiasis, alcoholism, diabetes. Associated findings:
- Esophageal stricture (usually below stricture), 90%
- Esophagitis

Radiographic features
- Thin flask-shaped structures in longitudinal rows parallel to the long axis of the esophagus
- Diffuse distribution or localized clusters near peptic strictures
- Much smaller than true diverticula

- When viewed en face, the pseudodiverticula can sometimes be mistaken for ulcers. When viewed in profile, however, they often seem to be "floating" outside the esophageal wall with barely perceptible channel to the lumen; esophageal ulcers almost always visibly communicate with the lumen.

ESOPHAGITIS

Esophagitis may present with erosions, ulcers, strictures; rarely, perforations and fistulas.

Types
Infectious (common in debilitated patients)
- Herpes
- Candidiasis
- Cytomegalovirus (CMV)

Chemical
- Reflux esophagitis
- Corrosives (lye)

Iatrogenic
- Radiotherapy
- Extended use of nasogastric tubes
- Drugs: tetracycline, antiinflammatory drugs, potassium, iron

Other
- HIV
- Scleroderma
- Crohn's disease (rare)
- Dermatological manifestations (pemphigoid, dermatomyositis bullosa)

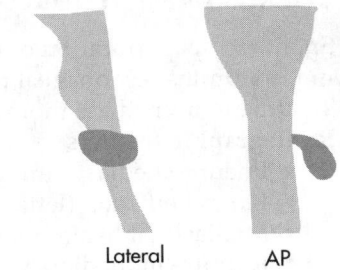

Killian Jamieson diverticulum

Lateral   AP

Radiographic features
- Thickening, nodularity of esophageal folds
- Irregularity of mucosa: granularity, ulcerations
- Retraction, luminal narrowing, stricture

Infectious esophagitis
Herpes simplex
- Abnormal motility
- Small ulcers, < 5 mm

Candidiasis
- Plaquelike, reticular
- Abnormal motility

CMV and HIV
- Typically large ulcers
- Etiological distinction between CMV and HIV ulcers is important because therapies are different.

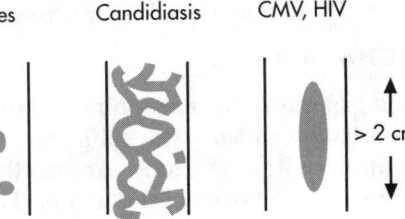

Herpes   Candidiasis   CMV, HIV

< 5 mm   > 2 cm

BARRETT'S ESOPHAGUS

Esophagus is abnormally lined with columnar, acid-secreting gastric mucosa. Usually due to chronic reflux esophagitis. Because there is an increased risk of esophageal cancer, close follow-up and repeated biopsies are recommended.

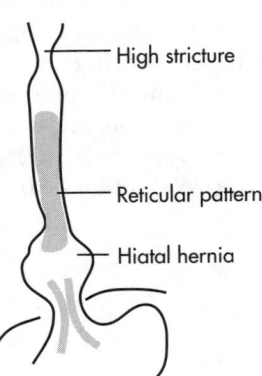

High stricture

Reticular pattern

Hiatal hernia

Radiographic features
- A reticular mucosal pattern, which may be discontinuous in the distal esophagus (short segment), is the most sensitive finding.
- Suspect the diagnosis if there is:
    High esophageal stricture accompanied by reticular mucosal pattern (long segment) below transition or ulcer
    Low strictures: the majority cannot be differentiated from simple reflux esophagitis strictures, and biopsies are required

BOERHAAVE'S SYNDROME

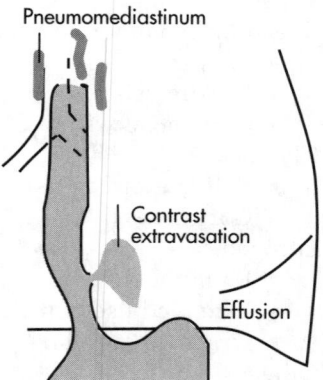

Spontaneous perforation of the thoracic esophagus due to a sudden increase in intraluminal esophageal pressure. Clinical: severe epigastric pain. Treatment: immediate thoracotomy. Mortality, 25%.

Radiographic features
- Pneumomediastinum
- Pleural effusion (left >> right)
- Mediastinal hematoma
- Rupture immediately above diaphragm, usually on left posterolateral side (90%)

MALLORY-WEISS TEAR

Mucosal tear in proximal stomach, across GEJ or distal esophagus (10%) usually due to prolonged vomiting (alcoholics) or increased intraluminal pressure. Because the tear is not transmural, there is no pneumomediastinum.

Radiographic features
- Radiographs are usually normal.
- Extravasation per se is rare.
- There may be subtle mucosal irregularity.

ACHALASIA

The gastroesophageal sphincter fails to relax because of Wallerian degeneration of Auerbach's plexus. The sphincter relaxes only when the hydrostatic pressure of the column of liquid or food exceeds that of the sphincter; emptying occurs more in the upright than horizontal position. Types:
- Primary (idiopathic)
- Secondary (destruction of myenteric plexus by tumor cells)
    Metastases
    Adenocarcinoma invasion from cardia
- Infectious: Chagas' disease

Clinical findings
- Primarily predominant in young patients (in contradistinction to esophageal tumors); onset: 20-40 years
- Dysphagia, 100% to both liquids and solids when symptoms begin
- Weight loss, 90%

Diagnosis

- Need to exclude malignancy (fundal carcinoma and lymphoma destroying Auerbach's plexus)
- Need to exclude esophageal spasm
- Manometry is the most sensitive to diagnose elevated lower esophageal sphincter (LES) pressure and incomplete relaxation.

DIFFERENTIATING SPASM FROM ACHALASIA

Parameter	Esophageal Spasm	Achalasia
SYMPTOMS		
Dysphagia	Midstream	Xiphoid or suprasternal notch
Pain	Common	Rare
Weight loss	Rare	Common
Emotional	Common	Common
MOTILITY		
Waves	Simultaneous	Tertiary
LES relaxation	Present	Absent
RADIOGRAPHIC FEATURES		
Esophageal contraction	Vigorous	Discoordinated
Esophageal emptying	Efficient	Poor
RESPONSE TO THERAPY		
Pneumostatic dilation	Not indicated	Good
Surgery	Long myotomy	Low cardioesophageal myotomy

Radiographic features

- Two diagnostic criteria must be met:
  - Primary and secondary peristalsis absent throughout esophagus.
  - LES fails to relax in response to swallowing.
- Dilated esophagus typically curves to right and then back to left when passing through diaphragm.
- There may be minimal esophageal dilation in the early stage of disease.
- Beaked tapering at GEJ
- Tertiary waves
- Air-fluid level in esophagus on plain film

Complications

- Recurrent aspiration and pneumonias, 10%
- Increased incidence of esophageal cancer

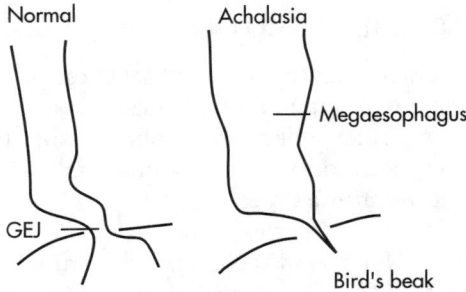

Treatment
- Drugs: nitrates, beta agonists, calcium blockers (effective in < 50%)
- Balloon dilatation (effective in 70%)
- Myotomy: procedure of choice

SCLERODERMA

Collagen vascular disease that involves the smooth muscle of esophagus, stomach, and small bowel.

Radiographic features
- Lack of primary waves in distal two-thirds
- GEJ patulous unless stricture supervenes
- Reflux esophagitis (common)
- Strictures occur late in disease
- Esophagus dilates most when stricture supervenes

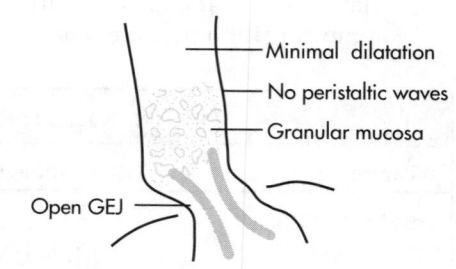

DIFFERENTIATING ACHALASIA FROM SCLERODERMA		
	Achalasia	**Scleroderma**
Esophagus	Massively dilated	Mildly dilated
GEJ	Closed, tapers to beak shape	Open; stricture late
Horizontal swallow	Tertiary contractions	Primary in proximal ⅓, tertiary contraction in distal ⅔
Reflux	No	Yes
Complications	Aspiration pneumonia	Early: esophagitis
		Late: stricture, interstitial lung disease

DIFFUSE DYSMOTILITY

Characterized by intermittent chest pain, dysphagia, and forceful contractions. Diagnosis: manometry. Types:
- Primary neurogenic abnormality (vagus)
- Secondary reflux esophagitis

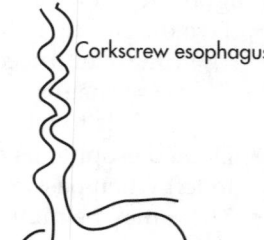

Radiographic types
- Nutcracker esophagus
- Nonspecific esophageal dysmotility disorders
- Diffuse esophageal spasm: corkscrew esophagus

CHAGAS' DISEASE (AMERICAN TRYPANOSOMIASIS)

Caused by *Trypanosoma cruzi*, which multiply in reticuloendothelial system (RES), muscle, and glia cells. When these cells rupture and organisms are destroyed, a neurotoxin is released that destroys ganglion cells in the myenteric plexus. Mortality, 5% (myocarditis, encephalitis).

Radiographic features
Esophagus
- Early findings: hypercontractility, distal muscular spasm; normal caliber
- Classic late findings (denervation): megaesophagus, aperistalsis: bird's beak appearance at GEJ (achalasia look-alike)

- Esophageal complications:
  Ulcers, hemorrhage
  Perforation into mediastinum, abscess formation
  Carcinoma, 7%

Colon
- Megacolon (anal sphincter neuropathy)
- Sigmoid volvulus, 10%

Other GI tract
- Megastomach
- Megaduodenum

Heart
- Cardiomyopathy (cardiomegaly)
- Clear lungs, no pericardial effusions

Central nervous system (CNS)
- Encephalitis

BENIGN ESOPHAGEAL NEOPLASM

- Leiomyoma, 50%
- Fibrovascular polyp (may be large and mobile attached to upper esophagus, 25%)
- Cysts, 10%
- Papilloma, 3%
- Fibroma, 3%
- Hemangioma, 2%

MALIGNANT ESOPHAGEAL NEOPLASM

Types
- Squamous cell carcinoma, 95% (5% multifocal)
- Adenocarcinoma, 5%; usually in lower esophagus at GEJ: increasing in frequency
- Lymphoma
- Leiomyosarcoma
- Metastasis

Associations
Squamous cell carcinomas are associated with:
- Head and neck cancers
- Smoking
- Alcohol
- Achalasia
- Lye ingestion

Adenocarcinoma is associated with:
- Barrett's esophagus

Radiographic features
Staging (CT)
- Invasion into mediastinum, aorta
- Local lymph node enlargement
- Metastases: liver, lung, lymphadenopathy, gastrohepatic ligament

Staging (endoscopic US)
- Extension through wall
- Lymph node metastases

Spectrum of appearance
- Infiltrative, shelflike margins
- Annular, constricting
- Polypoid
- Ulcerative
- Varicoid
- Unusual bulky forms: carcinosarcoma, fibrovascular polyp, leiomyosarcoma, metastases

Infiltrative	Polypoid	Annular stenotic	Ulcerative	Varicoid
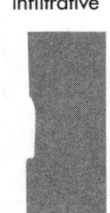	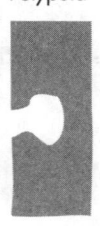	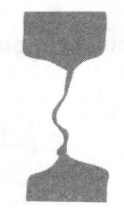	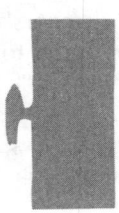	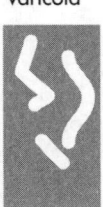

LYMPHOMA

Because the esophagus and stomach do not normally have lymphocytes, primary lymphoma is rare unless present from inflammation. Secondary metastatic lymphoma is more common. Secondary esophageal lymphoma accounts for < 2% of all gastrointestinal (GI) tract lymphomas (stomach >> small bowel). Four radiographic presentations: infiltrative, ulcerating, polypoid, and endoexophytic.

ESOPHAGEAL FOREIGN BODY

Radiographic features
- Foreign body usually lodges in coronal orientation.
- Important to exclude underlying Schatzki's ring or esophageal carcinoma once the foreign body is removed.

Stomach

TYPES OF BARIUM STUDIES

DOUBLE- VS. SINGLE-CONTRAST BARIUM STUDIES		
	Single Contrast	**Double Contrast**
Contrast agent	Thin barium (40% weight/weight)	Thick barium (85% weight/weight) Effervescent granules
Differences	Opaque distention	Translucent distention ("see through")
	Compression is necessary to allow penetration of beam	Compression less important
	Fluoroscopy emphasized	Filming emphasized
Indication	Acute setting, uncooperative patient, obstruction	All elective barium studies

UPPER GI SERIES (UGI)

Patient preparation
- Nothing by mouth for 8 hours before examination
- If a barium enema has been performed within the last 48 hours, give 4 tablespoons of milk of magnesia 12 hours before examination (cathartic)

Single-contrast technique

1. Patient is in upright position and drinks thin barium. Spot GEJ.
2. Prone position to observe esophageal motility. Spot GEJ, antrum, and bulb.
3. Turn supine under fluoroscopic control.
4. Turn LPO for air contrast of antrum, bulb. Evaluate duodenum and proximal small bowel.
5. Overhead films: LPO, RAO of stomach, PA of abdomen

Double contrast

X-ray beam ↓

Single contrast

Double-contrast technique

1. Patient upright in slight LPO position. Administer effervescent granules with 20 ml of water. Start patient drinking thick barium (120 cc) and obtain air-contrast spot films of esophagus.
2. Table down with patient in prone position (compression view may be obtained here). Patient rolls to supine position through the left side. Check mucosal coating: if not adequate, turn patient to prone again and back to supine position, roll to keep left side dependent (so that emptying of barium into the duodenum is delayed).
3. Obtain views of the stomach. This is generally the most important part of the study. The patient is turned to get air into different regions of the stomach.
   - Patient supine (for body of stomach)
   - Patient LPO (for antrum)
   - Patient RPO (for Schatzki view for lesser curvature)
   - Patient RAO (for fundus)
4. Study of esophagus. Patient RAO drinking regular "thin" barium. Observe entire esophagus and evaluate motility. Take spot films (routinely of distended GEJ).
5. Views of bulb with contrast and air filling. First leave the patient in RAO view and then turn to LPO view. Include some C-loop.
6. Upright compression. Compression of antrum, lesser curve, duodenum.
7. Overhead films:
   - RAO, drinking esophagus (optional)
   - AP, PA of abdomen
   - LPO and RAO stomach

PERCUTANEOUS GASTROSTOMY

Success rate 95%, minor complications 1%-2%, major complications 2%-4%.

Indications:
- Decompression in terminally ill patients with gastric outlet or small bowel obstruction (SBO): gastrostomy is sufficient
- Feeding: gastrojejunostomy preferred

Technique
1. Half cup of barium the night before to opacify colon. Nasogastric (NG) tube placement.
2. Distend stomach by insufflating air through NG tube; mark entry high in midbody pointing towards pylorus.
3. Anesthesia through four 25-g needles about 1-2 cm away from insertion point. Leave needles in.
4. Gastropexy with T-tacks is not universally accepted. If they are placed, deploy them with 0.35 ring wire under fluoroscopic guidance. Crimp T-tacks in place.

5. Place needle with guidewire into stomach through central insertion point.
6. Dilators 8, 10, 12, 14, 16 Fr, place 15-Fr peel-away sheath.
7. Place 14-Fr ultrathane gastrostomy catheter. Gastric decompression can be achieved with smaller bore catheters (>10 Fr). Secure catheter in place.

Contraindications
- Organs overlying stomach: liver, colon, ribs (high position of stomach)
- Massive ascites (perform therapeutic paracentesis before gastrostomy)
- Abnormal gastric wall (ulcer, tumor): hemorrhage is common
- Elevated bleeding time

NORMAL APPEARANCE

Anatomy
- Fundus
- Body
- Antrum
- Pylorus
- Curvatures: lesser, greater

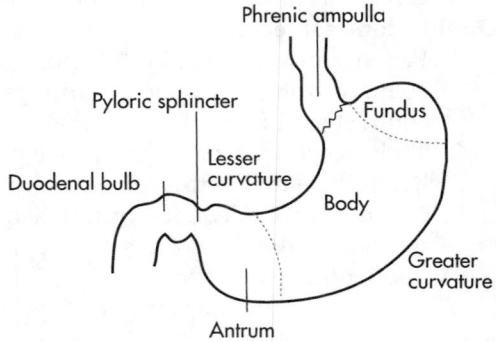

Muscosal relief
- Gastric rugae ("macromucosal" pattern) are seen in single-contrast barium studies; in double-contrast studies rugae are often effaced by gaseous distention
- Area gastricae (normal gastric mucosal pattern) is most prominent in antrum and body; ectopic duodenal area gastricae present in 20%

TYPES OF GASTRIC LESIONS

There are 3 morphological types of lesions:
- Ulcer: abnormal accumulation of contrast media
- Polypoid lesion (masses): filling defect
- Coexistent pattern: ulcerated mass

The above lesions have different appearances depending on whether they are imaged with single- or double-contrast techniques, whether they exist on dependent or nondependent walls, and whether they are imaged in profile or en face.

Mucosal vs. extramucosal location of mass

The location of a lesion can be evaluated by observing the angle the lesion forms with the wall:
- Acute angle (looks like an *a*): mucosal (polyp, cancer)
- Obtuse angle (looks like an *o*): extramucosal (intramural or extramural)

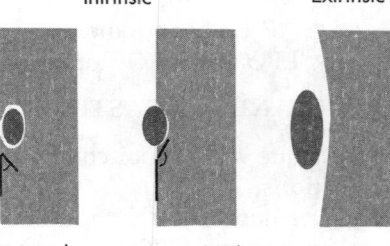

Preservation of mucosal pattern is also a hint to location of lesions:
- Disruption of normal pattern: mucosal
- Presence of normal pattern: intramural or extramural location

Distinction of outline:
- Smooth distinct: extramucosal
- Irregular, fuzzy: mucosal

PEPTIC ULCER DISEASE (PUD)

Cause

PUD was previously believed to be due to oversecretion of acid. More recently, *Helicobacter pylori* (gram-negative) has been shown to play a causal role in the development of peptic ulcer.

- Not all individuals with *H. pylori* will develop ulcers. Prevalence of *H. pylori*: 10% of population < 30 years, 60% of population > 60 years.
- Prevalence of *H. pylori* in duodenal and gastric ulcers: 80%-90%
- Implications:
  Precaution against infection should be taken by all GI personnel.
  H. pylori serology may become useful for diganosis of PUD.
  PUD heals faster with antibiotics and antacids than with antacids alone.

Detection

Detection rate of ulcers by double-contrast barium is 60%-80%. This low sensitivity is due to the fact that (1) craters are often too superficial, (2) craters are often too small (erosions in gastritis), (3) craters are so big that they are occasionally overlooked as an abnormality, (4) extensive gaseous distention has effaced the crater; or (5) treatment began before UGI.

Radiographic features

Benign   Malignant

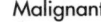
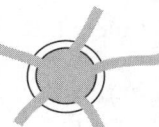
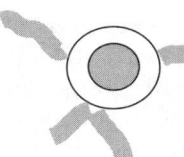

- Ulcer crater seen en face: distinct collection of barium that persists on different views; the collection is most often round but can be linear
- Ulcer crater seen in profile: barium collection extends outside the projected margin of the gastric or duodenal wall
- Double-contrast studies: the crater has a black center with a rim coated with barium: target sign
- Greater curvature ulcers are commonly due to malignancy or NSAID ingestion. (Aspirin-induced ulcers are also called sump ulcers because of their typical location on greater curvature.)
- Multiple ulcers are usually due to NSAID ingestion.
- Multiple superficial erosions (gastritis):
  Pinpoint size surrounded by small mound of edema (aphthous-like)
  Tend to appear on top nondistorted rugal folds
- Signs of benign and malignant ulcers

Benign ulcers (95% of all ulcers)

- PUD, 90%
- Other: hormonal, steroids, NSAID, gastritis

Malignant ulcers (5% of all ulcers)

- Carcinoma, 90%
- Lymphoma, 5%
- Rare malignancies (sarcoma, carcinoid, metastases)

DIFFERENTIAL DIAGNOSIS OF ULCERS		
Parameter	Benign Ulcer	Malignant Ulcer
Mucosal folds	Thin, regular, extend up to crater edge	Thick, irregular, do not extend to edge
Penetration	Margin of ulcer crater extends beyond projected luminal surface	Ulcers project within (projected) luminal surface; Carman's (meniscus) sign*
Location	Centrally within mound of edema	Eccentrically in tumor mound
Collar	Hampton's line: 1-2 mm lucent line around the ulcer†	Thick, nodular, irregular
Other	Normal peristalsis	Abnormal peristalsis
	Incisura: invagination of opposite wall	Limited distensibility

*Results from the fluroscopically induced apposition of rolled halves of the tumor margin forming the periphery of the ulcerated carcinoma; meniscus refers to meniscoid shape of ulcer.
†This line is caused by thin mucosa overhanging the crater mouth seen in tangent; it is a reliable sign of a benign ulcer, but present in very few patients.

Complications of gastric ulcer
- Obstruction
- Posterior penetration of ulcer into pancreas
- Perforation
- Bleeding: filling defect in the ulcer crater may represent blood clots.
- Gastroduodenal fistulas: double channel pylorus

Pearls
- Categorize all gastric ulcers as definite/probable/unlikely benign or malignant.
- All patients, except for those with de novo definitely benign gastric ulcers, should proceed to endoscopy with biopsy.
- Benign ulcers decrease 50% in size within 3 weeks and show complete healing within 6 weeks with successful medical treatment.
- Benign ulcers may heal with local scarring.

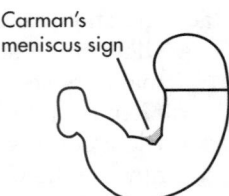

Carman's meniscus sign

MÉNÉTRIER'S DISEASE (GIANT HYPERTROPHIC GASTRITIS)

Large gastric rugal folds (hypertrophic gastritis) with protein-losing enteropathy. Clinical triad: achlorhydria, hypoproteinemia, edema. Typically occurs in middle-age men. Complication: gastric carcinoma, 10%.

Radiographic features
- Giant gastric rugal folds, usually proximal half of stomach
- Hypersecretion: poor coating, dilution of barium
- Gastric wall thickening
- Small intestinal fold thickening due to hypoproteinemia
- Peptic ulcers are uncommon

EOSINOPHILIC GASTROENTERITIS

Inflammatory disease of unknown etiology characterized by focal or diffuse eosinophilic infiltration of the GI tract. An allergic or immunological disorder is suspected because 50% of patients have another allergic disease (asthma, allergic rhinitis, hay fever). Clinical: abdominal pain, 80%; diarrhea, 40%; eosinophilia. Only 300 cases have been reported to date. Treatment: steroids.

Radiographic features

Esophagus
- Strictures

Stomach, 50%
- Antral stenosis (common)
- Pyloric stenosis (common)
- Gastric rigidity
- Gastric fold thickening

Small bowel, 50%
- Fold thickening (common)
- Dilatation
- Stenosis

GASTRODUODENAL CROHN'S DISEASE

Pseudo-Billroth I appearance on barium studies
- Aphthous ulcers
- Stricture
- Fistulization

ZOLLINGER-ELLISON SYNDROME

Syndrome caused by excessive gastrin production. Clinical: diarrhea, recurrent PUD, pain.

Causes

Gastrinoma, 90%
- Islet cell tumor in pancreas or duodenal wall (90%)
- 50% of tumors are malignant
- 10% of tumors are associated with multiple endocrine neoplasia (MEN) I

Antral G cell hyperplasia, 10%

Radiographic features
- Ulcers
    Location: duodenal bulb > stomach > postbulbar duodenum
    Multiple ulcers, 10%
- Thickened gastric and duodenal folds
- Increased gastric secretions
- Reflux esophagitis

GASTRIC POLYPS

Gastric polyps are far less common than colonic polyps. Classification:
- Hyperplastic polyps (80% of all gastric polyps; < 1 cm, sessile; not premalignant)
    Associated with chronic atrophic gastritis
    Typically multiple and clustered in the fundus and body
    5%-25% of patients have synchronous gastric carcinoma

- Adenomatous polyps (20% of all gastric polyps; > 2 cm, sessile)
    True tumors (familial polyposis, Gardner's syndrome)
    Malignant transformation in 50%
    35% of patients have synchronous gastric carcinoma
- Villous polyps (uncommon; cauliflower-like, sessile)
    Strong malignant potential
- Hamartomatous polyps (rare; Peutz-Jeghers syndrome)

GASTRIC CARCINOMA

Third most common GI malignancy (colon > pancreas > stomach). Risk factors:
- Pernicious anemia
- Adenomatous polyps
- Chronic atrophic gastritis
- Billroth II > Billroth I

Location
- Greater curvature fundus antrum, 30%
- Body curvature, 30%
- Fundus, 40%

Staging
- T1: limited to mucosa, submucosa (5-year survival, 85%)
- T2: muscle, serosa involved (5-year survival, 50%)
- T3: penetration through serosa
- T4: adjacent organs invaded

Radiographic features
Features of early gastric cancers:
- Polydoid lesions (type 1)
    > 0.5 cm (normal peristalsis does not pass through lesion)
    Difficult to detect radiographically
- Superficial lesions (type 2)
    2A: < 0.5 cm
    2B: most difficult to diagnose (mucosal irregularity only)
    2C: 75% of all gastric carcinoma (folds tend to stop
        abruptly at lesion)
- Excavated lesion (type 3) = malignant ulcer

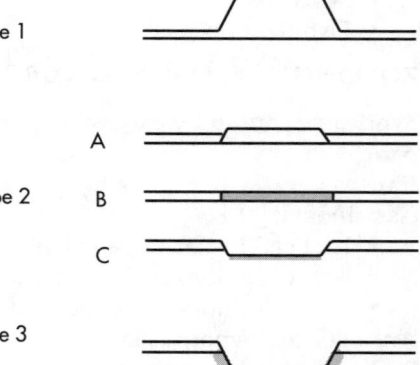

Features of advanced gastric cancer
- Malignant ulcer
- Ulcerated luminal mass
- Rigidity, diffuse narrowing linitis plastica
- Thickened wall > 1 cm by CT
- Lymphadenopathy
    Gastrohepatic ligament
    Gastrocolic ligament
    Perigastric nodes
- Hepatic metastases

GASTRIC LYMPHOMA

3% of all gastric malignancies. NHL (common) >> Hodgkin's lymphoma (uncommon). Types:
- Primary gastric lymphoma (arise from lymphatic tissue in lamina propria mucosae), 10%
- Secondary (gastric involvement in generalized lymphoma), 90%

Radiographic features
- Diffuse infiltrating disease
    Normal gastric wall 2-5 mm (distended stomach)
    $\geq$ 6 mm is abnormal except at GEJ
- Thick folds
- Ulcerating mass
- More often than carcinoma, lymphomas spread across the pylorus into the duodenum
- Hodgkin's lymphoma of the stomach mimics scirrhous carcinoma (strong desmoplastic reaction)

METASTASES

Contiguous spread
- From colon (gastrocolic ligament)
- From liver (gastrohepatic ligament)
- From pancreas

Hematogenous spread to stomach (target lesions)
- Melanoma (most common)
- Breast
- Lung

Radiographic features
- Multiple lesions
- Bull's eye lesions: sharply demarcated lesions with central ulcer (bigger than aphthoid ulcer)

CARNEY'S TRIAD (RARE)

- Gastric leiomyosarcoma
- Functioning extraadrenal paraganglioma
- Pulmonary chondroma

BENIGN TUMORS

Benign tumors are usually submucosal in location. Types:
- Leiomyoma. Most common benign tumor; may ulcerate, 10% malignant
- Lipoma, fibroma, schwannoma, hemangioma, lymphangioma
- Carcinoid (malignant transformation in 20%)

GASTRIC VOLVULUS

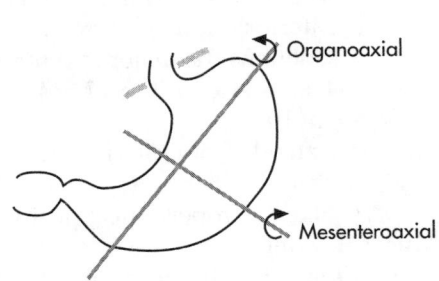

Abnormal rotation of stomach. Two types:
Organoaxial
- Rotation around the long axis of stomach
- Stomach rotates 180° so that greater curvature is cranially located; upside-down stomach
- Observed in adults with large hiatus hernia
- Complications rare

Mesenteroaxial
- Stomach rotates around its short axis (perpendicular to long axis).
- Fundus is caudal to antrum.
- More common when large portions of stomach are above diaphragm (traumatic diaphragmatic rupture in children).
- Obstruction, ischemia likely

GASTRIC VARICES

Fundal varices represent dilated peripheral branches of short gastric and left gastric veins. Fundal varices are usually associated with esophageal varices; the combination is almost always due to portal hypertension.

Presence of isolated gastric varices, without esophageal varices, is often caused by splenic vein obstruction and is most commonly secondary to pancreatitis or pancreatic carcinoma. Gastric varices appear as multiple, smooth, serpiginous filling defects. Occasionally, a conglomerate of varices may simulate a fundal mass.

BENIGN GASTRIC EMPHYSEMA

Gas in wall of stomach is usually due to:
- Trauma from endoscopy
- Infection
- Ischemia
- Increased intraluminal pressure
- Vomiting
- Spontaneous or traumatic rupture of a pulmonary bulla into areolar tissue surrounding the esophagus
- No discernible underlying disease

Duodenum and Small Bowel

Duodenum

NORMAL APPEARANCE

The duodenum has three segments:
Segment I
- Begins at pylorus and extends to the superior duodenal flexure
- Contains the duodenal bulb
- Intraperitoneal position: freely movable

Segment II
- Begins at superior duodenal flexure and extends to inferior duodenal flexure
- Contains the major and minor papilla and the promontory
- Fixed retroperitoneal position

Segment III
- Extends from inferior duodenal flexure to ligament of Treitz
- Fixed retroperitoneal position

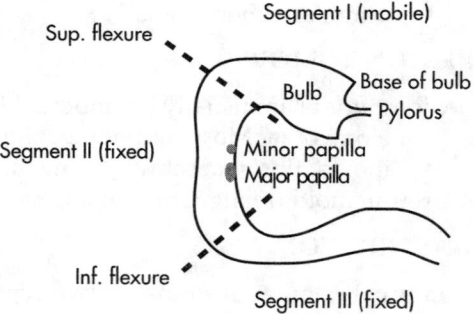

Mucosal relief
- Folds in the duodenal bulb are longitudinally oriented.
- In the descending portion of the duodenum, Kerkring's folds are transversely oriented.
- These folds are usually visible despite complete duodenal distention.

Papilla

Major papilla (Vater's papilla): orifice for ducts
- Appears as round filling defect
- Located below the promontory
- 8-10 mm in length
- Abnormal if > 15 mm

Minor papilla (accessory papilla, Santorini's papilla)
- Located superiorly and ventral to major papilla
- Mean distance from major papilla 20 mm
- Not usually visualized

Promontory
- Shoulderlike luminal projection along medial aspect of the 2nd portion of the duodenum
- Begins superior to major papilla

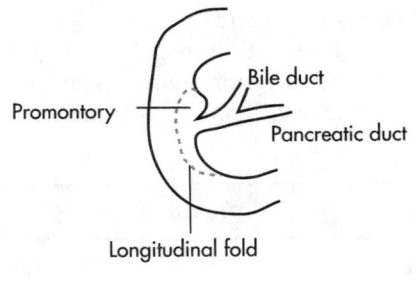

DUODENAL ULCER

Duodenal ulcers are 2-3 times more common than gastric ulcers. All bulbar duodenal ulcers are considered benign. Postbulbar or multiple ulcers raise the suspicion for Zollinger-Ellison syndrome. Locations:

Bulbar, 95%
- Anterior wall: most common site, perforate
- Posterior wall: penetration into pancreas

Postbulbar, 5%

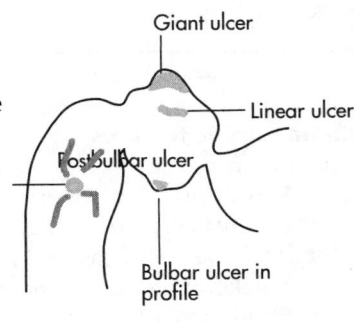

Predisposing factors
- Chronic obstructive pulmonary disease
- Severe stress: injury, surgery, burn
- Steroids

Radiographic features
- Persistent round or elliptical collection; radiating folds, spasm
- Linear ulcers, 25%
- Kissing ulcers: 2 or more ulcers located opposite each other
- Giant ulcers
    Crater is > 2 cm
    Ulcer largely replaces the duodenal bulb
    A large ulcer crater is easily mistaken for a deformed bulb; does not change shape during upper gastrointestinal (UGI) examination
- Duodenal ulcers often heal with a scar; this can lead to deformity and contraction of the duodenal bulb: cloverleaf deformity, hourglass deformity
- Postbulbar ulcers: Any ulcer distal to the first portion of the duodenum should be considered malignant until proven otherwise (only 5% are benign ulcers, mostly secondary to Zollinger-Ellison syndrome).

DUODENAL TRAUMA

Duodenal injuries are due either to penetrating (stab, gunshot) wounds or blunt trauma (motor vehicle accident). Because duodenum is immobile in retroperitoneum, most perforations occur there. Mortality of untreated duodenal rupture is 65%.

Location of intestinal trauma
- Duodenum, proximal jejunum 95%
- Colon, 5%

Types of injuries
- Perforation (requires surgery)
- Transection (requires surgery)
- Hematoma (nonsurgical treatment)

ORGAN INJURIES ASSOCIATED WITH DUODENAL TRAUMA		
	Blunt Trauma (%)	Penetrating Trauma (%)
Liver	30	55
Pancreas	45	35
Spleen	25	2
Colon	15	10
Small bowel	10	25
Kidney	10	20

Radiographic features
Perforation
- Extraluminal retroperitoneal gas
- Extravasation of oral contrast material

Other less specific signs that may occur with perforation or hematoma:
- Thickening of duodenal wall or mass effect narrowing lumen
- Fluid in right anterior pararenal space
- Fluid in right peripararenal space
- Fluid or oral contrast in duodenum that does not pass into small bowel (not to be confused with a duodenal diverticulum)
- Peritoneal fluid

Surgical treatment
- Simple repair
- Pyloric exclusion for complex injuries
- Whipple's procedure is rarely necessary
- Surgical complications:
    Intraabdominal abscess, 15%
    Duodenal fistula, 4%
    Duodenal dehiscence, 4%
    Pancreatic fistula, 1%

BENIGN TUMORS

More common than malignant duodenal tumors. Types:
- Lipoma, leiomyoma (most common)
- Villous adenoma, adenomatous polyp
- Brunner's gland adenoma
- Ectopic pancreas

ANTRAL MUCOSAL PROLAPSE

Rare "disorder" characterized by movement of gastric mucosa bulging into the base of the duodenal bulb. Movement is secondary to discoordination of muscularis mucosa and muscularis propria.

Radiographic features

- Lobulated filling defect in the duodenal bulb
- The filling defect has to be in contiguity with antral rugal folds
- The radiographic appearance can (but does not have to) vary with peristaltic activity, (i.e., the prolapse may move back and forth from the antrum)

MALIGNANT TUMORS

Infrequent. The most common locations of malignant tumors are in the periampullary and infraampullary areas. Types:

- Adenocarcinoma (most common)
- Leiomyosarcoma
- Lymphoma (see below)
- Metastases
- Benign tumors with malignant potential: villous and adenomatous polyps, carcinoid

UPPER GI SURGERY

Complications of surgery

Immediate

- Anastomotic leak
- Abscess
- Gastric outlet obstruction (edema)
- Bile reflux
- Ileus

Late complications

- Bowel dysmotility: dumping, postvagotomy hypotomia
- Ulcer
- Bowel obstruction: outlet obstruction, adhesions, stricture
- Prolapse, intususception
- Gastric carcinoma (in 5% of patients 15 years after surgery) Billroth II > Billroth I
- Metabolic effects: malabsorption
- Afferent loop syndrome
- Small pouch syndrome

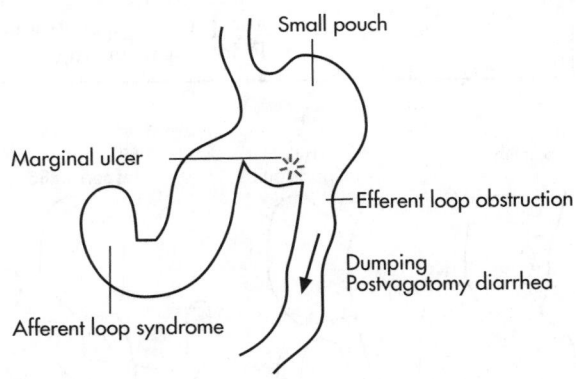

TYPES OF SURGERY		
Type	**Anastomosis/Surgery**	**Common Indication**
Antireflux	Nissen fundoplication	Hiatal hernia
	Angelchik procedure	
Gastrectomy	Gastroduodenostomy (Billroth I)	Gastroduodenal ulcer
	Gastrojejunostomy (Billroth II)	Gastroduodenal ulcer
	• Isoperistaltic (Whipple)	
	• Antiperistaltic	
	• Roux-en-Y	
	Total gastrectomy	Gastric cancer
Vagotomy	Truncal vagotomy	
	Selective vagotomy	
	Parietal cell vagotomy	
	Drainage procedures	Facilitate gastric emptying after
	• Gastroenterostomy	vagotomy
	• Jaboulay	
	• Finney	
	• Heineke-Mikulicz	
Complex	Pancreaticoduodenectomy (Whipple)	Pancreatic cancer
	• Standard: Roux-en-Y choledochojejunostomy and pancreaticojejunostomy	
	• Pylorus preserving	

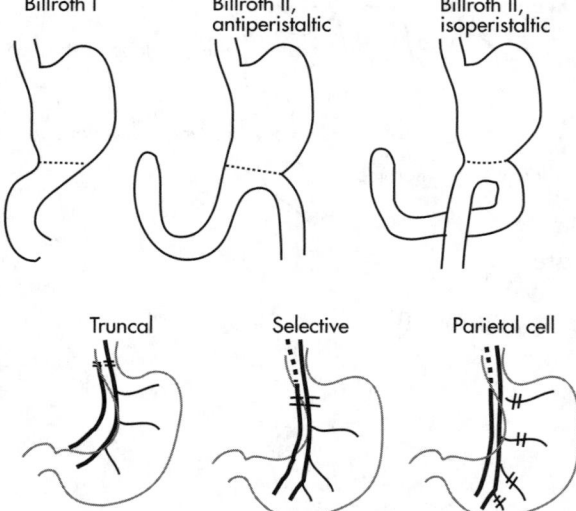

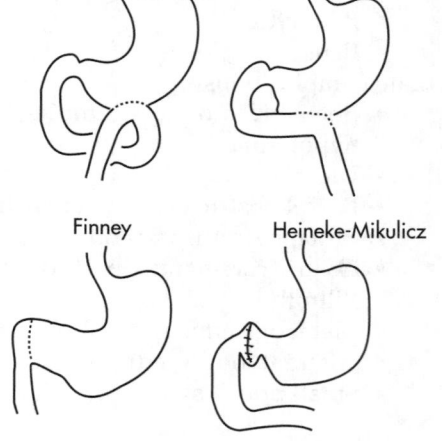

GASTRIC BYPASS SURGERY

In gastric bypass surgery, a small gastric pouch is constructed and anastomosed to the jejunum via a narrow channel in a standard loop or Roux-en-Y configuration. The distal stomach is intact but functionally separate from food pathway.

Complications
- Outlet obstruction. Gastric outlet obstruction is not uncommon in the early postsurgical period. Early outlet problems due to edema at anastomotic site. When channel lumen is less than 6-8 mm wide, chronic problems appear. The stenosis usually occurs more than 6 weeks after surgery. Because weight loss is dramatic, patients often do not seek prompt follow-up.
- Perforation

Jejunum and Ileum

NORMAL APPEARANCE

The small bowel is examined by conventional small bowel follow-through (SBFT), enteroclysis, and/or CT. The specific indications for enteroclysis are:
- Occult bleeding
- Recurrent obstructive symptoms
- Malabsorption
- Determine extent of Crohn's disease

Normal appearance of small bowel on conventional SBFT

Luminal diameter
- > 3 cm is abnormal

Fold thickness
- Valvulae conniventes measure 1-2 mm
- > 3 mm is abnormal

Wall thickness
- Normal 1-1.5 mm

Secretions
- There should normally be no appreciable fluid in small bowel.
- Excess secretions cause dilution of barium column.

BLIND LOOP SYNDROME

Syndrome develops after bypassing small bowel by an enteroanastomosis with subsequent stagnation of bowel contents. Clinical: malabsorption in large diverticula may cause similar dynamics.

MALABSORPTION

Abnormal absorption of fat, water, protein, carbohydrates from small bowel.

Radiographic features
- Dilatation of bowel loops
- Diluted barium (mixes with watery bowel content)
- Flocculated barium: barium aggregates into particles (mainly seen with older barium suspensions)
- Slow transit
- Segmentation of barium (lack of continuous column) rarely occurs with new agents
- Moulage pattern: featureless barium collection (rarely occurs with new agents)
- Hidebound pattern: valvulae thinner, closer together, wrinkled-look

SPRUE

Three entities:

- Tropical sprue (unknown etiology; responds to antibiotics)
- Nontropical (adults; intolerance to gluten in wheat and other grains; HLA DR3, IgA, IgM antibodies)
- Celiac disease (children)

Radiographic features

- Dilatation of small bowel is the most typical finding (caliber increases with severity of disease)
- Nodular changes in duodenum (bubbly duodenum)
- Reversal of jejunal and ileal fold patterns: "The jejunum looks like the ileum, the ileum looks like the jejunum, and the duodenum looks like hell"
- Segmentation
- Hypersecretion and mucosal atrophy causes the Moulage sign (rare)
- Transient intussusception pattern (coiled spring) is typical
- Increased secretions: flocculation with older barium suspensions
- Increased incidence of malignancy, aggressive lymphoma, carcinoma

Associated disorders

- Dermatitis herpetiformis
- Selective immunoglobulin A deficiency
- Hyposplenism
- Adenopathy
- Cavitary mesenteric lymph node syndrome

Complications

- Ulcerative jejunoileitis: several segments of bowel wall thickening with irregularity and ulceration
- Enteropathy: associated T cell lymphoma
- Increased incidence of cancers of esophagus, pharynx, duodenum, and rectum
- Sprue, scleroderma, small bowel obstruction: dilated, prolonged motility, normal folds

OTHER DISEASES CAUSING MALABSORPTION PATTERN*		
Disease	**Primary Pattern**	**Comment**
Scleroderma	AM + D, hidebound folds	Muscularis replaced by fibrosis
Whipple	DFTN, adenopathy may occur	Intestinal lipodystrophy
Amyloidosis	DFTN	Tiny nodule filling defects
Lymphangiectasia	DFTN, MA	Dilated lymphatics in wall
IG deficiencies	DFTN	Nodular lymphoid hyperplasia
Mastocytosis	DFTN	Hepatomegaly, PUD, dense bones
Eosinophilic gastroenteritis	Very thick folds (polypoid)	Food allergy, 70%
Graft-vs.-host disease	Effaced folds (ribbonlike)	Bone marrow transplants
MAI infection	DFTN, MA, pseudo Whipples	Immunocompromised host

AM, Abnormal motility; *D*, dilatation; *DFTN*, diffuse fold thickening with fine nodularity; *MA*, mesenteric adenopathy; *MAI*, *Mycobacterium avium-intracellulare*.
*See also infectious enterities.

MASTOCYTOSIS

Systemic mast cell proliferation in reticuloendothelial system (RES) (small bowel, liver, spleen, lymph nodes, bone marrow); and skin (95%) with histamine release.
Clinical: diarrhea, steatorrhea, histamine effects (flushing, tachycardia, pruritus, PUD)
Radiographic features
Small bowel
- Irregular fold thickening
- Diffuse small nodules
Other
- Sclerotic bone lesions
- Hepatosplenomegaly
- Peptic ulcers (increased HCl secretion)

AMYLOIDOSIS

Heterogenous group of disorders characterized by abnormal extracellular deposition of insoluble fibrillar protein material. Diagnosis is established by biopsy of affected organs (birefringence, staining with Congo red). Clinical amyloidosis syndromes:
Systemic amyloidosis
- Immunocyte dyscrasia (myeloma, monoclonal gammopathy)
- Chronic active disease (see below)
- Hereditary syndromes
    Neuropathic form
    Nephropathic form
    Cardiomyopathic form
- Chronic hemodialysis
- Senile form
Localized amyloidosis
- Cerebral amyloid angiopathy (Alzheimer's, senile dementia)
- Cutaneous form
- Ocular form
- Others
Common chronic active diseases that are associated with systemic amyloidosis (there are many, less common causes):
Infections (recurrent and chronic)
- Tuberculosis (TB)
- Chronic osteomyleitis
- Decubitus ulcers
- Bronchiectasis
- Chronic pyelonephritis
Chronic inflammatory disease
- Rheumatoid arthritis (5%-20% of cases)
- Ankylosing spondylitis
- Crohn's disease
- Reiters
- Psoriasis

Neoplasm
- Hodgkin's disease (4% of cases)
- Renal cell carcinoma (3% of cases)

Radiographic features

Kidneys
- Nephrotic syndrome
- Renal insufficiency
- RTA
- Renal vein thrombosis

GI tract
- Diffuse thickening of small bowel folds
- Jejunization of ileum
- Small bowel dilatation
- Multiple nodular filling defects, > 2 mm
- Hepatosplenomegaly
- Macroglossia
- Colonic pseudodiverticulosis (may be unilateral and large)

Heart
- Cardiomyopathy (restrictive)
- Rhythm abnormalities

Nervous system
- Signs of dementia
- Carpal tunnel syndrome
- Peripheral neuropathy

INTESTINAL LYMPHANGIECTASIA

Spectrum of lymphatic abnormality (dilated lymphatics in lamina propria of small bowel) that clinically results in protein-losing enteropathy. Types:

Congenital (infantile) form presents with:
- Generalized lymphedema
- Chylous pleural effusions
- Diarrhea, steatorrhea
- Lymphocytopenia

Acquired (adult) form due to:
- Obstruction of thoracic duct (radiation, tumors, retroperitoneal fibrosis)
- Small bowel lymphoma
- Pancreatitis

Radiographic features
- Diffuse thickening of folds in jejunum and ileum due to dilated lymphatics and hypoalbuminemic edema
- Dilution of contrast material due to hypersecretion
- Lymphographic studies
    Hypoplastic lymphatics of lower extremity
    Tortuous thoracic duct
    Hypoplastic lymph nodes

GASTROINTESTINAL LYMPHOMA

Distinct subgroup of lymphoma that primarily arises in lymphoid tissue of the bowel rather than in lymph nodes. Categories:

GI-lymphoma in otherwise healthy patients
- Gastric lymphoma arising from mucosa-associated lymphoid tissue (MALT)
- Usually low-grade malignancy
- Represent 20% of malignant small bowel tumors; usual age: 5th-6th decade
- Radiographic features
     Mass, nodule, fold thickening (focal or diffuse) confined to GI tract in 50%
     Adenopathy, 30%
     Extraabdominal findings, 30%
- Large ulcerated mass presenting as endoenteric or exoenteric tumor (Differential diagnosis: gastrointestinal stromal tumor, metastatic melanoma, jejunal diverticulitis with abscess, ectopic pancreas)
- Aneurysmal dilatation: localized dilated, thick-walled, noncontractile lumen due to mural tumor. Auerback plexus neuropathy

GI lymphoma in HIV-positive or immunosuppressed patients
- Usually aggressive NHL with rapid spread, poor response to chemotherapy, short survival
- Widespread extraintestinal involvement, 80%
- Radiographic features
     GI abnormalities: nodules, fold thickening, mass
     Splenomegaly, 30%
     Adenopathy, 30%
     Ascites, 20%

GRAFT-VS.-HOST (GVH) REACTION

Donor lymphocytes react against organs (GI tract, skin, liver) of the recipient following bone marrow transplant. Pathology: granular necrosis of crypt epithelium.

Radiographic features
- Classic finding: small bowel loops, which are too narrow, and featureless margins (ribbon bowel)
- Luminal narrowing is due to edema of the bowel wall
- Flattening of mucosal folds (edema)
- Prolonged coating of barium for days

SCLERODERMA

Scleroderma or progressive systemic sclerosis (PSS) is a systemic disease that involves primarily skin, joints, and the GI tract (esophagus > small bowel > colon > stomach). Age: 30-50 years, female > male.

Radiographic features
Small bowel
- Dilation of bowel loops with hypomotility is a key feature.
- Mucosal folds are tight and closer together (fibrosis): hidebound appearance.
- Segmentation, fragmentation are absent.

Other
- Dilated dysmotile esophagus, eophagitis, incompetent LES, reflux, stricture
- Dilated duodenum and colon (pseudoobstruction)
- Pulmonary interstitial fibrosis
- Acroosteolysis
- Soft tissue calcification

WHIPPLE'S DISEASE

Rare multisystem disease, probably of bacterial origin. Organs primarily involved include: SI joints, joint capsule, heart valves, CNS, and jejunum. Clinical:
- Middle-aged men, USA, Northern Europe
- Diarrhea, steatorrhea
- Immune defects

Radiographic features
- 1-2 mm diffuse micronodules in jejunum
- No dilatation or increased secretions
- Nodal masses in mesentery (echogenic by US)
- Sacroileitis

WALDENSTRÖM'S MACROGLOBULINEMIA

Proliferation of malignant cells with lymphoplasmacytic morphology that secrete IgM components: lymph nodes; bone marrow, spleen. Intestinal involvement is rare, but tiny nodules ("sandlike") can be found in small bowel representing greatly distended villi.

ENTERIC FISTULAS

Fistulas of small bowel with adjacent structures are most common in Crohn's disease > colorectal cancer > postoperative diverticular disease. Types:
- Enteroenteric :   Small bowel → small bowel
- Enterocolonic: Small bowel → colon
- Enterocutaneous: Small bowel → skin
- Enterovesical: Small bowel → bladder
- Enterovaginal: Small bowel → vagina

Radiographic workup
- Fistulogram (enterocutaneous fistula): injection of water-soluble contrast material through small catheter inserted into fistula
- UGI and SBFT
- Barium enema

Therapy
- Total parenteral nutrition to achieve "bowel rest"
- Postoperative fistulas usually heal spontaneously with conservative measures
- Fistulas in active Crohn's disease usually require excision of diseased bowel
- Cyclosporin A and other immunosuppressants have been used to heal fistulas in Crohn's disease

INFECTIOUS ENTERITIS

COMMON RADIOGRAPHIC PRESENTATIONS	
Infection	**Common Radiographic Patterns**
PARASITES	
Hookworms (*Necator, Ancylostoma*)	TFN
Tapeworms	FD
Ascaris	FD, worms in GI tract visible; intestinal obstruction
INFECTIOUS	
Yersinia enterocolitica	TFN, ulcers, cobblestone in terminal ileum
TB	Stricture → obstruction
Histoplasmosis	TFN
Salmonellosis	TFN
Campylobacter	TFN, loss of haustration, may resemble Crohn's disease
COMMON IN AIDS	
Cytomegalovirus	TF in cecum, pancolitis
Tuberculosis	TF in cecum; adenopathy (low central attenuation)
MAI	TF in distal ileum, adenopathy (homogeneous)
Cryptosporidiosis	TFN, duodenum, jejunum, adenopathy
Giardiasis	TFN, largely jejunal, jejunal spasm

TFN, Thickened folds with nodularity; *TF,* thickened folds; *FD,* worm seen as filling defect in bowel; *MAI, Mycobacterium avium-intracellulare.*

Cryptosporidiosis
Protozoa that frequently causes enteritis in AIDS patients but rarely in immunocompetent patients. Diagnosis is made by examination of stool or duodenal aspirate.
Radiographic features
- Thickened small bowel folds
- Dilatation of small bowel

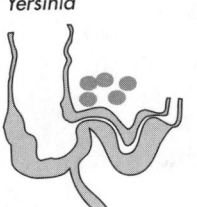 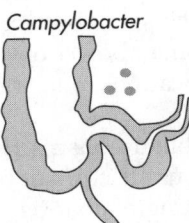 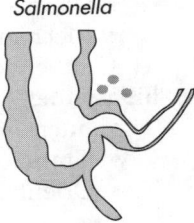

INTESTINAL HELMINTHS

OVERVIEW		
Organism (Treatment)	Route	Clinical
NEMATODE (MEBENDAZOLE)		
*Ascaris lumbricoides**	Fecal-oral	Intestinal, biliary obstruction, PIE
Ancylostoma duodenale	Skin penetration	Iron-deficiency anemia, PIE
Necator americanus	Skin penetration	Iron-deficiency anemia, PIE
Strongyloides stercoralis	Skin penetration	Malabsorption, PIE
Trichuris trichiura	Fecal-oral	Rectal prolapse
Enterobius vermicularis	Fecal-oral	
CESTODE (PRAZIQUANTEL)		
Beef tapeworm (*Taenia saginata*)	Raw beef	
Pork tapeworm (*Taenia solium*)	Raw pork	Cysticercosis: CNS
Fish tapeworm	Raw fish	Vitamin B_{12} deficiency
Dwarf tapeworm	Fecal-oral	Diarrhea
TREMATODE (PRAZIQUANTEL)		
Heterophyes heterophyes	Raw fish	Diarrhea
Metagonimus yokogawai	Raw fish	Diarrhea

PIE, Pulmonary infiltrates with eosinophilia; *CNS*, central nervous system.
*Worms in GI tract visible by barium studies.

Ascariasis

Ascaris lumbricoides (roundworm, 15-35 cm long) is the most common parasitic infection worldwide. Radiographic features:

GI tract
- Jejunum > ileum, duodenum, stomach
- Worms visible on SBFT as longitudinal filling defects
- Enteric canal of worm is filled with barium
- Worms may cluster: "bolus of worm"
- Mechanical small bowel obstruction (SBO)
- Other complications: perforation, volvulus

Biliary tract
- Intermittent biliary obstruction
- Granulomatous stricture of bile duct (rare)
- Oriental cholangiohepatitis

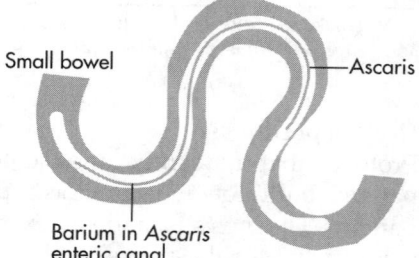

CARCINOID TUMORS

Carcinoid tumors arise from enterochromaffin cells. Location:

GI tract, 80%
- Appendix, 60% > small bowel, particularly distal 2 feet of ileum, 20%
- Uncommon: rectum, stomach
- Virtually never occur in esophagus

Bronchial tree, 15%
- 90% central, 10% peripheral

Other rare locations
- Thyroid
- Teratomas (ovarian, testicular)

Symptoms of GI carcinoids:
- Asymptomatic, 70%
- Obstruction, 20%
- Weight loss, 15%
- Palpable mass, 15%

Carcinoid syndrome

90% of patients with carcinoid syndrome have liver metastases. The tumor produces ACTH, histamine, bradykinin, kallikrein, serotonin (excreted as 5-HIAA in urine), causing:
- Recurrent diarrhea, 70%
- Right-sided endocardial fibroelastosis → tricuspid insufficiency, pulmonary valvular stenosis (left heart is spared because of metabolism by monoamine oxidase inhibitor in lung)
- Wheezing, bronchospasm, 15%
- Flushing of face and neck

Radiographic features
- Mass lesion in appendix or small bowel: filling defect
- Strong desmoplastic reaction causes angulation, kinking of bowel loops (tethered appearance), mesenteric venous congestion
- Mesenteric mass on CT with spoke wheel pattern is virtually pathognomonic; the only other disease that causes this appearance is mesenteric lipodystrophy (very rare)
- Stippled calcification in mesenteric mass
- Obstruction secondary to desmoplastic reaction
- Very vascular tumors (tumor blush at angiography, very hyperintense on T2-weighted images)
- Liver metastases (strong enhancement at CT)

Complications
- Ischemia with mesenteric venous compromise
- Hemorrhage
- Malignant degeneration
  Gastric and appendiceal tumors rarely metastasize.
  Small bowel tumors metastasize commonly.

Colon

General

BARIUM ENEMA (BE)

Patient preparation
- Clear liquid diet day before examination
- 300 cc magnesium citrate afternoon before examination
- 50 cc castor oil evening before examination
- Cleansing enema morning of examination

Single-contrast technique
1. Insert tube with patient in lateral position.
2. Decide if need to inflate balloon for retention; if so, inflate under fluoroscopic control, being sure that balloon is in the rectum.
3. Fluoroscopy as the barium goes in.
4. Patient in supine position (as opposed to double-contrast study). Instill barium just beyond sigmoid colon. Take AP and two oblique spot films of sigmoid.
5. Try to follow head of column fluoroscopically.
6. Take spot views of both splenic flexure and hepatic flexure.
7. Spot cecum and terminal ileum. If a filling defect is encountered, palpate to see if it is sessile or floating.
8. Obtain overhead views and postevacuation films.

Double-contrast technique
1. Patient is in lateral position. Insert tube.
2. Patient supine: administer glucagon IV. Turn patient prone: this helps barium flow to the descending colon, decreases pooling in the rectum and sigmoid and thereby is less uncomfortable. Instill barium beyond the splenic flexure. Stand patient up, bag to the floor, and let barium drain.
3. Place patient in horizontal prone position. Start slow inflation with air and rotate patient towards you into a supine position. Take spot views of the sigmoid in different obliquities (take spots of any air-filled loop). When patient is supine, check to see if barium has already coated the ascending colon.
4. Stand patient up to facilitate coating of ascending colon. Drain as much barium as possible through rectal tube. Insufflate more air.
5. Spot views of splenic and hepatic flexure in upright position. Take spots in slightly different obliquities of both flexures.
6. Patient prone, put table down. Take spot views of the cecum and sigmoid.
7. Obtain overhead views:
   AP, PA
   Prone, cross-table lateral
   Decubitus
   Postevacuation films

Contraindications to BE
- Suspected colonic perforation (use Gastrografin)
- Patients at risk for intraperitoneal leakage (use Gastrografin):
   Severe colitis
   Toxic megacolon
   Recent deep biopsy
- Colonoscopy *needs* to follow enema (use Gastrografin)
- Severe recent disease: myocardial infarction, cerebrovascular accident (CVA)

Complications of BE
- Perforation (incidence 1:5000), typically due to overinflation or traumatic insertion of balloon or fragile colonic walls
- Appearance of gas in portal venous system in patients with inflammatory bowel disease (no significant ill effects)
- Allergy to latex tips

Glucagon
Glucagon is a 29-aminoacid peptide produced in A cells of the pancreas. Physiologically, the main stimulus for glucagon release is hunger (hypoglycemia). Effects:
- Antagonist to insulin (increases blood glucose)
- Relaxation of smooth muscle cells
- Relaxation of gallbladder sphincter and sphincter of Oddi; increased bile flow

Glucagon is a useful adjunct (0.1-1 mg IV) to barium enema, or whenever smooth muscle spasm is present that may produce "pseudostenotic lesion." Thus it can be used in evaluation of the esophagus, stomach, duodenum, small intestine, common bile duct, and colon. Contraindications:

- Pheochromocytoma
- Insulinoma
- Glaucoma

Virtual colonscopy

- Abdominal axial CT images of air-distended colon taken in seconds during breath-holding are used to create two-dimensional multiplanar reformats and three-dimensional images of colon.
- Supine and prone images obtained during a single 35-40 second breath-hold continuous CT screening with low mA.
- Recent series report sensitivity and specificity ranging from 75%-91% and 90%-93%, respectively, for polyps $\geq$ 1 cm.
- Adequate bowel preparation similar to optical colonoscopy preferred.
- Examination begins by inflation of the colon with 1-2 L of either air or carbon dioxide.

Polyps

A wide variety of colonic polyps exist. Nonneoplastic, hyperplastic polyps have been cited as the most frequent type for a long time. More recently, however, neoplastic adenomas have become more common.

OVERVIEW		
	Single Polyp	**Multiple Polyps**
NEOPLASTIC		
Epithelial	Tubular adenoma	Familial polyposis
	Tubulovillous adenoma	Gardner's syndrome
	Villous adenoma	
	Turcot's syndrome	
Nonepithelial	Carcinoid	
	Leiomyoma	
	Lipoma	
	Fibroma	
NONNEOPLASTIC		
Hamartomas	Juvenile polyposis	
	Peutz-Jeghers syndrome	Cronkhite-Canada syndrome
Inflammatory	Benign lymphoid polyp	Juvenile polyp, benign lymphoid polyp
	Fibroid granulation polyp	Granulomatous colitis
Unclassified	Hyperplastic polyp	Hyperplastic polyposis

ADENOMATOUS POLYPS

Most common true colonic tumor (in up to 10% of the population by the 7th decade). Up to 50% of polyps are multiple. Symptoms: asymptomatic, diarrhea, pain, hemorrhage.

TYPES OF ADENOMATOUS POLYPS			
	Tubular	Tubulovillous	Villous
Frequency	75%	15%	10%
Malignancy potential			
< 10 mm	1%	5%	10%
> 20 mm	30%	40%	50%

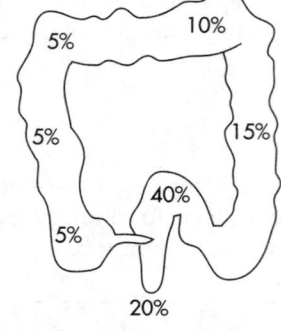

Location
- Rectum and sigmoid, 60%
- Descending colon, 15%
- Transverse colon, 15%
- Ascending colon, 10%

Differentiation of benign and malignant polyps

Histological differentiation of polyps is invariably difficult radiographically, so the majority of lesions require endoscopical sampling.

BENIGN VS. MALIGNANT POLYP		
Feature	Benign	Malignant
Size*	< 1 cm	> 2 cm
Stalk	Present (pedunculated, thin)	Absent (sessile)
Contour	Smooth	Irregular, lobulated
Number	Single	Multiple
Underlying colonic wall	Smooth	Indented, retracted

*The larger the size of any polyp, the more likely it is malignant: < 1 cm: 1%, 1-2 cm: 25%, > 2 cm: > 40%.

HYPERPLASTIC POLYPS

Focal proliferation of normal mucosa, hence not a true tumor. Hyperplastic polyps have no malignant potential. Hyperplastic polyps are due to excessive cellular proliferation in Lieberkühn's crypts. 75% of polyps occur distal to the splenic flexure mostly in the rectosigmoid area.

Radiographic appearance
- Stalked polyp
- Sessile but < 5 mm

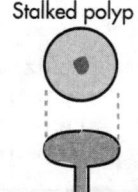

Stalked polyp

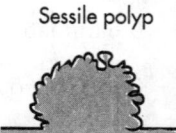

Sessile polyp

POSTINFLAMMATORY POLYPS (PIP)

Postinflammatory polyposis (pseudopolypopsis, filiform polyps) represent a benign condition, not associated with cancer. PIP occur most commonly in Crohn's disease, ulcerative colitis.

Radiographic features
- Filiform polyps: thin, short, branching structures

DIFFERENTIATION OF TRUE POLYPS FROM PSEUDOPOLYPS		
	Polyp	**Pseudopolyp**
Size	Uniform in size	Uniform in size
Form	Round, stalked, sessile	Y-shaped, filiform, irregular
Margins	Well delineated	Fuzzy (inflammation)
Colonic haustra	Preserved	Distorted (inflammation)

POLYPOSIS SYNDROMES

OVERVIEW							
Type	**Trait**	**Gastric**	**SB**	**Colon**	**Histology**	**GI Malignancy**	**Extraintestinal**
Familial polyposis	AD	< 5%	< 5%	100%	Adenoma	100%	—
Gardner's	AD	5%	5%	100%	Adenoma	100%	Osteoma, others*
Peutz-Jeghers	AD	25%	95%	30%	Hamartoma	Rare	Perioral pigmentation
Juvenile polyposis	AD	—	—	100%	Inflammatory	?	—
Turcot's†	AR	—	—	100%	Adenoma	100%	Glioma
Cronkhite-Canada	NH	100%	50%	100%	Inflammatory	None	Ectodermal changes
Cowden†	AD	—	—	—	Hamartoma	None	Oral papilloma‡
Ruvalcaba-Myhre†	AD	yes	yes	yes	Hamartoma	None	Macrocephaly, penile macules, mental retardation, SC lipomas

AD, Autosomal dominant; *AR*, autosomal recessive; *NH*, nonhereditary; *SB*, small bowel.
*Soft tissue tumors, sarcomas, ampullary carcinoma, ovarian carcinoma.
†Extremely rare.
‡Gingival hyperplasia, breast cancer, thyroid cancer.

Familial polyposis
- Most common intestinal polyposis syndrome (incidence 1:8000)
- Screening of family members of familial polyposis should start at puberty: malignant degeneration by 40 years (treatment: prophylactic total proctocolectomy)
- Usually > 100 polyps
- Polyps may be sessile or stalked
- Familial adenomatous polyposis syndrome (FAPS) is a common umbrella name under which Gardner's and familial polyposis syndrome are included.

Gardner's syndrome
- Polyposis: colon 100%, duodenum 90%, other bowel segments < 10%
- Hamartomas of stomach
- Soft tissue tumors: inclusion cysts, desmoids (30%), fibrosis
- Osteoma in calvarium, mandible, sinuses
- Entrapment of cranial nerves
- Malignant transformation in 100% if untreated
- Small bowel and pancreaticoduodenal malignancies
- Total colectomy recommended

Peutz-Jeghers syndrome
- Second most common intestinal polyposis
- Autosomal dominant
- Hamartomas througout GI tract except the esophagus
- Mucocutaneous pigmentations (buccal mucosa, palm, sole)
- Polyps have virtually no malignant potential
- Slightly increased risk of stomach, duodenal, ovarian cancer; benign neoplasm of testes, thryoid and GU system

Juvenile polyposis
- Usually large polyps in rectum
- Usually single; 80% are located in the rectosigmoid
- Present in children with bleeding, prolapse, or obstruction

Cowden disease
- Multiple hamartoma syndrome
- Mucocutaneous pigmentations (buccal mucosa, palm, sole)
- Most commonly in rectosigmoid with lesions also present in esopahgus
- Mucocutaneous lesions → facial papules, oral mucosal papillomatosis, acral keratoses, sclerotic fibromas
- Thyroid gland abnormalities: goiter, adenomas
- Breast cancer (ductal), bilateral in 30%
- Uterine and cervical carcinomas
- Transitional cell carcinoma of bladder and ureter

Lhermite-Duclos disease
- Gangliocytoma of cerebellar cortex

Turcot's syndrome
- Gliomapolyposis syndrome
- Colonic adenomas with CNS gliomas and medulloblastomas

Colon Carcinoma

GENERAL

Second most common cancer (men most common: lung; women most common: breast). Risk factor: low-carbohydrate diet? Synchronous lesions 5%, metachronous lesions 3%.

High-risk groups
- Polyp: the larger the size of a polyp, the more likely it is malignant: < 1 cm: 1%, 1-2 cm: 25%, > 2 cm: > 40%
- Polyposis syndromes (especially familial polyposis, Gardner's)
- Ulcerative colitis, less commonly Crohn's disease
- Positive family history of colon cancer
- Positive family history of endometrial or breast cancer
- Ureterosigmoidostomy

Location
- Rectum, 35%
- Sigmoid, 25%
- Descending colon, 10%
- Ascending colon, 10%
- Transverse colon, 10%
- Cecum, 10%

Radiographic features
- Polypoid
- Ulcerative
- Annular constricting (apple core); < 5 cm long
- Plaquelike (e.g., cloacogenic tumor at anorectal junction)
- Scirrhous carcinoma (rare): long (> 5 cm) circumferential spread

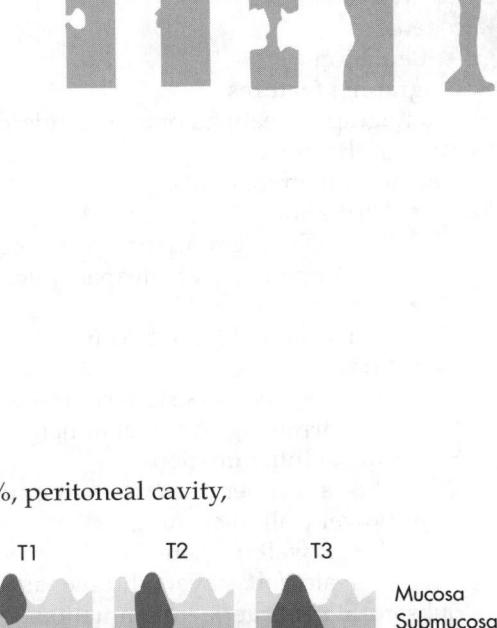

Complications
- Obstruction
- Intussusception (in polypoid lesions), rare
- Local perforation (simulates diverticulitis)
- Local tumor recurrence in 30%-50%
- Peritoneal spread

Staging

Dukes staging system
- Dukes A: limited to bowel wall, 15%
- Dukes B: extension into serosa or mesenteric fat, 35%
- Dukes C: lymph node metastases, 50%
- Dukes D: distant metastases: liver, 25%, hydronephrosis, 10%, peritoneal cavity, adrenal, 10%

TNM classification system
- T1: mucosa or submucosa only
- T2: invasion of muscularis propria
- T3: invasion into subserosa
- T4: invasion into adjacent structures, fistula
- N1: 1-3 regional (pericolic) lymph nodes
- N2: ≥ 4 regional nodes distant lymph nodes
- N3: lymph nodes along named vascular trunk
- M: metastases

Diagnostic accuracy

Detection of lymph node metastases
- CT: 50%-70%
- MR currently < CT

Detection of liver metastases
- Contrast enhanced CT: 60%-70%
- MRI: 70%-80%

Colitis

Etiology
Idiopathic inflammatory bowel disease
- Ulcerative colitis (UC)
- Crohn's disease
- Behçet's disease

Infectious colitis
Ischemic colitis
Iatrogenic
- Radiation

Radiographic features
The radiographic features of bowel inflammation (any etiology) depend mainly on the location of the process:

Mucosal inflammation
- Ulceration
    Shallow: granularity of mucosa, aphthoid
    Deeper: discrete deeper collections of barium: collar button
- Edema
    Displacement of barium: translucent halo around central ulcer
- Spasm
    Localized persistent contraction
    Narrowing of bowel lumen

Submucosal inflammation
- Ulcers (deeper linear than in mucosal inflammation): cobblestone appearance
- Bowel wall thickening
    CT: wall thickened (> 3 mm with lumen distended)
    Halo: fatty layer (chronic) and/or gray (acute) halo stratification

Subserosal mesenteric inflammation
- Stranding in surrounding fat
- Inflammatory mass
- Fistula
- Creeping fat: excessive fat deposited around serosal surface (Crohn's disease)

CROHN'S DISEASE (REGIONAL ENTERITIS)

Recurrent inflammatory condition of bowel of unknown etiology. Lesions may occur in the entire GI tract but are most common in:
- Small bowel (especially terminal ileum): 80%
    30% only small bowel involved
    50% small bowel and colon involved
- Colon 70%
    25% of patients with colonic disease have pancolitis
        (entire colon affected)
- Duodenum 20%

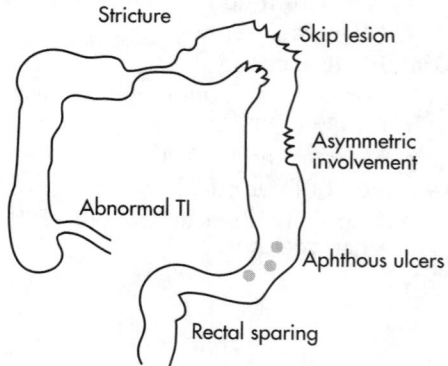

Pathological development of lesions: initial event → hyperplasia of lymphoid tissue in submucosa → lymphedema → aphthoid ulcerations → deeper ulcers → fistulas, abscesses → strictures

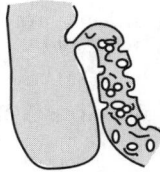 Nodular pattern ("cobblestone")

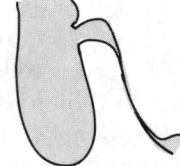 String sign

Radiographic features

Type of lesions

- Thickening of folds (edema)
- Nodular pattern (submucosal edema and inflammation)
- String sign: tubular narrowing of intestinal lumen (edema, spasm, scarring depending on chronicity)
- Ulcerations:
    - Aphthoid ulcers are early lesions and correspond to mucosal erosions (pinpoint ulcer in edematous mound up to 3 mm in diameter and 2 mm in depth).
    - Ulcers are irregularly scattered throughout GI tract and are interspersed with normal mucosa.
    - Ulcerations grow and fuse with each other in linear fashion and, with intervening edematous mucosa produce an ulceronodular pattern ("cobblestone" appearance).
- Filiform polyposis: thin, elongated, branching mucosal lesions; represents proliferative sequella of mucosa adjacent to denuded surface.
- Sinus tracts and fistulas originate in fissures or deep ulcers; characteristic of Crohn's disease at advanced stages.
- Fatty thickening and/or retraction of the mesentery. Mass (creeping fat, lymphadenopathy) effect may separate bowel loops or make loops display a concentric shape (omega sign).
- Fibrosis and scarring may result in:
    - Pseudodiverticula (fibrosis develops eccentrically)
    - Rigid, featureless bowel
    - Strictures and obstruction
    - Foreshortening of bowel

Spatial arrangement of lesions

- Transitional zones are typical; they occur between involved bowel loops and normal bowel
- Skip lesions are typical: discontinuous involvement of bowel
- Lesions appear preferentially at mesenteric side of intestine

Mural and extramural changes (CT findings)

Primary intestinal findings

- Bowel wall thickening
    - Normally < 3 mm if well distended
    - Mean diameter in Crohn's disease: 10 mm
    - If >> 10 mm include pseudomembranous, ischemic, or CMV colitis in differential diagnosis
- Circumferential submucosal low attenuation surrounded by higher outer attenuation: halo sign.
- Inner and outer layers surrounding low attenuation middle layer: target sign; middle layer of fat density: chronic, middle layer of water density

Peribowel inflammation ("dirty fat," "ground glass")

Mesentery

- Fat accumulates on serosal surfaces ("creeping fat")
- Inflamed mesentery fat (stranding, "misty")
- Adenopathy in small bowel mesentery common

Extraintestinal findings
- Gallstones
- Osseous complications (may cause pain)
  > Spondylitis
  > Sacroileitis
  > Steroid complications: osteomyelitis, osteoporosis, avascular necrosis
- Renal stones, 7%

Complications
- Recurrence of disease after surgery (in contrast to UC where proctocolectomy is curative)
- Increased incidence of malignancies:
  > GI tract tumors
  > Lymphoma
- Toxic megacolon
- Fistulas
- Abscess formation

ULCERATIVE COLITIS (UC)

Unknown etiology. Clinical: diarrhea, rectal bleeding. Disease affects primarily mucosa (crypt abscesses) and typically starts in rectum. Associated findings:

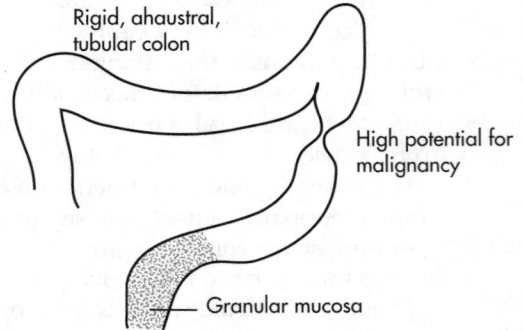

Rigid, ahaustral, tubular colon

High potential for malignancy

Granular mucosa

- Joints, 25%: arthritis, arthralgia, ankylosing spondylitis
- Liver, 10%: sclerosing cholangitis, chronic active hepatitis, cholangiocarcinoma
- Skin: pyoderma gangrenosum, erythema nodosum
- Uveitis, episcleritis

Radiographic features
Ahaustral, foreshortened colon (leadpipe)
Granular mucosa, shallow confluent ulcerations
Polyps:
- Pseudopolyps
- Filiform polyps (regenerative mucosa, small thin, branching polyps)

Spread:
- Disease first and worst in rectum
- Continuous spread from distal to proximal colon
- Circumferential bowel involvement
- Backwash ileitis: only short segment of terminal ileum unlike Crohn's disease, gaping ileocecal valve

Atypical radiographic features:
- Atypical pattern of distribution: sparing of rectum (which may be healing), 5%
- Crohn-like findings: discontinuous disease in 5%-10% of patients

Mural and extramural changes (CT findings)
- Bowel wall thickening less than Crohn's disease
- Distribution from rectum continuously proximal
- If pancolitus, terminal ilium may be affected for a very short length
- Halo, target signs may coexist
- Superimposed carcinoma: mass lesion or thick wall stricture
- Excessive fat surrounding rectum
- Local lymph node enlargement; rare in SB mesentery or retroperitoneum

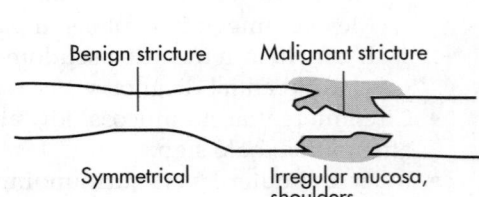

Crypt abscess   Sessile mucosal polyp   Mucosal bridge of deep ulcer

Mucosa
Submucosa
Muscularis

Collar button ulcer   Postinflammatory pseudopolyp

Benign stricture   Malignant stricture

Symmetrical   Irregular mucosa, shoulders

Complications

- Toxic megacolon: transverse colon: > 6 cm
- Strictures, obstruction: benign or malignant. Any stricture is suspicious for malignancy
- Malignancy (5- to 30-fold higher risk than general population)
- Annual incidence of 10% after the first decade
- Multiple in 25% of cases
- Often flat and scirrhous

SYNOPSIS		
	Crohn's Disease	**Ulcerative Colitis**
GENERAL FEATURES		
Distribution	Skip lesions, entire GI tract	Confined to colon, terminal ileum
Symmetry	Eccentric	Concentric
Ulcers	Early: aphthoid ulcers (mucosa) Late: deep ulcers (submucosa)	Superficial
Fistula	Common	Rare
Pseudopolyps	Yes	20%
Toxic dilatation	Uncommon	Common
Strictures	Yes	Yes
INVOLVEMENT		
Rectum	50%	95%
Anus	Perianal fistula and fissures	Normal
Terminal ileum	Narrowed, inflamed, fissured (cobblestone)	Dilated and wide open (backwash ileitis), gaping valve
OTHER		
Surgery	May exacerbate disease	Curative
Cancer risk	Uncommon	High
Recurrence	Common	Not after colectomy
CLINICAL FINDINGS		
Diarrhea	++++	++++
Rectal bleeding	+++	++++
Pain	++++	+++
Weight loss	++	++
Fever	+++	+
Abdominal mass	++++	−
Malnutrition	+++	+

INFECTIOUS COLITIS

Some agents more commonly cause superficial lesions (similar to UC), and some are more likely to cause transmural inflammation (similar to Crohn's disease). Infectious colitis is common in immunocompromised hosts.

ETIOLOGIES OF INFECTIOUS COLITIS		
Pathogen	**Pattern**	**Comments**
Campylobacter	SU	Usually in distal colon
Shigella	SU	Most severe in rectosigmoid
Salmonella	SU	Confined to colon
Gonococcus	SU	Rectum
Amebiasis	SU, DU	Diffuse but most severe in right colon, (ameboma), small bowel rarely affected
Tuberculosis	DU	Loss of demarcation between cecum and TI ileum (Stierlin sign); lymph nodes
Lymphogranuloma venereum	DU	Rectal strictures typical
Yersinia	DU	Typically terminal ileum, cecum
Strongyloides	DU	Duodenum, jejunum > colon
Trichuris trichiura (whipworm)		Rectal prolapse
Schistosomiasis		Hepatosplenomegaly
Chagas' disease		Megacolon, megaesophagus

SU, Superficial ulcers (UC-like); *DU,* deep ulcers (Crohn-like).

CYTOMEGALOVIRUS (CMV) COLITIS

Occurs mainly in immunocompromised hosts. Variable radiographic features:
- Superficial (aphthoid) or deep ulcers
- Thick wall: > 10 mm
- Localized distribution in cecum, terminal ileum or universal colitis
- Radiographically, may be indistinguishable from pseudomembranous colitis

TYPHLITIS (NEUTROPENIC COLITIS)

Acute necrotizing colitis involving the cecum, terminal ileum, and ascending colon in patients with leukemia undergoing therapy and/or immunosuppression. Incidence in autopsy series of young leukemia patients is 10%-25%. The disease may also involve the terminal ileum, ascending colon, and/or appendix. Clinical: RLQ pain 50%, diarrhea 40%, peritoneal signs in perforation. Cause: unknown pathogenesis (leukemic bowel infiltration, intramural hemorrhage, necrosis, local ischemia). Indications for surgery: failed medical therapy, perforation, hemorrhage, pericecal abscess, uncontrolled sepsis.

Radiographic features
- Marked thickening of cecum, terminal ileum and/or ascending colon
- Pericecal fluid, soft tissue stranding is more marked than in pseudomembranous colitis.
- Pneumatosis
- Complications
    Perforation
    Pericolonic abscess
    Pneumatosis

PSEUDOMEMBRANOUS COLITIS (PMC)

Colitis caused by colonic overgrowth of *Clostridium difficile* 1-6 weeks after administration of antibiotics (clindamycin , lincomycin > tetracycline, ampicillin; much less common causes: *Staphylococcus*, steroids, chemotherapeutic agents). Clinical: diarrhea, fever, pain, leukocytosis.

Radiographic features
Plain films, abnormal in 40%
- Thumbprinting, 40%
- Ileus, 40%
- Megacolon, <20%

CT, abnormal in 60%
- Very thick (average 15 mm) colonic wall but preserved, thickened haustra (plaques, ulcers, edema)
- Contrast between thickened folds (accordion sign)
- Usually starts in rectum and progresses retrograde
- Largely left-sided disease, may be pancolitic
- Pericolonic fat changes, 35%
- Ascites, 35%

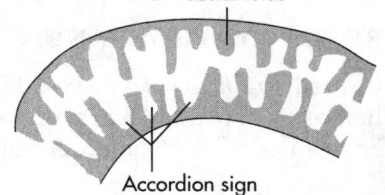

Thick haustal folds

Accordion sign

AMEBIASIS

Infection with *Entamoeba histolytica.* Common in Mexico, South America, Africa, and Asia. Clinical: diarrhea (bloody), fever, may be asymptomatic for long times.
Transmission: direct person to person, contaminated water or food.

Radiographic features
Colon
- Cecum, right colon > transverse colon > rectosigmoid
- Ulcers: initially punctate then confluent
- Coned cecum
- Stenosis from healing and fibrosis
- Ameboma: hyperplastic granuloma (in 1% of cases)
- Pericolic inflammation

Other
- Fistula formation
- Intussusception due to ameboma (children)
- Liver abscess (very painful)
- Pleuropulmonary abscess
- Brain abscess
- Cutaneous extension (perianal region)

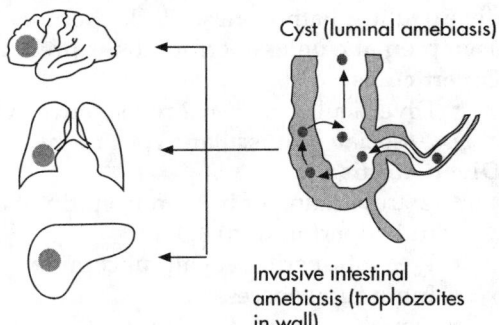

Extraintestinal amebiasis

Cyst (luminal amebiasis)

Invasive intestinal amebiasis (trophozoites in wall)

INTESTINAL TUBERCULOSIS (TB)

Types:
- Primary intestinal TB
    Mycobacterium avium-intracellulare (AIDS)
    M. bovis (cow milk)
- Hematogeneous spread from pulmonary TB
    Location: cecum > colon > jejunum > stomach

Radiographic features
- Narrowed terminal ileum (Stierlin's sign)
- Bowel wall thickening
- Ulcers, fissures, fistulas, stricture
- Marked hypertrophy: ileocecal valve (Fleischner sign)

COLITIS CYSTICA PROFUNDA

Benign disease characterized by the presence of submucosal, fluid-fillled cysts. The disease is most commonly localized to the rectum (85%). Cysts can be up to 3 cm in size. Diagnosis is made histologically by exclusion of malignancy (cystic mucinous adenocarcinoma).

RECTAL LYMPHOGRANULOMA VENERUM

Caused by *Chlamydia trachomatis*. Transmitted by sexual contact, usually in homosexual men. Major symptom is bleeding. Purulent inflammation of inguinal lymph nodes. Frei's intradermal test.

Other Colonic Diseases

DIVERTICULAR DISEASE

Colonic diverticulae represent mucosal and submucosal outpouchings through the muscularis. Outpouchings occur mainly where vessels pierce the muscularis, (i.e., between mesenteric and antimesenteric taenia). 95% of diverticula are located in sigmoid, in 20% the proximal colon also, never rectum. Perforation causes diverticulitis. Pathogenesis: lack of crude fiber in diet? Clinical: asymptomatic unless perforation is present: pain, fever > bleeding.

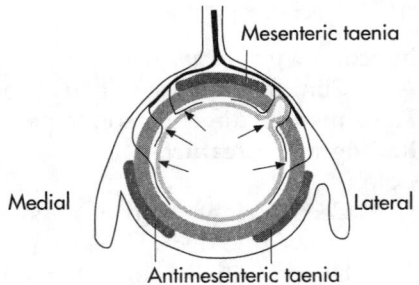

Diverticulosis
- Diverticula occur in 2 rows between taenia
- Associated muscular hypertrophy

Diverticulitis
- Extravasation of barium from tip of diverticulum (microperforation), 20%
- Free intraperitoneal air: uncommon
- Intramural abscess
- Double tracking (intramural fistula): uncommon
- Fistula to bladder, uterus 10%
- Pericolic mass (extrinsic compression)
- Muscular hypertrophy, 25%
- Local penetration may lead to coexistent small bowel obstruction

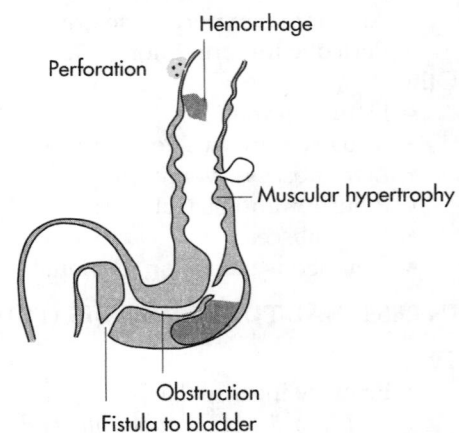

Pearls
- Disease common and worse in patients on steroids
- Isolated giant sigmoidal diverticulum is a rare entity caused by ball-valve mechanism
- Diverticulitis may be present without radiographically apparent diverticula

GIANT SIGMOID DIVERTICULUM

The characteristical radiological feature is a large balloonlike gas-filled structure in lower abdomen; located centrally with no obvious connection to the sigmoid. Although rare, it is important to differentiate from sigmoid and cecal volvulus.

Complications
- Diverticulitis
- Small bowel obstruction due to adhesions
- Perforation
- Volvulus of diverticulum

APPENDIX

The appendix is located about 3 cm below the ileocecal valve on the medial wall. Common abnormalities:

Inflammation
- Appendicitis

Tumor
- Mucocele (abnormal accumulation of mucus: rupture leads to pseudomyxoma peritonei)
- Cystadenoma, cystadenocarcinoma, adenocarcinoma
- Carcinoid (usually small tumor found incidentally at surgery)

APPENDICITIS

Appendicitis occurs secondary to obstruction of the appendiceal lumenvenous obstruction → ischemia → bacterial invasion → necrosis. Classic clinical signs are absent in one-third of adults. Common causes of obstruction are:
- Appendicolith
- Lymphoid hypertrophy
- Tumor
- Intestinal worms (usually *Ascaris*)

Radiographic features

Plain film
- Calcified appendicolith, 10%
- Focal ileus
- Abscess

Barium enema
- Nonfilling of appendix; complete filling excludes appendicitis
- Mass effect on cecum, terminal ileum

CT
- Appendix thickness > 6 mm
- Calcified appendicolith, 30%
- Stranding of fat (subtle important finding)
- Asymmetric cecal wall thickening
- Lymph nodes in mesoappendix

US
- Total appendiceal thickness > 6 mm
- Noncompressible appendix
- > 3 mm wall thickness
- Shadowing appendicolith

Choice of imaging study
- US (lower sensitivity than CT): children, pregnant women
- CT: all other patients, symptoms present > 48 hours

MUCOCELE OF THE APPENDIX

Accumulation of mucus within abnormally distended appendix. Most cases are due to tumor (mucinous cystadenocarcinoma), whereas other cases are due to an obstructed orifice.

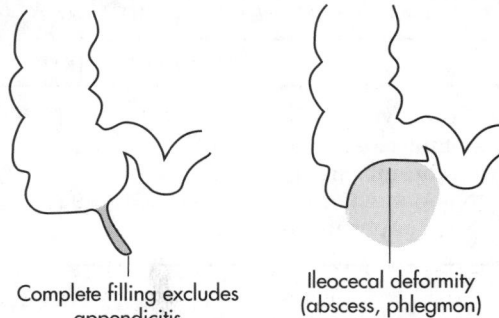

Normal   < 4 mm

Thick wall Noncompressible   > 4 mm

Appendicolith   >6 mm

Transducer

Radiographic features

- Nonfilling of appendix
- Smooth, rounded appendiceal mass
- Curvilinear calcification

ISCHEMIC BOWEL DISEASE

Basic underlying mechanism is hypoxemia that can be caused in small bowel by:

- Arterial occlusion (thrombotic, embolic, vasculitis), 40%
- Low flow states (reversible, nonocclusive), 50%
- Venous thrombosis, 10%

Ischemic bowel disease may occur in either superior mesenteric artery (SMA) or inferior mesenteric artery (IMA) distribution, or both.

CAUSES OF ISCHEMIC BOWEL DISEASE			
	SMA	IMA	SMV
Occlusive	40%	5%	
Embolus			
Thrombosis			10%
Nonocclusive	50%	95%	
Hypoperfusion			

Radiographic features

SMA distribution

- Sick patients, hypotension, acidosis: high mortality
- Requires surgery, resection
- Plain film findings similar to SBO; may see "pink-prints" in wall
- Submucosal edema > pneumatosis > portal vein gas, 5%

IMA distribution

- Patients not very sick (mimics diverticulitis)
- Usually affects 1-3 feet of colon (splenic flexure to sigmoid)
- Rectum involved: 15%
- Invariably nonocclusive etiology
- Thumbprinting: hemorrhage and edema in wall
- Rarely pancolonic in distribution
- May also cause ulceration
- Conservative treatment: heals spontaneously, strictures rare
- CT: halo or target signs

VOLVULUS

Location: sigmoid >> cecum >> transverse colon. Predisposing factors: redundant loops of bowel, elongated mesentery, chronic colonic distention. Diagnostic study: barium enema.

Sigmoid volvulus

- Massively dilated sigmoid loop (inverted U) projects from pelvis to upper quadrant
- Proximal colonic dilatation is typical, but not always present
- Typically occurs in elderly constipated patients

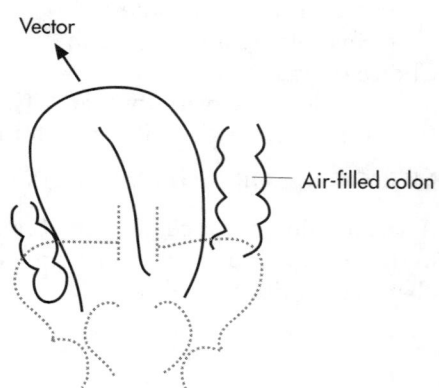

Radiographic features
- Massively dilated; devoid of haustra; U-shaped form
- Left flank overlap sign: overlies haustrated left colon
- Liver overlap sign: overlaps lower margin of liver
- Apex above T10
- Apex lies under left hemidiaphragm
- Inferior convergence on left

Cecal volvulus
- Massively dilated cecum rotates toward midabdomen and left upper quadrant (LUQ)
- Associated small bowel dilatation
- Through foramen of Winslow: lesser sac hernia

Cecal bascule
- Mobile cecum is folded across the lower midabdomen horizontally.
- May mimic cecal volvulus but more likely located in pelvis and small bowel not dilated.

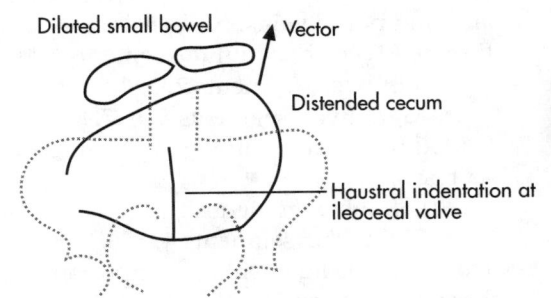

PSEUDOOBSTRUCTION OF THE LARGE BOWEL (OGILVIE'S SYNDROME)

Dilatation of colon in elderly patients. Often history of cathartic abuse, anti-parkinson's medication, or metabolic abnormalities.

Radiographic features
- Dilated, ahaustral colon
- Often affects just proximal colon
- No mechanical obstruction
- Barium enema is the diagnostic study of choice

TOXIC MEGACOLON (TMC)

Severe dilation of the transverse colon that occurs when inflammation spreads from the mucosa through other layers of the colon. The colon becomes a peristaltic and can perforate, carrying a 30% mortality rate. Treatment: anyone with UC or Crohn's disease serious enough to be at risk for toxic megacolon should be hospitalized and be closely monitored; many patients require surgery. Underlying causes:
- UC (most common cause)
- Other colitides (uncommon): Crohn's, pseudomembranous colitis, ischemic, infectious (CMV, amebiasis)

Radiographic features
- Dilated (> 6 cm), transverse colon
- Ahaustral irregular colonic contour; may show intraluminal soft tissue masses (pseudopolyps)
- BE contraindicated in TMC; proceed to proctoscopy; gravity maneuvers (patient in prone, decubitus position) for plain film assessment
- Diameter of transverse colon should reduce as successful treatment proceeds

Liver

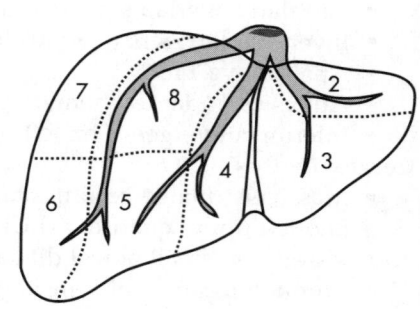

General

LIVER ANATOMY

The liver is anatomically subdivided into 8 segments, landmarked by hepatic and portal veins. Nomenclature:

Europe (liver divided into segments by hepatic veins)
- Left liver: segments 2, 3, 4
- Right liver: segments 5, 6, 7, 8

United States (liver divided by main lobar fissure 5, gallbladder fossa)
- Left lobe: segments 2, 3
- Right lobe: segments 4, 5, 6, 7, 8

Three hepatic ligaments are important because of their marker function (ligaments appear very hyperechoic relative to liver) in US.

HEPATIC LIGAMENTS

OVERVIEW		
Ligament	Location	Landmark
Falciform ligament	Extends from umbilicus to diaphragm	Divides medial and lateral segments of left lobe
Ligamentum teres (round ligament = obliterated umbilical vein)	Hyperechoic structure in left lobe	Gastroesophageal junction
Main lobar fissure (major fissure, interlobar fissure, oblique ligament)	Extends from GB to porta hepatis	Divides right and left hepatic lobe (United States)
Fissure of ligamentum venosum	Between caudate lobe and lateral segment of left lobe	Contains hepatogastric ligament

Ligaments and spaces

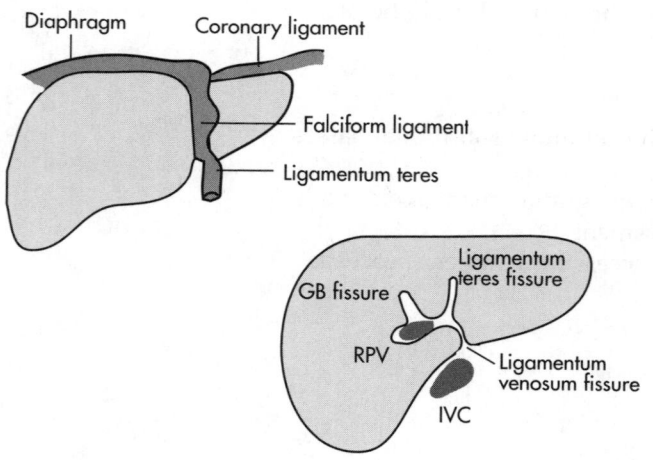

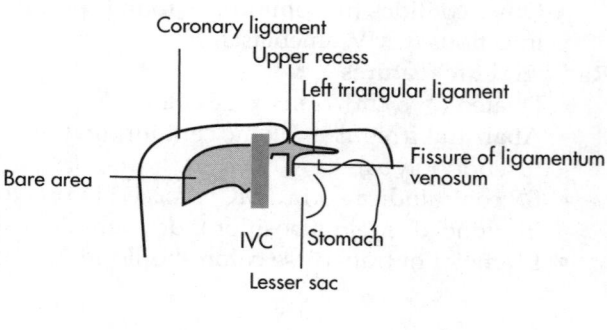

US Doppler waveforms

Hepatic veins
- Triphasic flow pattern
- Arterial contraction (right ventricle)

Portal vein
- Low velocity (10-20 cm/sec) flow pattern
- Respiratory variation present
- Pulsation in portal vein flow is seen in tricuspid regurgitation

Hepatic artery
- Low impedance
- Arterial flow pattern
- Same flow direction as portal vein

Types of contrast-enhanced CT techniques (CECT)

Blood flow and contrast material
- Hepatic artery, contributes 25% of blood flow to liver
- Portal vein, contributes 75% of blood flow to liver
- Most tumors have only arterial blood supply

Dynamic bolus CT (portal venous phase imaging for hypovascular lesions)
- 120-150 mL at 2 mL/sec
- 40-second delay for conventional CT
- 80-second delay for helical CT

Dynamic bolus CT (arterial phase imaging for hypervascular lesions)
- 20-second delay at 3-5 mL/sec
- Transient hyperattenuation of liver may be present (predominant arterial supply, decreased portal supply)
- Then 80-sec delay as in PVP

Delayed equilibrium CT
- 10-20 minutes after contrast administration
- Retention of contrast may be observed in cholangiocarcinoma, fibrous tumors or scars

Delayed high dose CT
- 60 g of iodine total
- 1%-2% of contrast material is excreted through liver
- 4-6 hrs after injection, liver parenchyma is 20 HU increased

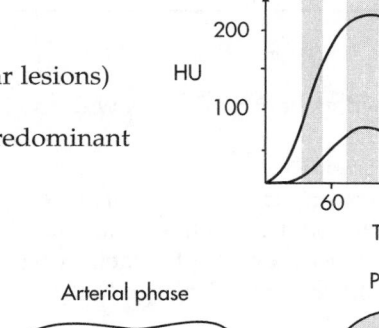

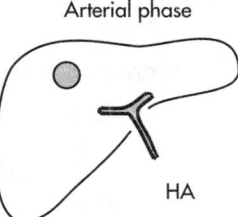

Arterial phase

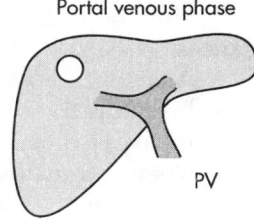

Portal venous phase

Diffuse Liver Disease

HEPATITIS

Causes

Viral hepatitis
- Hepatitis A, B, non-A non-B, delta
- Other viruses: cytomegalovirus, Epstein-Barr, herpes simplex, rubella, yellow fever

Chemical hepatitis
- Alcohol
- Drugs: INH, halothane, chlorpromazine, diphenylhydantoin, methyldopa, acetaminophen
- Toxins such as CCl_4

US features
- GB wall thickening may occur
- Increased echogenicity of portal triads in acute hepatitis, decreased echogenicity in chronic hepatitis
- Echogenicity: patterns are difficult to evaluate and there exists considerable interobserver variability; only fatty liver substantially increases echogenicity of the liver:

ECHOGENICITY OF LIVER	
Disease	Echogenicity
Hepatitis	±
Fatty liver	+++
Cirrhosis	±

CIRRHOSIS

Cirrhosis is defined as hepatic fibrosis with the formation of nodules that lack a central vein.

Types
- Chronic sclerosing cirrhosis: minimal regenerative activity of hepatocytes, little nodule formation, liver is hard and small
- Nodular cirrhosis: regenerative activity with presence of many small nodules, initially the liver may be enlarged

Causes
- Alcoholic (most common, Laënnec's cirrhosis)
- Hepatitis B
- Biliary cirrhosis
- Hemochromatosis
- Rare causes
     Wilson's disease
     Alpha$_1$-antitrypsin deficiency
     Drug induced

Radiographic features

Liver US features
- Small liver, increased echogenicity, coarse, heterogenous
- Nodular surface
- Regenerating nodules: hypoechoic
- Unequal distribution of cirrhosis in different segments (sparing):
     Left lobe appears larger than right lobe
     Lateral segment of left lobe (segments 2, 3) enlarges, medial segment (segments 4A, 4B) shrinks
     The ratio of the width of the caudate lobe (segment 1) to the right hepatic lobe (segments 5 and 6 or 7 and 8) is > 0.6

Portal hypertension (hepatic wedge pressure > 10 mm Hg)
- Collaterals: left gastric, paraesophageal, mesenteric, retroperitoneal veins, splenorenal
- Splenomegaly
- Ascites

Complications
- Hepatocellular carcinoma (HCC) occurs in 10% of patients with cirrhosis; hemangiomas are much less common: 2%. In cirrhotic livers, HCC is best detected by helical CT or dynamic contrast MRI during arterial phase; delayed CT or noncontrast MRI has much lower sensitivity in lesion detection
- Esophageal varices with bleeding

FATTY LIVER

Causes
- Obesity (most common cause)
- Alcohol
- Hyperalimentation
- Debilitation
- Chemotherapy
- Hepatitis
- Steroids, Cushing's syndrome

Radiographic findings

General
- Uniform decrease in density compared to vessels
- Fatty infiltration is usually geographical (straight borders) in distribution but may occasionally have all features of a tumor
- Focal fatty "mass" also occurs, most commonly adjacent to falciform ligament, usually anterolateral edge of medial segment
- Areas of fatty liver are interspersed with normal liver
- Lack of mass effect: vessel distribution and architecture are preserved in areas of fat
- Rapid change with time: fat appearance or resolution may be as fast as 6 days
- Common areas of fatty sparing:
  Segment 1 (periportal region)
  Segment 4 (medial segment of left lobe)

US
- Fat increases liver echogenicity
- Visual criteria (most commonly used)
  Renal cortex appears more hypointense relative to liver than normal
  Intrahepatic vessel borders become indistinct or cannot be visualized
  Nonvisualization of diaphragm (because of increased beam attenuation)
- Quantitative
  Method uses backscatter amplitude measurements

CT
- Fatty areas are hypodense; normal liver appears relatively hyperdense
- Normal liver is 8 HU denser than spleen; each milligram of triglyceride per gram of liver decreases density by 1.6 HU; visual: liver less dense than spleen
- Hepatic and portal veins appear dense relative to decreased parenchymal density
- Common focal fatty deposit: segments #, anteriorly near fissure for falciform ligament

MRI
- Use fat saturation techniques to verify presence of fat

GLYCOGEN STORAGE DISEASE

Enzyme deficiency resulting in accumulation of polysaccharides in liver and other organs.

GLYCOGEN STORAGE DISEASE		
Type of Disease	Enzyme Deficiency	Organ Involvement
von Gierke's	Glucose-6-phosphatase	Liver, kidney, intestine
Pompe's	Lysosomal glucosidase	All organs
Forbes', Cori's	Debrancher enzyme	Liver, muscle, heart
Andersen's	Brancher enzyme	Generalized amylopectin
McArdle's	Muscle phosphorylase	Muscle
Hers'	Liver phosphorylase	Liver
Tarui's	Phosphofructokinase	Muscle

Radiographic features
Primary liver finding
- Hepatomegaly
- US: increased echogenicity (looks like fatty liver)
- CT: increased density (55-90 HU)

Other organs
- Nephromegaly

Hepatic complications
- Hepatic adenoma
- Hepatocellular carcinoma (uncommon)

GAUCHER'S DISEASE

Glucocerebrosidase deficiency leads to accumulation of ceramide in cells of the RES.
Clinical findings
- Liver: hepatosplenomegaly, impaired liver function, hemachromatosis
- Bone marrow: anemia, leukopenia, thrombocytopenia, bone pain

Radiographic features

Liver
- Hepatomegaly

Spleen
- Splenomegaly (marked)
- Focal lesions (infarcts) typically have low density (CT) and are hyperechoic (US)

Musculoskeletal
- Erlenmeyer flask deformity of femur
- Generalized osteopenia
- Multiple lytic bone lesions
- Aseptic necrosis of femoral head

HEMACHROMATOSIS

Iron overload. Types:
- Primary hemachromatosis (defect in intestinal mucosa, increased iron absorption). Clinical: bronze diabetes: cirrhosis, diabetes mellitus, hyperpigmentation
- Secondary hemachromatosis: multiple transfusions in bleeders

Radiographic features

US
- Hyperechoic liver

CT
- Dense liver (> 75 HU), much denser than spleen
- Intrahepatic vessels stand out as low-density structures

MRI
- Liver and spleen are markedly hypointense on T2-weighted (T2W) images
- Other organs with decreased SI: LN, bone marrow, pituitary, heart, adrenals, bowel
- In primary hemachromatosis, pancreas also appears hypointense

Complication
- Hepatocellular carcinoma

Infections

PYOGENIC ABSCESS

Pathogens: *Escherichia coli*, aerobic streptococci, anaerobes. Causes:
- Ascending cholangitis
- Trauma, surgery
- Pylephlebitis

Radiographic features
- CT: hypodense mass or masses with peripheral enhancement, no fill-in
- Double target sign: wall enhancement with surrounding hypodense zone (edema)

- 30% contain gas
- Percutaneous abscess drainage: any abscess can be drained percutaneously, particularly:
    - Deep abscesses
    - No response to treatment
    - Nonsurgical candidates

AMEBIC ABSCESS

Pathogen: *Entamoeba histolytica.*
Radiographic features
- Abscesses do not contain gas unless secondarily superinfected
- Irregular, shaggy borders
- Internal septations, 30%
- Multiple abscesses, 25%

Treatment
- Conservative: metronidazole
- Abscess drainage indicated if:
    - No response to treatment
    - Nonsurgical candidates

ECHINOCOCCUS (HYDATID DISEASE)

Humans are intermediate hosts of the dog tapeworm *(Taenia echinococcus)*. The embryos penetrate the human intestinal mucosa and disseminate to liver and lungs >> spleen, kidney, bone, CNS. The disease is most prevalent in countries where dogs are used to herd livestock: (e.g., Greece, Argentina, New Zealand). Two forms:

- *Echinococcus granulosus* (hosts: dog, cattle): more common, few large cysts
- *E. multilocularis* (*alveolaris;* host: rodents): less common, more invasive

Most patients acquire disease in childhood. Initially cysts are 5 mm and then enlarge at a rate of 1 cm/yr until they become symptomatic.

Radiographic features
E. granulosus
- Well-delineated cysts (multilocular > unilocular)
- Size of cysts usually very large
- Daughter cysts within larger cysts (multiseptated cyst) pathognomonic
- Rimlike cyst calcification, 30%
- Double-rim sign: pericyst, endocyst
- Waterlily sign
- Enhancement of cyst wall

E. multilocularis
- Poorly marginated, multiple hypodense liver lesions
- Lesions infiltrative (chronic granulomatous reaction with necrosis, cavitation)
- Calcifications punctate and dystrophic, not rimlike

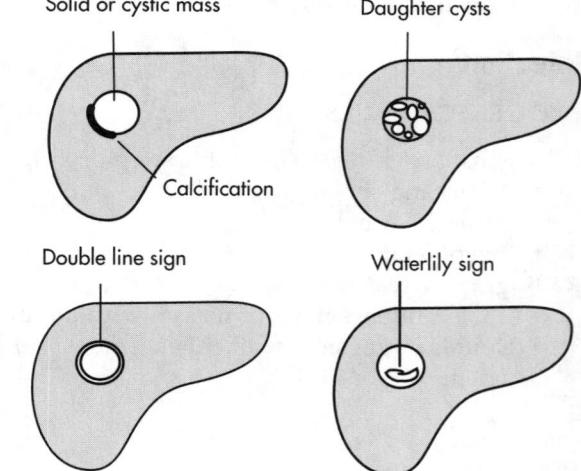

Classification of cysts

Type I: pure fluid collection, unilocular, well-defined cyst—amenable to percutaneous therapy

Type II: partial/complete detachment of membrane floating in cyst—amenable to percutaneous therapy

Type III: multiseptated or multilocular—amenable to percutaneous therapy

Type IV: heterogeneous cystic mass—not amenable to percutaneous therapy

Type V: calcified wall—not amenable to percutaneous therapy

Complications

- Rupture into peritoneal, pleural, pericardial cavity
- Obstructive jaundice due to external compression or intrinsic obstruction of biliary tree, biliary fistula
- Superinfection (bacterial) requiring prolonged drainage
- Anaphylaxis, shock, disseminated intravascular coagulation (DIC) < 1%

Percutaneous drainage

Surgical evacuation is procedure of choice. Percutaneous drainage is indicated in poor surgical candidates.

- < 6 cm aspiration with 19-G needle
- > 6 cms catheter placement 6 Fr for 1 day
    - Inject 15%-20% hypertonic NaCl (one-third cyst volume) or alcohol (one-half cyst volume) for 20 min with patient rotating during that period.
    - Followed by catheter to gravity drainage.
- Prophylactic albendazole 20 mg/kg q12h PO for 1 week
- Anesthesia standby in case of hypersensitivity reaction
- Prophylactic 200 mg hydrocortisone IV before procedure
- Complications
    - Anaphylaxis, shock, DIC < 1 %
    - Biliary fistula
    - Superinfection (bacterial) requiring longer drainage
- Fluid analysis is positive for hydatid fragments in only 70%

Tumors

TYPES OF HEPATIC TUMORS

OVERVIEW		
Origin	Benign	Malignant
Hepatocellular	Adenoma	HCC
	Focal nodular hyperplasia	Fibrolamellar HCC
	Regenerating nodule	Hepatoblastoma
Cholangiocellular	Biliary cystadenoma	Cholangiocarcinoma
	Bile duct adenoma	Cystadenocarcinoma
Mesenchymal	Hemangioma	Angiosarcoma (Thorotrast)
	Fibroma, lipoma, others	Primary lymphoma (AIDS)
Heterotopic tissue	Adrenal	Metastases
	Pancreatic	

LESION CHARACTERIZATION BY MODALITY*						
	Cyst	Hemangioma	FNH	Adenoma	HCC	Metastasis
Age	All ages	All ages	20-40	20-40	50-70	40-70
Sex	M = F	F > M	F >> M	F >> M	M > F	M = F
AFP	Nl	Nl	Nl	Nl	High	Nl
Scar	No	In giant	Common	Occasional	Occasional	No
Calcification	Occasional	Yes	No	No	Rare	Rare
Rupture	Yes (rare)	Yes (rare)	No	Yes	Yes	No
US	Anechoic	Hyperechoic	Variable	Variable	Variable	Variable
CT	Hypodense No enhancement	Enhancement† Early peripheral	Scar Arterial phase	Arterial enhancement	Capsule Arterial — enhancement	Variable
MRI	CSF intensity	CSF intensity	Liver intensity‡	Liver intensity	Liver intensity	Spleen
Angiography	Avascular	Hypervascular	Hypervascular	Hypervascular	Hypervascular	Variable
Scintigraphy§	Cold	Uptake	Uptake	Uptake	Cold	Cold

NI, Not indicated.
*Most frequent diagnostic pattern.
†Nodular peripheral with centripetal fill-in.
‡Arterial enhancement, with delayed enhancing central scar.
§Labeled RBC scan.

Whereas US is commonly used for the differentiation of solid and cystic masses, diagnostic modalities for further differentiation of solid tumors (> 1 cm) is usually assigned to MR or CECT (MR is preferable). Two criteria are used for lesion characterization: signal intensity and morphological features. Ultimately, the majority of lesions other than hemangiomas are biopsied. It is difficult to characterize lesions < 1 cm.

LESION CHARACTERIZATION BY MRI	
SIGNAL INTENSITY	
T1 hyperintense tumors	HCC
	Hemorrhagic tumors
	Melanoma
	Lesions in hemachromatosis livers
	Thrombosed portal vein
T2 hypointense tumors	Regenerating nodules
T2 lightbulb sign (lesion has CSF intensity)	Hemangioma
	Cysts
	Cystic metastases
	Cystadenocarcinoma
OTHER MORPHOLOGICAL FEATURES	
Scars	Focal nodular hyperplasia
	Adenoma
	Hemangioma
Capsule	HCC
	Adenoma

HEMANGIOMA

Frequency: 4%-7% of population. 80% in females. Hemangiomas may enlarge particularly during pregnancy or estrogen administration. Two types:
- Typical hemangioma (common): small, asymptomatic, discovered incidentally
- Giant hemangioma (> 5 cm, uncommon), may be:
    Symptomatic (hemorrhage, thrombosis)
    Kasabach-Merritt syndrome: sequestration of thrombocytes in hemangioma
        causes thrombocytopenia (rare)

Radiographic features
US
- Hyperechoic lesions, 80%
- Hypoechoic lesions, 10%; especially in fatty liver
- Giant hemangiomas are heterogenous
- Anechoic peripheral vessels may be demonstrated by color Doppler US
- Posterior acoustic enhancement is common (even in hypoechoic lesions)

CT
- Hypodense, well-circumscribed lesion on precontrast scan
- Globular or nodular intense peripheral enhancement during dynamic bolus phase, most characteristic findings on good bolus
- Fill-in occurs within minutes after administration of contrast (longer for giant hemangiomas) but also occurs often in metastases

MRI
- Hyperintense (similar to CSF) on heavily T2W sequences (lightbulb sign)
- Post gadolinium peripheral nodular enhancement with centripetal fill-in
- Imaging modality of choice

Nuclear imaging (SPECT with ^{99m}Tc-labeled RBC)
- Decreased activity on early dynamic images
- Increased activity on delayed (1-2 hours) blood pool images
- Only useful if lesion is > 3 cm (limited spatial resolution)

FOCAL NODULAR HYPERPLASIA (FNH)

Rare hepatic neoplasm, most common in young women (75%). Composed of hepatocytes, Kupffer cells, and bile ducts. Association with oral contraceptives is questionable. Conservative management; no malignant transformation. 20% are multiple.

Radiographic features
- Mass lesion, usually difficult to detect because it has similar density, intensity, echogenicity as surrounding liver (normal hepatocytes, Kupffer cells, bile ducts)
- Central fibrous scar is common
- 70% have normal or increased ^{99m}Tc sulfur colloid uptake, 30% have decreased uptake

MRI
- Lesion isointense to liver, central scar hyperintense on T2W image
- Arterial enhancement
- Delayed enhancement of central scar
- Angiography: hypervascular lesion

ADENOMA

Composed of hepatocytes; no bile ducts or Kupffer cells (cold on ^{99m}Tc sulfur colloid scan). Less common than FNH. Associated with oral contraceptives and glycogen storage disease (especially von Gierke's disease). May resolve completely after discontinuation of hormone therapy. Liver adenomatosis appears to be a distinct entity. Although the adenomas in liver adenomatosis are histologically similar to other adenomas, they are not steroid dependent but are multiple, progressive, symptomatic, and more likely to lead to impaired liver function, hemorrhage, and perhaps malignant degeneration.

Complications
- Hemorrhage
- Infarction
- Malignant degeneration

Radiographic features
- Usually solitary, encapsulated. Patients with glycogen storage disease and liver adenomatosis may have dozens of adenomas detected at imaging and even more at close examination of resected specimens.
- CT: peripherally hypodense (lipid accumulation in hepatocytes). Because adenomas consist almost entirely of uniform hepatocytes and a variable number of Kupffer cells, it is not surprising that most of the adenomas are nearly isoattenuating relative to normal liver on unenhanced, portal venous–phase, and delayed-phase images. In patients with fatty liver, adenomas are hyperattenuating at all phases of contrast enhancement and on unenhanced images as well.
- US features are nonspecific (may be isoechoic, hypoechoic, hyperechoic)
- MRI: Lesions may show fall in signal intensity on gradient echo out of phase images due to intralesional fat content. Arterially enhanced with capsule seen on delayed images
- Cold lesions by ^{99m}Tc sulfur colloid scan
- Angiography: varied appearance (hypervascular, hypovascular), no neovascularity, pooling, or AV shunting

HEPATOCELLULAR CARCINOMA (HCC)

Most common primary visceral malignancy worldwide. Incidence:
- Asia, Japan, Africa: 5%-20%
- Western hemisphere: 0.2%-0.8%

Risk factors
- Cirrhosis: 5% develop HCC
- Chronic hepatitis B: 10% develop HCC
- Hepatotoxins (aflatoxin, oral contraceptives, Thorotrast)
- Metabolic disease (galactosemia, glycogen storage disease) in pediatric patients

Radiographic features
General
- Three forms: solitary (25%), multiple (25%), diffuse (50%)
- Portal (35%) and hepatic vein (15%) invasion is common (rare in other malignancies)
- Metastases: lung > adrenal, lymph nodes > bone (10%-20% at autopsy, bone metastases may be painful)
- HCC typically occurs in abnormal livers (cirrhosis, hemochromatosis)

CT
- Hypodense mass lesion
- Lesion may appear hyperdense in fatty liver
- Enhancement: early arterial enhancement
  - Arterial supply, prominent AV shunting cause early enhancement, remains enhanced on PVP
  - Venous invasion, 50%
  - In cirrhotic livers, HCC are best detected by helical CT or dynamic contrast MRI during arterial phase
- Calcifications, 25%
  - More commonly seen in fibrolamellar HCC: 40% (better prognosis, younger patients, normal alpha-fetoprotein, central scar calcification)

US
- Most small HCC are hypoechoic
- Larger HCC are heterogenous
- Fibrolamellar HCC are hyperechoic
- High velocity Doppler pattern, feeding tumor vessels can be seen by color Doppler

MRI
- T1W: hyperintense, 50% (because of fat in lesions); iso-, hypointense, 50%
- Hypointense capsule in 25%-40%

Angiography
- Hypervascular
- AV shunting is typical
- Dilated arterial supply

FIRBROLAMELLAR HCC

- Malignant hepatocellular tumor with distinct clinical and pathological differences from hepatocellular carcinoma
- Lobulated heterogeneous mass with a central scar in an otherwise normal liver
- Radiologic evidence of cirrhosis, vascular invasion, or multifocal disease— findings typical of hepatocellular carcinoma—is uncommon
- Imaging features of fibrolamellar carcinoma overlap with those of other scar-producing lesions including FNH, hepatocellular adenoma and HCC, hemangioma, metastases, and cholangiocarcinoma
- The fibrous scar is usually hypointense on all MR sequences. This widely described imaging feature has been used to discriminate between fibrolamellar carcinoma and FNH. However, in rare cases, fibrolamellar carcinoma may demonstrate a hyperintense scar on T2W images, a finding that simulates the hyperintense scar characteristic of FNH.
- Dense heterogeneous enhancement in the arterial and portal phases. The scar usually does not enhance and is best visualized on delayed images.

METASTASES

30% of patients who die of malignancy have liver metastases. The liver is the most common site of metastatic disease from colorectal carcinoma: colon > stomach > pancreas > breast, lung. Up to 20% of patients die from liver metastases rather than the primary tumor.

Sensitivity for lesion detection
MR > CECT > US > noncontrast FDG PET
US features
Echogenic metastases
- GI malignancy
- HCC
- Vascular metastases

Hypoechoic metastases
- Most metastases are hypovascular
- Lymphoma
- Bull's eye pattern (hypoechoic halo around lesion)
      Nonspecific sign but frequently seen in bronchogenic carcinoma
      Hypoechoic rim represents compressed liver tissue, tumor fibrosis

Calcified metastases: hyperechoic with distal shadowing
- All mucinous metastases: colon > thyroid, ovary, kidney, stomach

Cystic metastases: necrotic leiomyosarcoma; mucinous metastases
CT features
Best seen on portal venous phase images except for hypervascular lesions (arterial phase). Small lesions may fill-in on delayed scans. Peripheral washout sign (when seen) is characteristic of metastases.

UNSUSPECTED HEPATIC LESIONS

Small lesions (< 15 mm) of the liver are frequently detected during routine CT, MRI, and US studies of the abdomen ("incidentaloma"). In larger series, 70% of such lesions are benign and 30% are malignant. In the subset of patients with lesions < 1 cm and no known primary, virtually all lesions are benign. In the subset of patients with known malignant neoplasm the percentage of malignant lesions is 50%.

ALCOHOL ABLATION OF LIVER TUMORS

Indication
HCC
- No extrahepatic spread
- ≤ 5 cm, single or multiple
- Child A or B cirrhosis

Metastases
- ≤ 5 cm, single lesion
- Vascular lesion (carcinoid, islet cell tumor)

Procedure
1. Localize hepatic lesion by US or CT.
2. Advance 20-G needle into tumor center avoiding multiple perforations.
3. Slowly instill ethanol into tumor. We usually use 15-30 ml/lesion/setting.
4. Withdraw needle.
5. Lesions are typically treated at least 3 times or until no tumor is apparent.

Complications
- Major complications for which admission is necessary (10% by patient, 3% by procedure): bleeding, chest tube placement
- Minor complications (virtually all patients): pain, fever

Outcome
- Efficacy similar to that of surgery for lesions
- The larger the lesion, the more difficult to treat
- Metastases are more difficult to treat (alcohol diffuses less well, tumors have no capsule)

Trauma

The liver is the most common intraabdominal site of injury; however, one must inspect other organs (spleen, bowel) for coexistent trauma.

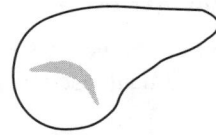
Simple intrahepatic laceration

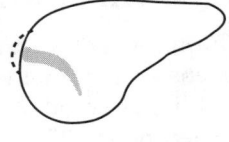
Laceration extending to capsule

Types
- Subcapsular hematoma: hypodense or hyperdense lenticular fluid collection contained by the liver capsule; usually caused by blunt trauma
- Laceration: single or multiple stellate configurations usually of low density relative to enhanced parenchyma. Clots may appear high density; usually caused by penetrating or blunt trauma

Complications
- Perihepatic hemorrhage
- Intraperitoneal or extraperitoneal hemorrhage

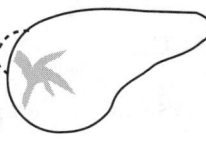
Complex injury, stellate laceration

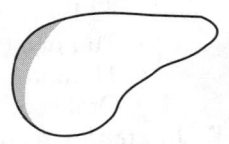
Subcapsular hematoma

Vascular Abnormalities

PORTAL HYPERTENSION

Criteria: hepatic wedge pressure > 10 mm Hg. Causes:
Presinusoidal
- Extrahepatic (obstruction of portal vein)
    Thrombosis
    Compression
- Intrahepatic (obstruction of portal venules)
    Hepatic fibrosis: congenital, toxic (copper, polyvinyl chloride), myelofibrosis, Wilson's disease, sarcoid
    Infection: malaria, schistosomiasis

Sinusoidal
- Cirrhosis (most common cause)
- Sclerosing cholangitis

Postsinusoidal
- Budd-Chiari syndrome
- Congestive heart failure

Radiographic features
- Portal vein diameter > 13 mm
- Collaterals
    Gastroesophageal varices via coronary vein, azygos
    SMV collateral: mesenteric varices
    Splenorenal varices
    IMV collateral: hemorrhoids
    Recanalization of umbilical vein: caput medusa
    Unnamed retroperitoneal collaterals that communicate with phrenic, adrenal, and renal veins
- Splenomegaly
- Ascites

BUDD-CHIARI SYNDROME (BCS)

Thrombosis of the main hepatic veins, branches of hepatic veins or IVC; with possible extension to portal vein. Clinical: ascites, pain, hepatomegaly, splenomegaly. Causes:

Idiopathic, 50%-75%

Secondary, 25%-50%

- Coagulation anomalies
    - Clotting disorders
    - Polycythemia
- Tumors: HCC, RCC
- Trauma
- Oral contraceptives, chemotherapy

Radiographic features

Veins

- Absent hepatic veins
- Flow in inferior vena cava (IVC) may be reversed, turbulent, diminished, absent
- Flow in portal vessels may be reversed, diminished
- Intrahepatic collateral vessels
- Narrowing of the intrahepatic IVC

Liver parenchyma

- Hemorrhagic infarction appears hypoechoic by US
- Caudate lobe is often spared (emissary veins drain directly into the IVC) and appears enlarged; small right lobe

CT

- Increased central (periportal) parenchymal enhancement
- Patchy peripheral enhancement: geographic zones of poorly opacified parenchyma interspersed with well-opacified zones

Pearls

- Hepatic venoocclusive disease, which causes progressive occlusion of small vessels, is clinically indistinguishable from BCS. Causes:
    - Toxins from bush tea (Jamaica)
    - Chemotherapy
    - Bone marrow transplantation (GVH)

PORTAL VEIN THROMBOSIS

Causes

- Malignancy (HCC)
- Chronic pancreatitis
- Hepatitis
- Trauma
- Shunts
- Hypercoagulable states (pregnancy)

US features

- Echogenic thrombus in vein
- Portal vein enlargement
- Hepatofugal flow

CT

- Clot in portal vein with collaterals: gastroesophageal umbilical collateral vessels
- Cavernous transformation: numerous wormlike vessels at the porta hepatis reconstituting intrahepatic portal venous system
- Splenomegaly, ascites

Pearls
- Flow in hepatic artery and portal vein should always be in the same direction: hepatopedal flow
- Opposite flow directions in portal vein and hepatic artery indicate hepatofugal flow

HEPATIC ARTERY ANEURYSM

Decreasing order of frequency of abdominal aneurysms: aorta > iliac artery > splenic artery > hepatic artery. 10% of patients with hepatic artery aneurysm have sudden rupture. Hepatic pseudoaneurysm may occur secondary to pancreatitis.

Transplant

Complications
- UGI bleeding (ulcer)
- Biliary: obstruction, leak, fistula, biloma, sludge
- Vascular complications
    - Hepatic artery thrombosis: most common serious vascular complication, more common in pediatric patients usually necessitating retransplantation. US reveals no arterial flow within the liver. Pediatric patients may develop extensive collaterization to the liver. The waveforms of these collateral vessels are abnormal showing parvus-tardus waveform, RI of less than 0.5, and systolic acceleration time of greater than 0.1 second.
    - Hepatic artery thrombosis: usually occurs at the anastomotic site within 3 months of transplantation. Nonanastomotic stenosis may indicate rejection or hepatic necrosis.
    - Portal vein thrombosis: less frequent then hepatic artery thrombosis. US echogenic thrombus can be seen within the lumen of the vessel.
    - Hepatic vein thrombosis: quite rare because no surgical anastomosis is involved.
- Rejection, 40%

CT findings (after transplantation)
- Atelectasis and pleural effusions are the most frequent CT findings
- Periportal increased attenuation (periportal collar), common (70%) and typical finding
- Ascites, 40%
- Splenomegaly
- Noninfected loculated intraperitoneal fluid collections
- Abscesses (hepatic, splenic, perihepatic, pancreatic)
- Hepatic infarction, 10%
- Hepatic hematoma
- Sludge (inspissated thick bile, 15%); may be extensive and cause "biliary casts"
- Splenic infarction
- Hepatic calcification
- Other
    - IVC thrombosis
    - Pseudoaneurysm of hepatic artery
    - Recurrent hepatic tumor

3

ERCP findings (after transplantation)
- Anormal cholangiograms are seen in 80% of patients with hepatic artery stenosis (bile duct ischemia) but only in 30% of patients with patent hepatic artery. Abnormalities include:
    Nonanastomotic strictures, 25% (up to 50% in hepatic artery stenosis)
    Anastomotic strictures, 5%
    Intraluminal filling defects (sludge, casts), 5%
    Bile leaks, 5%

Biliary System

General

DUCTAL ANATOMY

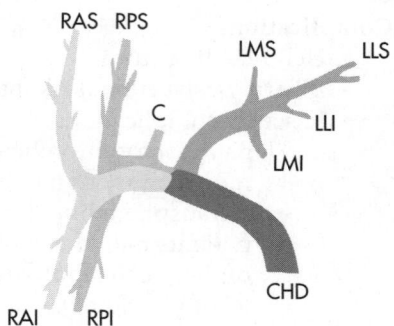

Right hepatic duct (RHD)
- Right anterior superior (RAS) segment
- Right anterior inferior (RAI) segment
- Right posterior superior (RPS) segment
- Right posterior inferior (RPI) segment
- Caudate (C) segment

Left hepatic duct (LHD)
- Left medial superior (LMS) segment
- Left medial inferior (LMI) segment
- Left lateral superior (LLS) segment
- Left lateral inferior (LLI) segment

RHD and LHD form the common hepatic duct (CHD), which receives the cystic duct (CD) from the GB to form the common bile duct (CBD).

Variations of intrahepatic biliary anatomy
- "Normal" anatomy as shown above, 60%
- Right posterior ducts drain directly into LHD, 20%
- Right posterior, right anterior and LHD form CHD, 10%

Variations of cystic duct insertion
- Normal insertion
- Low union
- Parallel course
- Anterior spiral course
- Posterior spiral course

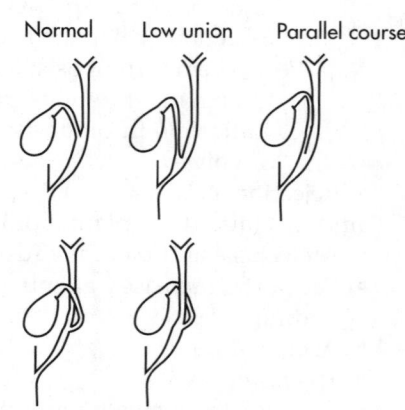

Variations of papillary insertion (ducts within papilla = ampulla)
The CBD drains into the duodenum through the ampulla. Variations of pancreatic duct (PD) and CBD insertion:
- Y type: CBD and PD combine before insertion into ampulla
- V type: CBD and PD insert jointly into ampulla
- U type: CBD and PD insert separately into ampulla

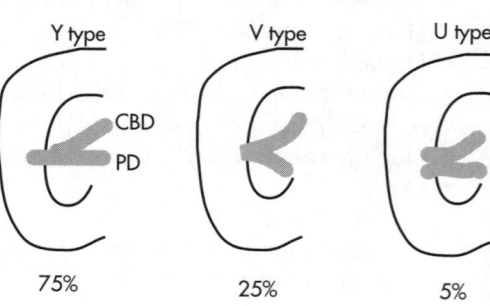

US measurements of CHD

CHD measurements (inner wall to inner wall) are performed at the level of hepatic artery. Normal measurements:

- < 7 mm in normal fasting patients < 60 years; in 95% the CHD is < 4 mm
- < 10 mm in normal fasting patients 60-100 years
- < 11 mm in patients with
    Previous surgery
    Previous CD obstruction
- Fatty meal challenge: if CHD enlarges more than 2 mm after fatty meal (Lipomul), it indicates obstruction

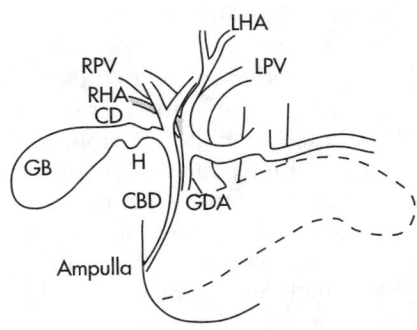

Location of the hepatic artery relative to the CBD:

Most common (80%)
- Hepatic artery between CBD and portal vein
- Hepatic artery medial to MPV
- CBD lateral to portal vein

Less common (20%)
- Hepatic artery anterior to CBD
- Hepatic artery posterior to portal vein

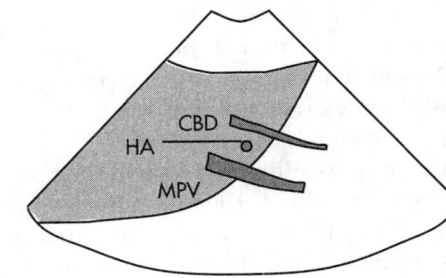

Long axis, left lateral decubitus

GALLBLADDER

US Measurements

- Wall ≤ 2 mm (distended GB)
- Maximum dimensions 5 × 10 cm

Variants

- Phrygian cap: fundal locule from septal-like invagination
- Junctional fold: fold between infundibulum and body; may be hyperechoic and cause posterior shadowing
- Agenesis of GB (rare); more common causes of nonvisualized GB
    Previous cholecystectomy
    Nonfasting
    Chronic cholecystitis

ERCP

Contrast-agent injection is performed through the endoscope after cannulation of the CBD. Complications:

- Pancreatitis, 5%
- Duodenal perforation
- Gastrointestinal bleeding

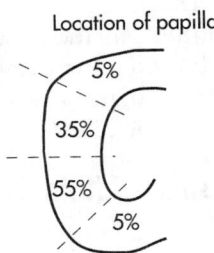

Location of papilla

MAGNETIC RESONANCE CHOLANGIOPANCREATICOGRAPHY (MRCP)

Fat-suppressed 2D or 3D heavily T2W sequences are obtained of the upper abdomen (e.g., fast spin echo, spin echo, echo planar, gradient echo). Bile appears hyperintense and images of the entire biliary and pancreatic ductal system can be rendered by maximum signal intensity projection reconstruction. Common indications for MRCP usually include unsuccessful ERCP or a contraindication to ERCP and the presence of biliary enteric anastomoses (e.g., choledochojejunostomy, Billroth II anastomosis).

Advantages of MRCP over ERCP

MRCP (1) is noninvasive, (2) is cheaper, (3) uses no radiation, (4) requires no anesthesia, (5) is less operator dependent, (6) allows better visualization of ducts proximal to obstruction, (7) when combined with conventional T1W and T2W sequences, allows detection of extraductal disease.

Disadvantages of MRCP
- Decreased spatial resolution, making MRCP less sensitive to abnormalities of the peripheral intrahepatic ducts (e.g., sclerosing cholangitis) and pancreatic ductal side branches (e.g., chronic pancreatitis).
- Imaging in the physiological, nondistended state, which decreases the sensitivity to detect subtle ductal abnormalities.
- Cannot perform therapeutic endoscopic or percutaneous intervention of obstructing bile duct lesions. Thus, in patients with high clinical suspicion for bile duct obstruction, ERCP should be the initial imaging modality to provide timely intervention (e.g., sphincterotomy, dilatation, stent placement, stone removal) if necessary.

Technique

MRCP is usually performed with heavily T2W sequences by using fast spin-echo or single-shot fast spin-echo pulse sequences and both a thick-collimation (single-section) and thin-collimation (multisection) technique with a torso phased–array coil. The coronal plane is used to provide a cholangiographic display, and the axial plane is used to evaluate the pancreatic duct and distal common bile duct. In addition, 3-dimensional reconstruction by using a maximum-intensity projection (MIP) algorithm on the thin-collimation source images can be performed. The patients fast 3 hours before the MRCP, thereby reducing unwanted signal from the intestine. Secretin (1 CU/kg IV) can be given to patients suspected of having pancreatic disease; this substance transiently distends the duct and allows better visualization of its morphological features. Maximum dilatation occurs 2 minutes after secretin injection, and then the duct relaxes to baseline. Persistent dilatation implies papillary stenosis, and dilatation of side branches suggests chronic pancreatitis.

MRCP is comparable with ERCP in detection of obstruction, with a sensitivity, specificity, and accuracy of 91%, 100%, and 94%, respectively. It is 94% sensitive and 93% specific for detection of dilatation. MRCP may also allow more accurate assessment of ductal caliber in the physiological state, unlike ERCP, with which ductal caliber may be overestimated because of injection pressure. MRCP is comparable with ERCP in detection of choledocholithiasis and superior to CT or US. Numerous studies have shown sensitivities of 81%-100% and specificities of 85%-100% for MRCP.

Pitfalls

Pitfalls include pseudo-filling defects, pseudo-dilatations, and nonvisualization of the ducts. Filling defects are usually due to stones, air, tumors, hemorrhage, or sludge. Infrequent causes of filling defects include susceptibility artifact from adjacent clips, metallic bile duct stents, folds, or flow voids.

Biliary Lithiasis

CHOLELITHIASIS

Gallstones occur in 10%-20% of the United States population. 30% are calcified. 30%-50% of patients are asymptomatic. Surgical removal is indicated in symptomatic and diabetic patients (high risk of acute cholecystitis). Types:
- Cholesterol stones are caused by precipitation of supersaturated bile (Western population, women > men, old age > young age)
- Pigment stones: precipitate of calcium bilirubinate (Asian population)
- Mixed stones (most common type)

Predisposing factors:
- Obesity
- Hemolytic anemia (pigment stones)
- Abnormal enterohepatic circulation of bile salts (Crohn's disease, SB resection)
- Diabetes
- Cirrhosis
- Hyperparathyroidism

US features
- Prominent posterior shadow (type I). Very small stones may not shadow: reposition the patient to heap up calculi.
- Mobility of stones; gravity-dependent movement; exception: stones impacted in neck or stones adherent to wall.
- Wall-echo-shadow (WES triad, double-arc sign) is seen if the GB is contracted (type M) and completely filled with stones; however, WES triad can also be seen with:
  Porcelain GB (calcification of GB)
  Emphysematous cholecystitis
- Highly reflective echo originating from the anterior surface of calculus

US SIGNS OF CHOLELITHIASIS			
	Type I	**Type II**	**Type III**
US appearance	Calculus / Gravel / Posterior shadowing	Contracted gallblader	
	Hyperechoic stone Posterior shadow Visible GB	Hyperechoic stone Posterior shadow Nonvisible GB	Hyperchoic stone No posterior shadow Visible GB
Sensitivity	100%	90%-100%	50%-80%

Clean vs. dirty shadows
The acoustic shadowing depends on:
- Size of stone (small stones may not shadow)
- Angle of beam
- Stone-beam focus distance
- Frequency of transducer

CLEAN VS. DIRTY SHADOWS	
Clean Shadow	**Dirty Shadow**
Hypoechoic shadow with no echoes in it	Comet tail with echoes in shadow
Rough surface Small radius of curvature Stones with calcification	Smooth surface Large radius of curvature Stones with high cholesterol content Bowel loops visualized rather than GB

CHOLEDOCHOLITHIASIS

Presence of stone or stones in the bile duct, typically associated with high grade obstruction and jaundice. Diagnostic accuracy with US, 75%.

SLUDGE

Sludge (echogenic bile) is a sonographic term that refers to layering particulate material (calcium bilirubinate and/or cholesterol crystals) within bile; no posterior shadowing. Cause:
- Fasting (decreased CCK)
    - 10 days: 30% of patients have sludge
    - 6 weeks: 100% of patients have sludge
- Hyperalimentation (decreased CCK)
- Infection, obstruction

Implications
- Sludge is a common finding of stasis in the GB.
- Sludge is associated with infection/obstruction (cholecystitis) in 20% of ICU patients.
- Symptomatic patients (unexplained fever, RUQ pain, dilated GB with sludge) may benefit from percutaneous cholecystostomy.

MILK OF CALCIUM BILE

Concentration of intravesicular calcium salts in long-standing CD obstruction. Radiographically, GB contents appear dense.

MIRIZZI SYNDROME

Impacted stone in the CD and surrounding inflammation causes compression and obstruction of CHD. The calculus may ultimately erode into the CHD or gut.

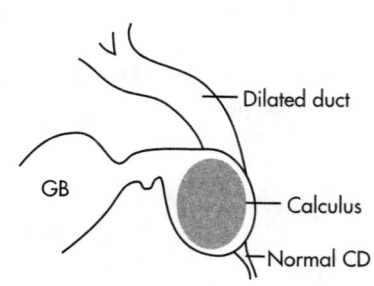

BILIARY-ENTERIC FISTULAS

Causes
- Chronic cholecystitis with erosion of a gallstone into the GI tract, 90%
- Penetration of posterior duodenal ulcer into CHD, 5%
- Tumor
- Trauma

Types
- Biliary-gastric (Bouveret's syndrome)
- Biliary-duodenal, 70% (most common; may cause gallstone ileus)
- Biliary-colonic
- Biliary-ileojejunal
- Bouveret's syndrome: obstruction of stomach or duodenum by stone
  Most common cause for biliary ductal air iatrogenic (ERCP, surgical)

Inflammation

ACUTE CHOLECYSTITIS

Causes
- Gallstone obstruction, 95%
- Acalculous cholecystitis, 5%

US features
- Luminal distention > 4 cm
- Wall thickening > 5 mm (edema, congestion); thickening is usually worse on the hepatic side
- Gallstones; CD stones may be difficult to detect if they are not surrounded by bile
- Positive Murphy's sign (sensitivity, 60%, specificity, 90%)
- Pericholecystic fluid

Complications
- Gangrenous cholecystitis: rupture of GB; mortality, 20%, gangrene causes nerve death so that 65% of patients have a negative Murphy's sign
- Emphysematous cholecystitis, rare (40% occur in diabetics)
- Empyema

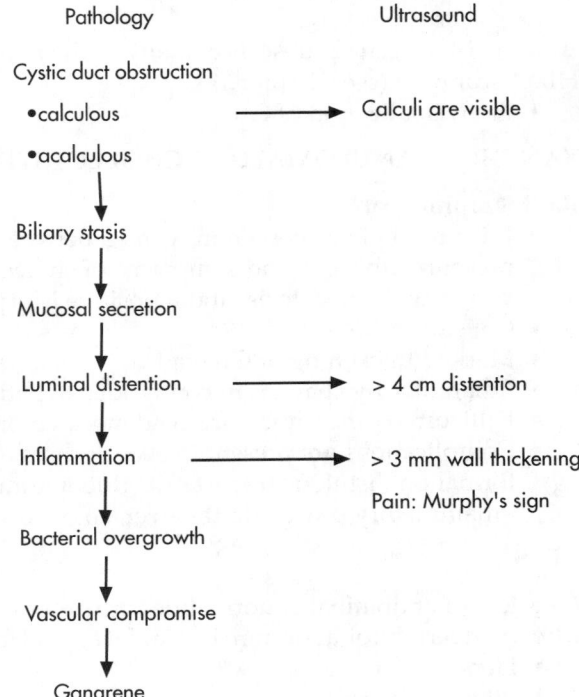

Pathology	Ultrasound
Cystic duct obstruction	
• calculous	→ Calculi are visible
• acalculous	
↓	
Biliary stasis	
↓	
Mucosal secretion	
↓	
Luminal distention	→ > 4 cm distention
↓	
Inflammation	→ > 3 mm wall thickening
	Pain: Murphy's sign
↓	
Bacterial overgrowth	
↓	
Vascular compromise	
↓	
Gangrene	

CHRONIC CHOLECYSTITIS

US features
- GB wall thickening (fibrosis, chronic inflammation)
- Intramural epithelial crypts (Rokitansky-Aschoff sinuses)
- Gallstones, 95%
- Failure of GB to contract in response to CCK

ACALCULOUS CHOLECYSTITIS

Clinical settings associated with acalculous cholecystitis:
- Trauma
- Burn patient
- Prolonged fasting (postoperative patients), hyperalimentation
- Diabetes
- AIDS
- Others: colitis, hepatic arterial chemotherapy, postpartum, vascular insufficiency

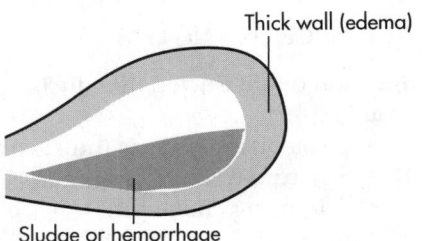

Thick wall (edema)

Sludge or hemorrhage

Radiographic features
US

- No calculi
- Sludge and debris
- Usually in critically ill patients
- Same findings as in calculous cholecystitis:
    Sonographic Murphy's sign
    GB wall thickening (> 2 mm)
    Pericholecystic fluid
    May occur in abscence of any of the above findings

HIDA scanning (see Chapter 12)

- Nonvisualization of GB

XANTHOGRANULOMATOUS CHOLECYSTITIS

Radiographic features

- It is predominantly seen in women between the ages of 60 and 70 years. Patients present with signs and symptoms of cholecystitis: right upper quadrant pain, vomiting, leukocytosis, and a positive Murphy's sign
- Gallstones
- Marked thickening of GB wall
- Inflammatory changes in contiguous hepatic parenchyma
- Difficult to differentiate from adenocarcinoma
- Complications are present in 30% of cases and include perforation, abscess formation, fistulous tracts to the duodenum or skin, and extension of the inflammatory process to the liver, colon, or surrounding soft tissues

AIDS

A variety of abdominal abnormalities are detected by US and/or CT in AIDS patients who are referred for abdominal pain, fever, and/or abnormal LFT:

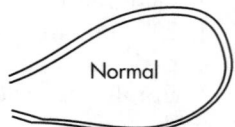

- Hepatosplenomegaly, 30%
- Biliary abnormalities, 20%
    GB wall thickening, 7%
    Cholelithiasis, 6%
    Sludge, 4%
    Biliary dilatation, 2%
- Lymphadenopathy, 20%
- Ascites, 15%

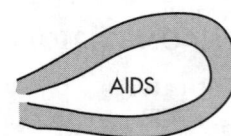

GB wall thickening is relatively common and may be marked, and its cause is often unknown. Only symptomatic patients should be treated for acalculus cholecystitis, which may be due to cryptosporidium and/or cytomegalovirus.

ACUTE CHOLANGITIS

Infection of obstructed bile ducts. *E. coli* > *Klebsiella* > *Pseudomonas*.
Causes

- Choledocholithiasis (most common cause)
- Stricture from prior surgery
- Sclerosing cholangitis
- Infected drainage catheter
- Ampullary carcinoma

Radiographic features
- Dilatation of intrahepatic ducts; dilated CBD, 70%
- Pigment stones and sludge in intrahepatic bile ducts (pathognomonic)
- Biliary strictures, 20%
- Segmental hepatic atrophy, 30%
- Liver abscess, pancreatitis (less common complications)

ORIENTAL CHOLANGIOHEPATITIS (OCH, RECURRENT PYOGENIC CHOLANGITIS)

Endemic disease in Asia characterized by recurrent attacks of fever, jaundice, and abdominal pain. Cause: *Clonorchis sinensis* and *Ascaris* infections; however, at time of diagnosis these infections are typically absent. Bacterial superinfection. Very common in Asia. Young adults.

Imaging features

Detection
- US is the primary screening modality of choice
- CT is commonly used to assess the extent of disease
- Cholangiography (hepatic, ERCP or intraoperative) is mandatory to delineate intrahepatic biliary anatomy and to exclude high biliary strictures

Morphologic features
- Biliary dilatation
    Extrahepatic biliary dilatation, 90%
    Intrahepatic biliary dilatation, 75%
    Left lobe and posterior right lobe most commonly affected
- Biliary strictures
- Intrahepatic calculi (hepatolithiasis)
    Contain calcium bilirubinate, cellular debris and mucinous substance
    Typically hyperechoic and cast shadows
    Stones may not be sufficiently hyperdense to be detectable by CT

Complications
- Intrahepatic abscess formation
- Hepatic atrophy due to portal vein occlusion
- Cholangiocarcinoma, 5%
- Pancreatic duct involvement, 20%
- GB disease is present in only 20%

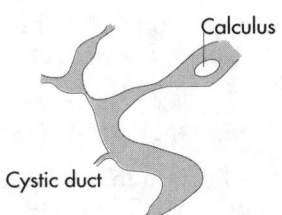

Calculus

Cystic duct

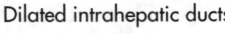

Dilated intrahepatic ducts

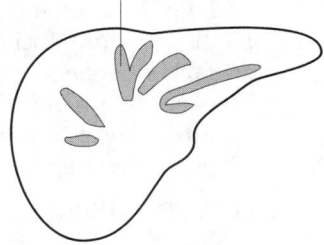

SCLEROSING CHOLANGITIS

Chronic inflammatory process of intrahepatic (20%) and extrahepatic (80%) bile ducts that causes progressive narrowing. Symptoms: chronic or intermittent obstructive jaundice. Two types:

Primary sclerosing cholangitis (idiopathic)
Secondary sclerosing cholangitis
- Inflammatory bowel disease (65%), usually ulcerative colitis
- Cirrhosis, chronic active hepatitis
- Retroperitoneal fibrosis
- Pancreatitis
- Some other rare diseases (e.g., Riedel's thyroiditis, Peyronie's disease)

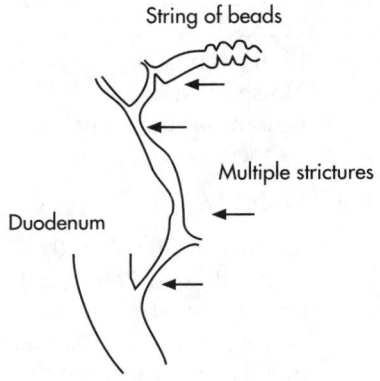

String of beads

Multiple strictures

Duodenum

Radiographic features
- Irregular dilatation, stenosis, beading of intrahepatic and extrahepatic bile ducts (seen best by cholangiogram): string-of-beads appearance
- Small "diverticulae" of biliary tree are pathognomonic
- Differential diagnosis:
    Primary biliary cirrhosis (normal extrahepatic ducts)
    Sclerosing cholangiocarcinoma

Complications
- Cholangiocarcinoma, 10%
- Biliary cirrhosis
- Portal hypertension

Hyperplastic Cholecystoses

Benign group of diseases with no neoplastic potential, uncertain clinical significance. Commonly seen in cholecystectomy specimen, less commonly identified by US or cholecystogram.

ADENOMYOMATOSIS

Most common form of hyperplastic cholesterolosis. There is marked hyperplasia of the GB wall. Epithelium herniates into the wall, forming Rokitansky-Aschoff sinuses. Findings may be focal (more common) or diffuse.

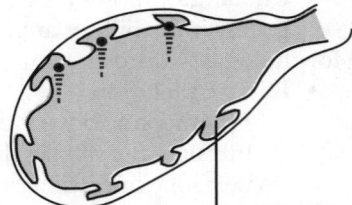

Rokitansky-Aschoff sinuses

US features
- Large Rokitansky-Aschoff sinuses
    Hypoechoic sinuses if they contain bile
    Hyperechoic sinuses if they contain sludge or calculi
- High amplitude foci in the wall (cholesterol crystals) that produce comet tail artifacts (V-shaped, ring-down artifacts)
- Thickening of GB wall is common but nonspecific
- Inflammation is not typical
- Hypercontractility

CHOLESTEROSIS (STRAWBERRY GB)

Triglycerides and cholesterol are deposited in macrophages of GB wall. The cholesterol nodules stud the wall and give the GB the appearance of a strawberry.
US features
- Lipid deposits (usually < 1 mm) are echogenic
- No shadowing
- Inflammation is not a prominent feature
- Associated with multiple (0.5 mm polyps), which should be followed up.

GB ADENOMA

- Single or multiple (10%) 5-20 mm in size. 60% of the cases are associated with cholelithiasis. Found in 0.5% of cholecystectomy specimens (F > M) in normal population and to a higher degree in familial adenomatous polyposis and Peutz-Jeghers syndrome. Adenomas are usually asymptomatic and discovered incidentally during a radiological evaluation of abdominal pain.

- Polyps > 1 cm require a careful search for features associated with malignancy, such as thickening or nodularity of the GB wall; evidence of hepatic invasion, such as an indistinct margin between the liver and GB; biliary duct dilatation; and peripancreatic or hepatoduodenal ligament adenopathy.
- US: gallbladder adenomas are typically smoothly marginated. Intraluminal polypoid masses. Should raise concern for malignancy. The echo-texture of adenomas is typically homogeneously hyperechoic; however, adenomas tend to be less echogenic and more heterogeneous as they increase in size. The additional finding of gallstones is common in patients with GB adenomas.
- CT: intraluminal soft-tissue masses, isoattenuating or hypoattenuating relative to liver. They may be difficult to distinguish from noncalcified gallstones.

Tumors

GB CARCINOMA

Biliary cancers (adenocarcinoma of the GB, cholangiocarcinoma) are the fifth most common GI malignancy. Associations:
- Cholelithiasis in 90% (cholelithiasis per se is not carcinogenic)
- IBD (UC > Crohn's disease)
- Porcelain GB, 15%
- Familial polyposis
- Chronic cholecystitis

Radiographic features
- Intraluminal soft tissue density (polypoid or fungating mass)
- Asymmetrically thickened GB wall
- Usually no biliary dilatation
- Cholelithiasis
- Direct invasion of liver
    Direct extension, 50%
    Distant liver metastases, 5%
- Gastrohepatic and hepatoduodenal ligaments
    Ligamentous extension, 75%
    Direct invasion into duodenum, 50%
    Lymph node metastases, 70%
- Lymph nodes
    Foramen of Winslow node
    Superior and posterior pancreaticoduodenal nodes
    Hepatic and celiac nodes
    Peritoneal spread
    Carcinomatosis, 50%
    Intestinal obstruction, 25%

CHOLANGIOCARCINOMA

Adenocarcinoma of the biliary tree. Clinical: jaundice, pruritus, weight loss. Treatment: pancreaticoduodenectomy (Whipple procedure) or palliative procedures (stent placement, biliary bypass procedure). Locations:
- Hilar: originates from epithelium of main hepatic ducts or junction: Klatskin tumor
- Peripheral: originates from epithelium of intralobular ducts

Associations
- UC
- *Clonorchis* exposure in Asian population
- Caroli's disease
- Benzene, toluene exposure

Radiographic features
- Dilated intrahepatic ducts with normal extrahepatic ducts
- Hilar lesions
    Central obstruction
    Lesions are usually infiltrative so that a mass is not usually apparent
    Encasement of portal veins causes irregular enhancement by CT
- Peripheral lesions
    May present as a focal mass or be diffusely infiltrative
    Retains contrast materials on delayed scans
    Occasionally invades veins
- ERCP patterns
    Short annular constricting lesion, 75%
    Long stricture, 10%
    Intraluminal polypoid mass, 5%

BILIARY CYSTADENOMA

Biliary cystadenoma is an uncommon, multilocular cystic liver mass that originates in the bile duct and usually occurs in the right hepatic lobe. It typically occurs in women; many women complain of chronic abdominal pain. May represent a congenital anomaly of the biliary anlage. Malignant transformation to cystadenocarcinoma occurs.

Radiographic features
- CT: lesions appear well defined and cystic. The wall and internal septations are often visible and help distinguish this lesion from a simple cyst. The cyst walls and any other soft-tissue components typically enhance with contrast.
- MR: variable appearance, depending on the protein content of the fluid and the presence of an intracystic soft-tissue component.

BILE DUCT HAMARTOMA OR ADENOMA (MEYENBURG'S COMPLEX)

Benign tumor composed of disorganized bile ducts and ductules and fibrocollagenous stroma. The tumor is usually small (1-5 mm), although the nodules may coalesce into larger masses. Although bile duct hamartoma is benign, there have been reports of an association of cholangiocarcinoma with multiple bile duct hamartomas.

Radiographic features
- Nonspecific imaging appearance can simulate metastases or microabscesses, therefore histological diagnosis is required. Multiple bile duct hamartomas may simulate metastases or hepatic abscesses.
- CT: small, well-defined hypoattenuating or isoattenuating mass. Little if any enhancement.
- MR usually hypointense on T1W images, isointense or slightly hyperintense on T2W images, and hypointense after administration of Gd-DTPA.

Cystic Diseases

Cystic disease of the biliary tree can take several forms:
- Cyst in the main duct (choledochal cyst)
- Cysts in the main duct at the duodenal opening (choledochocele)
- Cysts in the small biliary branches within the liver (Caroli's syndrome)
- Other cysts

CHOLEDOCHAL CYST

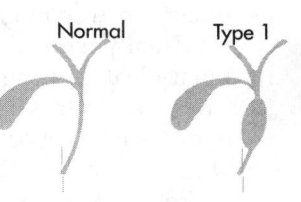

Cystic dilatation of CBD (types 1, 2). Choledochal cysts are often lined with duodenal mucosa. They typically occur in children and young adults (congenital?). Most common in Asia (Japan), uncommon in United States. Because there is a 20-fold increased risk of bile duct malignancy, choledochal cysts are usually excised. Classic triad:
- Jaundice
- Abdominal pain (infection of bile)
- Palpable mass

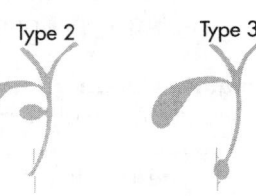

CAROLI'S DISEASE SUBSET

Segmental cystic dilatation of intrahepatic (only) bile ducts (type 5, subset of choledochal cyst). Etiology unknown. Autosomal recessive. Sequence of events:
- Bile stasis predisposes to intrahepatic calculi
- Secondary pyogenic cholangitis
- Intrahepatic abscesses
- Increased risk of cholangiocarcinoma

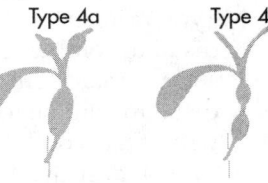

Associations
- Medullary sponge kidney, 80%
- Infantile polycystic kidney disease

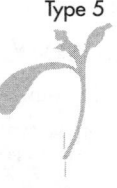

Radiographic features
- Multiple cystic structures converging toward porta hepatis
- Beaded appearance of intrahepatic bile ducts
- Most of the cysts arranged in a branching pattern
- The "central dot sign" is a very specific sign of Caroli's disease in which portal radicals are partially or completely surrounded by abnormally dilated and ectatic bile ducts on both sonography and CT scanning.
- Sludge, calculi in dilated ducts

Intervention

LAPAROSCOPIC CHOLECYSTECTOMY

Technique
1. First trocar is placed blindly in supraumbilical region (most common site of complications).
2. CO_2 is used to inflate the abdomen. Postoperatively, CO_2 is resorbed quickly and persistent gas may indicate bowel perforation.
3. CD is dissected and clipped at both ends.
4. GB is removed via supraumbilical cannula.

Contraindications to laparoscopic cholecystectomy
- Acute cholecystitis, cholangitis
- Peritonitis, sepsis
- Pancreatitis
- Bowel distention
- Portal hypertension
- Morbid obesity

Complications (0.5%-5%)
- Biliary obstruction (clipping or thermal injury to CBD, postoperative fibrosis)
    Usually requires percutaneous drainage
- Biliary leak causing peritonitis and/or biloma (cystic duct stump leak, injury to CBD, leak from small Luschka bile ducts draining directly into GB). Detection of bile leaks: HIDA scan, ERCP, transhepatic cholangiogram
- Other
    Retained stones, stones dropped in peritoneal cavity (Morrison's pouch)
    Bowel perforation
    Hemorrhage, infection

Bismuth classification of bile duct injury

Based on the level of traumatic injury in relation to the confluence of LHD and RHD.

- Type 1: injury > 2 cm distal to confluence
- Type 2: injury < 2 cm distal to confluence
- Type 3: injury immediately distal to confluence but with intact confluence
- Type 4: destroyed confluence

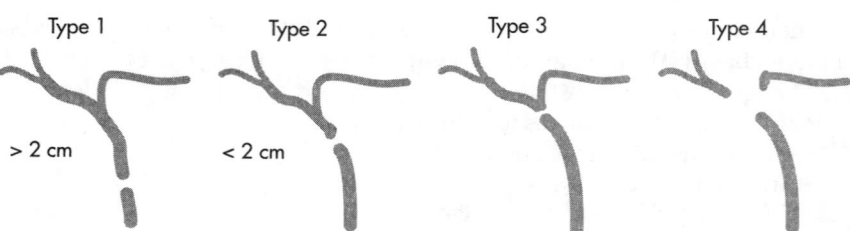

CHOLECYSTOSTOMY

Percutaneous cholecystostomy is often performed for acalculous cholecystitis in ICU patients with unexplained sepsis. In these patients, sonographic findings are not helpful in making the diagnosis of acute cholecystitis and a "trial" of cholecystostomy is often warranted (clinical response is typically seen in 60% of patients).

Indications
- Unexplained fever, suspected cholecystitis. Rationale for catheter placement is to decompress an inflammed GB
- GB must be distended
- GB wall may be thickened, GB may contain sludge

Technique
1. Scan liver by US and choose appropriate entry site. Go through liver to minimize the occurrence of a bile leak.
2. Anesthetize skin.
3. Place 22-G spinal needle into GB under US guidance.
4. Place catheter into GB in tandem. Visualize catheter tip by US before deploying catheter.
5. Aspirate bile for culture. Connect catheter to collecting bag.

Management
- If there is no cholelithiasis the catheter is usually left for ~ 3 weeks. At this point the catheter is clamped to make sure that there is adequate internal drainage. If the patient tolerates clamping, the catheter can be removed.

- If there is cholecystitis, the catheter is left in place until the patient is stable and can undergo a surgical cholecystectomy
- Patients with cholelithiasis have an irritant in the GB and thus a reason for inflammation to recur unlike the patient with acalculous cholecystitis

PERCUTANEOUS BILIARY PROCEDURES

Three types of percutaneous procedures are frequently performed:
- Transhepatic cholangiogram
- Biliary drainage
- Biliary stent placement

Transhepatic cholangiogram
Indication: demonstration of biliary anatomy, first step before biliary drainage or stent placement. Steps in procedure:
1. Antibiotic coverage (particularly if biliary obstruction)
2. Using a lateral midaxillary approach, advance one-stick system into liver
3. Attach extension tubing and syringe filled with contrast. Slowly inject contrast while retracting the needle under fluoroscopy. Repeat until opacification of bile ducts.

Biliary drainage
Indication: biliary obstruction. Steps after transhepatic cholangiogram:

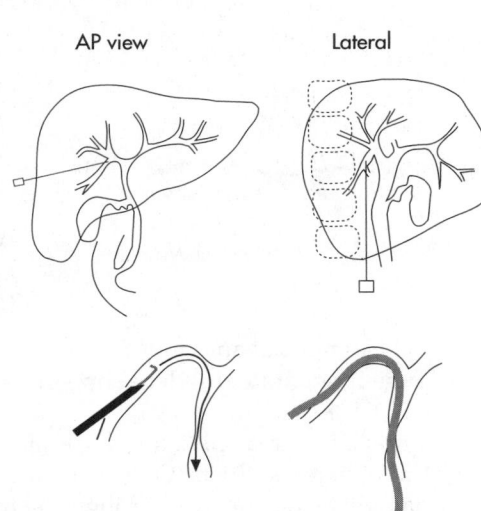

AP view   Lateral

1. After cannulation of bile duct advance a Nitinol guide wire (or the guide wire that comes with the one-stick access set) through the needle into the biliary system. Obtain as much purchase as possible. Remove needle.
2. Pass plastic catheter over guidewire. Exchange guidewire for a 0.038 metal wire or Terumo; pass guidewire into duodenum.
3. Dilate skin tract up to 12 Fr.
4. Place drainage catheter over guidewire (Cope, Ring catheters).
5. Perform catheter injection with contrast material to adjust placement of sideholes.

Biliary stent placement
Indication: (malignant) biliary stricture; inability to place endoscopic stent. Steps:
1. Inject existing catheter to determine exact site of stricture.
2. Choose appropriate stent lengths.
3. Place ultrastiff guidewire, remove indwelling catheter.
4. Place 8 Fr peel-away sheath.
5. Deploy expandable stent (e.g., Wallstent).
6. Inject to confirm location. Leave safety catheter in. Remove guidewire.

Pancreas

General

PANCREATIC ANATOMY

Pancreatic duct

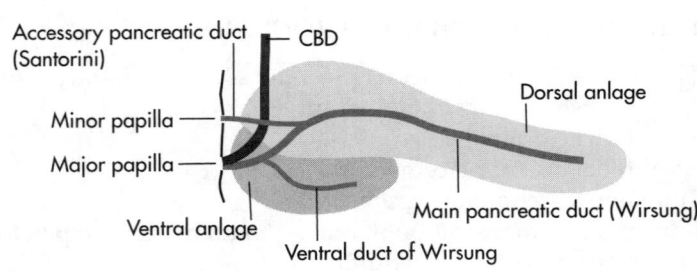

- Duct of Wirsung enters into major papilla together with the CBD
- Duct of Santorini empties into minor papilla
- Both pancreatic ducts communicate with each other near the neck of the pancreas, forming a single remaining duct that runs through the center of the body and tail of the pancreas
- Upper limit size of main duct in young adults: 3 mm, elderly: 5 mm

Variations

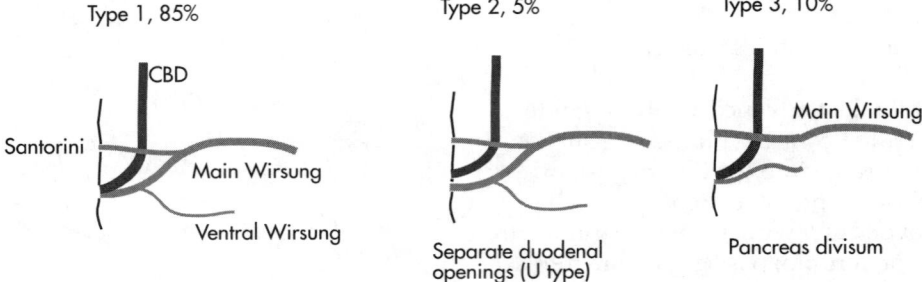

- Type 1: normal anatomy, 85%
- Type 2: separate duodenal openings for pancreatic duct and CBD, 5%
- Type 3: pancreas divisum. Lack of fusion of dorsal and ventral pancreatic ducts. Occurs in 10% of population. Main pancreatic drainage is through the minor papilla. Up to 25% of patients with recurrent idiopathic pancreatitis have pancreas divisum. Pathophysiology of pancreatitis: orifice of duct of Santorini is relatively too small to handle secretions.

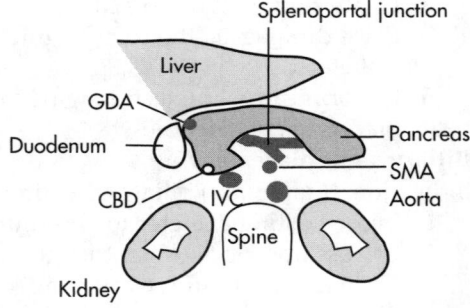

Pancreas dimensions

- Head 2 cm
- Neck (anterior to portal vein) < 1.0 cm
- Body and tail 1-2 cm
- Cephalocaudate diameter 3-4 cm

FATTY INFILTRATION

Fatty infiltration of the pancreas is common normal finding with increasing age.
- Fatty distribution is often uniform
- Focal sparing around CBD is common
- Lobulated external contour

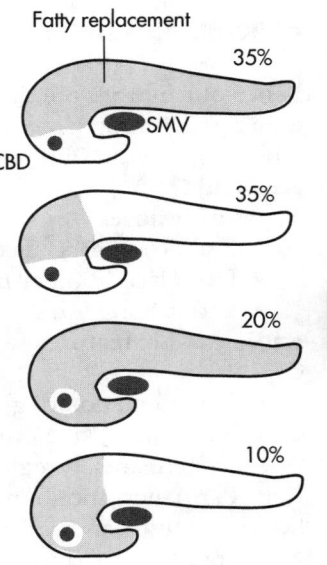

SECRETIN STIMULATION TEST

Secretin (1 CU/kg body weight) is given IV, and the pancreatic and CBD size are measured before and at 1, 5, 15, and 30 minutes. Secretin increases the volume and bicarbonate content of secreted pancreatic juice. Changes in duct diameter:

Normal volunteers
- Baseline duct size 1.9 mm (range 1-3 mm)
- 70%-100% increase in duct size is normal
- Return to baseline duct size within 30 minutes

Chronic pancreatitis
- No significant increase in pancreatic duct size

Functional ductal obstruction
- Pancreatic duct remains dilated 15-30 minutes after administration of secretin

Congenital Anomalies in Adults

CYSTIC FIBROSIS

Pancreatic tissue largely nonexistent; often total fatty replacement is seen. Endstage disease: pancreatic insufficiency.

US features
- Increased echogenicity (fatty replacement)
- Small cysts are rarely visualized, although they are very common (1-3 mm)
- Large cysts (< 5 cm) have been reported but are uncommon

CT features
- Pancreatic tissue totally missing; may see duct
- Small bowel may be dilated with "fecal appearing" contents
- Fibrosing colonopathy: wall thickening predominately proximal colon complication of enzyme replacement therapy

ANNULAR PANCREAS

- Results from abnormal migration of the ventral pancreas
- The pancreas surrounds and obstructs the duodenum
- Appears as annular constriction of second portion of duodenum
- ERCP is the imaging study of choice
- Increased incidence of pancreatitis and peptic ulcer disease

ECTOPIC PANCREATIC TISSUE

- Present in 1%-10% of population
- Sites
  - Stomach (antrum)
  - Duodenum
- Smooth, submucosal mass often with central umbilication (remnant of pancreatic duct)

Pancreatic Trauma

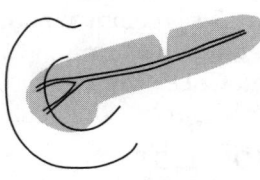

Contusion

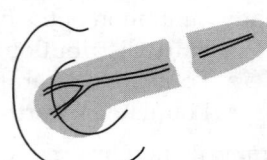

Laceration Complete Transection

Pancreatic injuries are due to either penetrating (stab, gunshot wounds) or blunt (motor vehicle accident) trauma.

Types of injuries
- Simple superficial contusion with minimal parenchymal hemorrhage
- Deep laceration or perforation without duct injury
- Laceration with duct transection

Radiographic features

CT
- Fragmentation of gland
- Pancreatic hematoma
- Nonenhancing regions
- Peripancreatic stranding, exudate

Intraoperative pancreaticography
- Should be performed to evaluate integrity of pancreatic duct (injury to the duct requires different surgery)

Delayed complications
- Pancreatic fistula, 10%-20%
- Abscess, 10%-20%
- Pancreatitis
- Pseudocyst, 2%

Pancreatitis

GENERAL

Pancreatitis classification

Acute pancreatitis
- Mild acute pancreatitis (interstitial edema)
- Severe acute pancreatitis (necrosis, fluid collections)

Chronic pancreatitis

Causes

Common, 70%
- Alcoholic pancreatitis
- Cholelithiasis

Less common, 30%
- Postoperative, post-ERCP, abdominal trauma
- Hyperlipidemia, hypercalcemia
- Drugs: azathioprine, thiazides, sulfonamides
- Inflammation: PUD
- Hyperparathyroidism
- Pregnancy

Clinical

Mild pancreatitis usually presents with pain, vomiting, and tenderness, and progression to severe, acute pancreatitis is not common. Severe, acute pancreatitis is manifested by more dramatic symptoms and signs: shock, pulmonary insufficiency, renal failure, GI hemorrhage, metabolic abnormalities, flank ecchymosis (Grey Turner's sign), and/or periumbilical ecchymosis (Cullen's sign). The severity of acute pancreatitis can be assessed using Ranson (severe pancreatitis: > 3 signs at onset) or APACHE II criteria (severe pancreatitis: > 8 criteria during time of pancreatitis)

IMAGING OF ACUTE PANCREATITIS

CT staging (value of predicting clinical outcome is in dispute)
- Grade A: normal pancreatic appearance
- Grade B: focal or diffuse enlargement of pancreas
- Grade C: pancreatic abnormalities and peripancreatic inflammation
- Grade D: 1 peripancreatic fluid collection
- Grade E: > 2 peripancreatic fluid collections and/or gas in or adjacent to the pancreas

Pearls
- By US, an inflamed pancreas appears hypoechoic relative to liver (reversal of normal pattern) because of edema.
- US is mainly used for investigation of gallstones and/or to follow the size of pseudocysts.

TERMINOLOGY AND COMPLICATIONS

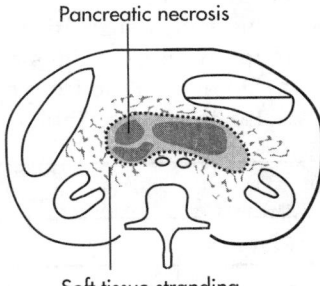

Pancreatic necrosis

Soft tissue stranding

Pancreatic necrosis
- Diffuse parenchymal (> 30% of pancreatic area) or focal areas (> 3 cm) of nonviable parenchyma, peripancreatic fat necrosis and fluid accumulation
- Accuracy of CECT for detection of pancreatic necrosis: 80%-90%
- Presence and extent of fluid associated with fat necrosis can not be accurately determined by CT attenuations #s.
- Prognosis: 30% necrosis = 8% mortality; 50% necrosis = 24% mortality; > 90% necrosis = 50% mortality

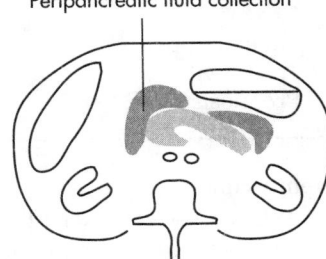

Peripancreatic fluid collection

Acute fluid collections (formerly called phlegmon)
- Collections of enzyme rich pancreatic fluid occur in 40% of patients.
- No fibrous capsule (in contradistinction to pseudocysts).
- Most common location is within and around the periphery of the pancreas. Fluid collections are not limited to the anatomical space in which they arise and may dissect into mediastinum, pararenal space, or organs (spleen, kidney, liver).
- Prognosis: 50% resolve spontaneously; the rest evolve into pseudocysts or are associated with other complications (infection, hemorrhage).
- Differentiation from pseudocyst difficult: test of time

Pseudocyst

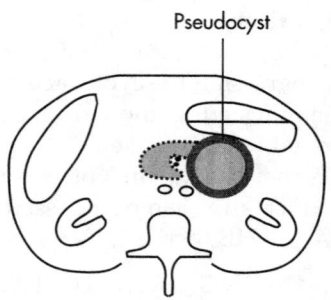

Pseudocyst

- Encapsulated collection of pancreatic fluid which is typically round or oval. The capsule is usually indistinguishable but may occasionally be identified. Caused by microperforation of the pancreatic duct; such a communication can be identified by ERCP in 50% of patients
- Surgical definiton of pseudocyst requires persistence at least 6 weeks from the onset of pancreatitis
- Occurs in 40% of patients with acute pancreatitis and in 30% of patients with chronic pancreatitis
- Bacteria may be present but are often of no clinical significance; if pus is present the lesion is termed a *pancreatic abscess*
- Prognosis: 50% resolve spontaneously and are not clinically significant; 20% are stable and 30% cause complications such as:
    - Dissection into adjacent organs: liver, spleen, kidney, stomach
    - Hemorrhage (erosion into vessel, thrombosis, pseudoaneurysm)
    - Peritonitis: rupture into peritoneal cavity
    - Obstruction of duodenum, bile ducts (jaundice, cholangitis)
    - Infection

Pancreatic abscess

- Intrabadominal fluid collection in or adjacent to the pancreas that contains pus
    - Effectively treated by percutaneous drainage
- Usually occurs > 4 weeks after onset of acute pancreatitis

Infected necrosis

- Necrotic pancreatic (and/or peripancreatic) tissue that can become infected; rarely specific signs of infection; precipitates surgical drainage if infected.
- Differentiation from pancreatic abscess is crucial for appropriate clinical treatment (see Table).

COMPARISON		
Features	Pancreatic Abscess	Infected Necrosis
Location	In or adjacent to pancreas	In pancreas
Pancreas enhancement	Enhancement of periphery	Nonenhancement of necrotic pancreas
Gas	Very infrequent	Very infrequent
Time of appearance	> 4 weeks after onset	Any time
Treatment	Percutaneous drainage	Surgical debridement
Prognosis	Better	Worse

Hemorrhage

- Usually occurs as a late consequence of vascular injury, commonly erosion into splenic or pancreaticoduodenal arteries
- May result from rupture of pseudoaneurysm

PERCUTANEOUS THERAPY

Needle aspiration

- May be performed on any fluid collection, necrotic tissue, or hemorrhage to determine if infected
- Pseudocysts < 5 cm should be monitored rather than aspirated because pseudocysts commonly resolve spontaneously; aspiration risks superinfection (in 10% of cases)

Percutaneous drainage

- Fluid collections are amenable to drainage if clinically suspect of infection: success rate 70%
- Pseudocysts > 5 cm are good candidates for drainage; smaller pseudocysts should be monitored
- Necrotic pancreatic tissue, soft tissue (peri)pancreatic collections and hematomas are a contraindication to drainage; these entities usually require surgery

CHRONIC PANCREATITIS

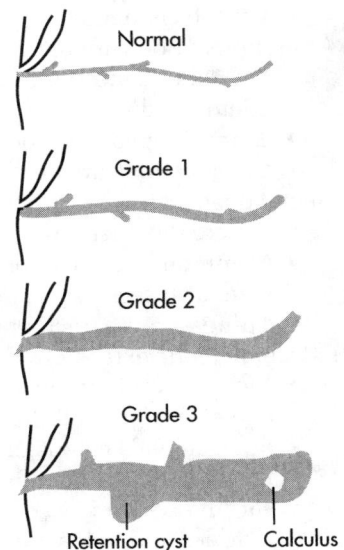

ERCP grading of chronic pancreatitis

Progressive, irreversible destruction of pancreatic parenchyma by repeated episodes of mild or subclinical pancreatitis. Etiology: alcohol, hyperparathyroidism, hyperlipidemia, hereditary.

Radiographic features

Size
- Commonly small, uniformly atrophic pancreas
- Focal enlargement from normal or inflamed pancreas may be coexistent, 40%

Tissue
- Fatty replacement
- Fibrosis
- Parenchymal calcifications, intraductal calculi

Irregular dilatation of pancreatic duct by ERCP: grade 1-3 (see figure)

Complications
- Pseudocysts, 30%
- Obstructed CBD, 10%
- Venous thrombosis (splenic, portal, mesenteric veins), 5%
- Increased incidence of carcinoma
- Malabsorption, steatorrhea, 50%

Neoplasm

TYPES

Exocrine pancreatic tumor
- Adenocarcinoma represents 95% of all pancreatic cancers
- Cystic neoplasm (microcystic adenoma, macrocystic adenoma), 1%
- Intraductal papillary mucinous tumor (IPMT), 1%
- Rare tumors (acinar cell carcinoma, pleomorphic carcinoma, epithelial neoplasm)

Endocrine pancreatic tumor (islet cell neoplasm)
- Insulinoma
- Gastrinoma
- Nonfunctioning islet cell tumor

Other tumors
- Lymphoma
- Metastases
- Connective tissue tumors

ADENOCARCINOMA

Poor prognosis (1-year mean survival rate, 8%). 65% > 60 years. Clinical: jaundice, weight loss, Courvoisier's sign (enlarged, nontender GB), 25%.

Radiographic features
Mass effect
- 65% of tumors occur in head (5% curable), 35% in body and tail (incurable)
- Only part of pancreas is enlarged; global enlargement from associated pancreatitis is uncommon (15%)
- Compression of duodenum
- Enlargement may be subtle
- Sensitivity: contrast-enhanced-high resolution CT > US
- Some small pancreatic tumors are better resolved by US than by CT because of texture changes

Alterations of density (clue to diagnosis)
- On nonenhanced CT scans tumors may appear subtly hypodense because of edema and necrosis
- Tumor appears hypodense on bolus contrast enhanced scans
- Calcifications are very uncommon in contrast to cystic and islet cell tumors

Ductal obstruction
- Pancreatic duct obstruction; pseudocysts are rare
- Common bile duct obstruction with pancreatic duct obstruction (double duct sign: also seen with pancreatis)
- Tumors in the uncinate process may not cause ductal obstruction

Extrapancreatic extension
- Most commonly retropancreatic (obliteration of fat around celiac axis or SMA one sign of incurability)
- Porta hepatis extension
- Direct invasion of stomach, small bowel, etc.

Vascular involvement
- Arteries and veins are best evaluated by angiography or helical CT; rule out replaced right HA pre-Whipples
- Criteria for unresectability
    - SMA encased
    - Portal vein or proximal superior mesenteric vein (SMV) obstructed or largely encased
    - Tumors are still resectable if smaller branches (MCV, RCV, arcades) encased
    - Dilatation of smaller venous branches (> 5 mm): an indirect sign of venous encasement

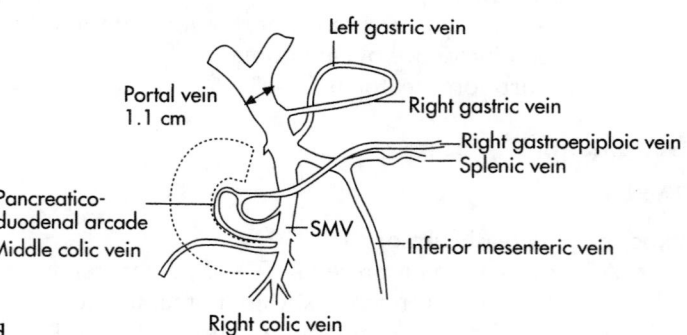

Metastases
- Liver (very common) > lymph nodes > peritoneal and serosal > lung

CYSTIC NEOPLASM

Mucin-producing cystic tumors should be considered when cystic lesions arise in the pancreas. Of all cystic pancreatic lesions, 10% are neoplastic, whereas the remainder represent benign lesions (simple cysts, VHL, pseudocysts). Classification:

- Mucin-producing tumors: malignant potential
    Intraductal papillary mucinous neoplasm (IPMT)
    Mucinous cystic neoplasm
- Serous cystadenoma: no malignant potential

	OVERVIEW	
Features	Serous Microcystic Adenoma (Benign)	Mucinous Cystic Neoplasm (Malignant Potential)
Number of cysts	> 6	< 6
Size of individual cysts	< 20 mm	> 20 mm
Calcification	40%: amorphous, starbursts	20%: rim calcification
Enhancement	Hypervascular	Hypovascular
Cyst content (aspiration)	Glycogen ++++	Mucin ++++
Other features	Central scar (15%)	Peripheral enhancement Spread: local, LN, liver
Demographics	Older patients (> 60 years) 70% in head of pancreas	Younger patients (40-60 years) 95% in body or tail of pancreas

DIFFERENTIATION OF CYSTIC LESIONS BY FLUID CONTENT

	CYST ASPIRATION			
Parameter	Pseudocyst	Serous Cystadenoma	Mucinous Cystadenoma	Mucinous Cystadenocarcinoma
Cytology	Inflammatory	50% positive	Usually positive	Usually positive
CEA	Low	Low	High	High
CA 15-3	Low	Low	Low	High
Viscosity	Low	Low	High	High
Amylase	High	Low	Variable	Variable

INTRADUCTAL PAPILLARY MUCINOUS TUMOR (IPMT) OF PANCREAS

Rare pancreatic cystic neoplasms that arise from the epithelial lining of the pancreatic ducts and secrete thick mucin, which leads to ductal dilatation and obstruction. Synonyms: duct ectatic cystadenocarcinoma, intraductal papillary tumor, duct ectatic mucinous cystadenocarinoma. Types:

- Side branch lesions
- Main duct lesions

Associated with:

- Adenocarcinoma, 25%
- Hyperplasia, 25%
- Dysplasia, 50%

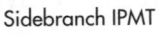
Sidebranch IPMT

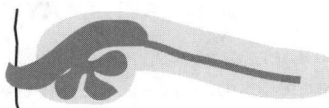

Main duct IPMT

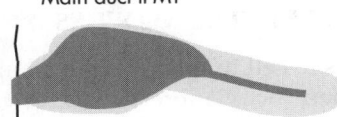

Radiographic features

Location

- Head, uncinate, 55%
- Body, tail, 10%
- Diffuse, multifocal 35%

Ductal abnormalities

- Combined main/side branch duct type, 70%
- Isolated side branch duct type, 30%
- Ductal dilatation, 97%
- "Masses of mucin"
- Clusters of small cysts from 1-2 cm in diameter

Signs of malignancy

- Solid mass
- Main pancreatic duct > 10 mm
- Intraluminal calcified content
- Diffuse or multifocal; involvement
- Presence of diabetes

MUCINOUS CYSTIC NEOPLASMS

Large peripheral tumors surrounded by thick fibrous capsule. The cyst cavity is filled mucinous material. Unlike IPMT, there is no connection to the pancreatic duct. Synonyms: mucinous macrocystic neoplasm, mucinous cystadenoma, mucinous cystadenocarcinoma, macrocystic adenoma.

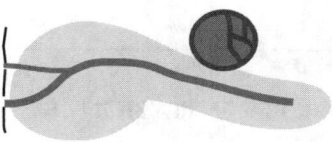

PANCREATOBLASTOMA

- Rare primary pancreatic neoplasm of childhood
- Usually affects patients between 1-8 years of age but has been reported in neonates and in adults
- A congenital form is associated with Beckwith-Wiedemann syndrome
- Slow growing and usually large at presentation
- Large, well-defined, multilobulated masses with enhancing septa by CT; mixed echotexture at US.
- The tumors are soft and gelatinous in consistency, and if arising in pancreatic head, do not usually produce obstructive symptoms.

SOLID AND PAPILLARY EPITHELIAL NEOPLASM

Women < 50 years old

Large lesions of epithelial tissue with slightly more common in body/tail. Well-demarcated, mixed solid and cystic hemorrhagic mass. Solid components with increased enhancement. Prognosis: good with surgical resection.

ISLET CELL NEOPLASM

Islet cell tumors arise from multipotential stem cells: *a*mine *p*recursor *u*ptake and *d*ecarboxylation (APUD) system. Classification:

- Functional (85%): secretion of one or more hormones
- Nonfunctional

Insulinoma (most common functional tumor)
- Single, 70%; multiple, 10%; diffuse hyperplasia or extrapancreatic, 10%
- Malignant transformation, 10%
- 90% < 2 cm
- Hypervascular, 70%
- Diagnostic accuracy: intraoperative US > pancreatic venous sampling > angiography > MRI > other
- Main symptoms: hypoglycemia

Gastrinoma (second most common)
- Solitary, 25%; multiple, ectopic, in stomach, duodenum, etc.
- 60% malignant transformation
- Mean tumor size 35 mm
- Hypervascular, 70%
- Main symptoms: Zollinger-Ellison syndrome (diarrhea, PUD)

Nonfunctioning islet cell tumors (third most common)
- Most common in pancreatic head
- 80%-90% malignant transformation (5-year survival 45%)
- Usually large (> 5 cm) and cause symptoms by exerting mass effect: jaundice, palpable
- Calcification, 20%
- Hypervascular at angiography
- Liver metastases enhance brightly on CT
- Less aggressive than adenocarcinoma
- Better response to chemotherapy

Rare islet cell tumors
- Less aggressive than adenocarcinoma
- Better response to chemotherapy
- Vipoma (vasoactive intestinal peptide)
  WDHA syndrome (*w*atery *d*iarrhea, *h*ypokalemia, *a*chlorhydria)
  60% malignant transformation
- Somatostatinoma
  Suppression of insulin, thyroid-stimulating hormone, growth hormone secretion (hyperglycemia)
  90% malignant transformation
- Glucagonoma
  Diarrhea, diabetes, glossitis, necrolytic erythema migrans
  80% malignant transformation

Transplant

Normal radiographic features
- Pancreas is attached to bladder by duodenal interposition
- Stent may be in place

Complications
- Rejection, 35%
- Pancreatitis, 35%
- Peripancreatic abscess, 35%
- Peripancreatic hemorrhage, 35%
- Vascular thrombosis, 20%

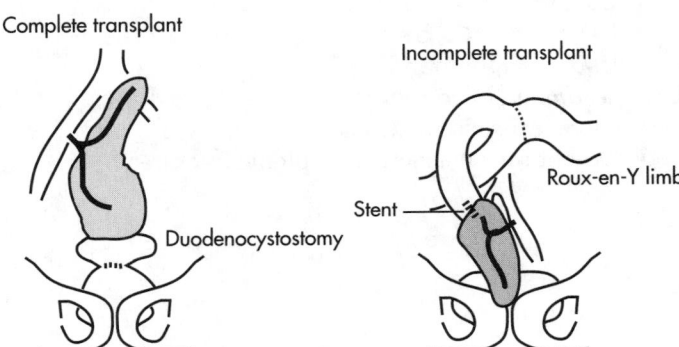

Complete transplant

Duodenocystostomy

Incomplete transplant

Roux-en-Y limb

Stent

WHIPPLE SURGERY

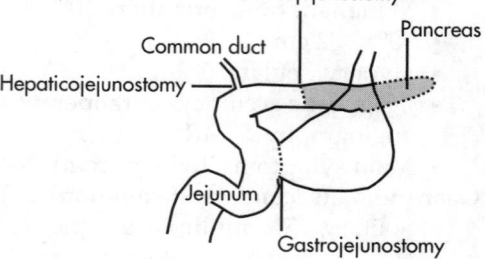

Traditional Whipple
Pancreaticojejunostomy
Pancreas
Common duct
Hepaticojejunostomy
Jejunum
Gastrojejunostomy

- The conventional standard Whipple procedure involves resection of the pancreatic head, duodenum, and gastric antrum. The GB is almost always removed. A jejunal loop is brought up to the right upper quadrant for gastrojejunal, choledochojejunal, or hepaticojejunal, and pancreatojejunal anastomosis.
- Some surgeons prefer to perform pancreatoduodenectomy to preserve the pylorus when possible. In pylorus-preserving pancreatoduodenectomy, the stomach is left intact and the proximal duodenum is used for a duodenojejunal anastomosis.

Complications of pancreatoduodenectomy:

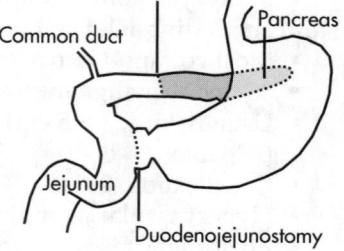

Pylorus sparing Whipple
Pancreaticojejunostomy
Pancreas
Common duct
Jejunum
Duodenojejunostomy

- *Delayed gastric emptying* is defined as the persistent need for a nasogastric tube for longer than 10 days and is seen in 11%-29% of patients.
- *Pancreatic fistula* is defined as surgical drain output of amylase-rich fluid greater than 5 ml/day at or beyond 7 to 10 days. Patients with the clinical diagnosis of pancreatic fistula usually undergo CT to assess for associated abscess formation, but approximately 80% of fistulas heal with conservative management. 10%-15% of patients with pancreatic fistulas require percutaneous drainage, and 5% require repeat surgery.
- Wound infection
- Hemorrhage (can occur if replaced right hepatic artery is severed)
- Pancreatitis
- Abscess formation
- Biliary complications

Spleen

General

ANATOMICAL VARIATIONS

Accessory spleen (in 40% of patients)
- Arise from failure of fusion
- Usually near hilum of spleen
- Usual size: < 3 cm
- Usual shape: round

Lobulations (very common)
- Clefts cause lobulations
- Do not mistake clefts for splenic fractures

Wandering spleen
- Abnormal congenital development of the dorsal mesogastrium. Normally the posterior leaf of dorsal mesogastrium fuses with the parietal peritoneum anterior to the left kidney to form the lienorenal ligament, the most important stabilizer of splenic position. Failure of complete fusion of these structures allows for abnormal mobility of the spleen with a long splenic vascular pedicle. Because of the long pedicle, excessive intraperitoneal movement and torsion can occur. Laxity of suspensory ligaments allows spleen to move in abdomen.
- Confirm with ^{99m}Tc sulphur colloid scan

Polysplenia
- Multiple splenic nodules
- Left-sided liver
- Absence of gallbladder
- Cardiac anomalies
- Incomplete development of inferior vena cava

ASPLENIA

- Absence of spleen (exclude splenectomy)

CT APPEARANCE

- CT density of spleen is slightly less than liver
- Inhomogenous enhancement may normally occur early during contrast administration

Splenomegaly

Defined as splenic length: > 12 cm longest diameter on transverse image. The splenic index (multiply the 3 dimensions) is more accurate for determining splenic size. Normal: 120-480 cm^3. Most radiologists eyeball the size.

Common causes
Tumor
- Leukemia
- Lymphoma

Infection
- AIDS related
- Infectious mononucleosis

Metabolic disorders
- Gaucher's disease
- Vascular
- Portal hypertension

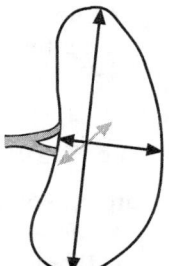

Tumor

HAMARTOMA

Rare, benign tumors primarily composed of vascular elements. Clinical: asymptomatic, anemia, thrombocytopenia.

HEMANGIOMA

Incidence: most common benign splenic tumor (14% of autopsy series).
Radiographic features
- Hyperechoic by US features (similar appearance as liver hemangioma)
- Well delineated, small
- Foci of calcification occur occasionally

METASTASES

- Breast
- Lung
- Stomach
- Melanoma
- Endstage ovarian cancer

Trauma

INJURY

Mechanism
- Blunt trauma
- Penetrating trauma

Spectrum of injuries
- Subcapsular hematoma (crescentic fluid collection)
- Intraparenchymal hematoma
- Laceration
- Fragmented spleen
- Delayed rupture (rare)

Radiographic features
- High density (> 30 HU in acute stage, i.e., < 48 hours) blood in abdomen
- Blood clot is of high CT density and often located near source of bleeding: sentinel clot sign
- Splenic contour abnormality
- Associated other trauma

SPLENOSIS

Autotransplantation of splenic fragments after trauma. Location
- Mesentery, peritoneum, omentum
- Pleura
- Diaphragm

Radiographic features
- Small, enhancing implants
- Best imaged with ^{99m}RBC or ^{99m}Tc sulfur colloid
- Accumulation in most dependent portions: Morrison's pouch, perihepatic space, paracolic gutter

Vascular

Splenic infarct

Common cause of focal filling defects on contrast-enhanced CT. Classically wedge-shaped and peripheral, but more commonly rounded, irregularly shaped and random in distribution. Cause:

Cardiovascular
- Bacterial endocarditis, 50%
- Atheroma
- Valve vegetations
- Mitral stenosis

Tumor
- Lymphoproliferative
- Pancreas
- Inflammatory
- Pancreatitis

Other
- Sickle cell disease
- Polycythemia vera

AIDS

Splenic involvement is common in AIDS. CT has high sensitivity for detection (> 90%) of splenic lesions and identification of associated findings in retroperitoneum, mesentery and/or bowel. Causes of splenic lesions:

Tumor
- Kaposi's sarcoma
- Lymphoma

Infectious
- *Mycobacterium tuberculosis:* low density, abnormal ileocecal region
- MAI: lymph nodes, jejunal wall thickening
- Fungus: *Candida, Aspergillus, Cryptococcus*
- Bacterial: *Staphylococcus, Streptococcus, E. coli*
- Protozoa: *Pneumocystis carinii;* progressively enlarging lesions, calcification in spleen, liver, and lymph nodes

Peritoneum and Abdominal Wall

General

PERITONEAL SPACES

- Subphrenic (suprahepatic) space; divided by the falciform ligament into:
   Right subphrenic space between diaphragm and liver
   Left subphrenic space between diaphragm and spleen
- Morrison's pouch is formed by:
   Right subhepatic recess
   Hepatorenal recess

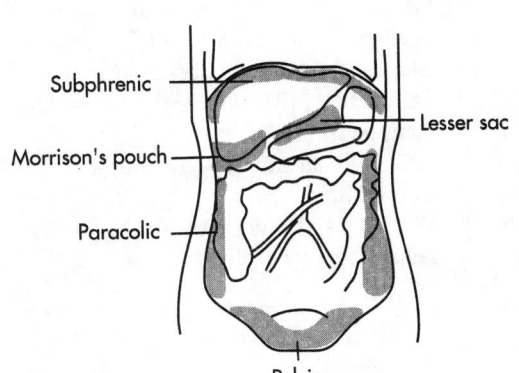

- Morrison's pouch communicates the lesser sac (via the epiploic foramen), the subphrenic space and the right paracolic gutter. In supine position Morrison's pouch is the most dependent portion of the abdominal cavity and collects fluid (it is the most frequently infected space); the pelvic cul-de-sac is the other dependent space.
- Lesser sac (omental bursa): posterior to stomach and anterior to pancreas. Medial cephalad extent between lesser curvature and left hepatic lobe; roofed by gastrohepatic ligament. Access is by the epiploic foramen (Winslow).

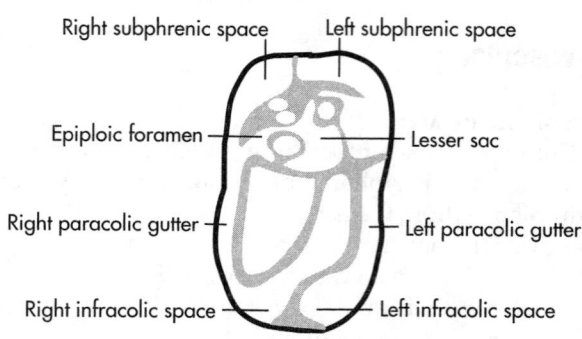

Peritoneum

ABSCESS DRAINAGE

Two techniques are frequently used to percutaneously treat abdominal and pelvic abscesses: trocar technique and Seldinger technique.

Trocar technique

Commonly performed for large abscesses or collections with easy access.

1. Localize abscess by CT or US.
2. Anesthetize skin. Advance 20-G needle into abscess under imaging guidance. Obtain 2-5 mL of fluid for culture. Do not aspirate more because cavity will collapse.
3. Make skin nick and perforate subcutaneous tissues.
4. Place 8-16 Fr abscess drainage catheter in tandem. Remove stylette.
5. Aspirate all fluid; wash cavity with saline.

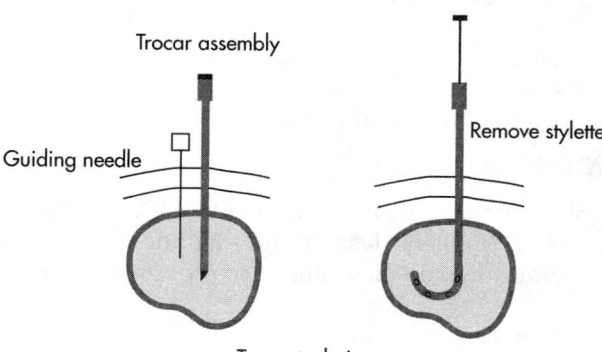

Seldinger technique

Commonly performed for abscesses with difficult access or for necrotic tumors with hard rims.

1. Localize abscess.
2. Anesthetize skin. Localize abscess with 4, 6, or 8 inch Seldinger needle under imaging guidance.
3. Remove needle, leave outer plastic sheath. Pass guidewire (3J) through plastic sheath into abscess cavity.
4. Dilate tract (8, 10, 12 Fr) over stiff guidewire.
5. Pass 8-16 Fr abscess drainage catheter over guidewire.
6. Remove stiffener and guide wire. Aspirate abscess.

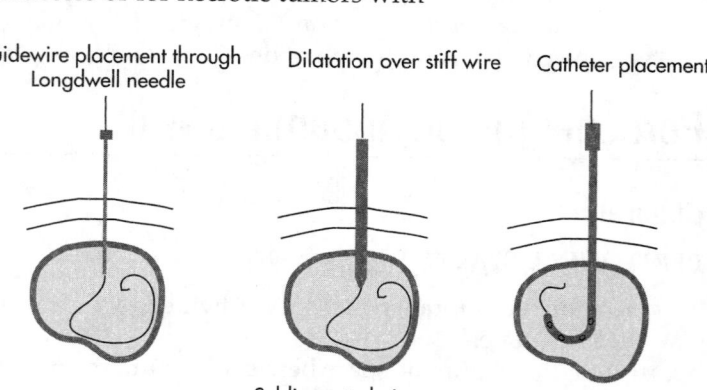

PERITONEAL METASTASES

Most common origin: ovarian cancer, gastrointestinal cancer

Radiographic features
- Greater omentum overlying small bowel: "omental cake"
- Masses on peritoneal surfaces (superior surface of sigmoid colon pouch of Douglas, terminal ileum, Morrison's pouch), gastrocolic ligament
- Malignant ascites (may enhance with Gd-DTPA due to increased permeability of peritoneum)

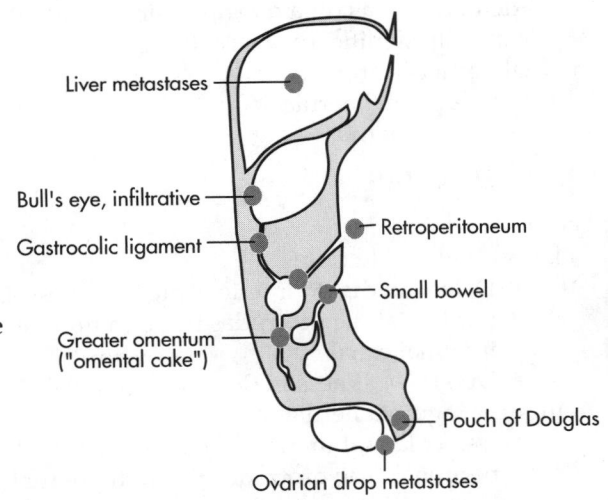

PSEUDOMYXOMA PERITONEI

Accumulation of gelatinous substance in peritoneal cavity due to widespread mucinous cystadenocarcinoma (especially from the appendix or ovary, rarely from other sites).

Radiographic findings
- Scalloped indentations of liver with or without calcification
- Thickening of peritoneal surfaces
- Septated "pseudo" ascites
- Thin-walled cystic masses

ABDOMINAL HERNIAS

Terminology:
- Incarceration: a hernia that cannot be manually reduced
- Strangulation: occlusion of blood supply to the herniated bowel leading to infarction. Findings include bowel wall thickening, hemorrhage, and pneumatosis, as well as venous engorgement and mesenteric edema.

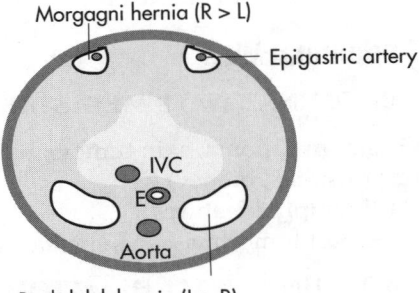

Diaphragmatic hernias
- Congenital diaphragmatic hernias (see also pediatric chapter)
  Bochdalek hernia (posterior)
  Morgagni hernia (anterior)
- Traumatic hernia (left > right)

Abdominal wall hernias
- Spigelian hernias occur along lateral margin of rectus muscle through the hiatus semilunaris. Although these hernias protrude beyond the transverse abdominal and internal oblique muscles, they are contained within the external oblique muscle, thus they may be difficult to detect on physical examination.
- Groin hernias
- Lumbar hernias occur through either superior (Grynfelt) or inferior (Petit) lumbar triangle. The superior lumbar triangle is formed by the 12th rib, internal oblique, serratus posterior, and erector spinae muscles. The iliac crest, lattissmus dorsi, and external oblique muscles form the inferior lumbar triangle. The inferior lumbar triangle is a site of laproscopic nephrectomy ports.

- Richter hernia contains only a single wall of a bowel loop but may still represent clinically significant obstruction.

Internal hernias (rare)
- Paraduodenal hernia
- Lesser sac hernia

GROIN HERNIAS

Types:

Direct inguinal hernia
- Defect medial to inferior epigastric vessels, peritoneal sac protrudes through floor of inguinal canal
- Due to weakness in floor of inguinal canal

Indirect inguinal hernia
- Defect lateral to inferior epigastric vessels, peritoneal sac protrudes through internal inguinal canal
- Due to persistence of processus vaginalis

Femoral hernia
- Enlargement of femoral ring, peritoneal sac protrudes medial to femoral sheath
- Due to increased intraabdominal pressure

Obturator canal hernia occurs through the obturator canal, adjacent to the obturator externus muscle

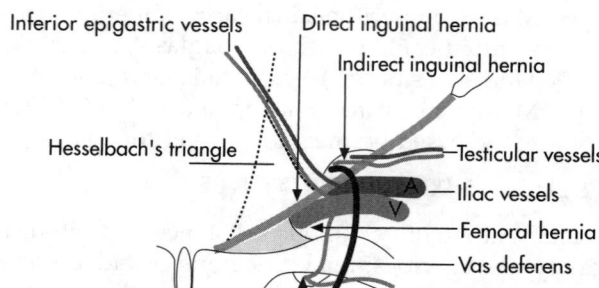

Abdominal Wall

ABDOMINAL WALL METASTASES

Origin: melanoma, skin tumors, neurofibromatosis, iatrogenic seeding, lymphoma (gastrostomy, biopsy)

Radiographic features
- Soft tumor mass in subcutaneous fat with or without focal bulging

ABDOMINAL WALL HEMATOMA

Cause: anticoagulant therapy, femoral catheterization, trauma

Radiographic features
- High attenuation fluid collection: first several days with or without fluid-fluid level (hematocrit level). If there is no further bleeding, the high density RBCs decompose to reduced density fluid.
- Fluid-fluid level (hematocrit level)
- Usually confined to rectus muscle. About 2 cm below the umbilicus (arcuate line), the posterior portion of the rectus sheath disappears, and fibers of all three lateral muscle groups (external oblique, internal oblique and transversus abdominis) pass anterior to rectus muscle. This arrangement has imaging significance in that rectus sheath hematomas above the line are confined within the rectus sheath; inferior to the arcuate line, they are directly opposed to the transversalis fascia and can dissect across the midline or laterally into the flank.

MESENTERIC PANNICULITIS

Rare disorder characterized by chronic nonspecific inflammation involving the adipose tissue of the small bowel mesentry. When the predominant component is inflammatory or fatty, the disease is called *mesenteric panniculitis*. When fibrosis is dominant component, the disease is called *retractile mesenteritis.* The latter is considered the final, more invasive stage of mesenteric panniculitis. The cause of this condition is unclear.

Radiographic features
- Well-circumscribed, inhomogeneous fatty small bowel mesentery displaying higher attenuation than normal retroperitoneal fat. The mass is usually directed toward left abdomen where it extends from mesenteric root to jejunum.
- Speculated, soft tissue mass: a carcinoid mesenteric mass look-alike.

SCLEROSING PERITONITIS

Uncommon but important complication of chronic ambulatory peritoneal dialysis (CAPD). Incidence increases with duration of CAPD. Exact etiology is not known. Clinical onset is heralded by abdominal pain, anorexia, weight loss, and eventually partial or complete small bowel obstruction. Loss of ultrafiltration is common as is bloody dialysis effluent.

Radiographic features
- Plain radiographs normal early in disease. Later curvilinear peritoneal calcification can be seen within the abdomen.
- Plain radiographs may also show centrally located, dilated loops of bowel with wall thickening, edema, and thumb printing.
- CT shows peritoneal enhancement, thickening, calcification, as well as loculated intraperitoneal fluid collection. Adherent and dilated loops of bowel.
- Early diagnosis is essential , as cessation of CAPD and treatment with total parenteral nutrition, hemodialysis, immunosuppression, and/or renal transplantation may result in recovery.

DESMOPLASTIC SMALL ROUND CELL TUMOR

Aggressive malignancy usually occurring in adolescents and young adults.

Radiographic features
- CT shows multiple peritoneal based soft tissue masses with necrosis and hemorrhage
- Hematogenous or serosal liver metastases can be present without detectable primary tumor.

Differential Diagnosis

Esophagus

DIVERTICULAR DISEASE

- Pharyngocele: usually lateral in hypopharynx
- Zenker's diverticulum (pulsion diverticulum)
- Traction diverticula; all layers involved: pulling usually by adhesions to mediastinal structures due to malignancy or TB; typically at level of bifurcation
- Pulsion: all layers, secondary to increased intraluminal pressure
- Pseudodiverticula: small outpouchings due to dilated mucus glands; associated with diabetes, alcoholism, candidiasis, obstruction, cancer
- Epiphrenic diverticulum
- Mimicking lesions:
    Paraesophageal hernia
    Esophageal perforation with contrast extravasation

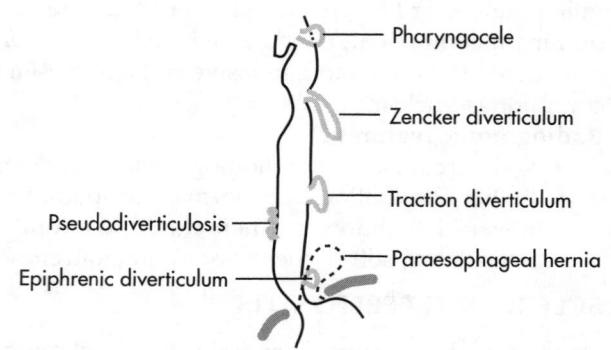

LUMINAL NARROWING

Webs
- Idiopathic
- Plummer-Vinson syndrome

Rings
- Congenital: vascular, muscular rings
- Schatzki's ring

Strictures
- Skin lesions (epidermolysis, pemphigoid): proximal one third of esophagus
- Tumor
- Esophagitis (lye, Barrett's esophagus, infection)
- Achalasia, scleroderma, Chagas' disease

Extrinsic compression
- Vascular aortic arch, arch anomalies, aneurysm, left atrium
- Left bronchus
- Mediastinal tumors

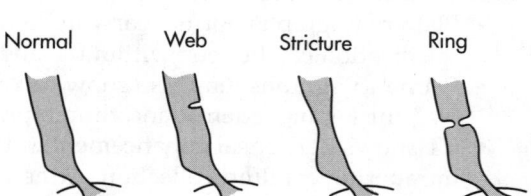

MEGAESOPHAGUS

- Achalasia
- Scleroderma
- Dilatation secondary to distal narrowing
    Tumor
    Stricture
- Chagas's disease
- Diabetic or alcoholic neuropathy
- Bulbar palsy

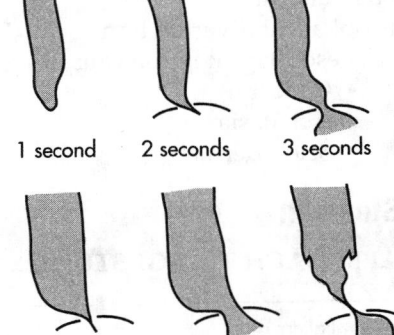

Normal swallowing

1 second   2 seconds   3 seconds

Achalasia   Scleroderma   Tumor

ESOPHAGEAL TEARS (CONTRAST EXTRAVASATION, FISTULA)

- Esophagitis
- Tumor
- Vomiting
    Mallory-Weiss syndrome: only mucosa is disrupted (longitudinal, superficial tear), rarely visualized
    Boerhaave's syndrome: entire wall is ruptured (pneumomediastinum, extravasation of contrast)
- Tracheoesophageal fistulae (pediatric)
- Bronchopulmonary foregut malformation with communication to esophagus
    Bronchogenic cysts
    Extralobar sequestration (pediatric)

SOLITARY FILLING DEFECTS (MASS LESIONS)

Neoplasm
- Benign
    Leiomyoma, 50%
    Pedunculated fibrovascular polyp (especially upper esophagus), 25%
    Cysts, papilloma, fibroma, hemangioma
- Malignant
    Squamous cell carcinoma, 95%
    Adenocarcinoma, 5%
    Carcinosarcoma
    Lymphoma
    Metastases

Foreign bodies

Varices
- Uphill varices (portal hypertension), predominantly inferior location
- Downhill varices (superior vena cava obstruction), predominantly superior location

Extrinsic lesions (lymph nodes, engorged vessels, aneurysms, cysts)

THICKENED FOLDS

- Early forms of esophagitis
- Neoplasm
    Lymphoma
    Varicoid carcinoma
- Varices

AIR-FLUID LEVEL

Hiatal hernia

Esophageal diverticulum

Any esophageal lesion caused by a motility disorder or a stricture

- Cancer
- Achalasia
- Scleroderma

Stomach

APPROACH TO UGI STUDIES

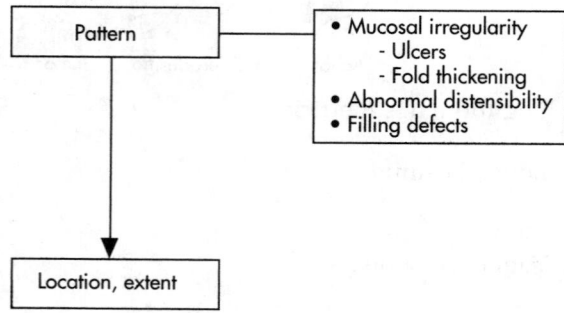

GASTRITIS

- Erosive gastritis (corrosives, alcohol, stress, drugs)
- Granulomatous gastritis (Crohn's, sarcoid, syphilis, TB, histoplasmosis)
- Eosinophilic gastritis (peripheral eosinophilia, 60%, hypoalbuminemia, hypogammaglobulinemia; hyperplastic polyps)
- Hypertrophic gastritis
    Ménétrier's disease
    Zollinger-Ellison syndrome
    Idiopathic
- Recurrent gastric ulcer
    Zollinger-Ellison syndrome
    Peptic ulcer disease
    Retained gastric antrum
    Drugs
- Miscellaneous
    Radiation (> 4000 rad; gastritis occurs 6 months to 2 years after radiation)
    Ulcer
    Corrosives
    Rare causes of gastritis:
        Pseudolymphoma
        Suture line ulceration
        Intraarterial chemotherapy

TARGET (BULL'S EYE) LESIONS

Ulcer surrounded by a radiolucent halo, multiple
Gastritis (aphthoid type, tiny ulcer)

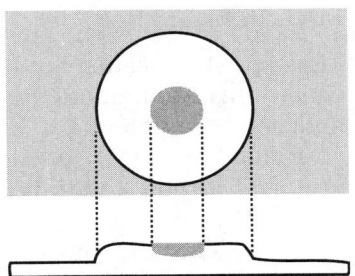

- Erosive: NSAID, alcohol
- Granulomatous: Crohn's disease
- Infections: candidiasis, herpes, syphilis CMV

Submucosal metastases (large ulcer)
- Melanoma, Kaposi's sarcoma >> all other metastases (breast, lung, pancreas)
- Lymphoma

Solitary, giant bull's eye (very large ulcer)
- Leiomyoma
- Sarcoma

FILLING DEFECT (MASS LESION)

Any ingested material may cause a filling defect in the stomach; however, it should move from gastric wall with gravity. If it becomes very large it may be confused with an immobile mass: bezoar. Phytobezoar: undigested vegetable material. Trichobezoar: mass of matted hair. Trichophytobezoar: both. Fixed filling defects:

Neoplasm
- Adenocarcinoma
- Lymphoma
- Leiomyosarcoma
- Metastases
- Kaposi sarcoma

Other
- Endometriosis
- Carcinoid
- Benign tumors: leiomyoma > lipoma, fibroma, schwannoma
- Polyps
- Varices
- Extramedullary hematopoiesis
- Ectopic pancreas

Extrinsic compression
- Spleen
- Pancreas
- Liver

GIANT RUGAL FOLDS

Tumor
- Lymphoma

Inflammation
- Ménétrier's disease
- Zollinger-Ellison syndrome
- Gastritis associated with pancreatitis
- Bile reflux gastritis
- Eosinophilic gastroenteritis

LINITIS PLASTICA

Linitis plastica (leather bottle stomach): marked thickening and irregularity of gastric wall (diffuse infiltration), rigidity, narrowing, and nondistensibility; peristalsis does not pass through linitis.

Tumor
- Scirrhous cancer is the most common cause
- Lymphoma
- Metastases (most common breast cancer)
- Pancreatic carcinoma (direct invasion)

Inflammation
- Erosive gastritis
- Radiotherapy

Infiltrative disease
- Sarcoid
- Amyloid (rare)
- Intramural gastric hematoma (rare)

Infection
- TB, syphilis

ANTRAL LESIONS

Tumor
- Adenocarcinoma
- Lymphoma
- Metastases

Inflammatory
- Crohn's disease
- Peptic ulcer disease
- TB
- Sarcoid

Other (less extensive)
- Hypertrophic pyloric stenosis
- Pylorospasm
- Antral web

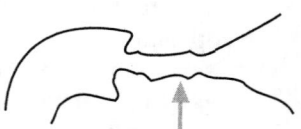

Narrow, rigid, irregular

FREE INTRAPERITONEAL AIR

- Surgery and laparoscopy and other radiologic interventions (most common cause)
- Perforated gastric or duodenal ulcer (second most common cause)
- Cecal perforation from colonic obstruction
- Pneumatosis coli
- Air through genital tract in females
- Perforated distal bowel (e.g., inflammatory bowel disease, diverticulitis, tumor) is usually associated with abscess and lesser amounts of free air

Duodenum

FILLING DEFECTS

Neoplastic filling defects

Benign (often in first portion, asymptomatic)
- Adenoma (usually < 1 cm)
- Leiomyoma
- Carcinoid
- Villous adenoma—near papilla, high malignant potential

Malignant (often distal to first portion, symptomatic)
- Adenocarcinoma at or distal to papilla (90% of malignant tumors)
- Metastases (direct invasion from stomach, pancreas, colon, kidney, etc. or hematogenous such as melanoma)

Other filling defects

Bulb
- Ectopic gastric mucosa
- Prolapsed antral mucosa
- Brunner gland hyperplasia
- Varices

Distal
- Benign lymphoid hyperplasia
- Ectopic pancreas
- Annular pancreas
- Papilla of Vater
- Tumor
- Edema with impacted or passed gallstone
- Choledochocele

Malignancy of duodenal lesions depending on location
- Duodenal bulb: 90% are benign
- 2nd and 3rd portion: 50% are malignant
- 4th portion: 90% are malignant

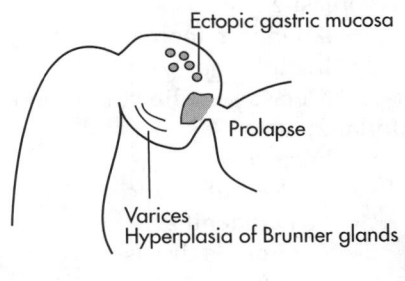

Ectopic gastric mucosa
Prolapse
Varices
Hyperplasia of Brunner glands

LUMINAL OUTPOUCHINGS

Ulcer
- Ulcer with contained perforation
- Malignant ulcer (rarely primary)

Diverticulum
- Pseudodiverticulum: ulcer scarring
- Choledochoduodenal or cholecystoduodenal fistula
- True diverticulum medial, 2nd part duodenum

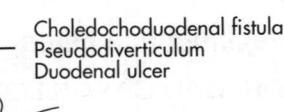

Choledochoduodenal fistula
Pseudodiverticulum
Duodenal ulcer

ULCER VS. DIVERTICULUM		
Finding	Ulcer	Diverticulum*
Opposite incisura	Yes	No
Mucosal folds	Thickened	Normal
Spasm	Present	Absent
Symptoms	Yes	Possible

*Duodenal bulb; pseudodiverticulum; postbulbar duodenum: true diverticulum.

POSTBULBAR NARROWING

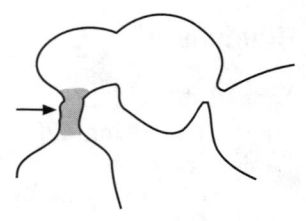

Neoplastic
- Adenocarcinoma
- Lymphoma
- Metastases (direct invasion from colon, kidney, pancreas, GB)

Inflammatory
- Intrinsic
    Postbulbar ulcer
    Duodenitis
    Crohn's disease
- Extrinsic
    Pancreatitis

Other
- Annular pancreas
- Intramural diverticulum
- Duodenal duplication cyst
- Duodenal hematoma
- Aortic aneurysm (3rd portion)
- SMA syndrome (supine position causes partial obstruction of 3rd portion of duodenum by SMA)

PAPILLARY ENLARGEMENT

- Normal variant
- Choledochocele
- Papillary edema
    Pancreatitis
    Acute duodenal ulcer
    Impacted stone
- Ampullary cancer
    Adenomatous polyp
    CA

Jejunum and Ileum

DILATED GAS-FILLED BOWEL LOOPS

The following approach will ensure a correct determination of presence and level of obstruction in 80%.

Approach
1. Is there too much gas in dilated intestine (small bowel > 3 cm, large bowel > 6 cm)?
2. Where is the gas located (large or small bowel or both)?
3. Is the distribution of gas and/or fluid disproportionate between small and large bowel?
4. Is the cecum dilated?
5. Is there free peritoneal air (perforation)?

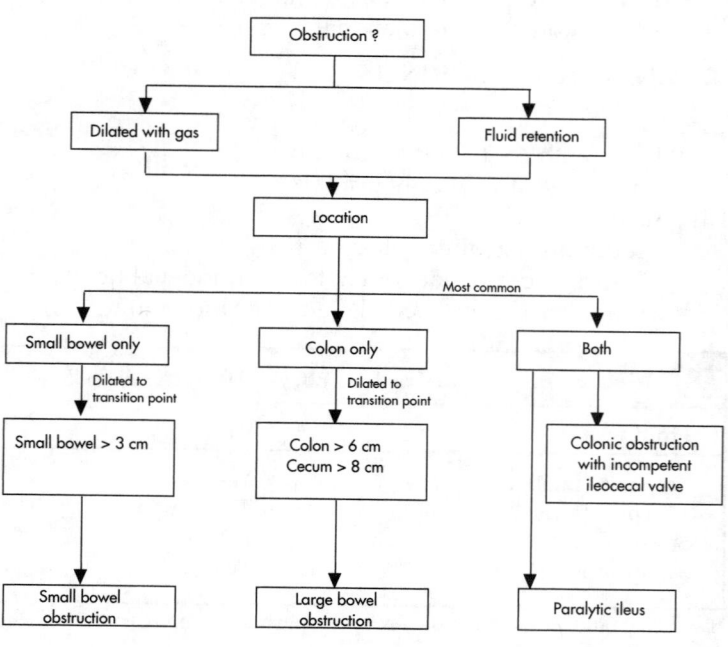

Small bowel obstruction (SBO)

Normal

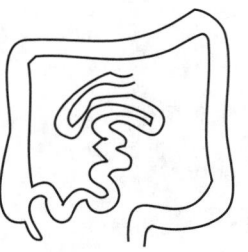

Small bowel obstruction

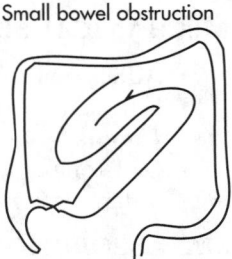

Disproportionate distribution of gas is the key radiographic finding:
- Much more gas and fluid in small bowel compared to colon
- Much more gas in proximal small bowel compared to distal small bowel

Fluid retention parallels gas distribution: no fluid, no obstruction.

Additional examinations in presumed acute SBO:
- If very dilated or abundant fluid: CT (fluid acts as an intrinsic contrast material)
- If mild dilatation: CT with oral contrast or small bowel follow-through
- Enteroclysis: need to decompress bowel before study, best applied to nonacute situations

Colonic obstruction

Colonic obstruction or ileus

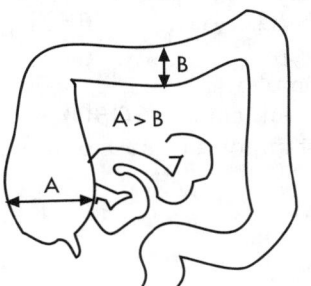

Ileus

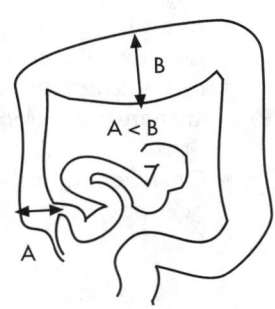

Cecal dilatation is the key radiographic finding:
- Cecum is invariably most dilated in colonic obstruction; however, it may also be very dilated in paralytic ileus (A > B).
- If the transverse colon is more dilated than the cecum (A < B), there is rarely an obstruction (exception: concomitant disease that intrinsically narrows the cecum, such as IBD).
- Fluid retention *not* necessarily seen in colonic obstruction.

A useful initial screening procedure to rule out distal colonic obstruction is a prone KUB: if there is no obstruction, gas passes to the rectum. Barium enema is the definitive study. Do not perform UGI series in a patient with possible colonic obstruction (contraindicated because barium impacts in the colon).

PARALYTIC (ADYNAMIC) ILEUS

Postoperative (most common)
Vascular
- IBD

Inflammatory (often localized ileus: sentinel loop)
- Pancreatitis
- Appendicitis
- Cholecystitis
- Diverticulitis
- Peritonitis

Metabolic
- Hypokalemia
- Hypocalcemia
- Hypomagnesemia

Medication
- Morphine, diphenoxylate (Lomotil)

MECHANICAL SBO

- Adhesions
- Hernias
- Tumors
- Gallstones
- Inflammation with strictures

MALABSORPTION PATTERNS

Signs: dilution of barium (hypersecretion), flocculation of barium, moulage, segmentation of barium column, delay in transit.

Predominantly thick/irregular folds (mnemonic WAG CLEM):

- **W**hipple's disease
- **A**myloid
- **G**iardiasis (largely affects jejunum), graft vs. host reaction, gammaglobulinopathy
- **C**ryptosporidiosis (largely affects jejunum)
- **L**ymphoma, lymphangiectasia, lactase deficiency
- **E**osinophilic gastroenteritis
- *Mycobacterium avium* complex

Predominantly dilated loops (mnemonic SOSO), normal folds

- **S**prue is the single most important cause of true malabsorption
- **O**bstruction or ileus
- **S**cleroderma
- **O**ther
    - Medication
        - Morphine
        - Lomotil
        - Atropine
        - Pro-Banthine
    - Vagotomy

THICK FOLDS WITHOUT MALABSORPTION PATTERN (EDEMA, TUMOR HEMORRHAGE)

Criteria: folds > 3 mm. By CT, the edema in small bowel wall may appear as ring or halo sign. Two types:

- Diffuse: uniformly thickened folds
- Focal: nodular thickening ("pinky printing"), analogous to "thumbprinting" in ischemic colitis, stack-of-coins appearance, picket fence appearance.

Causes

Submucosal edema

- Ischemia
- Enteritis
    - Infectious
    - Radiation
- Hypoproteinemia
- GVH reaction

Submucosal tumor

- Lymphoma, leukemia
- Infiltrating carcinoid causing venous stasis

Normal

Thick folds

Submucosal hemorrhage
- Henoch-Schönlein disease
- Hemolytic uremic syndrome
- Coagulopathies (e.g., hemophilia, vitamin K, anticoagulants)
- Thrombocytopenia, disseminated intravascular coagulation

NODULES

- Mastocytosis
- Lymphoid hyperplasia
- Lymphoma
- Metastases
- Polyps
- Crohn's disease

SMALL BOWEL TUMORS

Benign tumors
- Adenoma (most common)
- Leiomyoma (second most common)
- Lipoma
- Hemangioma
- Neurogenic tumors (usually in neurofibromatosis)
- Other
    Brunner gland hyperplasia
    Heterotopic pancreatic tissue

Malignant tumors
- Metastases
    Melanoma
    Kidney
    Breast
    Kaposi sarcoma
- Lymphoma, very variable appearance
- Carcinoid (most common primary; 50% are malignant and have metastases at time of diagnosis)
- Sarcoma (sarcomatous degeneration of benign tumors: e.g., leiomyosarcoma, lymphosarcoma); usually large ulcerating tumors
- Adenocarcinoma (rare)

Polyposis syndromes

MESENTERIC BOWEL ISCHEMIA

Occlusive disease
- Emboli (atrial fibrillation, ventricular aneurysm)
- Arterial thrombosis (atherosclerosis)
- Venous thrombosis (portal hypertension, pancreatitis, tumor)

Nonocclusive disease (low flow)
- Hypotension
- Hypovolemia

SHORTENED TRANSIT TIME

- Anxiety
- Hyperthyroidism
- Medication
  - Metoclopramide
  - Neostigmine
  - Quinidine
  - Methacholine
- Partial SBO (paradoxical rapid propulsion to point of obstruction)

Colon

MASS LESIONS

Nonneoplastic polypoid abnormalities
- Normal lymphofollicular pattern
- Pneumatosis coli
- Colitis cystica profunda
- Amyloidosis
- Endometriosis
- Ischemic colitis

Polyps
Polyposis syndromes
Benign neoplasm
- Lipoma (common)
- Leiomyoma (rare)

Malignant neoplasm
- Adenocarcinoma
- Metastases
- Lymphoma

POLYPS

Hyperplastic polyps (90% of colonic polyps)
- Not true tumors
- No malignant potential

Adenomatous polyps (second most common type; 25% multiple)
- True tumors
- Malignant transformation
- Types
  - Tubular
  - Villous
  - Tubulovillous

Hamartomatous polyps (rare; Peutz-Jeghers syndrome)

ULCERS

Aphthoid ulcers (superficial)
- Crohn's disease (in 50% of patients)
- Amebiasis
- Behçet's syndrome
- CMV
- Herpes

Deep ulcers

Inflammatory colitis
- Ulcerative colitis
- Crohn's colitis
- Behçet's syndrome

Infectious colitis
- Amebiasis
- TB
- *Salmonella*
- *Shigella*
- Histoplasmosis
- AIDS: *Candida*, herpes, CMV

Ischemic colitis

Radiation colitis

BOWEL WALL THICKENING (THUMBPRINTING)

Thumbprinting refers to luminal indentations the size of a thumb (due to edema, tumor, or hemorrhage). Morphology of accompanying haustral folds may be a clue to underlying diagnosis: preserved haustral folds: infection, ischemia; effaced haustral folds: tumor, IBD.

Edema
- Infectious colitis

    Pseudomembranous colitis (*Clostridium difficile*)

    CMV colitis

    E. coli, Shigella, Salmonella, amebiasis

    Neutropenic colitis (typhlitis)
- IBD

Tumor
- Lymphoma, leukemia

Hemorrhage
- Ischemia
- Schönlein-Henoch disease, thrombocytopenia, DIC
- Coagulopathies (e.g., hemophilia, vitamin K, anticoagulants)

TUMORLIKE COLONIC DEFORMITY

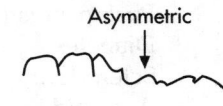

Deformities may be symmetrical (circumferential, apple core) or asymmetrical.

Tumor
- Adenocarcinoma

    Saddle-shaped if asymmetrical

    Apple core if circumferential
- Metastases (common serosal implants: gastric, ovarian)

Inflammation
- Diverticulitis
- Focal inflammation

    IBD: Crohn's disease, UC

    Infectious: ameboma, TB

Other
- Endometriosis
- Pelvic abscess
- Epiploic appendagitis

LONG (> 10 CM) COLONIC NARROWING

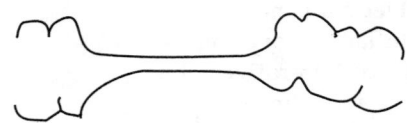

- Scirrhous adenocarcinoma
- Lymphoma
- UC (with or without carcinoma)
- Crohn's disease
- Ischemic stricture
- Radiation

AHAUSTRAL COLON

- Cathartic abuse (often right colon)
- UC, Crohn's disease
- Amebiasis
- Aging (usually left colon)

COLONIC OBSTRUCTION

- Carcinoma, 65%
- Diverticulitis, 20%
- Volvulus, 5%
- Other
    - Impaction
    - Hernia

MEGACOLON

Descriptive term for abnormally distended transverse colon (> 6 cm); most commonly used in conjunction with toxic megacolon.
Toxic megacolon (haustral deformity, pseudopolyps; risk of perforation; systemic signs)
- UC, Crohn's disease
- Infectious: amebiasis, shigellosis, clostridium difficile

Acute colonic distention (risk of perforation with cecum > 9 cm)
- Obstructive: cancer
- Paralytic ileus
- Volvulus

Chronic megacolon (no or small risk of perforation)
- Cathartic colon (chronic laxative abuse)
- Colonic pseudoobstruction (Ogilvie's syndrome, colonic ileus)
- Psychogenic
- Congenital (Hirschsprung's disease)
- Chagas' disease
- Neuromuscular disorders
    - Parkinsonism
    - Diabetes
    - Scleroderma
    - Amyloid
- Metabolic, drugs
    - Hypothyroidism
    - Electrolyte imbalances

ADULT INTUSSUSCEPTION

Ileoileal (40%) > ileocolic (15%) > other locations.
  Idiopathic, 20%
  Tumors, 35%
    • Polyps, lipoma, 25%
    • Malignant tumors (metastases, lymphoma, carcinoid), 10%
  Other
    • Meckel's diverticulum
    • Adhesions
    • Aberrant pancreas

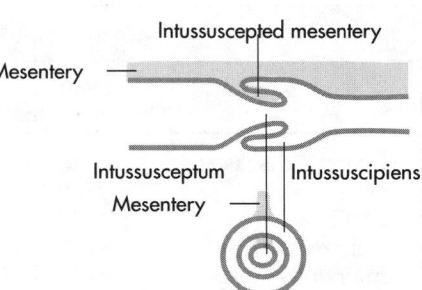

PNEUMATOSIS COLI

Pneumatosis cystoides (large, cystlike collection of air, few symptoms); associated
with benign etiologies:
  • Chronic obstructive pulmonary disease
  • Patients on ventilator
  • Mucosal injury (rectal tube insertion, colonoscopy, surgery)
  • Scleroderma
  • Steroids
  • Chemotherapy
Pneumatosis intestinalis (symptomatic); associated with serious etiologies:
  • Infarcted bowel (tiny bubbles, linear gas collections)
  • Necrotizing enterocolitis (neonates)
  • Toxic megacolon
  • Typhlitis

ILEOCECAL DEFORMITIES

Inflammation (coned cecum)
  • Crohn's disease: aphthous ulcers → linear fissures → nodules → cobblestone →
    stricture, spasm (string sign), fistula
  • UC: valve is wide open (gaping), labia are atrophied, terminal ileum dilated
  • Amebiasis (predominantly affects cecum, not terminal ileum)
  • TB: narrow cecum (Fleischner sign), narrow Crohn's may produce same
    appearance, terminal ileum (Stierlin's sign)
  • Typhlitis: inflammatory changes of cecum and/or ascending colon in
    neutropenic (immunosuppressed, leukemia, lymphoma) patients; caused by
    infection, bleeding, ischemia)
Tumor
  • Lymphoma
  • Adenocarcinoma
  • Carcinoid of ileum (desmoplastic response) or appendix
  • Intussusception

DIFFERENTIAL DIAGNOSES OF COLITIS BY CT					
	Wall Thickness (mm)	Submucosal Fat	SB Involvement	Left Colonic Involvement Only %	Ascites	Abscess
Crohn's disease	> 10	10%	60%	50	10%	35%
UC	< 10	60%	5%	30	0%	0%
PMC	> 10	5%	5%	30	50%	0%
Ischemic colitis	< 10	0%	Uncommon	80	15%	0%
Infectious colitis	< 10	0%	0%	0	50%	0%

PROCTITIS

- Condylomata acuminata
- Lymphogranuloma venereum
- Gonococcal proctitis
- UC, Crohn's disease

Liver

LIVER MASSES

Solid masses
- Neoplasm
    Benign: hemangioma
    Malignant: primary, secondary
- Focal fatty liver (pseudotumor)
- Regenerating nodules in cirrhosis

Cystic masses
- Infectious
    Echinococcus
    Amebiasis
    Other abscesses (often complex and have debris)
- Benign masses
    Simple liver cysts
    Polycystic disease of the liver
    Biliary cystadenoma
    Obstructed intrahepatic GB
    Biloma
- Malignant masses
    Cystadenocarcinoma
    Cystic metastases: ovarian tumors
    Necrotic tumors
    Cholangiocarcinoma

ABNORMAL LIVER DENSITY (CT)

Increased liver density
- Hemachromatosis
- Glycogen storage disease
- Wilson's disease
- Drugs: amiodarone, cisplatin
- Apparent increased density of liver parenchyma in patients with anemia (relative decreased blood density)

Decreased liver density
- Fatty liver (common)
    - Obesity, nutritional
    - Alcohol
    - Diabetes
    - Steroids
    - Chemotherapy

HYPERVASCULAR LIVER LESIONS

- Hemangioma
- Hemangioendothelioma, hemangiopericytoma, angiosarcoma (all rare), intrahepatic cholangiocarcinoma
- Metastases
    - Islet cell
    - Melanoma
    - Carcinoid
    - Renal cell cancer
    - Thyroid
    - Breast
    - Sarcoma

HYPERECHOIC LIVER LESIONS

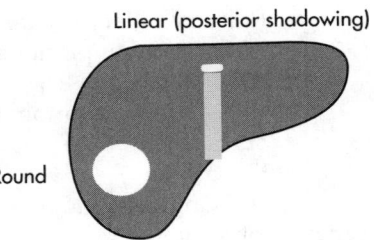

Round lesions
- Hemangioma
- Hyperechoic metastases
    - Hypervascular metastases, sarcoma
    - Calcified metastases
- Primary liver tumors (contain fat)
    - HCC
    - Fibrolamellar HCC
- Focal fat, lipoma, angiomyolipoma (tuberous sclerosis)
- Gaucher's disease

Linear lesions
- Air in biliary tree
- Air in portal veins
- Biliary ascariasis

MULTIPLE HYPOECHOIC LIVER LESIONS

Tumor
- Metastases
- Lymphoma
- Multifocal HCC

Infection
- Multiple pyogenic abscesses
- Amebic abscesses
- *Echinococcus*
- Candidiasis
- Schistosomiasis

Other

- Regenerating nodules, cirrhosis
- Sarcoid
- Extramedullary hematopoiesis
- Hematomas
- Hemangioma

GAS IN LIVER

- Biliary gas (ERCP, surgery)
- Portal venous gas (bowel necrosis, diverticulitis)
- Abscess
- Emphysematous cholecystitis

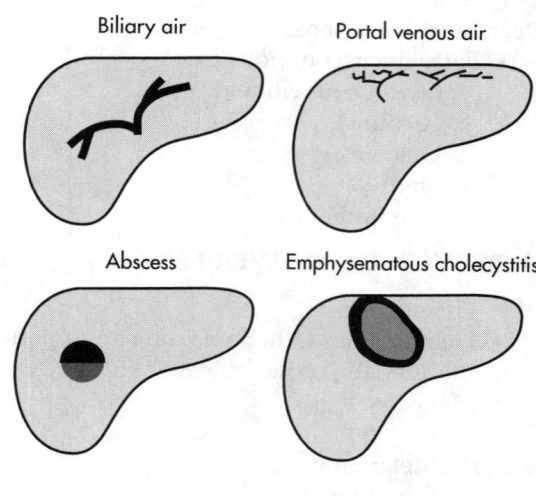

Biliary System

EXTRAHEPATIC BILIARY DILATATION

The obstruction may occur at any of three levels:

Intrapancreatic (most common)
- Pancreatic cancer
- Calculus
- Chronic pancreatitis

Suprapancreatic
- Primary biliary ductal carcinoma
- Metastatic lymph nodes

Portal
- Invasive GB carcinoma
- Surgical strictures
- Hepatoma
- Cholangiocarcinoma

Types of obstruction

Tumor
- Abrupt termination of duct
- Mass adjacent to duct

Pancreatitis
- Smooth, long tapering

Lithiasis-related disease
- Calculus visible
- Mensicus sign (ERCP, CT) intrahepatic dilatation

Cholangitis
- Sclerosing cholangitis (50% have ulcerative colitis)
- AIDS cholangitis
- Intrahepatic biliary calculi (oriental cholangiohepatitis)

Caroli's disease

Intrahepatic biliary neoplasm (rare)
- Cystadenoma
- Cystadenocarcinoma

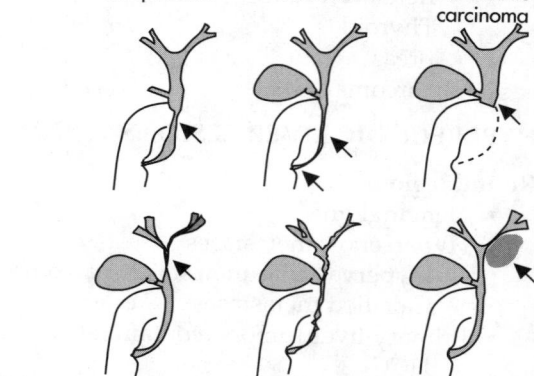

Ultrasound signs of intrahepatic dilatation

- Color Doppler flow absent in dilated ducts
- Acoustic enhancement behind dilated ducts; blood, in contrast, attenuates acoustic beam (high protein content)
- Double duct sign: dilated biliary vessel accompanies portal veins
- Caliber irregularity and tortuosity of dilated bile ducts; veins are always smooth and taper gradually
- Spoke-wheel appearance at points of conversion of ducts

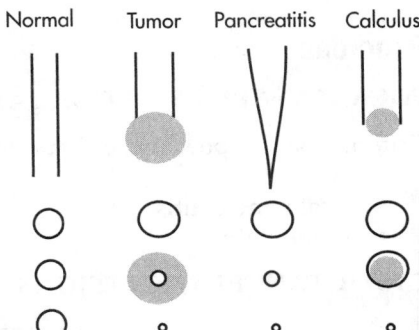

GALLBLADDER WALL THICKENING

GB wall thickening: > 3 mm. Wall thickening typically appears as a hypoechoic region between two echogenic lines. When measuring wall thickening by US, a 5-Mhz transducer should be used.

Diffuse (concentric) thickening (in order of decreasing frequency)
- Nonfasting GB (GB is usually < 2 cm in size)
- Acute cholecystitis (50%-75% of patients have thickening)
- Chronic cholecystitis (< 25% of patients have thickening)
- Portal venous hypertension (cystic vein dilatation causes edema)
- Hypoalbuminemia (must be < 2.5 g/dl)
- Hepatitis
- AIDS (cryptosporidiosis, CMV, MAI)
- Ascites
    Benign ascites → GB wall thickening
    Malignant ascites → no GB wall thickening

Focal (eccentric) thickening
- GB carcinoma (40% present with focal thickening; mass typically fills the GB)
- Metastases (melanoma >> gastric, pancreas)
- Benign tumors
    Polyps (cholesterol, adenomatous)
    Adenomyomatosis
- Tumefactive sludge adherent to GB wall
- AIDS

HYPERECHOIC FOCI IN GALLBLADDER WALL

- Calculus
- Polyp
- Cholesterol
- Emphysematous cholecystitis
- Porcelain GB

DENSE GALLBADDER (CT)

- Hepatobiliary (vicarious) excretion of contrast material
- Calculi
- Milk of calcium bile
- Reflux of oral contrast agent after surgery
- Oral cholecystogram
- Hemorrhage (hematocrit effect)

Pancreas

FOCAL PANCREATIC SIGNAL ABNORMALITY

Criteria: focal hypoechoic or hypodense pancreatic lesion
- Tumor
- Focal pancreatitis
- Adenopathy

CYSTIC PANCREATIC LESIONS

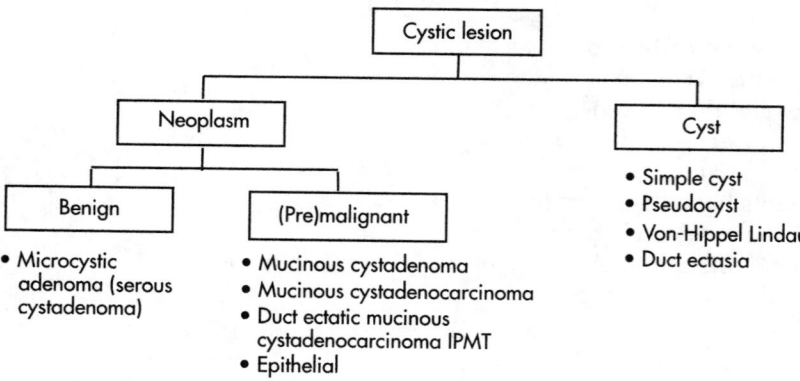

HYPERECHOIC PANCREAS

The normal pancreas appears slightly hyperechoic relative to liver. Marked hyper-echogenicity is seen in:
- Cystic fibrosis
- Pancreatic lipomatosis

Spleen

FOCAL SPLENIC LESIONS

Tumor
- Metastases (usually in endstage disease); lymphoma, melanoma, ovary
- Hemangioma (common benign lesion)
- Lymphangioma
- Hamartoma
- Rare lesions: myxoma, chondroma, osteoma, hemangiosarcoma, fibrosarcoma

Infection (often calcified)
- Abscess
- Candidiasis (common in AIDS)
- TB, MAI
- Schistosomiasis (splenic nodules in 10%)
- *Pneumocystis carinii*

Other
- Infarcts
- Hematoma (trauma)
- Cysts: simple, hydatid
- Fatty nodules in Gaucher's disease

SPLENOMEGALY

Tumor
- Leukemia
- Lymphoma

Infection
- Infectious mononucleosis
- Histoplasmosis

Metabolic disorders
- Gaucher's disease
- Amyloid
- Hemochromatosis

Trauma

Vascular
- Portal hypertension
- Hematological disorders (anemias, sickle cell, thalassemia, myelofibrosis, myelosclerosis)

Peritoneal Cavity

PERITONEAL FLUID COLLECTIONS

Water density
- Ascites
- Urinoma
- Biloma
- Seroma
- Lymphocele (after lymph node resection)
- Pancreatic pseudocyst
- Cerebrospinal fluid pseudocyst from VP shunt

Complex (may be loculated, noncommunicating, heterogenous signal intensity)
- Abscess
- Hematoma
- Pseudomyxoma peritonei
- Pancreatic necrosis

INTRAPERITONEAL CALCIFICATIONS

- Arterial calcification
- Appendicolith
- Mesenteric node
- Cholelithiasis
- Pancreatic calcification
- Porcelain GB
- Renal/ureteral calculi
- Old hematoma, abscess
- Uterine leiomyoma
- Fetal skeletal part
- Pelvic phlebolith
- Teratoma
- Liver: echinococcal cyst

Other

AIDS

Common gastrointestinal manifestations by cause
Infection
- CMV
- *Candida*
- Herpes
- *Cryptococcus*
- MAI

Tumor
- Kaposi
- Lymphoma

Common gastrointestinal manifestations by organ system
Esophagus
- Ulcers: *Candida,* CMV, herpes
- Sinus tracts: TB, actinomycosis

Proximal small bowel
- Ulcers: cryptococcosis
- Nodules: Kaposi's sarcoma, MAI

Distal small bowel
- Enteritis: TB, MAI, CMV

Colon
- Colitis: CMV, pseudomembranous colitis
- Typhlitis

Biliary
- Strictures: CMV, cryptococcosis

ABDOMINAL TRAUMA

Injuries in decreasing order of frequency:
- Liver laceration (most common)
- Splenic laceration
- Renal trauma
- Bowel hematoma
- Pancreatic fracture
- Rare: GB injury, adrenal hemorrhage

ABDOMINAL COMPLICATIONS AFTER CARDIAC SURGERY

Incidence 0.2%-2%. Most commonly, complications are related to ischemia (e.g., intraoperative hypotension, hemorrhage, vasculopathy, emboli, clotting abnormalities).
- GI hemorrhage, 50%
- Cholecystitis (emphysematous, acalculous, or calculous), 20%
- Pancreatitis, 10%
- Perforated peptic ulcer, 10%
- Mesenteric ischemia, 5%
- Perforated diverticular disease, 5%

SUGGESTED READINGS

Eisenberg RL: *Gastrointestinal radiology: a pattern approach*, Philadelphia, 1990, JB Lippincott.

Gedgaudas-McClees R: *Handbook of gastrointestinal imaging*, New York, 1987, Churchill Livingstone.

Gore RM, Levine MS, Laufer I: *Textbook of gastrointestinal radiology*, Philadelphia, 2000, WB Saunders.

Halpert RD, Goodman P: *Gastrointestinal radiology: the requisites*, St Louis, 1999, Mosby.

Jones B, Braver JM: *Essentials of gastrointestinal radiology*, Philadelphia, 1982, WB Saunders.

Marguilis AR, Burhenne HJ, editors: *Alimenatry tract radiology*, ed 4, St Louis, 1989, Mosby

Meyer MA : *Dynamic radiology of the abdomen: normal and pathologic anatomy*, New York, 2000, Springer-Verlag.

Moss AA, Gamsu G, Genant HK: *Computed tomography of the body with magnetic resonance imaging*, Philadelphia, 1992, WB Saunders.

Rifkin M, Charboneau J, Laing F: *Syllabus special course: ultrasound*, Oak Brook, Ill, 1991, Radiological Society of North America.

Rumack CM, Wilson M: *Diagnostic ultrasound*, St Louis, 1997, Mosby.

Taylor KJW: *Atlas of ultrasonography*, New York, 1985, Churchill Livingstone.

Weissleder R, Stark DD: *MRI atlas of the abdomen*, London, 1989, Martin Dunitz Publishers.

3

Chapter 4

Genitourinary Imaging

Chapter Outline

Kidneys

General

ANATOMY

The kidneys, renal pedicle, and adrenal glands are located in the perirenal space, which is bound by the anterior and posterior renal fascia (Gerota's fascia; for anatomy, see the section titled Retroperitoneum).

Renal pedicle
- Renal artery
- Renal vein
- Collecting system and ureter
- Lymphatics

Collecting system
- Minor calyces: most kidneys have between 10-14 minor calyces
- Major calyces
- Renal pelvis: may be completely within the renal sinus or partially "extrarenal"

Orientation and size of kidneys
- Kidneys are 3 to 4 lumbar vertebral bodies in length, 12-14 cm long, 5-7 cm wide
- Intravenous pyelograms (IVPs) overestimate the true renal length because of magnification and renal engorgement from osmotic diuresis. Ultrasound (US) often underestimates the true renal length because of technical difficulties in imaging the entire kidney
- Left and right kidney size should not vary more than 1 cm
- Right kidney is 1-2 cm lower than left kidney and slightly more lateral
- Renal axis parallels axis of psoas muscles

Techniques

BOLUS IVP

Bolus administration assures maximum concentration of contrast media in the kidney. Indication: healthy ambulatory patients (screening type urography, e.g., for urinary tract infection), trauma. Technique:
1. Kidney, ureter, bladder (KUB).
2. Inject 100 mL of 30% contrast.
3. 1-min and 5-min film of both kidneys.
4. 10-min KUB and both obliques.
5. Coned bladder view.
6. Postvoid KUB.

DRIP-INFUSION NEPHROTOMOGRAM

With drip infusion, the nephrogram persists longer allowing more time for nephrotomography and special views, if necessary. Today, this is much less commonly performed than bolus technique or computed tomography (CT). If calcifications are seen on the renal outlines, scout oblique films can be obtained to determine the exact location relative to the kidneys. Technique:

1. KUB and preliminary tomogram of kidneys (starting at 8 cm from back)
2. Drip infusion of 300 mL of Urovist 14% (or Conray-30) or 150 mL of Isovue 300 (or Omnipaque 300)
3. Obtain tomograms after 150 mL has been given. Usually 7-9 cuts are obtained.
4. Postinfusion KUB and both oblique views
5. Coned bladder view
6. Postvoid KUB

SUMMARY OF CONTRAST DOSAGE		
	Body Weight	Dose of Contrast
Bolus injection		
Children	5-25 kg	0.5 mL/kg
	25-50 kg	50 mL
Adult	> 50 kg	100 mL (28-40 g iodine)
Infusion technique		
Children		Contraindicated
Adult		300 mL (33-45 g iodine)

CT PROTOCOLS OF THE KIDNEY/URETERS

Patients with hematuria:
- Phase 1: Noncontrast CT of abdomen and pelvis from top of kidney to pubic symphysis. Administer 30 mL of IV contrast and wait 5-10 min.
- Phase 2: Place patient back on scanner and inject 100 mL of IV contrast at 2-3 mL/sec and scan patient prone from top of kidneys to pubic symphysis at 100 sec.
- Delayed phase (5 minutes) through the kidneys

Patients with suspected stone disease:
- Noncontrast CT of the abdomen and pelvis

PERCUTANEOUS NEPHROSTOMY (PCN)

Refers to percutaneous drainage of renal collecting system by catheter placement.
Complications: 2%-4% (extravasation of contrast, bleeding).

Indications
- Hydronephrosis (acute, subacute obstruction)
- Pyonephrosis

Technique
1. Preprocedure workup:
   - Check bleeding status.
   - Antibiotic coverage: ampicillin 1 g, gentamicin 80 mg.
   - Review all films and determine on plain film where kidneys are located, especially in relation to colon and pleural reflections.
   - US or IV contrast opacification of kidneys may be helpful in difficult approaches or nondilated collecting systems. IV contrast is less useful with severe obstruction because opacification may not occur or may be impractically delayed.

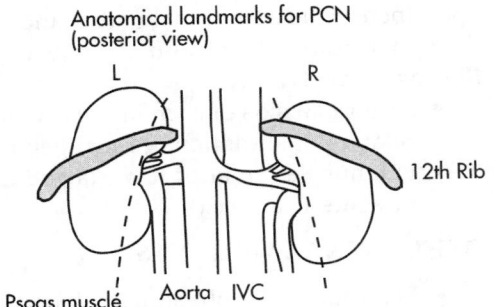

Anatomical landmarks for PCN (posterior view)

2. Local anesthesia, aiming for upper pole calyx with Turner biopsy needle or spinal needle (20 G). Aspirate urine to check for position and for partial decompression of collecting system before contrast opacification.
3. Using a second needle/sheath system, aim for middle pole calyx. Skin insertion point is inferior and slightly lateral to calyx. When positive urine returns, advance 0.038 guidewire as far as possible. If wire coils in calyceal system, a Kumpe catheter may be useful for manipulation.
4. Dilate skin up to 12 Fr.
5. Pass 10 Fr PCN tube over guidewire. Remove stiffener and guidewire. Coil pigtail. Inject contrast to check position of catheter. Cut thread.
6. In the setting of infection, complete evaluation of the ureter via an antegrade injection is best deferred to a second visit.

Congenital Anomalies

DUPLICATED COLLECTING SYSTEM

Bifid renal pelvis
One pelvis drains upper pole calyces; the other drains the middle and lower pole calyces. The two pelvises join proximally to the ureteropelvic junction (UPJ). Incidence: 10% of population. No complications.

Incomplete ureteral duplication
Duplications join distal to UPJ and proximal to bladder: "Y-shaped ureters." No complications.

Complete ureteral duplication
See pediatric chapter.

HORSESHOE KIDNEY

The two kidneys are connected across the midline by an isthmus. This is the most common fusion anomaly (other fusion anomalies: cross-fused ectopia, pancake kidney). The isthmus may contain parenchymal tissue with its own blood supply or consist of fibrous tissue.

Associations
- UPJ obstruction, 30%
- Ureteral duplication, 10%
- Genital anomalies
- Other anomalies: anorectal, cardiovascular, musculoskeletal anomalies

Complications
- Obstruction, infection, calculus formation in 30%
- Increased risk of renal malignancies, especially Wilms' tumor
- Increased risk of traumatic injury

Radiographic features
- Abnormal axis of each kidney with lower calyx more medial than upper calyx
- Bilateral malrotation of renal pelvises in anterior position
- Isthmus lies anterior to aorta and inferior vena cava (IVC) but behind inferior mesenteric artery (IMA)

OTHER RENAL VARIANTS

- Persistent fetal lobation: scalloped appearance of renal outline; adjacent calyx is normal
- Junctional parenchymal defect: fusion defect in upper pole of kidney that does not represent a scar; echogenic linear defect extends from sinus; commonly seen in pediatric patients

- Septum of Bertin (upper pole 90%, bilateral 60%); associated with bifid renal pelvis
- Dromedary hump: parenchymal prominence in left kidney; results from compression of adjacent spleen
- Lobar dysmorphism: abnormally oriented lobe between upper and middle calyces; always points to posterior calyx, which is key to diagnosis on CT or IVP. By US this entity is indistinguishable from column of Bertin.
- Aberrant papilla: papilla indents infundibulum or pelvis rather than minor calyx
- Linear vascular impressions on renal pelvis and infundibula
- Ureteral spindle: dilatation of middle third of ureter at crossing of iliac vessels
- Sinus lipomatosis: large amount of fat in renal sinus
- Cross-fused ectopia; the ectopic kidney is inferior

Cystic Disease

CLASSIFICATION

Cortical cysts
- Simple cysts
- Complicated (complex) cysts

Medullary cystic disease

Polycystic renal disease
- Infantile polycystic disease
- Adult polycystic disease

Multicystic dysplastic kidney

Multilocular cystic nephroma

Cysts associated with systemic disease
- Tuberous sclerosis
- Von Hippel-Lindau disease

Miscellaneous cysts
- Hydatid
- Acquired cysts in uremia
- Extraparenchymal cysts
    - Parapelvic cysts
    - Perinephric cysts

SIMPLE CYSTS

Simple cysts (in > 50% of population > 50 years) probably arise from obstructed tubules or ducts. They do not, however, communicate with collecting system. Clinical: most commonly asymptomatic; rare: hematuria (from cyst rupture), HTN, cyst infection. Mass effect from large cysts may cause dull ache or discomfort.

Radiographic features

IVP
- Lucent defect
- Cortical bulge
- Round indentations on collecting system
- "Beak sign" can be seen with large cysts.

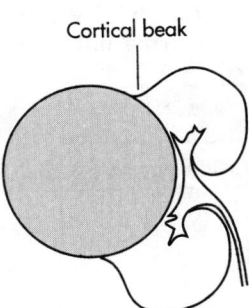

Cortical beak

Simple cyst

US
- Anechoic
- Enhanced through-transmission
- Sharply marginated, smooth walls
- Very thin septations may occasionally be seen.

CT
- Smooth cyst wall
- Sharp demarcation from surrounding renal parenchyma
- Water density (< 10-15 HU) that is homogenous throughout lesion
- No significant enhancement after IV contrast administration (small increases of < 5 HU, however, can be seen—likely due to technical factors, not true enhancement)
- Cyst wall too thin to be seen by CT (with small cysts, volume-averaging may create the false appearance of a thick wall)

Pearls
- True renal cysts should always be differentiated from hydronephrosis, calyceal diverticulum, and peripelvic cysts.
- Differentiate renal cyst from hypoechoic renal artery aneurysm using color Doppler US.
- Cysts that contain calcium, septations, and irregular margins (complicated cysts) need further workup.

COMPLICATED CYSTS

Complicated cysts are cysts that do not meet the criteria of simple cysts and thus require further workup. Bosniak classification:
- Category 1 lesions: benign simple cyst (see previous section)
- Category 2 lesions: these minimally complicated cysts are benign but have certain radiologic findings of concern. This category includes septated (paper-thin septations) cysts, minimally calcified cysts, high-density cysts.
- Category 3 lesions: complicated cystic lesions that exhibit some radiologic features also seen in malignancy. This category includes multiloculated cystic nephroma, multiloculated cysts, complex septated cysts, chronically infected cysts, heavily calcified cysts, and cystic renal cell carcinoma (RCC). Because these entities are difficult to separate radiologically, surgery is usually performed.
- Category 4 lesion: clearly malignant lesions with large cystic component. Irregular margins, solid vascular elements.

CYST CATEGORIES (BOSNIAK)		
Category (Bosniak)	US Features	Workup
Type 1: Simple cyst	Round, anechoic, thin wall, enhanced through transmission	None
Type 2: Mildly complicated cyst	Thin septation, calcium in wall	CT or US follow-up
Type 3: Indeterminate lesion	Multiple septae, internal echos, mural nodules	Partial nephrectomy, biopsy
	Thick septae	CT follow-up if surgery is high risk
Type 4: Clearly malignant	Solid mass component	Nephrectomy

Radiographic features
Septations
- Thin septa within cysts are usually benign.
- Thick or irregular septa require workup.

Calcifications
- Thin calcifications in cyst walls are usually benign.
- Milk of calcium: collection of small calcific granules in cyst fluid: usually benign

Thick wall
- These lesions usually require surgical exploration.

Increased CT density (> 15 HU) of cyst content
- Vast majority of these lesions are benign.
- High density is usually due to hemorrhage, high protein content, and/or calcium.
- 50% appear as simple cysts by US.

The remainder of patients require further imaging workup (to exclude soft tissue mass) or occasionally cyst puncture (analyze fluid, inject contrast).

CYST ASPIRATION

Indications for cyst aspiration
Diagnosis
- Complex, high-density cyst (type 2) ≥ 3 cm
- Evaluate fluid for character, as well as cytology.
- After aspiration, inject contrast ("cystogram") and obtain multiple projections so that all surfaces of the wall are smooth.

Therapy
- Most commonly performed for large cyst obstructing collecting system or causing dull, aching pain or, rarely, HTN (Page kidney)
- If the cyst is simple and the fluid is clear, yellow, and free-flowing, laboratory analysis is not necessary. Bloody or brownish fluid should be sent for cytology.

Cyst ablation
If a symptomatic cyst recurs after aspiration, percutaneous ablation may be considered to avoid surgery.
1. Place 20-G needle into cyst and measure total volume aspirated. Some interventional radiologists prefer a small pigtail catheter.
2. Inject contrast to exclude communication with the collecting system, which would preclude alcohol ablation.
3. Inject absolute ethanol, 25% of the total volume of cyst fluid aspirated.
4. Leave ethanol in place 15-20 min, turning the patient to different positions to maximize wall contact of alcohol with different surfaces.
5. Aspirate residual ethanol.

OTHER CYSTIC STRUCTURES

Milk of calcium cyst
- Not a true cyst but a calyceal diverticulum, which may be communicating or be closed off
- Contains layering calcific granules (calcium carbonate)
- No pathological consequence

Parapelvic cyst
- Originates from renal parenchyma but expands into the renal sinus
- May cause compression of the collecting system

Peripelvic cyst
- Originates from sinus structures, most likely lymphatic in origin
- May be indistinguishable from hydronephrosis on US, requiring an IVP or CT for definitive diagnosis
- Attenuated, stretched infundibula
- IVP differential diagnosis: renal sinus lipomatosis

Perinephric cyst
- Located beneath the renal capsule
- Not true cysts; represent extravasated urine trapped beneath renal capsule (pseudocysts, uriniferous cysts, urinoma)

MEDULLARY CYSTIC DISEASE (MCD)

Spectrum of diseases characterized by medullary cysts and tubulointerstitial fibrosis. Patients usually present with azotemia and anemia and subsequently progress to endstage renal failure. Types:

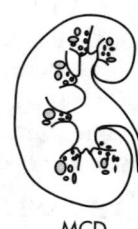

MCD

- Familial nephronophthisis, 70%, autosomal recessive
    Juvenile type, onset 3-5 years (most common)
    Adult type
- Adult medullary cystic disease, 15%, autosomal dominant
- Renal-retinal dysplasia, 15%, recessive; associated with retinitis pigmentosa

Radiographic features
- Small kidneys (as opposed to large kidneys in polycystic disease)
- Multiple small (< 2 cm) cysts in medulla
- Cysts may be too small to resolve by imaging, but their multiplicity will result in increased medullary echogenicity and apparent widening of central sinus echoes.
- Cortex is thin and does not contain cysts.
- No calcifications

ADULT POLYCYSTIC KIDNEY DISEASE (APKD)

Cystic dilatation of collecting tubules, as well as nephrons (unlike MCD and infantile polycystic kidney disease in which only the collecting tubules are involved). Autosomal dominant trait (childhood type is autosomal recessive). Incidence: 0.1% (most common form of cystic kidney disease; accounts for 10% of patients on chronic dialysis). Clinical: slowly progressive renal failure. Symptoms usually begin in 3rd or 4th decade, but clinical onset is extremely variable, ranging from palpable cystic kidneys at birth to multiple cysts without symptoms in old age. Enlarged kidneys may be palpable. Treatment: dialysis, transplant.

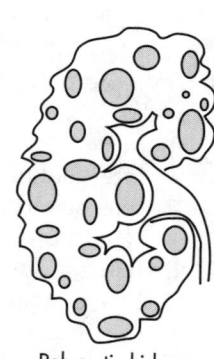

Polycystic kidney

Associated findings
- Hepatic cysts, 70%
- Intracranial berry aneurysm, 20%
- Cysts in pancreas and spleen, < 5%

Radiographic features
- Kidneys are enlarged and contain innumerable cysts, creating a bosselated surface.
- Calcification of cyst walls are common.
- Pressure deformities of calyces and infundibula
- IVP: "swiss-cheese" nephrogram

- Cysts have variable signal characteristics
    CT: hypodense, hyperdense (hemorrhage, protein, calcium)
    T1-weighted (T1W): some cysts contain clear watery fluid (hypointense),
        others contain blood and protein (hyperintense); layering in some cysts is
        caused by cellular debris
- Hepatic cysts

UREMIC CYSTIC DISEASE (UCD)

40% of patients with endstage renal disease develop renal cysts. Incidence increases with time on dialysis so that incidence of UCD is 90% in patients 5 years on dialysis. Associated complications:
- Incidence of malignancy is not as high as previously believed.
- Hemorrhage of cysts
- Cysts can regress following successful transplantation.

Tumors

CLASSIFICATION

Renal parenchymal tumors
- Renal cell adenocarcinoma, 80%
- Wilms' tumor, 5%
- Adenoma (thought to represent early RCC)
- Oncocytoma
- Nephroblastomatosis
- Mesoblastic nephroma

Mesenchymal tumors
- Angiomyolipoma
- Malignant fibrous histiocytoma
- Hemangioma
- Other rare tumors

Renal pelvis tumors
- Transitional cell carcinoma, < 10%
- Squamous cell carcinoma
- Other malignant tumors: undifferentiated adenocarcinoma tumors
- Benign tumors: papilloma > angioma, fibroma, myoma, polyp

Secondary tumors
- Metastases
- Lymphoma

RENAL CELL CARCINOMA (RCC)

Synonyms: renal adenocarcinoma, hypernephroma, clear cell carcinoma, malignant nephroma. Clinical: hematuria, 50%; flank pain, 40%; palpable mass, 35%; weight loss, 25%; paraneoplastic syndrome: hypertension (renin), erythrocytosis (erythropoietin), hypercalcemia (PTH), gynecomastia (gonadotropin), Cushing's syndrome (ACTH).

Risk factors
- Tobacco
- Phenacetin, long-term use
- Von Hippel-Lindau disease (bilateral tumors)
- Chronic dialysis (> 3 years)
- Family history

Prognosis

5-year survival: stage 1, 2 = 50%, stage 3 = 35%, stage 4 = 15%

Tumors often have atypical behavior:

- Late recurrence of metastases: 10% recur 10 years after nephrectomy.
- Some patients survive for years with untreated tumor.
- Spontaneous regression of tumor has been reported but is very rare.

Radiographic features

Imaging findings

- Mass lesion: renal contour abnormality, calyceal displacement
- Large variability in signal characteristics on noncontrast CT and MRI scans depending on the degree of hemorrhage and necrosis
- Contrast enhancement is usually heterogeneous; strong contrast enhancement (> 15 HU)
- Calcification, 10%
- Cystic areas (2%-5% are predominantly cystic)
- Filling defects (clots, tumor thrombus) in collecting system and renal veins
- US appearance
  Hyperechoic: 70% of tumors > 3 cm, 30% of tumors < 3 cm
  Hypoechoic

Angiography

- 95% of tumors are hypervascular.
  Caliber irregularities of tumor vessels are typical (encasement).
  Prominent AV shunting, venous lakes
- Angiography may be useful for detection in complicated and equivocal cases:
  Small tumors
  Underlying abnormal renal parenchyma
  VHL disease
- Preoperative embolization with alcohol or Ivalon

Staging

- Stage I: tumor confined to kidney
- Stage II: extrarenal (may involve adrenal gland) but confined to Gerota's fascia
- Stage III: A: venous invasion (renal vein); B: lymph node metastases; C: both
- Stage IV: A: direct extension into adjacent organs through Gerota's fascia, B: metastases
  Lungs, 55%
  Liver, 25%
  Bone, 20% (classic lesions are lytic, expansile)
  Adrenal, 20%
  Contralateral kidney, 10%
  Other organs, < 5%

Therapy

- Radical nephrectomy (entire contents of Gerota's fascia is removed)
- Radiofrequencing ablation for smaller (< 5 cm) RCCs in inoperable, aged
- Chemotherapy
- Radiotherapy is used for palliation only.

LYMPHOMA

Incidence of renal involvement in lymphoma is 5% (non-Hodgkin's lymphoma >> Hodgkin's disease) at diagnosis and 30% at autopsy. Three patterns of involvement:
- Direct extension from retroperitoneal disease (common)
- Hematogenous dissemination (common)
- Primary renal lymphoma (i.e., no other organ involvements) is rare because kidneys do not have primary lymphatic tissue.

Radiographic features
- Multiple lymphomatous masses (hypoechoic, hypodense), 50%
- Diffuse involvement of one or both kidneys
- Adenopathy

METASTASES

Incidence: 20% of cancer patients at autopsy. Common primaries:
- Lung
- Breast
- Colon
- Melanoma

ANGIOMYOLIPOMA (AML)

Hamartomas containing fat, smooth muscle and blood vessels. Treatment: small lesions are not treated; large and symptomatic lesions are resected or embolized. Unlikely to bleed if < 4 cm. Complication: tumors may spontaneously bleed because of their vascular elements. Associations:
- Tuberous sclerosis: 80% of patients with tuberous sclerosis have AML, typically multiple, bilateral lesions. However, < 40% of patients with AML have tuberous sclerosis. In the absence of tuberous sclerosis, 5% of all AMLs, patients will have multiple, bilateral AML.
- Lymphangiomyomatosis

Radiographic features
- Fat appears hypodense (CT), hyperechoic (US), hyperintense (T1W). The presence of fat in a renal lesion is virtually diagnostic of AML. There have been only a few case reports of fat in RCC or in oncocytomas. Caveat: be certain that fat associated with a large mass is not trapped renal sinus or peripheral fat
- Predominance of blood vessels
     Strong contrast enhancement
     T2-weighted (T2W) hyperintensity
- Predominance of muscle: signal intensity similar to RCC
- AMLs do not contain calcifications; if a lesion does contain calcification, consider other diagnosis such as RCC.
- Angiography: tortuous, irregular, aneurysmally dilated vessels are seen in 3%. Presence depends on the amount of angiomatous tissue. Predominantly myxomatous AMLs may be hypovascular.

ADENOMA

Best described as adenocarcinoma with no metastatic potential. Usually detected at autopsy.

ONCOCYTOMA

These tumors arise from oncocytes (epithelial cell) of the proximal tubule. Although the majority of lesions are well differentiated and benign, these tumors need to be resected because of their malignant potential and the inability to differentiate from RCC preoperatively. Represent 5% of renal tumors.

Radiographic features

- Central stellate scar (CT) and spoke-wheel appearance (angiography) are typical but not specific (also seen in adenocarcinoma).
- Well-defined, sharp borders
- Radiographically impossible to differentiate from RCC

JUXTAGLOMERULAR TUMOR (RENINOMA)

Secretion of renin causes HTN, hypernatremia, hypokalemia (secondary aldosteronism). Most patients undergo angiography as part of the workup for hypertension. Tumors appear as small hypovascular masses. Rare.

RENAL PELVIS TUMORS

Most tumors arising from the renal pelvis are malignant with transitional cell cancer being the most common tumor. Papillomas are the most common benign tumor.

Inverted papilloma

- No malignant potential
- 20% are associated with uroepithelial malignancies elsewhere, most commonly in bladder.

Transitional cell carcinoma (TCC)

- Tumors are often multifocal: 40%-80% of patients have bladder TCC. However, only 3% of patients with bladder TCC later develop upper tract TCC.
- Radiographic finding: irregular filling defect
- 60% recurrence on ipsilateral side
- 50% have lung metastases.
- Staging

  Stage I: mucosal lamina propria involved
  Stage II: into but not beyond muscular layer
  Stage III: invasion of adjacent fat/renal parenchynma
  Stage IV: metastases

Squamous cell carcinoma (SCC)

- Represent 5% of renal pelvis tumors and < 1% of all renal tumors
- Frequently associated with leukoplakia or chronic irritation (nephrolithiasis, schistosomiasis)

Collecting duct carcinoma

- Uncommon yet distinct epithelial neoplasm of the kidney.
- Aggressive malignancy derived from the renal medulla, possibly from the distal collecting ducts of Bellini.
- Propensity for showing infiltrative growth, which differs from the typical expansible pattern of growth exhibited by most renal malignancies.
- Radiographic findings:

  By US, cortical renal cell carcinoma may be hypoechoic to normal renal parenchyma, isoechoic to renal parenchyma, hyperechoic to renal parenchyma but hypoechoic to renal sinus fat, or isoechoic to renal sinus fat.

By CT, the lesions are medullary in location and have an infiltrative
appearance. The reniform contour of the kidney is maintained.
By renal angiography, the tumors are usually hypovascular.
By MR imaging, the tumors are hypointense on T2W images.

Inflammation

URINARY TRACT INFECTION (UTI)

Most common pathogen is *Escherichia coli*. Less common organisms include other
gram-negative bacteria: *Proteus, Klebsiella, Enterobacter, Pseudomonas, Neisseria*, and
Trichomonas vaginalis. "Sterile pyuria" refers to increased urinary white blood cell
count (WBC) without being able to culture pathogens. Common causes of sterile
pyuria:

- Tuberculosis (TB)
- Fungal infections
- Interstitial nephritis
- Glomerulonephritis

Risk factors for UTI
- Urinary obstruction (e.g., benign prostatic hyperplasia, calculi)
- Vesicoureteral reflux
- Pregnancy (dilatation of ureters)
- Diabetes mellitus
- Immune deficiency
- Instrumentation

Complications
- Abscess formation
- Xanthogranulomatous pyelonephritis
- Emphysematous pyelonephritis
- Scarring and renal failure

ACUTE PYELONEPHRITIS

Acute bacterial infection of the kidney and urinary tract (*Proteus, Klebsiella, E. coli*).
Medical treatment is usually initiated without imaging studies. Role of imaging
studies:

Define underlying pathology
- Obstruction
- Reflux
- Calculus

Rule out complications
- Abscess
- Emphysematous pyelonephritis
- Determine presence of chronic changes such as scarring

Common underlying conditions
- Diabetes mellitus
- Immunosuppresion
- Obstruction

Types
- Focal type (lobar nephronia)
- Diffuse type: more severe and extensive

Radiographic features

Imaging studies (IVP, CT, US) are normal in 75%. In the remaining 25% there are non-specific findings:

- Renal enlargement (edema)
- Loss of the corticomedullary differentiation (edema)
- IVP findings:
    Delay of contrast excretion
    Narrowing of collecting system (edema)
    Striated nephrogram
    Ridging of uroepithelium
- Areas of decreased perfusion by contrast-enhanced CT
- Focal areas of hypodensity in lobar nephronia
- Complications: abscess, scarring

PYONEPHROSIS

Infected renal collecting system usually due to obstruction, calculi, 50% > tumor strictures > postoperative strictures. Treatment: penicillin and other antibiotics sufficient in 35% of cases; remainder of patients require nephrectomy (depending on underlying cause).

Radiographic features

US

- Best study to differentiate pyonephrosis from uninfected hydronephrosis
- Echoes within collecting system
- Urine/debris levels
- Dense shadowing due to gas in collecting system
- Poor through-transmission

CT

- Best study to show cause and level of obstruction, as well as complications
- Dilated collecting system
- Allows detection of perinephric or renal abscess

Interventional procedures

- Aspiration for culture and sensitivity (definitive diagnostic study)
- Penicillin
- Formal antegrade pyelography should be deferred to a 2nd visit so as not to cause sepsis.

RENAL ABSCESS

Usually caused by gram-negative bacteria, less commonly by *Staphylococcus* or fungus (candidiasis). Underlying disease: calculi, obstruction, diabetes, AIDS.

Radiographic features

- Well-delineated focal renal lesion
- Central necrosis (no enhancement with IV contrast)
- Thickened, hyperemic abscess wall with contrast enhancement
- Perinephric inflammatory involvement:
    Thickening of Gerota's fascia
    Stranding of perirenal fat

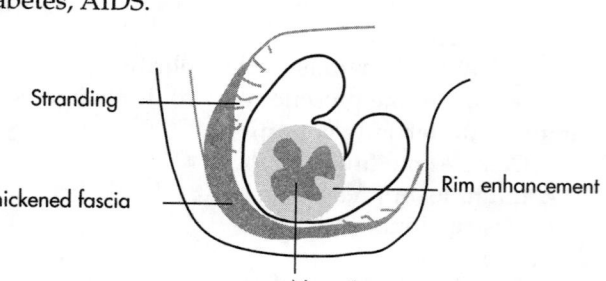

Complications

- Retroperitoneal spread of abscess
- Renocolic fistula

PERINEPHRIC ABSCESS

Results most commonly from high-grade ureteral obstruction and infected kidney. Nonrenal etiologies include duodenal perforation, diverticular abscess, Crohn's disease, infected pancreatic fluid collections, and spinal TB, which may spread and cause perirenal as well as psoas abscess. Treatment: percutaneous drainage.

EMPHYSEMATOUS PYELONEPHRITIS

Most commonly caused by gram-negative bacteria in patients with diabetes mellitus, less commonly in nondiabetics with obstruction. Spectrum:
- Emphysematous pyelonephritis: gas in renal parenchyma and collecting system Mortality 60%-80%
- Emphysematous pyelitis: gas in collecting system ("air pyelogram"). Mortality: 20%

Radiographic features
- Gas in collecting system and/or renal parenchyma
- Gas air may extend to Gerota's fascia (high mortality)

Treatment
- Nephrectomy
- In poor surgical candidates or in patients with focal disease, percutaneous drainage has been used as a temporizing or, occasionally, definitive therapy.

XANTHOGRANULOMATOUS PYELONEPHRITIS (XGP)

Chronic suppurative form of renal infection characterized by parenchymal destruction and replacement of parenchyma with lipid laden macrophages. Diffuse form 90%, focal form 10%. 10% of patients have diabetes mellitus. Rare.

Radiographic findings
- Large or staghorn calculus (thought to cause obstruction and inflammatory response), 75%; in the remaining 25% of patients, XGP is due to UPJ obstruction or ureteral tumors.
- Enlarged, nonexcreting kidney
- Multiple nonenhancing low attenuation masses (−10-30 HU): xanthomatous masses. The masses may extend beyond the kidney into the perinephric space. There may be a thin peripheral ring of enhancement.
- Fine calcifications may be present in xanthomatous masses.
- Thickened Gerota's fascia

REPLACEMENT LIPOMATOSIS

Also known as *replacement fibrolipomatosis*, replacement represents extreme form of renal sinus lipomatosis in which infection, long-term hydronephrosis, and calculi are associated with severe renal parenchymal atrophy. Calculi and inflammation are present in > 70% of cases.

Radiographic findings
- Enlarged renal outline, fatty lucent mass, and staghorn calculus
- IVP shows poorly or nonfunctioning kidney.
- By US kidney is enlarged but has a preserved shape. Residual hypoechoic renal parenchymal rim surrounded by hyperechoic areas of fatty proliferation in both renal hilum and perinephric space.
- CT is the imaging modality of choice to best demonstrate fatty characteristics.

Differential diagnoses for this condition include XGP, fat-containing tumors such as angiomyolipomas, lipoma, and liposarcoma. CT can aid in differentiating XGP as CT shows attenuation values of −5 to +15 HU in XGP, in contrast to replacement lipomatosis where the fatty tissues measure −100 HU. Fat-containing tumors usually produce a mass effect and show renal function, unlike replacement lipomatosis.

TUBERCULOSIS

Genitourinary (GU) tract is the second most common site of tuberculous involvement after the lung. GU disease is typically due to hematogenous spread. Clinical: history of pulmonary TB, pyuria, hematuria, dysuria. Sites of involvement:

- Renal
- Ureteral
- Bladder
- Seminal vesicles, epidydimis

Radiographic features of renal tuberculosis
Distribution

- Unilateral involvement is more common (70%) than bilateral (30%).

Size

- Early kidneys are enlarged.
- Later kidneys are small.
- Autonephrectomy (nonfunctioning kidney)

Parenchyma

- Parenchymal calcifications, 70%
- Calcification may take multiple forms: curvilinear, mottled, or amorphous; "putty kidney" results when calcification has homogeneous, ground-glass appearance.
- Papillary necrosis, papillae may be irregular, necrotic, or sloughed.
- Tuberculoma
- Parenchymal scarring, 20%

Collecting system

- Mucosal irregularity
- Infundibular stenosis
- Amputated calyx
- Corkscrew ureter: multiple infundibular and ureteral stenoses (hallmark finding)
- "Purse-string" stenosis of renal pelvis
- "Pipestem ureter" refers to a narrow, rigid, aperistaltic segment.
- Renal calculi, 10%

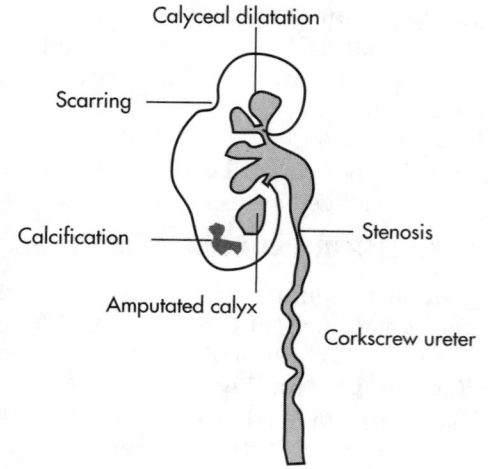

CANDIDIASIS

Most common renal fungal infections (coccidioidomycosis, cryptococcosis less common). Commonly in patients with diabetes mellitus.
Radiographic features

- Multiple medullary and cortical abscesses
- Papillary necrosis due to diffuse fungal infiltration
- Fungus balls in collecting system (mycetoma) cause filling defects on IVP; nonshadowing echogenic foci on US
- Hydronephrosis secondary to mycetoma
- Scalloping of ureters (submucosal edema)

RENAL MANIFESTATION OF AIDS

AIDS-related renal abnormalities are seen in most AIDS patients during the course of their illness. AIDS nephropathy refers to irreversible renal failure in 10% of patients and is seen in endstage disease.

Radiographic features
- Increased cortical US echogenicity, 70%; (tubulointerstitial abnormalities)
- Renal enlargement without hydronephrosis, 40%
- Focal hypoechoic (US)/low attenuation (CT) lesions (infection, tumor), 30%

Other renal abnormalities
- Acute tubular necrosis (ATN)
- Interstitial nephritis
- Focal nephrocalcinosis
- Infection: Cytomegalovirus (CMV), aspergillus, toxoplasmosis, *Pneumocystis carinii*, histoplasmosis, *Mycobacterium avium-intracellulare* (MAI)
- Tumors: increased incidence of RCC, lymphoma, Kaposi's sarcoma

Prostate abnormalities
- Prostatitis: bacterial, fungal, viral
- Prostate abscess

Testicular abnormalities
- Testicular atrophy: common
- Infection: bacterial, fungal, viral
- Tumors: germ cell tumors, lymphoma

Nephrocalcinosis and Lithiasis

Renal calcifications can be located in renal parenchyma (nephrocalcinosis), abnormal tissue (e.g., dystrophic calcification in cysts, tumors) or in the collecting system (e.g., nephrolithiasis, calculi).

CALCULI

Incidence: 5% of population; 20% at autopsy. Recurrence of stone disease: 50%. Symptoms in 50% of patients during first 5 years of stone presence. Predisposing conditions: calyceal diverticuli, Crohn's disease, some diversions, stents, renal tubular acidosis, hypercalcemia, hypercalciuria. The radiographic density of a calculus depends mainly on its calcium content:

Calcium calculi (opaque), 75%
- Calcium oxalate
- Calcium phosphate

Struvite calculi (opaque), 15%
- Magnesium ammonium phosphate: "infection stones" (represent 70% of staghorn calculi, remainder are cystine or uric acid calculi); struvite is usually mixed with calcium phosphate to create "triple phosphate" calculi

Cystine calculi (less opaque)
- Cystinuria, 2%

Nonopaque calculi
- Uric acid (gout, treatment of myeloproliferative disorders), 10%
- Xanthine (rare)
- Mucoprotein matrix calculi in poorly functioning, infected urinary tracts; rare
- Protease inhibitor indinavir used in HIV treatment can result in radiolucent stones.

Radiographic features
Calculus (determine size, number, location)
- Radiopaque calculus, (90%) are best detected on KUB or CT and confirmed by IVP.
- Radiolucent calculi are best detected by IVP.
- Renal calculi can be detected by US: hyperechoic focus (calculus), posterior shadowing; calculi 3 mm or less may not be detected.

	Calculus	Phlebolith
Shape	Any shape 90% homogenously opaque	Round, smooth Central lucency
Location	Along projected tract of ureter	In true pelvis (below distal ureter)

IVP
- Delayed and persistent nephrogram due to ureteral obstruction
- Column of opacified urine extends in ureter from renal pelvis to lodged calculus (diminished or absent peristalsis).
- Ureter distal to calculus is narrowed (edema, inflammation); may create false impression of stricture.
- Ureter proximal to calculus is minimally dilated and straightened: columnization; degree of dilatation has no relationship to stone size
- "Steinstrasse": several calculi are bunched up along the ureter (commonly seen after lithotripsy)
- Halo appearance (edema) around distal ureter may resemble appearance of ureterocele (pseudoureterocele) or bladder carcinoma.

CT
- CT detects most calculi regardless of calcium content. The exception are matrix stones.
- Contiguous sections should be used to avoid gaps so as not to miss small stones; helical CT is very helpful in this regard.
- Dedicated CT protocol for stone search is performed; may need to follow with contrast-enhanced CT (CECT) to differentiate stone in ureter from phlebolith. Contrast-only CT may obscure a calcified ureteral calculus because it may blend in with high-density contrast material.

Location: 3 narrow sites in the ureter at which calculi often lodge
- UPJ: junction of renal pelvis and ureter proper
- At crossing of ureter with iliac vessels
- Ureterovesical junction (UVJ): insertion of ureters into bladder

Complications
- Forniceal rupture (pyelosinus backflow); inconsequential in isolation if urine is uninfected; chronic leak may result in periureteral/retroperitoneal fibrosis
- Chronic calculous pyelonephritis
- XGP in the presence of staghorn calculus
- Squamous metaplasia (leukoplakia); more common in pyelocalyceal system and upper ureter than lower ureter or bladder. Cholesteatoma may result from desquamation of keratinized epithelium.
- SCC

Treatment options
- Small renal calculi, (< 2.5 cm): extracoporeal lithotripsy
- Large renal calculi, (> 2.5 cm): percutaneous removal
- Upper ureteral calculi: extracoporeal lithotripsy
- Lower ureteral calculi: ureteroscopy

Extracorporeal shock wave lithotripsy (ESWL)
- Best results with calcium oxalate and uric acid stones and calculi < 2.5 cm
  Larger calculi are better treated by percutaneous removal.
- Contraindiations for ESWL include:
  - Patient not eligible for anesthesia
  - Severe bleeding
  - Pregnancy
  - Urinary tract infections
  - Nonfunctioning kidneys
  - Gross obesity
  - Small children
  - Tall patients (> 200 cm)
  - Distal obstruction
  - Calyceal neck stensosis
  - UPJ obstruction
  - Prostatic enlargement
  - Renal artery anerusym
- Complications of ESWL
  - Intrarenal; subscapsular and perinephric hematoma
  - Decrease in effective renal plasma flow

Indications for PCN
- Large stones requiring initial debulking (e.g., staghorn calculus)
- Calculi not responding to ESWL (e.g., cysteine stones)
- Body habitus precludes ESWL
- When patient has certain type of pacemaker
- Renal artery aneurysms
- Calculi > 5 cm

CORTICAL NEPHROCALCINOSIS

Usually dystrophic calcification
Causes
- Chronic glomerulonephritis
- Cortical necrosis (due to ischemia)
  - Pregnancy
  - Shock
  - Infection
  - Toxins: methoxyfluorane, ethylene glycol
- AIDS-related nephropathy
  - Glomerular sclerosis
  - Punctate calcifications
  - MAI
- Uncommon causes
  - Rejected renal transplants
  - Chronic hypercalcemia
  - Oxalosis
  - Alport syndrome

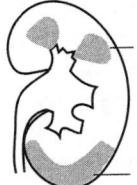

Medullary nephrocalcinosis

Cortical nephrocalcinosis

Radiographic features
- Peripheral calcifications (medullary pyramids are spared)
- Tramline calcifications are classic: interface of necrotic cortex and viable subcapsular cortex
- Columns of Bertin may be calcified.
- US: hyperechoic cortex

MEDULLARY NEPHROCALCINOSIS

Causes
- Hyperparathyroidism (hypercalciuria, hypercalcemia), 40%
- Renal tubular acidosis, 20%
- Medullary sponge kidney, 20%
- Papillary necrosis
- Other causes
    Nephrotoxic drugs (amphotericin B)
    Chronic pyelonephritis

Radiographic features
- Bilateral, stippled calcification of medullary pyramids
- Calcifications may extend peripherally.
- US: hyperechoic medulla

Pelvicalyceal System

CONGENITAL MEGACALYCES

Congenital condition in which there are too many (20-25; normal is 10-14) calyces that are enlarged. Associated with hypoplastic pyramids resulting in polyconal, faceted calyces rather than the blunting that is seen with obstruction. There is no obstruction, and the remainder of the collecting system is normal. Renal parenchyma and renal function are normal. Etiology is not known; congenital underdevelopment of pyramids, "burnt-out" fetal obstruction or reflux or abnormal branching of collecting system. Associated with megaureter.

INFUNDIBULOPELVIC DYSGENESIS

Spectrum of diseases characterized by hypoplasia or aplasia of the upper collecting system. Spectrum:
- Calyceal diverticulum
- Pyelogenous cyst
- Multiinfundibular stenosis
- UPJ stenosis
- Infundibulopelvic stenosis
- Multicystic kidney

(PYELO) CALYCEAL DIVERTICULUM

Outpouching of calyx into corticomedulary region. May also arise from renal pelvis or an infundibulum. Usually asymptomatic but patients may develop calculi.
- Type I : originates from minor calyx
- Type II: originates from infundibulum
- Type III : originates from renal pelvis

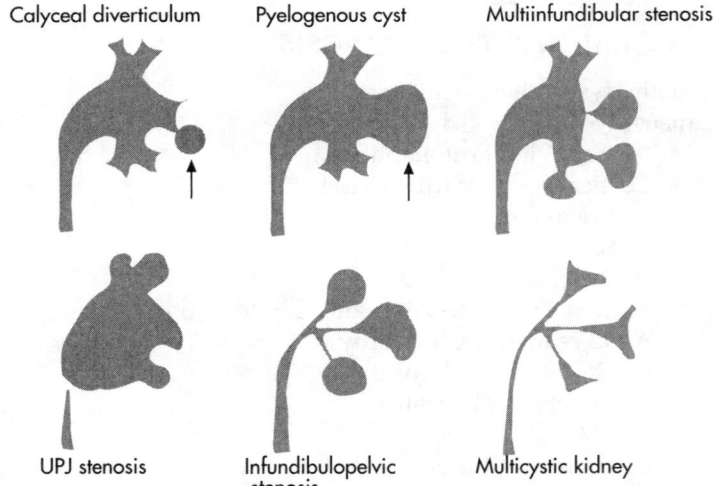

Calyceal diverticulum   Pyelogenous cyst   Multiinfundibular stenosis

UPJ stenosis   Infundibulopelvic stenosis   Multicystic kidney

Radiographic features
- Cystic lesion connects through channel with collecting system
- If the neck is not obstructed, diverticuli opacify retrograde from the collecting system on delayed IVP films.
- May contain calculi or milk of calcium, 50%
- Fragmented calculi after ESWL may fail to pass because of a narrow neck. Percutaneous stone retrieval may be indicated.

RENAL PAPILLARY NECROSIS (RPN)

RPN represents an ischemic coagulative necrosis involving variable amounts of pyramids and medullary papillae. RPN never extends to the renal cortex. Etiological factors:

Ischemic necrosis
- Diabetes mellitus
- Chronic obstruction, calculus
- Sickle cell disease
- Analgesics

Necrosis due to infections
- TB
- Fungal

Radiographic features
Papillae
- Enlargement (early)
- Small collection of contrast medium extends outside the interpapillary line in partial necrosis.
- Contrast may extend into central portion of papilla in "medullary type" RPN.
- Eventually contrast curves around papilla from both fomices resulting in "lobster-claw" deformity
- Sequestered, sloughed papillae cause filling defects in collecting system: "ring sign"
- Tissue necrosis leads to blunted or clubbed calyces

Multiple papillae affected in 85%.
Rimlike calcification of necrotic papilla

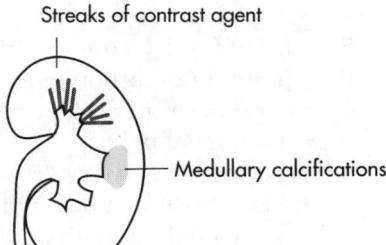

Extension of contrast from fornix

Lobster-claw deformity

Ring shadow around sequestered tissue

Sloughed tissue has passed into calyx

Clubbed calyx after absorption

MEDULLARY SPONGE KIDNEY (BENIGN RENAL TUBULAR ECTASIA)

Dysplastic dilatation of renal collecting tubules (ducts of Bellini). Cause: developmental? Usually detected in young adults (20-40 years) as an incidental finding. Clinical: usually no signs, urine stasis: UTI, calculi hematuria. 10% may develop progressive renal failure. Relatively common (0.5% of IVP). May involve one or both kidneys or be confined to a single papilla. Associations (rare):
- Hemihypertrophy
- Congenital pyloric stenosis
- Ehlers-Danlos syndrome
- Other renal abnormalities: cortical renal cysts, horseshoe kidney, renal ectopia, APKD, RTA

Streaks of contrast agent

Medullary calcifications

Radiographic features

- Striated nephrogram (contrast in dilated collecting ducts), "brushlike" appearance
- Cystic tubular dilatation usually 1-3 mm: occasionally larger, usually too small for CT resolution
- Punctuate calcifications in medullary distribution (located in dilated tubules), 50%
- Differentiate on IVP from "papillary blush," a normal variant, representing amorphous enhancement without tubular dilation, streaks or globules, nephrocalcinosis, or pyramidal enlargement. Papillary blush is an also inconstant finding on successive IVPs.

OBSTRUCTION OF COLLECTING SYSTEM

Common causes:
- Calculi
- Tumor
- Previous surgery (ligation, edema, clot)

Radiographic findings

IVP

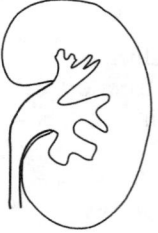
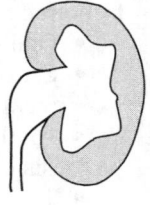

Normal
< 15 cm H$_2$O

Acute obstruction
> 20 cm H$_2$O

Chronic obstruction
< 15 cm H$_2$O

Kidney
- Delayed nephrogram (peak enhancement at > 30 minutes after IV injection, slow fading)
- Delayed renal (peak) density may be higher than in normal kidney.
- Faint radial striations of nephrogram
- Negative pyelogram: nephrogram with delayed pyelogram resulting in dilated unopacified calyces outlined by opacified parenchyma
- Dunbar's crescents (caliceal cresents): thin rings or crescents at interface with cali and parenchyma resulting from contrast in dilated collecting ducts; disappear when collecting system is completely opacified
- Atrophy of renal parenchyma in chronic obstruction: "rim nephrogram" or "shell nephrogram"

Collecting system
- Blunting of forniceal angles
- Dilatation of ureter and pelvis; decreased or absent peristalisis
- Backflow

US

Sensitivity for detection of chronic obstruction: 90%

Sensitivity for detection of acute obstruction: 60%

Common causes of false positive examinations:
- Extrarenal pelvis
- Peripelvic cyst
- Vessels: differentiate with color Doppler
- Vesicoureteral reflux, full bladder
- High urine flow (overhydration, furosemide)
- Corrected long-standing obstruction with residual dilatation
- Prune-belly syndrome

Common causes of false negative examinations:
- US performed early in disease before dilatation has occurred.
- Distal obstruction

WHITAKER TEST

Pressure-flow study for determining ureteral obstruction or resistance in dilated, non-refluxing upper urinary tracts. Useful test particularly in patients with surgically corrected obstruction having residual dilatation and/or symptoms. Because the test is invasive and time-consuming, it is usually reserved for cases with equivocal diuretic renograms.

1. Catheterize bladder and inject contrast to exclude refluxing megaureter.
2. Percutaneous access to collecting system with 20-G needle.
3. Connect extension tubing, 3-way stopcock, and manometer to both antegrade needle and bladder catheter. The bases of both manometers have to be set at the same level as the tip of the antegrade needle.
4. Connect perfusion pump to antegrade needle and bladder catheter.
5. Spot and overhead films obtained during perfusion (intermittent fluoroscopic monitoring).
6. Pressures in collecting system and bladder are recorded during delivery of known flow rates (5, 10, 15 mL/min), and pressure differences are calculated.
7. Pressure difference of > 15 mm is abnormal, and test should be terminated.

PYELORENAL BACKFLOW

Backflow of contrast material from collecting system into renal or perirenal spaces. Usually due to increased pressure in collecting system from retrograde pyelography or ureteral obstruction. Types:

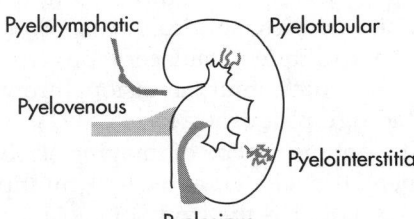

- Pyelosinus backflow (forniceal rupture): extravasation along infundibula, renal pelvis, ureter
- Pyelotubular backflow (no rupture): backflow into terminal collecting ducts; thin streaks with fanlike radiation from the papillae
- Pyelointerstitial backflow: extravasation into parenchyma and subcapsular structures; more amorphous than pyelotubular backflow
- Pyelolymphatic backflow: dilated lymphatic vessels (may occasionally rupture): thin irregular bands extending from hilum or calices
- Pyelovenous backflow: contrast in interlobar or arcuate veins; rarely seen because venous flow clears contrast material rapidly: renal vein extends superiorly from renal hilum

Trauma

RENAL INJURY

Spectrum of renal injury in trauma:
Renal infarction
- Segmental branch
- Vascular pedicle avulsion

Hemorrhage (renal laceration, rupture)
- Intraparenchymal
- Extraparenchymal

Ruptured collecting system

Mechanism
- Blunt trauma: 70%-80%
- Penetrating trauma: 20%-30%

Classification
Minor injuries (conservative treatment), 85%
- Hematomas
- Contusion (any injury that results in hematuria)
- Small lacerations
- Subsegmental renal infarcts

Moderate injuries (management controversial, 15%-50% will eventually require surgery), 10%
- Urine leak
- Laceration communicating with collecting system

Major injuries (surgical tratment), 15%
- Multiple renal lacerations (rupture)
- Pedicle injury avulsion, thrombosis

Radiographic features
The optimum type of imaging study depends on stability of patient and symptoms (hematuria, blood at meatus, multiple bony fractures):
- CECT is the study of choice.
- One-shot IVP: visualization of both kidneys excludes pedicle avulsion
- Indications for angiography:
    Nonvisualization of kidney on IVP in patient with abdominal trauma
    Persistent hematuria in a patient with abdominal trauma
    Hypotension or hypertension or persistent hematuria after an interventional urological procedure

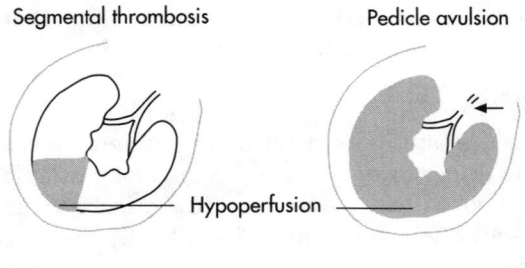

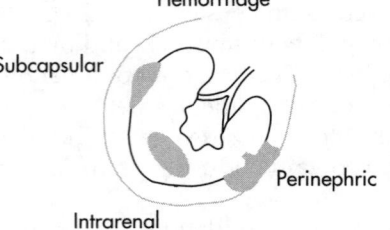

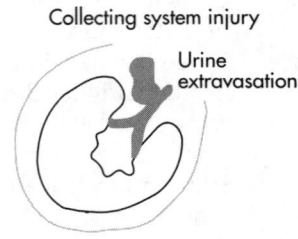

Vascular Abnormalities

RENAL VEIN THROMBOSIS (RVT)

RVT may be caused by many conditions:
- Adults: tumor > renal disease > other causes (nephrotic syndrome, postpartum, hypercoagulable states)
- Infants: dehydration, shock, trauma, sepsis, sickle cell disease

Radiographic features

Renal vein

- Absence of flow (US, CT, MRI)
- Intraluminal thrombus
- Renal vein dilatation proximal to occlusion
- Renal venography: amputation of renal vein
- MRV or conventional venography: studies of choice

Kidneys

- Renal enlargement
- US: hypoechoic cortex (early edema); hyperechoic cortex after 10 days (fibrosis, cellular infiltrates) with preserved corticomedullary differentiation; late phase (several weeks): decreased size, hyperechoic kidney with loss of corticomedullary differentiation
- IVP: little opacification, prolonged nephrogram, striated nephrogram (stasis in collecting tubules); intrarenal collecting system is stretched and compressed by edema
- CT may show low-attenuation thrombus in renal vein, or simple renal enlargement with collaterals; prolongation of corticomedullary differentiation (CMD)
- Loss of CMD
- Scintigraphy (^{99m}Tc DTPA): absent or delayed renal perfusion and excretion, alternatively may be delayed and reveal a large kidney

Chronic thrombosis

- Small kidneys
- Collateral veins may cause pelvic and ureteral notches by extrinsic compression

RENAL INFARCTS

Renal infarcts may be focal and wedge shaped or larger, involving the anterior or posterior kidney or entire kidney. CECT or IVP may show thin, enhancing rim from capsular arteries.

Causes

- Trauma to renal vessels
- Embolism
    Cardiac causes: e.g., atrial fibrillation, endocarditis
    Catheter
- Thrombosis
    Arterial
    Venous

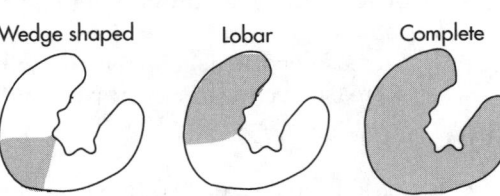

Renal Transplant

NORMAL RENAL TRANSPLANT

Morphology of normal transplanted kidney:

- Well-defined kidney, elliptical contour (i.e., not swollen)
- CMD should be present but may not always be very well-defined.
- Cortical echogenicity should be similar to liver echogenicity.
- The central echo complex should be well-defined.

FUNCTIONAL EVALUATION OF TRANSPLANTED KIDNEY

- Normal perfusion and excretion by scintigraphy (MAG_3, DTPA)
- Resistive index (P_{sys}-P_{diast}/P_{sys}) should be < 0.7 by Doppler US

COMMON TRANSPLANT COMPLICATIONS

- ATN
- Rejection
- Cyclosporine toxicity
- Arterial or venous occlusion
- Urinary leak
- Urinary obstruction

ACUTE TUBULAR NECROSIS (ATN)

Most common form of acute, reversible renal failure in transplant patients, usually seen within 24 hours. Other causes of ATN are:

Renal ischemia, 60%
- Surgery, transplant, other causes
- Pregnancy related

Nephrotoxins, 40%
- Radiographic contrast material, particularly in patients with diabetes
- Aminoglycosides
- Antineoplastic agents
- Hemoglobin, myoglobin
- Chemicals: organic solvents, $HgCl_2$

Radiographic features
- Smooth large kidneys
- Normal renal perfusion (MAG_3, angiography)
- Diminished or absent opacification after IV contrast administration
- Persistent dense nephrogram at late time points, 75%
- Variable US features:
    Increased cortical echogenicity with normal corticomedullary junction
    Increased echogenicity of pyramids

REJECTION

- Increased renal size, 90% (in chronic rejection, size is decreased)
- Thickened cortex may be hypoechoic or hyperechoic
- Large renal pyramids, edematous uroepithelium
- Indistinct corticomedullary junction
- Focal hypoechoic areas in cortex and/or medulla, 20%
- Increased cortical echogenicity, 15%
- Decrease or complete absence of central echo complex echogenicity
- Resistive index > 0.7 by Doppler US; nonspecific

EVALUATION OF TRANSPLANT COMPLICATIONS (NUCS, IVP)		
Cause	Flow	Excretion
ATN	Normal	Reduced
Rejection	Reduced	Reduced
Vascular compromise	Reduced	Reduced

Pearls

- ATN is the only renal process with normal renal flow but reduced excretion.
- Hyperacute rejection has decreased flow but excretion on delayed images (opposite to ATN).
- Cyclosporine toxicity has similar pattern as ATN but occurs later in the posttransplant period.
- ATN rarely occurs beyond 1 month after transplant.
- Cyclosporine toxicity is uncommon within first month after transplant.
- MAG$_3$ results in better quality images in transplant patients with renal insufficiency compared to DTPA.

VASCULAR COMPLICATIONS

- Renal vein thrombosis: most occur in first 3 days after transplantation
- Renal artery occlusion or stenosis. Anastomotic stenosis is treated with angioplasty with up to 87% success rates.
- Infarction
- Pseudoaneurysm of anastomosis. surgical treatment
- AV fistula: usually from renal biopsy; if symptomatic, embolization is performed
- Ureterovesical anastomosis obstruction may result from edema, stricture, ischemia, rejection, extrinsic compression or compromised position of kidney.

PERIRENAL FLUID COLLECTIONS

Perirenal fluid collections occur in 40% of transplants. The collections persist in 15%. Causes:

- Lymphocele: in 10%-20% of transplants at 1-4 months posttransplant. Usually inferomedial to kidney; linear septations are detectable in 80%. Most lymphoceles are inconsequential; if large and symtomatic or obstructing percutaneous sclerosis with tetracycline or povidone-iodine may be tried.
- Abscess: develops within weeks; complex fluid collection; fever
- Urinoma: develops during 1st month; near UVJ; may be "cold" on nuclear medicine study if leak is not active at time of examination; may be associated with hydronephrosis
- Hematoma: hyperechoic by US; pain, hematocrit drop

Bladder and Urethra

Ureter

ECTOPIC URETER

Ureter does not insert in the normal location in the trigone of the bladder (see also Chapter 11). Incidence: M:F = 1:6. Clinical: UTI, obstruction, incontinence. Associations:

- 80% have complete ureteral duplication.
- 30% have a ureterocele ("cobra head" appearance on IVP).

Insertion sites

- Males: ureter inserts ectopically into the bladder > prostatic urethra > seminal vesicles, vas deferens, ejaculatory ducts
- Females: ectopic ureter commonly empties into postsphincteric urethra, vagina, tubes, perineum

RETROCAVAL URETER

Ureter passes behind inferior vena cava (IVC) and exits between aorta and IVC. Medial looping at L2-3 level is seen on IVP. May result in ureteral narrowing and obstruction.

OVARIAN VEIN SYNDROME

Ureteral notching (vascular impression), dilatation, or obstruction as a result of ovarian vein thrombosis or varices. Usually associated with pregnancy. Normally the right gonadal vein crosses the ureter to drain into the IVC; the left gonadal vein drains into the left renal vein.

PYELOURETERITIS CYSTICA

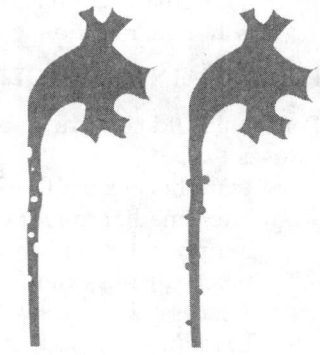

Asymptomatic ureteral and/or pyelocalyceal cysts 2-4 mm in diameter (may be up to 2 cm), usually related to infection or calculi. Radiographically, there are small multiple intraluminal filling defects (cysts originate from degenerated uroepithelial cells). Most common in 6th decade, usually unilateral. May resolve with treatment of underlying infection or remain unchanged for months or years. Not a premalignant condition.

URETERAL PSEUDODIVERTICULOSIS

1-2 mm outpouchings produced by outward proliferation of epithelium into lamina propria. Associated with inflammation. 50% eventually develop a uroepithelial malignancy.

URETERAL DIVERTICULUM

Congenital blind-ending ureter. Probably due to aborted attempt at duplication.

MALACOPLAKIA

Rare inflammatory condition which most commonly affects the bladder. Yellow-brown subepithelial plaques consist of mononuclear histiocytes that contain Michaelis-Gutmann bodies. On IVP, multiple mural filling defects with flat or convex border are seen, giving a cobblestone appearance. Obstruction is a rare complication.

LEUKOPLAKIA

Ureteral involvement is less common than bladder and collecting system involvement.

URETERAL TUMORS

Types:
  Benign tumors
  - Epithelial: inverted papilloma, polyp, adenoma
  - Mesodermal: fibroma, hemangioma, myoma, lymphangioma
  Malignant tumors
  - Epithelial: transitional cell carcinoma, squamous cell carcinoma, adenocarcinoma
  - Mesodermal: sarcoma, angiosarcoma, carcinosarcoma

Prognosis
- 50% of patients will develop bladder cancer.
- 75% of tumors are unilateral.
- 5% of patients with bladder cancer will develop ureteral cancer.

Radiographic features
- Intraluminal filling defect
- Bergman's (goblet) sign: on retrograde ureterography, catheter coiled in dilated portion of ureter just distal to the lesion

Sites of metastatic spread of primary ureteral neoplasm (at autopsy):
- Retroperitoneal lymph nodes, 75%
- Liver, 60%
- Lung, 60%
- Bone, 40%
- Gastrointestinal tract, 20%
- Peritoneum, 20%
- Other (< 15%): adrenal glands, ovary, uterus

4

URETERAL DIVERSIONS

Ileal loop

Ureter(s) drain into isolated ileal segment, which serves as an isoperistaltic conduit (not as a reservoir). May or may not have a surgical "intussusception" of conduit. 50% of patients have hydronephrosis immediately postoperatively; the hydronephrosis should resolve by 3 months. Common locations of strictures are at the ureteroileal anastomosis and where the left ureter enters the peritoneum.

Colon conduit

Ureter(s) drain into isolated colon segment. Ureters are tunneled submucosally for antireflux.

Ureterosigmoidostomy

Distal ureter(s) drain into sigmoid colon; ureters are tunneled for antiperistalsis. Largely surpassed by ileal conduit nowadays because of complications: pyelonephritis, reflux, hyperchloremic acidosis, high risk of colon cancer.

Loopogram

1. 18-24 Fr Foley catheter with 5-mL balloon inflated in conduit.
2. Administer 30-50 mL of 30% water-soluble contrast by gravity (< 30 cm H_2O). Reflux in an ileal loop is a normal finding.
3. Search for: drainage, stasis, stenosis, extravasation, calculi, tumor.

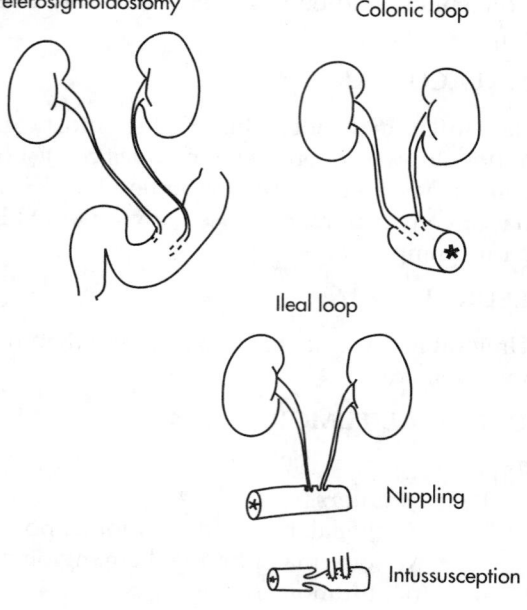

Bladder

CONGENITAL URACHAL ANOMALIES

Congenital urachal anomalies are twice as common in men as in women. There are four types of congenital urachal anomalies:

- Patent urachus
- Umbilical-urachal sinus
- Vesicourachal diverticulum
- Urachal cyst

The majority of patients with urachal abnormalities (except those with a patent urachus) are asymptomatic. However, these patients may become symptomatic if these abnormalities are associated with infection.

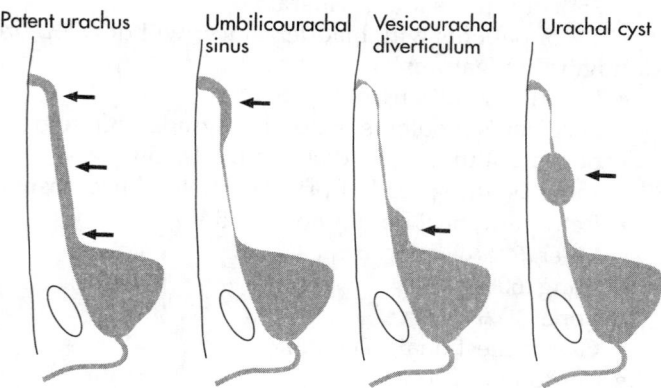

BACTERIAL CYSTITIS

Acute cystitis

Pathogens: *E. coli* > *Staphylococcus* > *Streptococcus* > *Pseudomonas*. Predisposing factors:

- Instrumentation, trauma
- Bladder outlet obstruction, neurogenic bladder
- Calculus
- Cystitis
- Tumor

Radiographic features
- Mucosal thickening (cobblestone appearance)
- Reduced bladder capacity
- Stranding of perivesical fat

CHRONIC CYSTITIS

Repeated bacterial infections usually due to such causes as reflux, diverticulum, bladder outlet obstruction. Radiographic features:
- Cystitis cystica: serous fluid–filled cysts; multiple smooth round filling defects
- Cystitis glandularis: mucin-secreting glandular hypertophy: multiple cystlike filling defects along mucosa
- Same findings as in acute cystitis

EMPHYSEMATOUS CYSTITIS

Infection (most commonly *E. coli*) that causes gas within the bladder and bladder wall. Predisposing diseases:
- Diabetes mellitus (most common)
- Long-standing urinary obstruction (neurogenic bladder, diverticulum, outlet obstruction)

Radiographic features
- Gas in bladder wall
- Gas may enter the ureter
- Air-fluid level in bladder

TUBERCULOSIS

Chronic interstitial cystitis that usually ends in fibrosis. Typically coexists with renal TB.

Radiographic features
- Cystitis cystica or glandularis often coexists, causing filling defects in bladder.
- Small, contracted thick-walled bladder
- Mural calcification (less common)

SCHISTOSOMIASIS (BILHARZIOSIS)

Caused by *Schistosoma haematobium* (*S. japonicum* and *S. mansoni* affect GI tract). Infected humans excrete eggs in urinary tract; eggs become trapped in mucosa and cause a severe granulomatous reaction.

Radiographic findings
- Extensive calcifications in bladder wall and ureter (hallmark)
- Inflammatory pseudopolyps: "bilharziomas"
- Ureteral strictures, fistulas
- SCC (suspect when previously identified calcifications have changed in appearance)

OTHER TYPES OF CYSTITIS

- Radiation cystitis occurs in 15% of patients receiving 6500 rad for pelvic malignancies.
- Cyclophosphamide treatment results in hemorrhagic cystitis in 40% of patients.
- Eosinophilic cystitis: severe allergic reactions
- Interstitial cystitis: most common in women; small, painful bladder

NEUROGENIC BLADDER

The detrusor muscle is innervated by S2-S4 parasympathetic nerves. Types of neurogenic bladder:
- Spastic bladder: upper motor neuron defect
- Atonic bladder: lower motor neuron defect

BLADDER FISTULAS

Types and common causes
- Vesicovaginal fistula: surgery, catheters, cancer, radiation
- Vesicoenteric fistula: diverticular disease (most common cause), Crohn's disease, cancer
- Vesicocutaneous fistula: trauma, surgery
- Vesicouterine fistula: C-section
- Vesicoureteral fistula: hysterectomy

LEUKOPLAKIA

Squamous metaplasia of transitional cell epithelium (keratinization). Associated with chronic infection (80%) and calculi (40%). Bladder > renal pelvis > ureter. Premalignant? Symptoms: hematuria, 30%, passage of desquamated keratinized epithelial layers.

Radiographic features
- Mucosal thickening
- Filling defect

MALACOPLAKIA

Chronic inflammatory response to gram-negative infection. More prevalent in patients with diabetes mellitus. Michaelis-Guttman bodies in biopsy specimen are diagnostic.

Radiographic features
- Single or multiple filling defects
- Requires cystoscopy and biopsy to differentiate from TCC

BLADDER DIVERTICULUM

Types
Hutch diverticulum: congenital weakness of musculature near UVJ
- Usually associated with reflux

Acquired diverticulum in bladder outlet obstruction
- Usually multiple
- Not associated with reflux
- Complications
  Infection
  Calculi, 25%
  Tumor, 3%

MALIGNANT BLADDER NEOPLASM

Clinical: painless hematuria.

Types and underlying causes

Transitional cell carcinoma, 90%
- Aniline dyes
- Phenacetin
- Pelvic radiation
- Tobacco
- Interstitial nephritis

Squamous cell carcinoma, 5%
- Calculi
- Chronic infection, leukoplakia
- Schistosomiasis

Adenocarcinoma, 2%
- Bladder exstrophy
- Urachal remnant
- Cystitis glandularis. 10% pass mucus in urine.

Radiographic features

Imaging findings
- Mass in bladder wall: US > contrast CT, MRI
- Obstructive uropathy due to involvement of ureteric orifices

Staging
- T1 = mucosal and submucosal tumors
- T2 = superficial muscle layer is involved
- T3a = deep muscular wall involved
- T3b = perivesicular fat involved
- T4 = other organs invaded

URACHAL CARCINOMA

Rare tumor (0.4% of bladder cancers, 40% of bladder adenocarcinomas) arising from urachus (fibrous band extending from bladder dome to umbilicus; remnant of allantois and cloaca). Tumors are usually located anterior and superior to dome of bladder in midline (90%). In contradistinction to bladder tumors, calcifications occur in 70%. 70% occur before the age of 20. Poor prognosis. Histologically, this tumor is classified as:
- Adenocarcinoma, 90%
- SCC, TCC, sarcoma

BENIGN BLADDER TUMORS

- Primary leiomyoma (most common); ulcerated leiomyomas may cause hematuria
- Hemangioma associated with cutaneous hemangiomas
- Neurofibromatosis
- Nephrogenic adenoma
- Endometriosis
- Pheochromocytoma

BLADDER CALCULI

Usually seen in patients with bladder outlet obstruction. Calculi usually form around a foreign body nidus (catheter, surgical clip). Calcium oxalate stones may have an irregular border (mulberry stones) or spiculated appearance (jack stones).

BLADDER OUTLET OBSTRUCTION

CAUSES	
Adults	**Children***
Benign prostatic hypertrophy	Posterior urethral valves (most common in males)
Bladder lesions	Ectopic ureterocele (most common in females)
Tumor	Bladder neck obstruction
Calculus	
Ureterocele	
Urethral stricture	Urethral stricture
Postoperative, traumatic	Prune belly syndrome
Detrusor/sphincter dyssynergy	

*See pediatric chapter.

Radiographic features

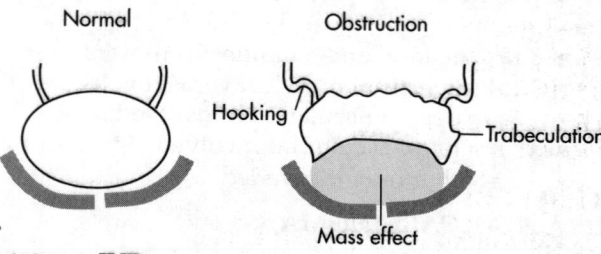

- Distended bladder with incomplete emptying (postvoid residual); best seen by US or IVP
- Increased bladder pressure causes formation of trabeculae and diverticulae
- Enlarged prostate:
  - Rounded central filling defect at base of bladder
  - Hooking of ureters with massively enlarged prostate on IVP
- Upper urinary tract changes
  - Reflux
  - Dilated ureter

BLADDER INJURIES

Bladder injuries occur in 10% of patients with pelvic fractures; instrumentation and penetrating trauma are less common causes. There are two types of ruptures: extraperitoneal and intraperitoneal. The likelihood of rupture increases with degree of distention of the bladder at time of injury.

TYPES OF BLADDER RUPTURE		
	Extraperitoneal, 45%	**Intraperitoneal, 45%***
Cause	Pelvic fractures (bone spicule), avulsion tear	Blunt trauma, stab wounds, invasive procedures
Location	Base of bladder, anterolateral	Dome of bladder (weakest point)
Imaging	Pear-shaped bladder	Contrast extravasation into paracolic gutters
	Fluid around bladder with displaced bowel loops	Urine ascites
	Paralytic ileus	

*Combined ruptures: 10%.

Classification of bladder injury
- Type 1: Bladder contusion
- Type 2: Intraperitoneal rupture
- Type 3: Interstitial bladder injury
- Type 4: Extraperitoneal rupture
- Type 4a: Simple extraperitoneal rupture
- Type 4b: Complex extraperitoneal rupture
- Type 5: Combined bladder injury

Radiographic examinations in suspected bladder injury
Retrograde urethrogram
- Should precede cystogram if there is suspicion of uretheral injury such as blood at meatus, "high-riding" prostate, or inability to void

Cystogram
- 350 mL of 30% water-soluble contrast is administered.
- Obtain scout view, AP, both obliques and postvoid films
- 10% of ruptures will become evident on postvoid films.

CT Cystogram
- Retrograde bladder distention is required before CT cystography.
- After Foley catheter insertion, adequate bladder distention is achieved by instilling at least 350 mL of a diluted mixture of contrast material under gravity control.
- Obtain contiguous 10-mm axial images from the dome of the diaphragm to the perineum, including the upper thighs.
- Obtain postdrainage images through the decompressed bladder.
- The normal CT cystogram will demonstrate a uniformly hyperattenuating, well-distended urinary bladder with thin walls. The adjacent fat planes will be distinct, with no evidence of extravasated contrast material.

CYSTOSTOMY

Indication:
- Bladder outlet obstruction

Technique
1. Preprocedure workup:
   - Check bleeding status.
   - Antibiotic coverage: ampicillin 1 g, gentamicin 80 mg
   - Review all films and determine whether bowel loops lie anterior to bladder.
   - Place Foley catheter to distend bladder with contrast.

2. Local anesthesia with Xylocaine. Place Longdwell needle into bladder and aspirate urine to check for position.
3. Advance stiff 0.038 guidewire and coil in bladder.
4. Dilate skin up to 16 Fr and then use a balloon catheter for further dilatation.
5. Place 16 Fr peel-away sheath. Pass 12 Fr Foley over guidewire. Remove guidewire. Inject contrast to check position of catheter.

Male Urethra

RETROGRADE URETHROGRAM (RUG)

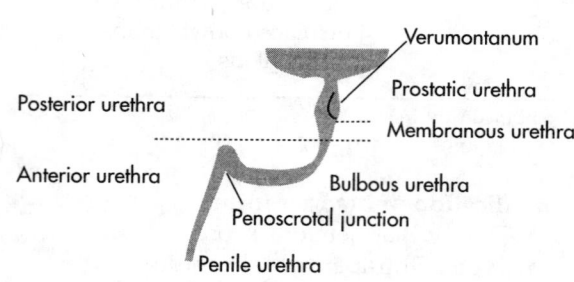

- Posterior urethra = prostatic + membranous portions
- Anterior urethra = bulbous and penile portions
- Verumontanum: dorsal elevation in prostatic urethra that receives paired ejaculatory ducts and the utricle
- Membranous urethra demarcates urogenital diaphragm; radiographically defined as the portion between the distal verumontanum and the cone of bulbous urethra
- Cowper glands in urogenital diaphragm; ducts empty into proximal bulbous urethra
- Littre glands in anterior urethra
- Utricle: Müllerian duct remnant. Blind ending pouch in midline
- Fossa navicularis: 1-cm long dilatation of distal anterior urethra

URETHRAL INJURIES

Complications: strictures, impotence.

Types

Complex trauma with pelvic fractures

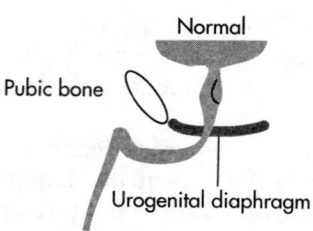

- Type 1: urethra intact but narrowed, stretched by periurethral hematoma
- Type 2: rupture above urogenital diaphragm; extraperitoneal contrast, none in perineum
  Partial rupture: contrast seen in bladder; complete rupture: no contrast seen in bladder
- Type 3: rupture below urogenital diaphragm; contrast in extraperitoneal space and perineum

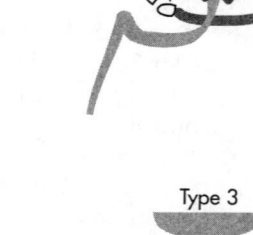

Soft tissue injury

- Straddle injury: injuries to penile or bulbous urethra

URETHRAL STRICTURES AND FILLING DEFECTS

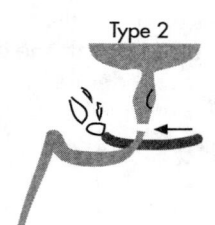
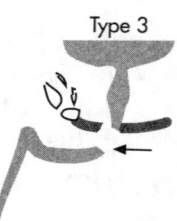

Infection

- Gonococcal (most common, 40% of all strictures in United States), most common in bulbopenile urethra. Radiographic features: beaded appearance, retrograde filling glands of Littré
- TB: fistulas result in "watering can" perineum

Trauma
- Instrumentation, e.g., transurethral resection of the prostate (TURP): short, well-defined stricture in bulbomembranous urethra or penoscrotal junction
- Catheters: long, irregular, penoscrotal junction
- Injuries (straddle injury: bulbous urethra; pelvic fracture: prostatomembranous urethra)

Tumor (rare)
- Polyps: inflammatory, transitional cell papilloma
- Malignant primaries: TCC, 15%, SCC, 80%; often associated with history of stricture
- Prostate cancer

Female Urethra

ANATOMY

- 2.5-4.0 cm long, ovoid or tubular
- Sphincter seen on US as a hypoechoic structure 1.0-1.3 cm in diameter
- Skene's glands, periurethral glands

INFECTION

- Usually seen in conjuction with cystitis
- Chronic irritation may result in polyps in the region of the bladder neck.
- Female urethral syndrome: chronic irritation on voiding. Radiographically, there is increased thickness of hypoechoic tissue by US; elevation of bladder on IVP

CARCINOMA

- Incidence in females 5 times that of males
- 90% in distal two-thirds, 70% are SCC
- TCC is usually posterior.

DIVERTICULA

- Female urethral diverticula usually acquired after infection, followed by obstruction of Skene's glands.
- If nonobstructed, 75% will be seen on postvoid IVP film, 90% on VCUG, remainder require double-balloon catheter positive pressure urethrography.
- Calculi, 5%-10%
- Most common tumor is adenocarcinoma.

Retroperitoneum

General

Retromesenteric anterior interfascial space (RMS), retrorenal posterior interfascial space (RRS), anterior pararenal space (APS), anterior renal fascia (ARF), dorsal pleural sinus (DPS), lateroconal fascia (LCF), parietal peritoneum (PP), posterior pararenal space (PPS), posterior renal fascia (PRF), transversalis fascia (TF)

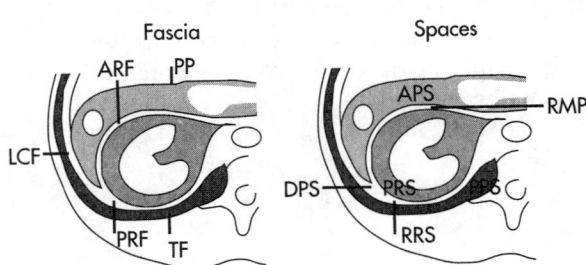

ANATOMICAL TERMS

- Interfascial plane: Potential space between layers of renal, lateroconal, or transversalis fascia; result of fusion of embryonic mesentery
- Anterior interfascial retromesenteric plane: Potentially expansile plane between the anterior pararenal and perinephric spaces; continuous across the midline, it is an important potential route of contralateral spread of retroperitoneal collections
- Posterior interfascial retrorenal plane: Potentially expansile plane between the perinephric space and posterior pararenal space; anterior pararenal, peritoneal, or intrafascial fluid may reside within the retrorenal space
- Lateroconal interfascial plane: Potentially expansile plane between layers of lateroconal fascia; communicates with anterior and posterior interfascial planes at the fascial trifurcation
- Combined interfascial plane: Potentially expansile plane formed by the inferior blending of the anterior renal, posterior renal, and lateroconal fasciae; continues into the pelvis, providing a route of disease spread from the abdominal retroperitoneum into the pelvis
- Fascial trifurcation: Site at which the lateroconal fascia emerges from Gerota's fascia; anterior, posterior, and lateroconal interfascial planes communicate at the fascial trifurcation, usually located laterally to the kidney
- Anterior pararenal space: between posterior peritoneum and anterior renal fascia; contains pancreas and bowel
- Posterior pararenal space: between posterior renal fascia and transveralis fascia; contains no organs. Fat continues laterally as properitoneal flank stripe
- Perirenal space: between anterior and posterior renal fascia; contains kidney, adrenal gland, proximal collecting systems, renal vessels, and a variable amount of fat
- Renal fascia (Gerota's fascia) has an anterior and a posterior part. Renal and lateroconal fasciae are laminated planes composed of apposed layers of embryonic mesentery.
- Lateroconal fascia formed by lateral fusion of anterior and posterior renal fascia
- Transversalis fascia
- The perinephric spaces (PRS) are closed medially.
- The retromesenteric space is continuous across midline.

Peritoneum   Transversalis fascia

PERINEPHRIC SPACE

The perinephric space contains a rich network of bridging septa, lymphatics, arteries, and veins. The perirenal lymphatics communicate with small lymph nodes at the renal hilum, and these, in turn, connect with periaortic and pericaval lymph nodes. This lymphatic network provides potential route of spread for metastatic tumor into perinephric space.

Benign Conditions

RETROPERITONEAL HEMATOMA

Common causes:
- Anticoagulation
- Trauma
- Iatrogenic
- Ruptured abdominal aortic aneurysm (particularly if > 6 cm)
- Tumor: renal cell carcinoma, large angiomyolipoma

Radiographic findings
- Dissection through retroperitoneal spaces
- Acute hemorrhage: 40-60 HU
- Hematocrit level

ABSCESS

Location and common causes:
- Anterior pararenal space (> 50%): pancreatitis
- Perirenal space: renal inflammatory disease
- Posterior pararenal space: osteomyelitis

RETROPERITONEAL AIR

Causes
- Trauma (perforation)
- ERCP
- Emphysematous pyelonephritis

RETROPERITONEAL FIBROSIS

Fibrotic retroperitoneal process that can lead to ureteral and vascular obstruction.

Causes

Idiopathic (Ormond's disease), 70%

Benign
- Medication: methysergide, ergotamine, methyldopa
- Radiation, surgery
- Inflammation extending from other organs
- Retroperitoneal fluid: hematoma, urine

Malignant
- Desmoplastic reaction to tumors: HD > NHL > anaplastic carcinoma, metastases

Radiographic features
- Fibrotic tissue envelopes retroperitoneal structures.
- Fibrosis may enhance after contrast administration.
- Extrinsic compression of ureter
- Medial deviation of ureters
- Extrinsic compression of IVC, aorta, iliac vessels
- On T1W MRI, fibrous tissue appears hypointense. Active inflammation has an intermediate to hyperintense SI on T2W.
- Differential diagnosis: inflammatory aneurysm of the aorta, enhancing perianeurysmal soft tissue, which may obstruct ureters and IVC

PELVIC LIPOMATOSIS

Abnormal large amount of fatty tissue in pelvis compressing normal structures. Unrelated to obesity or race. May occur with IBD of rectum.

Radiographic features

- Elongation and narrowing of urinary bladder (pear shape)
- Elongation and narrowing of rectosigmoid
- Large amount of fat in pelvis

Tumors

Retroperitoneal tumors may arise from muscle, fascia, connective tissue fat, vessels, nerves or remnants of the embryonic urogenital ridge. 90% of retroperitoneal tumors are malignant and are usually very large (10-20 cm) at diagnosis.

Types

Mesodermal tumors

- Lipoma, liposarcoma
- Leiomyosarcoma
- Fibrosarcoma
- Malignant fibrous histiocytoma
- Lymphangiosarcoma
- Lymphoma

Neural tumors

- Neurofibroma, schwannoma
- Neuroblastoma
- Pheochromocytoma

Embryonic tumors

- Teratoma
- Primary germ-cell tumor

LIPOSARCOMA

Fat-containing retroperitoneal tumors range in spectrum from lipomas (benign) to liposarcoma (malignant).

Radiographic features

- Nonhomogeneity with focal higher density structures (i.e., > -25 HU) is strong evidence of a liposarcoma.
- Tumors are classified histologically as lipogenic, myxoid, or pleomorphic. Myxoid and pleomorphic tumors are most common and may demonstrate little or no fat on CT.

LEIOMYOSARCOMA

Radiographic features

- Large mass
- Typically large areas of central necrosis
- Heterogeneous enhancement

Adrenal Glands

General

Arterial supply
- Superior adrenal artery: branch of inferior phrenic artery
- Middle adrenal artery: branch of the aorta
- Inferior adrenal artery: branch of the renal artery

Venous drainage
Each gland is drained by a single vein which enters into the:
- Inferior vena cava on the right
- Renal vein on the left

Physiology
Cortex divided into 3 zones:
- Zona glomerulosa (aldosterone)
- Zona fasciculata (ACTH dependent)
- Zona reticularis (cortisol)

Medulla (adrenaline, noradrenaline)

Imaging appearance
- "Y" configuration: each adrenal gland consists of an anteromedial ridge (body) and two posterior limbs best seen by CT/MR.
- Posterior limbs are close together superiorly but spread out inferiorly (angle 120 degrees).
- Right adrenal lies adjacent to IVC throughout its extent.
- Left adrenal lies adjacent to splenic vessels at its cephalad margin.
- Size:
    Limbs: 3-6 mm thick
    Length of entire adrenal: 4-6 cm
    Width of entire adrenal: < 1 cm
    Weight: 4-5 g/gland

Medullary Tumors

PHEOCHROMOCYTOMA

Pheochromocytoma is a subtype of a paraganglioma, a neuroendocrine tumor that arises from paraganglionic tissue. Rule of "10s": 10% of pheochromocytomas are extraadrenal, 10% are bilateral, and 10% are malignant. The most common location of an extraadrenal pheochromocytoma is the organ's of Zuckerkandl (near aortic bifurcation).

Classification of paraganglioma
Paraganglioma arising from adrenal medulla = pheochromocytoma
Aortosympathetic paraganglioma arising from the sympathetic chains and
    retroperitoneal ganglia = extraadrenal pheochromocytoma

Parasympathetic paragangliomas including chemodectomas (nonchromaffin paraganglioma)

- Glomus tympanicum
- Glomus jugulare
- Glomus vagale
- Carotid body tumor
- Others, not specified

Paraganglioma cells belong to the amine precursors uptake and decarboxylation (APUD) system. Cells may secrete catecholamines (epinephrine, dopamine, norepinephrine) or be nonfunctional.

Clinical (excess catecholamines)

- Episodic (50%) or sustained (50%) hypertension, tachycardia, diaphoresis, headache (catecholamine-producing tumors); however, only 0.1% of hypertension is caused by pheochromocytomas.
- Elevated VMA in 24-hour urine in 50%
- Elevated serum catecholamines, urine metanephrines

Pharmacological testing

Diagnostic pharmacological tests are potentially hazardous and may result in acute hypertension (stimulation tests) or hypotension (suppression tests). Careful monitoring is therefore necessary.

- Stimulators: glucagon, histamine, contrast material during arteriography
- Suppressors: clonidine, phentolamine.

Associations

- Multiple endocrine neoplasia in 5%; pheochromocytomas are usually bilateral and almost always intraadrenal.
- Neurofibromatosis (10% of patients have pheochromocytomas)
- Von Hippel-Lindau disease (10% of patients have pheochromocytomas)
- Familial pheochromocytosis, (10% of all pheochromocytomas)

Radiographic features

Sensitivity for detection of functional tumors

- CT or MRI: 90%
- MIBG scintigraphy: 80%
- Octreotide scintigraphy

Appearance

- Adrenal mass
- Strong contrast enhancement (CT, angiography)
- Calcification
- MRI: very high signal intensity (SI) on T2W images. The SI is usually considerable higher when compared with adenomas or metatsases.
- Percutaneous biopsy: method of choice for tissue diagnosis; biopsy of pheochromocytoma may precipitate acute hypertensive crisis and pharmacological prophylaxis is therefore indicated.

MULTIPLE ENDOCRINE NEOPLASIA (MEN)

MEN II (mucosal neuroma syndrome, multiple endocrine adenomatosis) is a rare autosomal dominant cancer syndrome.

Types

- MEN IIa: medullary thyroid carcinoma, pheochromocytoma, parathyroid adenoma
- MEN IIb: medullary thyroid carcinoma, pheochromocytoma, oral ganglioneuromas, other soft tissue tumors

Clinically, MEN IIb is characterized by marfanoid habitus, coarse facial features with prognathism, and gastrointestinal (GI) tract abnormalities (constipation, diarrhea, feeding difficulties).

Cortical Tumors

APPROACH TO ADRENAL MASSES

Adrenal masses are best evaluated first by noncontrast CT according to the flow diagram on the right. Points to remember:

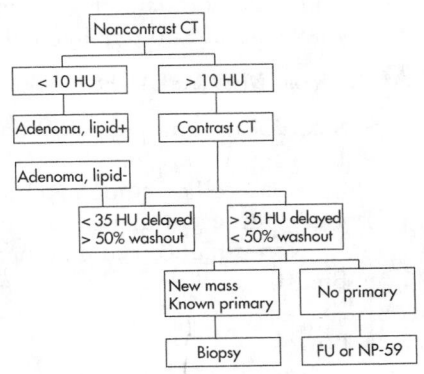

- Masses with attenuation averaging ≤ 10 HU all considered adenomas
- If the attenuation is more than 10 HU, the mass is considered indeterminate and an enhanced and 15-min delayed enhanced CT scan is obtained. If the enhancement washout is more than 50%, especially if the delayed attenuation value is less than 35 HU, a diagnosis of lipid-poor adenoma is made with no further evaluation.
- If the enhancement washout is less than about 50%, especially if the delayed attenuation value is more than 35 HU, the mass is considered indeterminate. If the patient has a new extraadrenal primary neoplasm with no other evidence of metastases, percutaneous adrenal biopsy is recommended to confirm adrenal metastasis. In a patient without cancer, surgery, follow-up CT, or adrenal scintigraphy with the use of radioiodinated norcholesterol (NP-59) is recommended, depending on the size of the mass and the other specific clinical features.
- Using 10 HU as a cut-off for diagnosis, the test has a sensitivity of 71% and a specificity of 98%.
- 30% of adenomas have an attenuation value of more than 10 HU and are thus indistinguishable from other masses. 98% of homogeneous adrenal masses with a nonenhanced CT attenuation value of 10 HU or less will be benign (most will be adenomas).
- For the occasional adrenal mass that is detected at enhanced CT before the patient leaves the scanning table, a 15-min delayed scan should be obtained and the above criteria applied.
- It is useful to refer to adenomas with nonenhanced CT attenuation values of 10 HU or less as lipid-rich and to refer to those with values of more than 10 HU as lipid-poor. The lipid-poor adenomas are an important subgroup because it is precisely these adenomas that cannot be characterized with nonenhanced CT densitometry
- Although chemical shift MR imaging can be used to characterize lipid-rich adenomas with accuracy similar to that of nonenhanced CT, adenomas with only small amounts of lipid will not be detected.
- Most adrenal cortical carcinomas are larger than 5 cm at presentation and often have demonstrable metastases. Typically, these tumors also have large amounts of necrosis, which would invalidate attempts to assess enhancement washout.

ADRENOCORTICAL CARCINOMA

50% of adrenocortical carcinomas are functioning (Cushing's syndrome most common clinical manifestation). Poor prognosis because tumor is usually large at time of diagnosis.

Radiographic features

- Mass usually > 5 cm at time of diagnosis
- CT: heterogeneous enhancement because of areas of necrosis, hemorrhage; 50% have calcifications
- MRI: tumor appears hyperintense relative to liver T2W but is less hyperintense and usually much larger than pheochromocytoma
- May extend into renal vein, IVC, or right atrium

ADRENAL METASTASES

Incidence: 25% at autopsy. Most common primary sites:
- Lung
  - Small cell carcinoma: 90% of adrenal masses detected by CT screening represent metastases
  - Non–small cell carcinoma: 60% of adrenal masses metastases
- Breast
- Kidney
- Bowel
- Ovary
- Melanoma

Radiographic features

- Adrenal mass
- Bilateral masses
- Heterogeneous enhancement
- Indistinct, irregular margins
- SI of metastases by MRI is similar to that of spleen on T1W and T2W images. However, there is considerable overlap in SI between metastases and adenomas; the typical adenoma has an SI similar to that of adrenal tissue on T1W and T2W images.
- CT biopsy usually performed in equivocal cases

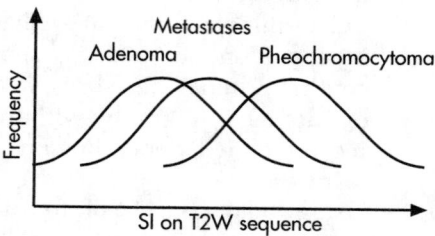

ADENOMA

Benign nonfunctioning adrenal adenomas are common (detected in 1%-3% of CT scans). Higher incidence in diabetes, hypertension, old age.

Radiographic features

CT

- Mass 1-5 cm
- < 0 HU: diagnostic of adenoma (due to fat)
- 0-10 HU: diagnosis almost certain, (F/U or MRI)
- Calcification rare
- Slight enhancement with IV contrast

MRI

- Fat-suppression techniques are used to determine if a given lesion contains fat, (e.g., in phase/out of phase imaging, spin echo fat–suppression imaging). If a lesion contains fat, it is considered an adenoma.

MYELOLIPOMA

Rare (250 cases reported up to 1994) benign tumors composed of adipose and hematopoietic tissue. Most common in the adrenal gland but extraadrenal tumors (retroperitoneum, pelvis, liver) have been reported. Usually very small and discovered incidentally at autopsy.

Radiographic features
- Area of obvious fat mass (low negative attenuation)
- May enhance with contrast administration
- Calcification, 20%

ADRENAL CYST

Rare lesions. Classification:
- Endothelial cyst (lymphangiectatic or angiomatous), 40%
- Pseudocyst (hemorrhage), 40%; may contain calcified rim
- Epithelial cyst, 10%
    Cystic adenoma
    Retention cyst
    Cystic transformation of embryonal remnant
- Parasitic cysts (echinococcus), 5%

Radiographic features
- Mural calcification (15%), especially in pseudocysts and parasitic cysts
- Imaging findings of adrenal cyst are similar to those seen in cysts in other locations.

ADRENAL HEMORRHAGE

More common in neonates than adults. Causes of hemorrhage:
- Hemorrhagic tumors
- Perinatal (common cause of calcification in later life)
- Severe trauma, traumatic hemorrhage, shock, postoperative, burn (traumatic hemorrhage is more common on the right)
- Anticoagulation, hemorrhagic diseases. Adrenal hemorrhage related to anticoagulation; usually occurs within the first month of treatment.
- Sepsis (disseminated intravascular coagulation, Waterhouse-Friderichsen syndrome)
- Adrenal venography (hemorrhage occurs in 10% of studies)
- Addison's disease

Radiographic features
Acute hematoma
- High CT density (> 40 HU)
- Enlarged adrenal gland

Old hematoma
- Liquefaction
- Fluid/fluid level
- May evolve into pseudocyst
- Typical MRI appearance of blood (see Chapter 6)

INFECTION

Most common causes are TB, histoplasmosis, blastomycosis, meningococcus, and echinococcus.
- TB may cause calcification and/or a soft tissue mass, which may have hypodense necrotic regions.
- Histoplasmosis usually preserves shape and may calcify.

Functional Diseases

CUSHING'S SYNDROME

Excess steroid causes truncal obesity, HTN, hirsutism, cutaneous striae, amenorrhea. Diagnostic studies: elevated plasma cortisol levels in 50%, elevated urinary 24-hour cortisol levels, abnormal dexamethasone suppression test (suppresses pituitary, not ectopic ACTH production).

Causes of Cushing's syndrome

Adrenal hyperplasia, 70%

- Cushing's disease (90% of adrenal hyperplasia): pituitary adenoma (ACTH hypersecretion). By imaging, 50% of patients will have normal adrenals, and 50% will be diffusely enlarged. A small number will show macronodular enlargement.
- Ectopic ACTH (10% of adrenal hyperplasia): carcinoma of lung, ovary, pancreas.
- Nonspecific hyperplasia is also associated with:
    Acromegaly, 100%
    Hyperthyroidism, 40%
    Hypertension, 15%

Adenoma, 20%

Cortical carcinoma, 10%

HYPERALDOSTERONISM

Clinical: HTN, hypokalemia.

Types

Primary (Conn's disease)

- Adenoma, 75%
- Hyperplasia, 25%

Secondary (renal artery stenosis, reninoma)

Radiographic features

- Small tumors usually < 2 cm
- Usually requires thin (1.5-3.0 mm.) sections through the adrenal glands

ADRENAL INSUFFICIENCY

Clinical

Hyperpigmentation.

Types

Primary (Addison's disease; adrenal destruction)

- Autoimmune, idiopathic
- Infarction, hemorrhage
- Bilateral tumors: metastases
- Fungal

Secondary (hypopituitarism)

Radiographic features

- May be difficult to visualize small limbs
- Evidence of prior bilateral adrenal disease:
    Metastases
    TB
    Hemorrhage

Male Pelvis

Prostate

NORMAL ANATOMY

- Peripheral gland: peripheral zone and central zone
- Central gland: transitional zone and periurethral zone

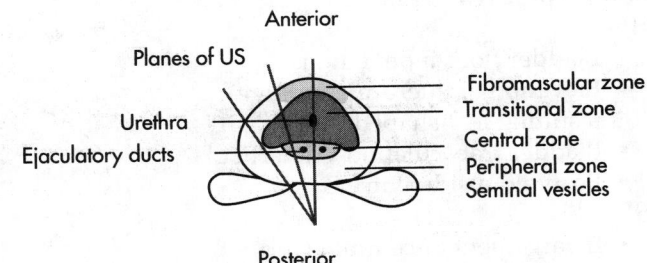

US-GUIDED PROSTATE BIOPSY

Indications

- Elevated prostate-specific antigen (PSA)

Technique

1. Obtain PSA, family history, and results of urological examination.

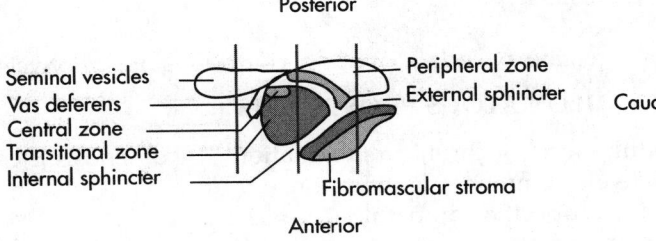

2. 3 days of oral antibiotics, 80 mg gentamicin IM immediately before biopsy.
3. Insert US probe with notch up (transverse view). Obtain the following views before biopsy (see lines in above diagram):
   - Seminal vesicles midline
   - Prostate gland superior
   - Prostate gland midgland
   - Prostate gland apex
   - Obtain above views from the right and then the left gland rather than in midline
4. Rotate notch 90 degrees counterclockwise (saggital view). Obtain the following views before biopsy (see lines in above diagram):
   - Find urethra at apex (white lines of mucosa) and orient probe
   - Base views: midline, left, right
   - Apex views: midline, left, right
   - Measure volume of gland
5. Perform biopsy through guide. Line up right and left peripheral zones on transverse view. Usually multiple biopsies (6-8) are obtained. 18-G cutting needle (e.g., Biopty gun).

PROSTATE MRI

Indications

- Staging of known prostate cancer

Technique

- Glucagon, 1 mg IV
- Endorectal surface coil
- Fully inflate coil
- Avoid rotation of coil
- T1W imaging of pelvis/abdomen for adenopathy

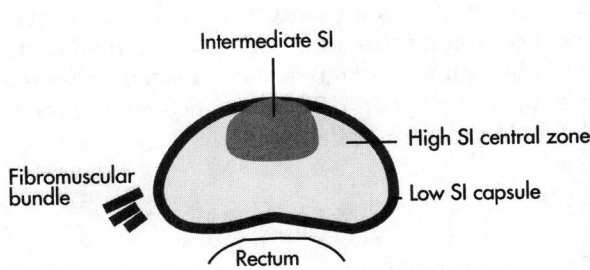

BENIGN PROSTATIC HYPERPLASIA (BPH)

Radiographic features
IVP
- Bladder floor indentation
- Elevation of interureteric ridge resulting in J-shaped ureters
- Bladder trabeculations, diverticula
- Postvoid residual urine

US
- Enlargement of central gland
- Hypoechoic or mixed echogenic nodules
- Calcifications within the central gland or surgical capsule
- Prostate volume > 30 cc

CT
- Prostate extends above superior ramus of symphysis pubis

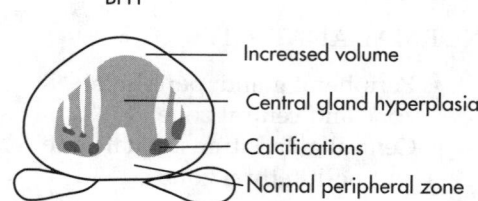

GRANULOMATOUS PROSTATITIS

Nodular form of chronic inflammation. The diagnosis is established by biopsy. Relatively common. Classification:
- Nonspecific, idiopathic
- Infectious
    Bacterial (tuberculosis [TB], brucella)
    Fungal
    Parasitic
    Viral
- Iatrogenic
    BCG induced
    Postsurgical, postradiation
- Systemic diseases
    Allergic
    Sarcoidosis
    Autoimmune diseases

Radiographic features
US
- Hypoechoic nodules, 70%
- Diffuse hypoechoic peripheral zone, 30%

MRI
- Hypointense gland on T2W, 95%
- No enhancement with Gd-DTPA

PROSTATE CANCER

Represents 18% of all cancers in the United States (50,000 new cases a year). Second most common cause of cancer death in men in the United States; 30% are potentially curable at time of diagnosis. Incidence increases with age (uncommon before 50 years, median age 72 years). BPH does not predispose to cancer.
Screening (controversial):

Prostate-specific antigen (PSA)
- Normal 2-4 U
- Cancer elevates PSA 10 times more than does BPH (per gram of tissue)
- Cancer: 1.8 ng/ml PSA/gram of tissue (i.e., the higher, the more tumor)

Digital rectal exam:
- Only 20% of palpable lesions are curable.
- False negative rate of 25%-45%

Ultrasound
- Most cancers are hypoechoic lesions in peripheral gland; however, only 20% of hypoechoic lesions are cancers.
- Isoechoic cancers, 40% (i.e., not detectable)

Origin
- Outer gland tumors (posterior and peripheral location), 70%
- Inner gland tumors (anterior and central location), 30%; inner gland tumors are not as rapidly invasive because of the presence of the surgical capsule and because there is no neurovascular bundle supply.

Radiographic features

US

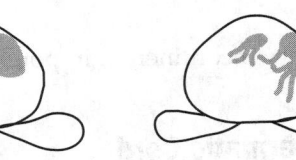
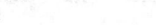
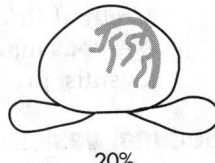

- Sensitivity for detection of cancers is low with a specificity of approximately 60%; US is therefore mainly used to guide sextant biopsies.
- Appearance
    Majority of tumors are hypoechoic
    Tumors may be hypervascular by Doppler US
    Suspect cancer if there are calcifications in the peripheral zone
- Pattern of spread
    Nodular
    Nodular infiltrative
    Infiltrative, spread along capsule, nonpalpable, nondetectable by US

CT
- Limited value in cancer detection and local staging; valuable for staging in abdomen

Bone scan
- Most commonly used technique to detect bone metastases
- Only 0.2% of patients with PSA< 20 will have bone metastases in the absence of bone pain.

MRI
- Cancers are hypointense relative to peripheral zone on T2W images. 30% of all prostate cancers are undetectable by MRI.
- Diagnostic uncertainty arises when peripheral zone is hypointense because of fibrosis. Positive predictive value: 70%.
- Capsular bulge can be indicative of capsular penetration of tumor
    Smooth bulge: 50% penetration
    Irregular bulge: 75% penetration
- Other signs have variable prognostic value
    Retraction
    Stranding of fat outside prostate

- Pitfalls of MRI
    Postbiopsy changes can mimic cancer.
    BPH can extend into peripheral zone, simulating cancer.
    Apical lesions are usually difficult to detect.
    "Pseudolesions" are often present at gland base.
    Image degradation by motion artifact
- MRI is a staging, not a screening tool. It allows determination of the extension into seminal vesicles, bladder, and periprostatic fat.

OUTCOME BY MRI	
MRI Findings	**3-Year Recurrence (%)**
Tumor confined to gland	25
Bulge of capsule	25
Definitely stage C	100

Staging (Jewett system)
- Stage A: nonpalpable tumor found at biopsy: radical prostatectomy
    A1 = well-differentiated: low morbidity, follow-up examination
    A2 = poorly differentiated (radiotherapy)
- Stage B: palpable tumor, confined to prostate (radical prostatectomy)
- Stage C: extension through prostatic capsule but no metastases (radiation therapy)
- Stage D: metastases (hormonal therapy, radiotherapy, chemotherapy)

Treatment complications
- Urethral stricture
- Nervous injury (urinary incontinence, impotence)
- Cystitis, proctitis

Seminal Vesicle and Spermatic Cord

SEMINAL VESICLE CYSTS

- Common, usually < 3 cm
- Associated with renal agenesis

OTHER SEMINAL VESICLE DISEASE

- Abscess (usually due to prostatitis)
- Primary carcinoma (rare)
- Hypospermia due to strictures, reflux

SPERMATIC CORD

Spermatic cord contains the draining spermatic veins, the testicular artery, the vas deferens, and the draining lymphatics and nerves. Calcification of the vas deferens is associated with diabetes.

Testis and Epididymis

GENERAL

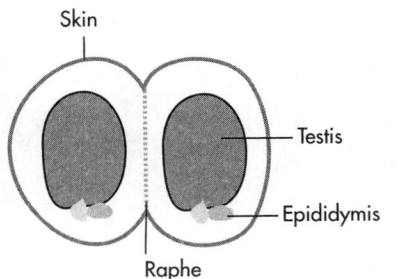

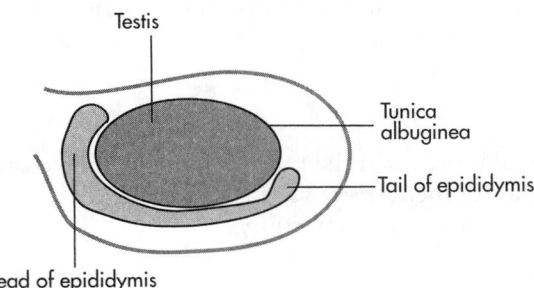

- Testes (5 × 3 × 3 cm) contain 250 pyramidal lobulations. There are 1-4 seminiferous tubules (30-70 cm long) per lobule, which converge into the rete testis. The rete testis communicates with the head of the epididymis via 10-15 efferent ductules.
- Epididymis contains 6 m of coiled tubules; the head is < 10 mm in diameter and lies lateral to the superior pole of the testis; the body and tail are smaller (2 mm).
- Mediastinum testis: invagination of the tunica albuginea (fibrous capsule that envelops the testis)

Arterial supply
- Main supply via testicular artery (from aorta)
- Cremasteric artery (via inferior epigastric)
- Differential artery (via inferior vesicle branch of internal iliac arteries, supplies the epididymis and vas deferens)

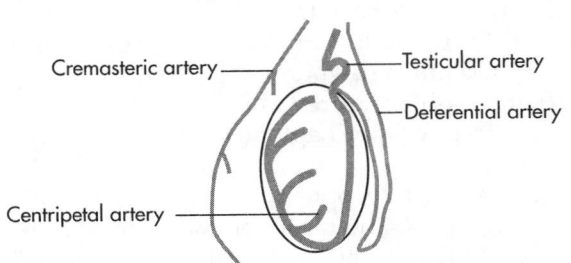

MRI EVALUATION OF TESTIS

- Surface coil
- Towel is placed under scrotum to raise testis between the thighs, second towel draped over scrotum and coil placed on towel; towels should be warm to prevent scrotal muscular contractions.
- Coronal T1W; axial, coronal, and sagittal T2W images acquired. Although not generally needed, gadolinium can be administered to characterize intermediate scrotal masses. T1W axial images of abdomen done to search for adenopathy.
- Normal testis has homogeneous intermediate signal intensity on T1W images and high signal intensity on T2W images. The epididymis is isointense or slightly hypointense relative to testis on T1W and hypointense on T2W images.

CRYPTORCHISM

Undescended testes are present in 0.3% of adult men. 20% of these testes lie within the abdomen or pelvis. Unilateral maldescent in the adult is usually treated by surgical removal of the testes. Bilateral maldescent is treated with orchiopexy and biopsy (to exclude malignancy). Early orchiopexy reduces the risk of tumor later in life.

Complications
- Torsion
- Malignancy: 30-fold increased risk; the malignancy rate correlates with increasing distance of the testis from the scrotal sac
- Testicular atrophy, resulting in infertility

TORSION

Types
Intravaginal torsion (common)
- Bell-clapper anomalous suspension: tunica vaginalis completely surrounds testis, epididymis and spermatic cord so that they are freely suspended in scrotal sac
- Testes twist within tunica vaginalis.
- 50%-80% are bilateral.

Extravaginal torsion (rare)
- Testis and its tunic twist at the external ring
- Occurs in newborns

Radiographic features
Scintigraphy (see Chapter 6)
  US
- Color Doppler
  < 4 hours: absent or decreased flow
  Late: peritesticular inflammation: hypervascularity
- Gray-scale imaging
  > 4 hours: enlargement, heterogenous echogenicity
  Late: reactive hydrocele, atrophy

Treatment
- < 4 hours: testes are usually salvageable
- > 24 hours: testes are usually nonsalvageable (orchiectomy)
- Long-standing torsion: orchiectomy and contralateral orchipexy

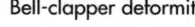
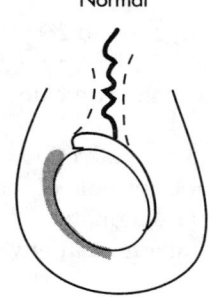
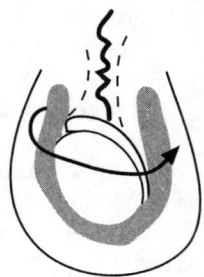

Normal   Bell-clapper deformity

EPIDIDYMOORCHITIS

Results from retrograde spread of organism from bladder or prostate via the vas deferens. Common pathogens:
- Gonococcus
- Pyogenic (E. coli, Pseudomonas)
- Mumps
- TB

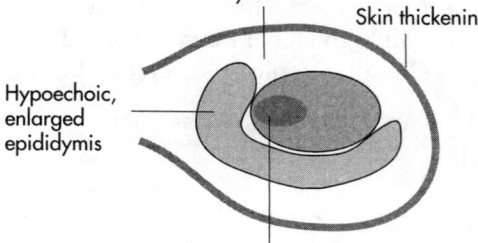

Hydrocele
Skin thickening
Hypoechoic, enlarged epididymis
Focal orchitis

Radiographic features
- Epididymis and spermatic cord enlargement
- Decreased echogenicity of epididymis and cord
- Focal orchitis: peripheral hypoechoic region; all hypoechoic testicular lesions need to be followed by ultrasound until resolution; 10% of patients with testicular tumors present with orchitis
- Reactive hydrocele or pyocele
- Thickening of the skin
- Calcification in chronic inflammation
- Color Doppler: hypervascularity in affected epididymis and/or testis

TESTICULAR ABSCESS

Abscesses occur most commonly in patients with diabetes, genitourinary tuberculosis, or mumps. Usually preceded or accompanied by epididymoorchitis
US features
- Testicular enlargement
- Hypoechoic lesion
- Fluid/fluid level

VARICOCELE

Varicoceles represent dilated veins of the pampiniform plexus. They result from incompetent or absent valves in the spermatic vein. Varicoceles occur in 15% of adult males.
Clinical findings
- Infertility
- Pain
- Scrotal enlargement

Location
- 90% of all varicoceles occur on the left side (drainage of left spermatic vein into the left renal vein at a right angle).
- 25% of varicoceles are bilateral.
- A solitary right-sided varicocele requires the exclusion of an underlying malignancy (tumor obstruction).

US features
- Hypoechoic veins ("bag of worms")
- Veins > 2 mm in diameter
- Dilated veins are easily compressed by transducer.
- Increase in venous size when patient is upright or performs Valsalva maneuver
- Color Doppler: flow is easily seen within varicocele and increases with Valsalva

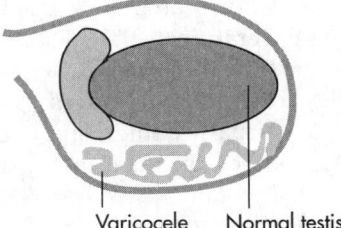
Varicocele   Normal testis

HYDROCELE

Simple fluid collection in scrotum. Most common cause of scrotal swelling.
Types
- Congenital: incomplete closure of processus vaginalis; spontaneous resolution by 18 months, associated with hernia
- Acquired:
    Obstruction
    Infection
    Idiopathic

TRAUMA

Types

- Testicular contusion
- Testicular rupture: requires emergency surgery to salvage testicle and to prevent antibody formation against sperm
- Testicular fracture: fracture line (detectable in 30%) or loss of sharpness of tunica albuginea (70%)
- Hematoma: complex cystic mass ("Swiss cheese")
- Hematocele (blood-stained hydrocele)

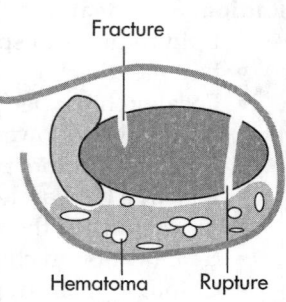

CYSTS

Causes: idiopathic, postinflammatory, posttraumatic

Types

- Epididymal cysts are very common; may be difficult to differentiate from spermatocele.
- Tunical cysts (mesothelial cysts) are common.
- Intratesticular cysts are uncommon (exclude malignancy).
- Rete testes dilatation is usually associated with epididymal cysts, older patients.

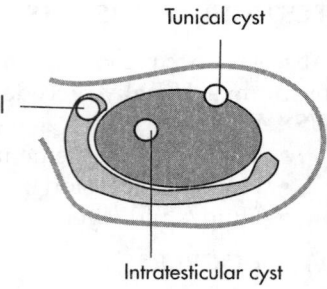

TESTICULAR MICROLITHIASIS

Multiple highly echogenic foci in testicles. No known underlying disease. Associated with crytorchidism and malignancy.

MALIGNANT TESTICULAR TUMORS

In the United States, there are 2500 new cases of testicular tumors per year. Testicular tumors are the most common malignancy in the age group 15-35 years. Tumor markers (AFP, HCG) aid in the early diagnosis and are important in follow-up.

Types

Germ cell tumors (mnemonic "SECT"), 95%

- **S**eminoma, 40%; extremely radiosensitive; good prognosis
- **E**mbryonal carcinoma, 10%; more aggressive than seminoma
- **C**horiocarcinoma, 1%; very aggressive
- **T**eratoma, 10%
- Mixed tumors, 40%

Sex cord–stromal tumors

- Usually benign and endocrinologically active (e.g., Leydig cell tumor)

Metastases, 5%. Common primaries:

- Prostate
- Kidney
- Lymphoma (most common testicular cancer in patients > 60 years of age)
- Leukemia

Radiographic features

US

- High sensitivity (95%) for detection
- Tissue diagnosis is made by biopsy/removal of testis; only some tumors have more typical imaging features:
  - Seminoma: homogenously hypoechoic
  - Embryonal cell carcinomas: cystic, heterogenous, wild
  - Lymphoma: diffuse or multifocal testicular enlargement

Staging
- Retroperitoneal nodes (20% at presentation): CT > lymphangiography

Pearls
- Rule of thumb:
    Intratesticular masses = malignant
    Extratesticular masses = benign
- Seminoma presents later than other tumors (4th-5th decade, may have two peak ages), most common in cryptorchidism
- Embryonal cancers (20%) are smaller and more aggressive than seminoma
- Choriocarcinomas (1%) are the most aggressive tumors
- Teratomas occur at younger age (10-20 years), good prognosis

BENIGN EPIDERMOID TUMOR

Represents 1% of all testicular tumors. Mean age: 20-40 years. US findings include well-circumscribed hypoechoic lesions with echogenic capsule; may have "onion-skin" appearance; internal shadowing is due to calcifications.

Penis

PEYRONIE'S DISEASE

Calcified plaques in the two corpora cavernosa.
Radiographic features
- Plaque usually located in periphery
- Hyperechoic, posterior shadowing of plaques
- Calcified plaques can also be seen by plain film.
- Septum between corpora may be thickened.

VASCULAR IMPOTENCE

50% of cases of impotence are due to vascular causes:
- Arterial insufficiency, 15%-35%
- Venous insufficiency, 15%
- Coexistent insufficiency, 50%-70%

Radiographic features
US
1. Inject papaverine into corpora cavernosa.
2. Scan with Doppler while erection develops.
3. Measure peak velocities:
    - < 25 cm/sec: severe arterial disease
    - 25-35 cm/sec: arterial disease
    - > 35 cm/sec: normal

Arteriography
Cavernosography and cavernosometry for venous leaks

Female Pelvis

General

PELVIC US

Uterus

- Endometrium appears hyperechoic (specular reflection from endometrial cavity); a hypoechoic halo surrounding the endometrium represents hypovascular myometrium (subendometrial halo).

CYCLICAL CHANGES OF ENDOMETRIUM		
Stage	Endometrium	Appearance
Menstrual	< 4 mm	
Proliferative	4-8 mm	
Secretory	7-14	

- Common age-related changes
  - Dilated peripheral uterine veins (hypoechoic)
  - Calcified arcuate arteries
- Version and flexion
  - Normal position (80%): anteversion and anteflexion
  - Retroversion: entire uterus is tilted backward (uterus and cervix)
  - Retroflexion: only body and fundus are flexed posteriorly
- Postmenopausal uterus (> 2 years following the last menstrual period [LMP]; perimenopausal < 2 years following LMP) may be difficult to see because of atrophy.
- Nabothian (retention) cysts of the cervix are common and usually insignificant.

Menstrual cycle

Follicular (Proliferative) phase

- Begins with day 1 of menses and continues until ovulation, usually on day 14 of a 28-day cycle
- Primordial follicles begin to grow under gonadotropin-releasing hormone—follicle-stimulating hormone (GnRH—FSH) stimulation (hypothalamic-pituitary axis); follicles may be visible sonographically as small cysts.
- Follicles secrete estrogen, which, through a negative feedback mechanism, causes a decrease in FSH; usually only one dominant follicle persists.
- Dominant follicle becomes visible by US at day 8-12; before ovulation, the dominant follicle undergoes rapid growth to reach a mean diameter of 20-24 mm by the time of ovulation.

Ovulation
- Ovulation occurs as a result of a luteinizing hormone (LH) surge, which is induced by rising estrogen levels.
- US signs of impending ovulation (within 36 hours):
  - Decreased echogenicity around the follicle
  - Irregularity of the follicle wall (crenation)
  - A small echogenic core of tissue (cumulus oophorus) occasionally projects into the follicle
- After ovulation there is sudden complete or partial collapse of the follicle; echoes appear within the cyst fluid.
- A small amount of free fluid may be noted in the cul-de-sac.

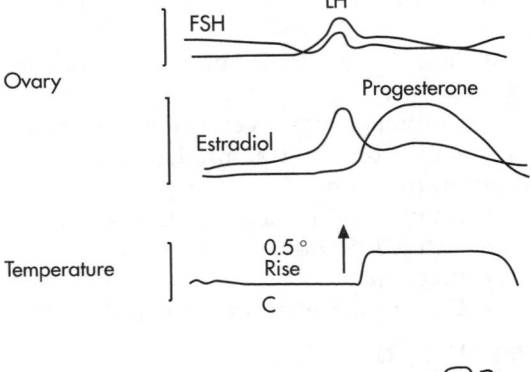

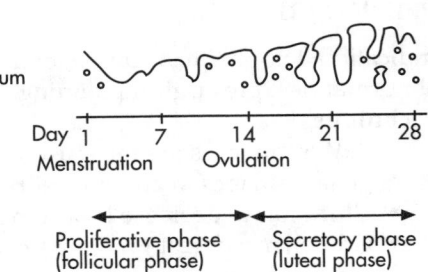

Secretory phase
- Granulosa cells (from the involuted follicle) form the corpus luteum, which synthesizes progesterone.
- Sonographically, the corpus luteum is a thin or irregular walled cyst (size 1-4 cm: "corpus luteum cyst").
- Progesterone maintains the secretory endometrium, which is necessary for successful implantation.
- Thick hyperechoic appearance due to engorged glands
- Endometrial thickness is greatest during the secretory phase (7-14 mm).

Ovary
- Normal volume: multiply the three diameters and divide by 2; normal volume < 18 cm^3 premenopausal, < 8 cm postmenopausal
- Cyst size up to 4 cm can be normal during the menstrual cycle (mean cyst size is 2.5 cm).
- Structures that may simulate ovaries:
  - Iliac vessel in cross-section
  - Bowel loops
  - Cervix containing multiple nabothian cysts
  - Lymph nodes
- Free fluid in the pelvis
  - Small amounts can be present during all phases of cycle (e.g., fluid from follicular rupture, estrogen-induced increased capillary permeability).
  - Large amounts of fluid are abnormal.

HYSTEROSALPINGOGRAM (HSG)

Indication: primarily used for infertility work-up, as an anatomical study prior to in vitro fertilization (IVF), and occasionally for evaluation of congenital anomalies.

Technique
1. HSG should be performed only on days 6-12 after LMP (4-week cycle).
2. Insert 6 Fr Foley catheter into cervical canal using speculum and inflate balloon.
3. Inject 4-30 ml of 28% contrast agent (water-soluble) under fluoroscopy until contrast agent passes into peritoneal cavity. Normal tubal length, 12-14 cm.
4. In dilated fallopian tubes administer doxycyclin (100 mg bid) for 10 days to prevent tuboovarian abscess. Patients with normal study do not require antibiotics.

Complications
- Pain
- Infection (< 3%), usually in patients with hydrosalpinx and pelvic inflammatory disease
- Contrast allergy (venous or lymphatic intravasation)
- Radiation: 100-600 mrad/ovary

Contraindications
- Active uterine bleeding/menses
- Active infection
- Pregnancy
- Uterine surgery within the last 3 days

PELVIC MRI

Indication: leiomyoma location, endometriosis, adenomyosis, congenital abnormalities, presurgical planning.

Techniques
- T2W sequences are most useful for imaging of uterus.
- Obtain images in anatomical planes of uterus.
- Glucagon to decrease bowel motility
- Gd-enhanced, fast gradient-echo sequences for evaluation of malignancies
- Fat-saturation sequences to diagnose dermoids

SI on T2W sequences
- Endometrium, high SI
- Junctional zone (inner layer of compact myometrium), low SI
- Myometrium, intermediate SI
- Cervix, low SI
- Serosal covering, low SI

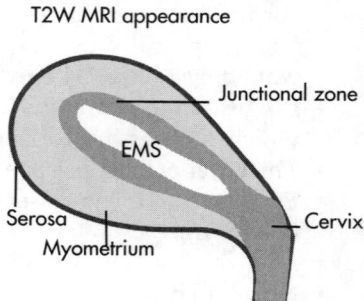

TRANSVAGINAL DRAINAGE PROCEDURES

The transvaginal approach is an ideal route for drainage of pelvic collections because of the proximity of the vaginal fornices to most pelvic lesions. The transvaginal approach allows use of endoluminal US probe needle guides to permit extremely accurate and speedy needle or catheter placement.

Indications
- Gynecological abscesses
- Nongynecological pelvic abscesses
- Incomplete therapeutic transvaginal aspiration
- Biopsies

Complications
- Bleeding
- Bowel injury
- Inadequate catheter positioning
- Potential for superinfection of sterile fluid collections because of the semisterile route of access

Uterus

UTERINE MALFORMATIONS

Incidence: 0.5%. Most often, duplication anomalies are discovered during pregnancy. Imaging modalities: US > MRI > HSG.

Types

Failure of fusion of the Müllerian ducts
- Complete: uterus didelphys
- Partial: uterus bicornis bicollis (2 cervices), uterus bicornis unicollis (1 cervix)

Arrested development of the Müllerian ducts
- Bilateral (very rare): uterine aplasia
- Unilateral: uterus unicornis unicollis ± rudimentary horn

Failure of resorption of the median septum
- Septate uterus
- Subseptate uterus

Complications

- Infertility and spontaneous abortions are common.
- Septate uterus: septum often consists of fibrous tissue rather than myometrium
    - Highest incidence of reproductive failure (zygote cannot implant on fibrous tissue)
    - Treatment: hysteroscopic excision of septum
- Hydrometrocolpos:
    - Rudimentary horn with no communication to uterine cavity
    - Uterine didelphys: one side may be obstructed by vaginal septum
- Premature labor or uterine size cannot accomodate full-grown fetus.
- Malpresentation: distorted uterine anatomy

Associations

- Congenital GU anomalies are common, 50%
    - Ipsilateral renal agenesis (most common)
    - Renal ectopia
- Mayer-Rokitansky-Kuster-Hauser syndrome
    - Dysgenesis of Müllerian ducts
    - Vaginal and/or uterine agenesis
    - Normal karyotype
    - Normal secondary sex characteristics
    - Renal anomalies

IN UTERO DIETHYLSTILBESTROL (DES) EXPOSURE

- Uterine hypoplasia
- T-shaped uterus
- Increased risk of clear cell cancer of vagina

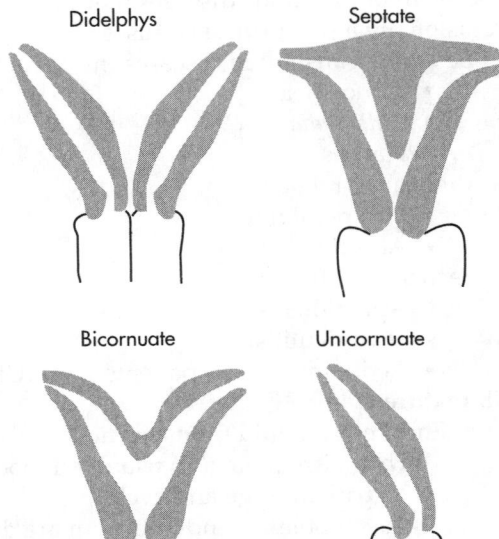

Didelphys Septate

Bicornuate Unicornuate

4

PELVIC INFLAMMATORY DISEASE (PID)

Spectrum of infectious diseases that present with pain, fever, discharge, and occasionally a pelvic mass. Causes:

Sexually transmitted diseases (most common)
- Gonorrhea
- *Chlamydia*
- Herpes

Pregnancy related
- Puerperal infection
- Abortion

Secondary PID
- Appendicitis
- Diverticulitis
- Actinomycosis in patients with IUD

US features
- Endometrial fluid (nonspecific)
  Thick, irregular, and usually hypoechoic endometrium (must correlate with patient's age and cycle)
  Gas bubbles in endometrium are diagnostic.
- Hydrosalpinx or pyosalpinx: cystic and tubular adnexal mass:
- Inflammatory pelvic mass lesion usually represents a tuboovarian abscess.
- Fibrosis and adhesions in end stage

PYOMETRA

Causes
- Malignancy
- Radiation
- Iatrogenic cervical stenosis

Radiographic features
- Endometrial canal filled with pus, blood
- Uterine enlargement

INTRAUTERINE DEVICE (IUD)

Complications
- Embedding
- Perforation
- 3-fold increased risk of PID (depends on IUD and string)
- Actinomycosis
- Associated pregnancy, spontaneous abortion

Radiographic feature
- Hyperechoic (shadowing) structures in endometrial canal or myometrium if embedded

ADENOMYOSIS

Heterotopic endometrial glands and stroma are located within the myometrium ("internal endometriosis"). Clinical: dysmenorrhea, bleeding, enlarged uterus, asymptomatic (5%-30%).

Radiographic features

MRI

- T2W MR imaging is study of choice.
- Focal or diffuse thickening of the junctional zone (> 12 mm) is the key finding.
- High SI endometrial foci within myometrium
- Enlargement of uterus

US

- US is nonspecific and less sensitive than MRI.
    Findings include heterogeneously increased echotexture, enlarged uterus

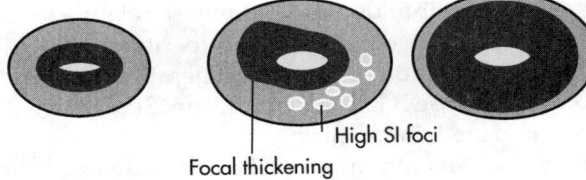

Normal   Focal form   Diffuse form

High SI foci

Focal thickening

LEIOMYOMA

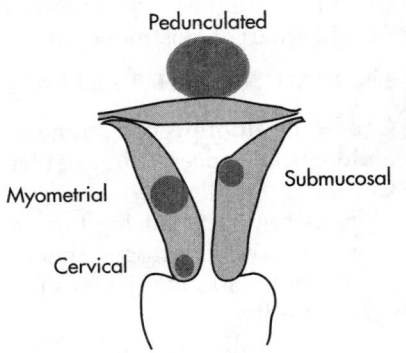

Pedunculated

Myometrial   Submucosal

Cervical

Uterine leiomyomas (fibroids) are the most common tumor of the uterus (in 25% of women > 35 years). Fibroids arise from smooth muscle cells. Clinical: asymptomatic (most common), uterine bleeding, pain, dysuria, and infertility (especially if located in lower segment or cervix). Fibroids are estrogen dependent:

- May grow during pregnancy
- Regression after menopause

Location

- Intramural (myometrial): most common
- Submucosal: least common but most likely to produce symptoms
- Subserosal: frequently pedunculated
- Broad ligament: may simulate adnexal mass
- Cervical: uncommon

Complications

- Torsion if pedunculated
- Cervical fibroids may interfere with vaginal delivery and require cesarean section (C-section).
- Infertility
- Sarcomatous degeneration (very rare)

Imaging features

US

- Fibroids are typically hypoechoic but may be heterogeneous:
    Calcification, 25%
    Degeneration: fatty (hyperechoic), cystic (hypoechoic)
    Rarely may contain cystic center
- Deformation of uterine contour
- Often multiple
- Lipoleiomyomas appear uniformly echogenic
- 20% of patients with fibroids have normal US.
- Transient muscular contraction (e.g., in abortion) may simulate the appearance of fibroid

CT

- Same density as uterus
- Same contrast enhancement as rest of myometrium
- Diagnosis is usually based on contour abnormalities of uterus.
- Often coarse calcification

MRI

- Allows accurate anatomical localization of fibroids prior to planned surgery.
- Simple fibroids are hypointense relative to uterus on T2W images.
- Atypical leiomyomas are hyperintense on T2W, which may be due to mucoid degeneration or cystic degeneration.
- Isointense relative to uterus on T1W images.

Extrauterine leiomyomas

Arise from smooth muscle cells in blood vessels (inferior vena cava), spermatic cord, Wolffian and Müllerian duct remnants, bladder, stomach, and esophagus. Very rare.

Uterine leiomyosarcomas

Usually present as large masses with homogenous SI. Suspect the diagnosis if a fibroid enlarges postmenopausally. Rare.

ENDOMETRIAL HYPERPLASIA

Caused by unopposed estrogen stimulation. Hyperplasia is a precursor to endometrial cancer. Clinical: bleeding.

Causes

- Estrogen-producing tumor
- Exogenous estrogen therapy (tamoxifen)
- Anovulation (any cause)
- Obesity
- Polycystic ovary (PCO)

Types

- Glandular-cystic (predominantly during reproductive years producing long menses and metrorrhagia). Hypoechoic spaces may be present within hyperechoic endometrium.
- Adenomatous (predominantly in menopause)

US features

- Thick endometrial stripe
    > 5 mm postmenopausal
    > 14 mm premenopausal or postmenopausal on tamoxifen
- Mandatory biopsy if endometrial stripe is > 15 mm to exclude cancer

Tamoxifen

Antiestrogen (binds to 17-β estrogen receptor) with weak estrogenic activity. Uses:

- Breast cancer adjuvant therapy
- Improves lipid profile
- Osteoporosis

Tamoxifen is associated with increased incidence of:

- Endometrial hyperplasia
- Endometrial polyps
- Endometrial cancer
- Subendometrial cystic atrophy (anechoic areas in the subendometrial myometrium)

GARTNER'S DUCT CYST

Inclusion cyst of the mesonephric tubules (Gartner's duct). Located lateral to uterus. Represents one type of paraovarian cysts.

ENDOMETRIAL CARCINOMA

Adenocarcinoma. Risk factors (increased estrogen): nulliparity, failure of ovulation, obesity, late menopause.

Radiographic features
- Prominent, thick echogenic endometrium (usually cannot be differentiated from endometrial hyperplasia or polyps)
- Obstruction of internal os may result in:
    Hydrometra
    Pyometra
    Hematometra
- Staging: (combined US and CT accuracy: 80%-90%)
    Stage 1, 2: confined to uterus (tumor enhancement < myometrial enhancement)
    Stage 3, 4: extrauterine
- MRI: variable appearance

CERVICAL CARCINOMA

Squamous cell carcinoma. Risk factors: condylomas, multiple sexual partners, sexually transmitted disease. Spread: local invasion of parametrium > lymph nodes > hematogenous spread.

Radiographic features
- Cervical stenosis with endometrial fluid collections (common)
- CT criteria for parametrial invasion (differentiates stage IIA from IIB, surgical vs. nonsurgical):
    Irregular or poorly defined margins of lateral cervix
    Prominent soft tissue stranding
    Obliteration of periureteral fat plane
- Accuracy for detecting pelvic nodal metastases by CT: 65%
- MRI: tumor appears hyperintense with respect to normal uterus on T2W images; additional findings in large (> 4 cm) tumors:
    Blurring and widening of the low-intensity uterine junctional band
    Broadening of the central uterine high-intensity zone

Transvaginal (TVUS)
- Equivocal: 5-8 mm / Abnormal: > 9 mm → Sonohysterography
  - Normal → Stop
  - Abnormal → Sample
    - Normal → Follow-up
    - Diagnosis
- Normal: < 5 mm → Stop

CERVICAL CARCINOMA STAGING	
FIGO Staging	**MR Imaging Staging**
0 Carcinoma in situ	Not visible
I Confined to cervix	
IA Microscopic	
IA-1 Stromal invasion < 3 mm	No tumor visible
IA-2 > 3 mm, < 5-mm invasion, < 7-mm width	Small enhancing tumor may be seen
IB Clinically visible (> 5 mm)	Tumor visible, intact stromal ring surrounding tumor
IB-1 < 4 cm	—
IB-2 > 4 cm	—
II Extends beyond uterus but not to pelvic wall or lower one-third of vagina	
IIA Vaginal extension, no parametrial invasion	Disruption of low-SI vaginal wall (upper two-thirds)
IIB Parametrial invasion	Complete disruption of stromal ring with tumor extending into the parametrium
III Extension to lower one-third of vagina or pelvic wall invasion with hydronephrosis	
IIIA Extension to lower one-third of vagina	Invasion of lower one-third of vagina
IIIB Pelvic wall invasion with hydronephrosis	Extension to pelvic muscles or dilated ureter
IV Located outside true pelvis	
IVA Bladder or rectal mucosa	Loss of low signal intensity in bladder or rectal wall
IVB Distant metastasis	—

- Staging
    Stage IA: confined to cervix
    Stage IB: may extend to uterus
    Stage IIA: extension into upper vagina
    Stage IIB: parametrial involvement
    Stage IIIA: extension into lower vagina
    Stage IIIB: pelvic wall (hydronephrosis)
    Stage IVA: spread to adjacent organs
    Stage IVB: spread to distant organs

Fallopian Tubes

The normal fallopian tubes are not seen by TVUS (< 4 mm). Visible fallopian tubes are always abnormal.

HYDROSALPINX

Causes
- PID
- Tumor
- Iatrogenic ligation
- Endometriosis

Radiographic features
- Convoluted cystic-appearing structure
- Echogenic wall
- Small polypoid excrescences along the wall
- Fluid/debris levels

SALPINGITIS ISTHMICA NODOSA (SIN)

Diverticula-like invaginations of the epithelial lining herniating into myosalpinx. Unknown etiology. Frequently there is a history of prior PID. SIN indicates a 10-fold increase for ectopic pregnancy.

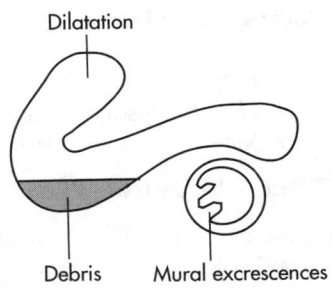

Ovaries

CLASSIFICATION OF CYSTIC OVARIAN STRUCTURES

A small cystic ovarian structure should be considered normal (ovarian follicle) unless the patient is prepubertal, postmenopausal, pregnant, or the mean diameter is > 25 mm (some authors use > 20 mm). Types of cysts:

Physiological cysts (mean diameter < 25 mm)
- Follicles
- Corpus luteum

Functional cysts (i.e., can produce hormones)
- Follicular cysts (estrogen), > 25 mm
- Corpus luteum cysts (progesterone)
- Theca lutein cyst (gestational trophoblastic disease)
- Complications in functional cysts:
    Hemorrhage
    Enlargement
    Rupture
    Torsion

Other cysts
- Postmenopausal cysts (serous inclusion cysts)
- Polycystic ovaries
- Ovarian torsion
- Cystic tumors

FOLLICULAR CYSTS

When a mature follicle fails to involute, a follicular cyst (> 2.5 cm in diameter) results. Clinical: asymptomatic (most common), pain, hemorrhage, rupture.

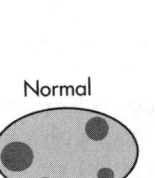
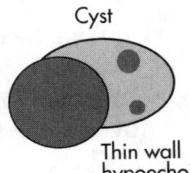

Radiographic features
- Usually anechoic, round, unilateral cyst ("simple cyst")
- If hemorrhage occurs, internal echoes are present.
- Size > 25 mm at time of ovulation
- Usually resolve spontaneously (repeat US in 2 weeks [½ cycle] or 6 weeks [1½ cycle] later)

CORPUS LUTEUM CYST (CLC)

A corpus luteum is a residual follicle after ovulation and normally involutes within 14 days. CLCs result from bleeding into or failed resorption of the corpus luteum. If an ovum is fertilized, the corpus luteum becomes the corpus luteum of pregnancy (maximum size at 8-10 weeks). Clinical: pain; more prone to hemorrhage and rupture.

Radiographic features

- Unilateral, large lesions (5-10 cm)
- Hypoechoic with low-level echoes (hemorrhage)
- Usually resolve spontaneously
- Most common in first trimester of pregnancy

THECA LUTEIN CYSTS

These cysts develop in conditions with elevated βHCG levels:

- Mole
- Choriocarcinoma
- Rh incompatibility (erythroblastosis fetalis)
- Twins
- Ovarian hyperstimulation syndrome

Radiographic features

- Largest of all ovarian cysts (may measure up to 20 cm)
- Usually bilateral and multilocular

PARAOVARIAN CYSTS

Arise from embryonic remnants in the broad ligament. Relatively common (10% of all adnexal masses).

Radiographic features

- May undergo torsion and rupture
- Show no cyclic changes
- Specific diagnosis only possible if the ipsilateral ovary is demonstrated as separate structure

PERITONEAL INCLUSION CYSTS

These cysts represent nonneoplastic reactive mesothelial proliferations. Abnormal functioning ovaries and peritoneal adhesions are usually present. These cysts occur exclusively in premenopausal women with a history of previous abdominal surgery, trauma, PID, or endometriosis. Patients usually present with pelvic pain or mass.

Radiographic features

- Extraovarian location
- Spider web pattern (entrapped ovary): peritoneal adhesions extend to surface of ovary distorting ovarian contour
- Oblong loculated collection simulating hydro- or pyosalpinx
- Complex cystic appearance simulating paraovarian cyst
- Irregular thick septations accompanied by complex cystic mass, simulating ovarian neoplasm

OVARIAN REMNANT SYNDROME

Residual ovarian tissue after bilateral oophorectomy.

- Tissue left after surgery is hormonally stimulated.
- May result in functional hemorrhagic cysts
- Usually occurs after complicated pelvic surgeries

POSTMENOPAUSAL CYSTS

Postmenopausal cysts are not physiological cysts, since there is not sufficient estrogen activity. Approach:

- TVUS should always be performed to determine that a cystic lesion is a simple, unilocular cyst. The incidence of malignancy in simple cysts < 5 cm is low.

- Management:
  - < 5 cm: US follow-up
  - > 5 cm or change in size of smaller lesion: surgery
- Cysts that are not simple are neoplasms until proven otherwise.

POLYCYSTIC OVARIAN DISEASE (PCO, STEIN-LEVENTHAL SYNDROME)

PCO is a chronic anovulation syndrome presumably related to hypothalamic pituitary dysfunction. The diagnosis of PCO is made on the basis of clinical, biochemical, and sonographic findings; sonographic findings alone are nonspecific.

Clinical

Triad of Stein-Leventhal syndrome

- Oligomenorrhea
- Hirsutism
- Obesity

Hormones

- Increased LH
- Increased LH/FSH ratio
- Increased androgens

Radiographic features

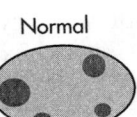
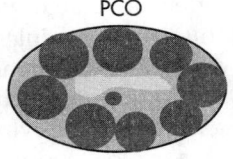

Normal   PCO

- Bilaterally enlarged ovaries with multiple small follicles, 50%
- Ovaries of similar size (key finding)
- > 5 cysts each of which are > 5 mm
- Peripheral location of cysts
- Hyperechoic central stroma (fibrous tissue)
- Hypoechoic ovary without individual cysts, 25%
- Normal ovaries, 25%

ENDOMETRIOSIS

Ectopic endometrial tissue in ovary (endometrioma), fallopian tube, pelvis, colon, bladder, etc. Endometrial implants undergo cyclical changes and hemorrhage occurs with subsequent local inflammation and adhesions.

MOST COMMON SITES FOR ENDOMETRIOTIC IMPLANTS AND ADHESIONS		
Location	Implants (%)	Adhesions (%)
Ovaries	75	40
Anterior and posterior cul-de-sac	70	15
Posterior broad ligament	45	45
Uterosacral ligament	35	5
Uterus	10	5
Fallopian tubes	5	25
Sigmoid colon	5	10
Ureter	3	2
Small intestine	1	3

Types
- Diffuse peritoneal and ligamentous implants
- Endometrioma ("chocolate cyst")

Radiographic features

Diffuse form
- Cannot be detected by US
- MR may be useful.
- High SI on T1W and low SI on T2W (shading) is caused by the high iron content of endometrioma.

Endometrioma
- Cystic mass with low level internal echoes
- May resemble a cystic neoplasm or hemorrhagic cyst

Uncommon manifestations
- Small bowel or colonic obstruction
- Bladder wall mass
- Anterior rectosigmoid abnormality

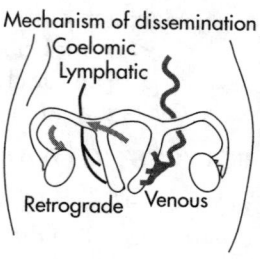

Mechanism of dissemination
Coelomic
Lymphatic
Retrograde   Venous

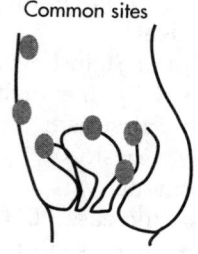

Common sites

OVARIAN TORSION

Often associated with neoplasm or cysts that act as lead points. Most common in children and adolescents. Clinical: Extreme pain (usually the finding that makes one consider this diagnosis).

Radiographic features
- Enlarged ovary with multiple cortical follicles
- Color Doppler: absence of flow to affected ovary has been shown not to be diagnostic of ovarian torsion
- Fluid in cul-de-sac
- Nonspecific ovarian mass (common)
- MRI: enlarged ovary with displaced follicles and low SI on T2W images due to interstitial hemorrhage. Peripheral enhancement may occur with gadolinium. Typical endometriomas and corpus luteal cysts do not have methemoglobin isolated to the rim and do not usually involve the entire ovary.

OVARIAN VEIN THROMBOSIS

Very rare cause of pulmonary thromboembolism. Causes:
- Infection (most common)
- Hypercoagulable states
- Delivery (especially C-section)

OVARIAN CANCER

Ovarian cancer (serous or mucinous cystadenocarcinoma) represents 25% of all gynecological malignancies, with 20,000 new cases a year in United States. Peak incidence is 6th decade. 65% of patients have distant metastases at time of diagnosis.
Survival:
- Stage 1: 80%-90%
- Stage 2: 60%
- Stage 3-4: <20%

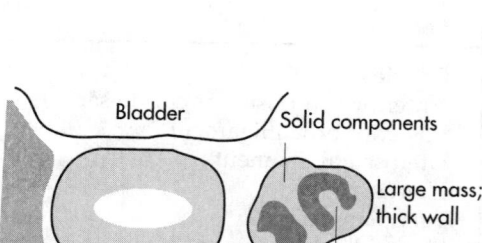

Bladder   Solid components

Large mass; thick wall

Mural nodule

Ascites

Types

OVARIAN NEOPLASIA			
Type	**Frequency (%)**	**Example**	**US Pattern**
Epithelial tumors (from surface epithelium that covers ovaries)	65-75	Serous or mucinous cystadenoma (carcinoma)	CCM
		Endometrioid carcinoma	CCM
		Clear cell carcinoma	CCM or SHM
		Brenner tumor	Small SHM
Germ cell tumors	15	Dysgerminoma	SEM
		Embryonal cell cancer	CCM
		Choriocarcinoma	CCM
		Teratoma	Mixed (fat, cyst, calc)
		Yolk sac (endodermal sinus) tumor	SEM
Sex chord–stromal tumors	5-10	Granulosa cell tumor	CCM
		Sertoli-Leydig cell tumor	CCM
		Thecoma and fibroma	SHM
Metastatic tumors	10	Primary uterine	
		Stomach, colon, breast	
		Lymphoma	

CCM, Complex cystic mass; *SHM*, solid hypoechoic mass; *SEM*, solid echogenic mass.

BILATERAL OVARIAN TUMORS		
	Serous Type	**Mucinous Type**
Benign cystadenoma	20% bilateral	5% bilateral
Malignant cystadenocarcinoma	50% bilateral	25% bilateral

Risk factors
- Family history
- Nulliparity
- High-fat diet, high-lactose diet

Screening

CA125 serum markers
- Normal value is <35 U/ml.
- CA125 is positive in 35% of patients with stage 1 ovarian cancer.
- CA125 is positive in 80% of patients with advanced ovarian cancer.
- 85% of patients < 50 years with elevated CA125 have benign disease (PID, endometriosis, early pregnancy, and fibroids), i.e., it is a useless screening test in patients under 50 years of age.
- More commonly elevated in serous than mucinous tumors

Who should be screened:

Patients with familial ovarian cancer; two types:

- Hereditary ovarian cancer syndrome; autosomal dominant; 50% lifetime chance to get ovarian cancer → prophylactic oophorectomy
- Familial history of ovarian cancer (first-degree relatives only); present in 7% of patients

Screening of general population is currently not recommended because of high-cost/low-benefit ratio (> $600,000 to detect one curable cancer).

Radiographic features

Adnexal mass

- Ovary

  Premenopausal volume > 18 cm^3 is abnormal

  Postmenopausal volume > 8 cm^3 is abnormal

- Findings suggestive of malignancy:

  Thick, irregular walls

  Septations > 2 mm

  Solid component

  Size of cystic structure

    < 5 cm: 1% malignant

    5-10 cm: 6% malignant

    > 10 cm: 40% malignant

  Ancillary features

    Ascites

    Hydronephrosis

    Metastases to liver, peritoneal cavity, lymph nodes

Peritoneal cavity

- Implants in omentum (omental cake) and other peritoneal surfaces
- Pseudomyxoma peritonei represents intraperitoneal spread of mucin-secreting tumor that fills the peritoneal cavity with gelatinous material (sonographic appearance similar to ascites with low-level echoes).

Staging

- Stage 1: limited to ovary
- Stage 2: both ovaries involved ± ascites
- Stage 3: intraperitoneal metastases
- Stage 4: metastases outside peritoneal cavity

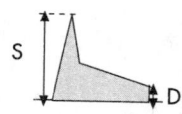

Pulsatility index (PI) = S – D/mean

Resistive index (RI) = S – D/S

Tumor vascularity (Doppler)

- Need both criteria to diagnose malignancy:

  High peak systolic velocity (> 25 cm/sec)

  Low-impedance diastolic flow

- Malignant tumors: resistive index (RI) < 0.4, pulsatility index (PI) < 1
- Tumor flow may be indistinguishable from normal luteal flow (repeat US within 14 days to differentiate)
- Problems:

  Overlap in Doppler findings between benign and malignant tumors

  Optimum cutoff value for malignant tumors has not been determined

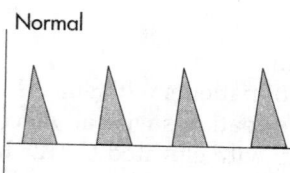

Normal

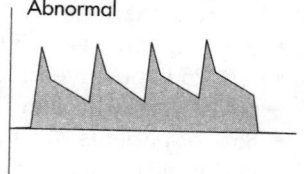

Abnormal

DERMOID, TERATOMA

GERM CELL TUMOR SPECTRUM		
Tumor	Origin	Content
Teratoma	Ectoderm + mesoderm + endoderm	Any tissue element*
Dermoid	Ectoderm	Hair, teeth, sebaceous glands
Epidermoid	Only epidermis	Secretes watery fluid; not a true tumor (CNS)

*Fat (echogenic), pancreas, muscle, calcification, teeth, thryoid, etc.

Radiographic features of dermoid
US
- Echogenic mass with acoustic shadowing
- May contain solid (isoechoic) and cystic (anechoic) components

CT
- Fatty mass with low HU
- Fat-fluid level
- Calcifications: tooth, rim calcification

MRI
- Protons from fat rotate near the Larmor frequency and are therefore very efficient T1-relaxation enhancers, which results in the high SI on T1W images seen with most ovarian dermoids and teratomas. Presence of fat within these masses is also the cause of chemical shift misregistration artifact in the frequency-encoding direction seen on SE images. The artifact occurs as a low signal intensity boundary at the fat water interface. Pre–fat and post–fat-saturation sequences may also help in identifying the fat.

Pearls
- Dermoids are common tumors in reproductive years.
- In the pelvis, dermoids have incorrectly been classified as cystic teratomas.
- Struma ovarii is a teratoma in which thyroid tissue predominates.

OTHER OVARIAN TUMORS

Dysgerminoma
5% of all ovarian neoplasms. These tumors are morphologically similar to seminomas in testicles and germinomas in pineal glands. Highly radiosensitive. 5-year survival, 80%. Peak incidence < 30 years.

Yolk sac tumors
Rare, highly malignant. Peak incidence < 20 years. Increased alpha-fetoprotein (AFP) levels.

Endometroid tumor
30%-50% are bilateral. Histologically similar to endometrial cancer. 30% of patients have concomitant endometrial adenocarcinoma.

Clear cell carcinoma
Müllerian duct origin. 40% bilateral.

Brenner tumor

Rare. Usually discovered incidentally. Patients are typically asymptomatic. Solid fibrous tumors. Associated with cystadenomas or cystic teratoma in ispilateral ovary in 30%. The high fibrous content account for the low SI on T2W images on MRI.

Granulosa cell tumors (estrogen)

2% of ovarian neoplasms; low malignant potential, most common estrogen active tumor; 95% bilateral. 10%-15% of patients will eventually develop endometrial carcinoma.

Sertoli-Leydig cell tumors

< 0.5% of ovarian neoplasms. Majority are androgen secreting.

Thecoma, fibroma

Both tumors arise from ovarian stroma and typically occur in postmenopausal women:

- Thecoma: predominantly thecal cells; 1% of ovarian neoplasms
- Fibroma: predominantly fibrous tissue; 4% of ovarian neoplasms

Ascites and pleural effusions (Meigs' syndrome) is present in 50% of patients with fibromas > 5 cm. A widened endometrial stripe accompanied by an ovarian mass with low SI on T2W images can suggest a diagnosis of functional fibrothecoma with endometrial hyperplasia.

Krukenberg tumor

Ovarian metastases from stomach or colon primary (signet ring cell types).

Meigs' syndrome

Pleural effusion and ascites from fibroma (original description) or other ovarian tumors and metastases (more recent use of terminology).

Pearls

- The approach to unilocular cysts depends on the age of the patient: in younger patients they are usually functional cysts, which may be hormonally active; in older woman a cystic neoplasm is more common.
- A complex adnexal mass in a young woman usually represents a hemorrhagic cyst, endometrioma, tuboovarian abscess (TOA), or ectopic; clinical setting helps to differentiate etiologies.
- Dermoids are the most common ovarian tumors in young women (< 30 years). Tumors are often partially cystic, and contain fat or calcium.

Infertility

GENERAL

Affects 15% of couples. In most infertility programs, the current success rates of achieving a normal pregnancy are 10%-20%. The major causes (anatomical, functional) of infertility are:

Female (70%)
- Ovulatory dysfunction (hypothalamic-pituitary-ovarian axis), 25%
- Mechanical tubal problems, 25%
- Endometriosis, 40%
- Inadequate cervical mucus (poor estrogen response), 5%
- Luteal phase defects (poor progesterone response), 5%

Male (30%)
- Impotence
- Oligospermia, aspermia (many causes, including varicocele)
- Sperm dysfunction

Role of ultrasound
- Monitor response to hormonal stimulation
- Percutaneous retrieval of mature oocytes
- Determine mechanical cause of infertility

Sonographic signs during cycle
First part of cycle
- Early on several 5-mm cysts are seen; these cysts grow to 10 mm.
- Dominant follicle (> 14 mm) can usually be identified from 8th-12th day; follicles typically measure 18-28 mm.
- Follicles < 15 mm usually do not go on to pregnancy.
- 5%-10% of patients have > 2 dominant follicles.

Signs of impending (within 24 hours) ovulation (generally unreliable):
- Thickening and lack of distinction of follicular lining
- Thin hypoechoic layer surrounds follicle
- Folding in granulosa cell layer (crenation)

Signs of ovulation (generally reliable)
- Disappearance of follicle
- Collapsed follicle
- Follicle filled with low-level echoes
- Fluid in cul-de-sac

DRUG TREATMENT FOR OVULATION INDUCTION

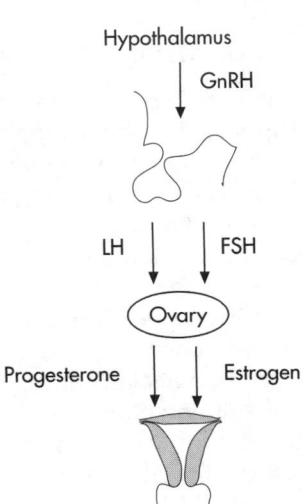

Human chorionic gonadotropin
Used to induce ovulation once follicular development is complete. HCG has a biologic effect similar to LH but a longer blood half-life. Ovulation occurs 36 hours after administration of 10,000 IU (as opposed to 24 hours after LH).

Clomiphene citrate (Clomid)
Nonsteroidal, synthetic weak estrogen agonist that binds to estrogen receptors in hypothalamus. Hypothalamus then releases GnRH, which produces FSH and LH. Requires an intact hypothalamic-pituitary-ovarian axis.

Pergonal
Used if Clomid is not successful after 3-4 cycles. Pergonal contains human menopausal gonadotropins: 75% FSH and 25% LH. Used in conjunction with βHCG to cause oocyte maturation and to trigger ovulation.

Leuprolide acetate (Lupron)
GnRH analog used to shut off the hypothalamic-pituitary-gonadal axis. Used in conjunction with Pergonal to manage ovarian stimulation and ovulation.

Urofollitropin (Metrodin)
Pure FSH, an alternative/additive to pergonal therapy. Originally used in patients with PCO and excess of LH.

PROTOCOLS

Baseline US
- Use transabdominal ultrasound (TAS) and TVS
- Performed on day 8
- Exclude endometriosis, fibroids, paraovarian cysts, hydrosalpinx, unruptured cysts

Subsequent scans

- Performed daily with estrogen level determination (400-500 pg/ml per ovulatory follicle suggests oocyte maturity). US is useful to determine whether elevated estrogen levels are due to one large follicle or numerous small follicles.
- Growth rate of follicles is 1-2 mm/day.
- Measurement of follicular diameter (> 18 mm) is used to time βHCG administration.
- Determine endometrial thickness.

COMPLICATIONS OF HORMONAL TREATMENT

Ovarian hyperstimulation

- Occurs in up to 40% of cycles
- Ovaries enlarge and contain multiple large lutein cysts; more commonly seen with pergonal than with Clomid therapy.
- Typically begins 3-10 days following βHCG administration
- May last for 6-8 weeks
- Symptoms: lower abdominal pain, weight gain, ascites, DIC; severe side effects (rare): renal failure, hypotension, death

Multiple pregnancies

Rate of multiple pregnancies is 25%.

Other

NORMAL PEVIC FLOOR ANATOMY

The female pelvic floor can be divided into three compartments with each being supported by the endopelvic fascia and the levator ani muscle:

- Anterior containing the bladder and urethra
- Middle containing the vagina
- Posterior containing the rectum

The levator ani muscle complex consists of three muscle groups:

- Iliococcygeal muscle, which arises from the junction of the arcus tendineus fascia pelvis and the fascia of the internal obturator muscle
- Pubococcygeal muscle, which arises from the superior ramus of the pubis
- Puborectalis muscle, which arises from the superior and inferior pubic rami

In healthy women at rest, the levator ani muscles are in contraction, thereby keeping the rectum, vagina, and urethra elevated and closed by pressing them anteriorly toward the pubic symphysis. The components of the levator ani muscles are clearly seen on T2W MR images.

PELVIC FLOOR PROLAPSE

- Results from specific defects in the endopelvic fascia and may involve the urethra, bladder, vaginal vault, rectum, and small bowel (typically multiple)
- Patients present with pain, pressure, urinary and fecal incontinence, constipation, urinary retention, and defecatory dysfunction.
- Diagnosis is made primarily on the basis of findings at physical pelvic examination.
- Imaging is useful in patients in whom findings at physical examination are equivocal.
- Fluoroscopy, US, and MR imaging have been used for diagnosis, with MR currently favored.

MR interpretation
- In healthy women, there is minimal movement of pelvic organs, even with maximal strain.
- Floor laxity: organ descent of 1-2 cm below the pubococcyggeal line. Both H and M line become elongated with Valsalva maneuver.
- Prolapse requiring surgical intervention: organ descent of > 2 cm below the pubococcyggeal line
- Enterocele: descent of small bowel > 2 cm between vagina and rectum
- Anterior rectocele: anterior bulging of rectum
- Cystocele: bladder > 1 cm below pubococcygeal line

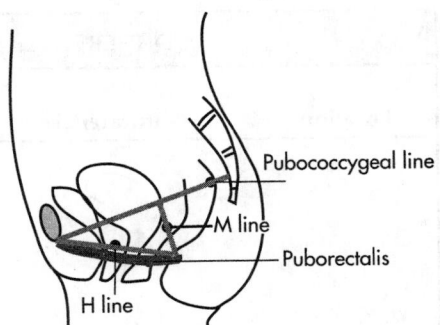

Differential Diagnosis

Kidneys

RENAL MASS LESIONS

Tumor
- Solid
- Cyst

Infection
- Lobar nephronia
- Abscess
- XGP

Congenital
- Duplicated collecting system
- Pseudotumors
  - Fetal lobulation
  - Dromedary hump
  - Column of Bertin
  - Suprahilar (less commonly infrahilar) "bump"
  - Lobar dysmorphism: doughnut sign on IVP or angiography

Trauma
- Hematoma

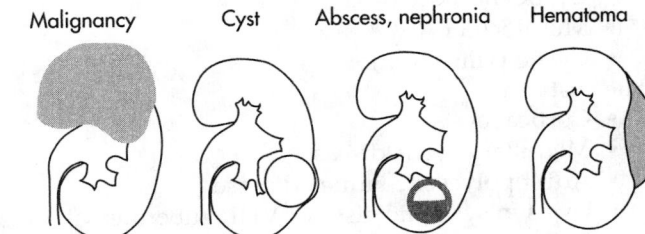

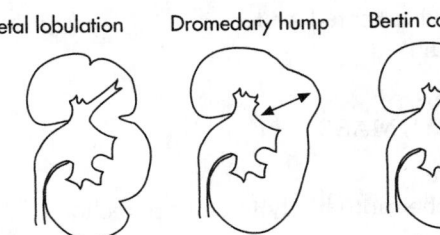
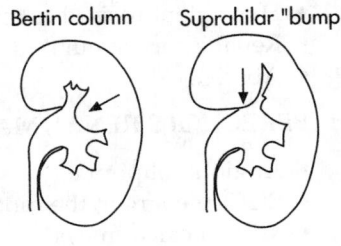

SOLID RENAL NEOPLASM

- RCC
- Wilms' tumor
- Oncocytoma
- Adenoma
- Angiomyolipoma (fat density, hamartoma)
- Transitional cell carcinoma of the renal pelvis or calyces
- Metastases (multiple): lung, colon, melanoma, RCC
- Lymphoma

DIFFERENTIAL DIAGNOSIS OF RENAL MASSES BY LOCATION

Location	Intrarenal	< 50% Protrusion	> 50% Protrusion	In Collecting System
RCC	15%	15%	65%	5%
Metastases	55%	20%	25%	< 5%
Renal TCC	80%	0%	0%	20%

CYSTIC RENAL MASSES

Tumors
- Cystic/necrotic RCC
- Multilocular RCC
- Cystic Wilms' tumor

True cysts
- Cortical cysts
- Medullary cystic disease
- Adult polycystic kidney disease
- Cysts in systemic disease: VHL, tuberous sclerosis
- Endstage renal failure
- Infectious cysts

Other (use Doppler or color US for differentiation)
- Hydronephrosis/duplicated system
- Renal artery aneurysm
- Abscess

HYPERECHOIC RENAL MASS

- Angiomyolipoma
- RCC (the larger, the more likely to be hyperechoic)
- Milk of calcium cyst
- Nephritis
    XGP
    Emphysematous pyelonephritis
    Focal nephritis
    Candidiasis
- Hematoma
- Infarction
- Lesions that mimic true hyperechoic masses
    Renal sinus fat
    Duplicated collecting system

RENAL SINUS MASS

Tumors
- TCC
- RCC
- Lymphoma
- Bellini duct carcinoma

Other
- Renal artery aneurysm
- Renal sinus hemorrhage
- Complicated parapelvic cyst

WEDGE-SHAPED RENAL LESION

- Renal metastasis
- Infarction
- Lobar nephritis

DIFFUSELY HYPERECHOIC KIDNEYS

- Inflammation
    - Glomerulonephritis
    - Glomerulosclerosis: HTN, DM
    - AIDS-related nephropathy
    - Interstitial nephritis: systemic lupus erythematosus (SLE), vasculitis
- Acute tubular necrosis
- Hemolytic uremic syndrome
- Multiple myeloma
- Endstage renal disease
- Medullary or cortical nephrocalcinosis
- Infantile polycystic kidney disease

RENAL CALCIFICATIONS

Tumors
- Cysts
- RCC

Infection
- Tuberculosis

"Metastastic" calcification
- Medullary nephrocalcinosis
- Cortical nephrocalcinosis

Collecting system
- Calculi

FAT IN KIDNEY

- Angiomyolipoma
- Lipoma
- Replacement lipomatosis

4

HYPOECHOIC PERIRENAL FAT

- Normal variant (in 10% of asymptomatic renal allografts)
- Perirenal hemorrhage (trauma, anticoagulants, adrenal hemorrhage)
- Cyst rupture
- SLE
- Polyarteriitis nodosa

FILLING DEFECT IN COLLECTING SYSTEM

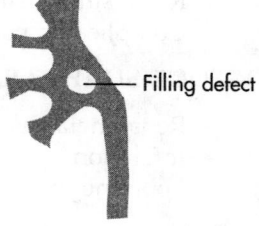
Filling defect

Tumor
- TCC
- Papilloma
- Leukoplakia, malacoplakia

Mobile filling defect
- Blood clot
- Sloughed papilla
- Calculus
- Fungus ball

Other
- Vascular impression, collateral vessels
- Artificial overlying bowel gas shadows mimicking filling defect

PAPILLARY NECROSIS

Mnemonic: "POSTCARD"
- **P**yelonephritis
- **O**bstruction (chronic)
- **S**ickle cell disease
- **T**B
- **C**irrhosis, ethanol
- **A**nalgesics: phenacetin
- **R**enal vein thrombosis
- **D**iabetes

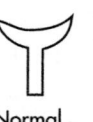 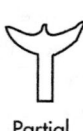 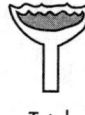 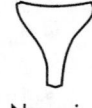

Normal   Partial   Total   Necrosis

DELAYED (PERSISTENT) NEPHROGRAM (SAME DIFFERENTIAL DIAGNOSIS AS RENAL FAILURE)

Prerenal causes (15%)
- Renal artery stenosis
- Hypotension

Renal causes (70%)
- Acute glomerulonephritis
- Acute tubular necrosis: radiographic iodinated contrast agents, antibiotics, anesthesia, ischemia, transplants
- Acute cortical necrosis: pregnancy related, 70%; sepsis; dehydration
- Tubular precipitation: uric acid, hemolysis, myeloma
- Acute interstitial nephritis: antibiotics
- Papillary necrosis: analgesic, sickle cell, DM
- Renal vein thrombosis

Postrenal causes (15%)
- Obstruction: stone, stricture

Rule of thumb
- Symmetrical, bilateral: medical disease
- Asymmetrical, unilateral: surgical disease

EXTRACALYCEAL CONTRAST AGENT

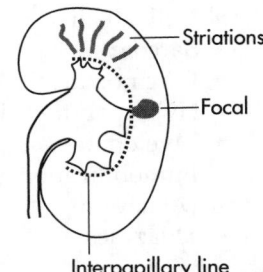

Striations
- Medullary sponge kidney
- Early papillary necrosis
- Pyelosinus or pyelovenous backflow in obstruction
- Interstitial edema

Focal collections
- Late papillary necrosis
- Calyceal diverticulum
- Cavity from cyst rupture
- Abscess

DILATED CALYCES/COLLECTING SYSTEM

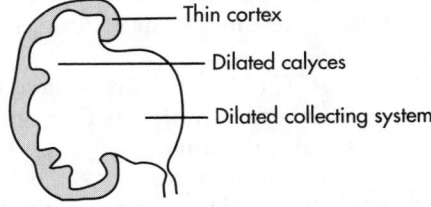

- Obstruction (calculi, tumor, acute, chronic)
- Papillary necrosis
- Congenital megacalyces
- Calyceal diverticulum
- Reflux

BILATERALLY ENLARGED KIDNEYS

Tumor
- Cystic disease (APCKD)
- Malignancy
  - Leukemia
  - Lymphoma
  - Multiple myeloma (protein deposition)

Inflammation (acute)
- Glomerulonephritis
- Interstitial nephritis
- Collagen vascular disease
- ATN

Metabolic
- Amyloid
- Diabetes mellitus
- Storage diseases, acromegaly

Vascular
- Bilateral renal vein thrombosis

BILATERALLY SMALL KIDNEYS

- Chronic inflammation: pyelonephritis, glomerulonephritis, interstitial nephritis
- Bilateral renal artery stenosis
- Reflux (chronic infection)

HYPERCALCEMIA

Mnemonic: "PAM SCHMIDT"
- **Parathyroid** adenoma, hyperplasia
- **Addison** disease
- **Milk** alkali
- **Sarcoid**
- **Carcinomatosis**
- **Hyperparathyroidism**, secondary
- **Myeloma**
- **Immobilization**
- **D** vitamin
- **Thiazides**

RENAL VEIN THROMBOSIS (RVT)

Acute thrombosis causes renal enlargement (congestion, hemorrhage). Chronic thrombosis results in small kidneys (infarction). Causes:

Tumor
- RCC (10% of patients have thrombosis)
- Other renal tumors (lymphoma, TCC, Wilms' tumor)
- Adrenal tumors
- Gonadal tumors
- Pancreatic carcinoma
- Extraluminal compression of renal vein by retroperitoneal tumors

Renal disease (often with nephrotic syndrome)
- Membranous glomerulonephritis
- SLE
- Amyloidosis

Other
- Hypercoaguable states
- Extension of ovarian vein, IVC thrombosis
- Trauma, surgery
- Transplant rejection

Ureter

DILATED URETER

Criteria: > 8 mm, ureter visible in entire length, no peristaltic waves. Differentiation between mechanical obstruction and dilatation is possible by performing a Whitaker test or furosemide scintigraphy.

Obstruction
- Functional: primary megaureter
- Mechanical stenosis
  - Ureteral stricture
  - Bladder outlet obstruction
  - Urethral stricture

Reflux

Other
- Diuresis (e.g., furosemide, diabetes insipidus)

URETERAL STRICTURE

Wide differential (mnemonic "TIC MTV"). Use IVP/retrograde pyelography to determine if there is a mass or a stricture and how long the narrowing is. CT/IVP (IVP reconstructed from CT) now combined.

Tumor
- TCC
- Metastases
- Lymphadenopathy

Inflammatory
- TB (corkscrew appearance)
- Schistosomiasis
- Pelvic disease
  - Crohn's disease
  - Pelvic inflammatory disease

Congenital
- Ectopic ureterocele
- Primary megaureter
- Congenital stenosis

Metabolic, drugs
- Morphine
- Methysergide: retroperitoneal fibrosis

Trauma
- Iatrogenic
- Radiation

Vascular
- Aortic, iliac artery aneurysm
- Ovarian vein syndrome
- Lymphocele

MULTIPLE URETERAL FILLING DEFECTS

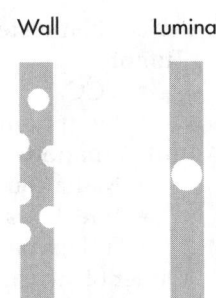

Wall
- Ureteritis cystica (more common in upper ureter)
- Allergic mucosal bullae
- Pseudodiverticulosis
- Vascular impressions (collateral veins in IVC obstruction)
- Multiple papillomas (more common in lower ureter)
- Melanoma metastases
- Suburothelial hemorrhage (less discrete than ureteritis cystica and associated with acoagulopathy)

Luminal
- Calculi (lucent, opaque)
- Blood clot
- Sloughed papillae
- Fungus ball
- Air bubbles

URETERAL DIVERTICULA

- Congenital
- Ureteritis cystica
- TB (also strictures)

DEVIATED URETERS

Normal ureters project over the transverse processes of the vertebral bodies. Deviations occur laterally or medially.

Lateral deviation
- Bulky retroperitoneal adenopathy
- Primary retroperitonal tumors
- Aortic aneurysm
- Retroperitoneal fluid collection
- Malrotated kidney
- Ovarian/uterine masses

Medial deviation
- Posterior bladder diverticulum (most common cause of distal medial deviation)
- Uterine fibroids
- Retroperitoneal fibrosis; associated with:
    Aortic aneurysm: chronic leakage?
    Methysergide
    Idiopathic
    Malignancy-related
- Postoperative (node dissection)
- Enlarged prostate (J-shaped ureter)
- Retrocaval ureter (only on right side)

Bladder

BLADDER WALL THICKENING

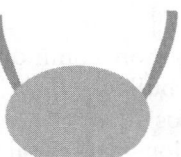 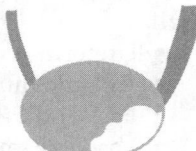

Normal   Focal filling defect

Criteria when distended: > 5 mm, trabeculations, small bladder.
Tumor
- TCC
- Lymphoma

Inflammation
- Radiation cystitis
- Infectious cystitis
- Inflammatory bowel disease, appendicitis, focal diverticulitis

Outlet obstruction
- Benign prostatic hyperplasia
- Urethral stricture

Neurogenic

BLADDER FILLING DEFECT

Tumor
- Primary: TCC, SCC
- Metastases
- Endometriosis
- Polyps

Infection
- PID
- Parasitic infection: schistosomiasis
- Related to infection:
    Leukoplakia, malacoplakia
    Cystitis cystica, cystitis glandularis

Luminal
- Calculi
- Blood clot
- Foreign bodies
- BPH

BLADDER NEOPLASM

Primary
- TCC
- SCC
- Adenocarcinoma
- Pheochromocytoma from bladder wall paraganglia (10% are malignant)
- Rare tumors: rhabdomyosarcoma, leiomyosarcoma, primary lymphoma

Secondary
- Metastases
    Hematogenous: melanoma > stomach > breast
    Direct extension: prostate, uterus, colon
- Lymphoma

BLADDER CALCULI

- Chronic bacterial infection, 30%
- Chronic bladder catheterization (struvite stones)
- Bladder outlet obstruction, 70%
- Schistosomiasis
- Renal calculi (usually pass through urethra)

BLADDER WALL CALCIFICATION

Mnemonic "SCRITT"
- **S**chistosomiasis
- **C**ytoxan
- **R**adiation
- **I**nterstitial cystitis
- **T**B
- **T**CC

AIR IN BLADDER

- Instrumentation, catheter
- Bladder fistula: diverticultis, Crohn's disease, colon carcinoma
- Emphysematous cystitis in patients with diabetes

TEARDROP BLADDER

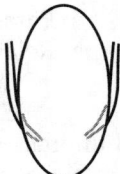

Criteria: Pear-shaped or teardrop-shaped contrast-filled bladder: circumferential extrinsic compression.

Physiological
- Normal variant
- Iliopsoas hypertrophy

Fluid
- Hematoma (usually from pelvic fracture)
- Abscess

Masses
- Pelvic lymphoma
- Pelvic lipomatosis (black males, hypertension)
- Retroperitoneal fibrosis

THE "FEMALE PROSTATE"

Criteria: Central filling defect at base of bladder in female patients
- Urethral diverticulum
- Urethral tumor
- Periurethritis
- Pubic bone lesion

Adrenal Glands

ADRENAL MASSES

Tumor
- Adenoma, 50%
- Metastases, 30%
- Pheochromocytoma, 10%
- Lymphoma
- Neuroblastoma if < 2 years
- Fatty lesions
  - Myelolipoma
  - Lipoma
- Cystic tumors
  - Simple cyst, 10%
  - Pseudocyst after previous hemorrhage

Other lesions
- Hemorrhage
- TB
- Wolman's disease (acid cholesteryl ester hydrolase deficiency, very rare)

Bilateral masses
- Metastases
- Lymphoma
- Bilateral pheochromocytoma in:
  - Multiple endocrine neoplasia type II
  - VHL
  - Neurofibromatosis
- Granulomatous masses: TB, histoplasmosis

ADRENAL CALCIFICATIONS

- Tumor: neuroblastoma, pheochromocytoma
- Infection: TB, histoplasmosis, Waterhouse-Friederichson syndrome
- Trauma: hemorrhage
- Congenital: Wolman's disease

ADRENAL PSEUDOTUMORS

Criteria: soft tissue density in location of adrenal glands on plain films of abdomen.
- Gastric fundus
- Accessory spleen
- Retroperitoneal varices
- Other lesions
  - Liver mass
  - Gallbladder mass
  - Renal mass

Adrenal pseudotumor by CT
- Gastric fundus or fundal diverticulum
- Varices
- Tortuous splenic artery
- Pancreatic tail
- Medial splenic lobulation

Testicles

SOLID TESTICULAR MASSES

Tumor
- Primary: germinal, 95%, nongerminal, 5%
- Metastases: prostate, kidney, leukemia, lymphoma

Infection
- Orchitis
- Abscess
- Granuloma

Trauma: fracture, rupture, hemorrhage, torsion

Other
- Atrophy
- Dilated rete testes

EXTRATESTICULAR ABNORMALITIES

- Epididymitis, diffuse or focal
- Spermatocele, epididymal cyst
- Hydrocele, hematocele, varicocele
- Tunical or mesothelial cyst
- Paratesticular hemorrhage, abscess
- Hernia
- Neoplasm (primary or metastatic)
  - Benign: adenomatoid tumor, fibroma, leiomyoma
  - Malignant: mesothelioma, sarcoma

Prostate

CYSTIC LESIONS

- Utricle cyst
- Cowper's duct cyst
- Ejaculatory duct cyst
- Prostatic retention cyst
- Seminal vesicle cyst
- Vas deferens cyst
- Müllerian duct cyst

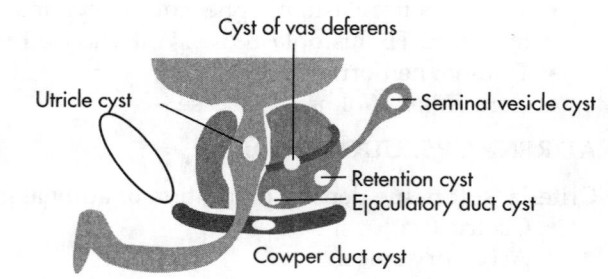

Female Pelvis

APPROACH

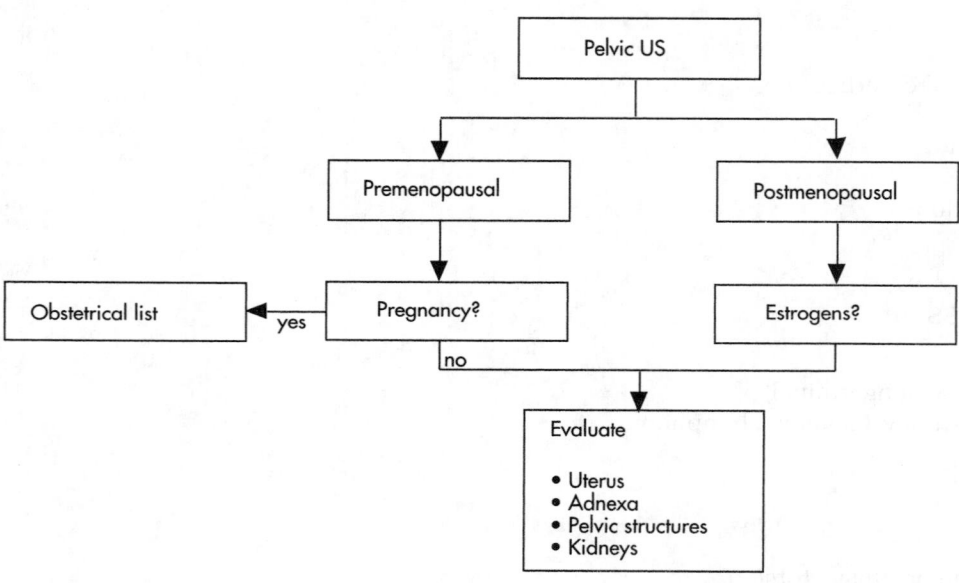

Uterus

THICK HYPERECHOIC ENDOMETRIAL STRIPE (EMS)

Criteria: > 5 mm in postmenopausal patients not taking hormone replacement therapy; > 14 mm in premenopausal patients (varies with stage in cycle).

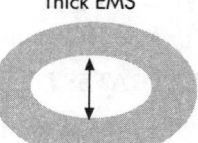

Thick EMS

CAUSES OF THICK HYPERECHOIC ENDOMETRIAL STRIPE	
Pregnancy Related	**Postmenopausal**
Normal early pregnancy	Hyperplasia
Ectopic	Tamoxifen, estrogen replacement
Incomplete abortion	Polyps
Molar pregnancy (cystic spaces can be missing early on)	Endometrial cancer

Pearls
- Endometrial cancer may be indistinguishable from other benign causes of thickened EMS; therefore curettage is indicated in postmenopausal patient.
- A sonographically normal endometrium in a postmenopausal woman excludes significant pathology.
- Approach in postmenopausal patient
  EMS ≤ 5: no further work-up
  EMS ≥ 5 (no hormone therapy): sonohysterogram to characterize must sample endometrium
  EMS ≥ 5 (hormonal therapy): sonohysterogram to characterize stop hormones and obtain follow up by US

HYPOECHOIC STRUCTURES IN HYPERECHOIC ENDOMETRIUM

Premenopausal
- Molar pregnancy
- Retained placenta, abortus
- Degenerated placenta
- Degenerated fibroid

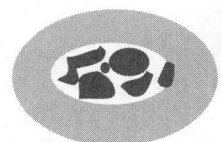

Postmenopausal
- Cystic glandular hyperplasia
- Endometrial polyps
- Endometrial carcinoma

FLUID IN UTERINE CAVITY

Acquired (cervical stenosis)
- Tumors: cervical cancer, endometrial cancer
- Inflammatory: endometritis, PID, radiation

Pregnancy related
- Early IUP
- Pseudogestational sac
- Blighted ovum

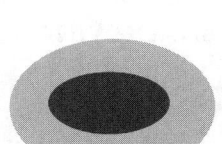

Congenital
- Imperforate hymen
- Vaginal septum
- Vaginal atresia
- Rudimentary uterine horn

UTERINE ENLARGEMENT OR DISTORTION

- Fibroids (most common cause)
- Adenomyosis
- Less common causes
  Congenital uterine anomalies
  Inflammation: PID, surgery
  Endometriosis
  Malignant tumors

UTERINE BLEEDING

- Endometrial hyperplasia or polyp (most common cause)
- Endometrial cancer
- Estrogen withdrawal
- Adenomyosis
- Submucosal fibroid
- Cervical cancer

UTERINE SIZE

Small uterus
- Hypoplasia
- Nulliparity
- Synechiae
- DES exposure

Large uterus
- Multiparity
- Pregnancy
- Molar pregnancy
- Neoplasm

UTERINE AND VAGINAL CYSTIC MASSES

- Nabothian cyst: retention cyst of the cervix
- Gartner's duct cyst: mesonephric duct remnants (vaginal wall)
- Bartholin cyst: perineal cyst
- Hydrometrocolpos

SHADOWING STRUCTURES IN ENDOMETRIAL CAVITY (US)

- IUD
- Calcifications: fibroids, TB
- Pyometra (gas)

Ovaries and Adnexa

CYSTIC MASSES

Ovary
- Normal ovarian cysts (physiological)
  Follicle (mean diameter < 25 mm), follicular cyst (mean diameter > 25 mm)
  Corpus luteum cyst
- Too many follicles: polycystic ovary, hyperstimulation syndrome
- Theca lutein cyst (with high levels of βHCG)
- Cystic adnexal masses
  Hemorrhagic cyst
  Endometrioma ("chocolate cyst")
  Ectopic pregnancy
  Cystadenocarcinoma
  TOA

Tube
- Hydrosalpinx

Other
- Paraovarian cyst
- Fluid in cul-de-sac
- Pelvic varices
- Lymphocele
- Bowel
- Pelvic abscess

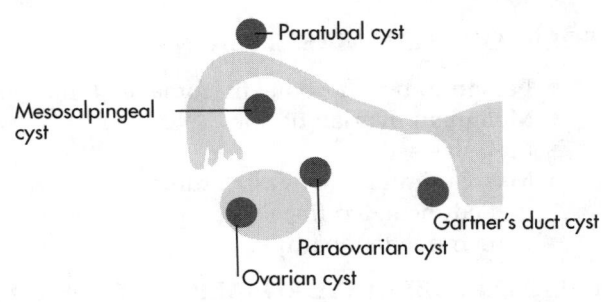

COMPLEX PELVIC MASSES

Ovarian, paraovarian (the "big 5")
- Ectopic pregnancy
- TOA
- Endometrioma, hemorrhagic cyst
- Ovarian torsion
- Tumor:
  - Benign: dermoid
  - Malignant: adenocarcinoma

Tubal
- Pyosalpinx

Uterine
- Pedunculated fibroid
- Extruded IUD
- Endometrial, cervical carcinoma (rare)

Other
- Pelvic abscess
- Appendicitis
- Diverticulitis
- Hematoma
- Pelvic kidneys
- Iliac aneurysm

Pearls
- US (gray scale or Doppler) cannot reliably distinguish benign from malignant ovarian tumors.
- MR useful to define etiology of solid, not cystic masses
- If a malignant lesion is suspected, scan the rest of the abdomen for metastases (liver, spleen, ascites).
- Always Doppler cystic-appearing structures to exclude vascular origin (i.e., aneurysm)

MASSES WITH HOMOGENOUS LOW-LEVEL ECHOES

- TOA
- Endometrioma
- Hemorrhagic cyst

SOLID OVARIAN MASS LESIONS

- Benign tumor: fibroma, thecoma, endometrioma, germ cell tumor
- Malignant ovarian tumors
- Metastasis
- Masses simulating ovarian tumor
    Pedunculated fibroid
    Lymphadenopathy

DILATED TUBES (HYDROSALPINX, PYOSALPINX, HEMATOSALPINX)

- Infection
- Tumor: endometrial or tubal carcinoma
- Endometriosis
- Iatrogenic ligation

TUBAL FILLING DEFECTS (HSG)

- Polyp
- Neoplasm
- Silicone implant
- Tubal pregnancy
- Air bubble from injection

TUBAL IRREGULARITY

- SIN
- Tubal diverticula
- Endometriosis
- Postoperative changes
- TB

PSEUDOKIDNEY SIGN (US)

Elliptical structure in pelvis or abdomen with an echogenic center (blood, prominent mucosa, infiltrated bowel wall) resembling the US appearance of a kidney.

- Inflammatory bowel disease
    Crohn's disease
    Infectious colitis
- Tumor
- Intussusception
- Always exclude pelvic kidney

SUGGESTED READINGS

Callen PW: *Ultrasonography in obstetrics and gynecology,* Philadelphia, 2000, WB Saunders.
Dunnick NR, Sandler CM, Newhouse JH, et al: *Textbook of uroradiology,* Philadelphia, 2000, Lippincott Williams & Wilkins.
Pollack HM: *Clinical urography: an atlas and textbook of urological imaging,* Philadelphia, 2000, WB Saunders.
Rumack CM: *Diagnostic ultrasound,* 1997, St Louis, Mosby.
Yoder IC: *Hysterosalpingography and pelvic ultrasound,* Baltimore, 1988, Lippincott Williams & Wilkins.
Zagoria RJ: *Genitourinary radiology: the requisites,* 1997, St Louis, Mosby.

Chapter 5

Musculoskeletal Imaging

Chapter Outline

Trauma

General

FRACTURE

FRACTURE SYNOPSIS	
Fracture	**Finding**
SPINE	
Jefferson's	Ring fracture of C1
Hangman's	Bilateral pedicle or pars fractures of C2
Teardrop (flexion)	Unstable flexion fracture
Clay-shoveler's	Avulsion fracture of spinous process lower cervical, high thoracic spine
Chance	Horizontal fracture through soft tissues and/or bone of thoracolumbar spine
FACE	
Le Fort I	Floating palate
Le Fort II	Floating maxilla
Le Fort III	Floating face
UPPER EXTREMITY	
Hill-Sachs lesion (anterior dislocation)	Impaction fracture of posterolateral humeral head
Bankart lesion (anterior dislocation)	Fracture of anterior glenoid rim
Trough sign (posterior dislocation)	Linear impaction fracture of anterior humeral head
Reverse Bankart lesion (posterior dislocation)	Fracture of posterior glenoid rim
Monteggia fracture-dislocation	Ulnar fracture, proximal radial dislocation
Galeazzi fracture-dislocation	Radial fracture, distal radioulnar dislocation
Essex-Lopresti	Radial head fracture and distal radioulnar subluxation
Colles'	Distal radius fracture, dorsal angulation
Smith's	Distal radius fracture, volar angulation
Barton's	Intraarticular distal radial fracture/dislocation
Bennett's	Fracture-dislocation of base of first metacarpal
Rolando	Comminuted Bennett's fracture
Boxer's	5th MCP shaft or neck fracture
Gamekeeper's thumb (skiers)	Ulnar collateral ligament injury of 1st MCP joint
Chauffeur's	Intraarticular fracture of radial styloid
PELVIS	
Duverney's	Iliac wing fracture
Malgaigne's	Sacroiliac (SI) joint or sacrum and both ipsilateral pubic rami
Bucket-handle	SI joint or sacrum and contralateral pubic rami
Straddle	Fracture of both obturator rings (all four pubic rami)

FRACTURE SYNOPSIS—cont'd	
Fracture	**Finding**
LOWER EXTREMITY	
Segond	Avulsion fracture of lateral tibial condyle; associated with anterior cruciate ligament (ACL) injury
Bumper	Intraarticular fracture of tibial condyle
Pilon	Intraarticular comminuted distal tibia fracture
Tillaux	Salter-Harris III of lateral distal tibia (due to later epiphyseal fusion)
Triplane	Salter III/IV fracture of distal tibial
Wagstaffe-Le Fort	Avulsion of the medial margin distal fibula
Dupuytren's	Fracture of fibula above tibiofibular ligament
Maisonneuve's	Proximal fibular fracture and disrupted ankle mortise or medial malleolar fracture
Lover's	Calcaneal fracture
Jones (dancer's)	Fracture of proximal 5th metatarsal shaft
Lisfranc's	Tarsometatarsal fracture-dislocation
March	Stress fracture of metatarsal neck

5

Fracture healing

Phases of healing:

Inflammatory phase
- Torn periosteum
- Blood clots in fracture line
- Inflammatory reaction

Reparative phase
- Granulation tissue replaces clot.
- Periosteum forms immature callus.
- Internal callus forms within granulation tissue.
- Cartilage forms around fracture.

Remodeling phase
- Woven bone in callus is replaced by compact bone (cortex) and cancellous bone (medullary cavity).

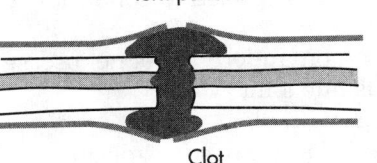

Inflammatory phase

Torn periosteum

Clot

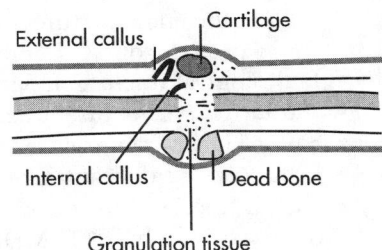

Reparative phase

External callus

Cartilage

Internal callus

Dead bone

Granulation tissue

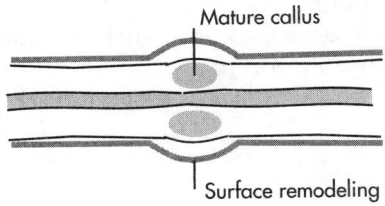

Remodeling phase

Mature callus

Surface remodeling

Terminology for description of fractures
Anatomical site of fracture
- In long bones, divide the shaft into thirds (e.g., fracture distal third of femur)
- Use anatomical landmarks for description (e.g., fracture near greater tuberosity)

Pattern of fracture
- Simple fracture: no fragments. Describe the direction of the fracture line: transverse, oblique, spiral, longitudinal
- Comminuted fracture (more than 2 fragments): T-, V-, Y-shaped patterns, butterfly fragments, segmental
- Complete or incomplete fractures

Apposition and alignment: defined in relation to distal fragments
- Displacement (e.g., medial, lateral, posterior, anterior)
- Angulation (e.g., medial, lateral, posterior, anterior)
- Rotation (internal, external)
- Overriding: overlap of fragments (bayonet apposition)
- Distracted: separated fragments

Adjacent joints
- Normal
- Dislocation
- Subluxation
- Intraarticular extension of fracture line

Specific fractures
- Stress fractures:
    - Fatigue fracture: abnormal muscular stress applied to normal bone (e.g., march fracture)
    - Insufficiency fracture: normal muscular stress applied to abnormal bone (e.g., osteoporotic vertebral fracture)
- Pathological fracture: fracture superimposed on underlying bone disease
- Intraarticular fracture: fracture line extends into joint
- Salter-Harris fracture: fractures involving growth plate
- Pseudofracture: fissurelike defects in osteomalacia (Looser's zones)
- Occult fracture: suspected but nonvisualized fracture on plain film; demonstrated by ^{99m}Tc MDP scintigraphy or magnetic resonance imaging (MRI)
- Hairline fracture: nondisplaced fracture with minimal separation
- Avulsion fracture: fragment pulled away from bone at tendinous and ligament insertion (commonly at tuberosity)
- Apophyseal fracture: at growth centers such as ischial tuberosity and medial epicondyle; commonly avulsion fractures

RELEVANT ANATOMY

Long bones
- Epiphysis
- Metaphysis
- Diaphysis

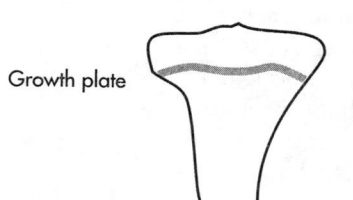

Types of joints
Synovial joint (diarthrosis)
- Appendicular skeleton
- Facet joints of spine
- Atlantoaxial joints
- Lower two thirds of SI joints
- Acromioclavicular (AC) joint
- Uncovertebral joints

Cartilaginous joint (amphiarthrosis)
- Synchondroses
- Pubic symphysis
- Intervertebral disks

Fibrous joint (synarthrosis)
- Interosseous membranes
- Tibiofibular syndesmosis
- Sutures

Synovial joint
In contradistinction to fibrous and cartilaginous joints, synovial joints allow wide ranges of motions and are classified according to axes of movement. The articular cartilage is hyaline. The most superficial layer has collagen fibrils parallel to the surface with microscopic pores to allow passage of electrolytes. This is also referred to as the *armor plate*. Deeper in the cartilage, collagen fibrils are arranged in arcades to give flexibility and allow for compression. Proteoglycans within the cartilage bind water to give a cushion effect.

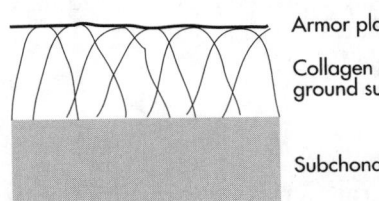

Armor plate

Collagen arcades, ground substance

Subchondral bone

FRACTURE COMPLICATIONS

Immediate
- Hemorrhage, shock
- Fat embolism
- Acute ischemia (5 "Ps": **p**ulselessness, **p**ain, **p**allor, **p**aresthesia, **p**aralysis)
- Spinal cord injury, epidural hematoma

Delayed
- Nonunion
- Osteoporosis due to disuse
- Secondary osteoarthritis
- Myositis ossificans
- Osteomyelitis
- Osteonecrosis
- Sudeck's atrophy
- Volkman's ischemic contracture

ORTHOPEDIC PROCEDURES

Types of repair
Reduction
- Closed: skin intact; may be performed in surgery under general anesthesia
- Open: requires exposing the fracture site in surgery

Fixation
- Internal: using fixation devices such as plates, screws, rods; a subsequent operation is usually necessary to remove hardware
- External: cast or external fixator

Orthopedic hardware
- Intramedullary rods: most of the intramedullary rods are hollow, closed nails; proximal and distal interlocking screws prevent rotation and shortening of bone fragments
- Kirschner wires (K-wires): unthreaded segments of wires drilled into cancellous bone; if more than one wire is placed, rotational stability can be achieved; the protruding ends of the K-wire are bent to prevent injury; K-wires are most frequently used for:
  - Provisional fixation
  - Fixation of small fragments
  - Pediatric metaphyseal fractures
- Cerclage wires are used to contain bone fragments.
- Staples are commonly used for osteotomies.
- Plates
- Nails
- Screws

Spine

CLASSIFICATION OF C-SPINE INJURIES

CLASSIFICATION		
Type of Injury	**Condition**	**Stability***
Flexion	Anterior subluxation	Stable†
	Unilateral facet dislocation	Stable
	Bilateral facet dislocation	Unstable
	Wedge compression fracture	Stable†
	Flexion teardrop fracture	Unstable
	Clay-shoveler's fracture	Stable
Extension	Posterior arch of C1 fracture	Stable
	Hangman's fracture	Unstable
	Laminar fracture	Stable
	Pillar fracture	Stable
	Extension teardrop fracture	Stable
	Hyperextension dislocation-fracture	Unstable
Compression	Jefferson's fracture	Unstable
	Burst fracture	Stable
Complex	Odontoid fractures	Unstable
	Atlantooccipital disassociation	Unstable

*Stability is a function of ligamentous injury. Plain films in neutral position allow one to infer *instability* when certain fractures or dislocations are present. However, *stability* may not be inferred with 100% accuracy. The anterior subluxation injury in which films may appear within normal limits is an example. Clinical judgment is necessary to decide whether to do nothing, obtain flexion/extension films, or obtain an MRI.
†Possible delayed instability.

Biomechanics

Nonangular stress translation

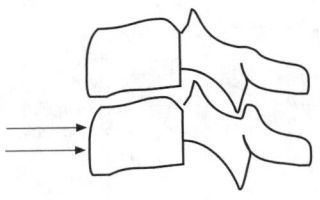

AP-shear

Angular stress translation

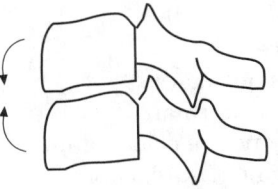

Flexion

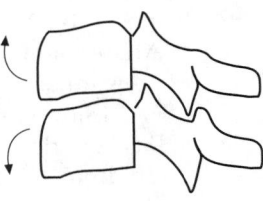

Extension

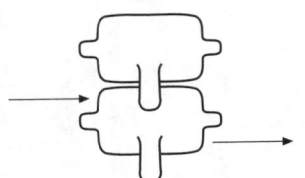

Lateral shear   Distraction-compression

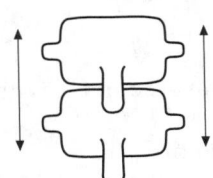

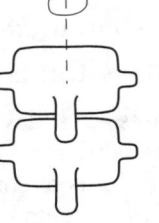

Torsion

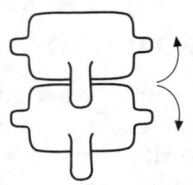

Lateral bending

Pearls

- 20% of spinal fractures are multiple.
- 5% of spinal fractures are at discontinous levels.
- Spinal cord injury occurs:
    At time of trauma, 85%
    As a late complication, 15%
- Cause of spinal fractures
    Motor vehicle accident (MVA), 50%
    Falls, 25%
    Sports related, 10%
- Most spinal fractures occur in upper (C1-C2) or lower (C5-C7) cervical spine and thoracolumbar (T10-L2) region.

APPROACH TO C-SPINE PLAIN FILM

1. Are all 7 cervical vertebrae well seen? If not, obtain additional views such as swimmer's view, computed tomography (CT), etc.
2. Is cervical lordosis maintained? If not consider
   - Positional
   - Spasm
   - Fracture/injury
3. Evaluate 5 parallel lines for step-offs and/or discontinuity
   - Prevertebral soft tissues
       C3-C4: 5 mm from vertebral body is normal (nonportable film)
       C4-C7: 20 mm from vertebral body is normal (not as reliable)
       Contour of soft tissues is as important as absolute measurements; a localized bulging anterior convex border usually indicates pathology.

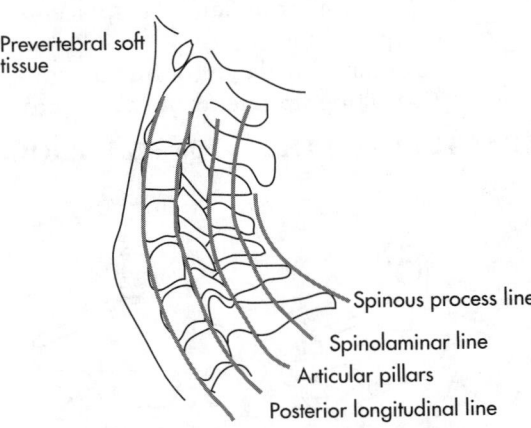

Prevertebral soft tissue

Spinous process line
Spinolaminar line
Articular pillars
Posterior longitudinal line
Anterior longitudinal line

5

- Anterior longitudinal line
- Posterior longitudinal line
- Spinolaminar line
- Posterior spinous process line

4. Inspect C1-C2 area
   - Atlantodental distance
     - Adults: < 3 mm is normal
     - Children: < 5 mm is normal
   - Base of odontoid may not be calcified in children (subdental synchondrosis).
5. Inspect disk spaces
   - Narrowing of disk spaces?
6. Transverse processes: C7 points downward, T1 points upward

APPROACH TO CERVICAL-SPINE INJURIES

1. Most suspected C-spine fractures are followed with thin section CT with reformation for most accurate evaluation.
2. All individuals with signs/symptoms of cord injury require MRI.
3. It is also prudent to obtain CT in patients with unexplained prevertebral soft tissue swelling.

JEFFERSON FRACTURES

Compression force to C1 that usually results from blow to the vertex of the head (diving injury). Consists of unilateral or bilateral fractures of both the anterior and posterior arches of C1. Treatment: halo placement for 3 months.

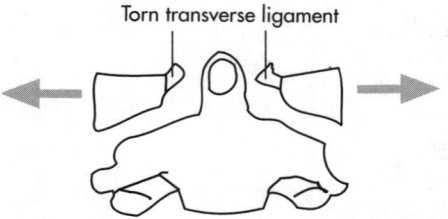
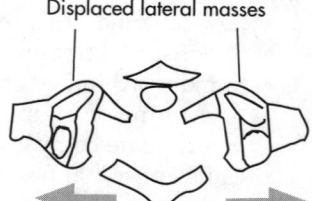

Radiographic features

- Key radiographic view: AP open-mouth
- Displacement of C1 lateral masses
  - > 2 mm bilateral is always abnormal
  - < 1-2 mm or unilateral displacement can be due to head tilt/rotation
- CT required for:
  - Defining full extent of fracture
  - Detecting fragments in spinal cord

FRACTURES OF THE ODONTOID PROCESS (DENS)

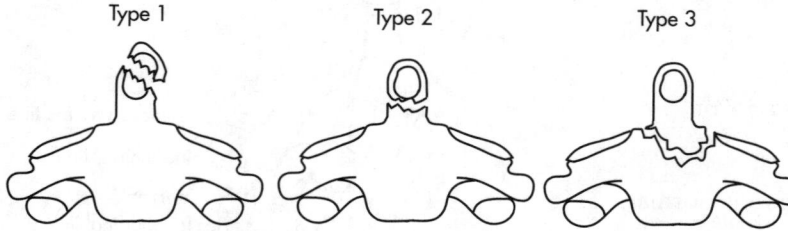

Various mechanisms: Anderson/D'Alonzo classification:
- Type I: fracture in the upper part of the odontoid (potentially unstable; rare fracture)
- Type II: fracture at base of the odontoid (unstable)
- Type III: fracture through base of odontoid into body of axis; best prognosis for healing because of larger surface area (unstable)

Radiographic features
- Anterior tilt of odontoid on lateral view is highly suspicious for fracture
- Plain film tomograms or CT with reformations is helpful to delineate fracture line
- Prevertebral soft tissue swelling (may be the only sign)
- Os odontoideum (type 1)
  Congenital or posttraumatic
  May be mechanically unstable

HANGMAN'S FRACTURE

Hyperextension and traction injury of C2. Causes:
- Hanging
- MVA (chin hits dashboard)

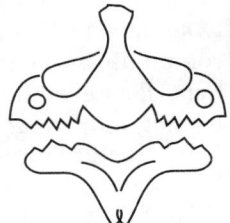

Lateral view   Axial view

Radiographic features
- Best demonstrated on lateral view
- Bilateral C2 pars (common) or pedicle (less common) fractures
- Anterior dislocation or subluxation of C2 vertebral body
- Avulsion of anterior inferior corner of C2 (ruptured anterior longitudinal ligament)
- Prevertebral soft tissue swelling

BURST (COMPRESSION) FRACTURE

Same mechanism as in Jefferson's fracture but located at C3-C7. Injury to spinal cord (displacement of posterior fragments) is common. All patients require CT to evaluate full extent of injury, to detect associated fractures, and to identify fragments in relation to spinal canal.

FLEXION TEARDROP FRACTURE (FLEXION FRACTURE-DISLOCATION)

The most severe C-spine injury. Results from severe flexion force and presents with clinical "acute anterior cord syndrome" (quadriplegia, loss of anterior column senses, retention of posterior column senses). Completely unstable.

Radiographic features

- Teardrop fragment is major shear fragment from anteroinferior vertebral body.
- All ligaments are disrupted.
- Posterior subluxation of vertebral body
- Bilateral subluxated or dislocated facets
- Severe compromise of spinal canal secondary to subluxation of body and facets
- Not to be confused with:
    Extension teardrop fracture (stable avulsive injury)
    Burst fracture (stable comminuted fracture of centrum with variable neurological involvement).

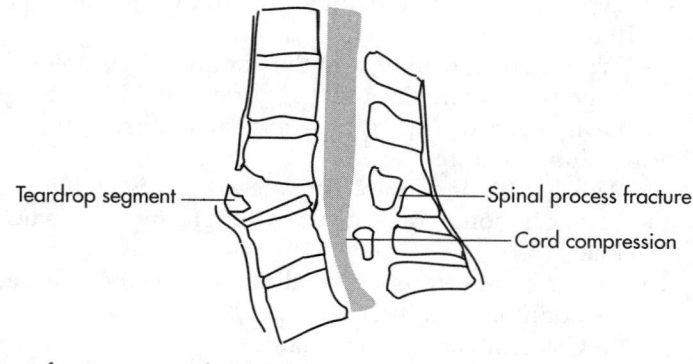

Posterior subluxation

Teardrop segment

Spinal process fracture

Cord compression

CLAY-SHOVELER'S FRACTURE

Oblique avulsive fracture of a lower spinous process, most commonly at C6-T1 levels (C7 > C6 > T1). Cause: powerful hyperflexion (shoveling).

Radiographic features

- Fracture through spinous process, best seen on lateral view
- If C6-C7 is not demonstrated on lateral view, obtain Swimmer's view and/or CT
- AP view: ghost sign (double-spinous process on C6-C7 caused by caudal displacement of the fractured tip of the spinous process)

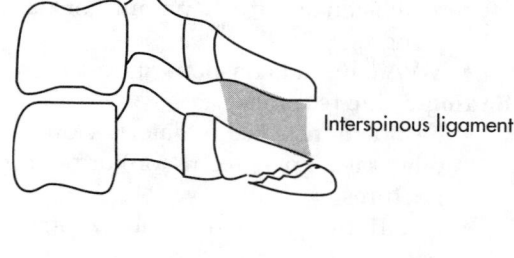

Interspinous ligament

WEDGE FRACTURE

Compression fracture resulting from flexion. Most fractures are stable.

Radiographic features

- Loss of height of anterior vertebral body
- Buckled anterior cortex
- Anterosuperior fracture of vertebral body
- Differentiate from burst fracture
    Lack of vertical fracture component
    Posterior cortex intact

EXTENSION TEARDROP FRACTURE

Avulsion fracture of anteroinferior corner of the axis resulting from hyperextension.

Radiographic features

- Teardrop fragment: avulsion by the anterior longitudinal ligament
- Vertical height of fragment ≥ horizontal width

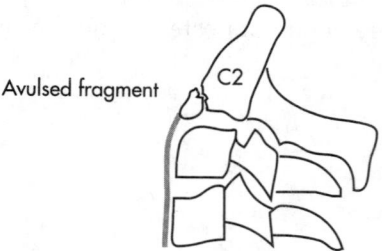

Avulsed fragment   C2

FACET DISLOCATION

Bilateral facet dislocation (unstable)
Results from extreme flexion of head and neck without axial compression.

Radiographic features
- Complete anterior dislocation of the affected vertebral body by half or more of the vertebral body AP diameter
- Batwing or bowtie configuration of locked facets
- Disruption of posterior ligament complex, intervertebral disk, and anterior longitudinal ligament

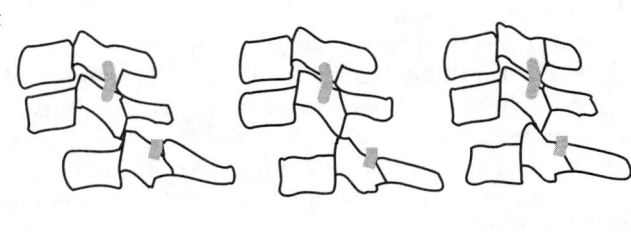

Locked facets   Perched facets   Subluxated facets

Unilateral facet dislocation (stable)
Results from simultaneous flexion and rotation.

Radiographic features
- Anterior dislocation of vertebral body less than half the AP diameter of the vertebral body
- Evidence of discordant rotation above and below involved level
- Disrupted "shingles-on-a-roof" on oblique view
- Facet within intervertebral foramen on oblique view
- Disrupted posterior ligament complex
- Best demonstrated on lateral and oblique views

ANTERIOR SUBLUXATION (HYPERFLEXION SPRAIN)

Anterior subluxation occurs when the posterior ligament complex is disrupted. Radiographic diagnosis can be difficult because muscle spasm may cause similar findings. Initially stable. 20%-50% show delayed instability.

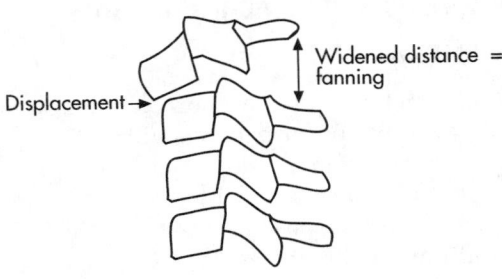

Widened distance = fanning

Displacement →

Radiographic features
- Localized kyphotic angulation
- Widened interspinous/interlaminar distance (fanning)
- Posterior widening of disk space
- Subluxation at facet joints
- Anterior vertebral body may be displaced
- In equivocal findings, voluntary flexion/extension views are helpful.

HYPEREXTENSION FRACTURE-DISLOCATION

Results from severe circular hyper-extending force (e.g., impact on forehead). Characteristically results in anterior vertebral displacement, a finding more commonly seen in flexion injuries. Unstable.

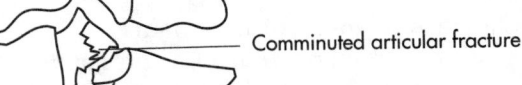

Comminuted articular fracture

Facet subluxation

Anterior displacement

Radiographic features
- Mild anterior vertebral displacement
- Comminuted articular mass fracture
- Contralateral facet subluxation
- Disrupted anterior longitudinal ligament and partial posterior ligamentous disruption

5

ATLANTOOCCIPITAL DISSOCIATION

Complex mechanism of injury. Complete dislocation is usually fatal.

Radiographic features

- Prevertebral soft tissue swelling
- The traditional methods used to identify occipitoatlantal articulation injury included the Power ratio and the "X" line of Lee. Each is dependent on identifying the opisthion and the spinolaminar line of C1. Anatomical variation and inconsistent visualization preclude consistent use of these methods.
- The current method uses the basion-axial interval (BAI) and is an easy and reliable method for assessing the occipitoatlantal relationship in patients of all ages. BAI is the distance between the basion and upward extension of the posterior axial line. Normally the BAI should not exceed 12 mm as determined on a lateral radiograph of the cervicocranium obtained at a target film distance of 1 meter.
- The vertical basion dens distance should also be less than 12 mm.
- Anterior dissociation is more common.
- Posterior dissociation (subluxation) can be very subtle, especially if partial.

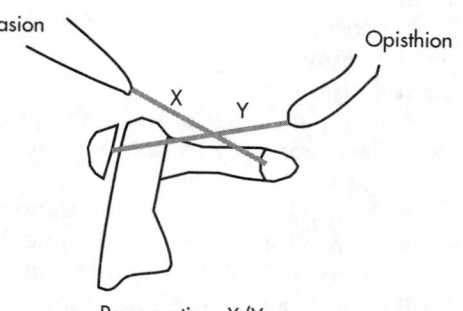

Power ratio = X/Y

Thoracic and Lumbar Fractures

GENERAL

Most fractures occur at thoracolumbar junction (90% at T11-L4). All patients should have CT except for patients with:

- Stable compression fractures
- Isolated spinous or transverse process fractures
- Spondylolysis

Radiographic features

- Widened interpedicular distance
- Paraspinal hematoma
- Unstable fractures:

  Compression fracture > 50%
  Widened interlaminar space
  Disrupted posterior elements
  All fracture-dislocations

TYPES OF FRACTURES

Classified by mechanism or injury:

Compression or wedge fractures: anterior or lateral flexion
- Wedge-shaped deformity of vertebral body
- Decreased vertebral body height

Burst fracture: axial compression
- Comminution of vertebral body
- Bone fragments in spinal canal are common

Chance fractures (lap seatbelt fracture, usually at L2 or L3): distraction from anterior hyperflexion across a restraining lap seatbelt
- Horizontal splitting of vertebra
- Horizontal disruption of intervertebral disk
- Rupture of ligaments
- More than 50% of patients have associated small bowel and colon injuries.

Fracture-dislocations: combined shearing and flexion forces
- Spinal cord injury is common

Minor fractures
- Transverse process fractures
- Spinous process fractures
- Pars interarticularis fractures

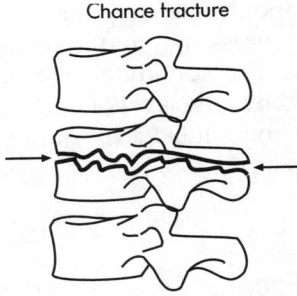

Chance fracture

SPONDYLOLYSIS

Defect in the pars interarticularis (neck of the "Scottie dog"). Chronic stress fracture with nonunion. Typically in adolescents involved in sports. Most commonly at the L4 or L5 level.

Radiographic features
- Separation of pars interarticularis
- Spondylolithesis common in bilateral spondylolysis
- If patient looks to right, the left pars is visualized by x-ray.
- Oblique view is usually diagnostic.
- CT or SPECT may be helpful in confirming diagnosis.

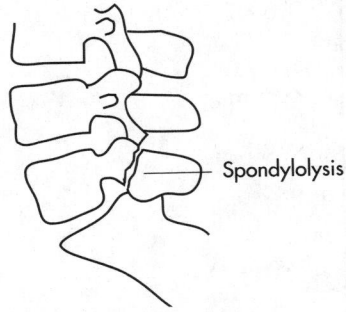

Spondylolysis

SPONDYLOLISTHESIS

Ventral subluxation of a vertebral body due to bilateral pars defects.
- Four grades based on degree of anterior displacement
- 95% of spondylolistheses occur at L4-L5 and L5-S1.

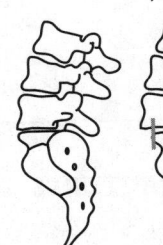
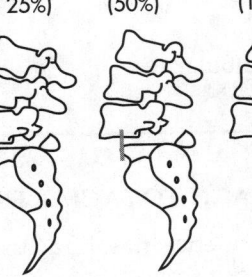

Normal Grade 1 (< 25%) Grade 2 (50%) Grade 4 (100%)

5

PSEUDOSPONDYLOLISTHESIS

Secondary to degenerative disk disease and/or apophyseal degenerative joint disease. Use spinous process sign to differentiate from true spondylolisthesis. In true spondylolisthesis the spinous process step off is above the level of vertebral slip, whereas in pseudospondylolisthesis the step-off is below the level of the slip.

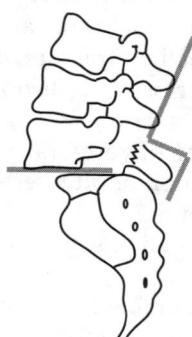

Spondylolisthesis

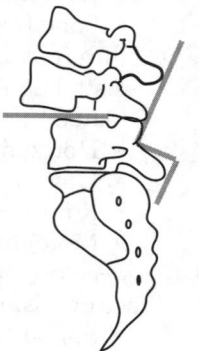

Pseudospondylolisthesis

Face

CLASSIFICATION OF FACIAL FRACTURES		
General Category	Types	Need for CT
Orbital	Pure blow-out	Yes
	Impure blowout	Yes
	Blow-in	Yes
Zygoma	Tripod fracture	Yes
	Isolated zygomatic arch	No
Nasal	Nondisplaced	No
	Comminuted	Variable
	Nasal-orbital-ethmoid	Yes
	Septal fracture/dislocation	Yes
Maxillary	Dentoalveolar	Yes
	Sagittal	Yes
	LeFort fractures	Yes
Craniofacial (smash fractures)	Central craniofacial	Yes
	Lateral craniofacial	Yes
	Frontal sinus	Yes
Mandibular	Defined by site	Variable
	Flail mandible	Variable

APPROACH TO FACIAL FRACTURES

1. Incidence: nasal fractures > zygoma > other fractures
2. Facial series
   - Waters view: three lines of the "elephant" should be traceable
     - Maxillary sinuses
     - Orbital floor and rim
     - Nasal septum
     - Zygoma
   - Caldwell view
     - Orbital rim
     - Medial orbital wall
     - Sphenoid wings
   - Lateral view
     - Paranasal sinuses
     - Pterygoid plates

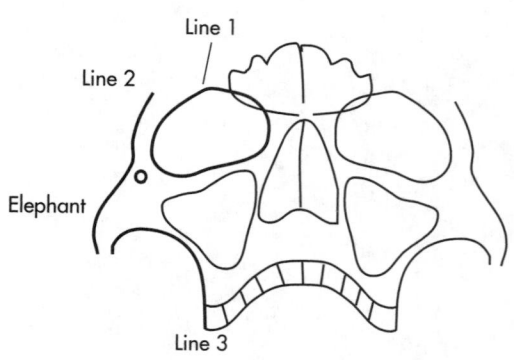

- Towne view
    - Mandible
- Base view (C-spine must be cleared first)
    - Zygoma
    - Mandible
3. Facial series is not adequate for nasal fractures:
    - Lateral (coned and soft tissue technique) views
    - Waters view
    - Occlusal view
4. Mandibular fractures require specific mandibular series:
    - Lateral, Towne, bilateral oblique views
5. Direct signs of fracture:
    - Cortical disruption, overlap, displacement
6. Indirect signs of fracture:
    - Asymmetry
    - Soft tissue swelling
    - Sinus abnormality (opacification, polypoid mass, air-fluid levels)
    - Orbital emphysema

ORBITAL FRACTURES

Pure orbital blow-out fracture
Isolated fracture of the orbital floor or less commonly the medial wall; the orbital rim is intact. Mechanism: sudden increase in intraorbital pressure (e.g., baseball, fist). Clinical: diplopia on upward gaze (inferior rectus muscle entrapment) and enophthalmos (may be masked by edema).

Radiographic findings
- Displacement of bone fragments into maxillary sinus (trap door sign)
- Opacification of maxillary sinus (hematoma)
- Orbital emphysema
- Caldwell and Waters views best demonstrate fractures

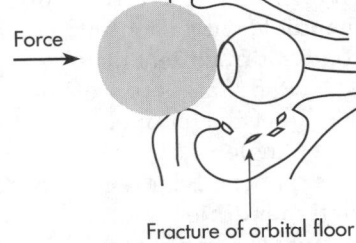

Fracture of orbital floor

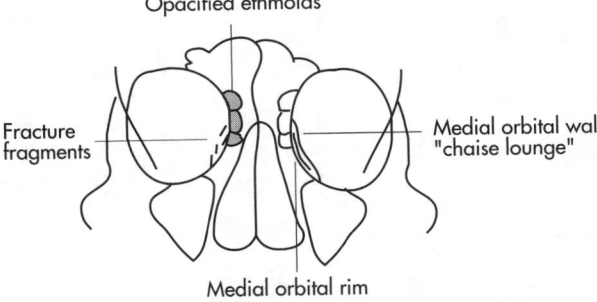

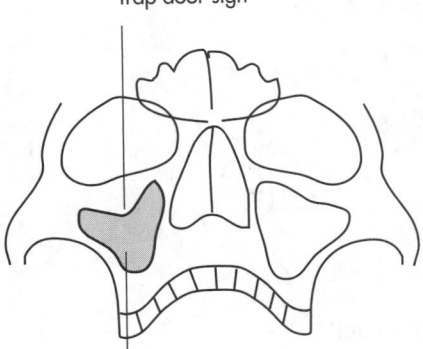

- Evaluate by CT for muscle entrapment and orbital content herniation

Impure orbital blow-out fracture
Associated with fracture of orbital rim and other facial fractures.

Orbital blow-in fracture
Impact to frontal bone causes blow-in of orbital roof. Associated with craniofacial fractures and frontal lobe contusion.

NASAL FRACTURES

Isolated nasal fractures are linear and transverse, result from a direct frontal impact, and usually occur in the lower one third of the nasal bone. More complex fractures result from lateral blows or more severe trauma and are often accompanied by other facial fractures.

Radiographic findings

- Most fractures are transverse and are depressed or displaced.
- Dislocation of septal cartilage is diagnosed by occlusal view or CT.
- Anterior nasal spine fracture is best evaluated by occlusal view.
- Do not mistake sutures and nasociliary grooves for fractures.

Normal

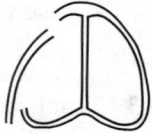

Nasal bone fracture

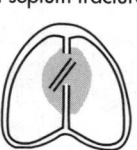

Nasal septum fracture

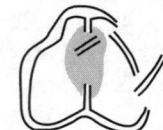

Comminuted fracture

MANDIBULAR FRACTURES

The type of fracture depends on the site of impact. Most fractures are multiple and bilateral. The most common type of mandibular fracture is an ipsilateral fracture through the body of the mandible with a contralateral angle or sub-condylar fracture. Fractures typically occur in:

- Body (areas of weakness include mental or incisive foramen)
- Angle
- Subcondylar region (condylar neck)

Flail mandible

Symphysis fracture with bilateral subcondylar, angle, or ramus fracture. Tongue may prolapse and obstruct airway.

Coronoid process

20%

Condyloid process

Ramus

35%

35%

Angle

Mental protuberance

Body

Parasymphaseal area

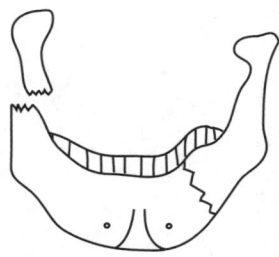

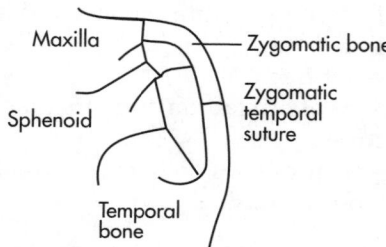

ZYGOMA FRACTURES

Best view to demonstrate zygoma fracture is the base view to demonstrate the "jug handle."

Simple arch fractures

Simple fractures of the zygomatic arch are less common than complex fractures. Fracture lines occur most commonly:

- Anteriorly at temporal process
- In midportion near zygomaticotemporal suture
- Posterior and anteriorly to condylar eminence

Normal

Maxilla

Zygomatic bone

Sphenoid

Zygomatic temporal suture

Temporal bone

Fracture

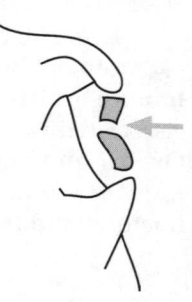

Complex arch fractures (tripod fracture)
- Diastasis of zygomaticofrontal suture
- Posterior zygomatic arch fracture
- Fracture of inferior orbital rim and lateral maxillary wall

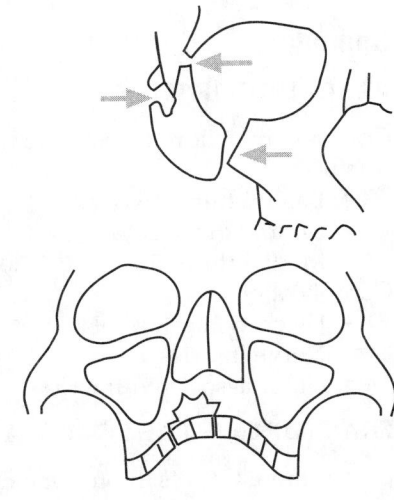

MAXILLARY FRACTURES

Dentoalveolar fracture
Fracture of the alveolar process of maxilla secondary to direct blow. May present clinically as loose teeth; managed as open fracture.
Sagittal maxillary fracture
Usually occurs with other injuries such as Le Fort fracture.

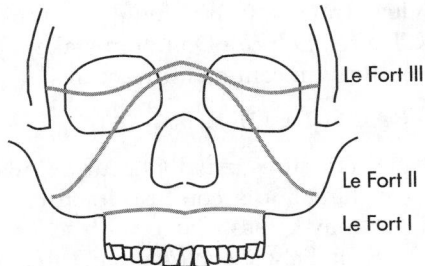

LE FORT FRACTURES

Fracture patterns that occur along lines of weakness in the face. Mechanism: severe force to face as would occur in motor vehicle accident. All LeFort fractures involve the ptyergoid plates of the sphenoid.
Lefort type I fracture
This fracture produces a floating palate; fracture lines extend through:
- Nasal septum (vomer and septal cartilage)
- Medial, anterior, lateral, posterior walls of maxillary sinus
- Pterygoid plates of sphenoid

Lefort type II
This fracture produces a floating maxilla; zygomatic arches are *not* included in this fracture; fracture line extends through:
- Nasal bone and nasal septum
- Frontal process of maxilla
- Medial orbital wall (ethmoid, lacrimal, palatine)
- Floor of orbit (inferior orbital fissure and canal)
- Infraorbital rim
- Anterior, lateral, posterior wall of maxillary sinus
- Pterygoid plates of sphenoid

Lefort type III
This fracture separates face from cranial vault and produces a floating face; the fracture line extends through:
- Nasal bone and septum
- Frontal process of maxilla
- Medial wall of orbit (lacrimal, ethmoid, palatine)
- Infraorbital fissure
- Lateral wall of orbit
- Zygomaticofrontal suture
- Zygomatic arch
- Pterygoid plates of sphenoid

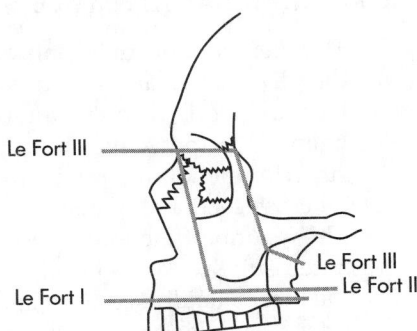

Shoulder

FRACTURE OF THE CLAVICLE

Common in children. Distal fragment is displaced inferior and medial. Sites of fracture:
- Lateral third: 15%
- Middle third: 80%
- Medial third: 5%

Complications
- Laceration of vessels
- Nerve injuries
- Other associated fracture

FRACTURE OF THE SCAPULA

Uncommon. Causes: motor vehicle accident, fall from height (direct impact injuries). Best radiographic view: transscapular view (Y-view), CT often helpful. Do not mistake ossification centers for fractures.

FRACTURE OF RIBS

- Fractures usually occur in lower 10 ribs.
- First and second rib fractures can occur after high energy trauma to chest and may be associated with severe mediastinal and vascular injury.
- Flail chest occurs when three or more ribs fracture and each rib fractures in two places. (segmental fractures). Commonly associated with pulmonary contusion, laceration, pneumothorax, hemothorax, etc.

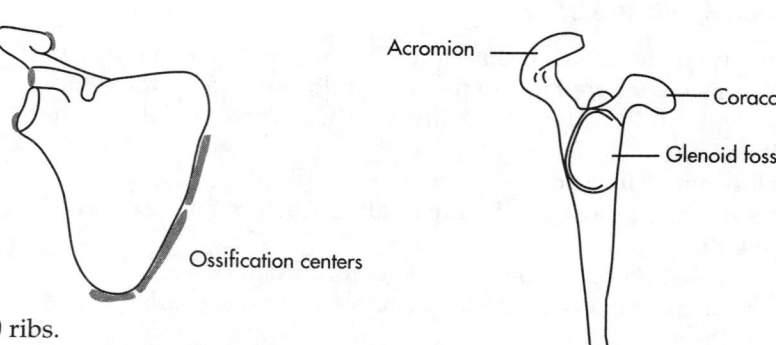

NORMAL MRI ANATOMY OF SHOULDER JOINT

- The glenoid labrum is a fibrocartilaginous structure that attaches to the glenoid rim and is about 4 mm wide. Anteriorly, the glenoid labrum blends with the anterior band of the inferior glenohumeral ligament. Superiorly, it blends with the biceps tendon and the superior glenohumeral ligament. It is usually rounded or triangular on cross-sectional images.
- The tendon of the long head of the biceps muscle attaches to the anterosuperior aspect of the glenoid rim. From its site of attachment, the biceps tendon courses laterally and exits the glenohumeral joint through the intertubercular groove where it is secured by the transverse ligament. In the adjacent diagram the biceps tendon attaches at the level of the superior labrum and glenoid illustrates attachments to the (1) superior glenoid rim, (2) the posterior labrum, (3) the anterior labrum, and (4) the base of the coracoid process.
- The labral-bicipital complex is well visualized on transverse CT or MR arthrograms, as well as on coronal MR arthrograms and reconstructed images from coronal CT arthrograms.

- The glenohumeral ligaments play a role as shoulder stabilizers and consist of thickened bands of the joint capsule. The superior glenohumeral ligament is the most consistently identified capsular ligament. It can arise from the anterosuperior labrum, the attachment of the tendon of the long head of the biceps muscle, or the middle glenohumeral ligament.
- The middle glenohumeral ligament varies most in size and site of attachment to the glenoid. It typically has an oblique orientation from superomedial to inferolateral. It may attach to the superior portion of the anterior glenoid but more frequently attaches medially on the glenoid neck.
- The middle glenohumeral ligament may be absent or may appear thick and cordlike (e.g., Buford complex).
- The inferior glenohumeral ligament is an important stabilizer of the anterior shoulder joint and consists of the axillary pouch and anterior and posterior bands. The anterior band inserts along the inferior two thirds of the anterior glenoid labrum.

DISLOCATIONS OF THE GLENOHUMERAL JOINT

Dislocation: separation of articular surface of glenoid fossa and humeral head that will not reduce spontaneously. Subluxation: transient incomplete separation that reduces spontaneously.

Anterior dislocation

Most common type (95%) of dislocation. Usually due to indirect force from abduction, external rotation, and extension.

Radiographic findings

- Humeral head lies inferior and medial to glenoid
- Two lesions can occur as humeral head strikes the glenoid:
  Hill-Sachs lesion (posterior-superior and lateral) of humeral head, (best seen on AP view with internal rotation)
  Bankart lesion (antero-inferior) of glenoid (may require CT)
- Bulbous distortion of the scapulohumeral arch (Moloney's arch)

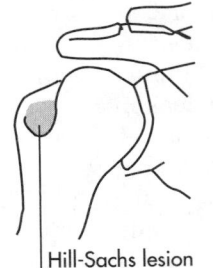
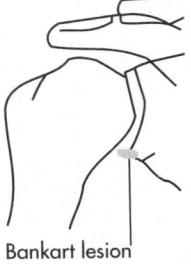

Hill-Sachs lesion   Bankart lesion

Posterior dislocation

Less common (5%); usually due to direct or indirect force. Associated with seizures or electrical shock.

Radiographic findings

- Humeral head lies superior to glenoid
- Trough sign: compression fracture of the anterior humeral surface, 15% (best seen on AP view with external rotation or axillary view)
- Sharp angle of the scapulohumeral arch (Moloney's arch)
- Posterior displacement is best seen on axillary view.
- 40-degree posterior oblique (Grashey view) may be needed: loss of glenohumeral space is diagnostic
- Fixed in internal rotation

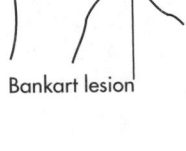
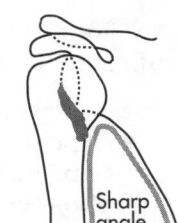

Inferior dislocation

Also called *luxatio erecta:* the humeral head is located below the glenoid and the shaft of the humerus is fixed in extreme abduction. Compllications of luxatio erecta include injuries to the brachial plexus and axillary artery.

PSEUDODISLOCATION OF GLENOHUMERAL JOINT

Inferior and lateral displacement of humeral head due to hemarthrosis that often occurs in fractures of humeral head or neck. Not a true inferior dislocation.

ROTATOR CUFF TEAR

Causes of rotator cuff tear: degeneration, trauma, impingement.

The rotator cuff (inserts into anatomical neck and tuberosities of humerus) consists of four muscles ("SITS"):

- **S**upraspinatus
- **I**nfraspinatus
- **T**eres minor
- **S**ubscapularis

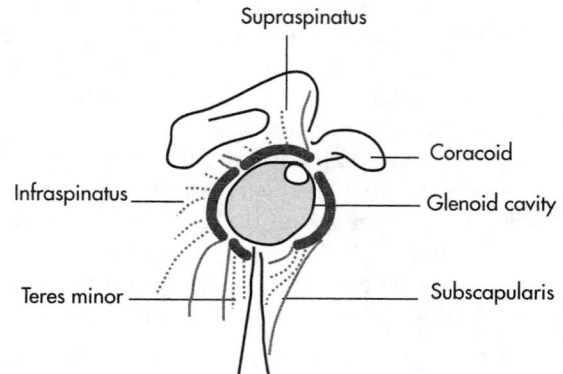

Radiographic features

- Narrowing of acromiohumeral space to less than 6 mm (chronic rupture)
- Eroded inferior aspect of acromion (chronic rupture)
- Flattening and atrophy of the greater tuberosity of the humeral head
- Arthrogram
    - Opacification of subacromial-subdeltoid bursae
    - Contrast may leak into the cuff in partial tears
- MR arthrography is most accurate diagnostic study
    - Abnormal contrast/signal in supraspinatous tendon
    - Supraspinatus atrophy with tendon retraction
    - Accurate delineation of size/extent of tear possible
    - Allows evaluation of glenoid labrum

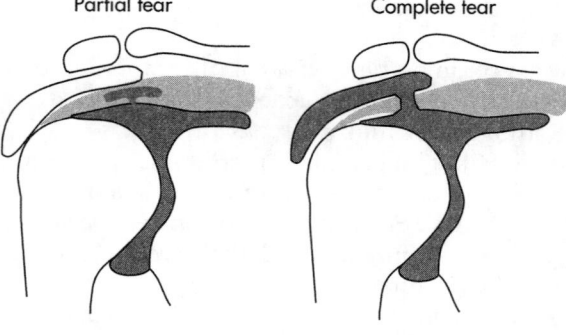

ANTERIOR-TO-POSTERIOR LESIONS OF THE SUPERIOR LABRUM (SLAP LESIONS)

- Type I: fraying or tear of the superior labrum
- Type II: detachment of the labral-bicipital complex from the superior glenoid
- Type III: bucket handle tear of the superior labrum
- Type IV: bucket handle tear with extension into the biceps tendon

ADHESIVE CAPSULITIS (FROZEN SHOULDER)

Pain, stiffness, and limited range of motion from posttraumatic adhesive inflammation of the joint capsule.

Radiographic findings

- Decreased size of joint capsule
- Obliteration of axillary and subscapular recesses
- Disuse osteoporosis
- Arthrogram if persistent

ACROMIOCLAVICULAR SEPARATION

Most commonly result from athletic injury to AC joint
- Direct blow to AC joint (e.g., football)
- Severe arm traction
- Fall on hand or elbow with arm flexed 90 degrees

Radiographic features

Technique
- AP view with 15-degree cephalad angulation is the preferred view for diagnosis.
- May need opposite shoulder for comparison
- May need stress views (10-20 lb weights)

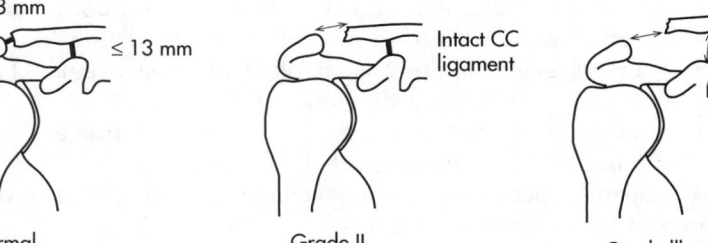

Normal (Grade 1)   Grade II   Grade III

Normal
- Acromioclavicular distance ≤ 8 mm
- Coracoclavicular distance ≤ 13 mm
- Inferior margin of clavicle lines up with inferior acromion

AC joint injury
- Downward displacement of scapula/extremity
- Downward displacement and AC separation worsen with stress weights.
- AC widening = disrupted AC ligament
- Craniocaudad (CC) widening due to disrupted CC ligament

6 grade classifications (Rockwood)
- Grade I (mild sprain): normal radiograph
- Grade II (moderate sprain): increased AC distance; normal CC distance
- Grade III (severe sprain): increased AC and CC distance
- Grade IV: total dislocation; clavicle displaced superoposteriorly into the trapezius
- Grade V: total dislocation; clavicle displaced superiorly into neck
- Grade VI: total dislocation; clavicle displaced inferiorly to subacromial or subcoracoid position

STERNOCLAVICULAR (SC) JOINT INJURY

Most injuries of the SC joint are dislocations resulting from a direct forceful impact. Although anterior dislocations are more common, posterior dislocations are more serious because the great vessels or trachea may be injured.

Radiographic features
- Superior displacement of clavicle
- Many injuries occur as Salter fractures of medial clavicular epiphysis.
- CT is the examination of choice: thin section with coronal reformation.
- Angled AP plain film (serendipidity view) is not as helpful.

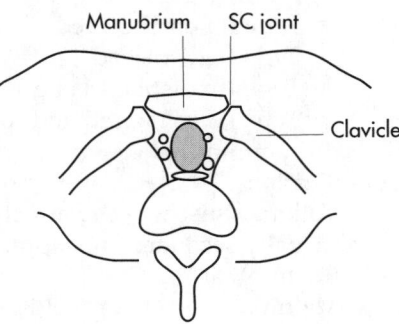

Normal axial view

Manubrium   SC joint   Clavicle

Arm

FRACTURES OF PROXIMAL HUMERUS

These fractures are common in osteoporotic elderly patients secondary to fall on outstretched hand. 85% are nondisplaced; 4-segment Neer classification aids in treatment and prognosis.

4-segment Neer classification
Based on number and type of displaced segments. 4 segments: anatomical neck, surgical neck, greater tuberosity, lesser tuberosity. Displacement defined as (a) > 1 cm separation of fragments or (b) > 45-degree angulation.

- 1-part: no displacement (regardless of comminution); treated with sling
- 2-part: displacement of 1 segment; closed reduction
- 3-part: displacement of 2 segments, 1 tuberosity remains in continuity with the head; closed reduction
- 4-part: displacement of 3 segments; open reduction and internal fixation or humeral head replacement
- 2, 3, and 4-part fractures may have anterior or posterior dislocation

Radiographic features

- Fracture lines according to Neer classification
- Pseudosubluxation: inferior displacement of humeral head due to hemarthrosis
- Subacromial fat-fluid level: lipohemarthrosis
- Transthoracic or transscapular views useful to accurately determine angulation

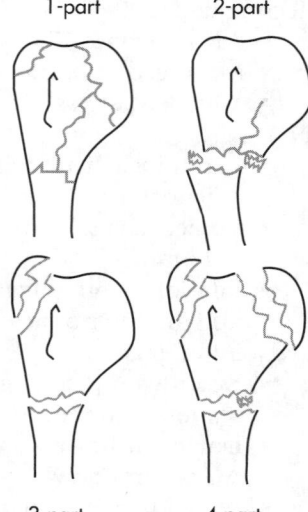

FRACTURE OF DISTAL HUMERUS

Classification:
Supracondylar-extraarticular fracture (3 types)
- Type I: nondisplaced
- Type II: displaced with posterior cortical continuity
- Type III: totally displaced

Transcondylar-intraarticular fracture
Intercondylar (bicondylar)-intraarticular fracture (4 types)
- Type I: nondisplaced
- Type II: displaced
- Type III: displaced and rotated
- Type IV: displaced and rotated and comminuted

Complications:
- Volkman's ischemic contracture (usually secondary to supracondylar fracture)
- Malunion (results in "cubitus varus" deformity)

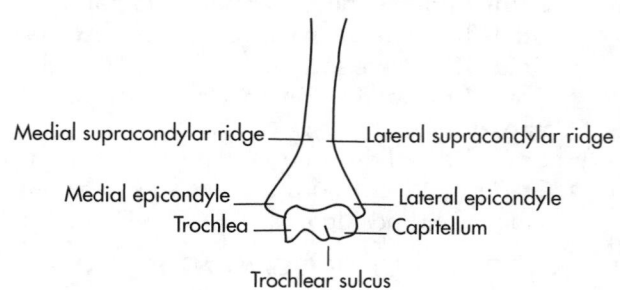

Normal distal humerus

Medial supracondylar ridge — Lateral supracondylar ridge
Medial epicondyle — Lateral epicondyle
Trochlea — Capitellum
Trochlear sulcus

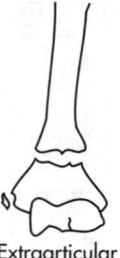 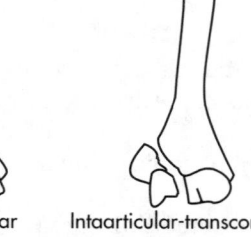 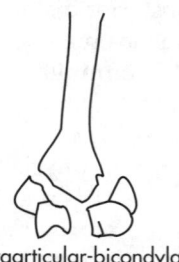

Extraarticular   Intaarticular-transcondylar   Intraarticular-bicondylar

RADIAL HEAD FRACTURES

Common fracture that results from a fall on oustretched hand. Treatment:
- No displacement: splint, cast
- > 3 mm displacement on lateral view: open reduction and internal fixation (ORIF)
- Comminuted: exicision of radial head

Radiographic features
- Positive fat pad sign
  > Anterior fat pad has the appearance of a sail (sail sign).
  > A positive posterior fat pad is a good indicator of a fracture since not normally seen.
- Fracture line may be difficult to see on standard projections. If in doubt, obtain radial head view, oblique views, or tomograms.

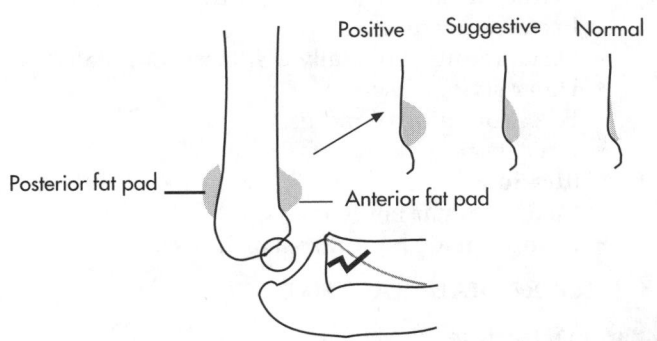

ULNAR FRACTURES

Isolated ulnar fractures are uncommon. Most fractures of the ulna also involve the radius (see below).

Olecranon fracture
Result from direct fall on flexed elbow. Treated conservatively if nondisplaced. ORIF if displaced (by pull of triceps). Best view: lateral.

Coronoid fracture
Usually in association with posterior elbow dislocations. Best view: radial head or oblique views.

ELBOW DISLOCATIONS

Different types of dislocations are defined by the relation of radius/ulna to distal humerus. Posterior dislocations of both the radius and ulna are the most common type (90%). Often associated with coronoid process or radial head fractures. Complication: myositis ossificans. Three types:
- Ulna and radius dislocation (most common)
- Ulna dislocation only
- Radial dislocation only (rare in adults)

COMBINED RADIUS-ULNA FRACTURES AND DISLOCATIONS

Most (60%) forearm fractures involve both the radius and ulna.

Monteggia fracture-dislocation
Ulnar shaft fracture and radial head dislocation.

Galeazzi fracture-dislocation
Distal radial shaft fracture and distal radioulnar dislocation.

Essex-Lopresti fracture-dislocation
Comminuted radial head fracture and distal radioulnar subluxation/dislocation.

COLLES' FRACTURE

Mechanism of injury: fall on the outstreched hand with the forearm pronated in dorsiflexion. Most common injury to distal forearm, especially in osteoporotic females.

Radiographic features

- Extraarticular fracture (in contradistinction to Barton's fracture)
- Distal radius is dorsally displaced/angulated
- Ulnar styloid fracture, 50%
- Foreshortening of radius
- Impaction

Complications

- Median, ulnar nerve injury
- Posttraumatic radiocarpal arthritis

OTHER RADIAL FRACTURES

Barton's fracture

Intraarticular fracture of the dorsal margin of the distal radius. The carpus usually follows the distal fragment. Unstable fracture requiring open reduction and internal fixation and/or external fixation.

Smith's fracture

- Same as a Colles' fracture except there is volar displacement and angulation of the distal fragment
- 3 types

    Type 1: horizontal fracture line
    Type 2: oblique fracture line
    Type 3: intraarticular oblique fracture = reverse Barton's fracture

Hutchinson's fracture

Intraarticular fracture of the radial styloid process. Also known as *chauffeur's fracture.*

Undisplaced   Colles' fracture   Impacted Colles' fracture

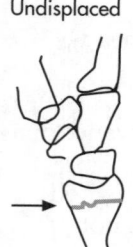 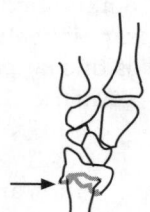

Barton's fracture

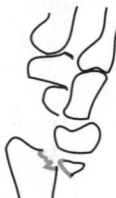

Smith's fracture

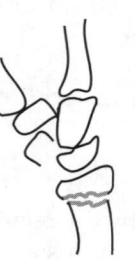 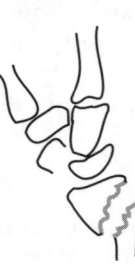 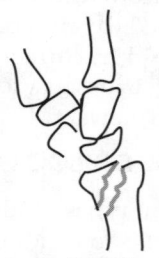

Type 1   Type 2   Type 3 (reverse Barton's fracture)

Hutchinson's fracture

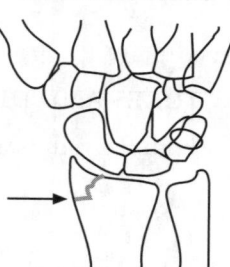

Wrist/Hand

WRIST ANATOMY

- Lunate
- Scaphoid
- Trapezium
- Trapezoid
- Capitate
- Hamate
- Triquetrum
- Pisiform

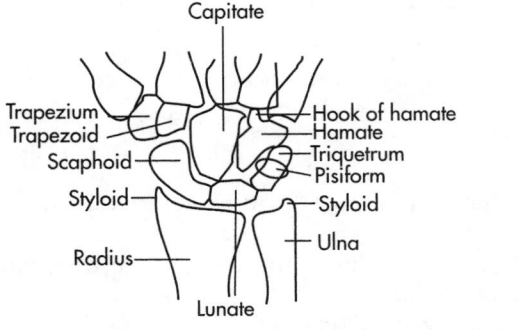
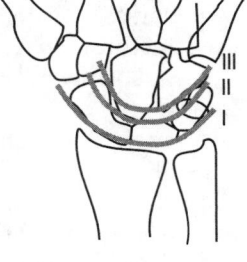

LINES OF ARTICULATIONS

Ulnar variance
- Neutral ulnar variance (normal)
- Negative ulnar variance (abnormal)
- Positive ulnar variance (abnormal)

Normal alignment
- Ulnar tilt of radius: 15°-25°
- Volar tilt of radius: 10°-25°

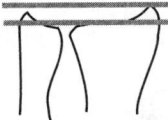
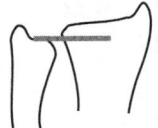
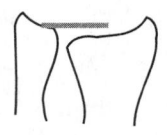

Normal: 9-12 mm Negative ulnar variance Positive ulnar variance

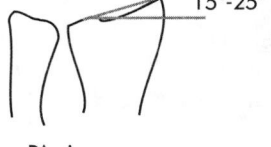
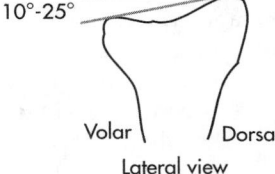

Ulnar tilt Volar tilt

PA view Lateral view

SCAPHOID FRACTURE

Most common fracture of carpus. Mechanism: fall on outstretched hand in young adults.
Locations:
- Waist, 70%
- Proximal pole, 20%
- Distal pole, 10%

Blood supply to the proximal pole enters at the waist; therefore the proximal pole is at high risk for nonunion and osteonecrosis.

Radiographic features
- Fracture may be difficult to detect on plain film.
- Scaphoid views (PA view in ulnar deviation) may be useful to demonstrate fracture.
- Loss of navicular fat stripe on PA view
- If a fracture is clinically suspected but not radiographically detected use:
    CT
    Bone scan
    MRI
    Cast and repeat plain films in one week.

Prognosis
- Waist fracture: 90% heal eventually; 10% nonunion or proximal avascular necrosis (AVN)
- Proximal fracture: high incidence of nonunion or AVN
- Distal fracture: usually heals without complications

FRACTURES OF OTHER CARPAL BONES

Triquetrum
- Dorsal avulsion at attachment of radiocarpal ligament (most common type of fracture)
- Best seen on lateral view

Hamate
- Hook of hamate fracture: diagnosis requires tomography, carpal tunnel view, or CT
- Other fractures are usually part of complex fracture/dislocations.

Kienböck's disease (lunatomalacia)
- AVN of lunate secondary to (usually trivial) trauma
- Associated with ulnar minus variant
- Acute lunate fractures are rare.

WRIST DISLOCATIONS

The continuum of perilunate injuries ranges from disassociation to dislocation. Mechanism: backwards fall on extended hand. Each of the four successive stages progresses from radial to ulnar side and indicates increased carpal instability.

Scapholunate dissociation (stage 1)
- Rupture of scaphoid ligaments
- > 3-mm gap between lunate and scaphoid (Terry-Thomas sign)
- Ring sign on PA view secondary to rotary subluxation of scaphoid

Perilunate dislocation (stage 2)
- Capitate dislocated dorsally
- Lunate maintains normal articulation with radius.
- May be accompanied by transcaphoid fracture, triquetrum fracture; capitate fracture and radial styloid process fracture

Midcarpal dislocation (stage 3)
- Rupture of triquetral ligaments
- Capitate and carpus dislocated dorsally

Lunate dislocation (stage 4)
- Lunate dislocates volarly.
- Capitate appears aligned with the radius.

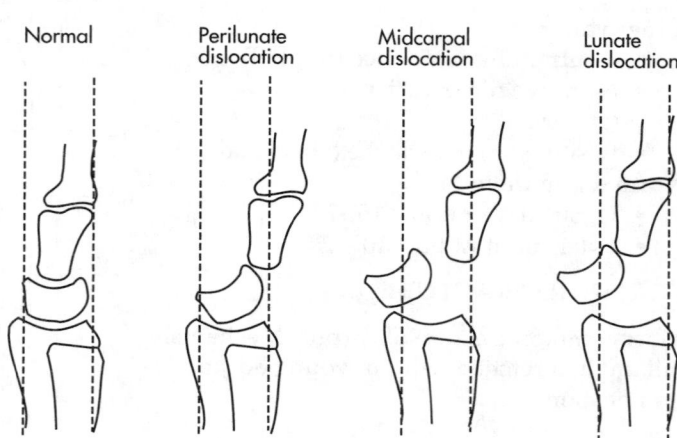

Normal   Perilunate dislocation   Midcarpal dislocation   Lunate dislocation

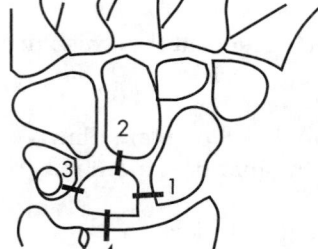

Stage 1—Scapholunate disruption
Stage 2—Capitolunate disruption
Stage 3—Triquetrolunate disruption
Stage 4—Dorsal radiocarpal disruption

CARPAL INSTABILITY

Most commonly due to ligamentous injury of the proximal carpal row (trauma or arthritis). Best diagnosed by stress fluoroscopy and/or plain film evaluation of the scapholunate and capitolunate relationships.

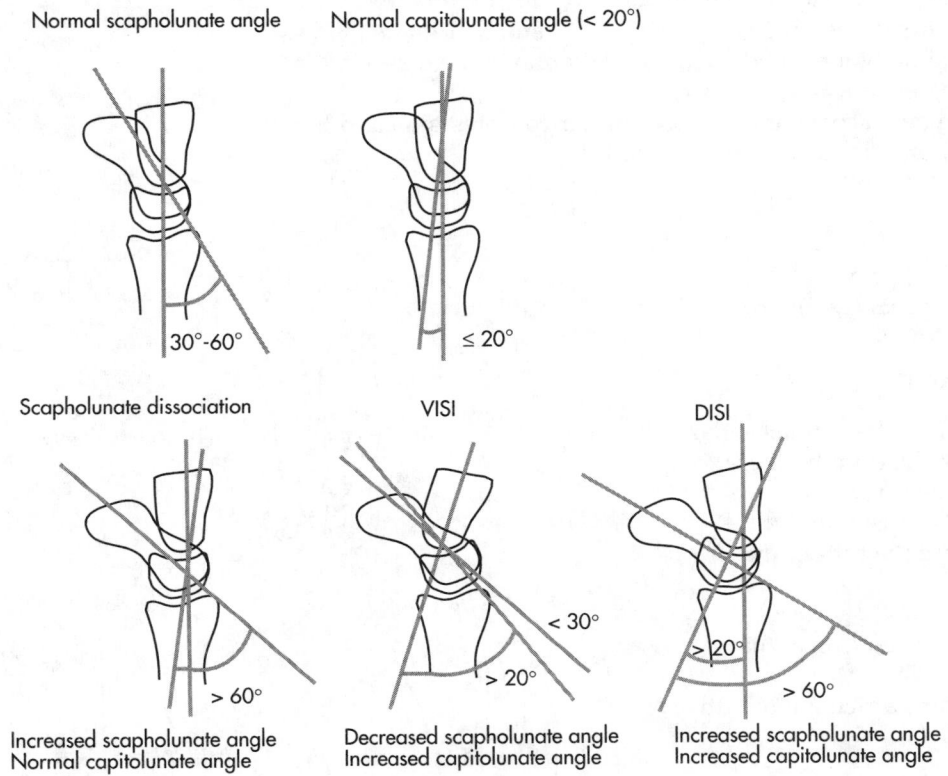

Normal scapholunate angle   Normal capitolunate angle (< 20°)

30°-60°   ≤ 20°

Scapholunate dissociation   VISI   DISI

> 60°   < 30°   > 20°
> 20°   > 60°

Increased scapholunate angle   Decreased scapholunate angle   Increased scapholunate angle
Normal capitolunate angle   Increased capitolunate angle   Increased capitolunate angle

Schapholunate dissociation
- Scapholunate angle > 60°

Volar intercalated segment instability (VISI)
- Increased capitolunate angle
- Volar tilt of lunate
- Scapholunate angle sometimes decreased
- Much less common than DISI

Dorsal intercalated segment instability (DISI)
- Increased scapholunate and capitolunate angles
- Dorsal tilt of lunate

SCALPHOLUNATE ADVANCED COLLAPSE (SLAC)

Specific pattern of osteoarthritis (OA) associated with chronic scapholunate dissociation and chronic scaphoid nonunion. CPPD is the most common etiology.

- Radial-scaphoid joint is intially involved, followed by degeneration in the unstable lunatocapitate joint as capitate subluxates dorsally on lunate.
- Radioscaphoid joint is first to be involved; capitolunate and STT joints follow.
- Capitate migrates proximally into space created by scapholunate dissociation.
- Radiolunate joint is spared.
- In end-stage SLAC the midcarpal joint collapses under compresssion and lunate assuming an extended or dorsiflexed position DISI.

HAND ANATOMY

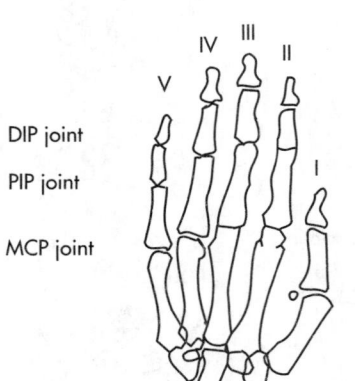

- Metacarpals
- Phalanges: distal, medial, proximal
- Joints: distal interphalangeal (DIP), proximal interphalangeal (PIP), MCP

FIRST METACARPAL FRACTURES

Bennett's and Rolando fractures are intraarticular MCP fracture dislocations of the thumb. These fractures must be distinguished from extraarticular fractures located distal to the carpometacarpal joint because the former may require open reduction.

Bennett's fracture

- Dorsal and radial dislocation (force from abductor pollicis longus)
- Small fragment maintains articulation with trapezium.

Rolando fracture

- Comminuted Bennett's fracture; the fracture line may have a Y, V, or T configuration.

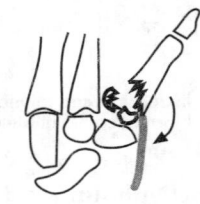

Bennett's fracture   Rolando fracture

BOXER'S FRACTURE

Fracture of the MCP neck (most commonly 5th MCP) with volar angulation and often external rotation of the distal fragment. Simple fractures are reduced externally, whereas volar comminution usually requires ORIF.

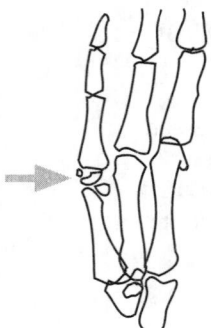

GAMEKEEPER'S THUMB (SKIER'S THUMB)

Results from disruption of ulnar collateral ligament. Often associated with a fracture of the base of the proximal phalanx. Common injury in downhill skiing (thumb gets hung up in ski pole). Stress views are required if no fracture is identified on routine plain films but is clinically suspected.

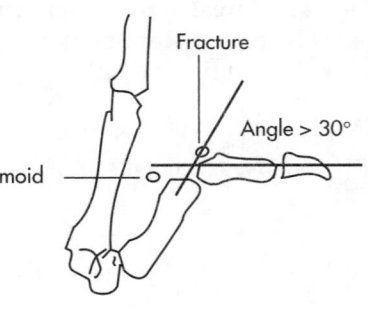

PHALANGEAL AVULSION INJURIES

Result from forceful pull at tendinous and ligamentous insertions.

Baseball (mallet) finger
- Avulsion of extensor mechanism
- DIP flexion with or without avulsion fragment

Mallet finger

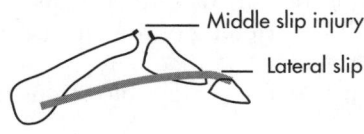

Volar plate fracture

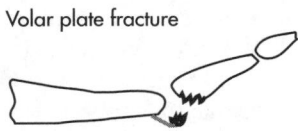

Boutonnière (buttonhole) finger
- Avulsion of middle extensor slip at base of middle phalanx
- PIP flexion and DIP extension with or without avulsion fragment

Boutonnière deformity

Middle slip injury

Lateral slip

Flexor digitorum profundus avulsion

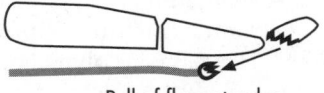

Pull of flexor tendon

Avulsion of flexor digitorum profundus
- Avulsion at volar distal phalanx
- DIP cannot be flexed.
- Fragment may retract to PIP joint.

Volar plate fracture
- Avulsion at base of middle phalanx
- PIP hyperextension

Lower Extremity

HIP ANATOMY

Acetabular lines and anatomy:
- Anterior column includes anterior aspect of the iliac wing, pelvic brim, superior pubic ramus, anterior wall of acetabulum, and teardrop. The column marker on plain radiographs are the iliopubic (iliopectineal line) and pelvic brim.
- Posterior column consists of posterior ilium, posterior wall of acetabulum, ischium, medial acetabular wall (quadrilateral plate). The marker on plain radiographs is the ilioischial line: posterior portion of quadrilateral plate of iliac bone.
- Teardrop: medial acetabular wall + acetabular notch + anterior portion of quadrilateral plate
- Roof of acetabulum
- Anterior rim of acetabulum
- Posterior rim of acetabulum

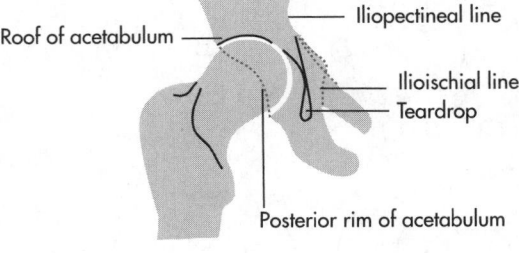

Roof of acetabulum · Iliopectineal line · Ilioischial line · Teardrop · Posterior rim of acetabulum

PELVIC FRACTURES

Classification
Stable fractures (single break of pelvic ring or peripheral fractures); more common
- Avulsion fractures
  - Anterosuperior iliac spine: sartorius avulsion
  - Anteroinferior iliac spine: rectus femoris avulsion
  - Ischial tuberosity: hamstring avulsion
  - Pubis: adductor avulsion

Other fractures
- Duverney's fracture of iliac wing
- Sacral fractures
- Fracture of ischiopubic rami: unilateral or bilateral
- Wide-swept pelvis: external rotation (anterior compression) injury to one side and an internal rotation (lateral compression) injury to contralateral side

Unstable fractures (pelvic ring interrupted in two places); less common
Significant risk of pelvic organ injury and hemorrhage. All unstable fractures require CT before fixation for more accurate evaluation; the extent of posterior ring disruption is often underestimated by plain film.

- Malgaigne fracture: SI joint (or paraarticular fracture) and ipsilateral ischiopubic ramus fracture. Clinically evident by shortening of the lower extremity.
- Straddle: involves both obturator rings
- Bucket-handle: SI fracture and contralateral ischiopubic ramus fracture
- Dislocations
- Pelvic ring disruptions and arterial injury
  - Sources of pelvic hemorrhage include arteries, veins, and osseous structures.
  - Arterial bleeding is usually from internal iliac artery branches. Frequency in descending order: gluteal, internal pudendal, lateral sacral, and obturator arteries.
  - High frequency of arterial hemorrhage in AP compression, vertical shear, crushed fracture of sacrum, and fractures extending into greater sciatic notch.

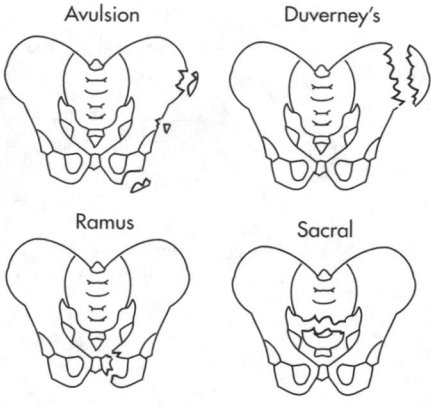

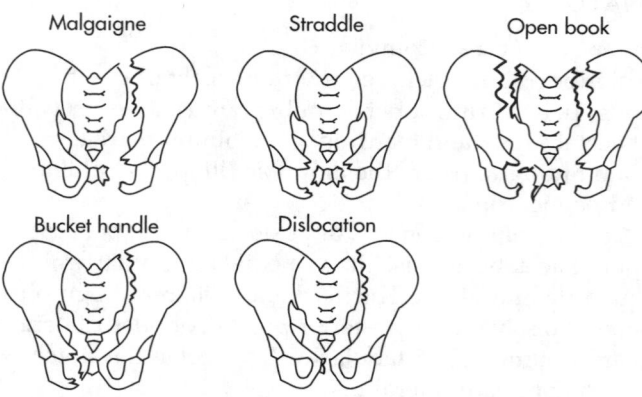

FRACTURE OF THE ACETABULUM

Classification (Letournel)
- Fracture of the anterior (iliopubic) column
- Fracture of the posterior (ilioischial) column
- Transverse fracture involving both columns
- Complex fracture: T-shaped, stellate

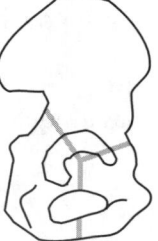
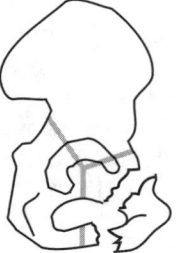
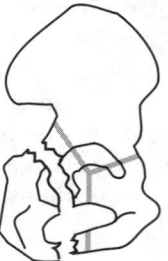

SACRAL FRACTURES

- Transverse fracture: direct trauma
- Vertical fracture: part of complex pelvic fracture
- Stress fractures: usually juxtaarticular and vertical
- One useful classification is Denis classification.
  - Zone I: lateral to foramina—50% of cases; 6% with neurological deficit
  - Zone II: Transforaminal—34% of cases; 28% with neurological deficit
  - Zone III: Central canal involvement—8% of cases; 57% with neurological deficit

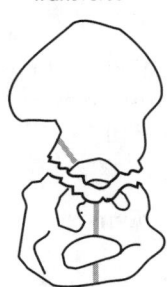
Transverse

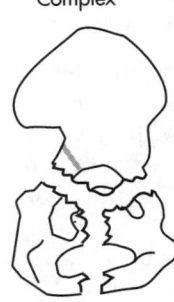
Complex

SOFT TISSUE INJURY

THIGH MUSCLES			
	Origin	Insertion	Nerve
FLEXORS (ANTERIOR)			
Iliopsoas	Vertebra/ilium	Lesser trochanter	Femoral, lumbar ventral rami
Rectus femoris	Anterior inferior iliac spine	Patellar ligament	Femoral
Vagh's group	Femur	Patellar ligament	Femoral
Sartorius	Anterior superior iliac spine	Medial tibial head	Femoral
Pectineus (adducts)	Iliopectineal line	Lesser trochanter	Femoral (obturator occasionally)
EXTENSORS (POSTERIOR)			
Adductors	Ischial tuberosity	Femur (adductor tubercle)	Obturator
Hamstrings			
Semitendinosus	Ischial tuberosity	Anteromedial tibial shaft	Tibial
Semimembranosus	Ischial tuberosity	Posteriomedial tibial condyle	Tibial
Long head biceps	Ischial tuberosity	Fibular head	Tibial
Gluteus	Ilium, sacrum, ligaments	Femur (gluteal tuberosity)	Gluteal

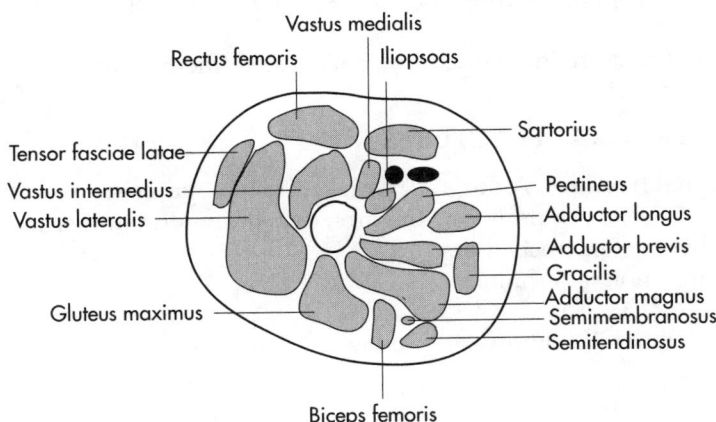

FRACTURES OF THE PROXIMAL FEMUR

Incidence: 200,000/year in the United States. Fracture incidence increases with age. In the old age group, mortality is nearly 20%.

Classification

Intracapsular fracture involving femoral head or neck

- Capital: uncommon
- Subcapital: common
- Transcervical: uncommon
- Basicervical: uncommon

Extracapsular fracture involving the trochanters

- Intertrochanteric
- Subtrochanteric

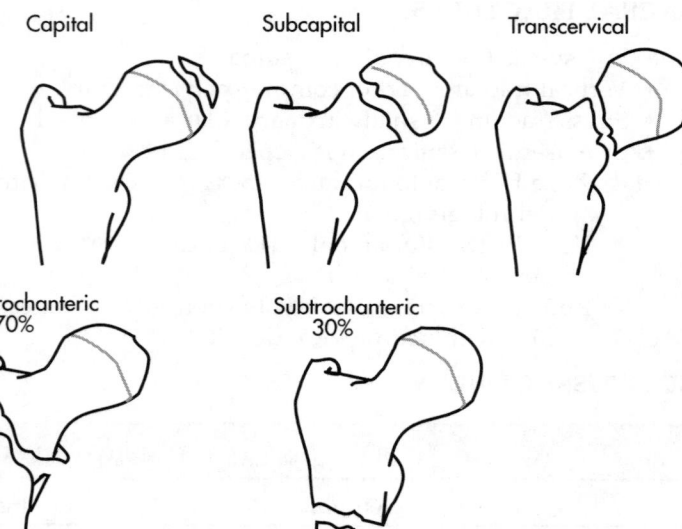

FEMORAL NECK FRACTURES

Associated with postmenopausal osteoporosis. Patients often have distal radius and/or proximal humeral fractures.

- Garden classification: based on displacement of femoral head; this classification best predicts risk of AVN and nonunion
- MRI or bone scan helpful if plain films are equivocal

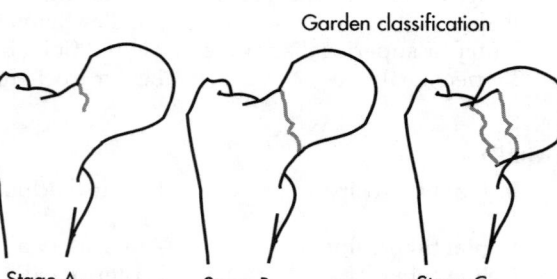
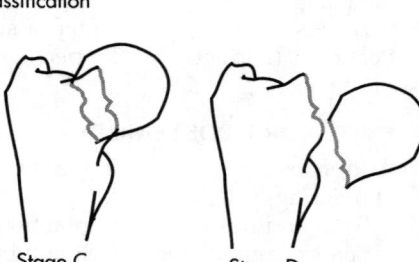

Treatment

- Bedrest: incomplete fractures
- Knowles pin
- Endoprosthesis if high risk of AVN or nonunion

Complications

- AVN (in 10%-30% of subcapital fractures) occurs secondary to disruption of femoral circumflex arteries
- Nonunion: obliquity of fracture influences prognosis (steep fractures have higher incidence of nonunion)

INTERTROCHANTERIC FEMORAL FRACTURES

Less common than subcapital fractures. Associated with senile osteoporosis.

- Simple classification: 2-, 3-, 4-, or multipart fracture, depending on number of fragments and involvement of trochanters
- Posteromedial comminution is common.

Treatment

- Internal fixation with dynamic compression screw
- Valgus osteotomy

Complications

- AVN is rare.
- Coxa vara deformity from failure of internal fixation
- Penetration of femoral head hardware as fragments collapse
- Arthritis

DISLOCATION OF THE HIP JOINT

Classification
Posterior dislocation, 90%
- Femoral head lateral and superior to the acetabulum
- Posterior rim of acetabulum is usually fractured
- Sciatic nerve injury, 10%

Anterior dislocation, 10%
- Femoral head displaced into the obturator, pubic, or iliac region

Internal dislocation
- Always associated with acetabular fracture
- Femoral head protrudes into pelvic cavity

FRACTURE OF THE DISTAL FEMUR

Classification
Supracondylar
- Nondisplaced
- Displaced
- Impacted
- Comminuted

Condylar

Intercondylar

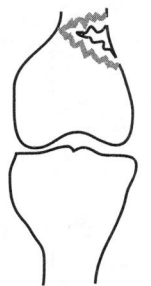 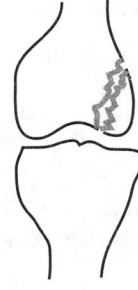 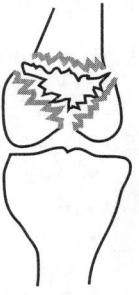

Stage A
Supracondylar

Stage B
Condylar

Stage C
Intercondylar

FRACTURE OF THE PROXIMAL TIBIA

Fender or bumper fracture: knee is struck by moving vehicle. Lateral (80%) plateau fracture is more common because most trauma results from valgus force; medial plateau fractures (10%); 10% combined medial and lateral fractures.

Classification (Müller)
- Type 1: split fracture of tibial condyle and proximal fibula (rare)
- Type 2: pure depression fracture of either plateau
- Type 3: combined types 1 and 2
- Type 4: comminuted fracture of both tibial condyles; lateral plateau is usually more severely damaged

Radiographic features
- Fractures of tibial plateau may not be obvious; plain films often underestimate the true extent of fractures; therefore CT or tomography in AP and lateral projection is often necessary
- Fat (marrow)-fluid (blood) interface sign (hemarthrosis) on cross-table lateral view
- Description of fractures:
    Type of fracture: split, depression, etc.
    Location: medial, lateral
    Number of fragments
    Displacement of fragments
    Degree of depression

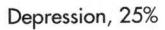 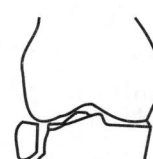 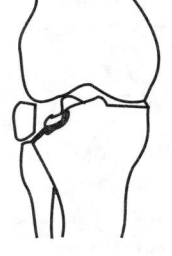

Depression, 25%   Split, 25%   Split depression, 25%

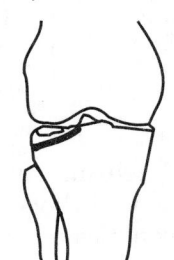

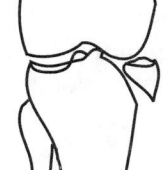 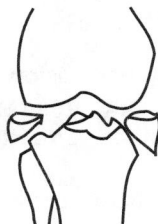

Medial condyle, 10%   Comminuted bicondylar, 10%

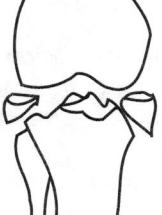

Complications
- Malunion (common)
- Secondary osteoarthritis (common)
- Concomitant ligament and meniscus injuries (i.e., MCL)
- Peroneal nerve injury

TIBIAL STRESS FRACTURE

Classic runner's fracture most commonly in proximal tibia.
- Zone of sclerosis with periosteal reaction
- Cortical thickening in posteromedial aspect of proximal tibia

FRACTURE OF THE PATELLA

Fracture classification (Hohl and Larson)
- Vertical fracture
- Transverse (most common)
- Comminuted
- Avulsed

Differentiation of multipartite patella from fractured patella:
- Bipartite or multipartite patella is typically located at the superolateral margin of the patella.
- Individual bones of a bipartite or multipartite patella do not fit together as do the fragments of a patellar fracture.
- The edges of bipartite or multipartite patella are well corticated.

OSTEOCHONDRAL AND CHONDRAL FRACTURE

Shearing, rotary, and tangential impaction forces may result in acute fracture of cartilage (chondral fracture) or cartilage and bone (osteochondral fracture).

Radiographic features
- Chondral fracture requires arthrography or MR for visualization.
- Osteochondral fracture may be seen by plain film.

OSTEOCHONDRITIS DISSECANS (CHRONIC OSTEOCHONDRAL FRACTURE)

Painful, usually unilateral, disease in children and young adults. Results from chronic trauma: a segment of articular cartilage and subchondral bone becomes partially or totally separated. Locations: lateral aspect of medial femoral condyle (75%), medial aspect of medial femoral condyle (10%), lateral aspect of lateral condyle (15%), anterior femoral condyle.

Radiographic features
- Earliest finding: joint effusion
- Radiolucent line separating osteochondral body from condyle (advanced stage)
- Normal ossification irregularity of posterior condyle may mimic osteochondritis dissecans
- Best evaluated by MRI

PATELLAR DISLOCATION

The patella normally sits in the trochlear sulcus of the distal femur. The mechanism of dislocation is usually an internal rotation of the femur on a fixed foot. Almost always lateral with disruption of medial retinaculum. Medial facet of patella impacts on anterior lateral femoral condyle.

Radiographic features
- Plain radiographs can be unremarkable except for joint effusion
- MRI is the imaging modality of choice and shows:
    Hemarthrosis
    Disruption or sprain of medial retinaculum
    Lateral patellar tilt or subluxation
    Bone contusions in lateral femoral condyle anteriorly and in medial facet of
      patella
    Osteochondral injuries of patella
    Associated injuries to ligaments and menisci in 30%

PATELLAR TENDINITIS (JUMPER'S KNEE)

Overuse syndrome occurring in athletes involved in sports that require kicking, jumping, and running. These activities can place a tremendous stress on the patellofemoral joint, with eventual necrosis, fibrosis, and degeneration of patellar tendon leading to rupture.
- MR imaging is the imaging modality of choice.
- Enlarged proximal patellar tendon with areas of increased signal intensity on T1-weighted (T1W) and T2-weighted (T2W) images

MENISCAL INJURY

The most common by injured meniscus is the medial one. The lateral meniscus is less commonly injured because it has a greater mobility. Injuries to the lateral meniscus are associated with discoid meniscus.

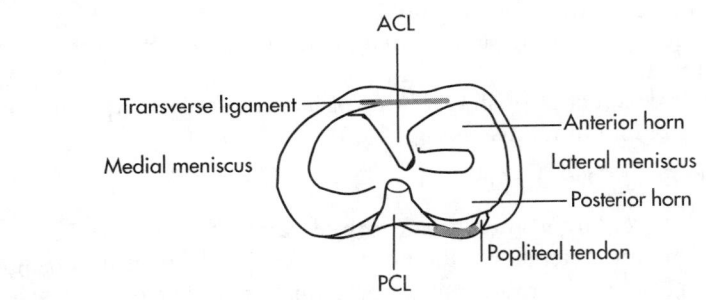

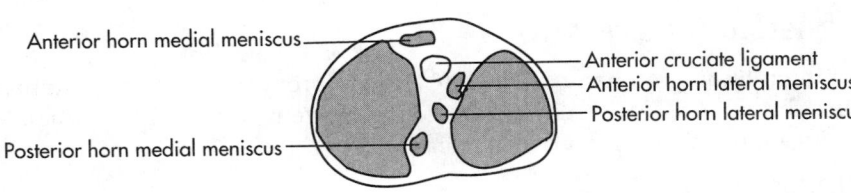

Types of meniscal injuries
- Vertical (longitudinal) tears; most commonly from acute trauma
- Horizontal tears (cleavage tears) in older patients: degenerative
- Oblique tears
- Bucket-handle: may become displaced or detached. There are characteristic signs by MRI: double posterior cruciate ligament (PCL) sign and flipped meniscus sign. The displaced fragment is typically seen within the intercondylar notch.
- Peripheral tear: meniscocapsular separation
- Truncated meniscus: resorbed or displaced fragment

MRI grading of tears

- Type 1: globular increased signal intensity, which does not communicate with articular surface. Pathology: mucinous, hyaline, or myxoid degeneration
- Type 2: linear increased signal intensity, which does not extend to articular surface. Pathology: collagen fragmentation with cleft formation
- Type 3: tapered apex of meniscus
- Type 4: blunted apex of meniscus
- Type 5: linear increased signal intensity, which extends to the articular surface. Pathology: tear
- Type 6: linear increased signal intensity, which extends to both articular surfaces
- Type 7: fragmented, comminuted meniscus

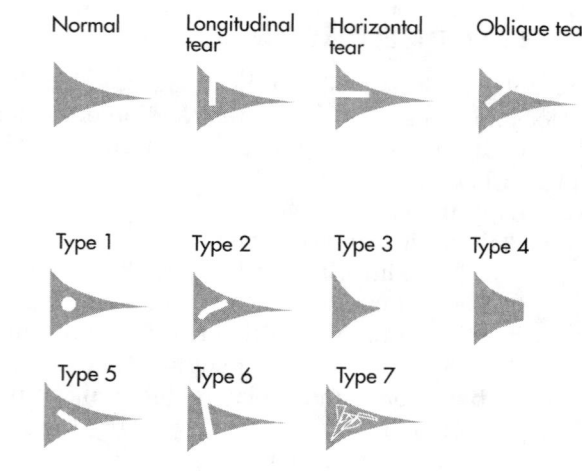

Pitfalls of diagnosing meniscal tears by MRI

- Fibrillatory degeneration of the free concave edge of the meniscal surface is often missed by MRI because of volume averaging.
- Normal transverse ligament courses through Hoffa's fat pad and may be mistaken for an anterior horn tear. The ligament connects the anterior horns of medial and lateral menisci.
- Postmeniscectomy menicis may have linear signal extending to articular surface as a result of intrameniscal signal.
- Pseudotears

    Lateral aspect of posterior horn of lateral meniscus (popliteus tendon)
    Medial lateral meniscus (ligament)

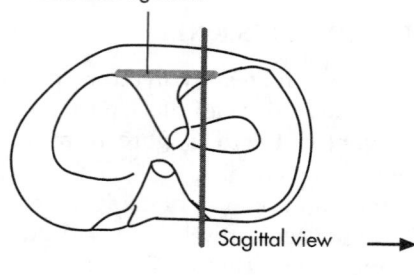
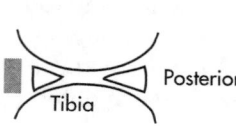

DISCOID MENISCUS

Morphologically enlarged meniscus (normal variant). Clinically presents as clicking of knee on flexion and extension. Diagnosed by MRI if three or more sagittal images show bridging between anterior and posterior horns. Prone to tears; almost always lateral.

MENISCAL CALCIFICATIONS

Common finding in many diseases (CPPD, hydroxyapatite, hyperparathyroidism, hemochromatosis, Wilson's disease, gout, collagen vascular, idiopathic). Meniscal calcification is usually not detectable by MRI.

MENISCAL CYSTS

Formed by insinuation of joint fluid through a meniscal tear into adjacent tissues; therefore meniscal cysts always occur with meniscal tears. Most common in lateral meniscus. Patient presents with knee pain and lateral joint swelling.

CRUCIATE LIGAMENT TEARS

The cruciate ligaments are intracapsular and extra-synovial. The anterior cruciate ligaments (ACL) limits anterior translation of the tibia and hyperextension. The PCL limits anterior translation of the femur and hyperflexion. ACL tears are far more common than PCL tears and are often associated with other injuries.

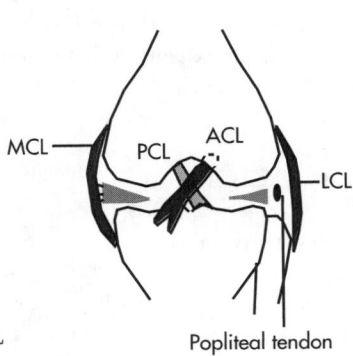

Anterior view

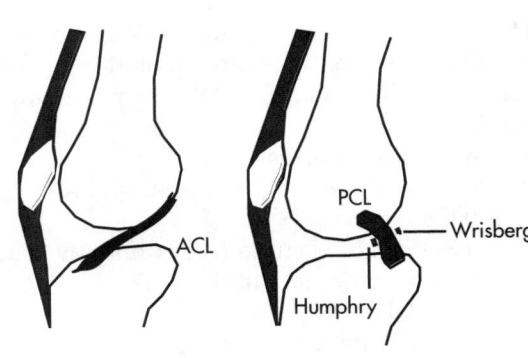

Sagittal view

Radiographic features

- Plain films may show avulsion fragment of intercondylar eminence.
- MRI is the study of choice for diagnosing ligamentous injury.
- PCL is larger than ACL and better seen by MRI.

MRI SIGNS OF ACL INJURY			
	Degree of Injury	**Direct Signs**	**Indirect Signs**
Mild sprain Moderate sprain	Ligament edema Partial tear Some fibers intact	T2 hyperintensity ACL edema/hemorrhage	Buckling of PCL ACL angulation Anterior tibial subluxation
Rupture	Complete tear	Wavy contour No ACL identified ACL discontinuity Edema/hemorrhagic mass	Lateral bone bruise MCL injury Medial meniscal injury
Chronic injury	Old mild/moderate sprains	Thickened ACL Thinned ACL Abnormal proton density signal No acute edema on T2-weighted images	Anterior tibial subluxation

SEGOND FRACTURE

Small avulsion fracture involving the superolateral surface of the proximal tibia. Frequently associated with tears of lateral capsular ligament, ACL, and menisci. Segond fracture is in midcoronal plane and must be differentiated from less common iliotibial band avulsion of Gerdy's tubercle seen more anteriorly on the tibia.

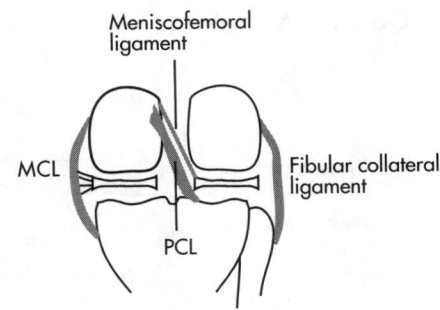

COLLATERAL LIGAMENTS

The medial collateral ligament (MCL) (injury common) is attached to medial meniscus and thus both are frequently injured together. The LCL complex (injury less common) consists of the fibular collateral ligament, the biceps femoris tendon, and the iliotibial band.

Radiographic features

- MRI criteria of injury are similar to those used for ACL and PCL tears
- O'Donoghue's triad (the "unhappy triad") results from valgus stress with rotation:
    ACL tear
    MCL injury
    Medial meniscal tear
    (lateral compartment bone bruise)
- Pelligrini-Steida lesion: curvilinear calcification or ossification at site of femoral attachment of MCL indicates old MCL injury

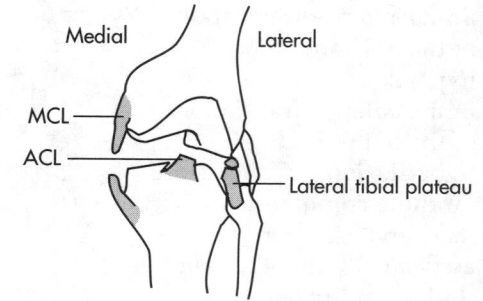

TENDON INJURY

Commonly occurs from acute trauma or overuse injury in athletes or degenerative tendinopathy in elderly.

Radiographic features

Acute tendinitis

- Tendon enlargement
- Fluid in synovial sheath (in tenosynovitis)
- Abnormal MRI signal within tendon may indicate partial tear

Chronic tendinitis

- Tendon thinning or thickening
- Intratendon signal does not increase on T2W images

KNEE DISLOCATION

- Posterior, 75%
- Anterior, 50%
- Serious vascular injury to popliteal vessels occurs in 35% and peroneal vessels in 25%.

Ankle

ANKLE ANATOMY

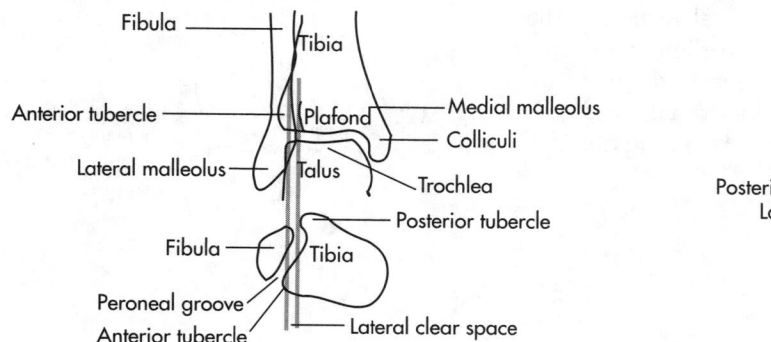

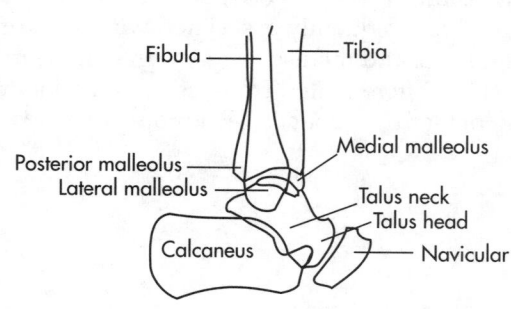

ANKLE FRACTURES

Classification

Of the different classifications of injuries available, the Weber classification is the most useful. It uses the level of fibular fracture to determine the extent of injury to the tibiofibular ligament complex. Types: Weber type A (below tibiofibular syndesmosis), Weber B (through tibiofibular syndesmosis), Weber C (above tibiofibular syndesmosis)

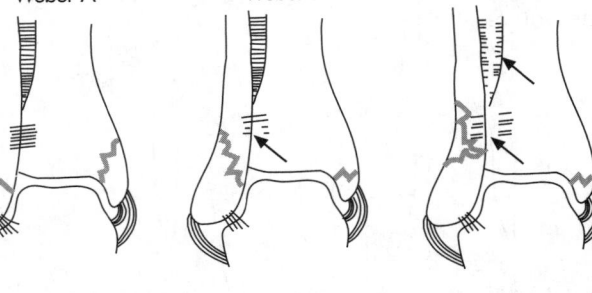

Weber A   Weber B   Weber C

Weber A
- Transverse fracture of lateral malleolus or rupture of lateral cruciate ligament (LCL)
- Oblique fracture of medial malleolus
- Tibiofibular ligament complex spared (stable)
- Results from supination-adduction (inversion)

Weber B
- Oblique or spiral fracture of lateral malleolus near the joint
- Transverse fracture of medial malleolus or rupture of deltoid ligament
- Partial disruption of tibiofibular ligament complex
- Results from supination-lateral rotation or pronation-abduction

Weber C
- Proximal fracture of fibula
- Transverse fracture of medial malleolus or rupture of deltoid ligament
- Rupture of tibiofibular ligament complex (lateral instability)
- Results from pronation-lateral rotation

Approach

1. Evaluate all three malleoli.
2. Assess ankle mortise stability (3-4 mm space over entire talus).
3. If an isolated medial malleolar injury is present, always look for proximal fibular fracture.
4. Obtain MRI or arthrography for accurate evaluation of ligaments.
5. Determine if the talar dome intact.

TIBIAL FRACTURES

Pilon fracture

Supramalleolar fractures of distal tibia that extend into tibial plafond. Usually associated with fractures of distal fibula and/or disruption of distal tibiofibular syndesmosis. Mechanism is usually due to vertical loading, e.g., in jumpers. Associated with intraarticular comminution. Complication: posttraumatic arthritis.

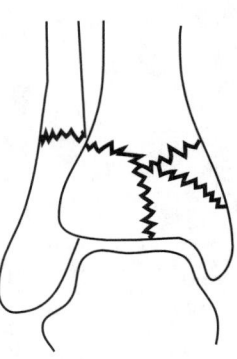

Pilon fracture

5

Tillaux fracture
Avulsion of the lateral tibial margin. In children, the juvenile Tillaux fracture is a Salter-Harris type III because the medial growth plate fuses earlier.

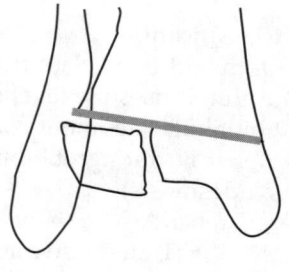

Tillaux fracture

Wagstaffe-Le Fort fracture
Avulsion of the medial margin of the fibula at the attachment of the anterior tibiofibular ligament.

Triplanar fracture
Childhood fracture with three fracture planes: vertical fracture of the epiphysis, horizontal fracture through the physis, and an oblique fracture through the metaphysis.

Triplanar fracture

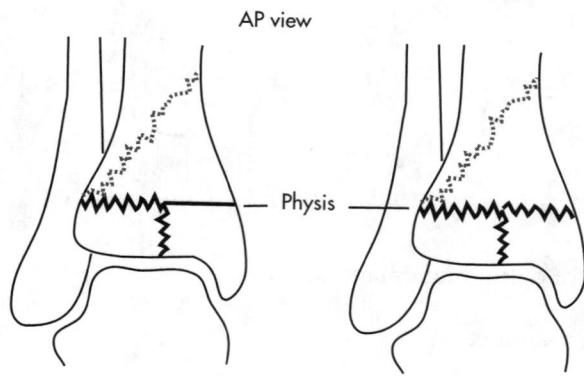

AP view

Physis

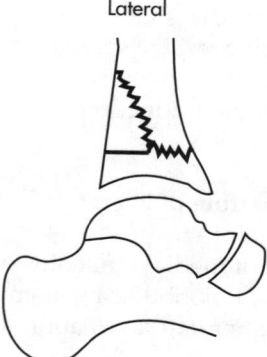

Lateral

Tibial insufficiency fracture
Occur in the distal tibia near plafond as opposed to tibial stress fractures, which occur in posterior proximal tibial diaphysis.

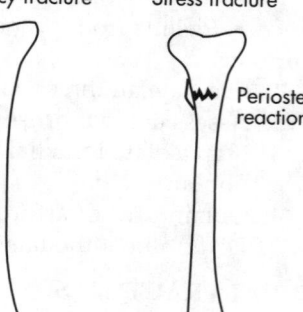

Insufficiency fracture   Stress fracture

Periosteal reaction

FIBULAR INJURY

Anatomy of ligaments

Three groups of ligaments stabilize the ankle:

Medial collateral ligament (deltoid ligament, four parts)
- Anterior tibiotalar ligament
- Posterior tibiotalar ligament
- Tibiocalcaneal ligament
- Tibionavicular ligament

Lateral-collateral ligament (three parts)
- Anterior talofibular ligament
- Posterior talofibular ligament
- Calcaneofibular ligament

Distal tibiofibular complex (most important for ankle stability)
- Anterior tibiofibular ligament
- Posterior tibiofibular ligament
- Tibiofibular syndesmosis

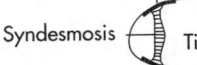

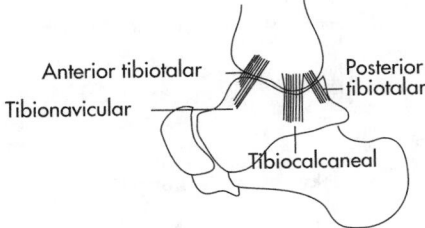

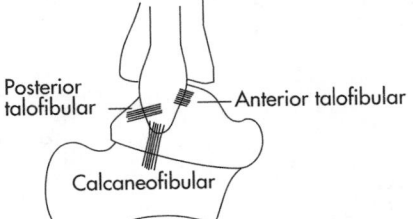

Tear of the medial collateral ligament
- Plain film: soft tissue swelling
- Lateral subluxation of the talus
- Eversion stress views (5-10 ml of 1% Xylocaine at site of maximum pain): > 20-degree talar tilt is abnormal (angle between plafond and dome of talus on AP film)
- Arthrogram: leak of contrast beneath the medial malleolus

Tear of the lateral collateral ligament
- Plain film: soft tissue swelling
- Medial subluxation of the talus
- Inversion stress views: < 15-degree talar tilt is normal
- Arthrogram: leak of contrast beneath the lateral malleolus
- The anterior talofibular ligament is the most frequently injured ankle ligament.

Tear of the distal anterior tibiofibular ligament
- Commonly associated with other ligament injuries
- Arthrogram: leak of contrast agent into the syndesmotic space

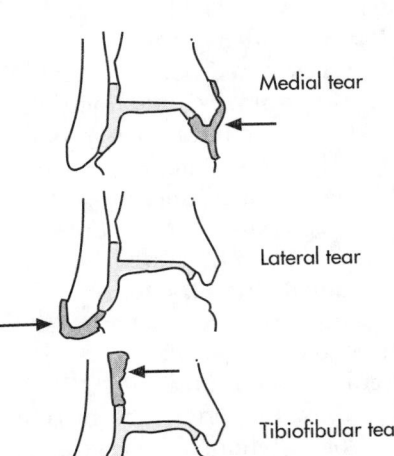

Maisonneuve's fracture

Maisonneuve's fracture is a spiral proximal fibular fracture associated with an ankle joint injury (named after a French surgeon). It is an important injury because it is easily overlooked clinically and occurs remote from the region covered by standard radiographs of ankle. The presence of this fracture type implies a ligamentous ankle injury and disruption of the syndesmosis. It is categorized as a Weber C category.

Foot

FOOT ANATOMY

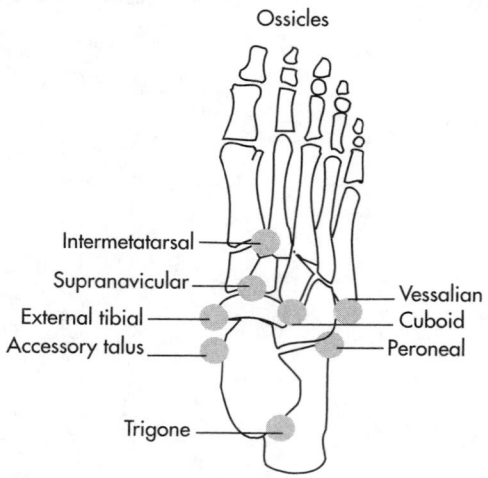

Ossicles

- Intermetatarsal
- Supranavicular
- External tibial
- Accessory talus
- Vessalian
- Cuboid
- Peroneal
- Trigone

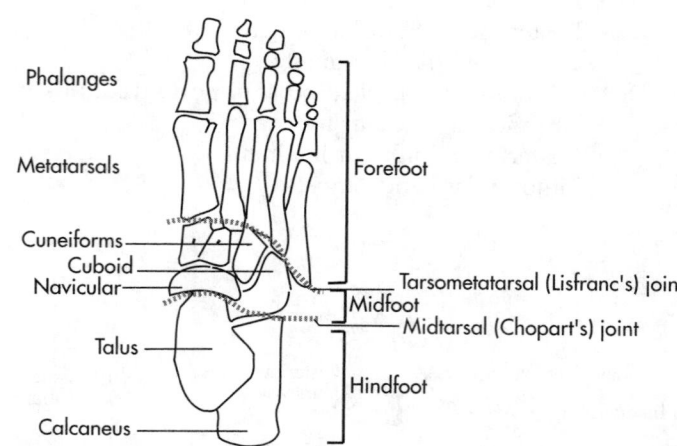

- Phalanges
- Metatarsals
- Cuneiforms
- Cuboid
- Navicular
- Talus
- Calcaneus
- Forefoot
- Tarsometatarsal (Lisfranc's) joint
- Midfoot
- Midtarsal (Chopart's) joint
- Hindfoot

CALCANEAL FRACTURES

Lover's fracture
Results from axial load (e.g., fall from height)

Radiographic features

- Decreased Boehler's angle (< 20%); normal Boehler's angle does not exclude fracture
- 75% are intraarticular (subtalar joint)
- 10% are bilateral
- Associated fractures:
    Thoracolumbar burst fracture (Don Juan fractures)
    Pilon fractures

Calcaneal stress fractures
Occurs in runners, diabetics, and elderly patients. Vertical linear appearance.

Achilles tendon tear
The Achilles tendon is formed by the confluence of the gastrocnemius and the soleus tendon. The critical zone, the site of most acute tears, is 2-6 cm proximal to its calcaneal insertion site.

- Plain radiographs show marked soft tissue swelling behind the distal tibial and ankle with obliteration of the pre-Achilles fat pad.
- MRI in partial tears shows tendon enlargement and edema, intratendinous areas of increased signal intensity on T2W and surrounding soft tissue edema.
- Incomplete tear; a tendinous gap is present and is filled with high signal blood and edema.

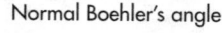

Normal Boehler's angle

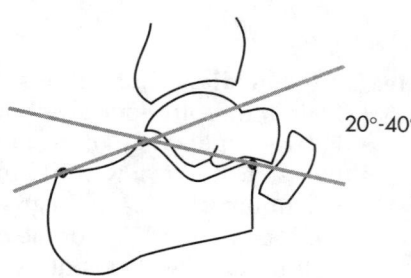

20°-40°

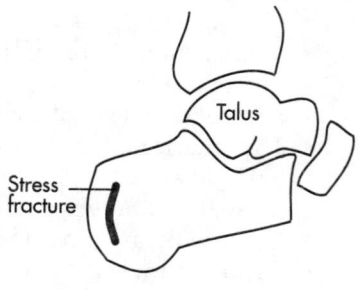

Talus

Stress fracture

Common fracture sites

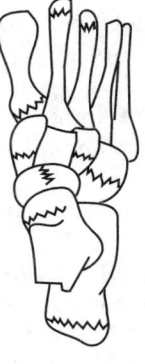

Talar fractures

Articular cartilage covers 60% of talus; there are no muscle or tendon insertions. Ligamentous avulsions are most common. Other types:

- Talar neck fracture (aviator's astralagus). Complication: proximal AVN
- Osteochondral fractures of talar dome
- Osteochondritis dissecans of talar dome

Jones fracture (dancer's fracture)

Fracture of proximal shaft of 5th metatarsal. Not due to peroneus brevis avulsion.

Nutcracker fracture of cuboid

- Cuboid fracture due to indirect compressive forces
- Occurs when abduction of forefoot compresses cuboid between bases of fourth and fifth metatarsal distally and calcaneus proximally (like nut in a nutcracker)

LISFRANC'S FRACTURE-DISLOCATION

Homolateral   Divergent

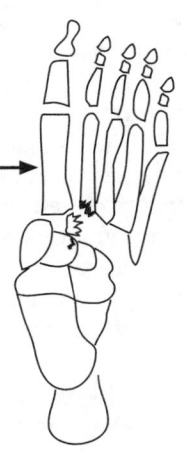
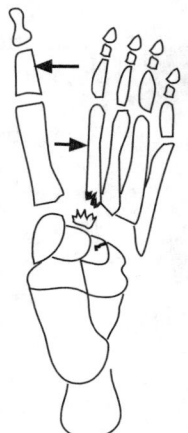

Named after Napoleon's surgeon, who described an amputation procedure at the tarsometatarsal joint. Dorsal dislocation of the tarsometatarsal joints. Most common dislocation of the foot. Usually a manifestation of a diabetic neuropathic joint (Charcot's joint). Two types: homolateral and divergent.

Radiographic features

- Homolateral: lateral dislocation of metatarsals 1-5 or 2-5
- Divergent: lateral dislocation of metatarsals 2-5 and medial dislocation of first metatarsal
- Associated fractures of base of metatarsal and cuneiform bones
- May be very subtle at early stage

Orthopedic Procedures

JOINT REPLACEMENTS

Four types of materials are used:

- Polyethylene is used for concave articular surfaces (acetabulum, tibial plateau). Usually backed by metal to provide support. Polyethylene is radiolucent.
- Silastic is used for arthroplasty implants in foot and hands. Made radiopaque during manufacture.
- Metal alloys (titanium, chromium)
- Methylmethacrylate is used as cement or is injected into the medullary space under high pressure. Made radiopaque during manufacture.

Constrained prostheses have inherent stability (ball-in-socket); unconstrained prostheses rely on normal extraarticular structures to provide stability. The more constrained a prosthesis, the higher the likelihood of loosening. The less constrained a prothesis, the more likely it will dislocate.

PROSTHETIC LOOSENING

Acute loosening is usually due to infection. Chronic loosening is due to mechanical factors, thus proper alignment is critical.

Radiographic features

- Immediate postoperative plain films are usually obtained to document position and alignment and as baseline to demonstrate progression of loosening over time.
- Widening of the radiolucency at bone-cement or metal-bone interfaces to > 2 mm indicates loosening.
- Migration of components
- Periosteal reaction
- Osteolysis is suggestive but not diagnostic of loosening.
- Cement fracture is a definite indicator of loosening.

Other complications

- Polyethylene wear
- Dislocation of prosthesis
- Hematoma
- Heterotopic bone formation
    - Frequently seen after hip surgery for degenerative disease
    - Excessive bone formation interferes with motion
- Thrombophlebitis is frequent in the immediate postoperative course.
- Foreign body granulomatous reaction
- Leakage of acrylic cement
    - Intrapelvic leakage of cement (polymerization heat induced) leads to:
        - Vascular and neurological damage
        - Necrosis
        - Genitourinary injury
    - To prevent accidental leaks, the following devices are used:
        - "Mexican hat" in acetabular drill holes
        - Wire mesh
- Infection
- Metal synovitis

HIP REPLACEMENT

Types of prosthesis

- Cemented (methyl-methacrylate) Charnely or Charnely/Miller prostheses are usually implanted in older patients; occasionally the acetabular component may be fixed with screws while the femoral compartment is cemented.
- Sintered prosthesis (bone ingrowth into porous-coated prosthesis without

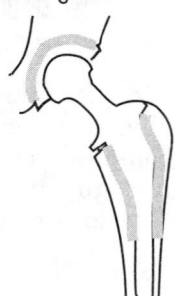

Noncemented with sintered surface for bone ingrowth

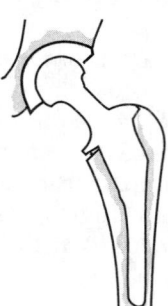

Cemented acetabular and femoral component

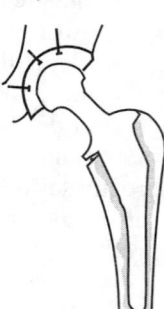

Cemented femoral component

cementing) is usually used for younger patients; loosening is difficult to assess other than by observing progressive motion of prosthesis.

- Modular prostheses are noncemented and consist of various components that optimize pressure distribution.

Types of replacements
- Total: replacement of acetabulum and femoral head
- Partial hip replacement:
    Bipolar (Bateman) prosthesis consists of cemented Charnely femoral stem with a double acetabular (bipolar) compartment; for most of the movement the femoral head articulates in the synthetic acetabulum; for extreme motion the synthetic acetabulum articulates with the real acetabulum; this prosthesis is used if the acetabulum is intact.
    Simple (unipolar) prosthesis: there is only one acetabular compartment; may have accelerated acetabular wear

Bipolar   Unipolar

Pearls
- Many prostheses, even from different manufacturers, have a similar radiographic appearance.
- When a complication is suspected and plain films are unrevealing, a bone scan should be obtained.
- Bone scans are usually positive for 6 months after surgery; after 6 months, a negative scan is good evidence against loosening, infection, or fracture. Noncemented prosthesis can remain "hot" on bone scan for up to 2 years.
- Femoral components usually loosen earlier than acetabular components.
- Infection cannot be excluded by radiographics. Joint aspiration is necessary.
- Cemented acetabular protheses almost always fail.

KNEE REPLACEMENT

Types
- Nonconstrained prostheses: replacement of articular surface; relies on intact collateral and cruciate ligaments for stability
- Semiconstrained prosthesis: provide some stability to the knee through the design of components
- Tibial component most likely to loosen

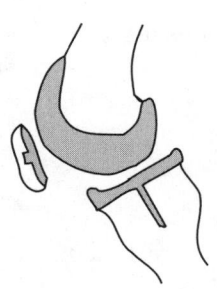

Tricompartment replacement

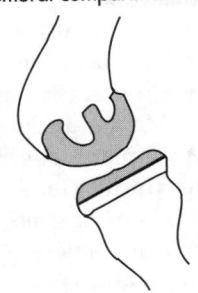

Unicondylar prosthesis with femoral compartment

OTHER PROCEDURES

Arthrodesis
- Surgical fusion of a joint
- Achieved by removing articular cartilage, internal fixation, and fixing ends of articulating bones
- Common arthrodesis: spinal fusion, wrist fusion, and knee fusion

Osteotomy
- Surgical cut through the bone to correct alignment or length
    Removal of bone for length discrepancy
    Interposition of bone for lengthening procedures
    Interposition of wedges
- Internal fixation is frequently used

Bone graft
- Used to stimulate bone growth and to provide mechanical stability
- Usually takes 1 year until the graft has been fully incorporated into the bone

SPINAL FUSION

Types

- Surgical fusion for fracture dislocation, disk disease, spondylolisthesis, scoliosis. Complications:

  Increased incidence of fracture/injury immediately above or below level of fusion

  Pseudoarthrosis

  Spinal stenosis due to bony or ligamentous overgrowth

  Osteomyelitis, diskitis
- Congenital fusion (Klippel-Feil)
- Inflammatory arthritis: juvenile rheumatoid arthritis, ankylosing spondylitis, psoriatic arthritis
- Short-term stability depends on rods; long-term stability depends on bony fusion.
- Types of Harrington rods:

  Distraction rods

  Compression rods

Arthrography

GENERAL

General principles

- Always obtain plain films before the arthrogram.
- All aspirated joint fluids should be sent for culture or other tests as indicated.
- Contrast agent is injected through long tubing.
- If the needle tip is intraarticular, the contrast should flow freely away from the needle tip.

Indications

- Ligamentous and tendinous tears
- Cartilage injuries
- Proliferative synovitis
- Masses and loose bodies
- Implant loosening

Contraindications

- Overlying skin infection
- Prior severe reaction to contrast media is a relative contraindication

Complications

- Postarthrography pain is the most common complication (sterile chemical synovitis); begins 4 hours after procedure, peaks at 12 hours, and then subsides
- Allergic reaction to contrast or lidocaine
- Infection
- Vasovagal reaction (may pretreat with atropine)

Preparation

Sterile preparation for arthrogram

- Determine puncture site fluoroscopically and mark skin.
- Scrub multiple times with povidone iodine (Betadine) and then with alcohol.
- Drape and puncture.

Sterile preparation for hip aspiration/hip replacements
- Determine puncture site fluoroscopically and mark skin.
- Patient and radiologist are fully gowned.
- Drape fluoroscopy tower.
- Scrub multiple times with povidone iodine (Betadine) and then with alcohol
- Surgical draping

Anesthesia
- Lidocaine 1%, SC
- Lidocaine is bacteriostatic: do not use if aspirating joint (i.e., total hip replacement)

Type of arthrogram
- Include epinephrine (1:1000) in contrast mixture to retard absorption (i.e., when subsequent CT is planned)
- Double-contrast arthrogram vs. single-contrast arthrogram
    Single-contrast: noncalcified loose body (calcified loose body may be missed)
    Double-contrast: cartilaginous injury (e.g., meniscus tear, labral tear)

Joint	Contrast Medium (ml)*	Epinephrine (ml)	Air (cc)	Comment
Shoulder	3	0.3	10	
Elbow	2†	For tomogram only	None	For loose body
Wrist	2†	None	None	
Hip	15	None	None	Single contrast
Knee	2	0.3	35	
Ankle	2	For tomogram only	None	

*30% lidocaine − 1% + 70% of Renografin-60 for single contrast, 1:1 mixture if followed by CT.
†For each of the three joint compartments.

SHOULDER ARTHROGRAM

Patient position
- Patient supine
- Arm externally rotated

Procedure
- 21-G spinal needle
- Aim lateral to the joint space over the medial margin of the humeral head.
- Guide needle medially off humeral head and into joint.
- Confirm intraarticular location by injection of lidocaine. An alternative way to ensure intraarticular needle placement is to have contrast material in tubing and keep air in the needle.
    Intraarticular: free flow
    Extraarticular: air bounces back

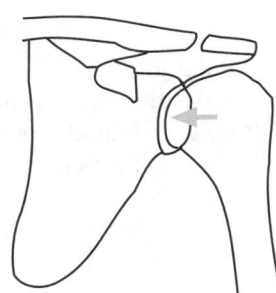

Pearls

- Elevation of contralateral side may open joint space more
- Most common problem is superficial needle placement
- Connective tissue anterior to the joint may feel very dense
- If needle is on humeral head in the correct position, it may be helpful to lessen the amount of external rotation (loosens the external capsule)

MR ARTHROGRAPHY OF THE SHOULDER

MR arthrography is performed by injecting 12 ml of a mixture of gadopentetate dimeglumine and saline (1:200 dilution) into the glenohumeral joint under fluoroscopic control. Coronal, transverse, and sagittal images are then obtained using T1W spin-echo sequences with or without fat saturation. The shoulder is placed in a neutral position or in slightly external rotation. Typical imaging parameters are as follows: section thickness, 2-3 mm; repetition time, 600 msec; echo time, < 15 msec; field of view, 130 × 180; matrix size, 180 × 256; and number of signals acquired, 2.

HIP ARTHROGRAM

Injection site

- Junction of femoral neck and head
- Puncture site is located 2 cm lateral to the femoral artery.

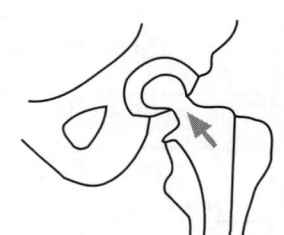

WRIST ARTHROGRAM

A complete arthrogram involves injection (25-G needle) of three separate compartments:

- Radiocarpal compartment (first injection); flexed wrist, localize midpoint of radioscaphoid space
- Midcarpal compartment (4-hour delay to allow resorption of contrast): inject space of Poirier
- Distal radioulnar joint

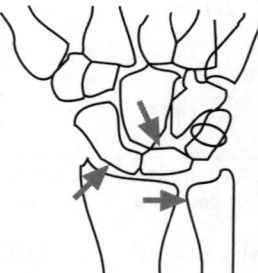

ANKLE ARTHROGRAM

- 25-G needle
- Mark midpoint tibiotalar joint and then turn the patient lateral.
- Angle 25-G needle under the anterior tibial margin (start 1 cm caudal to the tibiotalar joint on the lateral view).
- Identify and avoid the dorsalis pedis artery.

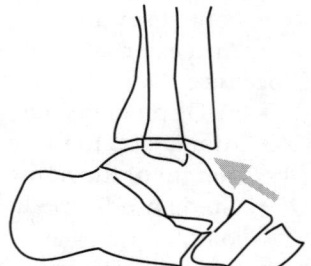

Biopsies of the Musculoskeletal System

INDICATIONS

- Primary or secondary bone tumors
- Osteitis
- Septic arthritis, diskitis

CONTRAINDICATIONS

- Bleeding diatheses
- Biopsies of inaccessible sites (odontoid process, anterior arch of C1)
- Soft-tissue infection

TECHNIQUE

A CT scan is initially performed to localize the lesion. The entry point and the pathway are determined, avoiding nerve, vascular, and visceral structures. For peripheral long-bone biopsy, the approach has to be orthogonal to the cortex. This approach angle avoids slippage with the tip of the needle. The shortest path should be chosen. For flat bones such as scapula, ribs, sternum, and skull an oblique approach angle of 30-60 degrees is used. For the pelvic girdle, a posterior approach is used avoiding the sacral canal and nerves. For vertebral body biopsy, different approach routes can be selected depending on vertebral level, the anterior route for cervical level, the transpedicular and intercostovertebral route for the thoracic level, and the posterolateral and transpedicular route for the lumbar level. For the neural posterior arch, a tangential approach is used to avoid damaging underlying neural structures.

COMPLICATIONS

- The major complication is septic osteitis. To avoid this complication, strict sterility during the intervention is mandatory.
- Hematoma
- Reflex sympathetic dystrophy
- Neural and vascular injuries
- Pneumothorax

Percutaneous Periradicular Steroid Injection

INDICATIONS

- Treatment of acute low back pain of diskogenic origin (without nerve paralysis) resistant to conventional medical therapy
- Postdiskectomy syndrome

TECHNIQUE

- Cervical level: The patient is placed in the supine position, head slightly turned and in hyperextension.
- Lumbar level: The patient is placed in prone position. The entry point and pathway are determined by CT. After local anesthesia of the skin, a 22-G spinal needle is placed under CT guidance via a posterior approach near the painful nerve root. In intracanalar infiltration, absence of cerebrospinal fluid (CSF) is verified by aspiration. Once the needle is in the epidural space, 1.5 ml of air is injected to confirm the extradural position of the needle tip. Then 2-3 ml of a long-acting steroid solution (cortivazol, 3.75 mg, is injected alone or mixed with 2 ml 0.5% lidocaine). Using precise CT guidance, dural sac perforation is avoided. However, if the dura is perforated because of an adhesion of the dural sac to the ligamentum flavum or because of a mistaken maneuver, the needle must be pulled back slightly and checked for CSF leakage. If there is none, the corticosteroid is injected without anesthetic. During injection, the patient may experience a spontaneous recurrence of pain lasting a few seconds, brought on by dural stretch.

COMPLICATIONS

- Meningitis with neurological damage (quadriplegia, multiple cranial nerve palsies, nystagmus) has been described after epidural or intrathecal injection of steroids if strict sterility is not respected. With precise CT monitoring, accidental intrathecal injection can be avoided.
- There is a risk of calcifications with use of triamcinolone hexacetonide as a long-acting steroid. This steroid is not recommended.
- At the cervical level, vertebral artery injury and intraarterial injection have been described. This can be avoided with precise CT guidance.

Percutaneous Cementoplasty

Percutaneous cementoplasty with acrylic cement (polymethylmethacrylate), also referred to as vertebral packing or vertebroplasty, is a procedure aimed at preventing vertebral body crushing and pain in patients with pathological vertebral bodies.

INDICATIONS

- Symptomatic vertebral angioma
- Painful vertebral body tumor (particularly metastasis and myeloma), especially when there is a risk of compression fracture
- Severe, painful osteoporosis with loss of height or compression fracture of the vertebral body or both

CONTRAINDICATIONS

- Hemorrhagic diathesis
- Infection
- Lesions with epidural extension require careful injection to prevent epidural overflow and spinal cord compression by the cement.

COMPLICATIONS

- The major complication is a cement leak.
- Infection
- Patients experience temporary pain after the procedure but are usually free of symptoms within 24 hours. The postprocedural pain is usually proportional to the volume of cement injected. The majority of the patients have good packing of the vertebral body with more than 4 ml of acrylic cement injected.
- Allergic reactions, hypertension

Bone Tumors

General

APPROACH TO TUMORS

1. Determine aggressiveness (pattern of destruction and repair)
2. Tissue characterization by matrix (usually by CT)
3. Location of lesion
4. Age of patient

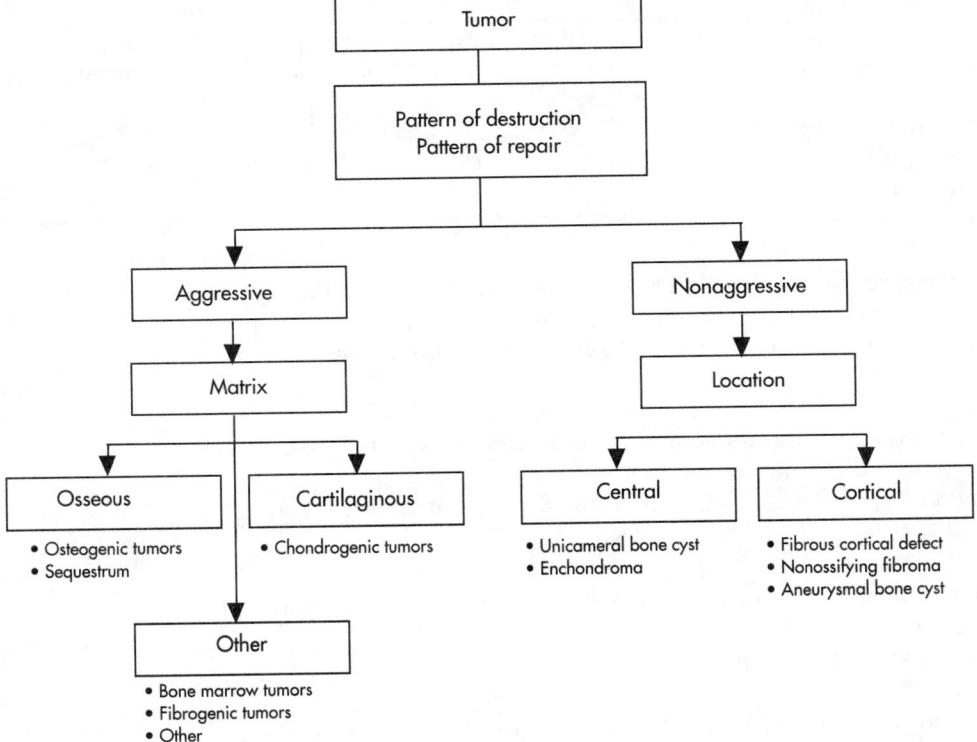

Some features have a higher diagnostic specificity than others. The most important ones are:

- Pattern of destruction (malignant vs benign)
- Pattern of matrix (to determine origin as osseous, cartilaginous, fibrous)

Pattern of bone destruction

Most important factor in determining the rate of growth or aggressiveness of the tumor. Cortical penetration is indicative of an aggressive lesion. Pattern types:

Geographic lytic pattern
- Well-delineated, circumscribed hole in the bone
- Sclerotic rim indicates relatively slow growth
- An ill-defined or wide transition zone indicates a moderately aggressive process.

Moth-eaten pattern
- Numerous small holes of varying size in cortical and trabecular bone
- Reflects aggressive behavior

Permeative pattern
- Numerous elongated holes along the cortex
- Occasionally, only a decrease in cortical bone density is visible.
- Reflects aggressive behavior

Pattern of bone repair

New bone (osteoblastic activity) is formed in response to destruction:

Periosteal response

Buttressing (wavy periostitis; benign lesion)
- Thick, single layer of periosteal reaction
- Indicates slow growth or benignity
- Nonspecific: hypertrophic pulmonary osteoarthropathy (HPO), atherosclerosis, benign tumors)

Aggressive patterns
- Seen with rapidly progressive lesions such as malignancy or osteomyelitis
  Lamination (onion-peel). Periosteum appears in layers.
  Codman's triangle. Periosteum forms bone only at the margin of the tumor.
- Spiculations
  Sunburst pattern is seen in aggressive malignant lesions; spiculations commonly point to the center of the lesion.
  Hair-on-end pattern is seen with lesions that invade the marrow cavity in long bones.

Endosteal response
- Thick rim of new bone indicates benign, slow growth (e.g., nonossifying fibroma [NOF], osteoma, Brodie abscess, fibrous dysplasia).
- Thin rim or no rim indicates a more active lesion.
- Mottled appearance
  Results from bone intermingled with a permeative or moth-eaten pattern of destruction
  Indicates invasiveness (malignant and nonmalignant causes)

Tissue characterization

Tumor matrix refers to the neoplastic intercellular substance produced by tumor cells. CT is often required to adequately define the matrix. For example, an increased tumor density on plain film may be due to osteoid matrix or periosteal/endosteal response.

TUMOR MATRIX DEFINITION		
Matrix	**Benign**	**Malignant**
OSTEOID MATRIX Does not always mineralize Mineralization is dense homogenous, cloudlike	Osteoid osteoma Osteoblastoma Osteochondroma Bone island	Osteosarcoma
CHONDROID MATRIX Does not always calcify Calcifications in the form of arcs or circles	Enchondroma Osteochondroma (cap) Chondroblastoma Chondromyxoid fibroma	Chondrosarcoma
INTERMEDIATE MATRIX Diffuse uniform mineralization: ground glass	Fibrous dysplasia Osteoblastoma	Osteosarcoma
CELLULAR MATRIX No calcification Radiolucent lesions	Fibrous tumors	Round cell tumors Fibrous tumors

Pearls

- Mineralization of chondroid and osteoid matrix in tumors is often central (mature center, peripheral growth).
- Mineralization in benign lesions (e.g., bone infarcts, myositis ossificans) is often peripheral.

Chondroid 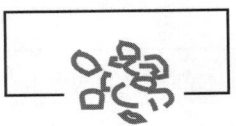   Osteoid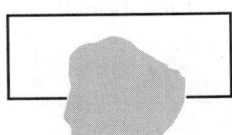

Location of a lesion in the skeleton

As a general rule, most primary tumors arise in areas of rapid growth (distal femur, proximal tibia, humerus), whereas metastases occur in well-vascularized red bone marrow (spine, iliac wings). The following tumors have a predilection for typical locations:

- Enchondromas: phalanges
- Osteosarcoma, giant cell tumor: around the knee
- Hemangioma: skull and spine
- Chondrosarcoma: innominate bone
- Chordoma: sacrum and clivus
- Adamantinoma: mid-tibia

Location within anatomical regions

- Epiphysis: typical are cartilaginous and articular lesions such as chondroblastoma or eosinophilic granuloma (EG)
- Metaphysis: lesions of different etiologies (e.g., neoplastic, inflammatory, metabolic) have a predilection for the metaphysis (rich blood supply); therefore this location alone is of limited differential diagnostic value
- Epiphyseal/metaphyseal region: giant cell tumors
- Diaphysis: after the 4th decade of life, most solitary diaphyseal bone lesions involve the bone marrow

Axial location within a bone

Refers to the position of the lesion with respect of the long axis of the bone.

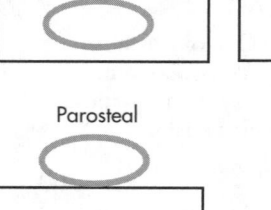

Central   Eccentric   Cortical

Parosteal

- Central lesions (usually benign)
    Enchondroma
    Unicameral bone cysts
    EG
- Eccentric lesions
    Aneurysmal bone cyst (ABC)
    Osteosarcoma
    NOF
    Giant cell tumor (GCT)
    Chondromyxoid fibroma
- Cortical lesions (most commonly benign)
    Cortical defect
    Cortical desmoid
    Osteoid osteoma
    Periosteal chondroma
- Parosteal lesions
    All osseous, cartilaginous and fibrous malignancies
    Osteochondroma
    Myositis ossificans (should be separate from bone)

INCIDENCE

The numbers in the following table indicate the approximate percentage of tumors in that location.

INCIDENCE OF TUMORS BY LOCATION*								
Tumor	Femur	Tibia	Foot	Humerus	Radius	Hand	Spine	Skull
Osteoid osteoma	30	25	10	5	1	10	5	1
Osteoblastoma	15	10	10	5	1	5	40	15
Osteosarcoma	40	15	1	15	< 1	< 1	2	5
Chondroma	10	3	5	5	2	55	1	1
Chondroblastoma	35	20	10	20	1	20	1	1
Chondrosarcoma	25	10	2	10	1	3	5	3
NOF	40	45	1	5	1	1	—	1
Fibrosarcoma	40	15	2	10	1	< 1	5	5
GCT	35	30	2	5	10	5	5	1
Malignant fibrous histiocytoma	45	20	2	10	1	—	2	5
Hemangioma	5	3	5	3	1	2	25	35
Hemangiopericytoma	10	—	5	15	5	2	10	5
Neurofibroma	—	5	—	2	—	—	5	75
Chordoma	—	—	—	—	—	—	75	25
Simple cyst	30	5	1	55	1	1	—	—
ABC	15	15	10	10	3	5	15	5
Adamantinoma	3	80	1	5	1	1	—	—
Ewing's tumor	40	30	3	10	2	1	5	1

*All numbers represent percentage of bone tumors in that location.

BONE BIOPSIES

- Two general types of needles are used:
    Needles to cut through cortical bone (Trephine, Turkell, Ackerman)
    Needles for predominantly soft tissue masses (True-Cut, spinal needle)
- Soft tissue biopsies are preferable over bone biopsies.
- The needle tip should hit the bone at a right angle, otherwise the needle tends to slide off the bone.
- Always biopsy the part of the lesion that will be resected. Likewise, the needle track should be within the surgical field (tumor seeding is rare but has been reported particularly with chondroid lesions and chordoma). Therefore all biopsies require consultation of orthopedic surgeon regarding surgical approach.
- Complications: 1%-10%

Bone-Forming Tumors

OSTEOID OSTEOMA

The clinical hallmark of the lesion is pain (increased prostaglandins), especially at night, that is improved with aspirin. Age: 5-25 years. Treatment: surgical excision, percutaneous thermal, or drill ablation. Preferred treatment currently is percutaneous radio frequency ablation. Failure to remove entire lesion may lead to recurrence. Location: femur and tibia 55%, hands and feet 20%; 80% intracortical.

Radiographic features
- Radiolucent nidus < 2 cm in diameter (may contain bone matrix)
- Nidus surrounded by sclerosis; the sclerosis may obscure the detection of the nidus on plain films
- Lesion located on concave side in patients with painful scoliosis
- Synovitis may occur with periarticular or intracapsular lesions.
- Limb overgrowth in children
- CT is the study of choice for identifying number and location of nidus.
- Bone scan: hot spot
- Angiography: nidus has dense blush
- MRI: may have extensive reactive marrow edema

OSTEOBLASTOMA

Histologically similar to osteoid osteoma but radiographically distinct. Age: < 30 years (80%). Treatment: curettage. Two appearances:
- Expansile lytic
- Sclerotic > 2 cm (giant osteoid osteoma)

DIFFERENTIATION OF OSTEOBLASTOMA VS OSTEOID OSTEOMA		
	Osteoblastoma	Osteoid Osteoma
Clinical	Rare	Common
	Rapidly increasing in size	Limited growth potential
	Pain inconsistent	Pain persistent (nocturnal)
Radiology	Expansile or > 2 cm	< 2 cm
	Variable sclerosis	Peripheral sclerosis sclerosis

5

Location
- Spine (posterior elements)   40%
- Long bones appendicular skeleton   30%
- Hand and feet   15%
- Skull and face   15%

Radiographic features
- Dense sclerotic bone reaction > 2 cm
- Expansile, well-circumscribed lesion similar to ABC
- Variable central calcification and matrix
- Malignant, aggressive osteoblastoma may disrupt cortex and have a soft tissue component (may mimic an osteosarcoma).

OTHER BENIGN BONE-FORMING LESIONS

Bone island (enostosis)
Cortical type bone within cancellous bone. Islands may be 1-4 cm in size. Homogeneously dense, well marginated. May be warm on bone scan.

Osteopoikilosis
Multiple epiphyseal enostoses.

Osteoma
Localized masses of mature bone on the endosteal or periosteal surface of cortex, commonly in the skull or paranasal sinuses. Associated with Gardner's syndrome.

OSTEOSARCOMA (OSA)

Second most frequent primary malignant bone tumor after multiple myeloma. Incidence: < 1000 new cases/year in United States. Age: 10-30 years. Clinical: pain, mass, fever. 5-year survival: parosteal 80% > periosteal 50% > conventional 20% > telangiectatic < 20%.

Types
Primary osseous OSA (95%)
- Conventional OSA
- Low-grade central OSA
- Telangiectatic OSA
- Small cell OSA
- Multicentric OSA

Juxtacortical OSA
- Parosteal OSA
- Periosteal OSA
- High-grade surface OSA

Secondary OSA
- Paget's disease
- Prior radiation (3-50 years after radiation)
- Dedifferentiated chondrosarcoma

Location of conventional OSA
- Tubular bones, 80%
    - Femur, 40% (75% of which occur around the knee)
    - Tibia, 15%
    - Humerus, 15%
- Other bones, 20%
    - Flat bones
    - Vertebral bodies

Radiographic features
- Poorly defined, intramedullary, metaphyseal mass lesion that extends through the cortex
- Matrix:
    Osteoid (osteoblastic OSA), 50%
    Chondroid matrix (chondroblastic OSA), 25%
    Spindle cell stroma (fibroblastic OSA), 25%
- Aggressive periosteal reaction: Codman's triangle, sunburst pattern
- Bone scan: increased uptake with activity extending beyond the true margins of the tumor (thought to be related to hyperemia)
- Skin lesions and metastases best detected by bone scan or MRI
- Pulmonary metastases best detected by high-resolution CT

Pearls
Role of imaging
- Presumptive diagnosis of OSA is made by plain film
- CT useful for evaluation of matrix, cortical penetration, and occasionally for biopsy
- MRI and bone scan are useful for staging.
- MRI may be better than CT for determining tumor margins.

Goals of cross-sectional imaging
- Determine extent of tumor within bone marrow and soft tissue
- Determine relationship to vessels and nerves
- Evaluate adjacent joints
- Detect skip lesions
- Provide measurements needed for surgery

Telangiectatic OSA
Purely lytic lesion that lacks the highly aggressive appearance of a conventional OSA (tumor matrix, periosteal reaction) but is actually much more malignant and carries a worse prognosis.

Radiographic features
- Large lytic lesion
- Cystic cavities filled with blood and/or necrosis
- May mimic ABC

Multicentric OSA
Synchronous osteoblastic OSA at multiple sites. Has a tendency to be metaphyseal and symmetrical. Occurs exclusively in children ages 5-10. Extremely poor prognosis.

Parosteal OSA
Low-grade OSA that occurs in an older age group (80% between 20-50 years). Locations similar to conventional OSA.

Radiographic features
- Posterior distal femur, 65%
- Attached to underlying cortex only at origin
- May wrap around bone
- Distinguishable from myositis ossificans by its zonal ossification; more mature ossification is located centrally but is located peripherally in myositis ossificans

Periosteal osteosarcoma
Intermediate grade OSA. Most commonly diaphyseal.
Radiographic features
- No medullary involvement
- Cortical thickening or "saucerization"
- Entire tumor closely apposed to cortex

Cartilage-Forming Tumors

ENCHONDROMA

Benign cartilaginous neoplasm in the medullary cavity. Most echondromas are asymptomatic but may present as pathological fractures. Peak age is 10-30 years.

Location
- Tubular bones (hand, foot): 50%
- Femur, tibia, humerus

Radiographic features
- Lytic lesion in bones of the hand or foot
- Chondroid calcifications: rings and arcs pattern ("O" and "C")
- Scalloped endosteum
- Expansion of cortex but no cortical breakthrough unless fractured
- No periosteal reaction or soft tissue mass

Pearls
- In the absence of a fracture, a painful enchondroma is considered malignant until proven otherwise.
- Malignant transformation occurs but is rare.
- Malignant transformation is more likely in central lesions.

ENCHONDROMATOSIS (OLLIER'S DISEASE)

Nonhereditary abnormality in which multiple enchondromas are present. Many lesions become stable at puberty. Risk of malignant transformation to chondrosarcoma is 25%.

Radiographic features
- Multiple radiolucent expansile masses in hand and feet
- Hand and foot deformity
- Tendency for unilaterality

MAFFUCCI'S SYNDROME

Enchondromatosis and multiple soft tissue hemangiomas. Unilateral involvement of hands and feet. Malignant transformation is much more common than in Ollier's disease.

OSTEOCHONDROMA (OSTEOCARTILAGINOUS EXOSTOSIS)

Cartilage-covered bony projection (exostosis) on the external surface of a bone. Most common benign bone lesion. Osteochondromas have their own growth plate and stop growing with skeletal maturity. Age: < 20 years (adolescence) in 80% (10-35 years; male:female = 2:1). Symptoms are those of a slowly growing painless tumor. Treatment: surgical resection if complications are present. Location: any bone with enchondral ossification but most commonly (85%): tibia, femur, humerus.

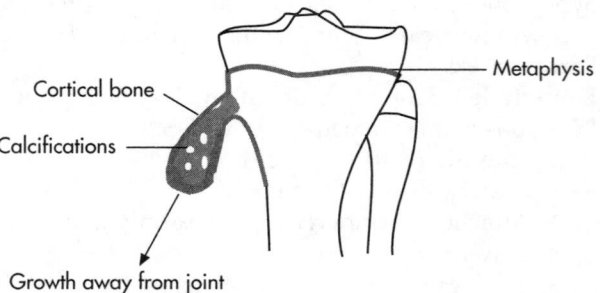

Radiographic features

Two types:

- Pedunculated: slender pedicle directed away from growth plate
- Sessile (broad base)

Characteristic findings:

- Continuous with parent bone:
    Uninterrupted cortex
    Continuous medullary bone
- Calcification in the chondrous portion of cap; may be cauliflower-like
- Metaphyseal location (cartilaginous origin)
- Lesion grows away from joint
- MR imaging demonstrates cortical and medullary continuity between the osteochondroma and the parent bone as a distinctive feature.
- MR imaging is the best imaging modality for visualizing the effect of the lesion on surrounding structures and for evaluating the hyaline cartilage cap. Mineralized areas in the cartilage cap remain low signal intensity with all MR pulse sequences, although as enchondral ossification proceeds, yellow marrow signal is ultimately apparent.

Complications

- Pressure on nerves and blood vessels
- Pressure on adjacent bone: deformation, fractures
- Overlying bursitis
- Malignant transformation (in < 1%). Suspect if:
    Pain in the absence of fracture, bursitis, or nerve compression
    Growth of lesion after skeletal maturation
    > 1 cm of cartilaginous cap by CT, > 2 cm by MRI
    Dispersed calcifications in the cap
    Enlargement of lesion
    Increased uptake on bone scan (unreliable)

MULTIPLE OSTEOCARTILAGINOUS EXOSTOSES (MOCE)

- Hereditary autosomal-dominant disease
- Knee, ankle, and shoulder are usually involved.
- Typically sessile and metaphyseal in location
- May simulate appearance of bone dysplasia
- Complications
    Severe growth abnormalities
    Malignant transformation is rare, but higher than in solitary osteochondromas (especially proximal lesions). Malignant transfomation is usually into chondrosarcoma.

DYSPLASIA EPIPHYSEALIS HEMIMELICA (TREVOR'S DISEASE)

Intraarticular epiphyseal osteochondromas. Usually unilateral.

CHONDROBLASTOMA (CODMAN TUMOR)

Uncommon benign neoplasm that occurs almost exclusively in the epiphysis in immature skeleton. Location: around knee, proximal humerus. Treatment: curettage.

CHONDROMYXOID FIBROMA

Uncommon benign neoplasm that consists mainly of fibrous tissue mixed with chondroid and myyoid tissue. Lesion typically appears geographic and lytic, cartilaginous matrix is rarely seen. Location: 50% around knee. Treatment: curettage.

CHONDROSARCOMA

Malignant cartilage-producing tumor. Mean age: 40-45 years. Most are low-grade asymptomatic tumors that are found incidentally. Location:
- 45% in long bones, especially the femur
- 25% innominate bone, ribs
- Most occur in the metaphysis but may extend to the epiphysis

Radiographic features
- Lytic mass that may or may not have chondroid matrix
- Medullary (central) chondrosarcomas arise within cancellous bone or the medullary cavity; may appear totally lytic.
- Exostotic (peripheral)) chondrosarcoma arises in the cartilage cap of a previously benign osteochondroma or exostoses; these tumors commonly have a chondroid matrix and an extraosseous soft tissue mass.
- Dedifferentiated chondrosarcoma is a high-grade tumor that frequently contains large areas of noncalcified tumor matrix.
- Degeneration to fibrosarcoma, MFH, or OSA in 10%

Fibrous Lesions

FIBROUS CORTICAL DEFECTS (FCD) AND NONOSSIFYING FIBROMA (NOF)

FCD and NOF are histologically identical (whorled bundles of connective tissue), cortically based lesions that differ only in the amount of medullary involvement. With time, lesions may sclerose and shrink.

DIFFERENTIAL DIAGNOSIS OF FCD AND NOF		
Parameter	**FCD**	**NOF**
Age	4-7 years	10-20 years
Location	Cortex	Medullary involvement
Size	1-4 cm (small)	1-7 cm (large)
Clinical	Clinically silent	May cause pain, fracture
Treatment	None	Curettage if symptomatic

Radiographic features
- Radiolucent cortical lesion with normal or sclerotic margins
- Well-demarcated peripheral osseous shell
- Metaphyseal location: close to the growth plate, usually posteromedially
- Tibia and fibula are most commonly affected (90%)

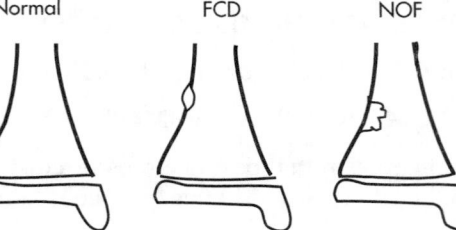
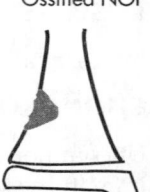

Normal   FCD   NOF   Ossified NOF

FIBROUS DYSPLASIA (LICHTENSTEIN-JAFFE DISEASE)

Benign, developmental anomaly in which the medullary cavity is replaced with fibrous material, woven bone, and spindle cells. Age: 5-20 years. Fibrous dysplasia does not spread or proliferate; malignant transformation is rare (0.5%).

Associations
- Endocrine disorders
  - Hyperthyroidism
  - Hyperparathryoidism
  - McCune-Albright syndrome (precocious puberty)
- Soft tissue myxomas (Mazabraud syndrome)

Types
- Monostotic form, 85%
  - Femur (most common)
  - Tibia, ribs
  - Craniofacial
- Polyostotic form, 15% (peak age 8 years)
  - Femur, 90%
  - Tibia, 80%
  - Pelvis, 80%
  - Craniofacial

Radiographic features
- Radiolucent expansile medullary lesions
- Degree of lucency depends on the amount of osteoid
- Typical ground-glass appearance is due to dysplastic microtrabeculae, which are not individually visible.
- Well-defined sclerotic margins, endosteal scalloping
- Bowing deformities: biomechanically insufficient bone (shepherd's crook deformity)
- Base-of-skull lesions tend to be sclerotic (in contrast to lucent lesions elsewhere).
- Frontal bossing, facial asymmetry
- Polyostotic form is often unilateral or monomelic.
- Bone scan: hot lesions

Variants
- Cherubism
  - Symmetrical involvement of mandible and maxilla
  - Familial inheritance
- McCune-Albright syndrome
  - Polyostotic unilateral fibrous dysplasia
  - Endocrine abnormalities (precocious puberty, hyperthryoidism)
  - Café au lait spots (coast of Maine)
  - Predominantly in girls
- Leontiasis ossea (craniofacial fibrous dysplasia)
  - Involvement of facial and frontal bones
  - Leonine facies (resembling a lion)
  - Cranial nerve palsies
- Fibrous dysplasia (pseudoarthrosis of the tibia)
  - Young infants
  - Anterior tibial bowing
  - Pathologic fracture and subsequent pseudoarthrosis

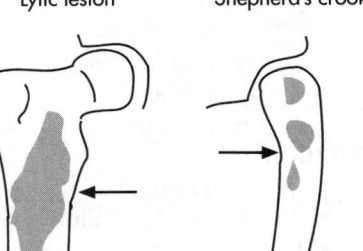

Lytic lesion   Shepherd's crook

Complications
- Pathological fractures
- Limb or growth deformity
- Sarcomatous transformation (very rare)

Pearls
- Fibrous dysplasia can mimic a variety of bone lesions.
- Pelvic involvement nearly always indicates polyostotic form; therefore the ipsilateral femur is usually also involved.
- Painful fibrous dysplasia usually indicates the presence of a fracture.

OSSIFYING FIBROMA

Histologically and radiologically in the spectrum of fibrous dysplasia, osteofibrous dysplasia, and adamantinoma. Diagnosis is established by pathology. The former ossifying fibroma of the jaw is now classified as an ameloblastoma.

Radiographic features
- Expansile cortical lesion of anterior tibial diaphysis
- Identical radiographic features of adamantinoma
- Occurs in younger age group than adamantinoma

DESMOPLASTIC FIBROMA (INTRAOSSEOUS DESMOID)

Histologically identical to soft tissue desmoid. Age: 50% occur in 2nd decade. Location: metaphyses, pelvis, mandible.

Radiographic features
- Expansile lytic lesion containing thick septations
- Difficult to distinguish from low-grade fibrosarcoma

MALIGNANT FIBROUS HISTIOCYTOMA (MFH)

Osseous MFH originate from histiocytes in the bone marrow. Although MFH is the most common soft tissue sarcoma in adults, osseous MFH is rare. Age: 40-60 years. The tumor has a poor prognosis because of the high frequency of local recurrence (up to 80%) and hematogenous metastases to regional lymph nodes and distant sites (lungs > liver > brain, heart, kidney, adrenal glands, GI tract, bone). Osseous MFH may be:
- Primary
- Secondary
    - Paget's disease
    - Dedifferentiation of a chondrosarcoma
    - Bone infarct
    - Postradiation

Location
- Bone MFH (rare): skeletal location of MFH is similar to that of osteosarcoma
- Soft tissues MFH: lower extremity > upper extremity > retroperitoneum
- Lung (extremely rare)

Radiographic features
- Tumors have aggressive features: permeative or moth-eaten.
- Calcifications or sclerotic margins are rarely present.
- Periostitis is limited, unless a pathological fracture is present.
- Density of tumor is similar to muscle (10-60 HU).
- Large soft tissue mass (common)

FIBROSARCOMA

Fibrosarcoma and malignant fibrous histiocytoma are clinically and radiographically indistinguishable.

LIPOSCLEROSING MYXOFIBROUS TUMOR (LSMFT)

LSFMT (mnemonic: **L**ucky **S**tripe **M**eans **F**ine **T**obacco) of bone is a benign fibroosseous lesion that is characterized by complex mixture of histological elements, including lipoma, fibroxanthoma, myxoma, myxofibroma, fibrous dysplasia like features, cyst formation, fat necrosis, ischemic ossification, and rarely cartilage. Despite its histological complexity, LSMFT has a relatively characteristic radiological appearance and skeletal distribution.

Radiographic features
- Predilection for femur
- Geographic lesion with well-defined and sclerotic margins
- Mineralization within lesion is common.
- Unlike an intraosseous lipoma, LSMFT does not show macroscopic fat by CT or MRI as the fatty component is small and is admixed with more prominent myxofibrous and/or fibroosseous tissue.
- Prevalence of malignant transformation is between 10%-16%.

Bone Marrow Tumors

EOSINOPHILIC GRANULOMA (EG)

Langerhans' cell histiocytosis is now the approved term for three diseases involving abnormal proliferation of histiocytes in organs of the reticuloendothelial system (RES):
- Letterer-Siwe: acute disseminated form, 10%
- Hand-Schüller-Christian: chronic disseminated form, 20%
- EG: only bone involvement, 70%

The radiological manifestation of Langerhans' cell histiocytosis may be skeletal or extraskeletal (involving any organ of the RES). Age: 1st to 3rd decade. Prognosis depends on degree of visceral involvement.

Radiographic features

Appendicular, 20%
- Permeative, metadiaphyseal lytic lesion
- Cortical destruction may be present: pathological fractures
- Aggressive tumors may mimic osteomyelitis or Ewing's sarcoma.
- Multifocal in 10%-20%

Skull, 50%
- Well-defined lytic lesions
- Beveled-edge appearance may produce hole-within-a-hole sign (outer table is more destroyed than inner table; button sequestrum); best seen by CT.
- Lesions may coalesce and form a geographical skull.
- In the healing phase, lesions may develop sclerotic borders.
- Floating tooth: lesion in aveolar portion of mandible

Spine and pelvis, 25%
- Vertebra plana: complete collapse of the vertebral body
- Vertebral lesions may produce scoliosis.

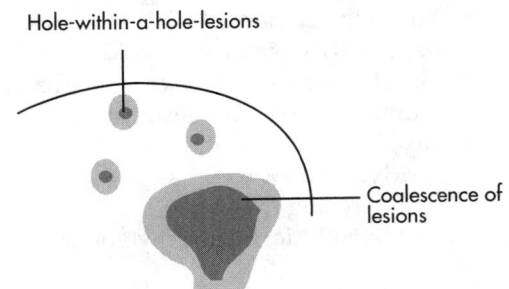

Hole-within-a-hole-lesions

Coalescence of lesions

Extraskeletal manifestation
Pulmonary involvement
- Alveolar disease (exudate of histiocytes)
- Interstitial pattern (upper lobe predominance)

Central nervous system involvement
- Meningeal involvement
- Pituitary involvement

Other RES organ involvement
- Liver
- Spleen
- Lymph nodes

MULTIPLE MYELOMA

Most common primary bone tumor (12,000 new cases/year in the United States). Age: 95% > age 40. Composed of plasmacytes (produce IgG) with a distribution identical to that of red marrow:
- Vertebral bodies are destroyed before the pedicles are, as opposed to metastases in which pedicles are destroyed first.
- Axial skeleton is most commonly affected (skull, spine, ribs, pelvis).

Clinical findings
- IgA and/or IgG peak (monoclonal gammopathy) by electrophoresis
- Bence-Jones proteins in urine (light chain Ig subunit)
- Reversed albumin/globulin ratio
- Bone pain
- Anemia

Types
- Multiple myeloma (multiple lesions)
    Vertebra, 65%
    Ribs, 45%
    Skull, 40%
    Shoulder, 40%
    Pelvis, 30%
    Long bones, 25%
- Solitary plasmacytoma. Common in vertebral body, pelvis, femur.

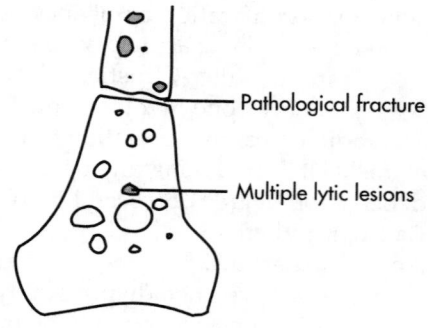

Pathological fracture

Multiple lytic lesions

Radiographic features
- Multiple myeloma has two common radiological appearances:
    Multiple, well-defined lytic lesions: punched-out lesions, 80%
    Generalized osteopenia with vertebral compression fractures, 20%
- Plasmacytoma: tends to be large and expansile
- MRI: replacement of normal marrow (sensitive)
- Bone scan: normal scan, cold or hot lesions
- Skeletal survey: more sensitive than bone scan but still misses significant number of myeloma lesions
- Atypical findings (rare)
    Myelomatosis
    Sclerosing myeloma
    Mixed lytic/blastic myeloma

DIFFERENTIATION OF MULTIPLE MYELOMA AND METASTASES		
Parameter	Multiple Myeloma	Metastases
Intervertebral disk	Yes	Rare
Mandible	Yes	Rare
Vertebral pedicles	No	Common
Large soft tissue mass	Yes	No
Bone scan	Cold, normal, hot	Hot, cold

Complications

- Pathological fractures
- Amyloidosis, 10%
- Most plasmacytoma progress to multiple myeloma

POEMS SYNDROME

Rare variant of sclerosing myeloma. Japanese predilection. Consists of:

- **P**olyneuropathy
- **O**rganomegaly
- **E**ndocrinopathy (gynecomastia, amenorrhea)
- **M** protein: sclerotic multple myeloma
- **S**kin changes (hyperpigmentation)

EWING'S TUMOR

Relatively common malignant tumor derived from undifferentiated mesenchymal cells of the bone marrow or primitive neuroectodermal cells (small, round cell tumor). Age: 5-15 years. Clinical: mass; 35% of patients have fever, leukocytosis, elevated ESR, and thus clinically mimic infection. 5-year survival: 40%. Very rare in black population.

Location

- Diaphysis of lower extremity, 70%
- Flat bones (sacrum, innominate bone, scapula), 25%
- Vertebral body, 5%

Radiographic features

- Aggressive tumor: permeative or moth-eaten osteolytic characteristics, cortical erosion, periostitis
- No tumor matrix
- Sclerotic reactive bone may be present
- Extraosseus soft tissue mass is typical
- Characteristically medullary in location, but usually only the cortical changes are apparent on plain radiograph
- Metastases (lung and bone): 30% at presentation

PRIMARY LYMPHOMA

Very rare; most osseous lymphomas are secondary. Primary osseous lymphoma is usually of the non-Hodgkin's type.

Radiographic features

- Permeative lytic lesion with similar appearance to other small, round cell tumors (e.g., Ewings tumor)

Metastases

GENERAL

BONE METASTASES		
Adult Male	**Adult Female**	**Children**
Prostate, 60%	Breast, 70%	Neuroblastoma
Lung, 15%	Lung, 5%	Leukemia, lymphoma
Kidney, 5%	Kidney, 5%	Medulloblastoma
Other, 20%	Other, 20%	Sarcomas
		Wilms' tumor

Spread of metastases
- Hematogenous spread through arterial circulation to vascular red marrow; common around shoulders and hip joints due to residual red marrow
- Hematogenous spread through retrograde venous flow (e.g., prostate)
- Direct extension (uncommon)
- Lymphangitic (rare)

Radiographic features

The radiographic feature reflects the aggressiveness of the primary tumor. Pattern of destruction may be moth-eaten, geographical, or permeated. Metastases may be lytic, blastic, or mixed. Pathological fractures are common.

Commonly lytic metastases
- Kidney
- Lung
- Thyroid
- Breast

Commonly sclerotic metastases
- Prostate
- Breast

Other sclerotic metastases (rare)
- Hodgkin's lymphoma
- Carcinoid
- Medulloblastoma
- Neuroblastoma
- Transitional cell cancer (TCC)

SECONDARY LYMPHOMA

Skeletal abnormalities occur in 5%-50% of all lymphomas. The more immature the cell line, the greater the frequency of bone involvement.

Radiographic features
- Usually aggressive tumors with no specific pathognomonic finding
- Suspect diagnosis in lymphoma patients
- Ivory vertebra is a manifestation of Hodgkin's lymphoma.

Other Bone Tumors

UNICAMERAL (SIMPLE) BONE CYST (UBC)

Common benign fluid filled lesion of childhood of unknown cause. Age: 10-20 years. Clinical: 50% of cysts present with pathological fractures and pain. Most resolve with bone maturity.

Location
- Most common location: proximal metaphysis of the humerus or femur
- Long tubular bones, 90%
- Less common location: calcaneus, ilium (older patients)

Radiographic features
- Central (intramedullary) location; metadiaphyseal
- Tumor respects the physis
- Expansile lesion
- Fluid-filled cavities (fluid/fluid levels)
- Fallen fragment sign secondary to pathological fracture is pathognomonic for UBC: fragment migrates to dependent portion of cyst
- No periosteal reaction unless fractured

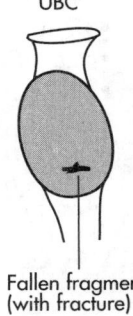

UBC

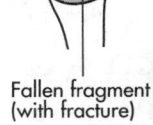

Fallen fragment (with fracture)

ANEURYSMAL BONE CYST (ABC)

ABC   Renal cell carcinoma

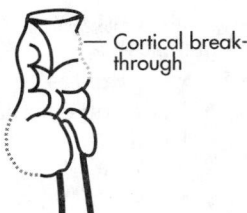

Cortical break-through

Expansile nonneoplastic lesion containing thin-walled, blood-filled cystic cavities. Age: 5-20 years. Clinical: rapid progression (2-6 months) with acute pain. Two types:
- Primary nonneoplastic lesion, 70%
- Secondary lesion arising in preexisting bone tumors, 30% (chondroblastoma, fibrous dysplasia, GCT, osteoblastoma)

Location
- Posterior elements of spine
- Metaphysis of long tubular bones
- Pelvis

Radiographic features
- Eccentric location (in contradistinction to UBC)
- Expansile
- Thin maintained cortex (best seen by CT) unlike in metastases (e.g., RCC) in which there is cortical breakthrough
- No periosteal reaction unless fractured
- Respects epiphyseal plate
- Large lesions may appear aggressive like lytic metastases
- Fluid-fluid levels in cystic components

HEMOPHILIAC PSEUDOTUMOR

Incidence: 2% of hemophiliacs. Pathologically, pseudotumors represent hematomas with thick fibrous capsules, caused by intraosseous, subperiosteal, or soft tissue hemorrhage. Clinical: painless expanding masses that may cause pressure on adjacent organs. Pseudotumors destroy soft tissue, erode bone, and cause neurovascular compromise. Location: femur, pelvis, tibia.

Radiographic features
- Large soft tissue mass with adjacent bone destruction
- Unresorbed hematoma increases in size over years.
- Calcifications are common.
- Periosteal elevation with new bone formation at the edge of the lesion
- Characteristic MRI appearance of hematoma (T1W):
  Hypointense rim: fibrous tissue, hemosiderin deposition
  Hyperintense center: paramagnetic breakdown products
- Fluid-blood levels may be present.

GIANT CELL TUMOR

Uncommon lesions thought to arise from osteoclasts. Typically occurs in epiphysis with metaphyseal extension. Age: after epiphyseal fusion. Location: 50% occur around knee. 10% are malignant (local spread, metastases).

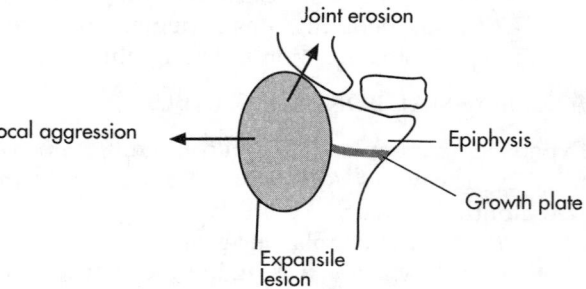

Radiographic features
- Lytic subarticular lesion
- Expansile
- Narrow transition; no sclerotic margin
- May erode into joint
- May be locally aggressive
- Pathological fracture, 30%

INTRAOSSEUS HEMANGIOMA

Asymptomatic unless a complication occurs: pathological fractures, rarely spinal cord compression (extension into epidural space, vertebral expansion and hemorrhage). Location: vertebral body > skull > face. Middle age predilection.

Radiographic features
- Corduroy appearance is pathognomonic: coarse, vertical trabecular pattern of vertebral body
- Radiolucent, slightly expansile intraosseous lesion in extraspinal sites

ADAMANTINOMA

Extremely rare locally aggressive tumor in the spectrum of osteofibrous dysplasia. Age: 20-50 years. Location: 90% in tibia.

Radiographic features
- Sharply circumscribed lytic lesions with marginal sclerosis
- Occurs in middle one third of diaphysis and can be central or eccentric, multilocular, slightly expansile
- Satellite foci may occur in fibula.

CHORDOMA

Rare, slow growing, locally aggressive tumor arising from notochord remnants. The notochord represents the early fetal axial skeleton, which is later surrounded by cartilaginous matrix. As the cartilage ossifies, the notochord is extruded into the intervertebral regions, where it evolves into the nucleus pulposus of the intervertebral disk. Remnants of the notochord may occur at any position along the neural axis. Age: 30-70 years. Clinical: morbidity is secondary to extensive local invasion and recurrence. Distant metastases occur late in the disease. Treatment: surgery and radiation.

Location
- Sacrum, 50%
- Clivus tumors, 35%
- Vertebral bodies, 15%

Radiographic features
- Nonspecific expansile lytic lesion
- Large soft tissue component
- Variable calcification

INTRAOSSEIOUS LIPOMA

Asymptomatic lytic lesion. Location: proximal femur, fibula, calcaneus. May have central calcified nidus.

HEMANGIOENDOTHELIOMA

Low-grade malignant lesion of adolescents. Multifocal lytic lesions involving multiple bones of a single extemity, usually the hands or feet. Locally aggressive; rarely metastasize.

ANGIOSARCOMA

Highly malignant vascular tumor of adolescents/young adults. One third are multifocal. Commonly metastasize.

MASSIVE OSTEOLYSIS (GORHAM'S DISEASE)

Extensive cystic angiomatosis (hemangiomatous and lymphangiomatous) of bone in children and young adults. Idiopathic but there frequently is a history of trauma. Location: shoulder and hip most common.

Radiographic features
- Rapid dissolution of bone
- Spreads contiguously and crosses joints
- No host reaction or periostitis

GLOMUS TUMOR

Benign vascular tumor of the terminal phalanx. Well-circumscribed, lytic, and painful. Clinical pain and terminal phalangeal location are characteristic.

Miscellaneous Lesions

MASTOCYTOSIS

Mast cell infiltration of skin, marrow, and other organs. Results in mixed lytic/sclerotic process (dense bones) with thickened trabecula; focal or diffuse. Organ involvement:

Bone, 60%
- Osteosclerosis, 20%
- Osteoporosis, fractures (heparin-like effect), 30%

GI, 35%
- Peptic ulcers
- Diffuse thickening of jejunal folds
- Hepatomegaly, splenomegaly
- Lymphadenopathy
- Ascites

Chest, 20%
- Skin: urticaria pigmentosum
- Fibrosis
- Pulmonary nodules

Other
- Reaction to contrast medium
- Associated malignancies, 30%: lymphoma, leukemia, adenocarcinoma

MYELOID METAPLASIA (MYELOFIBROSIS)

One of the myeloproliferative disorders in which neoplastic stem cells grow in multiple sites outside of the marrow and the hematopoietic marrow is replaced by fibrosis. Only 50% demonstrate radiographic findings on plain films.

Radiographic features
- Diffuse or patchy osteosclerosis
- Massive extramedullary hematopoeisis
    Massive splenomegaly (100%)
    Hepatomegaly
    Paraspinal mass

RADIATION-INDUCED CHANGES

Bone growth
The major effect of radiation is on chondroblasts in epiphyses:
- Epiphyseal growth arrest (limb length discrepancies)
- Slipped capital femoral epiphysis (damaged growth plate does not withstand shearing stress)
- Scoliosis (e.g., after radiation of Wilms' tumor)
- Hemihypoplasia (i.e., iliac wing)

Osteonecrosis
Radiotoxicity to osteoblasts results in decreased matrix production. Pathological fractures are not common. Radiation osteitis is most common in:
- Mandible, 30% (intraoral cancer)
- Clavicle, 20% (breast carcinoma)
- Humeral head, 14% (breast carcinoma)
- Ribs, 10% (breast carcinoma)
- Femur, 10%

Radiation-induced bone tumors
- Enchondroma (exostosis) is the most common lesion.
- OSA, chondrosarcoma, and MFH are the most common malignant lesions.

SOFT TISSUE TUMORS

Malignant fibrous histiocytoma
The most common soft tissue tumor in adults. Location: lower extremity is most common. Radiographic appearance is nonspecific (large mass); reactive pseudo-capsule may be seen.

Liposarcoma
Second most common soft tissue tumor in adults. Location: buttocks, lower extremity, retroperitoneum. Fatty component is progressively replaced by soft tissue while degree of malignancy increases: variable reactive pseudocapsule.

Synovial cell sarcoma
Soft tissue sarcoma of questionable synovial origin. Age: 15 to 35 years. Location: most commonly around the knee. Approximately one third contain calcifications.

Fibromatoses
A spectrum of fibrous soft tissue lesions that are infiltrative and prone to recurrence. Types: juvenile aponeurotic fibroma, infantile dermal fibromatosis, and aggressive fibromatosis (desmoid tumor).

PIGMENTED VILLONODULAR SYNOVITIS (PVNS)

PVNS predominantly affects adults in their second to fourth decade. Two forms: diffuse (within the joint) and focal. PVNS can affect any joint, bursa, or tendon sheath; however, the knee is the most commonly involved joint (followed by hip, elbow, and ankle).

Radiographic features
- PVNS almost never calcifies but can erode into bone, creating large cystic cavities. Joint space narrowing can occur only late in its course.
- MRI characteristics diffuse low signal masses on T1W and T2W sequences lining the joint synovium. The masses represent synovial hypertrophy with diffuse hemosiderin deposits. Joint effusion.
- The differential diagnosis for low signal intensity lesions on T1W and T2W in and around the joint includes PVNS, gout (the signal characteristics may be secondary to fibrous tissue, hemosiderin deposition, or calcification), amyloid (primary or secondary amyloidosis), fibrous lesions (fibromatosis, desmoid tumors included), and disorders causing hemosiderin deposition (hemophilia, synovial hemagioma, neuropathic osteoarthropathy). The deposition of hemosiderin from hemophilia is never as prominent as seen in PVNS.

Arthritis

General

APPROACH

ABCS APPROACH TO DIFFERENTIAL DIAGNOSIS OF ARTHRITIS	
Parameter	**Differential Diagnosis**
ALIGNMENT	Subluxation, dislocation: common in RA and SLE
BONE	
Osteoporosis	Normal mineralization: all arthritides except RA
	Juxtaarticular osteopenia: any arthropathy; subtle findings have no differential diagnosis value
	Diffuse osteoporosis: only in RA
Erosions	Aggressive erosion (no sclerotic borders, no reparative bone): RA, psoriasis
	Nonaggressive erosion (fine sclerotic border): gout
	Location: inflammatory erosions occur at margins (mouse ear), erosions in erosive OA occur in the central portion of the joint (seagull)
Bone production	Periosteal new bone formation: psoriasis, Reiter's syndrome (this is a feature that distinguishes RA from spondyloarthropathies, due to tenosynovitis)
	Ankylosis (bony bridging of a joint): inflammatory arthropathies
	Overhanging edges of cortex: typical of gout (tophus)
	Subchondral bone (reparative bone beneath cortex): typical of OA
	Osteophytes (occur where adjacent cartilage has undergone degeneration and loss): typical of OA
CARTILAGE	
Joint space	Maintenance of joint space: any early arthropathy; only gout and PVNS maintain normal joint space in progressive disease
	Uniform narrowing: all arthritis except OA
	Eccentric narrowing: typical of OA
	Wide joint space: early inflammatory process
DISTRIBUTION	
Monoarticular or polyarticular	Monarticular: infection, crystal deposition, or posttraumatic
Proximal/distal	Proximal joints: RA, CPPD, AS
	Distal joints: Reiter's, psoriatic
	Symmetrical: RA, multicentric reticulohistiocytosis
SOFT TISSUES	
Swelling	Symmetrical around joint: seen in all inflammatory arthropathies but most commonly in RA
	Asymmetrical: most commonly due to asymmetrical osteophytes rather than true soft tissue swelling; most common in OA
	Lumpy, bumpy soft tissue swelling: gout (tophus)
	Swelling of entire digit: psoriasis, Reiter's (sausage digit)
Calcification	Soft tissue: gout (calcified tophus)
	Cartilage: CPPD
	Subcutaneous tissue: scleroderma (typical)

RA, Rheumatoid arthritis; *OA*, osteoarthritis; *CPPD*, calcium pyrophosphate dihydrate; *AS*, ankylosing spondylitis.

TYPES OF ARTHRITIS

There are three types of arthritis (which often can be distinguished radiologically):

Degenerative joint disease
- Osteophytes
- Subchondral sclerosis
- Uneven loss of articular space

Inflammatory arthritis
- Unmarginated erosions
- Periarticular osteoporosis is common
- Soft tissue swelling
- Uniform loss of articular space

Metabolic arthritis
- Lumpy bumpy soft tissue swelling
- Marginated bony erosions with overhanging edges

Alignment	Ulnar deviation Subluxations
Bone	Osteoporosis Osteolysis (erosions, resorptions) Periosteal new bone
Cartilage	Joint space narrowing Calcification
Distribution	Proximal or peripheral Small or large joints Symmetry
Soft tissues	Diffuse swelling Focal soft tissue masses Calcification

Degenerative Arthritis

GENERAL

Degenerative joint disease (DJD) = osteoarthritis (OA). Early changes include disruption of the armor plate of the articular cartilage. Subsequently, there is a progressive loss of macromolecular components from the ground substance, eventually exposing subchondral bone. Incidence: > 40 million cases/year in United States; 80% of population > 50 years have radiological evidence of OA. There are two types:

Primary OA
- No underlying local etiological factors
- Abnormally high mechanical forces on normal joint
- Age related

Secondary OA
- Underlying etiological factors: calcium pyrophosphate dihydrate (CPPD) < trauma, inflammatory arthritis, hemochromatosis, acromegaly, congenital hip dysplasia, osteonecrosis, loose bodies
- Normal forces on abnormal joint

Clinical findings

Characteristics of joint discomfort
- Aggravated by joint use; relieved by rest
- Morning stiffness < 15 min

Joint examination
- Local tenderness
- Joint enlargement
- Crepitus
- Effusion
- Gross deformity
- Heberden's nodules
- Borchard's nodes

Joints most frequently involved: DIP, PIP, first carpometacarpal (CMC), hips, knees, spine, first metatarsal phalangeal (MTP)

Joints commonly spared: MCP, wrist, elbow, shoulder, ankles

No systemic manifestation
Synovial fluid
- High viscosity
- Normal mucin test
- Mild leukocytosis (< 2000/mm³)

Radiographic features
Five hallmarks:
- Narrowing of joint space, usually asymmetrical
- Subchondral sclerosis
- Subchondral cysts (true cysts or pseudocysts)
- Osteophytes
- Lack of osteoporosis

Treatment options
- Advanced OA: arthroplasty (e.g., total hip replacement [THR])
- Alternative surgical procedures:
    Osteotomy: sections of bone are excised to improve joint congruity and alignment, especially in young patients
    Excision arthroplasty: excision of femoral neck; leads to extremity shortening and joint instability. Indications: (1) salvage operation for failed THR; (2) patients with limited weight-bearing activities
    Arthrodesis: removal of articular cartilage with fusion of joint surfaces
- Antiinflammatory drugs: NSAIDs
- Experimental chondrocyte transplant

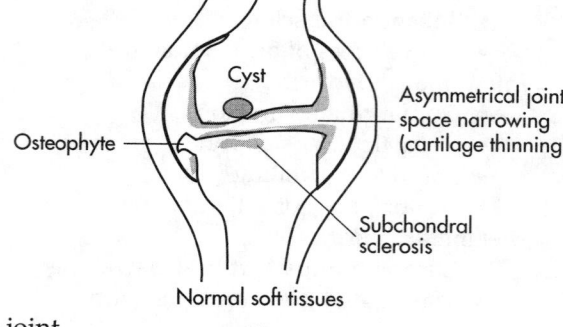

OSTEOARTHRITIS IN SPECIFIC LOCATIONS

Hip
- Joint space is narrowest superiorly at weight-bearing portion.
- Subchondral cyst formation (intrusion of synovium and synovial fluid into the altered bone); Egger's cysts: subchondral acetabular cysts
- Superolateral migration of the femoral head is common.
- Secondary OA of the hip is common and can be radiographically confusing.
- Postel's coxarthropathy: rapidly destructive OA of the hip joint that mimics Charcot's joint
- Protrusio acetabuli is uncommon.

Knee
- Medial femorotibial compartment most commonly narrowed.
- Weight-bearing views are often helpful for assessment of joint space narrowing.
- Osteochondral bodies
- Patellar tooth sign (enthesopathy at the patellar attachment of the quadriceps tendon)
- Secondary OA occurs commonly after trauma and meniscectomy.

Hand
- Heberden's nodes in DIP
- Bouchard's nodes in PIP
- Asymmetrical peripheral involvement

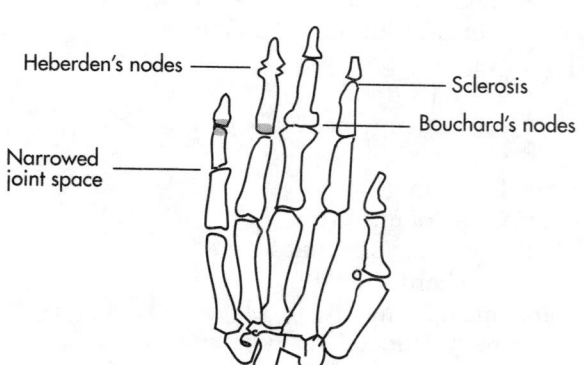

Spine

- OA of the spine occurs in the apophyseal joints (diarthroses).
- Lower cervical and low lumbar spine are most comonly affected.
- Osteophytes may encroach on neural foramina (best seen on oblique views).
- Vacuum phenomenon: gas (N_2) in apophyseal joints is pathognomonic of the degenerative process
- Degenerative spondylolisthesis (pseudospondylolithesis)

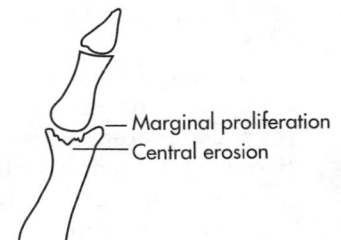

Subchondral sclerosis

Vacuum phenomenon

Oblique view

EROSIVE OSTEOARTHRITIS

OA with superimposed inflammatory, erosive changes. Characteristically affects middle-aged women.

Radiographic features

- Erosive and productive changes of DIP and PIP
- Gull-wing pattern: secondary to central erosions and marginal osteophytes
- Typical involvement of first CMC may help distinguish erosive OA from rheumatoid arthritis (RA), psoriatic arthritis, and adult Still's disease.
- Interphalangeal fusion may occur.

Gull-wing pattern

Marginal proliferation
Central erosion

DEGENERATIVE DISK DISEASE

Degenerative disk disease affects the intervertebral sympheses (amphiarthroses) and thus is not DJD (which affects diarthrodial joints). Degenerative disk disease and DJD often but not always occur together.

Radiographic features

- MRI is imaging modality of choice for evaluating intervertebral disks.
- Disk signal abnormalities (loss of T2 bright signal) indicate degeneration.
- Decreased disk height
- Endplate changes
    Modic I: dark T1/bright T2 (vascular tissue ingrowth)
    Modic II: bright T1/bright T2 (fatty change)
    Modic III: dark T1/dark T2 (sclerosis)
- Disk contour abnormalities
    Bulges
    Protrusions or herniations
- Plain film findings
    Disk space narrowing
    Vacuum phenomenon in disk space
    Endplate osteophytes and sclerosis

SPONDYLOSIS DEFORMANS

Degenerative changes of the annulus fibrosis result in anterior and anterolateral disk herniations. Traction osteophytes may form secondarily and project several millimeters from the endplate. Disk spaces are usually well preserved.

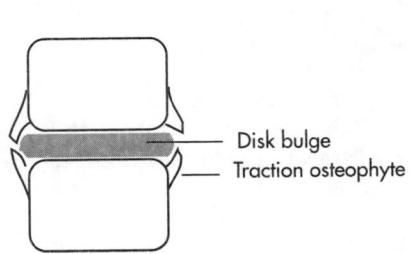

Disk bulge
Traction osteophyte

DIFFUSE IDIOPATHIC SKELETAL HYPEROSTOSIS (DISH, FORESTIER'S DISEASE)

Severe productive bone formation in the soft tissues around the spine, resulting in bulky flowing osteophytes. Most common site is thoracic spine. Unknown etiology. Clinical signs and symptoms are mild compared with radiographic appearance.

Radiographic features
- Flowing osteophytes of at least four contiguous vertebral bodies
- Preserved disk height
- No sacroiliitis or facet ankylosis
- Calcification of ligaments and tendons
- Associated with hypertrophic DJD

Inflammatory Arthritis

GENERAL

There are three types of inflammatory arthritis
    Autoimmune arthritis
- RA
- Scleroderma
- Systemic lupus erythematosus (SLE)
- Dermatomyositis

    Seronegative spondylarthropathies
- Ankylosing spondylitis
- Reiter's syndrome
- Psoriasis
- Enteropathic arthropathies

    Erosive OA

ADULT RHEUMATOID ARTHRITIS

Epidemiology
- Female:male = 3:1
- Incidence: 10^5 new cases/year in United States
- HLA-DW4 related

Diagnosis
- Classic RA: 7 criteria (from table below)
- Definite RA: 5 criteria
- Probable RA: 3 criteria

DIAGNOSTIC CRITERIA FOR RHEUMATOID ARTHRITIS	
Criterion	**Comment**
Morning stiffness	Indicator of inflammation
Pain on motion	In at least one joint
Swelling of one joint	No bony growth (indicates DJD)
Swelling of another joint	
Symmetrical swelling	DIP involvement excluded
Subcutaneous nodules	Exclude CPPD deposition disease
Typical radiological changes	See below
Positive rheumatoid factor	> 1:64
Synovial fluid	Poor mucin clot formation
Typical synovial histopathology	
Histopathology of rheumatoid nodules	

Radiographic features

Early changes

- Periarticular soft tissue swelling (edema, synovial congestion)
- Periarticular osteoporosis in symmetrical distribution (hallmark)
- Preferred sites of early involvement
  - Hands: 2nd and 3rd MCP joint
  - Feet: 4th and 5th MTP joint

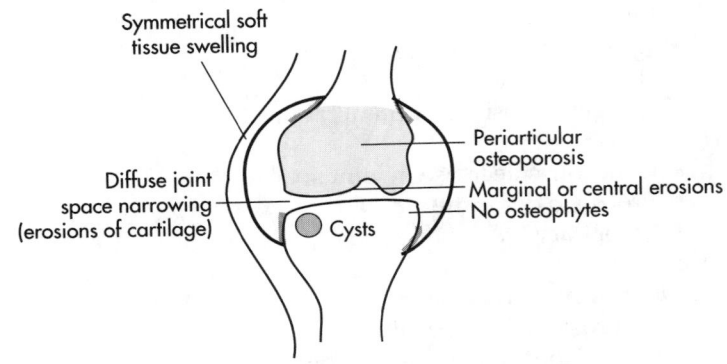

Late changes

- Erosions (pannus formation, granulation tissue) first attack joint portions in which protective cartilage is absent (i.e., capsular insertion site).
- Erosions of the ulnar styloid and triquetrum are characteristic.
- Subchondral cysts formation results from synovial fluid, which is pressed into bone marrow through destroyed cartilage.
- Subluxations
- Carpal instability
- Fibrous ankylosis is a late finding.

Extraarticular manifestations of rheumatoid arthritis

Abdominal

- Secondary renal disease: glomerulonephritis, amyloid, drug toxicity
- Arteritis: infarction, claudication

Pulmonary

- Pleural effusion
- Interstitial fibrosis
- Pulmonary nodules
- Caplan's syndrome: pneumoconiosis, rheumatoid lung nodules, RA
- Pneumonitis (very rare)

Cardiac

- Pericarditis and pericardial effusion, 30%
- Myocarditis

Felty syndrome

- RA
- Splenomegaly
- Neutropenia
- Thrombocytopenia

RHEUMATOID ARTHRITIS IN SPECIFIC LOCATIONS

Hand

- MCP ulnar deviation
- Boutonnière deformity: hyperextension of DIP, flexion of PIP
- Swan-neck deformity: hyperextension of PIP, flexion of DIP
- Hitchhiker's thumb
- Telescope fingers: shortening of phalanges due to dislocations
- Ulnar and radial styloid erosions are common.
- Wrist instability: ulnar translocation, scapholunate dissociation

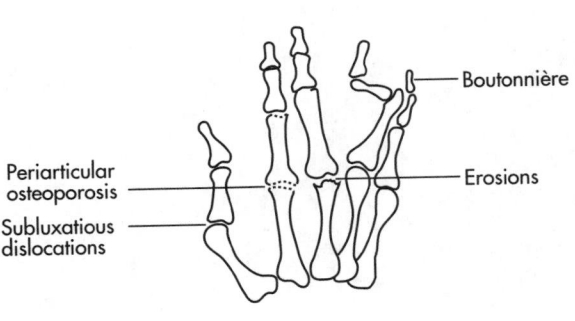

Shoulder
- Lysis of distal clavicle
- Rotator cuff tear
- Marginal erosions of humeral head

Hip
- Concentric decrease in joint space
- Protrusio deformity
- Secondary OA is common

Spine
- Synovial joint erosions
  - Erosions in odontoid
  - Erosions in apophyseal joints
- Atlantoaxial subluxation and impaction
  - \> 3 mm separation between odontoid and C1 in lateral flexion
  - Due to laxity of transverse cruciate ligament and joint destruction

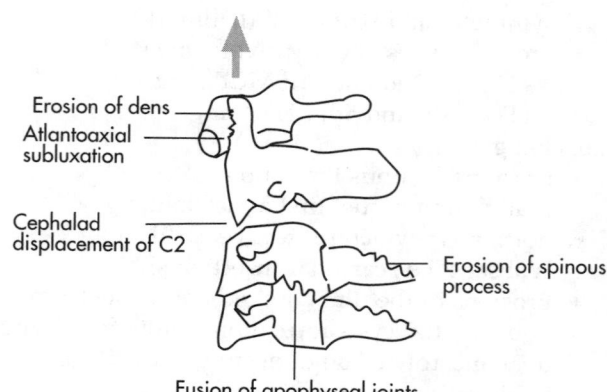

SCLERODERMA (SYSTEMIC SCLEROSIS)

Manifests as soft tissue abnormalities in addition to erosive arthritis.

Radiographic features
- Soft tissue calcification
- Acroosteolysis: tuft resorption results from pressure of tight and atrophic skin
- Soft tissue atrophy
- Erosive changes of DIP and PIP

SYSTEMIC LUPUS ERYTHEMATOSUS (SLE)

Nonerosive arthritis (in 90% of SLE) resulting from ligamentous laxity and joint deformity. Distribution is similar to that seen in RA.

Radiographic features
- Prominent subluxations of MCP
- Usually bilateral and symmetric
- No erosions
- Radiographically similar to Jaccoud's arthropathy
- Soft tissue swelling may be the only indicator.

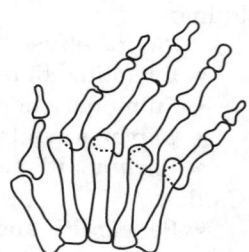

Dermatomyositis

DERMATOMYOSITIS

Widespread soft tissue calcification is the hallmark.

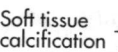
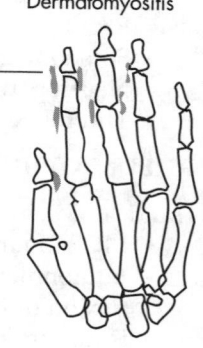

ANKYLOSING SPONDYLITIS (AS)

Seronegative spondyloarthropathy of the axial skeleton and proximal large joints.
Clinical: males >> females. HLA-B27 in 95%. Insiduous onset of back pain and
stiffness. Onset: 20 years.

Radiographic features

- SI joint is the initial site of involvement:
  bilateral, symmetrical
    - Erosions: early
    - Sclerosis: intermediate
    - Ankylosis: late
- Contiguous thoracolumbar involvement
    - Vertebral body "squaring": early
      osteitis
    - Syndesmophytes
    - Bamboo spine: late fusion and
      ligamentous ossification
- Anderson lesion and pseudoarthrosis of
  ankylosed spine (fracture)
- Enthesopathy is common
- Arthritis of proximal joints (hip > shoulder) in 50%
    - Erosions and osteophytes

Associations

- Inflammatory bowel disease (IBD)
- Iritis
- Aortitis
- Pulmonary fibrosis of upper lobes

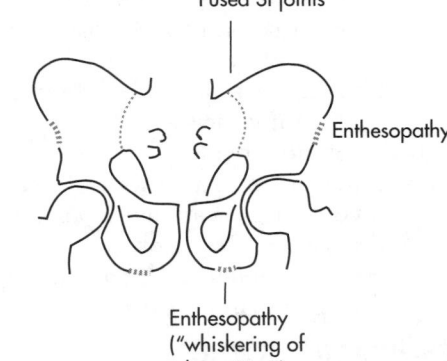

Bamboo spine

Fused SI joints

Enthesopathy

Enthesopathy
("whiskering of
tuberosities")

DIFFERENTIATION OF LUMBAR OSTEOPHYTES

Osteophytes
Extensions of the vertebral endplates in the horizontal direction. Osteophytes are
smaller in DJD and larger in psoriatic arthritis and Reiter's syndrome (calcifications of
periarticular soft tissues that become contiguous with the spine).

Syndesmophyte
Calcification of the outer portion of the anulus fibrosus such as in AS.

REITER'S SYNDROME

Seronegative spondyloarthropathy with lower extremity erosive joint disease. Clinical:
males >> females. HLA-B27 in 80%. Follows either nongonococcal urethritis or
bacillary dysentery (*Shigella, Yersinia, Salmonella*).

Clinical

- Classic triad occurs in minority of patients
    - Urethritis or cervicitis
    - Conjuctivitis
    - Arthritis
- Balanitis, keratoderma blennorrhagicum
- Back pain and heel pain are common.

Asymmetrical bridging

Fused SI joints

Radiographic features

- Predominant involvement of distal lower extremity
    MTP > calcaneus > ankle > knee
- Earliest changes (erosive arthropathy) are often in feet:
    MTP erosions
    Retrocalcaneal bursitis
    Enthesopathy and erosions at Achilles tendon and plantar aponeurosis insertion
- Bilateral sacroiliitis (less common than in AS), 30%
    Asymmetric: early
    Symmetric: late
- Bulky asymmetric thoracolumbar osteophytes with skip segments. Spine involvement is similar to psoriatic arthritis.
- Periostitis is common
- Hand involvement (pencil-in-cup deformity) may occur but is much less common than in psoriasis.

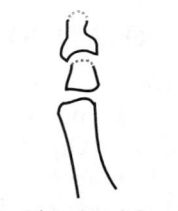

Pencil-in-cup deformity

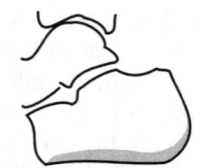

Heel enthesopathy
(periosteal new bone formation)

PSORIATIC ARTHRITIS

Seronegative spondyloarthropathy (inflammatory upper extremity polyarthritis) associated with psoriasis (approximately 10%-20% of patients with psoriasis will develop arthritis). In 90%, the skin changes procede the arthritis; 10% develop the arthritis first. HLA-B27 in 50%. Positive correlation between:
- Severity of skin lesions and joint disease
- Nail changes and DIP involvement

Types

- Asymmetrical oligoarthritis (most common type)
    DIP and PIP of hands
- Spondyloarthropathy of SI joints and spine, 50%
- Symmetrical polyarthritis that resembles RA
- Arthritis mutilans: marked deformity ("opera glass") hand
- Classic polyarthritis with nail changes and variable DIP abnormalities

Radiographic features

- Combination of productive and erosive changes (distinguishable feature from RA)
- Bone production
    Mouse ears: bone production adjacent to erosions
    Ivory phalanx: sclerosis of distal phalanx
- Erosions are aggressive.
    Pencil-in-cup deformity (this feature is not pathognomonic, however)
    Resorption of terminal tufts
- Ankylosis (10%): most common in hands and feet
- Soft tissue swelling of entire digit: sausage digit
- Joint space loss is usually severe.
- Sacroiliitis is usually bilateral.
- Periostitis is common.

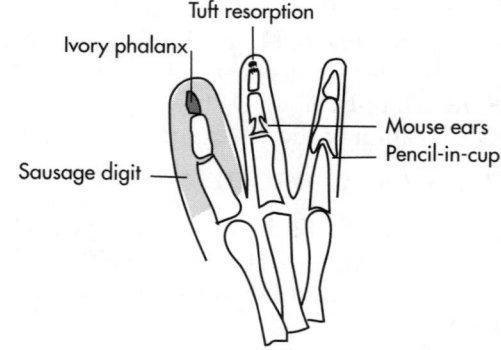

Tuft resorption

Ivory phalanx

Mouse ears
Pencil-in-cup

Sausage digit

Pearls
- SI and spine involvement of psoriatic arthritis is indistinguishable from Reiter's disease.
- Hand disease predominates in psoriasis; foot disease predominates in Reiter's disease.
- Spine disease can be differentiated from AS by asymmetrical osteophytes and lack of syndesmophytes.
- SI involvement is more common and tends to be more symmetrical in AS.
- In one third of patients, the diagnosis of psoriatic arthritis cannot be made on the basis of radiographs.

ENTEROPATHIC ARTHROPATHIES

Patients with IBD or infection may develop arthritis indistinguishable from Reiter's disease or AS. Often HLA-B27 positive. Underlying disease:
- Ulcerative colitis (10% have arthritis)
- Crohn's disease
- Whipple's disease
- *Salmonella, Shigella, Yersinia enteritis* infection

Metabolic Arthritis

GENERAL

Metabolic deposition diseases result in accumulation of crystals or other substances in cartilage and soft tissues. Depositions alter the mechanical properties of cartilage causing microfractures; crystals in the joint fluid elicit acute synovial inflammation. Ultimately secondary arthritis develops. Clinically there are two presentations:

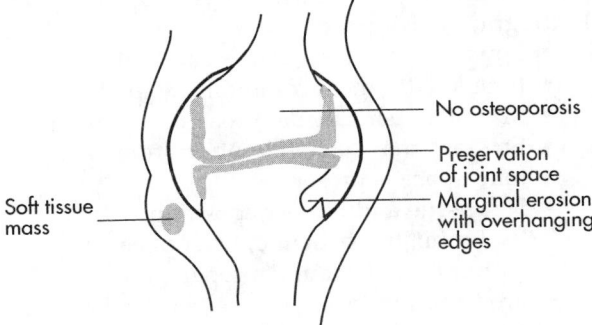

Soft tissue mass

No osteoporosis

Preservation of joint space

Marginal erosion with overhanging edges

- Acute inflammatory arthritis
- Chronic destructive arthropathy

Types
Crystal deposition diseases
- Sodium urate: gout
- CPPD
- Basic calcium phosphate (e.g., calcium hydroxypatite)

Other deposition diseases
- Hemochromatosis
- Wilson's disease
- Alkaptonuria
- Amyloidosis
- Multicentric reticulohistiocytosis
- Xanthomatosis

Endocrine
- Acromegaly

GOUT

Heterogeneous group of entities characterized by recurrent attacks of arthritis secondary to deposition of sodium urate crystals in and around joints. Hyperuricemia not always present; 90% of patients are male.

Urate crystals are strongly birefringent under polarized microscopy.

Causes

Uric acid overproduction, 10%
- Primary: enzyme defects in purine synthesis
- Secondary: increased turnover of nucleic acids
    Myeloproliferative and lymphoproliferative diseases
    Hemoglobinopathies, hemolytic anemias
    Chemotherapy
    Alcohol

Uric acid underexcretion, 90%
- Primary: reduced renal excretion of unknown cause
- Secondary
    Chronic renal failure (any cause)
    Diuretic therapy (thiazides)
    Alcohol, drugs
    Endocrine disorders (hyper-or hypoparathyroidism)

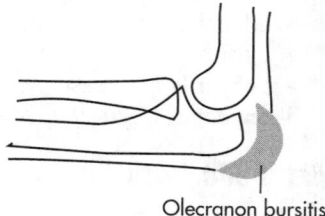

Olecranon bursitis

Radiographic features
- Lower extremity > upper extremity; small joints > large joints
- First MTP is most common site: podagra
- Marginal, pararticular erosions: overhanging edge
- Erosions may have sclerotic borders
- Joint space is preserved
- Soft tissue and bursa deposition
    Tophi: juxtaarticular, helix of ear
    Bursitis: olecranon, prepatellar
- Erosions and tophi only seen in longstanding disease
- Tophi calcification, 50%
- Chondrocalcinosis

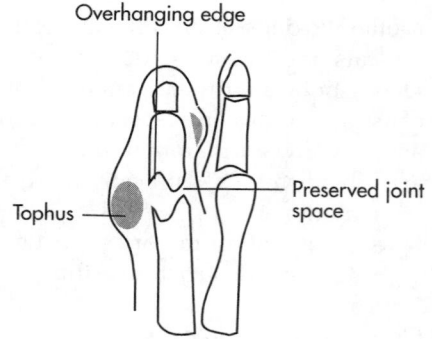

Overhanging edge

Tophus

Preserved joint space

CALCIUM PYROPHOSPHATE DIHYDRATE DEPOSITION (CPPD) DISEASE

Intraarticular deposition of CPPD ($Ca_2P_2O_7 \cdot H_2O$) resulting in chondrocalcinosis and a pattern of DJD in atypical joints. Terminology:
- Chondrocalcinosis: calcification of hydline and fibrocartilage, synovium, tendons, and ligaments. Chondrocalcinosis has many causes of which CPPD deposition is only one; not all patients with CPPD deposition have chondrocalcinosis.
- CPPD deposition: chondrocalcinosis secondary to CPPD. May or may not be associated with arthropathy.
- CPPD arthropathy: structural arthropathy secondary to CPPD
- Pseudogout: subset of patients with CPPD deposition disease who have a clinical presentation that resembles gout (i.e., acute intermittent attacks).

Radiographic features
- Two main features:
    Chondrocalcinosis
    Arthropathy resembling OA
- Chondrocalcinosis present in:
    Hyaline cartilage: linear calcification; especially
        in knee
    Fibrocartilage: menisci, triangular fibrocartilage
        complex of wrist, glenoid and acetabular
        labra, symphysis pubis, intervebral disks

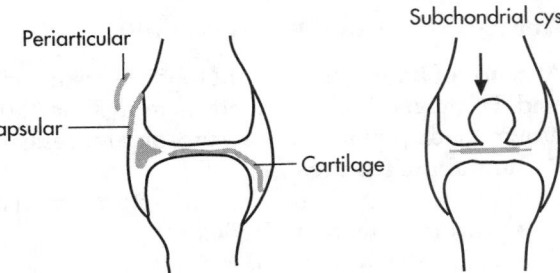

- Synovial, capsular, ligament, and tendon calcification may occur but are not common.
- Arthropathy differs from OA in distribution: predominance of knee (patellofemoral predilection), radiocarpal joint, second and third MCP involvement
- Subchondral cysts are common and a distinctive feature.

Associations
- Primary hyperparathyroidism
- Gout
- Hemochromatosis

BASIC CALCIUM PHOSPHATE (BCP) DEPOSITION DISEASE

BCP deposition is predominantly periarticular as opposed to intraarticular CPPD. The crystal deposition causes periarticular inflammation without structural joint abnormalities.

Radiographic features
Periarticular calcifications occur primarily:
- Near insertions of supraspinatus tendon
- In flexor carpi ulnaris tendon near pisiform bone
- In Milwaukee shoulder: rotator cuff, subacromial subdeltoid bursa
- In hand: MCP, interphalangeal joints

HEMOCHROMATOSIS ARTHROPATHY

Develops in 50% of patients with hemochromatosis. Secondary to iron deposition and/or concommitant CPPD deposition. Arthropathy changes are similar to those seen in CPPD.

Radiographic features
- Same distribution and productive changes as in CPPD
- Distinctive features:
    Beaklike osteophytes on MCP heads (4th and 5th)
    Generalized osteoporosis

WILSON'S DISEASE

Defect in the biliary excretion of copper results in accumulation of copper in basal ganglia, liver, joints and other tissues. Autosomal recessive.

Radiographic features
- Same distribution as CPPD
- Distinctive features:
    Subchondral fragmentation
    Generalized osteoporosis

ALKAPTONURIA (OCHRONOSIS)

Absence of homogentisic acid oxidase results in tissue accumulation of homogentisic acid. Homogentisic acid deposits in hyaline cartilage and fibrocartilage cause a brown-black pigmentation. Autosomal recessive.

Radiographic features
- Dystrophic calcification: intervertebral disks are most commonly affected
- Cartilage, tendons, ligaments
- Generalized osteoporosis
- OA of SI and large peripheral joints

AMYLOID ARTHROPATHY

10% of patients with amyloid have bone or joint involvement. Amyloid may cause a nodular synovitis with erosions, similar to that seen in RA.

Radiographic features
- Bulky soft tissue nodules (i.e., shoulder pad sign)
- Well-marginated erosions
- Preserved joint space
- Wrists, elbows, shoulders, hips

MULTICENTRIC RETICULOHISTIOCYTOSIS

Systemic disease of unknown origin. Similar radiographic features as gout and RA.

Radiographic features
- Nodular soft tissue swelling
- Sharply demarcated marginal erosions
- Mostly distal phalangeal joints
- Bilateral and symmetrical
- Absence of periarticular osteopenia

HEMOPHILIA

Arthropathy is secondary to repeated spontaneous hemarthroses, which occurs in 90% of hemophiliacs. 70% are monoarticular (knee > elbow > ankle > hip > shoulder).

Radiographic features
Acute episode
- Joint effusion (hemarthrosis)
- Periarticular osteoporosis

Chronic inflammation and synovial proliferation
- Epiphyseal overgrowth
- Subchondral cysts
- Secondary OA
- Distinct knee findings
    Widened intercondylar notch
    Squared patella
    Similar radiographic appearance as juvenile JRA
- Distinct elbow findings
    Enlarged radial head
    Enlarged trochlea notch

Infectious Arthritis

GENERAL

Infectious arthritis usually results from hematogenous spread to synovium and subsequent spread into the joint. Direct spread of osteomyelitis into the joint is much less common. The diagnosis is made by joint aspiration.

Organism

- *Staphylococcus aureus* (most common)
- β-*Streptococcus* in infants
- *Haemophilus* in preschoolers
- Gram negatives in diabetes mellitus, alcoholism
- Gonococcal arthritis in sexually active young patients (80% women)
- *Salmonella* is seen in sickle cell patients; however, the most common infection in sickle cell patients is *Staphylococcus.*
- Tuberuclosis: granulomatous infection
- Fungal infectious in immunocompromised patients
- Viral synovitis is transient and self-limited
- *Borrelia burgdorferi:* Lyme arthritis

Radiographic features

Plain film
- Joint effusion
- Juxtaarticular osteoporosis
- Destruction of subchondral bone on both sides of the joint

Bone scan
- Useful if underlying osteomyelitis is suspected

MRI
- Joint effusion
- Sensitive in detecting early cartilage damage

TUBERCULOUS ARTHRITIS

Radiographic features

- Phemister triad
      Cartilage destruction (occurs late)
      Marginal erosions
      Osteoporosis
- Kissing sequestra in bones adjacent to joints
- Location: hip, knee, tarsal joints, spine
- Spine: Pott's disease (see Chapter 6)

DISK SPACE INFECTION

Usually there is primary hematogenous spread to vertebral body endplate and subsequent spread to intervertebral disk.

Radiographic features

- Destruction of intervertebral disk space and endplates, process crosses the disk, unlike tumors (disk destruction occurs later compared with pypogenic infection)
- Paravertebral abscess
- MRI is most sensitive imaging modality

SPECTRUM OF OSTEOMYELITIS AND SEPTIC ARTHRITIS ON PLAIN FILM

Periosteal reaction
- Thin, linear periosteal reaction
- Thick periosteal reaction
- Laminated, ("onion peel")
- Codman's triangle

Bone destruction
- Permeating bone lesion
- Punched out bone
- Moth-eaten
- Geographic
- Aggressive osteolysis
- Well-defined osteolytic lesion with thick sclerotic border

Localized cortical thickening
Ground glass
Diffusely dense bones
Sequestrum
Septic arthritis
Disk space narrowing with endplate erosion

NEUROPATHIC ARTHRITIS (CHARCOT'S JOINT)

Primary loss of sensation in a joint leads to arthropathy. Distribution helps determine etiology.

Causes
- Diabetes neuropathy: usually foot
- Tertiary syphilis (tabes dorsalis): usually knee
- Syringomyelia: usually shoulder
- Other
    - Myelomeningocele
    - Spinal cord injury
    - Congenital insensitivity to pain
    - Any inherited or acquired neuropathy

Radiographic features
Common to all types
- Joint instability: subluxation or dislocation
- Prominent joint effusion
- Normal or increased bone density

Hypertrophic type, 20%
- Marked fragmentation of articular bone
- Much reactive bone

Atrophic type, 40%
- Bone resorption of articular portion

Combined type, 40%

Metabolic Bone Disease

General

Bone tissue consists of:
   Extracellular substance
   - Osteoid: collagen, mucopolysaccharide
   - Crystalline component: calcium phosphate, hydroxyapatite

   Cells
   - Osteoblasts
   - Osteoclasts

Bone is constantly absorbed and replaced with new bone. Disturbances in this equilibrium result in either too much bone (increased radiodensity, osteosclerosis) or too little bone (decreased density = osteopenia).

OSTEOPENIA

Osteopenia is a nonspecific radiographic finding that indicates increased radiolucency of bone. Bone density may be difficult to assess because of technical factors (kVp, mA) that influence the radiographic appearance.

Types
- Osteoporosis: decreased amount of normal bone
- Osteomalacia: decreased bone mineralization
- Marrow replacement: bone replaced by tumor, marrow hyperplasia, or metabolic products
- Hyperparathyroidism: increased bone resorption

OSTEOPOROSIS

Classification

Primary osteoporosis (most common): unassociated with an underlying illness
- Type I osteoporosis: postmenopausal
- Type II osteoporosis: senile
- Idiopathic juvenile osteoporosis

Secondary osteoporosis (less common)
- Endocrine disorders
   Hypogonadism
   Hyperthyroidism
   Cushing's disease
   Acromegaly
- Nutritional
   Malabsorption syndromes
   Alcoholism
   Scurvy
- Hereditary metabolic or collagen disorder
   Osteogenesis imperfecta
   Marfan syndrome
   Ehlers-Danlos syndrome
   Homocystinuria
   Hypophosphatasia
   Wilson's disease
   Alkaptonuria
   Menkes' syndrome

5

- Drugs
  - Heparin
  - Exogenous steroids

Radiographic features

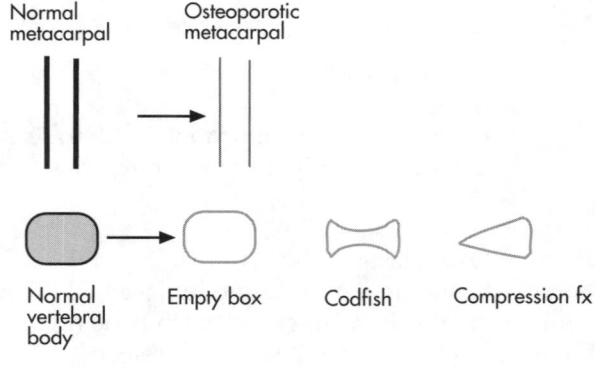

Normal metacarpal → Osteoporotic metacarpal

Normal vertebral body → Empty box   Codfish   Compression fx

- Osteopenia: 30%-50% of bone has to be lost to be detectable by plain film
- Diminution of cortical thickness: width of both MCP cortices should be less than half the shaft diameter
- Decrease in number and thickness of trabeculae in bone
- Vertebral bodies show earliest changes: resorption of horizontal trabeculae
- Empty box vertebra: apparent increased density of vertebral endplates due to resorption of spongy bone
- Vertebral body compression fractures: wedge, biconcave codfish bodies, true compression
- Pathological fractures
- Qualitative assessment: Singh index is based on trabecular pattern of proximal femur. Patterns:
  - Mild: loss of secondary trabeculae
  - Intermediate: loss of tensile trabeculae
  - Severe: loss of principal compressive trabecular

Quantitative bone densitometry
Predicts the risk for developing fractures. 3 methods are available:

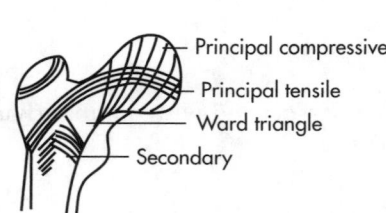

Normal

- Principal compressive
- Principal tensile
- Ward triangle
- Secondary

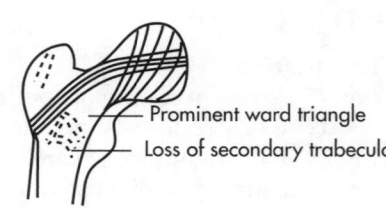

Early

- Prominent ward triangle
- Loss of secondary trabecula

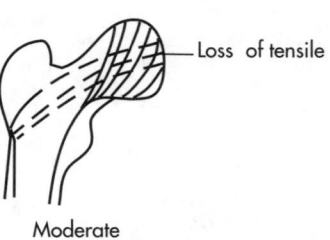

Moderate

- Loss of tensile

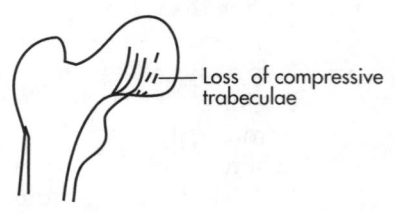

Severe

- Loss of compressive trabeculae

- Single-photon absorption
  - Measures cortical bone density of radial shaft
  - 2-3 mrem exposure
  - Precision 1%-3%
- Dual-photon absorption with radionuclide or dual-energy x-ray
  - Measures vertebral and hip done density (cortical and trabecular)
  - 5-10 mrem exposure
  - Precision 2%-4%
  - Cannot account for soft tissue contribution to x-ray absorption
- Quantitative CT with phantom
  - Measures vertebral body density (trabecular only)
  - 300-500 mrem exposure
  - Most effective technique for evaluation of bone density

Indications for measurements:

- Initiation of estrogen replacement therapy or phosphonate therapy
- Establish diagnosis of osteoporosis
- Assess severity of osteoporosis
- Monitor treatment efficacy

TRANSIENT OSTEOPOROSIS OF HIP JOINT

- Transient osteoporosis, which can be related to or be a variant of AVN
- Radiographs generally show osteopenia, whereas bone scanning demonstrates activities within the femoral head region.
- MRI usually shows diffuse marrow edema with decreased signal on T1W scans and more intense signal on T2W scans.
- Dual-energy x-ray absorptiometry is a good method to quantitatively assess bone density and the fracture risk of the proximal femur.

OSTEOMALACIA

Abnormal mineralization of bone is termed osteomalacia in adults and rickets in children. In the past, the most common cause was deficient intake of vitamin D. Today, absorption abnormalities and renal disorders are more common causes:

Nutritional deficiency of:
- Vitamin D
- Calcium
- Phosphorus

Absorption abnormalities
- Gastrointestinal (GI) surgery
- Malabsorption
- Biliary disease

Renal
- Chronic renal failure
- Renal tubular acidosis
- Proximal tubular lesions
- Dialysis induced

Abnormal vitamin D metabolism
- Liver disease
- Hereditary metabolic disorders

Drugs
- Dilantin
- Phenobarbitol

Radiographic features
- Generalized osteopenia
- Looser's zones (pseudofractures): cortical stress fractures filled with poorly mineralized osteoid tissue.
- Milkman's syndrome: osteomalacia with many Looser's zones
- Typical location of Looser's zones (often symmetrical)
    - Axillary margin of scapula
    - Inner margin of femoral neck
    - Rib
    - Pubic, ischial rami
- Osteomalacia may be indistinguishable from osteoporosis; however, Looser's zones are a reliable differentiating feature.

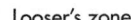
Looser's zones
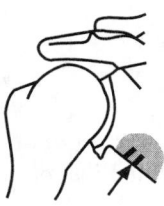
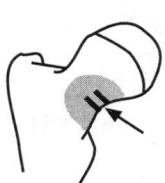
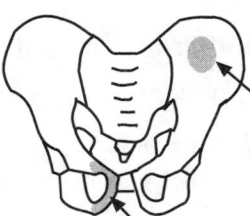

RENAL OSTEODYSTROPHY

Renal osteodystrophy is a general term that refers to a myriad of radiographic osseous changes in patients with renal failure. Radiographically, these changes are secondary to osteomalacia, secondary hyperparathyroidism, and aluminum intoxication.

Radiographic features

Changes of osteomalacia
- Osteopenia and cortical thinning
- Looser's zones occur but are uncommon

Changes of hyperparathyroidism
- Subperiosteal resorption (e.g., SI joint resorption)
- Rugger jersey spine
- Brown tumors
- Osteosclerosis
- Soft tissue calcification
- Chondrocalcinosis

SCURVY

Deficiency of vitamin C (ascorbic acid) impairs the ability of connective tissue to produce collagen. Never occurs before 6 months of age because maternal stores are transmitted to fetus. Findings are most evident at sites of rapid bone growth (long bones). Rare.

Radiographic features

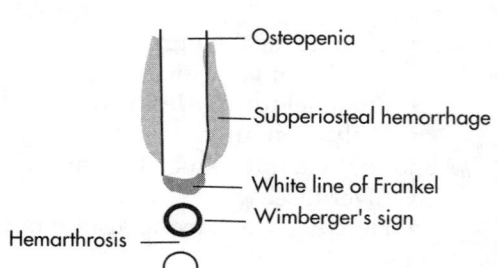

Children
- Generalized osteopenia
- Dense metaphyseal line (Frankel)
- Wimberger's sign: dense epiphyseal rim
- Corner sign: metaphyseal fractures (Pelkan spurs)
- Periosteal reaction (ossification) due to subperiosteal bleeding
- Hemarthrosis: bleeding into joint

Adults
- Osteopenia and pathologic fractures

Endocrine Bone Disease

HYPERPARATHYROIDISM (HPT)

Parathyroid hormone stimulates osteoclastic resorption of bone. HPT is usually detected by elevated serum calcium during routine biochemical screening. Three types:
- Primary HPT:
    - Adenoma, 85% (single 90%, multiple 10%)
    - Hyperplasia, 12%
    - Parathyroid carcinoma, 1%-3%
- Secondary HPT: most often secondary to renal failure; rarely seen with ectopic parathyroid production by hormonally active tumor
- Tertiary HPT: results from autonomous glandular function following longstanding renal failure

Radiographic features
- General osteopenia
- Bone resorption is virtually pathognomonic
    - Subperiosteal resorption
        - Radial aspect of middle phalanges
            (especially index and middle finger)
        - Phalangeal tufts
    - Trabecular resorption
        - Salt and pepper skull
    - Cortical resorption
        - Tunneling of MCP bones (nonspecific)
    - Subchondral resorption
        - Widened SI joint
        - Distal end of clavicle
        - Widened symphysis pubis
        - Can lead to articular disease
- Brown tumors (cystlike lesions) may be found anywhere in the skeleton but especially in the pelvis, jaw, and femur.
- Loss of the lamina dura
- Soft tissue calcification
- Chondrocalcinosis
- Complication: fractures

Clavicular lysis 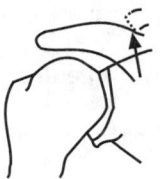   Subperiosteal resorption 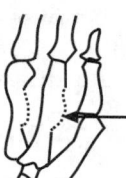   Brown tumors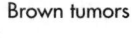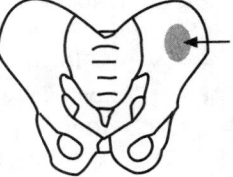

DIFFERENTIATION OF HYPERPARATHYROIDISM	
Primary HPT	**Secondary HPT**
Brown tumors Chondrocalcinosis	Osteosclerosis Rugger jersey spine (renal osteodystrophy) Soft tissue and vascular calcification

THYROID ACROPACHY

Occurs 1-2 years after surgical thyroidectomy or radioablation for hyperthyroidism. Incidence 5%.

Radiographic features
- Thick periosteal reaction of phalanges and metacarpals
- Soft tissue swelling

ACROMEGALY

Elevated growth hormone (adenoma, hyperplasia) results in:
- Children (open growth plates): gigantism
- Adults (closed growth plates): acromegaly = gradual enlargement of hands and feet and exaggeration of facial features

Radiographic features

The key feature is appositional bone growth: ends of bones, exostoses on toes, increase in size and number of sesamoid bones:

Hands
- Spade-shaped tufts due to overall enlargement
- Exostoses at tufts
- Widened joint spaces due to cartilage growth
- Secondary DJD

Feet
- Heel pad > 25 mm (typical)
- Increased number of sesamoid bones
- Exaggerated bony tuberosities at tendon insertion sites
- Exostoses on 1st toe

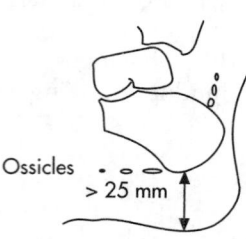
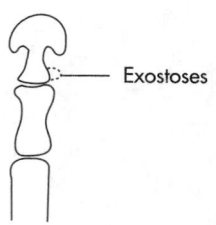

Skull
- Thickening of skull bones and increased density
- Prognathism: protrusion of jaw
- Overgrowth of frontal sinuses (frontal bossing)
- Accentuation of orbital ridges
- Enlargement of nose and soft tissues
- Enlarged sella

Spine
- Posterior vertebral scalloping
- Lordosis

Bone Marrow Disease

CLASSIFICATION

Malignant infiltration
- Myeloma
- Leukemia/lymphoma
- Metastases (small cell tumors)

Secondary marrow hyperplasia
- Hemoglobinopathies
- Hemolytic anemias

Lysosomal storage diseases
- Gaucher's disease
- Niemann-Pick disease: deficiency of sphingomyelinase; radiographically similar to Gaucher's disease except that AVN and cystic bone lesions do not occur

GAUCHER'S DISEASE

Deficiency of β-glucocerebrosidase leads to intracellular accumulation of glucosylceramide predominantly in cells of the RES. Autosomal recessive. Most common in Ashkenazi Jews. Forms:
- Infantile form: lethal
- Adult form: more benign (see below)

Clinical findings
- Liver: hepatosplenomegaly
- Spleen: focal lesions
- Bone marrow: pancytopenia, bone pain, characteristic foam cells

Radiographic features

- Osteopenia
- Focal lytic lesions (expansile, cortical scalloping, no periosteal response), 50%
- Osteonecrosis, 50%, usually occurs combined as:
    Medullary infarcts
    Osteoarticular infarcts
- Modeling deformities (Erlenmeyer flask), 50%
- Less common features
    Periosteal response: bone-within-bone
    H-shaped vertebra
    Hair-on-end appearance of the skull

Complications

- OA
- Fractures, often multiple
- Increased risk for osteomyelitis

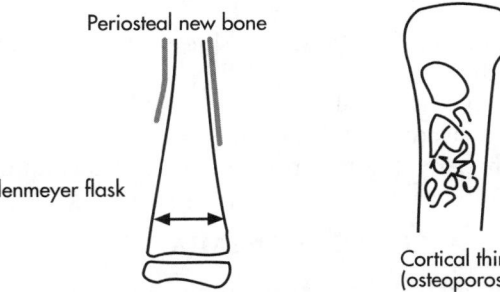

Periosteal new bone

Erlenmeyer flask

Honeycombing

Cortical thinning (osteoporosis)

SICKLE CELL ANEMIA

Structural defect in hemoglobin (hemoglobin S; point mutation). Most hemoglobinopathies (over 250 are known) result in rigid hemoglobin and hemolysis. Incidence: 1% of blacks. Diagnosis is confirmed by hemoglobin electrophoresis. Sickle cell disease (HbSS) has many bone findings, whereas sickle cell trait (HbAS) is only occasionally associated with bone infarcts. Hemoglobin sickle cell disease has same bone findings but the spleen is enlarged.

Clinical findings

- Hemolytic anemia, jaundice
- Skeletal pain (infarction, osteomyelitis)
- Abdominal pain
- High incidence of infections
- Chest pain: acute pulmonary crisis, infarcts

Radiographic features

Hyperplasia of marrow

- Hair-on-end appearance of skull
- Pathological fractures
- Biconcave H-shaped vertebra
- Osteopenia

Vascular occlusion

- AVN occurs primarily in medullary space of long bones, hands, growing epiphyses
- Bone sclerosis from infarctions
- H-shaped vertebral bodies
- Involvement of growing epiphyses leads to growth disturbances
- Dactylitis (hand-foot syndrome): bone infarcts of hands and feet

Osteomyelitis

- High incidence: most are caused by *Staphylococcus*
- *Salmonella* infection more common than in general population
- Most commonly at diaphysis of long bones
- Osteomyelitis and infarction may be difficult to distinguish.

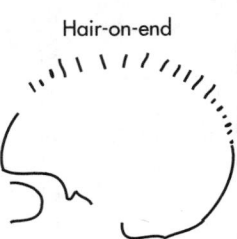

Hair-on-end

Other
- Small calcified fibrotic spleen due to autoinfarction
- Cholelithiasis
- Progressive renal failure
- Papillary necrosis
- Cardiomegaly: high output congestive heart failure (CHF)
- Pulmonary infarcts

THALASSEMIA (COOLEY'S ANEMIA)

Genetic disorder characterized by diminished synthesis of one of the globin chains. Thalassemias are classified according to the deficient chain:
- α-thalassemia: α-chain abnormality, Asian population
- β-thalassemia: β-chain abnormality
- β-thalassemia major (Cooley's anemia, Mediterranean anemia): usually fatal in 1st decade, transfusion dependent; 1% of American blacks, 7% Greeks
- β-thalassemia minor: non–transfusion dependent

Radiographic features

Hyperplasia of marrow is the dominant feature.
- Expands the marrow space: hair-on-end skull
- Modeling deformities of bone: Erlenmeyer flask deformity
- Premature closure of growth plates
- Paravertebral masses due to extramedullary hematopoiesis

Vascular occlusion
- Scattered bone sclerosis
- H-shaped vertebral bodies
- AVN less common than in sickle cell

Other
- Cardiomegaly and CHF
- Secondary hemochromatosis
- Cholelithiasis

SKELETAL MANIFESTATIONS OF ANEMIAS		
	Sickle Cell	**Thalassemia**
Skull	Hair-on-end appearance	Severe hair-on-end appearance
Spine	Fish vertebra	Less common
Other bones	Osteonecrosis	Erlenmeyer flask
	Osteomyelitis	Arthropathy (hemochromatosis, gout)
	Growth arrest (decreased flow)	Osteoporosis
Spleen	Small (autoinfarction)	Large (hepatosplenomegaly)
Kidney	Papillary necrosis	
Abdomen	Cholelithiasis	Cholelithiasis
Other	Pulmonary crisis	Transfusional hemachromatosis
	Cardiomegaly	Fatal 1st decade (homozygous)
		Extramedullary hematopoisis
		Cardiomegaly

MYELOFIBROSIS

Myeloproliferative disease in which bone marrow is replaced by fibrotic tissue.
Clinical:
- Splenomegaly (extramedullary hematopoiesis)
- Anemia (replacement of bone marrow)
- Changes in WBC, cell counts

Radiographic features

Plain film
- Dense bones, 50%
- Paraspinal masses and splenomegaly (marrow production sites)

Bone scan
- Increased uptake
- Superscan

PAGET'S DISEASE (OSTEITIS DEFORMANS)

Chronic progressive disease of osteoblasts and osteoclasts resulting in abnormal bone remodeling. Probable viral etiology. Age: unusual < 40 years. Usually polyostotic and asymmetric: pelvis, 75% > femur > skull > tibia > vertebra > clavicle > humerus > ribs.

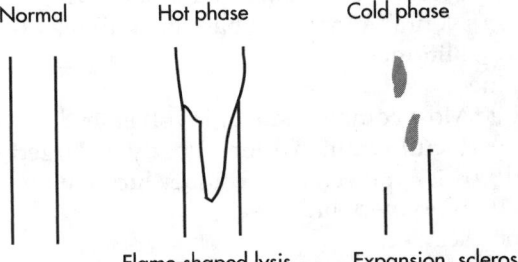

Stages

Active phase = lytic phase = "hot phase" ("hot phase" does not refer to bone scan)
- Aggressive bone resorption: lytic lesions with sharp borders that destroy cortex and advance along the shaft (candle flame, blade of grass)
- Characteristically, lesions start at one end of bone and slowly extend along the shaft.
- Bone marrow is replaced by fibrous tissue and disorganized, fragile trabecular.

Inactive phase = quiescent phase = "cold phase" ("cold phase" does not refer to bone scan)
- New bone formation and sclerosis: thickening of cortex and coarse trabeculations

Mixed pattern = lytic and sclerotic phases coexist
- Bowing of bones becomes a prominent feature.

Clinical findings
- Often asymptomatic
- Painful, warm extremities
- Bowed long bones
- Neurological disorders from nerve or spinal cord compression
- Enlarged hat size
- High-output CHF (increased perfusion of bone), increased metabolism
- Elevated serum alkaline phosphatase and urine hydroxyproline

Radiographic features

Long bones

- Thickening of cortex and enlargement of bone
- Bowing of tibia and femur
- Lysis begins in subarticular location
- Candle flame: V-shaped lytic lesion advancing into diaphysis

Pelvis

- Thickening of iliopubic, ilioischial lines (early signs)
- Thickening of trabeculae
- Acetabular protrusio

Skull

- Osteoporosis circumscripta: osteolytic phase, commonly seen in frontal bone
- Cotton-wool appearance: mixed lytic-sclerotic lesions
- Inner and outer table involved: diploic widening
- Basilar invagination with narrowing of foramen magnum: cord compression
- Neural foramen at base of skull may be narrowed: hearing loss, facial palsy, blindness

Spine

- Most common site of involvement
- Picture frame vertebral body: enlarged square vertebral body with peripheral thick trabeculae and inner lucency
- Ivory vertebra

Bone scan

- Extremely hot lesions in lytic phase
- Increased radiotracer uptake typically abuts one joint and extends distally
- Cold lesions if inactive (uncommon)

Complications

- Pathological fractures
    - Vertebral compression fractures
    - Small horizontal cortical stress fractures in long bones (banana fracture, usually along convex border)
- Malignant degeneration < 1% (osteosarcoma > fibrosarcoma > chondrosarcoma)
- Giant cell tumors in skull and face, often multiple
- Secondary OA (increased stress on cartilage)
- Bone deformity (chronic stress insufficiency)
- High-output

Pearls

- Bone scans are useful in determining the extent of the disease.
- Lesions in the lytic phase are very vascular: dense enhancement by CT.
- Always evaluate for sarcomatous degeneration.
- Treatment
    - Calcitonin (inhibits bone resorption)
    - Diphosphonate (inhibits demineralization)
    - Mithramycin (cytotoxin)

OSTEONECROSIS

Osteonecrosis (avascular necrosis, ischemic necrosis, aseptic necrosis) may be caused by two mechanisms:
- Interruption of arterial supply
- Intra/extraosseous venous insufficiency

The pathophysiology of all osteonecrosis is the same: ischemia → revascularization → repair → deformity → osteoarthrosis

PATHOPHYSIOLOGY OF OSTEONECROSIS	
Cause	Mechanism
Fractures (navicular bone, femoral neck)	Interruption of blood supply
Dislocation (talus, hip)	Ischemia (stretching of vessels)
Collagen vascular disease	Vasculitis
Sickle cell disease	Sludging of RBC
Gaucher's disease	Infiltration of red marrow and vascular compromise
Caisson disease	Nitrogen embolization
Radiation	Direct cytotoxic effect
Pancreatitis, alcoholism	Fat embolization
Hormonal (steroids, Cushing's disease)	Probable fat proliferation and vascular compromise
Idiopathic (Legg-Calvé-Perthes disease)	Unknown
Pregnancy	Unknown

Radiographic features

Plain films
- Findings lag several months behind time of injury. These findings include areas of radiolucency, sclerosis, bone collapse, joint space narrowing, and in the femoral head, a characteristic subchondral radiolucent crescent. Some of these represent late findings.
- Plain film staging system (Ficat)
    - Stage I: clinical symptoms of AVN but no radiographic findings
    - Stage II: osteoporosis, cystic areas and osteosclerosis
    - Stage III: translucent subcortical fracture line (crescent sign), flattening of femoral head
    - Stage IV: loss of bone contour with secondary osteoarthritis

MRI
- Most sensitive imaging modality: 95%-100% sensitivity
- Earliest sign is bone marrow edema (nonspecific)
- Early AVN: focal subchondral abnormalities (very specific)
    - Dark band on T1W/bright band on T2W
    - Double line sign (T2W): bright inner band/dark outerband occurs later in disease process after the start of osseous repair

- Late AVN: fibrosis of subchondral bone
    - Dark on T1W and T2W images
    - Femoral head collapse
- Mitchell classification
    - Class A (early disease): signal intensity analogous to fat (high on T1W and intermediate on T2W)
    - Class B: signal intensity analogous to blood (high on T1W and T2W)
    - Class C: signal intensity analogous to fluid (low on T1W and high on T2W)
    - Class D (late disease): signal intensity analogous to fibrous tissue (low on T1W and T2W)
- MR imaging is helpful in planning treatment for AVN. Treatment options include core decompression, used in early disease, bone grafts, osteotomy, and electric stimulation.

Bone scanning
- Less sensitive than MRI

Complications
- Fragmentation
- Cartilage destruction with secondary DJD
- Intraarticular fragments
- Malignant degeneration (malignant fibrous histiocytoma [MFH], fibrosarcoma, chondrosarcoma)

KIENBÖCK'S DISEASE

Osteonecrosis of the lunate bone. Mean age: 20-30 years. Rare under 15 years of age. Predilection for right wrist, males, heavy labor. High incidence of negative ulnar variance.

Radiographic features
- Sclerotic lunate
- Occasionally a subchondral fracture is seen along the radial surface.
- Most patients develop arthritic changes.

OSTEONECROSES: EPONYMS			
Location	Name	Age	Frequency
UPPER EXTREMITIES			
Humeral head	Haas	Adult	Rare
Humeral capitellum	Panner's	Adolescent	Rare
Distal ulnar epiphysis	Burns	Children	Rare
Scaphoid	Preiser's	Adolescent	+
Lunate	Kienböck's	Adult	+
Metacarpal head	Dietrich	Adolescent	Rare
Entire carpus	Caffey's	Children	Rare
LOWER EXTREMITIES			
Femoral head	Legg-Calvé-Perthes	4-10	+++
Idiopathic coxa vara		6-16	++
Inferior patella	Sinding-Larsen-Johansson	8-12	+
Tibial tubercle	Osgood-Schlatter	10-16	++
Proximal medial tibial epiphysis	Blount	2-14	+
Talus	Diaz	Children	Rare
Distal tibia	Liffert-Arkin	Children	Rare
Calcaneal apophysis	Sever's	5-15	Rare
Navicular	Köhler's bone	4-8	++
Middle cuneiform	Hicks	4-8	Rare
Metatarsal head	Frieberg's	11-18	Rare
Fifth metatarsal base	Iselin	Adolescent	Rare
Trochanters	Mancl		Rare
Os tibiale externum	Haglund's	Adult	Rare
PELVIS			
Ischiopubic synchondrosis	van Neck	Adolescent	Rare
Symphyseal synchondrosis	Pierson	Adolescent	Rare
Iliac crest	Buchman	Adolescent	Rare
Ischial tuberosity	Milch	Adolescent	Rare
SPINE			
Vertebral body	Kümmell's	4-8	Rare
Vertebral apophyses	Scheuermann's	10-18	++

These osteonecroses are usually idiopathic in origin. If an osteonecrosis occurs as a complication of trauma (i.e., scaphoid) it is not called by its eponym but simply referred to as a posttraumatic AVN. Many of the eponyms are archaic, and some are questionable. For instance, some authors believe that Kümmell's disease (manifests as vertebra plana and intervertebral vacuum phenomenon) may actually represent Langerhans' cell histiocytosis.

Differential Diagnosis

Focal Bone Lesions

FOCAL LESIONS

- Tumor
    Metastases (common)
    Primary (less common)
- Inflammation/infection/idiopathic
- Congenital
- Metabolic: brown tumors
- Trauma
    Stress fracture
    Insufficiency fracture
    Pathological fracture
- Vascular
    Osteonecrosis
    Infarct

BONE TUMORS

SYNOPSIS OF PRIMARY BONE TUMORS		
Origin	Benign	Malignant
Osteogenic	Osteoma Osteoid osteoma Osteoblastoma	Osteosarcoma
Chondrogenic	Enchondroma Chondroblastoma Osteochondroma Chondromyxoid fibroma	Chondrosarcoma
Fibrogenic	Fibrous cortical defect Nonossifying fibroma Ossifying fibroma (Sisson's) Desmoplastic fibroma Fibrous dysplasia	MFH Fibrosarcoma
Bone marrow	Eosinophilic granuloma	Ewing's sarcoma Myeloma Lymphoma Leukemia
Other	Simple bone cyst Aneurysmal bone cyst Intraosseous ganglion Intraosseous lipoma Giant cell tumor Brown tumor Pseudotomor	Adamantinoma Chordoma Malignant giant cell tumor
Vascular	Hemangioma Lymphangioma Angiomatosis	Hemangioendothelioma Hemangiopericytoma Angiosarcoma

MALIGNANT BONE TUMORS BY AGE

Up to age 10:
- Ewing's sarcoma
- OSA
- Leukemia, lymphoma

10-20:
- OSA
- Ewing's sarcoma
- Lymphoma, leukemia

20-30:
- OSA
- Lymphoma
- Ewing's sarcoma
- MFH

Over 30:
- Myeloma
- Metastases
- Lymphoma
- Chondrosarcoma
- MFH, fibrosarcoma
- OSA

BUBBLY LESIONS OF THE BONE (HELMS):

Mnemonic: FEGNOMASHIC
- **F**ibrous dysplasia, fibrous cortical defect
- **E**G, Enchondroma
- **G**CT
- **N**OF
- **O**steoblastoma
- **M**yeloma, metastases
- **A**neurysmal bone cyst (always eccentric)
- **S**imple unilocular bone cyst (always central)
- **H**yperparathyroidism (HPT), hemophilia
- **I**nfection
- **C**hondroblastoma

LYTIC EPIPHYSEAL LESIONS

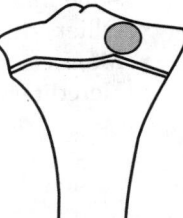

Tumor
- GCT
- EG
- Chondroblastoma
- Metastases (rare)

Infection
- Osteomyelitis
- Tuberculosis (TB)

Subchondral cyst
- Arthropathy (CPPD, OA, RA, hemophilia)

Interosseous ganglion

SCLEROTIC METASTASES

- Prostate
- Breast
- Hodgkin's lymphoma
- Other primaries
    Carcinoid
    Medulloblastoma
    Bladder
    Lung

PERMEATIVE LESION IN CHILDREN

- Round cell tumors (see above)
- Infection
- EG
- OSA (rare)

PERMEATIVE LESION IN ADULTS

- Metastases
- Multiple myeloma
- Lymphoma, leukemia
- Fibrosarcoma

BONY SEQUESTRUM

Criterion: calcified nidus in a bone lesion.
- Osteomyelitis
- EG (button sequestrum)
- Fibrosarcoma
- Osteoid osteoma (calcified nidus)

MALIGNANT TRANSFORMATION OF BONY LESIONS

- Fibrous dysplasia: fibrosarcoma, OSA, MFH
- Paget's disease: OSA >> chondrosarcoma, fibrosarcoma, MFH, lymphoma (rare)
- Osteomyelitis with draining sinus: squamous cell carcinoma (SCC)
- Radiation: OSA, chondrosarcoma, MFH
- Bone infarct: fibrosarcoma, MFH
- Olliers disease: chondrosarcoma
- Maffucci's syndrome: chondrosarcoma
- Hereditary osteochondromatosis: chondrosarcoma

FOCAL SCLEROTIC LESION

Mnemonic: TIC MTV

Tumor
- Benign
    Osteoma
    Osteoid osteoma, osteoblastoma
    Enchondroma
    Fibrous dysplasia
    Healing lesions: NOF, EG, brown tumor
- Malignant
    Metastasis
    Sarcomas
    Lymphoma, leukemia
- Any healing tumor (EG, brown tumor, treated metastases)

Infection
- Osteomyelitis
    Sequestration
    Sclerosing osteomyelitis of Garre

Congenital
- Bone island
- Melorheostosis
- Fibrous dysplasia

Metabolic
- Paget's disease

Trauma
- Stress fracture
- Healing fracture

Vascular
- Osteonecrosis
- Bone infarct

OSTEONECROSIS

Mnemonic: ASEPTIC
- Anemias (hereditary)
- Steroids
- Ethanol
- Pancreatitis, pregnancy
- Trauma
- Idiopathic
- Caisson disease, collagen vascular diseases

Joints

DEGENERATIVE JOINT DISEASE (DJD)

Primary DJD, 90%
Secondary DJD, 10%
- Mechanical joint abnormality
    Posttraumatic
    Osteonecrosis
    Injured menisci or ligaments
    Bone dysplasias
    Loose bodies
- Abnormal forces on a joint
    Occupational
    Postoperative
    Bone dysplasias
- Abnormal cartilage within joint
    Hemochromatosis
    Acromegaly
    Alkaptonuria
- Any inflammatory or metabolic arthritis

INFLAMMATORY ARTHRITIS

SYNOPSIS OF CLINICAL FEATURES				
	RA	AS	Psoriasis	Reiter
Sex	Female	Male	Both	Young male
Peripheral distribution	Hand	Hip	Hand	Feet
Asymmetry	No	Yes	Yes	Yes
Sausage digits	No	No	Yes	Yes
Periosteal reaction	No	No	Yes	Yes
Sacroiliitis	No	Yes	Yes	Yes
Clinical	RF+	IBD	Nail, skin changes	Urethritis, conjunctivitis
HLA-B27	No	< 90%	30%	80%

JACCOUD'S ARTHROPATHY

Ulnar and volar subluxation of metacarpals
- SLE
- Rheumatic fever
- Scleroderma

PERIARTICULAR OSTEOPENIA

- RA (also diffuse osteopenia)
- Scleroderma
- Hemophilia
- Osteomyelitis

SUBCHONDRAL CYSTS

Normal bone density
- DJD
- CPPD
- Seronegative spondyloarthropathies
- Gout
- Pigmented villonodular synovitis (PVNS)
- Synovial osteochondromatosis
- Neuropathic joint

Abnormal bone density
- Any of the above
- RA
- AVN

ACROOSTEOLYSIS

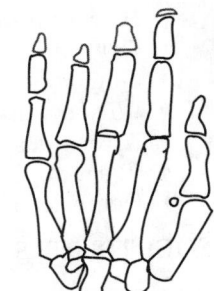

Mnemonic: PINCH FO
- **P**soriasis
- **I**njury (thermal burn, frostbite)
- **N**europathy
    Congenital insensitivity to pain
    Diabetes mellitus
    Leprosy
    Myelomeningocele
- **C**ollagen vascular
    Scleroderma
    Raynaud's disease
- **H**yperparathyroidism
- **F**amilial (Hadju-Cheney)
- **O**ther
    Polyvinyl chloride (PVC) exposure (midportion)
    Snake, scorpion venom

NEW BONE FORMATION IN ARTHRITIS

Periosteal new bone formation
- Psoriasis
- Reiter's syndrome

Osteophytes
- OA
- CPPD

CALCIFICATIONS AND ARTHROPATHY

Periarticular
- Scleroderma (common)
- SLE (uncommon)

Articular
- CPPD
- Chondrocalcinosis (see below)

Joint-space related
- Neuropathic arthropathy
- Synovial osteochondromatosis
- Osteochondritis dissecans
- Osteochondral fracture

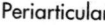
Periarticular

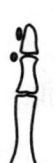

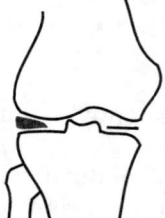
Chondrocalcinosis

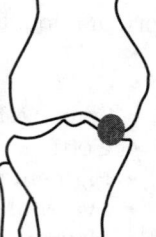
Joint-space related

CHONDROCALCINOSIS

Mnemonic: HOGWASH
- **H**yperparathyroidism
- **O**chronosis (alkaptonuria)
- **G**out
- **W**ilson's disease
- **A**rthritides (any)
- (**P**)seudogout: CPPD
- **H**emochromatosis

SOFT TISSUE SWELLING IN ARTHRITIS

Symmetric bilateral swelling
- RA (most common)
- Any inflammatory arthritis

Asymmetric swelling of one digit: sausage digit
- Psoriasis
- Reiter's syndrome

Lumpy-bumpy soft tissue swelling
- Gout (tophus)
- Amyloidosis
- Multicentric reticulohistiocytosis
- Sarcoid

DIFFERENTIAL DIAGNOSIS OF ARTHRITIS BY DISTRIBUTION

Distal (distal and proximal interphalangeal joints)
- OA
- Psoriasis
- Reiter's syndrome
- Multicentric reticulohistiocytosis

Proximal (MCP, carpus)
- RA
- CPPD
- Hemochromatosis
- Wilson's disease

Ulnar styloid
- RA

MONOARTICULAR ARTHRITIS

Mnemonic: CHRIST
- **C**rystal arthropathies
- **H**emophilia
- **R**A (atypical)
- **I**nfection (excluding Lyme disease and gonorrhea)
- **S**ynovial
    PVNS
    Synovial osteochondromatosis
- **T**rauma

NEUROPATHIC JOINT

Common
- Diabetes mellitus
- Spinal cord injury
- Myelomeningocele/syringomyelia
- Alcohol abuse

Uncommon
- Syphilis (tabes dorsalis)
- Congenital indifference to pain
- Neuropathies (e.g., Riley-Day)
- Amyloidosis

CLINICAL SYNDROMES ASSOCIATED WITH ARTHROPATHIES

- Behçet's disease: arthritis, orogenital ulcers, iritis, large artery, aneurysms, central nervous system (CNS) arteritis
- Reiter's disease: arthritis, urethritis, conjunctivitis
- Still's disease: juvenile RA (JRA), hepatosplenomegaly, lymphadenopathy
- Felty's syndrome: RA, splenomegaly, neutropenia
- Jaccoud's disease: arthritis following repeated episodes of rheumatic fever
- CREST syndrome: **c**alcinosis, **R**aynaud's disease, **e**sophageal dysmotility, **s**clerodactyly, **t**elangiectasia
- Phemister triad (TB arthritis): osteoporosis, marginal erosions, slow cartilage destruction

ATLANTOAXIAL SUBLUXATION

- RA, JRA
- Seronegative spondyloarthropathies
- SLE
- Down syndrome
- Morquio's syndrome
- Trauma

Bone Density

DIFFUSE OSTEOSCLEROSIS (DENSE BONES)

Tumor
- Metastases
- Lymphoma/leukemia
- Myelofibrosis
- Mastocytosis

Congenital
- Osteopetrosis
- Pyknodysostis
- Craniotubular dysplasias
- Sickle cell anemia
- Physiological newborn

Metabolic
- Paget's disesae
- Renal osteodystrophy
- Fluorosis
- Hypervitaminosis A and D

Alternative mnemonic: 3Ms PROOF
- **Metastases**
- **Myelofibrosis**
- **Mastocytosis**
- **Sickle cell anemia**
- **P**yknodysostosis, Paget's disease
- **R**enal osteodystrophy
- **O**steopetrosis
- **O**thers (dysplasias, hypothyroidism)
- **F**lurosis (heavy metal poisoning)

OSTEOPENIA

Localized osteopenia
- Disuse osteoporosis: pain, immobilization
- Arthritis
- Sudeck's atrophy, reflex sympathetic dystrophy
- Paget's disease (lytic phase)
- Transient osteoporosis
    Transient osteoporosis of the hip
    Regional migratory osteoporosis

Diffuse osteopenia
- Primary osteoporosis
- Secondary osteoporosis
    Endocrine diseases
    Nutritional deficiencies
    Hereditary metabolic and collagen disorders
    Medications

- Osteomalacia
    Nutritional deficiences
    Abnormal vitamin D metabolism (inherited, acquired)
    GI absorption disorders
    Renal disease
    Medications
- HPT
- Marrow replacement
    Malignancy (e.g., myeloma)
    Marrow hyperplasia (e.g., hemoglobinopathy)
    Lysosomal storage diseases (e.g., Gaucher's disease)

MULTIPLE SCLEROTIC LESIONS

Tumor
- Metastases
- Lymphoma/leukemia
- Osteomatosis (Gardner's syndrome)
- Healing lesions
- Sclerotic myeloma (very rare)

Congenital
- Fibrous dysplasia
- Osteopoikilosis
- Tuberous sclerosis
- Mastocytosis

Metabolic
- Paget's disease

Trauma
- Healing fractures

Vascular
- Bone infarcts

Periosteum

ASYMMETRIC PERIOSTEAL REACTION

- Tumor
- Infection (osteomyelitis, soft tissue infection, congenital infection)
- Inflammation (psoriatic, Reiter's disease, JRA)
- Trauma (fractures)
- Vascular (subperiosteal hemorrhage)

SYMMETRIC PERIOSTEAL REACTION IN ADULTS

- Vascular insufficiency (venous > arterial)
- Hypertrophic pulmonary osteoarthropathy
- Pachydermoperiostosis
- Fluorosis
- Thyroid acropathy

HYPERTROPHIC PULMONARY OSTEOARTHROPATHY (HPO)

Intrathoracic tumor (removal of malignancy produces relief of HPO pain)
- Bronchogenic carcinoma
- Benign fibrous tumor of the pleura
- Metastases
- Mesothelioma

Chronic pulmonary infection: bronchiectasis, abscess
Other entities that occasionally show periosteal bone formation but are more commonly associated with clubbing:
- Inflammatory bowel disease (ulcerative colitis, Crohn's disease)
- Dysentery
- Cirrhosis
- Cyanotic heart disease

Skull

SOLITARY LYTIC LESION

Tumors
- Metastases*
- Multiple myeloma*
- EG
- Epidermoid*
- Hemangioma*

Infections, inflammation
- Osteomyelitis (tuberculosis [TB], syphilis especially)
- Sarcoidosis*

Congenital
- Fibrous dysplasia
- Encephalocele

Metabolic
- Paget's disease*
- Hyperthyroidism

Trauma
- Leptomeningeal cyst

DIFFUSE SKULL LESIONS

- Sickle cell anemia and thalassemia (hair-on-end appearance)
- HPT (salt and pepper skull)
- Paget's disease (cotton wool appearance)
- Fibrous dysplasia (predominantely outer table)
- Tuberous sclerosis (increased density of both tables)

*Often present as multiple lesions.

MULTIPLE LYTIC LESIONS

Mnemonic: POEMS
- **P**aget's disease
- **P**arathyroid elevation (HPT)
- **O**steomyelitis
- **E**G
- **M**etastases
- **M**yeloma
- **S**arcoidosis

BASILAR INVAGINATION

Congenital
- Osteogenesis imperfecta
- Klippel-Feil syndrome
- Achondroplasia
- Chiari malformations
- Cleidocranial dysplasia

Acquired bone softening
- Paget's disease
- HPT
- Osteomalacia, rickets

Spine

VERTEBRAL BODY

Abnormal density
- Picture frame:
  - Paget's disease (cortex too prominent)
  - Osteoporosis (center too lucent)
- Rugger jersey:
  - Renal osteodystrophy
- Ivory vertebral body
  - Metastasis
  - Paget's disease
  - Lymphoma
  - Infection

Striated vertebral body
- Multiple myeloma
- Hemangioma
- Osteoporosis
- Paget's disease

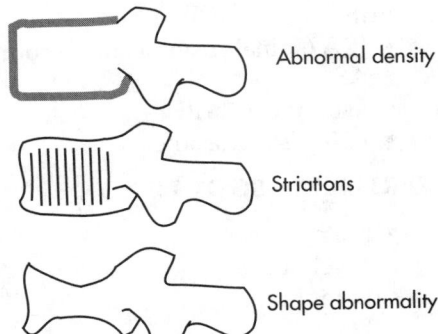
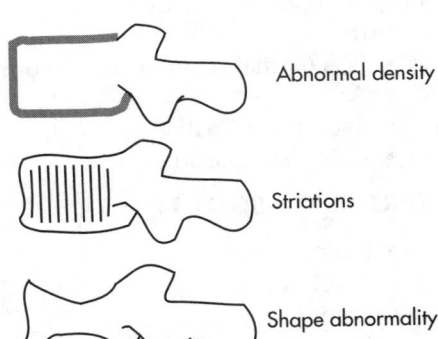

Abnormal density

Striations

Shape abnormality

Shape abnormalities
- Fish vertebra: sickle cell disease, thalassemias
- Squared vertebra: ankylosing spondylitis (AS), Paget's disease, psoriasis, Reiter's syndrome

IVORY VERTEBRAL BODY

- Metastasis
- Lymphoma (Hodgkin's > non-Hodgkin's)
- Paget's disease
- Infection

VERTEBRAL OUTGROWTHS

Syndesmophytes
- AS

Flowing paraspinal ossification
- DISH

Small osteophytes
- Degenerative disease
- Spondylosis deformans

Large osteophytes
- Psoriasis (common)
- Reiter's syndrome (uncommon)

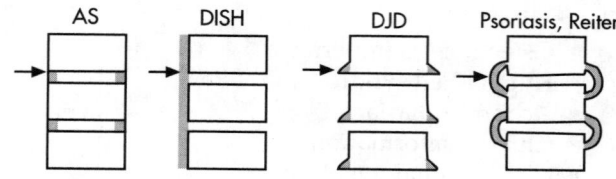

POSTERIOR SPINAL FUSION

Congenital (Klippel-Feil syndrome)
Surgical fusion
Arthritides
- JRA (spinal fusion is more common than in RA)
- AS
- Psoriatic arthritis
- Reiter's syndrome

VERTEBRAL BODY LESION

- Metastasis
- Myeloma
- Lymphoma
- EG
- GCT
- Hemangioma
- Sarcomas (rare)

POSTERIOR ELEMENT LESION

TYPES OF TUMORS	
Anterior: Malignant	**Posterior: Benign**
COMMON Lymphoma Myeloma Ewing's sarcoma Metastases	Osteoid osteoma Osteoblastoma ABC
EXCEPTIONS Hemangioma EG Giant cell tumor	

SOLITARY VERTEBRAL LESIONS

Mnemonic: A HOG
- **A**neurysmal bone cyst (ABC)
- **H**emangioma
- **O**steoblastoma/osteoid osteoma
- **G**iant cell tumor

POSTERIOR VERTEBRAL SCALLOPING

Increased intraspinal pressure
- Spinal canal tumors
- Syrinx
- Communicating hydrocephalus

Dural ectasia
- Neurofibromatosis
- Marfan syndrome
- Ehlers-Danlos syndrome

Congenital
- Achondroplasia
- Mucopolysaccharidoses (Morquio's, Hunter's, Hurler's)
- Osteogenesis imperfecta (tarda)

Bone resorption
- Acromegaly

ANTERIOR VERTEBRAL SCALLOPING

- Aortic aneurysm
- Lymphadenopathy
- TB spondylitis
- Delayed motor development

ANTERIOR VERTEBRAL BODY BEAK

- Morquio's syndrome (central beak)
- Hurler's syndrome
- Achondroplasia
- Cretinism
- Down syndrome
- Neuromuscular disease

Central beak (Morquio)

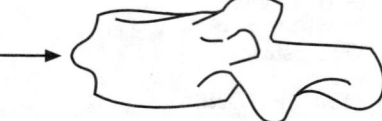

PLATYSPONDYLY

Diffuse
- Dwarf syndromes (thanatophoric, metatropic)
- Osteogenesis imperfecta
- Morquio's syndrome
- Spondyloepiphyseal dysplasia

Solitary or multifocal
- Leukemia
- EG
- Metastasis/myeloma
- Sickle cell disease

Inferior beak (others)

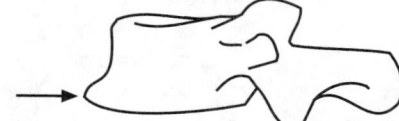

SPINAL OSTEOMYELITIS VS. TUMOR		
	Osteomyelitis	**Tumor**
Contiguity	Yes	No
Paraspinal soft tissue mass	Yes (abscess)	Less common
Disk space	Isocenter	Not involved

Paraspinal mass ——   > 2 vertebrae involved

Pelvis

PROTRUSIO ACETABULI

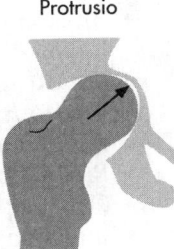

Protrusio

- Paget's disease
- RA
- Osteomalacia, rickets
- Trauma
- Marfan syndrome
- AS
- Idiopathic

SACROILIITIS

Bilateral symmetric
- AS
- Enteropathic spondyloarthropathy
- Psoriatic arthritis
- HPT
- DJD

Bilateral asymmetric
- Reiter's syndrome
- Psoriatic
- DJD

Unilateral
- Infection
- DJD
- Trauma
- RA

LYTIC LESIONS OF THE SACRUM

- Metastasis
- Chordoma
- Plasmacytoma
- Chondrosarcoma
- GCT

LYTIC LESION OF ILIUM

- Fibrous dysplasia
- ABC
- Unicameral bone cyst (UBC)
- Hemophiliac pseudotumor
- Malignant lesions
     Metastasis
     Plasmacytoma
     Ewing's sarcoma
     Chondrosarcoma
     Lymphoma

5

WIDENED PUBIC SYMPHYSIS

Congenital
- Bladder extrophy
- Epispadias
- Cleidocranial dysplasia
- Genitourinary or anorectal malformations

Bone resorption or destruction
- Pregnancy
- Osteitis pubis
- Infection
- Metastases
- HPT

Lower Extremity

ERLENMEYER FLASK DEFORMITY

Lack of modeling of tubular bones with flaring of the ends.
Mnemonic: CHONG
- **C**raniometaphyseal dysplasias
- **H**emoglobinopathies
    - Thalassemia
    - Sickle cell disease (often with AVN)
- **O**steopetrosis
- **N**iemann-Pick disease
- **G**aucher's disease (often with AVN)
- Other
    - Lead poisoning
    - Fibrous dysplasia
    - Osteochondromatosis
    - Enchondromatosis
    - Fibromatosis

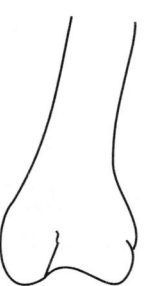
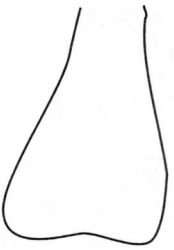

Normal   Erlenmeyer flask

GRACILE BONES

Overtubulation of the shaft with resultant prominent epiphyses. Mnemonic: NIMROD
- **N**eurofibromatosis
- **I**mmobilization or paralysis
    - Poliomyelitis
    - Birth palsies
    - Congenital CNS lesions
- **M**uscular dystrophies
- **R**A (juvenile)
- **O**steogenesis imperfecta
- **D**ysplasias (e.g., Marfan syndrome, homocystinuria)

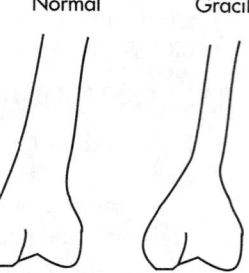

Normal   Gracile

FEMORAL HEAD AVN

Mnemonic: ASEPTIC LEG
- **Alcoholism**
- **Sickle cell disease**
- **Exogenous steroids or RT**
- **Pancreatitis**
- **Trauma**
  - Fracture/dislocation
  - Slipped capital femoral epiphysis
- **Infection**
- **Caisson disease**
- **Legg-Calvé-Perthes**
- **Epiphyseal dysplasia**
- **Gaucher's disease**

MEDIAL TIBIAL SPUR

- Osteochondroma
- Blount's disease
- Turner's syndrome
- Posttraumatic lesion

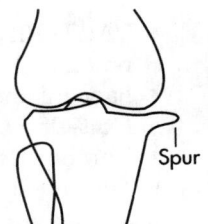

Spur

TIBIAL DIAPHYSEAL CORTICAL LESION

- Adamantinoma
- Osteofibrous dysplasia (ossifying fibroma)
- Fibrous dysplasia
- EG
- Metastasis (adult)

HEEL PAD THICKENING

Criteria: thickness > 25 mm. Mnemonic: MAD COP:
- **M**yxedema (hypothyroidism)
- **A**cromegaly
- **D**ilantin
- **C**allus
- **O**besity
- **P**eripheral edema

5

Upper Extremity

LYTIC LESION OF THE FINGER

- Enchondroma
    Solitary
    Multiple (Ollier's or Maffuci's)
- Glomus tumor (close to nail, painful)
- Foreign body reaction
- Epidermoid inclusion cyst (history of trauma)
- Metastasis (lung, breast)
- Sarcoidosis
- Infection
- Erosive arthropathy

RADIAL HYPOPLASIA

- VACTERL complex (vertebral body, anal, cardiovascular, traceoesophageal, renal, limb anomalies)
- Fanconi anemia
- Holt-Oram syndrome
- Cornelia de Lange syndrome
- Thrombocytopenia-absent radius (TAR syndrome)

SHORT 4TH/5TH METACARPALS

- Pseudohypoparathyroidism
- Pseudopseudohypoparathyroidism
- Idiopathic
- Chromosomal anomalies (Turner's, Klinefelter's)
- Basal cell nevus syndrome

MADELUNG'S DEFORMITY

Premature fusion of ulnar aspect of radial epiphysis. Results in:
- Ulnar angulation of distal radius
- Decreased carpal angle
- Dorsal subluxation of ulna
- Unilateral or bilateral

Mnemonic: HIT DOC
- **H**urler's syndrome
- **I**nfection
- **T**rauma
- **D**yschondrosteosis (Leri-Weil syndrome)
- **O**steochondromatosis
- **C**hromosomal XO (Turner's)

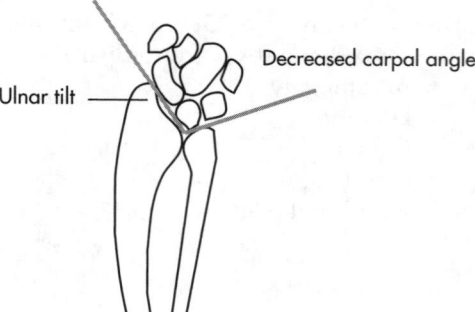

Decreased carpal angle

Ulnar tilt

MISSING DISTAL CLAVICLE

- Erosion RA
- HPT
- Posttraumatic osteolysis
- Infection
- Metastases/myeloma
- Gorham syndrome
- Absence cleidocranial dysplasia
- Pyknodysostosis

HIGH-RIDING SHOULDER

- RA
- CPPD
- Rotator cuff tear

Soft Tissues

SOFT TISSUE CALCIFICATION

Mnemonic: TIC MTV

Tumor
- Tumoral calcinosis
- Synovial osteochondromatosis
- Soft tissue tumor (sarcoma, hemangioma, lipoma)

Inflammation/infection
- Dermatomyositis
- Scleroderma
- Parasites
- Leprosy
- Pancreatitis (fat necrosis)
- Myonecrosis
- Bursitis/tendinitis

Congenital
- Ehlers-Danlos syndrome
- Myositis ossificans progressiva

Metabolic
- HPT (primary or secondary)
- Metastatic calcification (any cause)
- CPPD
- Calcium hydroxyapatite deposition

Trauma
- Myositis ossificans
- Burn injury
- Hematoma

Vascular calcification

SOFT TISSUE MASSES

Tumor
- Malignant fibrous histiocytoma
- Fatty tumors: lipoma, liposarcoma, fibromatoses
- Vascular tumors: hemangioma
- Nerve tumors: schwannoma, neurofibroma
- Metastasis
- Burns
- Hematoma
- Muscle: rhabdomyosarcoma, leiomyosarcoma

Other
- Mysositis ossificans
- Abscess
- Hematoma
- Aneurysm

SUGGESTED READINGS

Brower AC: *Arthritis in black and white,* Philadelphia, 1997, WB Saunders.

Chew F: *Skeletal radiology: the bare bones,* Philadelphia, 1997, Lippincott Williams & Wilkins.

Gerlock AJ, McBride KL, Sinn DP: *Clinical and radiographic interpretation of facial fractures,* Baltimore, 1981, Williams & Wilkins.

Greenspan A: *Orthopedic radiology: a practical approach,* Philadelphia, 1999, Lippincott Williams & Wilkins.

Harris JH, Harris WH, Noveline RA: *The radiology of emergency medicine,* ed 4, Philadelphia, 1999, Lippincott Williams & Wilkins.

Helms CA: *Fundamentals of skeletal radiology,* Philadelphia, 1994, WB Saunders.

Resnick D, Niwayama G: *Diagnosis of bone and joint disorders,* ed 3, Philadelphia, 1994, WB Saunders.

Rhea JT et al : *Emergency radiology: a manual of diagnosis and decisions,* Baltimore, 1988, Williams & Wilkins.

Schultz RJ: *The language of fractures,* Baltimore, 1990, Williams & Wilkins.

Chapter 6

Neurological Imaging

Chapter Outline

6

Imaging Anatomy

Parenchymal Anatomy

LOBAR ANATOMY

- Frontal lobe: anterior to central sulcus (Rolando)
- Parietal lobe: posterior to central sulcus
- Temporal lobe: inferior to lateral sulcus (Sylvius)
- Occipital lobe: posterior
- Limbic lobe
- Central (insular lobe)

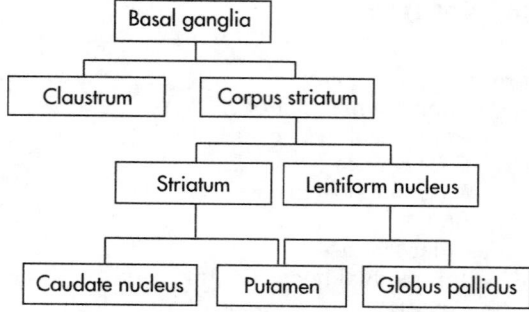

BASAL GANGLIA

- Lentiform nucleus: putamen + globus pallidus
- Striatum: putamen + caudate nucleus
- Claustrum
- Caudate nucleus consists of:
      Head (anterior)
      Body
      Tail (inferior)
- Subthalamic nucleus

THALAMUS

Contains over 25 separate nuclei and serves as a synaptic relay station. Organization:

Thalamus
- Lateral nuclei
- Medial nuclei
- Anterior nuclei

Subthalamus
- Subthalamic nucleus
- Substantia nigra

Hypothalamus

BRAIN MYELINIZATION

Neonatal and pediatric brains have a different computed tomography (CT) and magnetic resonance imaging (MRI) appearance because of:

- Increased water content (changes best seen with T2-weighted [T2W] sequences)
- Decreased myelinization (changes best seen with T1-weighted [T1W] sequences)
- Low iron deposits

Brain maturation begins in the brainstem and progresses to the cerebellum and then to the cerebrum.

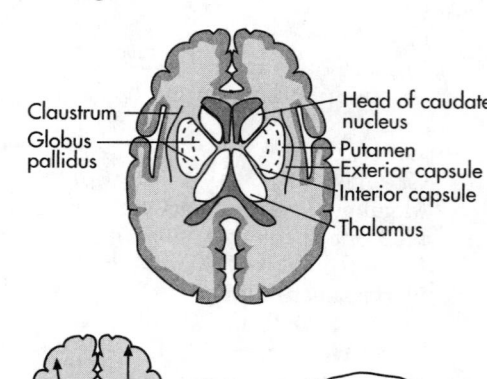

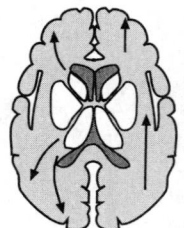

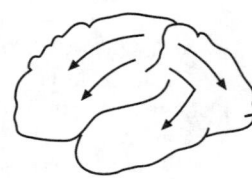

Characteristic MR appearance

Premature
- Smooth cortical surface, lacking cortical folding
- Gray-white matter (GWM) signal intensity reversal on T1W
    - Cortex is hyperintense
    - Basal ganglia are hyperintense

Neonate: myelinization of different structures depends on age

MR DETECTION OF MYELIN BY REGION AND AGE		
Region	T1W	T2W
Cerebellum	3 months	
Corpus callosum	5 months	7 months
Internal capsule		11 months
Frontal white matter		14 months
Adult pattern		18 months

Ventricular System

ANATOMY

Left and right lateral ventricles (1 and 2) connect to 3rd ventricle via a single T-shaped interventricular foramen (Monro's). Anatomical aspects:
- Frontal horn
- Temporal (inferior) horn
- Occipital (posterior) horn
- Central part

3rd ventricle connects to 4th ventricle via cerebral aqueduct of Sylvius. Anatomical aspects:
- Optic recess
- Infundibular recess
- Pineal recess
- Suprapineal recess
- Interthalamic adhesion (massa intermedia)

4th ventricle connects:
- Laterally to cerebrospinal fluid (CSF) via foramen of Luschka
- Posteriorly to CSF via foramen of Magendie
- Inferior to central canal of spinal cord

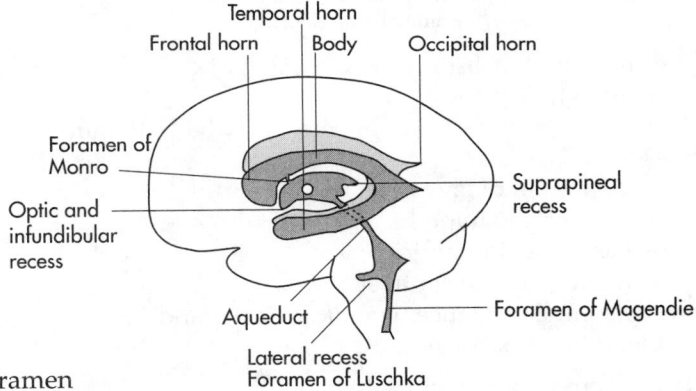

CAVUM VARIANTS

Cavum septum pellucidum
- Separates frontal horns of lateral ventricles (anterior to foramen of Monro)
- 80% of term infants; 15% of adults
- May dilate; rare cause of obstructive hydrocephalus

Cavum vergae
- Posterior continuation of cavum septum pellucidum; never exists without cavum septum pellucidum

Cavum velum interpositum
- Extension of quadrigeminal plate cistern to foramen of Monro

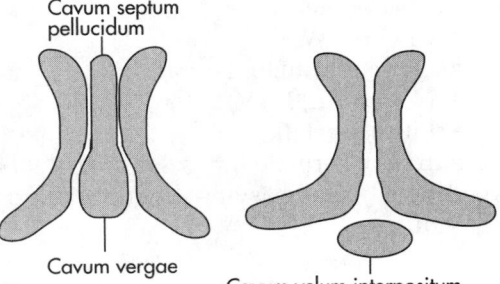

PINEAL REGION ANATOMY

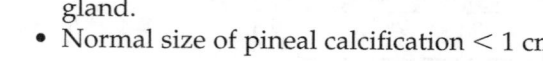

Location
- Posterior to 3rd ventricle
- Adjacent to thalamus

Normal pineal calcification
- 10% are calcified at 10 years of age
- 50% are calcified at 20 years of age
- Calcification should be approximately the size of the normal pineal gland.
- Normal size of pineal calcification < 1 cm

Sella Turcica

PITUITARY GLAND

COMPARTMENTS			
Lobe	Origin	Hormones	MRI Characteristics
Anterior (adenohypophysis)	Rathke's pouch*	PRL, ACTH, others	Intermediate signal
Intermediate	Rathke's pouch		Intermediate signal
Posterior (neurohyophysis)	Floor of 3rd ventricle	Oxytocin, vasopressin	Usually T2 hyperintense

PRL, Prolactin; *ACTH*, adrenocorticotropic hormone.
*Rathke's pouch: roof of primitive oral cavity.

Normal height measurements (coronal MRI)
- 3-8 mm in adults
- Up to 10 mm during puberty; may be > 10 mm during pregnancy

Stalk
- 2-5 mm in diameter
- Connects to hypothalamus
- Passes behind optic chiasm
- Enhances with contrast

Strong contrast enhancement of normal gland (no blood-brain barrier)

SUPRASELLAR CISTERN

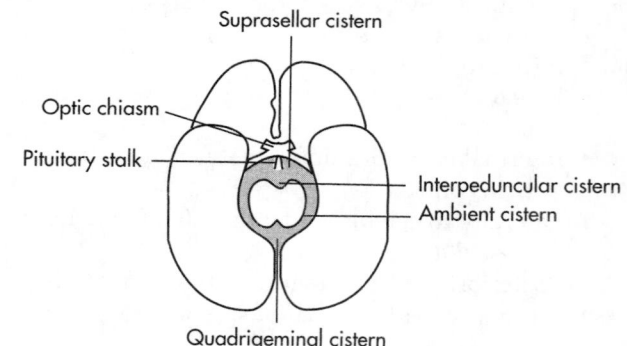

Located above the diaphragma sella. Shape on axial sections:
- 5-pointed star shape (pontine level)
- 6-pointed star shape (midbrain level)

Contents of cistern:
- Circle of Willis
- Optic chiasm, optic tracts
- Nerves (III, IV, V)
- Pituitary stalk

Cistern may herniate into sella: empty sella syndrome (usually asymptomatic with no consequence).

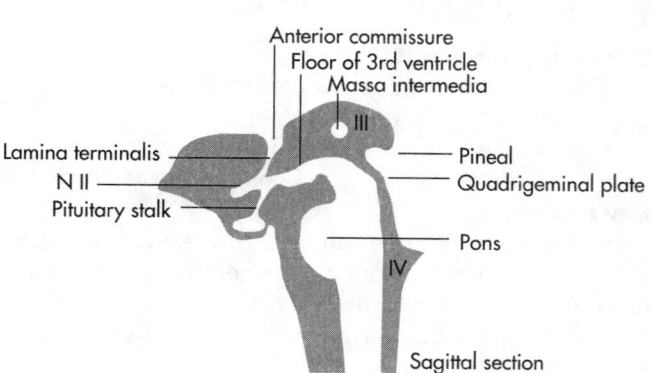

CAVERNOUS SINUS

Dura-enclosed venous channel containing:
- Internal carotid artery (ICA) and sympathetic plexus
- Cranial nerves: III, IV, V1, V2, VI

Connections of sinus:
- Ophthalmic veins
- Retinal veins
- Middle meningeal veins
- Pterygoid vein
- Petrosal sinuses
- Sphenoparietal sinus

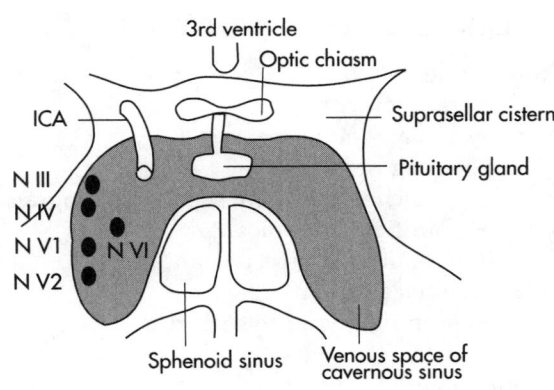

MECKEL'S CAVE (TRIGEMINAL CAVE)

Abuts the most posterior portion of the cavernous sinus (separate from cavernous sinus). Contains:
- Trigeminal nerve roots
- Trigeminal ganglion (Gasserian ganglion)
- CSF

Vascular System

EXTERNAL CAROTID ARTERY (ECA)

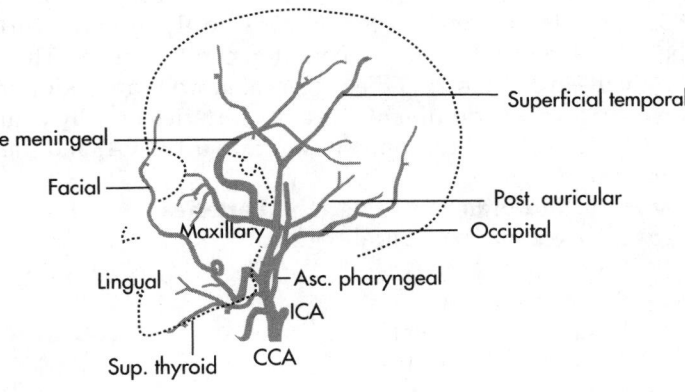

8-main branches (Mnemonic: SALFOPSM):
- **S**uperior thyroid artery
- **A**scending pharyngeal artery
- **L**ingual artery
- **F**acial artery
- **O**ccipital artery
- **P**osterior auricular artery
- **S**uperficial temporal artery
- **M**axillary artery

The major branches of the maxillary artery are:
- Middle meningeal artery through foramen spinosum
- Accessory middle meningeal artery through foramen ovale
- Descending palatine artery (greater palatine)
- Facial, sinus, and nasoorbital branches
- Sphenopalatine, infraorbital, post superior alveolar, artery of the Vidian canal

Meningeal artery supply is from:

ICA
- Inferolateral trunk (ILT)
- Meningohypophyseal trunk
- Ophthalmic branches

ECA
- Middle meningeal artery
- Accessory meningeal artery
- Sphenopalatine artery
- Branches of ascending pharyngeal artery
- Branches of occipital artery

Vertebral artery
- Posterior meningeal artery

INTERNAL CAROTID ARTERY (ICA)

Four segments:

Cervical segment
- Usually no branches

Petrous segment
- Branches are rarely seen on angiograms.
- Caroticotympanic artery
- Vidian artery (inconstant)

Cavernous segment
- Meningohypophyseal trunk
- ILT

Supraclinoid segment (cavernous and supraclinoid segments = carotid siphon)
- Ophthalmic artery
- Superior hypophyseal artery (not routinely visualized)
- Posterior communicating artery (PCOM)
- Anterior choroidal artery

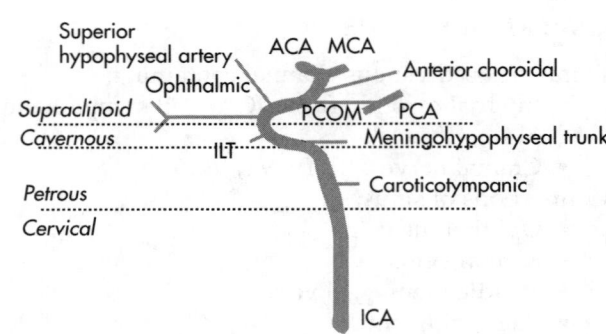

VERTEBROBASILAR SYSTEM

The vertebral arteries are the first branches of the subclavian arteries (95%). The left vertebral artery arises directly from the aortic arch (between left subclavian and common carotid) in 5%. The left artery is dominant in 50%; in 25% the vertebral arteries are codominant; in 25% the right artery is dominant. Vertebral arteries usually course through the C6-C1 vertebral foramina (but may start at C4) and then the foramen magnum.

Segments and branches of vertebral arteries

Cervical segment (extradural segment)
- Muscular branches
- Spinal branches
- Posterior meningeal artery

Intracranial segment (intradural)
- Anterior spinal artery (ASA)
- Posterior inferior cerebellar artery (PICA)

Basilar artery
- Anterior inferior cerebellar artery (AICA)
- Superior cerebellar artery (SCA)
- Brainstem perforating arteries
- Posterior cerebral arteries (PCA)

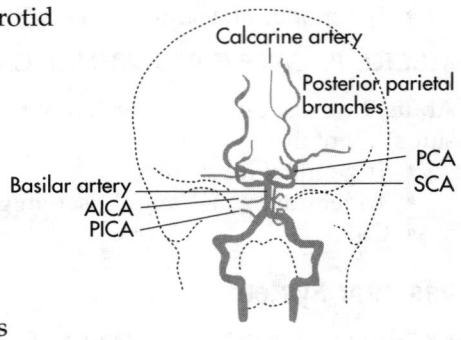

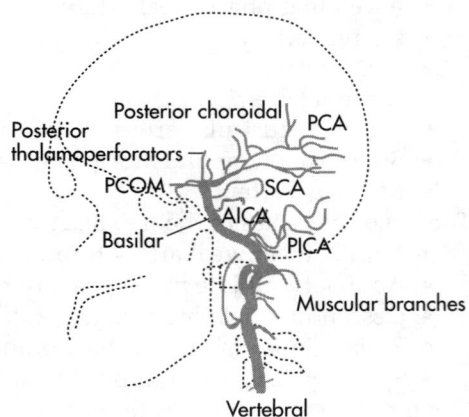

CIRCLE OF WILLIS

The circle is complete in 25% and incomplete in 75%. It consists of:
- Supraclinoid ICAs
- A1 segment of anterior cerebral arteries (ACAs)
- Anterior communicating arteries (ACOMs)
- PCOMs
- P1 segment of PCAs

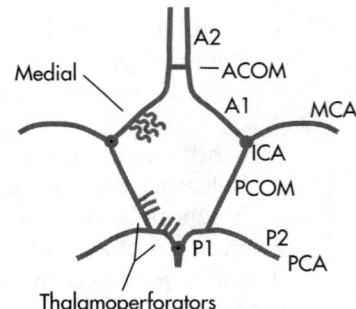

CEREBRAL ARTERIES

Anterior cerebral artery (ACA)
Represents one of the two ICA terminal branches
- A1 segment:
    Origin to ACOM
    Medial lenticulostriates
- A2 segment:
    From ACOM
    Recurrent artery of Heubner
    Frontal branches
- Terminal bifurcation
    Pericallosal artery
    Callosomarginal artery

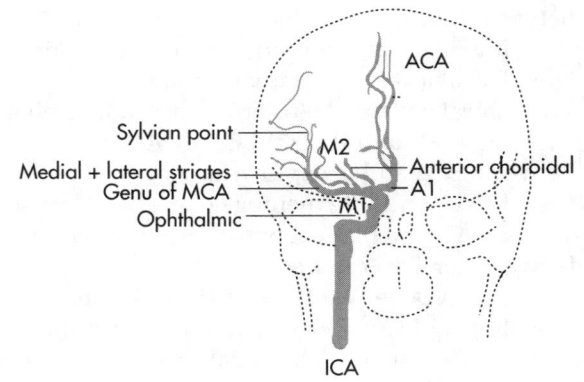

Middle cerebral artery (MCA)
Represents the larger of the two terminal ICA branches
- M1 segment:
    Origin to MCA bifurcation
    Lateral lenticulostriates
- M2 segment:
    Insular branches
- M3 segment:
    MCA branches beyond Sylvian fissure

Posterior cerebral artery (PCA)
- P1 segment:
    Origin to PCOM
    Posterior thalamoperforators
- P2 segment:
    Distal to the PCOM
    Thalamogeniculates
    Posterior choroidal arteries
- Terminal cortical branches

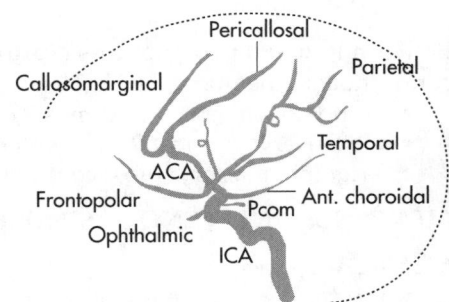

NORMAL VARIANTS OF VASCULAR ANATOMY

Internal carotid artery
- Persistent embryonic cervical ICA branches to vertebrobasilar system
    Proatlantal intersegmental artery
- Aberrant petrous ICA: courses posterolateral and traverses hypotympanum
- Persistent trigeminal artery: cavernous ICA to basilar artery
- Persistent hypoglossal artery: petrous ICA to basilar artery

External carotid artery
- Middle meningeal artery arises from ophthalmic artery
- Variation in order of branching

Circle of Willis
- Hypoplasia of PCOM
- Hypoplasia or absence of A1 segment
- Fetal PCA (originates from ICA) with atretic P1
- Hypoplastic ACOM

ANASTOMOSES BETWEEN ARTERIES

Between ICA and ECA via:
- Maxillary artery branches to ophthalmic artery
- Facial artery to ophthalmic artery
- Dural collaterals (occipital, ascending pharyngeal, middle meningeal)
- ECA → contralateral ECA → ICA

Between ECA and cerebral arteries
- ECA → middle meningeal artery → transdural → pial branches → ACA, MCA
- ECA → meningeal branches → vertebrobasilar artery

Between cerebral arteries
- Left ICA ↔ ACOM ↔ right ICA (circle of Willis)
- ICA ↔ PCOM ↔ basilar (circle of Willis)
- ICA ↔ anterior choroidal ↔ posterior choroidal ↔ basilar
- Leptomeningeal anastomoses: ACA ↔ MCA ↔ PCA ↔ ACA

Between ICA and posterior fossa (primitive embryonic connections; mnemonic: HOT)
- **H**ypoglossal artery: 2nd most common
- **O**tic artery: cervical ICA → vetebral artery; very rare
- **T**rigeminal artery: most common carotid vertebral anastomosis

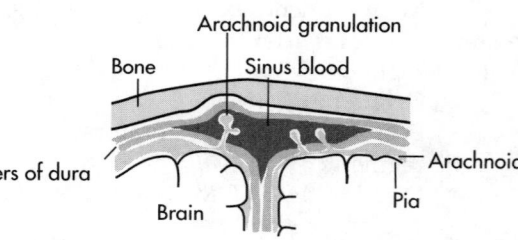

MENINGES AND VENOUS SINUSES

Meningial spaces
- Epidural space: potential space between dura mater (two layers) and bone
- Subdural space: space between dura and arachnoid
- Subarachnoid space: space between arachnoid and pia mater

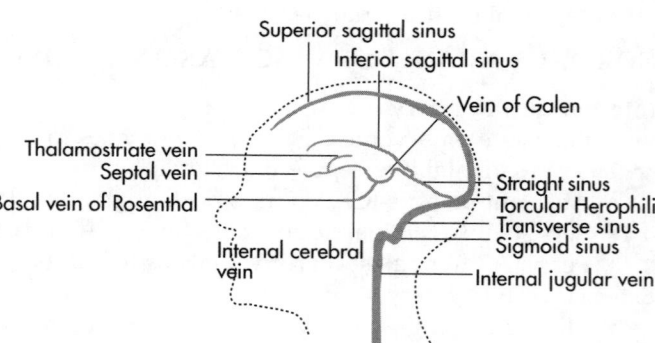

SINUSES
- Superior sagittal sinus: in root of falx
- Inferior sagittal sinus: in free edge of falx
- Straight sinus
- Great vein of Galen: drains into straight sinus
- Occipital sinus
- Confluence of sinuses (torcula of herophilus)
- Left and right transverse sinus: drain from confluence
- Sigmoid sinus: drains into IJV
- Superior petrosal sinus: enters into transverse sinus
- Inferior petrosal sinus

VASCULAR TERRITORIES

ACA
- Hemispheric
- Callosal
- Medial lenticulostriate (Heubner)
    - Caudate head
    - Anterior limb of internal capsule
    - Septum pellucidum

MCA
- Hemispheric
- Lateral lenticulostriate
    - Lentiform nucleus
    - Caudate capsule
    - Internal capsule

PCA
- Hemispheric
- Callosal
- Thalamic and midbrain perforators

SCA
- Superior cerebellum

AICA
- Inferolateral pons
- Middle cerebellar peduncle
- Anterior cerebellum

PICA
- Medulla
- Posterior and inferior cerebellum

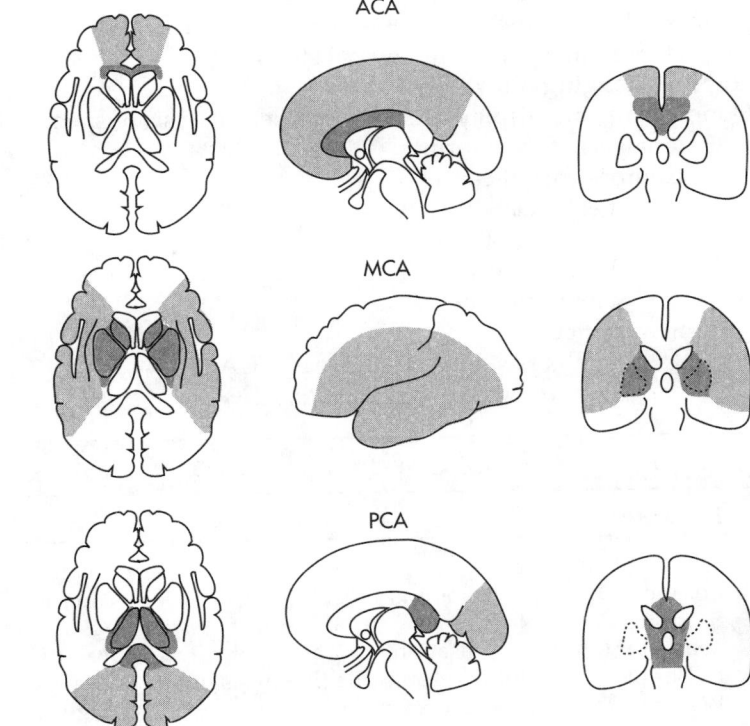

US OF CAROTID ARTERIES

B-mode imaging
Delineate CCA, ECA, ICA, bulb

Vessel wall thickness
- > 1.0 mm is abnormal
- All focal plaques are abnormal.

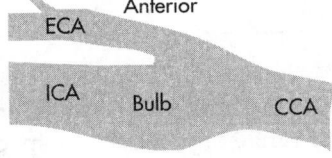

Plaque characterization
- Determine extent and location
- Plaque texture
    - Homogenous (dense fibrous connective tissue)
    - Heterogenous (intraplaque hemorrhage: echogenic center; unstable)
    - Calcified (stable)

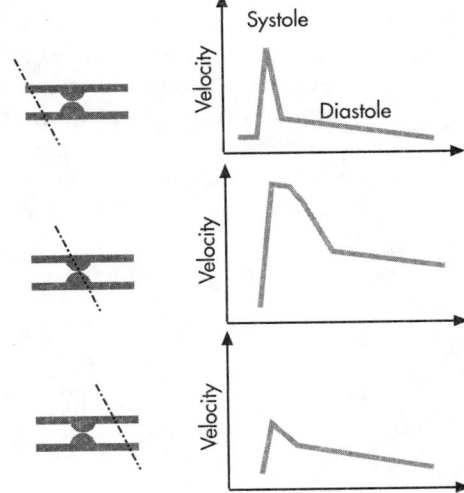

6

Evaluation of stenosis
- Measure visible stenosis in all three planes
- Symmetrical, asymmetrical stenosis

Doppler imaging (flow)

Doppler imaging displays velocity profile. Analysis of spectra:
1. Analysis of waveform
   Components of curve
   - Peak diastolic flow
   - Peak systolic flow
   - Peak broadness
   - Flow direction
   Shape of curves
   - High-resistance vessels (e.g., ECA)
   - Low-resistance vessels (e.g., ICA)

US DIFFERENTIATION OF ICA AND ECA		
Parameter	**ICA**	**ECA**
Size	Large	Small
Location	Posterior and lateral	Anterior and medial
Branches	No	Yes
Temporal tap	No pulsation	Pulsation
Pulsatility	Not very pulsatile (low resistance)	Very pulsatile (high resistance)
Waveform	Low resistance	High resistance
	Flow in systole and diastole	Flow in systole only

2. Spectral broadening
   When normal blood flow is disturbed (by plaques and/or stenoses), blood has a wider range of velocities = spectral broadening.
   Two ways to detect spectral broadening:
   - The spectral window is obliterated.
   - Automated determination of bandwidth = spread of maximum and minimum velocities.
3. Peak velocities
   Flow velocities increase proportionally with the degree of a stenosis: flow of > 225 cm/sec indicates a > 70% stenosis.

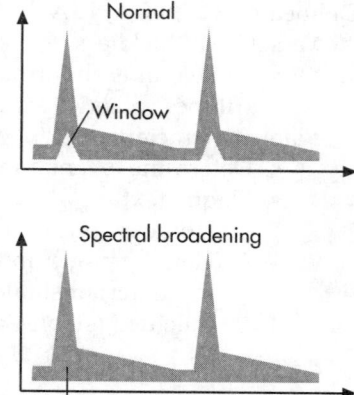

Color Doppler ultrasound

Color Doppler imaging (CDI) displays real-time velocity information in stationary soft tissues. The color assignment is arbitrary but conventionally displayed in the following manner:

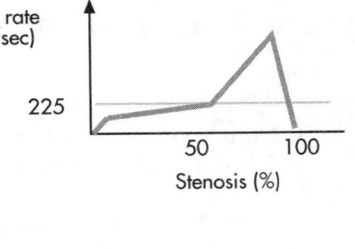

- Red: toward transducer
- Blue: away from transducer
- Green: high-velocity flow
- Color saturation indicates speed
    Deep shades: slow flow
    Light shades: fast flow

Pearls
- Perform CDI only with optimal gain and flow sensitivity settings.
    Ideally the vessel lumen should be filled with color.
    Color should not spill over to stationary tissues.
- Frame rates vary as a function of the area selected for CDI: the larger the area, the slower the frame rate.
- Laminar flow is disrupted at bifurcations.
- Do not equate color saturation with velocity: green-tagged flow in a vessel may represent abnormally high flow or simply a region in the vessel where flow is directed at a more acute angle relative to the transducer.

Spine

SPINAL CANAL

Vertebral elements:
- Body
- Posterior elements
    Neural ring
        Posterior margin of vertebral body
        Pedicles
        Laminae
    Articular facets
    Transverse process

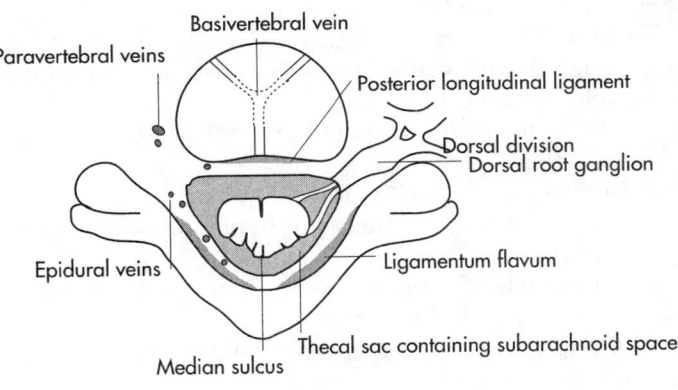

Disks
- Components:
    Nucleus pulposus (notochordal origin)
    Annulus fibrosus with peripheral Sharpey's fibers
- CT density (60-120 HU)
    Disk periphery is slightly denser than its center (Sharpey's fibers calcify).
    Disk is much denser than thecal sac (0-30 HU).
- MR signal intensity
    T1W: hypointense relative to marrow
    PDW, T2W: hyperintense relative to marrow with hypointense intranuclear cleft

Ligaments
- Ligametum flavum: attaches to lamina and facets
- Posterior longitudinal ligament: rarely seen by MRI except in herniations

Thecal sac
- Lined by dura and surrounded by epidural fat
- Normal AP diameter of thecal sac
    Cervical > 7 mm
    Lumbar > 10 mm
- MRI frequently shows CSF flow artifacts in thecal sac.

NEURAL STRUCTURES

Spinal cord
- AP diameter 7 mm
- Conus medullaris: 8 mm (tip at L1-L2)
- Filum terminale extends from L1 to S1

Nerve roots
- Ventral root, dorsal root, dorsal root ganglion
- The dorsal and ventral nerve roots join in the spinal canal to form the spinal nerve. The nerve splits into ventral and dorsal rami a short distance after exiting the neural foramen.
    - Below T1: spinal nerve courses under the pedicle for which they are named (e.g., L4 goes under L4 pedicle)
    - Above T1: spinal nerve courses above the pedicle for which they are named
- Nerve roots lie in the superior portion of the intervertebral neural foramen.

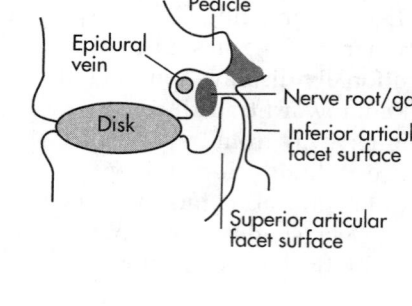

Vascular Disease

Intracranial Hemorrhage

CT APPEARANCE OF INTRACRANIAL HEMORRHAGE

Acute hemorrhage (< 3 days)
- Hyperdense (80-100 HU) relative to brain (40-50 HU)
- High density caused by protein-hemoglobin component (clot retraction)
- Acute hemorrhage is not hyperdense if the hematocrit is low (hemoglobin < 8 g/dl).

Subacute hemorrhage (3-14 days)
- Hyperintense, isointense, or hypointense relative to brain
- Degradation of protein-hemoglobin product evolves from peripheral to center
- Peripheral enhancement may be present.

Chronic hemorrhage (> 2 weeks)
- Hypodense

MR APPEARANCE OF INTRACRANIAL HEMORRHAGE

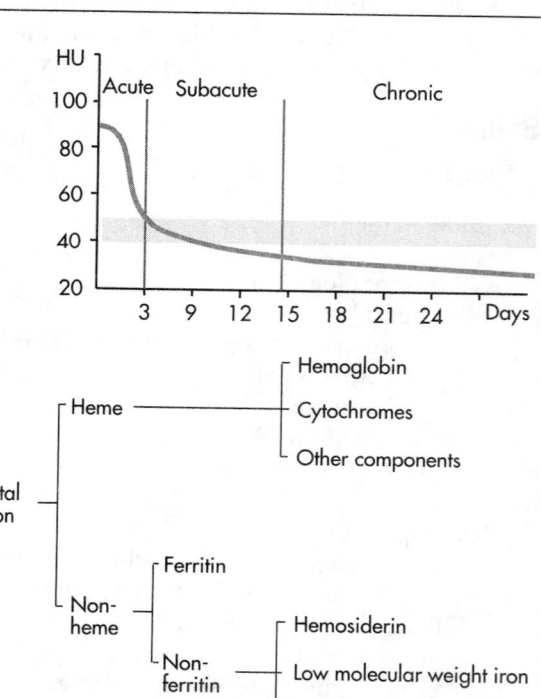

Different iron-containing substances have different magnetic effects (diamagnetic, paramagnetic, superparamagnetic) on surrounding brain tissue. In the circulating form, hemoglobin (Hb) alternates between oxy-Hb and deoxy-Hb as O_2 is exchanged. To bind O_2, the iron (Fe) must be in the reduced Fe (II) (ferrous) state. When Hb is removed from the circulation, the metabolic pathways fail to reduce iron, and Hb begins denaturation. The appearance of blood depends on the magnetic properties of blood products and compartmentalization.

			MRI APPEARANCE OF HEMORRHAGE			
Stage	Biochemistry	Pathophysiology	Location	Magnetism	Appearance T1W/T2W	
Hyperacute (hrs)	Oxy-Hb	Serum + RBCs	Intracellular	Diamagnetic	isointense	bright
Acute (1-2 days)	Deoxy-Hb	Deoxygenation	Intracellular	Paramagnetic	isointense	dark
Early subacute (2-7 days)	Met-Hb	Oxidation/ denaturation	Intracellular	Paramagnetic	bright	dark
Late subacute (1-4 wks)	Met-Hb	RBC lysis	Extracellular	Paramagnetic	bright	bright
Chronic	Hemosiderin Ferritin	Iron storage	Extracellular	Ferromagnetic	dark	dark rim

Isointense,   bright,   dark,   dark rim.

ETIOLOGIES OF INTRAAXIAL (INTRAPARENCHYMAL) HEMORRHAGE

- Hypertension (most common)
- Tumor
- Trauma
- Arteriovenous malformation (AVM)
- Aneurysm
- Coagulopathy
- Amyloid angiopathy
- Emboli
- Hemorrhagic infarction (especially venous)
- Vasculitis

HYPERTENSIVE HEMORRHAGE

Occurs most commonly in areas of penetrating arteries that come off the MCA and/or basilar artery. Depending on size and location of hemorrhage, the mortality is high.
Poor prognostic factors:
- Large size
- Brainstem location
- Intraventricular extension

Location
- Basal ganglia (putamen > thalamus), 80%
- Pons, 10%
- Deep gray matter, 5%
- Cerebellum, 5%

Radiographic features
- Typical location of hemorrhage (basal ganglia) in hypertensive patient
- Mass effect from hemorrhage and edema may cause herniation of brain
- If the patient survives, the hemorrhage heals and leaves a residual cavity that best demonstrated by MRI.

6

TUMOR HEMORRHAGE

Tumor-related intracranial hemorrhage may be due to coagulopathy (leukemia, anticoagulation) or spontaneous bleeding into a tumor. Most authors cite that the incidence of hemorrhage into tumors is roughly 5%-10%. Tumors that commonly hemorrhage include:

- Pituitary adenoma
- Glioblastoma multiforme, anaplastic astrocytoma
- Oligodendroglioma
- Ependymoma
- Primitive neuroectodermal tumors (PNETs)
- Epidermoid
- Metastases

DIFFERENTIAL DIAGNOSIS		
	Benign Hemorrhage	**Tumor Hemorrhage**
Pattern	Simple but may be complex on MR	Complex
Hemosiderin ring	Complete	Incomplete
Enhancement	Rarely (marginal)*	Yes; especially nonhemorrhagic areas
Course	Benign evolution	Persistent edema/mass
Location	Solitary	May be multifocal

*Depends on time after hemorrhage; after a few days, most benign hemorrhages enhance.

Aneurysm

TYPES

Saccular aneurysm ("berry aneurysm"), 80%
- Developmental or degenerative aneurysm (most common)
- Traumatic aneurysm
- Infectious (mycotic) aneurysm 3%
- Neoplastic (oncotic) aneurysm
- Flow-related aneurysm
- Vasculopathies (systemic lupus erythematosus [SLE], Takayasu's, fibromuscular dysplasia [FMDJ])

Fusiform aneurysm
Dissecting aneurysm

SACCULAR ANEURYSM

Berrylike outpouchings predominantly at arterial bifurcation points. Saccular aneurysm are true aneurysm where the sac consists of intima and adventitia. Etiology: degenerative vascular injury (previously thought to be congenital) > trauma, infection, tumor, vasculopathies. Present in approximately 2% of population; multiple in 20%; 25% are giant aneurysms (> 25 mm). Increased incidence of aneurysm in:

- Adult dominant polycystic kidney disease (ADPKD)
- Aortic coarctation
- FMD
- Structural collagen disorders (Marfan, Ehlers-Danlos)
- Spontaneous dissections

Radiographic features

Interpretation of conventional angiography

- Number of aneurysms: multiple in 20%
- Location, 90% in anterior circulation
- Size
- Relation to parent vessel
- Presence and size of aneurysm neck

MRA

- Usually combined with conventional MRI
- Used to screen patients with risk factors (e.g., APKD)
- Low sensitivity for aneurysms < 4 mm
- Need to verify presence of aneurysm by reviewing single slice raw images

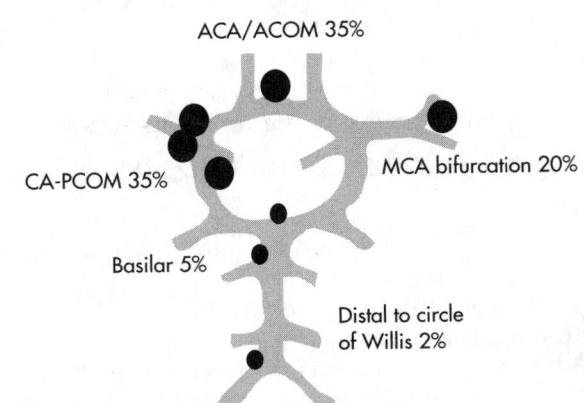

ACA/ACOM 35%

CA-PCOM 35%

MCA bifurcation 20%

Basilar 5%

Distal to circle of Willis 2%

Complications

Rupture

- Subarachnoid hemorrhage
- Parenchymal hematoma
- Hydrocephalus

Vasospasm

- Occurs 4-5 days after rupture
- Causes secondary infarctions
- Leading cause of death/morbidity from rupture

Mass effect

- Cranial nerve palsies
- Headache

Death, 30%

Rebleeding

- 50% rebleed within 6 months
- 50% mortality

In the presence of multiple aneurysms, one may identify the bleeding aneurysm using the following criteria:

- Location of subarachnoid hemorrhage (SAH) or hematoma adjacent to or around bleeding aneurysm
- Largest aneurysm is the one most likely to bleed
- Most irregular aneurysm is the one most likely to bleed
- Extravasation of contrast (rarely seen)
- Vasospasm adjacent to bleeding aneurysm

GIANT ANEURYSM

Aneurysm > 25 mm in diameter. Clinical: mass effect (cranial nerve palsies, retroorbital pain), hemorrhage.

Radiographic features
- Large mass lesion with internal blood degradation products
- Signet sign: eccentric vessel lumen with surrounding thrombus
- Curvilinear peripheral calcification
- Ring enhancement: fibrous outer wall enhances after complete thrombosis
- Mass effect on adjacent parenchyma
- Slow erosion of bone
    Sloping of sellar floor
    Undercutting of anterior clinoid
    Enlarged superior orbital fissure

INFECTIOUS (MYCOTIC) ANEURYSM

Cause:
- Bacterial endocarditis, intravenous drug abuse (IVDA), 80%
- Meningitis, 10%
- Septic thrombophlebitis, 10%

Radiographic features
- Aneurysm itself is rarely visualized by CT.
- Most often located peripherally and multiple
- Intense enhancement adjacent to vessel
- Conventional angiography is the imaging study of choice.

FUSIFORM (ATHEROSCLEROTIC) ANEURYSM

Elongated aneurysm caused by atherosclerotic disease. Most located in the vertebrobasilar system. Often associated with dolichoectasia (elongation and distention of the vertebrobasilar system).

Radiographic features
- Vertebrobasilar arteries are elongated, tortuous, and dilated.
- Tip of basilar artery may indent 3rd ventricle.
- Aneurysm may be thrombosed.
    CT: hyperdense
    T1W: hyperintense

Complications
- Brainstem infarction due to thrombosis
- Mass effect (cranial nerve palsies)

DISSECTING ANEURYSM

Following a dissection an intramural hematoma may organize and result in a saclike out-pouching. Etiology: trauma > vasculopathy (SLE, FMD) > spontaneous dissection. Location: extracranial ICA > vertebral artery.

Radiographic features
- Elongated contrast collections extending beyond the vessel lumen
- MRA is a useful screening modality.
- Angiography is sometimes required for imaging of vascular detail (dissection site).

SUBARACHNOID HEMORRHAGE (SAH)

Blood is present in the subarachnoid space, and sometimes also within ventricles. Secondary vasospasm and brain infarction is the leading cause of death in SAH.
Causes of SAH:

- Aneurysm (most common), 90%
- Trauma
- AVM
- Coagulopathy
- Extension of intraparenchymal bleed (hypertension, tumor)
- Idiopathic, 5%
- Spinal AVM

Radiographic features

- CT is the first imaging study of choice.
- Hyperdense cerebrospinal fluid (CSF) usually in basal cisterns, sylvian fissure (due to aneurysm location), and subarachnoid space
- Hematocrit effect in intraventricular hemorrhage.
- MRI is less sensitive than CT early on (deoxy-Hb and brain are isointense).
- MRI is more sensitive than CT for detecting subacute/chronic SAH.

Complications

- Hemorrhage-induced hydrocephalus is due to early ventricular obstruction and/or arachnoiditis.
- Vasospasm several days after SAH may lead to secondary infarctions.
- Leptomeningeal "superficial" siderosis (dark meninges on T2W): iron deposition in meninges secondary to chronic recurrent SAH. The location of siderosis corresponds to the extent of central myelin. Cranial nerves I, II, and VIII are preferentially affected because these have peripheral myelin envelope. Other cranial nerves have their transition points closer to the brain stem. If no etiology is identified, MRI of the spine should be performed to exclude a chronically bleeding spinal neoplasm such as an ependymoma or a paraganglioma.

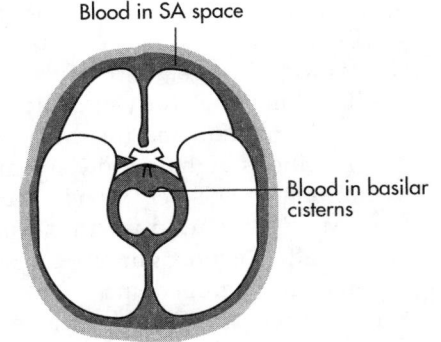

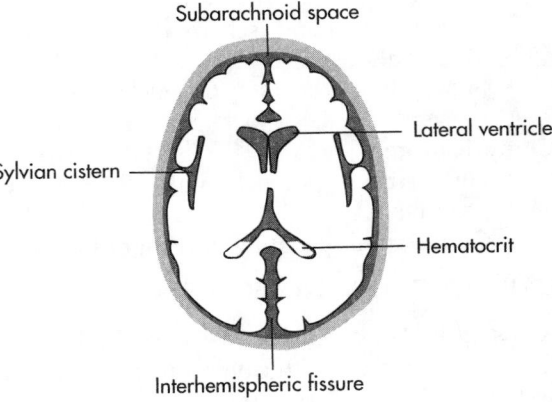

Vascular Malformation

TYPES OF VASCULAR MALFORMATIONS

There are four types of malformations:
AVM

- Parenchymal (pial) malformations
- Dural AVM and fistula
- Mixed pial/dural AVM

Capillary telangiectasia
Cavernous malformation
Venous malformations

- Venous anomaly
- Vein of Galen malformation
- Venous varix

ARTERIOVENOUS MALFORMATION (AVM)

Abnormal network of arteries and veins with no intervening capillary bed. 98% of AVM are solitary. Peak age is 20-40 years. Types:
- Parenchymal, 80% (ICA and vertebral artery supply; congenital lesions)
- Dural, 10% (ECA supply; mostly acquired lesions)
- Mixed, 10%

Radiographic features
- MRI is imaging study of choice for detection of AVM; arteriography superior for characterization and treatment planning.
- Serpiginous high and low signal (depending on flow rates) within feeding and draining vessels best seen by MRI/MRA
- AVM *re*places but does not *dis*place brain tissue (i.e., mass effect is uncommon) unless complicated by hemorrhage and edema
- Edema occurs only if there is recent hemorrhage or venous thrombosis with infarction
- Flow-related aneurysm, 10%
- Adjacent parenchymal atrophy is common due to vascular steal and ischemia
- Calcification, 25%
- Susceptibility artifacts on MRI if old hemorrhage is present

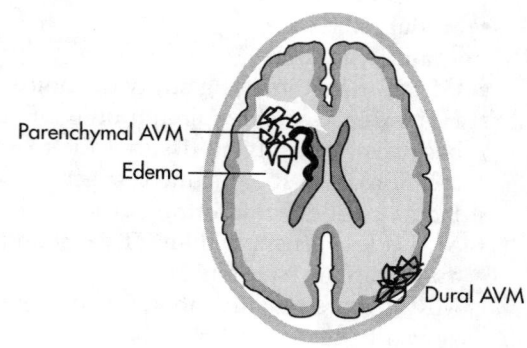

Complications
- Hemorrhage (parenchymal > SAH > intraventricular)
- Seizures
- Cumulative risk of hemorrhage is approximately 3% per year.

CAPILLARY TELANGIECTASIA

Nests of dilated capillaries with normal brain interspersed between dilated capillaries. Commonly coexist with cavernous malformation. Location: pons > cerebral cortex, spinal cord > other locations.

Radiographic features
- CT is often normal.
- MRI:
  Foci of increased signal intensity on contrast-enhanced studies
  T2 hypointense foci if hemorrhage has occurred
- Angiography is often normal but may show faint vascular stain.

CAVERNOUS MALFORMATION

Dilated endothelial-lined spaces with no normal brain within lesion. Usually detectable because cavernous malformation contains blood degradation products of different stages. Location: 80% supratentorial, 60%-80% multiple. All age groups. Clinical: seizures, focal deficits, headache secondary to occult hemorrhage.

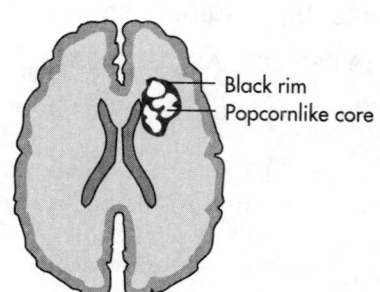

Radiographic features
- MRI is the imaging study of choice.
- Complex signal intensities due to blood products of varying age
- "Popcorn" lesion: bright lobulated center with black (hemosiderin) rim
- Always obtain susceptibility sequences to detect coexistent smaller lesions.
- Angiography is usually normal.

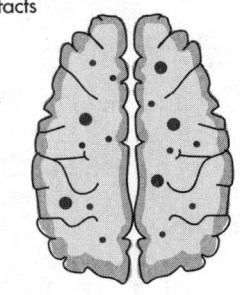

Multiple blooming susceptibility artifacts

VENOUS ANOMALY (ANOMALOUS VEIN)

Multiple small veins converge into a large transcortical draining vein. Typically discovered incidentally. Venous angiomas per se do not hemorrhage but are associated with cavernous malformation, which do bleed.

Radiographic features
Angiography
- Medusa head seen on venous phase (hallmark)
- Dilated medullary veins draining into a large transcortical vein

MRI
- Medusa head or large transcortical vein best seen on spin-echo images or after administration of gadolinium
- Location in deep cerebellar white matter or deep cerebral white matter
- Adjacent to the frontal horn (most common site)

Hemorrhage best detectable with MR susceptibility sequences, 10%.

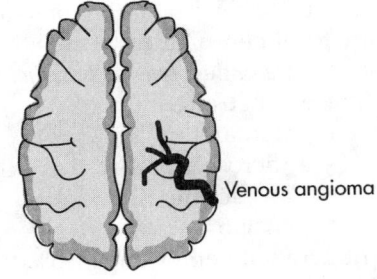

Venous angioma

VEIN OF GALEN AVM

Complex group of vascular anomalies that consist of a central AVM and resultant varix of the vein of Galen (incorrectly referred to as vein of Galen "aneurysm"). Two main types exist with the common feature of a dilated midline venous structure:

Vein of Galen AVM
- Primary malformation in development of vein of Galen
- AV shunts involving embryologic venous precursors (median vein of prosencephalon)
- Choroidal arteriovenous fistula with no nidus
- Absence of normal vein of Galen
- Median vein of prosencephalon does not drain normal brain tissue.
- Presents as high-output congestive heart failure (CHF) in infants and hydrocephalus in older children

Vein of Galen varix
- Primary parenchymal AVM drains into vein of Galen, which secondarily enlarges.
- Thalamic AVM with nidus is usually the primary AVM.
- Uncommon to present in neonates
- Higher risk of hemorrhage than the vein of Galen AVM

Radiographic features
US
- First choice imaging modality
- Sonolucent midline structure superior/posterior to 3rd ventricle
- Color Doppler ultrasound (US) to exclude arachnoid/developmental cyst

Anigography
- Used to determine type and therapy
- Endovascular embolization: therapy of choice

MRI
- Indicated to assess extent of brain damage that influences therapy

Chest X-ray
- High-output CHF, large heart

Stroke

Stroke is a term that describes an acute episode of neurological deficit. 80% of strokes are due to cerebral ischemia (embolic or thrombotic). Transient ischemic attacks (TIAs) are focal neurological events that resolve within 24 hours; those that resolve after 24 hours are called *reversible ischemic neurological deficits* (RINDS).

Causes of stroke

Cerebral infarction, 80%
- Atherosclerosis-related occlusion of vessels, 60%
- Cardiac emboli, 15%
- Other, 5%

Intracranial hemorrhage, 15%

Nontraumatic SAH, 5%

Venous occlusion, 1%

OVERVIEW OF COMMON CAUSES OF STROKE		
Old Patient	**Young Patient**	**Child**
Atherosclerosis Cardiac emboli	Emboli Arterial dissections Vasculopathy (FMD, vasculitis) Drug abuse	Emboli from congenital heart disease Venous thrombosis Blood dyscrasias (i.e., sickle cell)

ATHEROSCLEROTIC DISEASE

Atherosclerosis represents the most common cause of cerebral ischemia/infarction. Carotid atherosclerosis causes embolic ischemia; intracranial atherosclerosis causes in situ thrombotic or distal embolic ischemia. Location: ICA origin > distal basilar > carotid siphon, MCA.

Critical carotid stenosis is defined as a stenosis of > 70% in luminal diameter. Patients with critical stenosis and symptoms have an increased risk of stroke and benefit from carotid endarterectomy. Patients with stenosis < 70% or who are asymptomatic are usually treated medically.

Radiographic features

Gray scale imaging (B-scan) of carotid arteries
- Evaluate plaque morphology/extent
- Determine severity of stenosis (residual lumen)
- Other features
     "Slim sign": collapse of ICA above stenosis
     Collateral circulation

Doppler imaging of carotid arteries
- Severity of stenosis determined by measuring peak systolic velocity
    50%-75%: velocity 125-225 cm/sec
    75%-90%: velocity 225-350 cm/sec
    > 90%: velocity > 350 cm/sec
- Stenoses > 95% may result in decreased velocity (< 25 cm/sec)
- 90% accuracy for > 50% stenoses
- Other measures used for quantifying stenoses
    Peak diastolic velocity
    ICA/CCA peak systolic velocity ratio
    ICA/CCA peak end diastolic velocity ratio

Color Doppler flow imaging of carotid arteries
- High-grade stenosis with minimal flow (string sign in angiography) are detected more reliably than with conventional Doppler US.

MRA angiography
- At some institutions, carotid endarterectomy is performed on the basis of US and MRA if the results are concordant.
- Pitfalls of US and MRA in the diagnosis of carotid stenosis:
    Near occlusions (may be overdiagnosed as occluded)
    Postendarterectomy (complex flow, clip artifacts)
    Ulcerated plaques (suboptimal detection)
    Tandem lesions (easily missed)

Carotid arteriography (gold standard) is primariliy used for:
- Discordant MRA and US results
- Postendarterectomy patient
- Accurate evaluation of tandem lesions and collateral circulation
- Evaluation of aortic arch and great vessels

CEREBRAL ISCHEMIA AND INFARCTION

Cerebral ischemia refers to a diminished blood supply to the brain. Infarction refers to brain damage, being the result of ischemia. Causes of infarction:

Large vessel occlusion, 50%
Small vessel occlusion (lacunar infarcts), 20%
Emboli
- Cardiac, 15%
    Arrhythmia, atrial fibrillation
    Endocarditis
    Atrial myxoma
    Myocardial infarction (anterior infarction)
    Left ventricular aneurysm
- Noncardiac
    Atherosclerosis
    Fat, air embolism
Vasculitis
- SLE
- Polyarteritis nodosa

6

Other
- Hypoperfusion
- Vasospasm: ruptured aneurysm, SAH
- Hematologic abnormalities
    Hypercoagulable states
    Hb abnormalities (CO poisoning, sickle cell)
- Venous occlusion
- Moyamoya disease

Radiographic features

Angiographic signs of cerebral infarction
- Vessel occlusion, 50%
- Slow antegrade flow, delayed arterial emptying, 15%
- Collateral filling, 20%
- Nonperfused areas, 5%
- Vascular blush (luxury perfusion), 20%
- AV shunting, 10%
- Mass effect, 40%

Cross-sectional imaging
- CT is the first study of choice in acute stroke in order to:
    Exclude intracranial hemorrhage
    Exclude underlying mass/AVM
- Most CT examinations are normal in early stroke.
- Early CT signs of cerebral infarction include:
    Loss of gray-white interfaces (insular ribbon sign)
    Sulcal effacement
    Hyperdense clot in artery on noncontrast CT ("dense MCA sign")
- Edema
    Cytotoxic edema develops within 6 hours (detectable by MRI).
    Vasogenic edema develops later (first detectable by CT at 12-24 hours).
- Characteristic differences between distributions of infarcts
    Embolic: periphery, wedge shaped
    Hypoperfusion in watershed areas of ACA/MCA and MCA/PCA
    Border zone infarcts
    Basal ganglia infarcts
    Generalized cortical laminar necrosis
- Reperfusion hemorrhage is not uncommon after 48 hours.
    MRI much more sensitive than CT in detection
    Most hemorrhages are petechial or gyral.
- Mass effect in acute infarction
    Sulcal effacement
    Ventricular compression
- Subacute infarcts
    Hemorrhagic component, 40%
    Gyral or patchy contrast enhancement (1-3 weeks)
    GWM edema
- Chronic infarcts
    Focal tissue loss: atrophy, porencephaly, cavitation, focal ventricular
        dilatation
    Wallerian degeneration: distal axonal breakdown along white-matter tracks

CT AND MRI APPEARANCE OF INFARCTS				
	1st Day	**1st Week**	**1st Month**	**> 1 Month**
Stage	Acute	Acute	Subacute	Chronic
CT density*	Subtle decrease	Decrease	Hypodense	Hypodense
MRI	T2W: edema	T2W: edema	Varied	T1 dark, T2 bright
Mass effect	Mild	Maximum	Resolving	Atrophy
Hemorrhage	No	Most likely here	Variable	MR detectable
Enhancement	No	Yes; max at 2-3 weeks	Decreasing	No

*Due to cytotoxic and vasogenic edema.

Pearls

- Cerebral infarcts cannot be excluded on the basis of a negative CT in the first 12 hours. A follow-up CT or MRI is therefore indicated.
- Gross hemorrhage is a contraindication to anticoagulation.
- Contrast administration is reserved for clinical problem cases and should not be routinely given, particularly on the first examination.
- Luxury perfusion refers to hyperemia of an ischemic area. The increased blood flow is thought to be due to compensatory vasodilatation secondary to parenchymal lactic acidosis.
- Cerebral infarcts have a peripheral rim of viable but ischemic tissue (penumbra).
- Thrombotic and embolic infarcts occur in vascular distributions (i.e., MCA, ACA, PCA, etc.).
- MR perfusion/diffusion studies are imaging studies of choice in acute stroke.
    Diffusion-weighted imaging (DWI) detects reduced diffusion coefficient in acute infarction, which is thought to reflect cytotoxic edema.
    DWI is helpful in the early (6 hrs) detection of acute stroke.
    In patients with multiple T2 signal abnormalities of a variety of causes, DWI can identify those signal abnormalities that arise from acute infarction.

DIFFUSION AND PERFUSION IMAGING IN STROKE

Standard diffusion protocol includes a DWI and an apparent diffusion coefficient (ADC) image. These are usually interpreted side by side. DWI: summation of diffusion and T2 effects, abnormalities appear as high signal. ADC: diffusion effects only (T2 effects stripped out), abnormalities appear as low signal.

Perfusion imaging is performed using the susceptibility effects of a rapid bolus injection of gadolinium administered intravenously. Rapid continuous scanning during this injection allows the signal changes associated with the gadolinium to be plotted over time for a selected brain volume. These time-signal plots can be processed to yield several possible parameters relating to cerebral perfusion. Vascular parameters: mean transit time (MTT) is measured in seconds and is a measure of how long it takes blood to reach the particular region of the brain. Cerebral blood volume (CBV) is measured in relative units and correlates to the total volume of circulating blood in the voxel.

Cerebral blood flow (CBF) is measured in relative units and correlates to the flow of blood in the voxel.

Interpretation

- A typical infarct is DWI bright and ADC dark. Gliosis appears DWI bright due to T2 shine-through but is also bright on ADC, marking it as a T2 effect.
- DWI is very sensitive for detecting disease (will pick up infarcts from about 30 minutes onwards but is nonspecific and will also detect nonischemic disease).
- ADC is less sensitive than DWI, but dark signal is fairly specific for restricted diffusion, which usually means ischemia.
- Time course of imaging changes after cerebral infarction: DWI becomes bright very shortly after infarction and will stay bright, initially because of restricted diffusion, later due to T2 shine-through. ADC becomes dark very early and will stay dark for about 7 days, isointense to gray matter from about 7-10 days, and bright thereafter. This correlates to the transition of diffusion to T2 effects. Implies a window at about 1-2 weeks after the ictus (when ADC is isointense) when imaging findings might be harder to interpret without follow-up or good history.
- Significance of a DWI-bright, ADC-dark lesion: this tissue will almost certainly go on to infarct and full necrosis. Rare instances of reversible lesions have been reported (venous thrombosis, seizures, hemiplegic migraine, hyperacute arterial thrombosis).
- MTT is highly sensitive for disturbances in perfusion but not good for prediction of later events. For example, an asymptomatic carotid occlusion would have a dramatically abnormal MTT, without the patient being distressed.
- CBV is a parameter that changes late in the ischemic cascade, and usually reduced CBV is also accompanied by restricted diffusion. Reduced CBV (and restricted diffusion) correlate well with tissue that goes on to infarction.
- CBF in the experimental setting can be used to predict the likelihood of brain tissue infracting. In current clinical practice, a CBF abnormality exceeding the DWI abnormality (diffusion-perfusion mismatch) implies that there is brain at risk that has not infracted yet. This brain at risk is the target of therapeutic interventions.

ROLE OF CT/CTA IN ACUTE STROKE

Important in early stages of stroke evaluation to facilitate thrombolytic therapy. CT angiography (CTA) demonstrates the anatomical details of the neurovasculature from the great vessel origins at the aortic arch to their intracranial termination. Highly accurate in the identification of proximal large vessel circle of Willis occlusions and therefore in the rapid triage of patients to intraarterial (IA) or intravenous (IV) thrombolytic therapy.

TECHNIQUE

- Noncontrast CT is performed initially to exclude hemorrhage; an absolute contraindication to thrombolytic therapy. Large parenchymal hypodensity, typically indicating irreversible "core" of infarction, is a relative contraindication to thrombolysis.
- CTA/CTP imaging performed on a multislice scanner, which enables acquisition of imaging data from entire vascular territories in < 1 minute.
- The initial CT scan is performed at 140 kV, 170 mA, pitch = "high quality" (3:1), and a table speed of 7.5 mm/sec
- Images are obtained from the skull base to the vertex. Slice thickness can be set at 2.5 mm, at 5 mm, or at both.

- Initial image review is in "real-time," directly at the CT console. The use of narrow window-width settings, with a center level of about 30 HU (width of 5 to 30 HU), facilitates the detection of early, subtle, ischemic changes contiguous with normal parenchyma.
- Blood volume CTP is performed without repositioning the patient.
- Approximately 90-120 mL of nonionic, iso-osmolar contrast is used for CTA from the skull base to the vertex, with a 25-second scan delay.
- Initial scan parameters are as per the noncontrast CT scan described above. A second phase of scanning is performed immediately, with minimal possible delay, from the aortic arch to the skull base, with similar scan parameters except for an increase in the table speed to 15 mm/sec. Major advantages of first scanning the intracranial circulation include: (1) obtaining the most important data first, which can be reviewed during subsequent acquisition; and (2) allowing time for clearance of dense, IV contrast from the subclavian, axillary, and other veins at the thoracic inlet, reducing streak artifact.

THERAPEUTIC OPTIONS

- To date, the only FDA-approved treatment for acute stroke is IV thrombolysis with recombinant tissue plasminogen activator (IV rt-PA), administered within 3 hours of stroke onset. If thrombolysis is applied beyond this time window, the increased probability of intracranial hemorrhage is considered unacceptable.
- The time window for treatment with IA agents is twice as long for the anterior circulation and indefinite for the posterior circulation (depending on risk-to-benefit ratios); however, IA thrombolysis—although of proven benefit in preliminary trials—has not yet received FDA approval. For thrombosis localized to the posterior circulation, the time window for treatment may be extended beyond 6 hours due to the extreme consequences of loss of blood flow to the brainstem, despite the risk of hemorrhage.
- Advanced CTA/CTP imaging of acute stroke has the potential to not only help exclude patients at high risk for hemorrhage from thrombolysis, but also to identify those patients most likely to benefit from thrombolysis. Even without hemorrhage, treatment failure with thrombolytics is not uncommon.
- The choice between IA or IV thrombolysis depends on a variety of factors, including the time post-ictus, the clinical status of the patient, and whether the clot is proximal (IA) or distal (IV). When typical findings of occlusive thrombus on CTA and decreased tissue enhancement on CTP are not present, the differential diagnoses include lacunar infarct, early small distal embolic infarct, transient ischemic attack, complex migraine headaches, and seizure.

LACUNAR INFARCTS

Lacunar infarcts account for 20% of all strokes. The term refers to the occlusion of penetrating cerebral arterioles, most often caused by arteriolar lipohyalinosis (hypertensive vasculopathy). Commonly affected are:
- Thalamoperforators (thalamus)
- Lenticulostriates (caudate, putamen, internal capsule)
- Brainstem perforator (pons)

Lacunar infarcts usually cause characteristic clinical syndromes: pure motor hemiparesis, pure hemisensory deficit, hemiparetic ataxia, or dysarthria-hand deficit.

Radiographic features
- MRI is the imaging study of choice.
- Small ovoid lesion (< 1 cm): hyperintense on T2W and proton density–weighted (PDW) images
- Location of lesions is very helpful in differential diagnosis.

BASILAR ARTERY THROMBOEMBOLIC OCCLUSION

Risk factors
- Atherosclerosis
- Cardiac arrythmias
- Vertebral artery dissection
- Cocaine use
- Oral contraceptives

Top of basilar artery syndrome
- Occulomotor dysfunction
- Third nerve and vertical gaze palsies
- Hemiataxia
- Altered consciousness

Radiographic features
- Unlike anterior circulation infarction, the duration of symptoms before treatment, age of patient, neurological status at initiation of treatment do not predict the outcome of thrombolytic therapy.
- Basilar artery appears abnormally dense by CT.
- T2 hyperintensity is present in thalami, midbrain, pons, cerebellum, and occipital lobes.
- Absence of normal flow void in basilar artery and vertebral artery
- A T1W with fat saturation may be useful to look for associated dissection.

CENTRAL NERVOUS SYSTEM (CNS) VASCULITIS

CNS vasculitis may be caused by a large variety of underlying diseases. Differentiation may be possible by correlating systemic findings and clinical history, but a biopsy is often required for diagnosis.

Causes:

Infectious vasculitis
- Bacterial, viral, fungal, tuberculosis (TB), syphilis
- HIV-related

Systemic vasculitis
- Polyarteritis nodosa
- Giant cell arteritis/temporal arteritis
- Takayasu's arteritis
- Kawasaki syndrome
- Behçet's disease
- Collagen vascular diseases
- Serum sickness
- Allergic angiitis

Granulomatous vasculitis
- Sarcoidosis
- Wegener's granulomatosis
- Granulomatous angiitis (primary and secondary)

Drug-related vasculitis
- Cocaine
- Amphetamines
- Ergots
- Heroin

Radiographic features

MRI
- Most MRI findings are nonspecific.
- T2 hyperintensities
- Infarctions
- Hemorrhage

Angiography
- More definitive imaging study, but findings are often also nonspecific
- Vessel occlusions
- Stenoses
- Aneurysms

MOYAMOYA

Idiopathic progressive vascular occlusive disease. Common in Japanese (moyamoya = puff of smoke). Most commonly there is occlusion of supraclinoid ICA and numerous meningeal, lenticulostriate, thalamoperforate collaterals; occasionally the posterior circulation is involved.

Radiographic features
- Puff of smoke: numerous collaterals supplying ACA and MCA
- Stenosis or occlusion of supraclinoid ICA
- Similar radiographic findings can be seen in:
  - Sickle cell disease
  - Atherosclerosis
  - Radiation vasculopathy

AMYLOID ANGIOPATHY

Amyloid deposition in walls of small vessels. Common in elderly normotensive patients.

Radiographic features
- Usually multiple areas of hemorrhage sparing the basal ganglia
- Foci of hemorrhage at corticomedullary junction
- MRI is the imaging study of choice (susceptibility sequences).

VENOOCCLUSIVE DISEASE

Spectrum cerebral venous occlusion involving the following venous territories:
- Venous sinuses
- Cortical veins
- Deep cerebral veins (internal cerebral veins, basal vein of Rosenthal, vein of Galen)
- Unusual forms of venous stasis/occlusion (e.g., high-flow angiopathy associated with AVM)

VENOUS SINUS THROMBOSIS

Nonspecific clinical presentation. High mortality due to secondary infarction/hemorrhage. Causes:

- Pregnancy/puerperium
- Dehydration (particularly in children)
- Infection (mastoiditis, otitis, meningitis)
- Tumors with dural invasion
- L-asparaginase treatment
- Any hypercoagulable state
- Trauma
- Oral contraceptives
- Blood dyscrasias and coagulopathies

Radiographic features

General

- MRI with phase contrast MRA is the imaging study of choice.
- Location: superior sagittal sinus > transverse sinus > sigmoid sinus > cavernous sinus

Primary (sinus occlusion)

- Clot in sinus is hyperdense on noncontrast CT and hypodense on contrast-enhanced CT.
- Dural enhancement of sinus margin: delta sign
- MRI
    Bright sinus on T1W and T2W (depending on stage)
    Absence of flow void

Secondary (effects of venous infarction)

- Subcortical infarctions
- Corticomedullary hemorrhage is common.

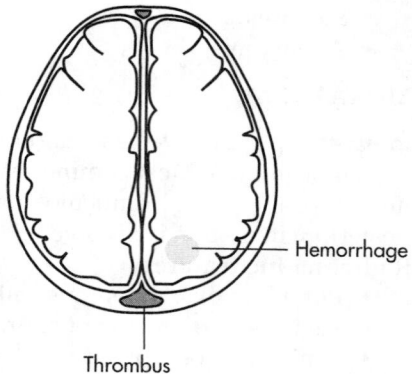

Trauma

General

CLASSIFICATION OF INJURY

Primary lesions

- Extraaxial hemorrhage
    Subarachnoid hemorrhage
    Subdural hematoma
    Epidural hematoma
- Intraaxial lesions
    Diffuse axonal injury
    Cortical contusion
    Deep cerebral gray matter injury
    Brainstem injury
    Intraventricular hemorrhage
- Fractures

Secondary lesions

- Brain herniations
- Traumatic ischemia
- Diffuse cerebral edema
- Hypoxic brain injury

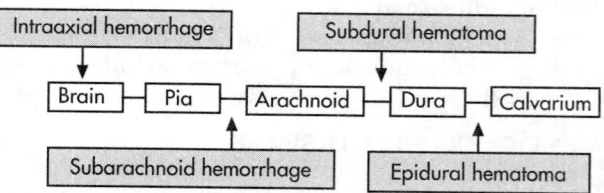

MECHANISM OF TRAUMATIC BRAIN INJURY (TBI)

Projectile (missile) injury
- Gunshot wounds
- Spear injury

Blunt injury (sudden deceleration or rotation)
- Automobile accident
- Fall from heights
- Direct blow

GLASGOW COMA SCALE

Minor head injury: score 13-15; moderate head injury: score 9-12; severe head injury: score ≤ 8.

Score

Eye opening
- Spontaneous = 4
- To sound = 3
- To pain = 2
- None = 1

Best motor response
- Obeys command = 6
- Localizes pain = 5
- Normal flexion = 4
- Abnormal flexion = 3
- Extension = 2
- None = 1

Best verbal response
- Oriented = 5
- Confused = 4
- Inappropriate words = 3
- Incomprehensible = 2
- None = 1

Primary Brain Injury

EPIDURAL HEMATOMA (EDH)

Types
- Arterial EDH, 90% (middle meningeal artery)
- Venous EDH, 10% (sinus laceration, meningeal vein)
    - Posterior fossa: transverse or sigmoid sinus laceration (common)
    - Parasagittal: tear of superior sagittal sinus

Large EDHs are neurosurgical emergencies. Small (< 5 mm thick) EDHs adjacent to fractures are common and do not represent a clinical emergency. 95% of all EDHs are associated with fractures.

Radiographic features

Arterial EDH
- 95% are unilateral, temporoparietal
- Biconvex, lenticular shape
- Does not cross suture lines
- May cross dural reflections (falx tentorium) in contradistinction to subdural hematoma (SDH)

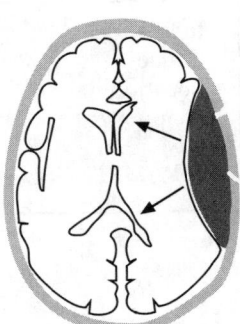

- Commonly associated with skull fractures
- Heterogeneity predicts rapid expansion of EDH, with areas of low density representing active bleeding.

Venous EDH

- More variable in shape (low pressure bleed)
- Often requires delayed imaging because of delayed onset of bleed after trauma

SUBDURAL HEMATOMA (SDH)

Caused by traumatic tear of bridging veins (rarely arteries). In contradistinction to EDH, there is no consistent relationship to the presence of skull fractures. Common in infants (child abuse; 80% are bilateral or interhemispheric) and elderly patients (20% are bilateral).

Radiographic features

Morphology of hematoma

- 95% supratentorial
- Crescentic shape along brain surface
- Crosses suture lines
- Does not cross dural reflections (falx, tentorium)
- MRI > CT particularly for:
    Bilateral hematomas
    Interhemispheric hematomas
    Hematomas along tentorium
    Subacute SDH

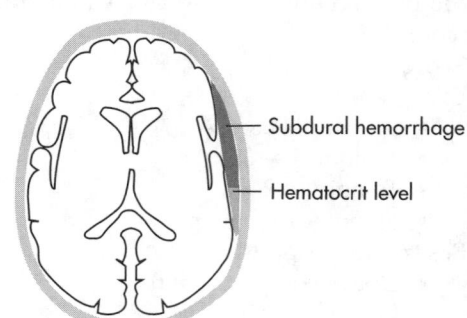

Other imaging findings

- Hematocrit level in subacute and early chronic hematomas
- Mass effect is present if SDH is large.

Acute SDH

- Hyperdense or mixed density

Subacute SDH (beyond 1 week)

- May be isointense and difficult to detect on CT
- Enhancing membrane and displaced cortical vessels (contrast administration is helpful)

Chronic SDH (beyond several weeks)

- Hypodense
- Mixed density with rebleeding
- Calcification, 1%

COMPARISON		
	Epidural Hematoma	Subdural Hematoma
Incidence	In < 5% of TBI	In 10%-20% of TBI
Cause	Fracture	Tear of cortical veins
Location	Between skull and dura	Between dura and arachnoid
Shape	Biconvex	Crescentic
CT	70% hyper, 30% isointense	Variable depending on age
T1W MRI	Isointense	Variable depending on age

SUBDURAL HYGROMA

Accumulation of CSF in subdural space after traumatic arachnoid tear.
Radiographic features
- CSF density
- Does not extend into sulci
- Vessels cross through lesion.
- Main differential diagnosis:
    Chronic SDH
    Focal atrophy with widened subarachnoid space

DIFFUSE AXONAL INJURY (DAI)

DAI is due to axonal disruption from shearing forces of acceleration/deceleration. It is most commonly seen in severe head injury. Clinical: loss of consciousness at time of injury. Cause: axonal disruption from shearing forces of acceleration/deceleration.
Radiographic features
- Characteristic location of lesions:
    Lobar gray matter (GM)/white matter (WM) junction
    Corpus callosum
    Dorsolateral brainstem
- Initial CT is often normal.
- Petechial hemorrhage develops later on.
- Multifocal T2 bright lesions
- Susceptibility-sensitive gradient echo sequences are most sensitive in detecting hemorrhagic shear injuries (acute or chronic) and can be helpful to document the extent of parenchymal injury (medicolegal implications) and to assess long-term prognosis (cognitive function) for patient and family.

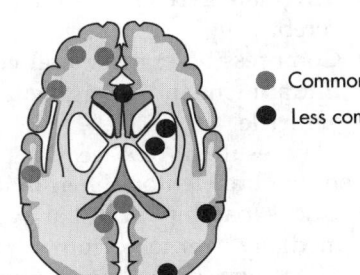

● Common
● Less common

6

CORTICAL CONTUSION

Focal hemorrhage/edema in gyri secondary to brain impacting (or rotational forces) on bone or dura.
Radiographic features
- Characteristic location of lesions
    Anterior temporal lobes, 50%
    Inferior frontal lobes, 30%
    Parasagittal hemisphere
    Brainstem
- Lesions evolve with time; delayed hemorrhage in 20%
- Initial CT is often normal; later on, low-density lesions with or without blood in them develop.

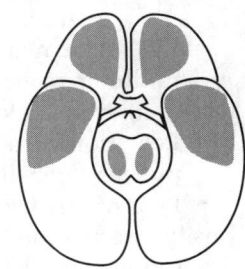

Common sites of contusions

Secondary Brain Injury

CEREBRAL HERNIATION

Mechanical displacement of brain secondary to mass effect. Herniation causes brain compression with neurological dysfunction and vascular compromise (ischemia).

Types

- Subfalcine herniation
- Transtentorial (uncal) herniation
    - Descending
    - Ascending
- Tonsillar herniation

Radiographic features

Subfalcine herniation

- Cingulate gyrus slips under free margin of falx cerebri.
- Compression of ipsilateral ventricle
- Entrapment and enlargment of contralateral ventricle
- May result in ACA ischemia

Descending transtentorial herniation(uncal)

- Uncus/parahippocampal gyrus displaced medially over tentorium
- Effacement of ipsilateral suprasellar cistern
- Enlargement of ipsilateral cerebellopontine angle (CPA) cistern
- Displaced midbrain impacts on contralateral tentorium.
    - Duret hemorrhage (anterior midbrain)
    - Kernohans notch (mass effect on penduncle)
- PCA ischemia: occipital lobe, thalami, midbrain

Ascending transtentorial herniation

- Posterior fossa mass (i.e., hemorrhage) pushes cerebellum up through incisura.
- Loss of quadrigeminal cistern

Tonsillar herniation

- Cerebellar tonsils pushed inferiorly

DIFFUSE CEREBRAL EDEMA

Massive brain swelling and intracranial hypertension secondary to dysfunction of cerebrovascular autoregulation and alterations of the blood-brain barrier. Underlying causes include ischemia and severe trauma. Ischemia may be primary (e.g., anoxic, drowning) or secondary to other brain injuries (e.g., large SDH) and may be followed by infarction. More common in children. High morbidity/mortality.

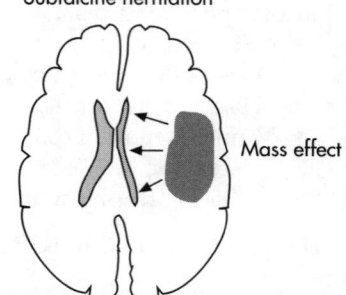

Subfalcine herniation

Mass effect

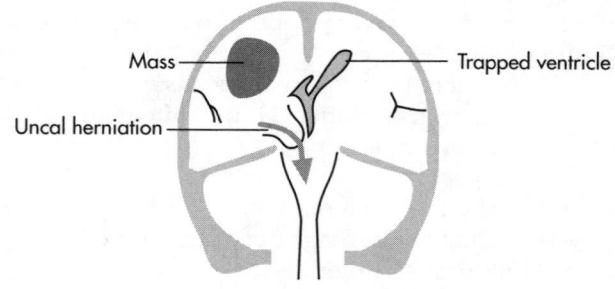

Mass

Uncal herniation

Trapped ventricle

Descending transtentorial (uncal) herniation

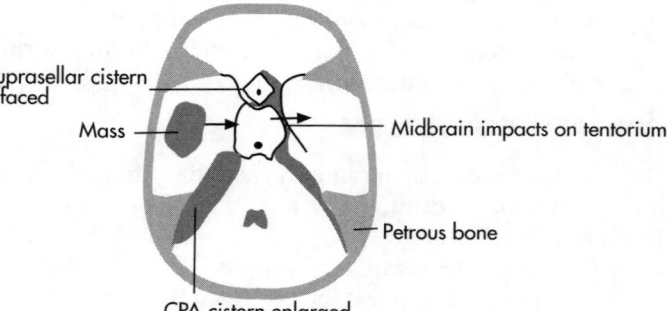

Suprasellar cistern effaced

Mass

Midbrain impacts on tentorium

Petrous bone

CPA cistern enlarged

Radiographic features
- Findings develop 24-48 hours after injury.
- Effacement of sulci and basilar cisterns
- Loss of perimesencephalic cisterns (hallmark)
- Loss of GM/WM interface (cerebral edema)
- White cerebellum sign: sparing of brainstem in comparison to hemispheres

ARTERIAL DISSECTION

Blood splits the media, creating a false lumen that dissects the arterial wall. Precise pathogenesis is unclear. Location: carotid artery (starts 2 cm distal to bulb and spares bulb) > ICA (petrous canal) > vertebral artery > others.

Underlying causes
- Spontaneous or with minimal trauma (strain, sports)
- Trauma
- Hypertension
- Vasculopathy (fibromuscular dysplasia [FMD], Marfan syndrome)
- Migraine headache
- Drug abuse

Radiographic features

MRI
- First study of choice; in unclear cases conventional angiography may establish the diagnosis and fully elucidate abnormal flow patterns
- T1 bright hematoma in vessel wall
- Long segment fusiform narrowing of affected artery
- MRA string sign

Complications
- Thrombosis
- Emboli and infarction
- Intramural hemorrhage
- False aneurysm

CAROTID CAVERNOUS SINUS FISTULA (CCF)

Abnormal connection between carotid artery and venous cavernous sinus. Clinical: ocular bruit. Types:
- Traumatic CCF (high flow)
- Spontaneous CCF
    Rupture of aneurysm in its cavernous segment (less common; high flow)
    Dural fistula (AVM) of the cavernous sinus (low flow); usually associated
        with venous thrombosis in older patients

Radiographic features
- Enlargement of cavernous sinus
- Enlargement of superior ophthalmic vein
- Angiographic embolization with detachable balloons (traumatic fistulas)

Neoplasm

General

CLASSIFICATION OF PRIMARY BRAIN TUMORS

Primary brain tumors constitute 70% of all intracranial mass lesions. The remaining 30% represents metastases. Classification of primary brain tumors:

Gliomas (most common primary brain tumors)
- Astrocytomas (most common glioma, 80%)
- Oligodendroglioma (5%-10%)
- Ependymoma
- Choroid plexus tumors

Meningeal and mesenchymal tumors
- Meningioma, 20%
- Hemangiopericytoma
- Hemangioblastoma

Neuronal and mixed glial/neuronal tumors
- Ganglioglioma
- Gangliocytoma
- Dysembryoplastic neuroepithelial tumor (DNET)
- Central neurocytoma

Germ cell tumors
- Germinoma
- Teratoma
- Mixed

PNETs
- Medulloblastoma
- Retinoblastoma
- Neuroblastoma
- Pineoblastoma
- Ependymoblastoma

Pineal region tumors
Pituitary tumors
Nerve sheath tumor
- Schwannoma
- Neurofibroma

Hematopoeitic tumors
- Lymphoma
- Leukemia

Tumorlike lesions
- Hamartoma
- Lipoma
- Dermoid

Pearls
- Glial cells have high potential for abnormal growth. There are three types of glial cells: astrocytes (astrocytoma), oligodendrocytes (oligodendroglioma), and ependymal cells (ependymoma).
- Choroid plexus cells are modified ependymal cells, and tumors derived from them are therefore classified with gliomas.

LOCATION

The differentiation of intracerebral masses into intraaxial or extraaxial location is the first step in narrowing the differential diagnosis.

DETERMINING TUMOR LOCATION		
Feature	Intraaxial Tumors	Extraaxial Tumors
Contiguity with bone or falx	Usually not	Yes
Bony changes	Usually not	Yes
CSF spaces, cisterns	Effaced	Often widened
Corticomedullary buckling	No	Yes
GM/WM junction	Destruction	Preservation
Vascular supply	Internal	External (dural branches)

FREQUENCY OF TUMORS

- Adults: metastases > hemangioblastoma > astrocytoma > lymphoma
- Children: astrocytoma > medulloblastoma > ependymoma

TUMOR EXTENT

Imaging modalities (see table below) are primarily used to diagnose the presence of a tumor. FDG-PET and MR blood volume maps can differentiate with fairly good reliability between low-grade and high-grade tumors. This can be helpful in recognizing transformation of low-grade to high-grade tumor and in identifying high grade components of otherwise lower grade tumors to guide stereotactic biopsy. Once tumors are diagnosed, evaluation of tumor extension is important to:

- Determine site of stereotactic biopsy
- Plan surgical resection
- Plan radiotherapy

For many tumors, no imaging technique identifies their total extent. Gliomas often infiltrate the surrounding brain; microscopic tumor foci can be seen in areas that are totally normal on all MR sequences, including gadolinium-enhanced MRI.

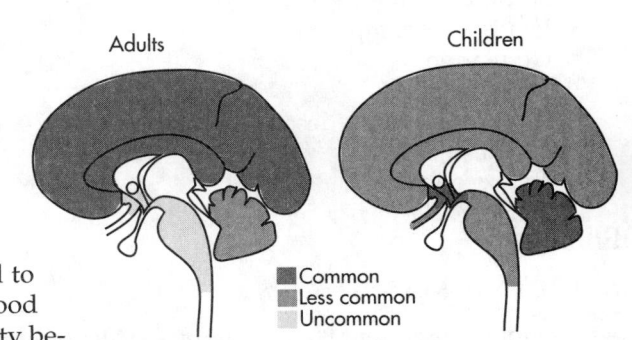

Adults   Children

Common
Less common
Uncommon

TECHNIQUES FOR DETERMINING TUMOR EXTENT/VIABILITY		
	Determine True Extent of Tumor	Differentiate Viable vs. Radiation Necrosis
Noncontrast CT	0	0
Contrast CT	++	0
T1W MRI	+	0
T2W MRI	+	0
Gd-DTPA MRI	+++	0
MR blood volume maps	+	+
PET	+	++
MR-guided biopsy	NA	+++

BRAIN EDEMA

TYPES OF BRAIN EDEMA		
	Vasogenic	Cytotoxic
Cause	Tumor, trauma, hemorrhage,	Ischemia, infection
Mechanism	Blood-brain barrier defect	Na-K pump defect
Substrate	Extracellular	Intracellular
Steroid response	Yes	No
Imaging	WM affected (cortical sparing)	GM and WM affected

MASS EFFECT

Radiographic signs of mass effect:
- Sulcal effacement
- Ventricular compression
- Herniation
     Subfalcine
     Transtentorial (descending, ascending)
     Tonsillar
- Hydrocephalus

Gliomas

ASTROCYTOMAS

Astrocytomas represent 80% of gliomas. Most tumors occur in cerebral hemispheres in adults. In children, posterior fossa and hypothalamus/optic chiasm are more common locations. The differentiation of types of astrocytoma is made histologically not by imaging. Classification:

Fibrillary astrocytomas
- Astrocytoma, WHO grade I (AI)
- Astrocytoma, WHO grade II (AII)
- Anaplastic astrocytoma, WHO grade III (AA III)
- Glioblastoma multiforme, WHO grade IV (GBM IV)

Other astrocytomas
- Multicentric glioma (multiple lesions)
- Gliomatosis cerebri
- Juvenile pilocytic astrocytoma (in the cerebellum these lesions are typically cystic and have a mural nodule; tumors in the hypothalamus, optic chiasm, and optic nerves are usually solid and lobulated)
- Giant cell astrocytoma (in tuberous sclerosis): subependymal tumor growth along caudothalamic groove
- Xanthoastrocytoma
- Gliosarcoma

Astrocytoma associations
- Tuberous sclerosis
- Neurofibromatosis

OVERVIEW OF ASTROCYTOMAS			
	Astrocytoma	Astrocytoma, Anaplastic	Glioblastoma Multiforme
Peak age	Younger patients	Middle age patients	50 years
Grade of malignancy	Low	High	High
Histology	Low-grade malignancy	Malignant	Very aggressive
Imaging features			
Multifocal	No	Occasionally	Occasionally
Enhancement (BBB)	±	++	+++
Edema	Little or no	Abundant edema	Abundant edema
Calcification	Frequent	Less	Uncommon
Other		Hemorrhagic, necrotic	Hemorrhagic, necrotic

LOW-GRADE ASTROCYTOMA (AI, AII)

Represent 20% of all astrocytomas. Peak age: 20-40 years. Primary location is in the cerebral hemispheres.

Radiographic features
- Focal or diffuse mass lesions
- Calcification, 20%
- Hemorrhage and extensive edema are rare.
- Mild enhancement

ANAPLASTIC ASTROCYTOMA (AAIII)

Represent 30% of all astrocytomas. Peak age: 40-60 years. Primary location is in the cerebral hemispheres.

Radiographic features
- Heterogenous mass
- Calcification uncommon
- Edema common
- Enhancement (reflects blood-brain barrier disruption [BBBD])

GLIOBLASTOMA MULTIFORME (GBM)

Most common primary brain tumor (represents 55% of astrocytomas). Age: > 50 years. Primary location is in the hemispheres. Tumor may spread along the following routes:
- WM tracts
- Across midline via commisures (e.g., corpus callosum)
- Subependymal seeding of ventricles
- CSF seeding of subarachnoid space

Radiographic features
- Usually heterogeneous low-density mass (CT)
- Strong contrast enhancement
- Hemorrhage, necrosis common
- Calcification is uncommon.
- Extensive vasogenic edema and mass effect
- Bihemispheric spread via corpus callosum or commissures (butterfly lesion)
- High-grade gliomas located peripherally can have a broad dural base and a dural tail, mimicking an extraaxial lesion.
- CSF seeding: leptomeningeal drop metastases

GLIOMATOSIS CEREBRI

Diffuse growth of glial neoplasm within brain. Usually there are no gross mass lesions but rather a diffuse infiltration of brain tissue by tumor cells. Age: 30-40 years. Rare. The MR appearances of gliomatosis may be similar to herpes encephalitis, but the clinical presentations differ.

Radiographic features
- Gliomatosis predominantly causes expansion of WM but may also involve cortex.
- Usually nonenhancing lesions
- Late in disease, small foci of enhancement become visible.
- Leptomeningeal gliomatosis can mimic meningeal carcinomatosis or leptomeningeal spread of primary central nervous system (CNS) tumors and cause marked enhancement.
- Important differential for gliomatosis include:
  Lymphomatosis cerebri
  Multicenteric glioma
  Viral encephalitis
  Vasculitis
  Extensive active demyelinating disease such as acute disseminated encephalomyelitis (ADEM)

BRAINSTEM GLIOMA

Common pediatric posterior fossa tumor. Mean age: 10 years. 80% are anaplastic high grade; 20% are low grade and grow slowly. Locations: pons >> midbrain > medulla. Clinical: cranial nerve VI and VII neuropathy, long track signs, hydrocephalus.

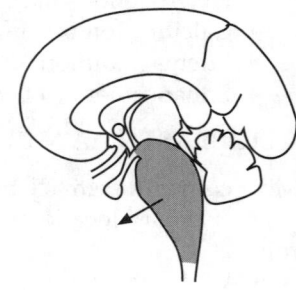

Radiographic features
- Enlargement of brainstem
- Posterior displacement of 4th ventricle (floor of the 4th ventricle should be in the middle of the Twining line: sella tuberculum–torcula)
- Cystic portions uncommon
- Hydrocephalus, 30%
- Enhancement occurs in 50% and is usually patchy and variable.
- Exophytic extension into basilar cisterns

- Focal tumors localized to the tectal plate are termed tectal gliomas. These consititute a distinct subset of brainstem gliomas. As these tumors have good long-term prognosis and are located deep, they are usually followed without biopsy and with serial imaging to document stability. If a lesion extends beyond the tectum but is still confined to the midbrain, it is referred to as a peritectal tumor. These have worse prognosis than purely tectal lesions. Peritectal tumors may be difficult to differentiate from pineal region tumors.
- Brainstem encephalitis may mimic a diffuse pontine glioma. Pontine gliomas have worse prognosis when compared with tectal gliomas.

PILOCYTIC ASTROCYTOMA

Most common in children (represents 30% of pediatric gliomas); second most common pediatric brain tumor. Indolent and slow growing. Location: optic chiasm/hypothalamus > cerebellum > brainstem.

Radiographic features
- Cerebellar tumors are usually cystic and have intense mural enhancement.
- Calcification, 10%
- Optic chiasm/hypothalamic tumors are solid and enhance.
- Most in brainstem show little enhancement.

OLIGODENDROGLIOMA

Uncommon slow-growing glioma that usually presents as a large mass. Oligodendroglioma represents 5%-10% of primary brain tumors. Peak age: 30-50 years. "Pure" oligodendrogliomas are rare; usually tumors are "mixed" (astrocytoma/oligodendroglioma). The vast majority of tumors are located in cerebral hemispheres, the frontal lobe being the most common location. Intraventricular oligodendrogliomas are rare lesions. Many intraventricular lesions that were previously called oligodendrogliomas are now recognized as neurocytomas.

Radiographic features
- Commonly involve cortex
- Typically hypodense mass lesions
- Cysts are common.
- Large nodular, clumpy calcifications are typical, 80%
- Hemorrhage and necrosis are uncommon.
- Enhancement depends on degree of histological differentiation.
- Pressure erosion of calvarium occurs occasionally.

EPENDYMAL TUMORS

The ependyma refers to a layer of ciliated cells lining the ventricular walls and the central canal. There are several histological variants of ependymal tumors:
- Ependymoma (children)
- Subependymoma (older patients)
- Anaplastic ependymoma
- Myxopapillary ependymoma of filum terminale
- Ependymoblastoma (PNET)

6

EPENDYMOMA

Slow-growing tumor of ependymal lining cells, usually located in or adjacent to ventricles within the parenchyma:
- 4th ventricle (70%): more common in children
- Lateral ventricle or periventricular parenchymal (30%): more common in adults

Most common in children. Age: 1-5 years. Spinal ependymomas are associated with neurofibromatosis, type 2 (NF2).

Radiographic features
- Growth pattern depends on location:
  - Supratentorial: tumors grow outside ventricle (i.e., resembles astrocytoma); remember to include ependymoma in the differential diagnosis of a supratentorial parenchymal mass lesion, particularly in a child.
  - Infratentorial: tumors grow inside 4th ventricle and extrude through foramen of Luschka into CPA and cisterna magna; this appearance is characteristic ("plastic ependymoma") and often helps to differentiate an ependymoma from a medulloblastoma.
- Hydrocephalus is virtually always present when in posterior fossa.
- Fine calcifications, 50%
- Cystic areas, 50%

Differential for supratentorial ependymoma:
- PNET: often peripheral and has more edema
- Malignant rhabdoid tumor: generally seen in infants and young children
- Gliomastoma multiforme: typically significant surrounding edema
- Anaplastic astrocytoma: may be indistinguishable but less likely to be in proximity of ventricular surface
- Metastatic disease: often multifocal with significant surrounding edema.

SUBEPENDYMOMA

- Asymptomatic fourth ventricular tumor found in elderly males
- 66% arise in the fourth ventricle; 33% in lateral ventricles
- Unlike ependymomas, these tumors tend not to seed the subarachnoid space.
- Lesions often are multiple.

DIFFERENTIAL DIAGNOSIS OF LATERAL VENTRICULAR MASS		
Location	**Adult**	**Child**
Atrium	Meningioma	CP papilloma
	Metastatses	CP carcinoma
	CP xanthogranuloma	Ependymoma
Body	Subependymoma	Astrocytoma
	Oligodendroglioma	PNET
	Central neurocytoma	Teratoma
	Astrocytoma	CP papilloma
Foramen of Monro	Giant cell astrocytoma	Giant cell astrocytoma

CP, Choroid plexus.

CHOROID PLEXUS PAPILLOMA/CARCINOMA

Rare tumors that arise from epithelium of choroid plexus. Peak age: < 5 years (85%). 90% represent choroid plexus papillomas, 10% choroid plexus carcinomas. Typical locations:

- Trigone of lateral ventricles (children)
- 4th ventricle and CPA (adults)
- Drop metastases to spinal canal

Radiographic features

- Intraventricular mass
- Ventricular dilatation due to CSF overproduction or obstruction
- Intense contrast enhancement
- Calcifications, 25%
- Supratentorial tumors are supplied by anterior and posterior choroidal arteries.
- Complications:
    Hydrocephalus
    Drop metastases to spinal dural space
- Papillomas and carcinomas are radiographically indistinguishable; both may invade brain and disseminate via CSF.

Meningeal and Mesenchymal Tumors

MENINGIOMA

Tumor originate from arachnoid cap cells. Age: 40-60 years. Three times more common in females. Represents 20% of all brain tumors. Meningiomas are uncommon in children and if present are commonly associated with NF2. 90% are supratentorial. Classification:

- Typical "benign" meningioma, 93%
- Atypical meningioma, 5%
- Anaplastic (malignant) meningioma, 1%-2%

Location

- Cerebral convexity along falx and lateral to it, 45%
- Sphenoid ridge, 20%
- Juxtasellar, 10%
- Olfactory groove, 10%
- Posterior fossa clivus, 10%
- Tentorium
- Uncommon locations:
    Lateral ventricles (pediatric age group)
    Optic nerve sheath (adult females)
- < 1% of meningiomas may arise extradurally. These sites include intradiploic space, outer table of skull, skin, paranasal sinuses, parotid gland, and parapharyngeal space.

6

Radiographic features

CT signal intensity

- Hyperdense (75%) or isodense (25%) on noncontrast CT
- Strong, homogenous enhancement, 90% (hallmark)
- Similar signal intensity as normal falx on enhanced and nonenhanced CT
- Calcifications, 20%
- Cystic areas, 15%

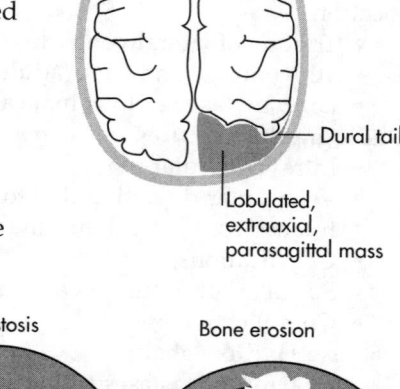

Dural tail

Lobulated, extraaxial, parasagittal mass

Morphology

- Round, unilobulated, sharp margin (most common)
- En plaque, pancake spread along dura (rare)
- Dural tail: extension of tumor or dural reaction along a dural surface
- Edema is absent in 40% because of the slow growth.

Bony abnormalities, 20%

- No changes (common)
- Hyperostosis (common)
- Bone erosion (rare; if present may indicate malignant meningioma)

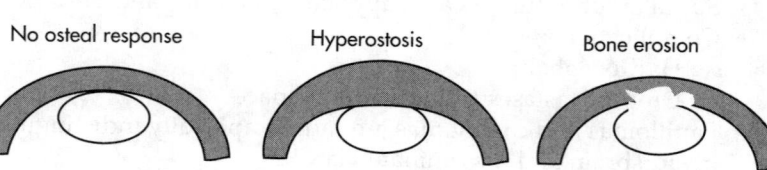

No osteal response   Hyperostosis   Bone erosion

MRI

- Tumors are typically isointense with GM.
- Strong gadolinium enhancement
- Best technique for detecting dural tail
- Dural tail (60%) is suggestive but not specific for meningioma.
- Increased vascular flow voids

Angiography

- Spoke-wheel appearance
- Dense venous filling
- Persistent tumor blush ("comes early and stays late")
- Well-demarcated margins
- Dural vascular supply

Arterial phase   Venous phase

Atypical meningiomas (15% of all meningiomas)

- Necrosis causing nonhomogenous enhancement, 15%
- Hemorrhage
- Peripheral low-density zones (trapped CSF in arachnoid cysts)

MALIGNANT MENINGIOMA

Presently there are no clear radiological signs to predict malignancy in a meningioma other than:

- Rapid growth
- Extensive brain or bone invasion
- Bright on T2W imaging relative to brain (indicating meningothelial, angioblastic, hemangiopericytic elements as opposed to T2 hypointense benign meningiomas containing primarily calcified or fibrous elements)

Histologically, malignant meningiomas include the following cell types:

- Hemangiopericytoma
- Malignant fibrous histiocytoma (MFH)
- Papillary meningioma
- "Benign" metastasizing meningioma

HEMANGIOBLASTOMA

Hemangioblastomas are benign neoplasms of endothelial origin. Overall, hemangioblastomas are uncommon; however, they represent the most common primary cerebellar tumor in the adult patients with VHL (hemangioblastomas occur in 35%-60% of VHL patients; the incidence of VHL in hemangioblastoma patients is 10%-20%). Multiple hemangioblastomas are pathognomic for VHL. Location: cerebellum >>> spinal cord > medulla.

Cerebellar hemangioblastoma, 80%
The tumor consists of a pial (mural) nodule with associated cysts. During surgery the nodule (not only the cystic contents) has to be removed entirely, otherwise tumor will recur. Angiography may be performed before surgery to demonstrate vascular supply. Three different appearances:

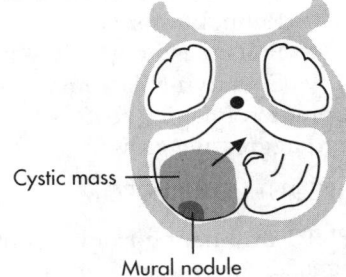

Cystic mass

Mural nodule

- Cystic lesion with an enhancing mural nodule, 75%. The cyst is generally not neoplastic and does not need to be resected unless there is evidence of tumor involvement (enhancement of cyst wall).
- Solid enhancing neoplasm, 10%
- Enhancing lesion with multiple cystic areas, 15%

Spinal hemangioblastoma, 10%
Commonly located on posterior aspect of spinal cord. 70% are associated with syringomyelia or cystic component. Contrast-enhanced MRI optimizes visualization of the small mural nodule.

Neuronal and Mixed Glial/Neuronal Tumors

GANGLIOGLIOMA/GANGLIONEUROMA

Benign neoplasm of children/young adults with glial and neural elements. Low grade and slow growing. Clinical presentations: seizures. Most tumors are located in cerebral hemispheres: temporal > frontal > parietal. This diagnosis should be suggested in a patient with long-standing seizure history and a cortically based lesion located in the temporal lobe. Nonspecific cystic mass, often calcified, with variable enhancement. Ganglioglioma may occasionally erode the inner table of the adjacent calvarium. Gangliogliomas may occasionally metastasize throughout CSF pathways, with a pattern of multiple small subarachnoid cysts. In the cerebellum a ganglioglioma may mimic Lhermitte-Duclos disease.

DYSEMBRYOPLASTIC NEUROEPITHELIAL TUMOR (DNET)

Newly recognized tumor with distinctive histological features. Like ganglioglioma, DNET is strongly associated with epilepsy. Younger patients. A well-circumscribed, often mixed cystic and solid cortically based lesion in a patient with long-standing seizure should bring DNET to mind. FLAIR imaging is helpful in identifying small peripheral lesions that are similar to CSF signal intensity. A temporal lobe location is common (> 60%), and the lesion often involves or lies close to mesial temporal structures; other locations include frontal lobe, followed by parietal and/or occipital lobes.

CENTRAL NEUROCYTOMA

Newly recognized tumor. Usually located in lateral ventricle, attached to ventricular wall. Calcification is common; mild to moderate enhancement. The tumor has feathery appearance on CT and MRI due to multiple cysts. It is usually attached to the septum pellucidum when arising from the lateral ventricle.

Primitive Neuroectodermal Tumors (PNETs)

Undifferentiated aggressive tumors that arise from multipotent embryonic neuroepithelial cells. They are common in children. Types:
- Medulloblastoma (infratentorial PNET)
- Primary cerebral neuroblastoma (supratentorial PNET)
- Retinoblastoma
- Pineoblastoma
- Ependymoblastoma

Common imaging features include intense contrast enhancement, dense cell packing, and aggressive growth.

MEDULLOBLASTOMA

PNET originating from roof of the 4th ventricle. Most common in childhood. Peak age: 2-8 years. Radiosensitive but metastasizes early via CSF. Associated with certain syndromes such as Gorlin's syndrome (basal cell nevi, odontogenic keratocysts, falx calficiation) or Turcot's syndrome (colonic polyps and CNS malignancy).

Radiographic features
- Typically intense and homogenous enhancement (hallmark)
- Cerebellar midline mass in 80%, lateral cerebellum 20%
- Dense cell packing (small cell tumor)
    Hyperdense on noncontrast CT
    May be intermediate signal intensity on T2W
- Hydrocephalus, 90%
- Rapid growth into cerebellar hemisphere, brainstem, and spine
- CSF seeding to spinal cord and meninges, 30%
- Systemic metastases can occur and appear as sclerotic lesions in bone. Metastases to abdominal cavity may occur via a VP shunt.
- Calcifications, 10%
- Atypical appearance and lateral cerebellar location are more common in older children.
- Strong enhancement

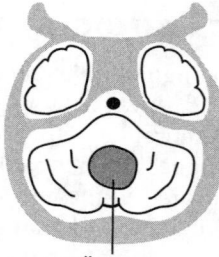

Midline tumor

PRIMARY CEREBRAL NEUROBLASTOMA

Rare, malignant tumor. 80% in first decade.
Radiographic features
- Large supratentorial mass
- Necrosis, hemorrhage cyst formation common
- Variable enhancement (neovascularity)

Nerve Sheath Tumors

SCHWANNOMA

Benign tumor of Schwann cell origin. Almost all intracranial schwannomas are related to cranial nerves. 90% are solitary; multiple schwannomas are commonly associated with NF2. 90% of intracranial schwannomas are located in the CPA originating from cranial nerve VIII (acoustic neuroma). Locations:

- CPA (VIII, most commonly from superior portion of vestibular nerve)
- Trigeminal nerve (V)
- Other intracranial sites (rare)
    - Intratemporal (VII)
    - Jugular foramen/bulb (IX, X, XI)
- Spinal cord schwannoma
- Peripheral nerve schwannoma
- Intracerebral schwannoma (very rare)

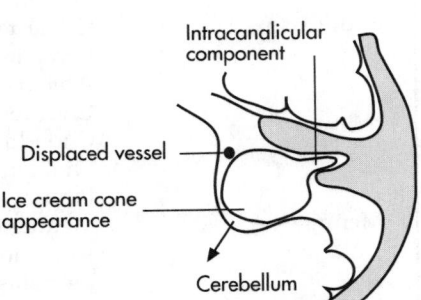

Radiographic features

Mass

- > 2 mm difference between left and right IAC
- Erosion and flaring of IAC
- IAC > 8 mm
- Extension into CPA (path of least resistance): ice cream cone appearance of extracanalicular portion

MRI/CT

- Isodense by CT
- MRI is more sensitive than CT.
- Dense enhancement, homogeneous if small, heterogeneous if large
- Gd-DTPA administration is necessary to detect small or intracanalicular tumors.
- May contain cystic degenerative areas
- Marginal arachnoid cysts
- Hyperintense on T2W

DIFFERENTIATION OF CPA TUMORS			
	Meningioma	Schwannoma	Epidermoid
Epicenter	Dural based	IAC	CPA
CT density	Hyper/isodense	Isodemse	Hypodense
Calcification	Frequent	None	Occasional
Porus acousticus/IAC	Normal	Widened	Normal
T2W signal intensity relative GM	50% isotense	Hyperintense	Hyperintense
Enhancement	Dense	Dense	None

SUMMARY OF COMMON MASSES BY LOCATION	
Cisters	Epidermoid cyst
	Dermoid cyst
	Lipoma
	Neurenteric cyst
	Neuroepithelial cyst
Arteries	Aneurysm
	Ectasia
Skull base	Cholesterol granuloma
	Paraganglioma
	Apicitis
	Chordoma
	Chondroma
	Endolymphatic sac tumor
	Pituitary adenoma
Meninges	Meningioma
	Arachnoid cyst
	Metastases
Nerves	Fifth to twelfth nerve schwanomas
Cerebellum	Glioma
Ventricle	Lymphoma
	Epndymoma
	Papilloma
	Hemangioblastoma
	Medulloblastoma
	DNET

Pearls

- Bilateral acoustic neuromas are pathognomic for NF2.
- Although 90% of CPA schwannomas are of cranial nerve VIII origin, hearing loss is the most common presentation, hence they are called *acoustic neuromas*.
- Meningiomas rarely extend into IAC but do not expand the IAC.

NEUROFIBROMA

Plexiform neurofibromas are unique to neurofibromatosis, type 1 (NF1). They do not occur primarily in the cranial cavity but may extend into it from posterior ganglia or as an extension of peripheral tumors.

DIFFERENTIATION OF SCHWANNOMA AND NEUROFIBROMA		
	Schwannoma	Neurofibroma
Origin	Schwann cells	Schwann cells and fibroblasts
Association	NF2	NF1
Incidence	Common	Uncommon
Location	NVIII > other CN	Cutaneous and spinal nerves
Malignant degeneration	No	5%-10%
Growth	Focal	Infiltrating
Enhancement	+++	++
T1W	70% hypo, 30% isointense	Isointense with muscle
T2W	Hyperintense	Hyperintense

Pineal Region Tumors

The pineal gland contributes to the circadian mechanism. Most pineal tumors occur in children and young adults. Patients may present with abnormal eye movement due to compression of the tectal plate (Parinaud's syndrome: inability to gaze upward) or hydrocephalus from compression of cerebral aqueduct. Types of tumors:

Germ cell tumors, > 50%
- Germinoma (most common tumor): equivalent to seminoma in testes and dysgerminoma in ovary
- Teratoma
- Embryonal cell carcinoma
- Choriocarcinoma

Pineal cell tumors, 25%
- Pineocytoma (benign)
- Pinealoblastoma (highly malignant, PNET)

Glioma

Other tumors
- Meningioma
- Metastases
- Epidermoid/dermoid
- Arachnoid cyst

TUMOR MARKERS		
	HCG	AFP
Germinoma	−	−
Embryonal cell carcinoma	+	+
Choriocarcinoma	+	−
Yolk sac tumor	−	+

GERMINOMA

- Pineal region is most common location.
- Males >> females, age 10-30 years
- Sharply circumscribed enlargement of pineal gland
- Hyperdense on noncontrast CT/isotense on T2W (dense cell packing)
- Homogenous intense enhancement
- Central calcification due to pineal engulfment (rare)
- May spread to ventricles and subarachnoid space via CSF
- In females, more commonly located in suprasellar location
- Sensitive to radiation therapy
- Germinomas located in the basal ganglia are often larger and more heterogeneous than those in pineal region.

6

TERATOMA

- Almost exclusively in male children
- Heterogeneous on CT and MR
- Presence of fat and calcification is diagnostically helpful
- Little-to-no enhancement

PINEALOBLASTOMA

- Highly malignant PNET
- In patients with trilateral retinoblastoma, pineoblastomas may develop in patients with familial and or bilateral retinoblastoma.
- "Exploded calcifications" along outside of mass
- Dense enhancement
- CSF dissemination

PINEOCYTOMA

- No male predilection
- Older age group, mean age 35 years
- Slow growing, dissemination is uncommon
- No helpful imaging features

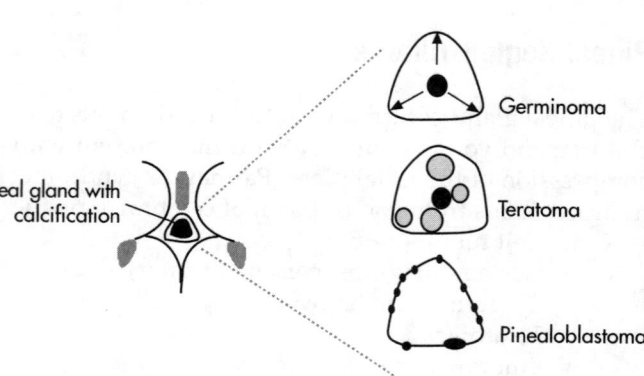

Normal pineal gland with calcification

Germinoma

Teratoma

Pinealoblastoma

Tumorlike Lesions

EPIDERMOID/DERMOID

Congenital tumor that arises from ectodermal elements in the neural tube before its closure. The concept of mesodermal elements within dermoids is probably incorrect; dermoids are of ectodermal origin.

SYNOPSIS		
	Epidermoid	**Dermoid**
Content	Squamous epithelium, keratin, cholesterol	Also has dermal appendages (hair, sebaceous fat, sweat glands)
Location	Off midline	Midline
	CPA most common	Spinal canal most common
	Parasellar, middle fossa	Parasellar, posterior fossa
	Intraventricular, diploic space (rare)	
Rupture	Rare	Common (chemical meningitis)
Age	Mean 40 years	Younger adults
CT density	CSF density	May have fat
Calcification	Uncommon	Common
Enhancement	Occasional peripherally	None
MRI	CSF-like signal	Proteinacious fluid
Other	5-10 times more common than dermoids	

DWI allows differentiation of epidermoid and arachnoid cysts. The ADC of an epidermoid cyst is significantly lower than that of an arachnoid cyst; therefore epidermoid cysts have high signal intensity on DWI, whereas arachnoid cysts, like CSF, have very low signal intensity.

HYPOTHALAMIC (TUBER CINEREUM) HAMARTOMA

Mature, disorganized ectopic tissue. Two clinical presentations:
- Isosexual, precocious puberty
- Associated with Pallister-Hall syndrome—nonspecific facial anomalies, polydactyly, imperforate anus, hypothalamic hamartoma
- No precocious puberty, gelastic seizures, intellectual impairment

Radiographic features
- CT: isodense, no enhancement (in contrast to hypothalamic gliomas)
- MR T1W: similar signal intensity of GM, T2W: hyperintense
- The floor of the third ventricle should be smooth from infundibulum to mammillary bodies. Any nodularity should raise suspicion for a hamartoma in the right clinical setting.

LIPOMA

Asymptomatic nonneoplastic tissue (malformation, not a true tumor). 50% are associated with other brain malformations. Location: midline 90%. 50% are pericallosal.

Radiographic features
- Fat density on CT (−50 to −100 HU)
- Calcification
- Avascular but callosal vessels may course through lesion
- MRI
   Chemical shift artifact
   Fat suppression sequences helpful
   T1 and T2 hypointense relative to brain on conventional spin-echo sequences.
      On fast-spin echo sequences fat appears hyperintense.

Hematopoietic Tumors

CENTRAL NERVOUS SYSTEM LYMPHOMA

Types
Primary lymphoma (1% of brain tumors), usually B-cell non-Hodgkin's lymphoma (NHL); high incidence in immunocompromised hosts.
- Basal ganglia, 50%
- Periventricular deep WM
- Corpus callosum

Secondary lymphoma (15% in patients with systemic lymphoma)
- Leptomeningeal spread

Radiographic features
Growth patterns
- Solitary or multiple masses in deep GM and WM, predominantly periventricular
- Diffuse meningeal or paraventricular ependymal involvement
- Diffusely infiltrative (mimics WM disease or gliomatosis cerebri)
- Spread along VR perivascular spaces
- Intraspinal

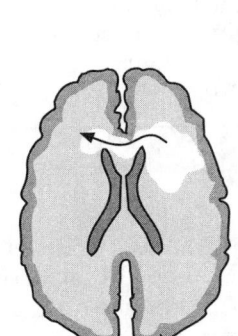
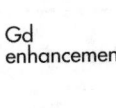

Nerve

Epidermoid

Gd enhancement

Signal characteristics
- Intrinsic hyperdensity, on noncontrast CT, with less mass effect than the size of the lesion
- Primary CNS lymphoma (PCNSL) often involves the corpus callosum and mimics butterfly glioma.
- Location in deep gray nuclei with extension to ependymal surfaces
- PCNSL rarely involves spine, whereas secondary CNS involvement with systemic lymphoma commonly involves both brain and spine.
- Isointense to GM on T2W (dense cell packing) or hyperintense
- Enhancement patterns
    Dense homogeneous enhancement is most common.
    Ringlike (central necrosis): more common in AIDS
    Meningeal enhancement in secondary lymphoma
    Fine feathery enhancement along VR spaces is typical.
- Calcification, hemorrhage, necrosis: multiple and large areas are typical in AIDS
- The tumor is very radiosensitive, and lesion may disappear after a short course of steroids. This may render the biopsy nondiagnostic.

AIDS-RELATED PRIMARY CNS LYMPHOMA

A solitary mass lesion in an AIDS patient is more often due to lymphoma than to infection. It may be difficult to distinguish PCNSL and toxoplasmosis in an AIDS patient with single- or multiple-enhancing lesions.

DIFFERENTIATION OF LYMPHOMA AND TOXOPLASMOSIS		
	Lymphoma	Toxoplasmosis
Single lesion	+	±
Deep gray nuclear involvement	+	+
Hyperdense on noncontrast CT	++	±
Eccenteric enhancing nodule	−	+
Callosal involvement	++	Rare
Ependymal spread	++	−
Subarachnoid spread	++	−
Thallium scanning	++	−
Spectroscopy	Elevated choline	Elevated lipid/lactate

Metastases

Metastases account for 30% of intracerebral tumors. Location in order of frequency: junction GM and WM (most common) > deep parenchymal structures (common) > brainstem (uncommon). Metastases also occur in dura, leptomeninges, and calvaria. The most common primaries are:
- Bronchogenic carcinoma, 50%
- Breast, 20%
- Colon, rectum, 15%
- Kidney, 10%
- Melanoma, 10%

Radiographic features

- Gadolinium-enhanced MRI is the most sensitive imaging study. Triple dose Gd-DTPA or magnetization-transfer increases sensitivity of lesion detection.
- 80% of lesions are multiple.
- Most metastases are T2 bright and enhance.
- Some metastases may be T2 isointense/hypointense relative to:
  - Hemorrhage (e.g., renal cell carcinoma)
  - Mucin (e.g., gastrointestinal adenocarcinoma)
  - Dense cell packing (e.g., germ cell tumor)
- Vasogenic edema is common.

Pearls

- Metastases and lymphoma are commonly multiple; gliomas are rarely multiple.
- A solitary enhancing brain tumor has a 50% chance of being a metastasis.
- Limbic encephalitis is a paraneoplastic syndrome associated with small cell lung cancer.

CARCINOMATOUS MENINGITIS

Leptomeningeal metastases are more common that dural metastases, although the two may coexist.

- Common primary neoplasms that cause carcinomatous meningitis include breast, lung, and skin (melanoma).
- MRI is more sensitive than CT for detection.
- Leptomeninges insinuate into cerebral sulci, which is a sign that helps distinguish a leptomeningeal process from a dural one.
- Subarachnoid tumor may be detected early by careful examination of cisternal segment of CNV and intracanalicular segment of cranial nerves VII and VIII.

Cystic Lesions

Various types of nonneoplastic, noninflammatory cysts are found intracranially:

- Arachnoid cyst
- Colloid cyst
- Rathke's cleft cyst
- Neuroepithelial cyst
- Enterogenous cyst
- Intraparenchymal cyst

ARACHNOID CYST (LEPTOMENINGEAL CYST)

Not a true neoplasm; probably arises from duplication or splitting of the arachnoid membrane (meningeal maldevelopment). 75% occur in children. Location:

- Middle cranial fossa (most common), 40%
- Suprasellar, quadrigeminal cisterns, 10%
- Posterior fossa, 50%
- CPA
- Cisterna magna

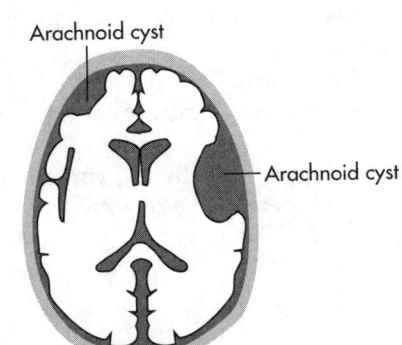

Arachnoid cyst

Arachnoid cyst

Radiographic features

- Extraaxial mass with CSF density (CT) and intensity (MRI)
- Slow enlargement with compression of subjacent parenchyma
- No communication with ventricles
- Pressure erosion of calvarium

DIFFERENTIATION OF ARACHNOID CYST AND EPIDERMOID		
	Arachnoid Cyst	Epidermoid
Signal intensity	Isointense to CSF on T1W	Mildly hyperintense to CSF
	Isointense to CSF on PDW	Hyperintense to CSF on PDW
	Isointense to CSF on T2W	Isointense to CSF on T2W
Enhancement	No	No
Margin of lesion	Smooth	Irregular
Effect on adjacent Structures	Displaces	Engulfs, insinuates
Pulsation artifact	Present	Absent
Diffusion imaging	Follows CSF	Hyperintense to CSF
FLAIR	Suppresses like CSF	Hyperintense to CSF
Calcification	No	May occur

COLLOID CYST

Cyst arises in foramen of Monro region. Peak age: adults. Clinical: intermittent headaches and ataxia from intermittent obstructive hydrocephalus.

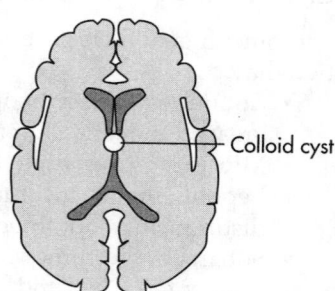

— Colloid cyst

- Typical location anterior to 3rd ventricle/foramen of Monro
- CT density: hyperdense 70%, hypodense (30%)
- MRI: variable signal intensity depending on paramagnetic content.
    T1 hyperintense
    T2 hypointense (most common)
- Differential of lesions in foramen of Monro
- Subependymoma (less dense on noncontrast CT)
- Astrocytoma (isointense or hypointense on T1W)
- Lymphoma
- Meningioma
- Choroid plexus papilloma
- Tumefactive intraventricular hemorrhage
- Intraventricular neurocysticercosis

RATHKE'S CLEFT CYST

Cyst arises from embryologic remnant of Rathke's pouch (rostral out-pouching during 4th week of embryogenesis; the precursor of anterior lobe and pars intermedia of pituitary gland).

Radiographic features

- Combined intrasellar and suprasellar location, 70%; purely intrasellar location, 20%
- Hypodense by CT, rim enhancement possible
- Hyperintense relative to brain on T1W imaging, variable signal intensity on T2W imaging

NEUROEPITHELIAL CYSTS

Heterogenous group of cysts comprising:
- Intraventricular ependymal cysts
- Choroid plexus cysts
- Choroid fissure cysts

Degenerative and White Matter Disease

General

CLASSIFICATION OF DEGENERATIVE DISEASES

WM disease
- Demyelinating disease: acquired disease in which normal myelin is destroyed
- Dysmyelinating disease: hereditary inborn errors of myelin synthesis, maintenance, or degradation

Gray matter disease
- Senile dementia, Alzheimer's type (SDAT)
- Pick's disease
- Vascular cortical dementia (multiinfarct dementia)
- Parkinson's disease
- Lysosomal storage diseases

Basal ganglia disorders
- Huntington's disease
- Wilson's disease
- Fahr's disease
- Leigh disease

DEGENERATION AND AGING

A variety of changes occur in the CNS with aging:

Diffuse cerebral atrophy
- Compensatory enlargement of ventricles, sulci, fissures, cisterns
- Loss of brain parenchyma

WM abnormalities
- Subcortical and central white matter abnormalities
- Periventricular WM abnormalities, in 30% of older population. Causes:
  Microvascular disease (ischemic demyelination), gliosis, protein deposits, occasionally lacunar infarction
  Periventricular and subcortical T2 bright signal abnormalities
  No contrast enhancement, no mass effect
- Virchow-Robin (VR) spaces; état criblé: dilated perivascular spaces
  Appearance:
  Perivascular demyelination causes an increase in perivascular subarachnoid space (filled with CSF)
  VR spaces always parallel CSF signal intensity (differentiate from WM lesions on PDW images)
  Common locations: anterior perforated substance (most common), basal ganglia, centrum semiovale

Iron deposition in basal ganglia
- T2 hypointensity

White Matter Disease

CLASSIFICATION

Demyelinating disease
- Multiple sclerosis (MS)
- ADEM
- Toxin related
    Central pontine myelinolysis
    Paraneoplastic syndromes
    Radiation therapy, chemotherapy
    Alcoholism

Dysmyelinating diseases (leukodystrophies)
- Lysosomal enzyme disorders
- Peroxisomal disorders
- Mitochondrial disorders
- Amino acidopathies
- Idiopathic

MULTIPLE SCLEROSIS (MS)

Idiopathic demyelinating disease characterized by edematous perivascular inflammation (acute plaques), which progresses to astroglial proliferation and demyelination (chronic plaques). Thought to be an autoimmune process influenced by genetic and environmental factors. Mainly affects young white adults; slightly more common in females (60%). Clinical: depends on anatomical location of lesions; monocular visual loss, gait difficulties, and sensory disturbances are most common. The diagnosis is based on a composite of clinical and laboratory data (evoked potentials, CSF oligoclonal bands) but not imaging studies. MRI aids in monitoring treatment.

Radiographic features

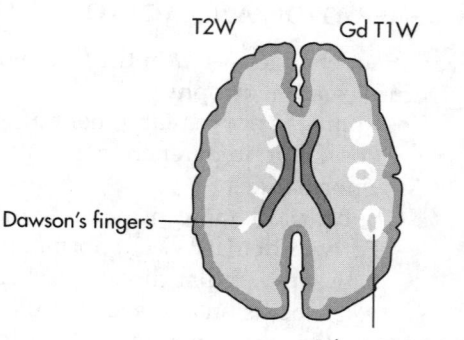

MRI appearance of plaques
- Plaques are most commonly multiple. To support the diagnosis of MS at least three plaques of > 5 mm should be present.
- Average size range: 0.5-3 cm
- Contrast enhancement may be homogeneous, ringlike, or patchy.
- Inactive plaques do not enhance.
- Bright signal intensity on T2W and PDW images
- Oblong, elliptical T2 bright structures at callososeptal interface
- Dawson's fingers: perivenular extension of elliptical structures into deep WM
- Tumefactive MS may mimic a brain tumor or infarct, but there is less mass effect then seen with a tumor.

Distribution of plaques
- Supratentorial
    Bilateral periventricular, 85%
    Corpus callosum, 70%
    Scattered in WM
    GM (uncommon)
- Brainstem
- Cerebellum
- Spinal cord, 50%
- Optic nerve, chiasm

Other findings
- Cortical central atrophy, 20%-80%
- Atrophy of corpus callosum, 40%
- Hypointense thalamus and putamen on T2W (increased ferritin)
- Mass effect of very large plaques (> 3 cm) may mimic tumors (uncommon)

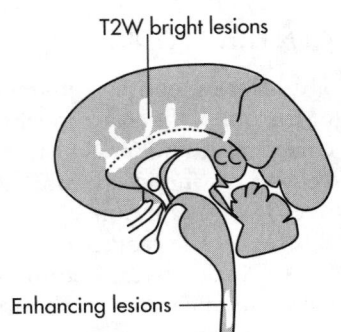

ACUTE DISSEMINATED ENCEPHALOMYELITIS (ADEM)

ADEM represents an immune response to a preceding viral illness or vaccination. Abrupt onset. More common in children. Indistinguishable from MS on imaging although less likely to be periventricular. Also, thalamic involvement is rare in MS but not uncommon in ADEM. Involves corpus callosum monophasic in contradistinction to multiple sclerosis, which is polyphasic. Although it is a monophasic illness, not all lesions enhance at the same time because some lesions may be developing while others are resolving.

RADIATION/CHEMOTHERAPY-INDUCED CNS ABNORMALITIES

Common causes
- Cyclosporine causes posterior confluent WM hyperintensity. Patients often present with blindness.
- Fluorouracil (5-FU), methotrexate (systemic)
- Intrathecal methotrexate
- Radiation and chemotherapy potentiate each other's toxic effects. Intrathecal methotroxate and whole brain radiation lead to diffuse deep WM T2 hyperintensity.

Two types of changes are observed:

Acute changes
- Occur during or immediately after course of radiation, resolve after therapy ends
- Changes usually represent mild edema, inflammation

Chronic changes
- Occurence:
    6-8 months after nonfractionated therapy: proton beam, stereotactical therapy
    2 years after fractionated conventional radiation
- May be permanent
- Pathology: occlusion of small vessels, focal demyelination, proliferation of glial elements and mononuclear cells, atrophy
- Signal intensity changes: T2 bright, CT hypodense

CENTRAL PONTINE MYELINOLYSIS (CPM)

This disease entity is characterized by symmetrical, noninflammatory demyelination of the pons, the exact mechanism of which is unknown. Osmotic shifts due to rapid correction in patients with hyponatremia have been implicated. CPM is also seen in chronic alcoholics and malnourished patients and in patients undergoing orthotopic liver transplantation.

Radiographic features

- Diffuse central pontine hyperintensity on T2W images without mass effect or enhancement and with sparing of corticospinal tracts
- Extra pontine lesions are commonly seen in putamina and thalami.
- MR may be negative initially on patient presentation but lesions become apparent on follow-up scans.
- Differential diagnosis
    Multiple sclerosis
    ADEM
    Ischemia/infarction
    Infiltrating neoplasm

LEUKODYSTROPHIES

A heterogeneous group of diseases characterized by enzyme defects that result in abnormal myelin production and turnover. In some disorders (e.g., idiopathic group), the biochemical abnormality is unknown. Imaging findings are nonspecific in many instances and non-WM regions can be involved (e.g., basal ganglia, cortex, vessels).

General categories

Lysosomal disorders

- Sphingolipidoses
- Mucolipidoses
- Mucopolysaccharidoses

Peroxisomal disorders

- Adrenoleukodystrophy
- Zellweger's syndrome

Mitochondrial disorders

- MELAS syndrome (**m**itochondrial myopathy, **e**ncephaloparthy, **la**ctic acidosis, **s**trokelike episodes)
- MERRF syndrome (**m**yoclonic **e**pilepsy with **r**agged **r**ed **f**ibers)
- Leigh syndrome

Aminoacidopathies

- Phenylketonuria (PKU)
- Homocystinuria
- Others

Idiopathic

- Alexander's disease
- Cockayne's disease
- Pelizaeus-Merzbacher disease
- Canavan's disease

Many entities have variable forms such as infantile, juvenile, and adult forms. Clinical manifestations overlap and include motor and intellectual deterioration, seizures, and progressive loss of function.

COMMON LEUKODYSTROPHIES			
Name	**Type**	**Deficiency**	**Comments**
Metachromatic leukodystrophy	Lysosomal (AR)	Aylsulfatase A	Most common type
Krabbe's disease	Lysosomal (AR)	Galactocerebroside β-Galactosidase	
Adrenoleukodystrophy	Peroxisomal (X-linked)	Acyl CoA synthetase	
Canavan's disease	Cytosol (AR)	Acetylaspartylase	Spongy degeneration
Alexander's disease	Unknown	Unknown	Sporadic
Pelizaeus-Merzbacher disease	Unknown	Proteolipid apoprotein	
Phenylketonuria	Amino acidopathy	Phenylalanine hydroxylase	Dietary treatment

Radiographic features
Macrocephaly
- Canavan's disease
- Alexander's disease

Frontal lobe predilection
- Alexander's disease

Occipital lobe predilection
- Adrenoleukodystrophy

Contrast enhancement
- Adrenoleukodystrophy
- Alexander's disease

Hyperdense basal ganglia
- Krabbe's disease

Ischemic infarctions
- Mitochondrial disorders (MELAS, MERRF)
- Homocystinuria

METACHROMATIC LEUKODYSTROPHY

Most common hereditary leukodystrophy; infantile form is most common. Age of presentation: < 2 years in 80%. Death in childhood.

Radiographic features
- Most common abnormality: periventricular WM abnormalities
    CT hypodense
    T2 hyperintense
- Prominent feature: cerebellar WM involvement
- Other nonspecific findings that do not allow differentiation from other dysmyelinating diseases

6

ADRENOLEUKODYSTROPHY (ALD)

Defective fatty acid oxidation (X-linked recessive is the most common). Accumulation of long-chain fatty acids in GM and WM and adrenal cortex. Age: preadolescent boys. Clinical: CNS manifestations and adrenal insufficiency. Definitive diagnosis made by detecting long-chain fatty acids in cultured fibroblasts, RBC, or plasma.

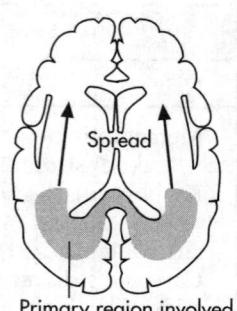

Primary region involved

Radiographic features

Distribution

- Common (80%): disease starts in occipital regions and spreads anterior to involve frontal lobes and across corpus callosum
- Less common: disease starts in frontal lobes and spreads posterior
- Symmetrical

Signal intensities

- CT

    Low attenuation (edema and gliosis)

    Enhancement of leading edge (inflammation)

- MRI

    T2 hyperintense with leading edge enhancement

    Pontomedullary corticospinal tract involvement is a common finding in ALD and is unusual in other leukodystrophies.

End-stage: atrophy

Gray Matter Disease

DEMENTIA

Dementia occurs in 5% of population > 65 years. Types:

- SDAT, 50%
- Multiinfarct dementia, 45%
- Less common causes (see table)

DIFFERENTIAL DIAGNOSIS OF DEMENTIA			
Disease	**Atrophy**	**Characteristics**	**Imaging**
SDAT	+	Temporal lobe, hippocampus	WM abnormalities not prominent
Multiinfarct dementia	+	Atrophy	Periventricular lacunae; cortical and subcortical infarction
NPH	−	Lacunae, basal ganglia	Hydrocephalus
Binswanger's*	+	Periventricular WM lesion	
Wernicke-Korsakoff†	+	Lacunae, basal ganglia, gyral and vermis atrophy	Medial thalamus T2 hyperintensity

*Subcortical arteriosclerotic encephalopathy.

†Clinically obvious (alcoholism, ataxia, ophthalmoparesis; thiamin deficiency).

SENILE DEMENTIA, ALZHEIMER'S TYPE (SDAT)

Most common degenerative brain disease and most common cortical dementia. Findings are nonspecific, so role of imaging is to exclude diseases that mimic SDAT: subdural hematoma, multi-infarct dementia, Binswanger's disease, primary brain tumor, and normal pressure hydrocephalus (NPH).

Radiographic features
- No reliable CT or MR findings that allow specific diagnosis
- Diffuse enlargement of sulci and ventricles is most common imaging finding.
- Disproportionate atrophy of anterior temporal lobes, hippocampi, and sylvian fissures
- WM hyperintensities may occur but are not a prominent feature.
- Regional bilateral temporoparietal abnormalities:
    SPECT: decreased HMPAO perfusion
    PET: decreased perfusion/metabolism ($^{15}O_2$/^{18}FDG)

PICK'S DISEASE

Rare cortical dementia that commonly presents before age 65 (presenile onset). Frontotemporal atrophy, frontal horn enlargement, and parietooccipital sparing are typical imaging features.

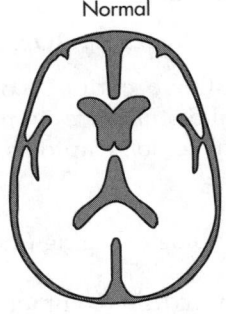 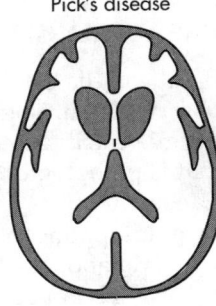

Normal   Pick's disease

VASCULAR CORTICAL DEMENTIAS

Ischemic dementia is the second most common form of dementia following SDAT. Types:

Multi-infarct dementia
- Cortical infarctions (territorial vascular infarctions)
- Enlarged sulci and ventricles
- Prominent T2 hyperintensities

Subcortical dementia (Binswanger's disease)
- Periventricular hyperintensity (penetrating vessel ischemia)
- Hypertension is common.

PARKINSON'S DISEASE

Idiopathic extrapyramidal disease of the striatonigral system. Hallmark is loss of melanin containing neurons in substantia nigra. Clinical: cogwheel rigidity, bradykinesia, tremor. Types:

Parkinson's disease
Secondary parkinsonism
- Neuroleptic drugs
- Trauma
- CO poisoning

Parkinson-plus syndrome (patients that respond poorly to Parkinson medication)
- Striatonigral degeneration
- Shy-Drager syndrome
- Olivopontocerebellar atrophy
- Progressive supranuclear palsy

6

Radiographic features
- MRI is commonly normal.
- Decreased width of T2 dark compacta
- Iron-induced signal loss in basal ganglia best seen on T2W spin echo and gradient echo images (black ganglia). Location of signal intensity change:
    Parkinson: globus pallidus
    Parkinson-plus: putamen
- Cerebral atrophy in chronic cases

AMYOTROPHIC LATERAL SCLEROSIS (ALS)

Progressive neurodegenerative illness. Unknown etiology, but 5% to 10% are familial.
- Abnormal high signal of corticospinal tracts on PDW images, best seen at level of middle or lower internal capsule
- Low signal intensity within motor cortex

Basal Ganglia Disorders

BASAL GANGLIA CALCIFICATION

Basal ganglia calcification occur in 1% of the general population. Unrelated to observed neurological disturbances in many instances. Most patients with basal ganglia calcification have no symptoms. No data exist as to the amount of calcification that is pathological.

Causes:
- Idiopathic/physiological aging (most common)
- Metabolic
    Hypoparathyroidism (common)
    Pseudohypoparathyroidism
    Pseudo-pseudohypoparathyroidism
    Hyperparathyroidism
- Infection (common)
    Toxoplasmosis
    HIV
- Toxin-related (uncommon)
    CO
    Lead poisoning
    Radiation/chemotherapy
- Ischemic/hypoxic injury
- Neurodegenerative diseases (rare)
    Fahr's disease
    Mitochondrial disorders
    Cockayne's disease
    Hallervorden-Spatz disease

HUNTINGTON'S CHOREA

Autosomal dominant inherited disease. Clinical: choreiform movements and dementia.

Radiographic features
- Caudate nucleus atrophy
- Boxcar appearance of frontal horns

WILSON'S DISEASE

Caused by abnormality in the copper transport protein, ceruloplasmin. Autosomal recessive.

Radiographic features
- MRI of the CNS may be normal.
- T2 hyperintense putamen and thalami
- Generalize atrophy
- Low-density basal ganglia on CT
- Hepatic cirrhosis

FAHR'S DISEASE

Historically, Fahr's disease was a term applied to a large group of disorders characterized by basal ganglia calcification. Fahr's disease is now used to describe a small category of patients with basal ganglia calcification and symptoms of late onset dementia with extrapyramidal motor dysfunction; predominantly autosomal dominant inheritance. A more precise name is familial idiopathic striopallidodentate calcification. Calcification in the dentate nuclei and cerebral WM can also be present.

LEIGH DISEASE

Mitochondrial disorder of oxidative phosphorylation (pyruvate carboxylase deficiency, thiamine pyrophosphate-ATP phosphoryl transferase inhibiting substance, pyruvate decarboxylase deficiency, cytochrome oxidase deficiency). Suspect the diagnosis in children with lactic acidosis and abnormal MRI or CT findings of the basal ganglia.

Diagnosis

Suggestive:
- Elevated serum pyruvate/lactate levels
- Typical findings by CT

Definitive:
- Cultured skin fibroblast assay for mitochondrial enzyme deficiency
- Histology

Radiographic features
- Location: putamen > globus pallidus > caudate nucleus
- Symmetric bilateral low attenuation areas in basal ganglia by CT
- Lesions are T2 hyperintense.
- MRI is more sensitive than CT in lesion detection.

NEUROSARCOIDOSIS

Symptomatic CNS involvement is seen in < 5% of cases. Serum or CSF ACE is elevated in 70% to 80% of patients with pulmonary sarcoidosis.

Radiologic features
- Plaquelike dural thickening on CT. These plaques are isointense on T1W and hypointense on T2W images.
- Homogeneous enhancement of involved dura and leptomeninges
- Underlying brain edema may be present.
- Parenchymal lesions show nodular enhancement.
- Sarcoid is a great mimic; enhancing lesions may involve dura, leptomeninges, brain parenchyma, hypothalamic pituitary axis, and cranial nerves.

6

Hydrocephalus

General

CLASSIFICATION

Noncommunicating hydrocephalus
- Intraventricular, foraminal, or aqueductal obstruction

Communicating hydrocephalus
- Obstruction at level of Pacchionian granulation (SAH, meningitis)
- Increased CSF production (rare): choroid plexus tumors
- NPH

APPROACH

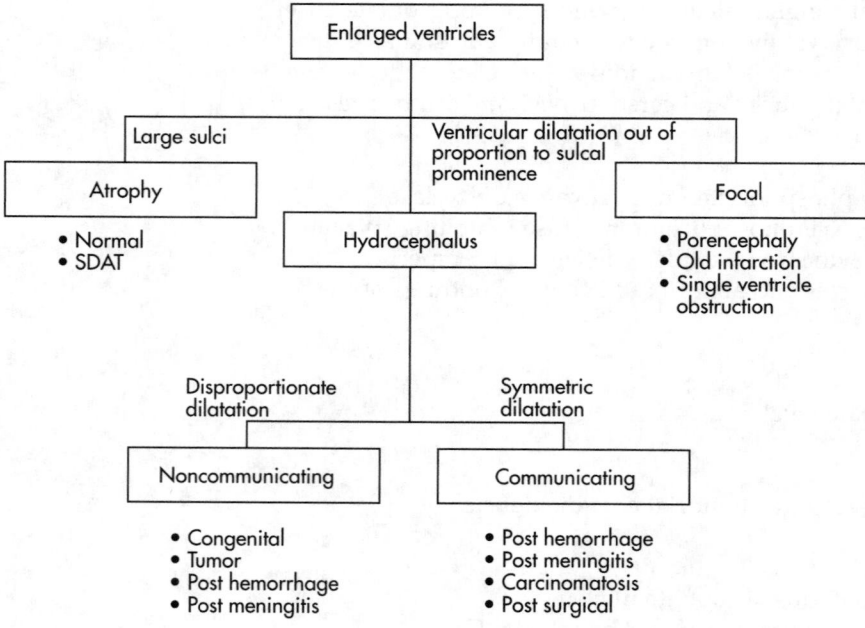

SHUNT COMPLICATIONS

- Ventriculitis/meningitis
- Obstruction (increase in amount of hydrocephalus)
- Subdural hematomas or effusions
- Meningeal fibrosis

Noncommunicating Hydrocephalus

Caused by obstruction of ventricles, foramina, or aqueduct. Ventricles are dilated proximal to the obstruction and normal in size distal to the obstruction.

Causes

Foramen of Monro obstruction
- 3rd ventricle tumors
    Colloid cyst
    Oligodendroglioma
    Central neurocytoma
    Giant cell astrocytoma in TS
    Ependymoma
    Meningioma (rare)
- Suprasellar tumors

Aqueduct obstruction
- Congenital aqueduct stenosis
- Ventriculitis
- Intraventricular hemorrhage
- Tumors
    Mesencephalic
    Pineal, posterior 3rd ventricular region

4th ventricle obstruction
- Congenital: Dandy-Walker (DW) malformation
- Intraventricular hemorrhage
- Infection (cysticercosis)
- Subependymoma
- Exophytic brainstem glioma
- Posterior fossa tumors: ependymoma, medulloblastoma, hemangioblastoma, metastasis, astrocytoma

Radiographic features
- Disproportionate dilatation of ventricles up to the point of obstruction
- Underlying abnormality causing the obstruction
- Ballooning of temporal horns ("Mickey Mouse ears") is a sensitive sign.
- Effaced sulci due to mass effect
- Periventricular interstitial edema due to elevated intraventricular pressure and transependymal CSF flow T2 bright halo in noncompensated cases
- Absence of normal flow void in aqueduct by MRI
- Direct measurement of increased intracranial pressure via CSF puncture is sometimes performed for diagnostic purposes.

Communicating Hydrocephalus

Results most commonly from extraventricular CSF pathway obstruction at the level of pacchionian granulations, basal cistern, or convexity. Causes:
- Meningitis
    Infectious
    Carcinomatous
- SAH and trauma
- Surgery
- Venous thrombosis

Radiographic features
- Following signs are the same as in noncommunicating hydrocephalus
    - Ballooning of temporal horns
    - Effaced sulci (mass effect)
    - Periventricular interstitial edema (T2 bright halo)
- Symmetrical dilatation of all ventricles
- The 4th ventricle is usually not very enlarged in convexity block hydrocephalus.

NORMAL PRESSURE HYDROCEPHALUS (NPH)

Form of communicating hydrocephalus in which there is no evidence of increased intracranial pressure. Clinical triad: gait incoordination, dementia, urinary incontinence. Clinical response to CSF tap is the gold standard for establishing the diagnosis.

Radiographic features
- No specific imaging findings
- Dilated ventricles in a patternlike communicating hydrocephalus
- Periventricular T2 bright halo is less common.
- Prominent cerebral aqueduct flow void

SPONTANEOUS INTRACRANIAL HYPOTENSION

The syndrome of intracranial hypotension results when CSF volume is lowered by leakage or by withdrawal of CSF in greater amounts than can be replenished by normal production. The syndrome is designated as spontaneous in absence of prior violation of dura. Manifests as postural headache exaceberated by upright position. Diffuse dural enhancement seen in 100% of cases. Other findings that may not always be present include:
- Downward displacement of cerebellar tonsils and midbrain
- Flattening of pons against the dorsal clivus
- Draping of optic chiasm over the sella
- Distention of major dural venous sinuses
- A fast spin-echo T2W image of spine is performed to look for a spinal source of leak.
- An epidural blood patch may be an effective way to treat this condition. This procedure involves mixing a few milliliters of contrast with blood and using fluoroscopy to insure instillation into the epidural space near suspected site of leak.

Infection

General

CLASSIFICATION BY INFECTIOUS AGENT

- Bacterial (purulent) infections
- Fungal infections
- Parasitic infections
- Viral infections

CLASSIFICATION BY LOCATION OF INFECTION

- Meningitis: pia or subarachnoid space and/or dura or arachnoid
- Empyema: epidural or subdural
- Cerebritis: intraparenchymal; early stage of abscess formation
- Intraparenchymal abscess
- Ventriculitis

Bacterial Infections

BACTERIAL MENINGITIS

Causes
- Neonates: Group B streptococcus, *Escherichia coli, Listeria*
- Children: *Hemophilus, E. coli, N. meningitidis*
- Adults: *Streptococcus pneumoniae, N. meningitidis*

Pathologically, meningitis can be separated into:
- Leptomeningitis (most common): arachnoid and pia involved
- Pachymeningitis: dura and outer layer of arachnoid involved

Predisposing factors:
- Sinusitis
- Chronic pulmonary infection
- Tetralogy of Fallot
- Transposition of great vessels
- Other cyanotic heart disease

Radiographic features
Meningeal contrast enhancement
- Normal CT examination is initially most common finding.
- Convexity enhancement occurring later on is a typical finding.
- Basilar meningeal enhancement alone is more commonly seen in granulomatous meningitis.

Cranial US in neonatal bacterial meningitis
- Subtle findings: abnormal parenchymal echogenicity
- Echogenic sulci, 40%
- Extraaxial fluid collections
- Ventricular dilatation
- Ventriculitis occurs in 70%-90% of bacterial meningitis
    - Normally thin ventricular wall thickens
    - Wall becomes hyperechoic
    - Debris in CSF

Complications
- Subdural effusion: common in infants and children
- Empyema
- Parenchymal extension: abscess and cerebritis
- Ventriculitis
- Hydrocephalus (communicating > noncommunicating)
- Venous infarctions secondary to venous thrombosis

TUBERCULOUS MENINGITIS

The most common CNS manifestation of TB followed by intraparenchymal tuberculoma. Spread is usually hematogenous from pulmonary TB. Basilar meningeal involvement by chronic granulomatous process leads to cranial nerve palsies.

Radiographic features

Basilar meningitis

- Intense contrast enhancement of basilar meninges (CT, MRI)
- Pituitary and parasellar involvement
- Pituitary or hypothalamic axis involvement
- T2 hypointense meninges
- Calcifications occur late in disease

Abscesses (tuberculoma)

- Rare unless immunocompromised or from endemic areas (Indian population)
- Usually solitary
- Nonspecific enhancing masslike lesions
- Cerebral hemispheres and basal ganglia
- Miliary form: multiple tiny intraparenchymal lesions

EMPYEMA

An empyema is an infected fluid collection in subdural (common) or epidural (uncommon) location. Empyemas are neurosurgical emergencies. Cause: sinusitis (most common), otitis, trauma, post-craniotomy.

Radiographic features

- Subdural or epidural low attenuation fluid collection with enhancement of adjacent brain
- Venous infarction → edema → mass effect → midline shift
- Thick, curvilinear enhancement of empyema
- Concomitant signs of sinusitis, otitis

BRAIN ABSCESS

Common organism

- Children: *Staphylococcus* (especially after trauma), *Streptococcus*, *Pneumococcus*
- Adults: mixed aerobic and anaerobic flora
- Immunosupression: toxoplasmosis, cryptococcosis, candidiasis, aspergillosis, nocardiosis, mucormycosis (diabetes), TB, atypical mycobacteria

Mechanism

Hematogenous dissemination (most common)

- Intravenous drug abuse
- Sepsis

Direct extension

- Sinusitis
- Otitis, mastoiditis
- Open injury (penetrating trauma, surgery)

Idiopathic

Radiographic features

Location

- Hematogenous seeding: multiple lesions at GM/WM junction
- Penetrating trauma or sinusitis: lesion around the entry site

Morphology

- Mass effect (abscess cavity, edema)
- Ring or wall enhancement, 90%
- Capsule forms in 7-14 days

    Capsule is thinner on WM side because of lower perfusion to WM than to
        GM. Because of the thinner capsule, daughter lesions (and
        intraventricular rupture) occur on the medial side.

    Capsule is hypointense on T2W images.

    Inner margin is often smooth.

    Capsule formation may be delayed by steroid administration

- Ventriculitis due to ventricular spread

    Increased CSF density (elevated protein concentration)

    Ependymal contrast enhancement

    May cause ventricular septations and hydrocephalus

- Daughter lesions

Fungal Infections

Causes

Immunocompetent patients

- Coccidioidomycosis, histoplasmosis, blastomycosis

Immunocompromised patients (AIDS, chemotherapy, steroids, transplant recipients)

- Nocardiosis, aspergillosis, candidiasis, cryptococcosis, mucormycosis

Radiographic features

Basilar meningitis

- Intense contrast enhancement of basilar meninges (similar to TB)

Abscesses

- Early: granuloma
- Late: abscess with ring enhancement and central necrosis

Helpful features:

- Aspergillosis

    Hemorrhagic infarcts from vascular invasion

    Often coexistent sinus disease that has extended to CNS

    T2 isointense/hypointense masslike lesions

- Mucormycosis: indistinguishable from aspergillosis
- Coccidioidomycosis: indistinguishable from TB
- Cryptococcosis: cystic lesions (gelatinous pseudocysts secondary to spread into
    Virchow-Robin spaces) in basal ganglia. Consider this diagnosis in an HIV
    positive patient with communicating hydrocephalus. "Lacunar infarct"-like
    appearance in an HIV-positive patient may be secondary to cryptococcal
    gelatinous pseudocysts.

Parasitic Infections

NEUROCYSTICERCOSIS

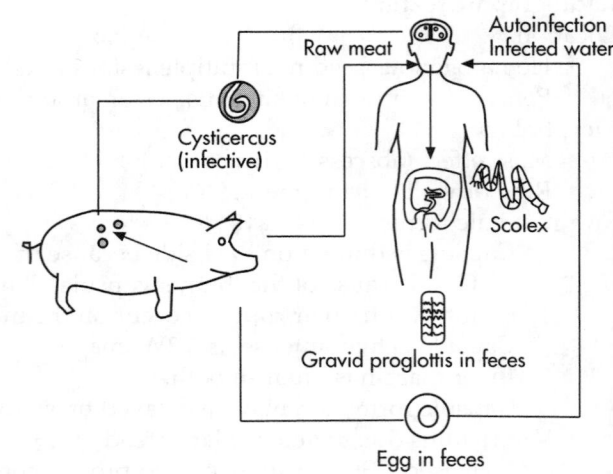

Caused by *Taenia solium* (pork tapeworm). Epidemiology: Central and South America, hispanic population in United States. Source: ingestion of contaminated water or pork. Ingested eggs penetrate intestine, disseminate hematogenously, and encyst in muscle, brain, and ocular tissue. Cysts first contain a living larva, which ultimately dies, causing inflammation (contrast enhancement) and calcifications. 75% of infected patients have CNS involvement. Seizures are the most common presentation. Treatment: praziquanatel, salbendezol, VP shunting for obstructive hydrocephalus. Evolution of lesions:

- Nonenhancing cyst: live larvae
- Ring-enhancing lesion: dying larvae cause inflammatory reaction
- Calcification: old lesion

Radiographic features

Four stages in brain parenchyma
- Vesicular stage—thin-walled vesicles (< 20 mm) present with CSF-like fluid and a mural nodule; inflammatory response is absent
- Colloid stage—viable cyst dies, cyst fluid becomes turbid, inflammatory reaction leads to breakdown of blood-brain barrier
- Nodular granular stage—lesion undergoes involution and begins to calcify
- Calcified stage

Typical appearance of cysts
- Multiple cystic lesions of water density
- Larvae (scolices) appear of variable signal intensity on T2W images
- Ring enhancement (inflammatory response caused by dying larvae)

Three locations
- Parenchymal (most common)
- Intraventricular (may cause obstruction)
- Subarachnoid

Other findings
- Hydrocephalus
- Chronic meningitis
- Calcification of skeletal muscle

LYME DISEASE

- Multisystem inflammatory disease caused by a spirochete *Borrelia burgdorferi*
- Single or multiple parenchymal abnormalities associated with meningeal and multiple cranial nerve enhancement
- May mimic multiple sclerosis by imaging

Viral Infections

HERPES SIMPLEX VIRUS ENCEPHALITIS (HSV)

Two general herpes types:

HSV-2, genital herpes
- Neonatal TORCH infection (see below)
- Acquired during parturition
- Manifests several weeks after birth
- Diffuse encephalitis (nonfocal)

HSV-1, oral herpes
- Children and adults
- Usually activation of latent virus in trigeminal ganglion
- Altered mental status; fulminant course
- Limbic system; frequently bilateral but asymmetrical

Radiographic features
- CT and MRI are usually normal early in disease.
- MRI is the imaging study of choice. The first imaging findings become apparent within 2-3 days after onset.
- Distribution: limbic system, temporal lobe > cingulate gyrus, subfrontal region
- Acute stage
    Gyral edema (T1 hypointense/T2 hyperintense)
    No enhancement
- Subacute stage
    Marked increase in edema
    Bilateral asymmetrical involvement
    Gyral enhancement
    Hemorrhage is common in this stage.

CONGENITAL INFECTIONS

Congenital CNS infections result in brain malformations, tissue destruction, and/or dystrophic calcification; the CNS manifestations depend on both the specific infectious agent and the timing of the infection during fetal development. Causes of congenital infections:

TORCH
- **To**xoplasmosis (second most common)
- **R**ubella
- **C**MV (most common)
- **H**erpes simplex

Other
- HIV
- Syphilis
- Varicella

Radiographic features

CMV

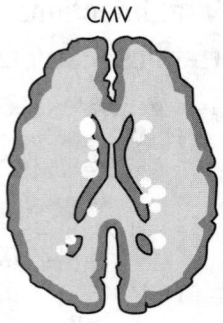

CMV

- Gestational age at time of infection predicts the nature and extent of abnormalities. In general, infection acquired during first two trimesters causes congenital malformations, whereas infection in the third trimester manifests as destructive lesions
- Periventricular calcification. CT is adequate for diagnosis in 40%-70% of cases with typical calcifications. However, calcifications may be in atypical locations such as basal ganglia or subcortical regions. In neonate, the calcifications may appear hyperintense on T1W and hyointense on T2W images in comparison to adjacent WM.
- Neuronal migration anomalies, especially polymicrogyria

Congenital toxoplasmosis

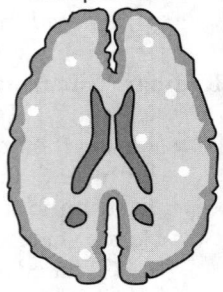

Toxoplasmosis

- Basal ganglia and parenchymal calcification (diffuse). Intracranial calcifications may regress or resolve over time in cases of treated toxoplasmosis.
- Hydrocephalus.
- Choriorentinitis.

Rubella

- Microcephaly
- Basal ganglia and parenchymal calcifications

HSV-2

- Multifocal GM and WM involvement
- Hemorrhagic infarction—consider this diagnosis in a neonate who presents in the second or third week of life with diffuse brain edema and leptomeningeal enhancement.
- Neonatal herpes encephalitis lacks the temporal and inferior frontal lobe predominance associated with adult herpes infection.

Congenital HIV (primary HIV encephalitis)

- Diffuse atrophy
- Basal ganglia calcification after 1 year

AIDS

HIV is a neurotropic virus that directly infects the CNS and is the most common CNS pathogen in AIDS. HIV-related infections:

- HIV encephalopathy (most common)
- Toxoplasmosis: most common opportunistic CNS infection
- Cryptococcosis
- Progressive multifocal leukocencephalopathy (PML)
- TB
- Syphilis
- Varicella
- CMV

HIV ENCEPHALOPATHY

Progressive subacute subcortical dementia secondary to HIV itself. Eventually develops in 60% of AIDS patients.

Radiographic features
- Atrophy is the most common finding.
- T2 bright WM lesions in frontal and occipital lobes and periventricular location (gliosis, demyelination)
- No enhancement or mass effect of WM lesions

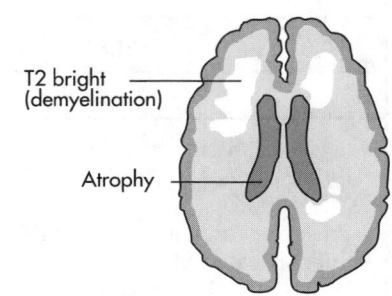

TOXOPLASMOSIS

Most common opportunistic CNS infection in AIDS. Caused by *Toxoplasma gondii* (reservoir: infected cats). Three manifestations:

Congenital
- Meningitis, encephalitis: calcifiaction
- Encephalomalacia, atrophy
- Chorioretinitis

Immunocompetent adults
- Systemic disease with lymphadenopathy and fever
- CNS is not involved (in contradistinction to AIDS)

Immunocompromised patients
- Fulminant CNS disease
- Predilection for basal ganglia and corticomedullary junction

Radiographic features
- Solitary or multiple ring-enhancing lesions with marked surrounding edema
- Target appearance of lesions is common.
- Treated lesions may calcify or hemorrhage.
- Major differential diagnosis is CNS lymphoma:
    Periventricular location and subependymal spread favors lymphoma.
    Empirical treatment with antiprotozoan drugs and reassessment of lesions is
        often used to distinguish between the two.
- SPECT thallium: lymphoma appears as hot lesions, toxoplasma appears as cold lesions

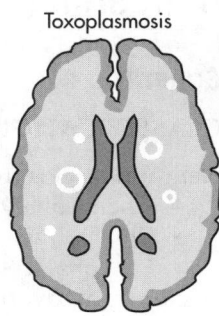
Toxoplasmosis

CRYPTOCOCCOSIS

Manifests as meningitis (more common) and intraparenchymal lesions. The most common intraparenchymal finding are multiple T2 bright foci in basal gelatinous pseudocysts ganglia and midbrain with variable enhancement (cryptococcomas).

PROGRESSIVE MULTIFOCAL LEUKOENCEPHALOPATHY (PML)

Demyelinating disease caused by reactivation of JC virus, a polyoma virus. The reactivated virus infects and destroys oligodendrocytes.

Radiographic features
- Posterior centrum semiovale is the most common site.
- Bilateral but asymmetrical
- Begins in subcortical WM; spreads to deep WM
- T2-bright lesions (parietooccipital)
- No enhancement (key distinguishing feature from infections and tumors)
- May cross corpus callosum
- No mass effect

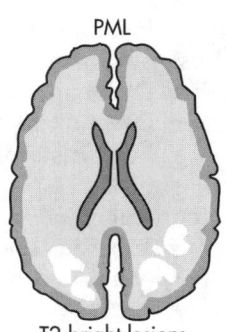
PML

T2-bright lesions

DIFFERENTIATION OF HIV ENCEPHALITIS AND PML		
	HIV Encephalitis	**PML**
Signal intensity on T1W images	Usually isointense	Commonly iso intense
Enhancement	—	May have mild enhancement
Mass effect	—	May have mild mass effect
Posterior fossa involvement	Uncommon	Common
Subcortical U fibers	Uncommon	Common
White matter lesions	Symmetrical	Asymmetrical
Hemorrhage	Never	Occasional

CMV ENCEPHALITIS

Indistinguishable imaging appearance from HIV encephalopathy. Shows perventricular hyperintensity on proton density or FLAIR images. Quantitative PCR of CSF may be useful in monitoring response to therapy.

Congenital Disease

General

CLASSIFICATION

Neural tube closure defects
- Anencephaly (most common anomaly)
- Chiari II, III
- Encephalocele

Disorders of diverticulation and cleavage
- Holoprosencephaly
- Septooptic dysplasia
- Corpus callosum anomalies

Neuronal migration and sulcation abnormalities
- Lissencephaly
- Pachygyria
- Polymicrogyria
- Schizencephaly
- Heterotopia
- Hemimegalencephaly

Posterior fossa malformations
- DW malformation
- DW variant
- Mega cisterna magna
- Chiari I

Neurocutaneous syndromes (phakomatoses)
- Tuberous sclerosis
- Neurofibromatosis
- Sturge-Weber syndrome (encephalotrigeminal angiomatosis)
- Von Hippel-Lindau (VHL) disease

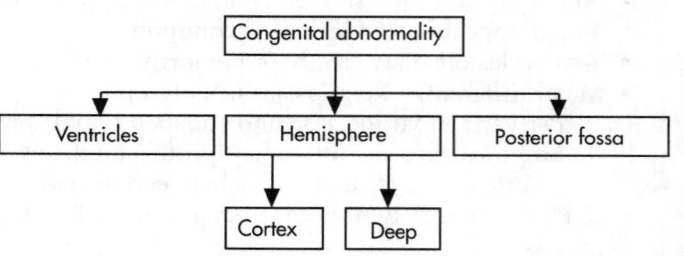

Neural Tube Closure Defects

CHIARI MALFORMATIONS

Overview of Chiari malformations
- Chiari I = downward displacement of cerebellar tonsils below foramen magnum (> 5 mm); unrelated to Chiari II malformation
- Chiari II = abnormal neurulation leads to a small posterior fossa, caudal displacement of brainstem and herniation of tonsils and vermis through the foramen magnum; myelomeningocele
- Chiari III = encephalocele and Chiari II findings (rare)
- Chiari IV = severe cerebellar hypoplasia (rare)

Chiari II malformation
Most common in newborns. Associations:
- Myelomeningocele, 90%
- Obstructive hydrocephalus, 90%
- Dysgenesis of corpus callosum
- Syringohydromyelia, 50%
- Abnormal cortical gyration
- Chiari II is not associated with Klippel-Feil anomaly or Chiari I.

Radiographic features
Posterior fossa
- Small posterior fossa
- Cerebellar vermis herniated through foramen (verminal peg)
- Upward herniation of cerebellum through widened incisure (towering cerebellum)
- Cerebellum wraps around pons (heart shape).
- Low widened tentorium
- Obliterated CPA cistern and cisterna magna
- Nonvisualization or very small 4th ventricle

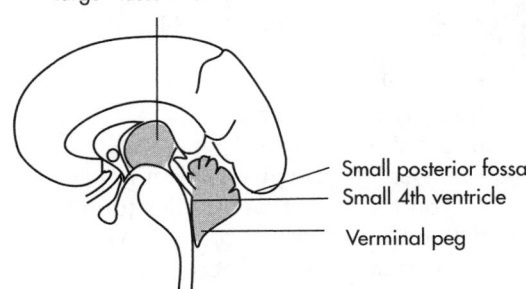

Large massa intermedia

Small posterior fossa
Small 4th ventricle

Verminal peg

Supratentorium
- Hypoplastic or fenestrated falx causes interdigitation of gyri (gyral interlocking).
- Small crowded gyri (stenogyria), 50%
- Hydrocephalus almost always present before shunting
- Batwing configuration of frontal horns (caused by impressions by caudate nucleus)
- Small biconcave 3rd ventricle (hourglass shape due to large massa intermedia)
- Beaked tectum

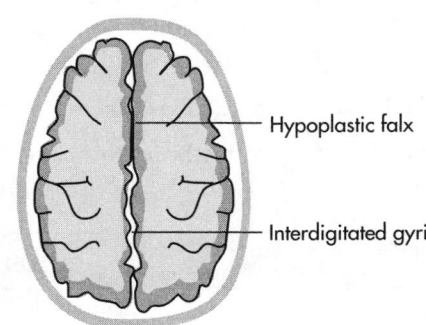

Hypoplastic falx

Interdigitated gyri

Osseous abnormalities
- Lückenschädel skull (present at birth, disappears later)
- Scalloped clivus and petrous ridge (pressure effect)
- Enlarged foramen magnum

Spinal cord
- Myelomeningocele, 90%
- Cervicomedullary kink at foramen magnum (pressure effect)
- Syringohydromyelia and diastematomyelia

6

CEPHALOCELE

Skull defect through which meninges, neural tissue, and/or CSF protrude. Usually midline and associated with other malformation (Chiari, callosal agenesis).
Location
- Occipital, 80%
- Frontal or nasoethmoidal
- Parietal, 10%
- Lateral from midline (suspect amniotic band syndrome)
- Sphenoidal (associated with sellar/endocrine anomalies)

Cerebral Hemisphere Defects

AGENESIS OF CORPUS CALLOSUM (ACC)

Fibers that usually cross through corpus callosum run in longitudinal bundles (bundles of Probst) along the medial walls of the lateral ventricles (lateral displacement) and end randomly in occipital and parietal lobes. The 3rd ventricle is pathologically elevated because of this abnormality. ACC may be complete or partial; when partial, the splenium and rostrum are absent. Associated CNS anomalies occur in 60%.
- DW malformation
- Lipoma (calcified in 10%)
- Chiari II
- Encephalocele
- Migration anomalies

Radiographic features
- Absence of corpus callosum
- Abnormal callosal bundles (bundles of Probst)
- Poor development of the WM around the atria and occipital horns: colpocephaly
- Compensatory abnormalities
  - Elevated 3rd ventricle (hallmark)
  - Parallel lateral ventricles
  - Frontal horns small (bull's horn appearance), occipital horns large

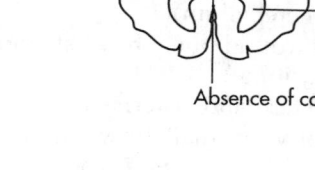

Interhemispheric cyst
Bundle of Probst
Small frontal horns, wide separation of ventricles
High and prominent 3rd ventricle
Large occipital, temporal horns
Absence of corpus

HOLOPROSENCEPHALY

Failure of primitive brain to cleave into left and right cerebral hemispheres. Commonly associated with midline facial anomalies ranging from cyclopia to hypotelorism.

THREE TYPES OF HOLOPROSENCEPHALY			
	Alobar	Semilobar	Lobar
Interhemispheric fissure and falx	Absent	Present posteriorly	Present*
Lateral ventricles	U-shaped monoventricle	Partially fused anteriorly	Near normal
Third ventricle	Absent	Rudimentary	Near normal
Cerebral hemisphere	One brain	Partial formation	Near normal
Thalamus	Fused	Variable fuison	Near normal
Facial anomalies	Severe	Less severe	None or mild
Septum pellucidum	Absent	Absent	Absent

*Nearly completely formed with most anteroinferior aspect absent.

Radiographic features

Alobar form

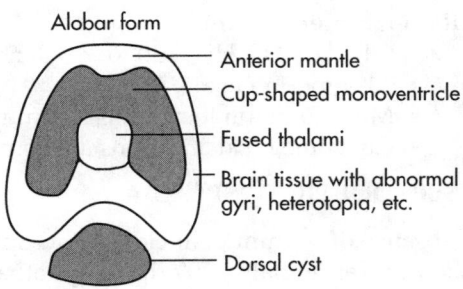

Alobar form

- No cleavage into two hemispheres: cup-shaped brain
- Single monoventricle
- Thalamic fusion
- Absent falx, corpus callosum, fornix, optic tracts, and olfactory bulbs
- Dorsal cysts common
- Midbrain, brainstem, and cerebellum are structurally normal.

Semilobar form

- Partial cleavage into hemispheres
- Partial occipital and temporal horns

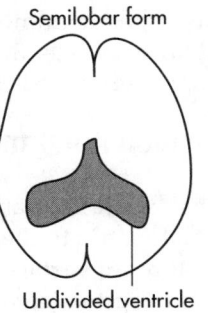

Lobar form

- Complete cleavage into two hemispheres, except for fusion in the rostral portion
- Lateral ventricles are normal or slightly dilated; frontal horns may be "squared."
- Absent septum pellucidum

Differential diagnosis

- Hydranencephaly
- Callosal agenesis with dorsal interhemispheric cyst
- Severe hydrocephalus

Facial abnormalities

- Facial abnormalities usually correlate with severity of brain abnormalities but not vice versa.
- Hypotelorism (eyes too close together)
- Midline maxillary cleft
- Cyclopia (single eye)
- Ethmocephaly, cebocephaly

Pearls

- 50% of patients with holoprosencephaly have trisomy 13.
- Presence of a septum pellucidum excludes the diagnosis of holoprosencephaly.
- Lobar holoprosencephaly is the anteroinferior fusion of frontal lobes and absence of septum pellucidum and can thus be differentiated from severe hydrocephalus.
- Hydranencephaly has no anterior cerebral mantle or facial anomalies; falx and thalami are normal.

CEREBRAL HEMIATROPHY (DYKE-DAVIDOFF)

Intrauterine and perinatal ICA infarction leads to hemiatrophy of a cerebral hemisphere.

Radiographic features

- Atrophy of a hemisphere causes midline shift.
- Compensatory ipsilateral skull thickening (key finding)
- Ipsilateral paranasal, mastoid sinus enlargement

INTERHEMISPHERIC LIPOMA

Collection of primitive fat within or adjacent to corpus callosum. Associations:

- Absence of corpus callosum, 50%
- Midline dysraphism
- Agenesis of cerebellar vermis
- Encephalocele, myelomeningocele, spina bifida

Radiographic features
- CT: pure fat (HU −50 to −100; no associated hair/debris) is pathognomonic
- T1 hyperintense
- Most common location is splenium and genu.
- Curvilinear calcifications are common.

SEPTOOPTIC DYSPLASIA

Absence of septum pellucidum and optic nerve hypoplasia (mild form of lobar holoprosencephaly). 70% have hypothalamic/pituitary dysfunction.
Radiographic findings
- Absence of septum pellucidum
- Squared frontal horns of lateral ventricles
- Hypoplasia of optic nerve and chiasm

Migration and Sulcation Abnormalities

Group of disorders that result from abnormal migration of neuroblasts from subependymal germinal matrix to their cortical location.
Lissencephaly (smooth brain surface)
Lack of sulcation leads to agyria (complete lissencephaly) or agyria-pachygyria (incomplete lissencephaly). May be secondary to in utero infections, especially CMV.
Schizencephaly (split brain)
GM-lined CSF cleft extends from ependyma to pia; high association with ACC.
Polymicrogyria
Excessive cerebral convolutions with increased cortical thickness. May be distinguished from pachygyria (thick flat cortex) by MRI.
Cortical heterotopia
Islands of normal GM in abnormal locations due to arrest of neuronal migration. May be nodular or laminar (bandlike). Occur most commonly in periventricular location and centrum semiovale (anywhere along path from germinal matrix to cortex). Clinical: childhood seizures.

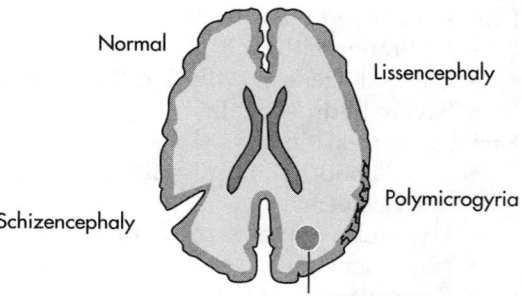

Posterior Fossa Malformations

DANDY-WALKER MALFORMATION

Exact etiology unknown: (1) insult to developing cerebellum and 4th ventricle, (2) congenital atresia of foramina of Magendie and Luschka. Mortality 25%-50%). Key findings:
- Large posterior fossa cyst
- Hydrocephalus, 75%
- Varying degrees of cerebellar hemispheric and vermian hypoplasia

Associated abnormalities:
- Agenesis of corpus callosum, 25%
- Lipoma of corpus callosum
- Malformation of cerebral gyri

- Holoprosencephaly, 25%
- Cerebellar heterotopia, 25%
- GM heterotopia
- Occipital cephalocele
- Tuber cinereum hamartoma
- Syringomyelia
- Cleft palate
- Polydactyly
- Cardiac abnormalities

Radiographic features
- Enlarged posterior fossa
- Large posterior fossa cyst communicates with the 4th ventricle.
- Absent or abnormal inferior cerebellar vermis (key finding)
- Elevation of vermian remnant
- Hypoplastic cerebellar hemispheres
- Hydrocephalus
- Elevation of torcular heterophils and tentorium

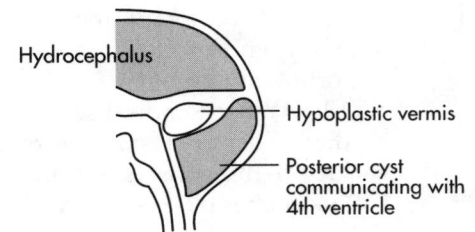

DANDY-WALKER VARIANT

Posterior fossa cyst with partially formed 4th ventricle and mild vermian hypoplasia. The 4th ventricle is not as dilated as in the DW malformation because it communicates freely with the basal cistern through a patent foramen of Magendie. The DW variant is more common than the DW malformation.

Radiographic features
- 4th ventricle communicates dorsally with enlarged cisterna magna: keyhole deformity
- Hydrocephalus not common

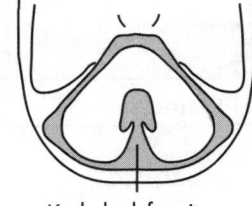

CHIARI I MALFORMATION

Downward displacement of cerebellar tonsils below foramen magnum (distance C from AB line > 5 mm). The 4th ventricle may be elongated but remains in a normal position. Chiari I malformation is not associated with mylomeningoceles and is unrelated to Chiari II and III malformations. Adult disease: 20 years. Clinical: intermittent compression of brainstem (nerve palsies, atypical facial pain, respiratory depression, long tract signs).

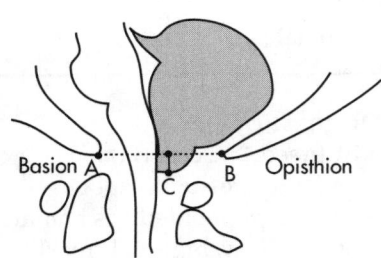

Associations
- Syringohydromyelia 50%; weakness of hands, arms, loss of tendon reflexes
- Hydrocephalus, 25%
- Basilar invagination, 30%
- Klippel-Feil anomaly: fusion of 2 or more cervical vertebrae, 10%
- Atlantooccipital fusion, 5%

Radiographic features
- Tonsillar herniation (ectopia is 3-5 mm, herniation is > 5 mm) is age dependent.
- Syringohydromyelia
- No brain anomalies

Phakomatoses

Group of neuroectodermal disorders characterized by coexistent skin and CNS tumors:

Common phakomatoses
- Neurofibromatosis
- Tuberous sclerosis
- VHL disease
- Sturge-Weber syndrome

Uncommon syndromes
- Gorlin's syndrome
- Osler-Weber-Rendu disease
- Ataxia telangiectasia syndrome
- Klippel-Trenaunay syndrome
- Blue rubber bleb nevus syndrome

NEUROFIBROMATOSIS

Most common phakomatosis (1:3000). 50% autosomal dominant, 50% spontaneous mutations. Dysplasia of mesodermal and neuroectodermal tissue.

TYPES OF NEUROFIBROMATOSIS		
Feature	**NF1**	**NF2**
Name	von Recklinghausen disease	Bilateral acoustic neuroma
Defect	Chromosome 17	Chromosome 22
Frequency	90%	10%
Skin (nodules, café au lait)	Prominent	Minimal
Tumors	Hamartomas, gliomas malignant nerve sheath tumor	Meningiomas, schwannoma, ependymoma
Spinal	Neurofibroma	Schwannoma

Diagnostic criteria

NF1 (need ≥ 2 criteria)
- ≥ 6 café au lait spots
- ≥ 2 pigmented iris hamartomas (Lisch nodules)
- Axillary, inguinal freckling
- ≥ 2 neurofibroma (or 1 plexiform neurofibroma)
- Optic nerve glioma
- First-degree relative with NF1
- Dysplasia of greater wing of sphenoid

NF2 (need ≥ 1 criterion)
- Bilateral acoustic neuromas
- First-degree relative and unilateral acoustic neuroma or meningioma, glioma, schwannoma, neurofibroma (any two)

Radiographic features of NF1

CNS

- Optic nerve gliomas, 15%
    Low-grade pilocytic astrocytoma
    Variable enhancement
- Low-grade brainstem gliomas
- Nonneoplastic hamartomas, 80%-90%
    T2 hyperintense, T1 not visible
    No mass effect or enhancement in 90%
    Basal ganglia, white matter, dentate nuclei
- Moyamoya cerebral occlusive disease
- Aneurysms

Spinal cord/canal

- Neurofibromas of exiting nerves
    Enlarged neural foramen
    Intradural extramedullary tumors (classic "dumbbell tumors")
- Dural ectasia
    Enlarged neural foramen
    Posterior vertebral scalloping
- Low-grade cord astrocytomas
- Lateral meningoceles

Skull

- Hypoplastic sphenoid wing
- Macrocrania
- Lambdoid suture defect

Plexiform neurofibromas, 33%

- Diagnostic of NF1
- Common along cranial nerve V peripherally
    Head and neck
    Intense enhancement
    Sarcomatous degeneration in 10%

Skeletal findings, 50%-80%

- Erosion of bones and foramina by slow-growing neuromas
- Bowing of tibia and fibula; pseudarthroses
- Unilateral overgrowth of limbs: focal gigantism
- Twisted ribs (ribbon ribs)

Chest

- Progressive pulmonary fibrosis
- Intrathoracic meningoceles
- Lung and mediastinal neurofibromas

Vascular

- Renal artery stenosis
- Renal artery aneurysm
- Abdominal coarctation

Other

- Pheochromocytoma

Radiographic features of NF2
CNS
- Bilateral acoustic schwannoma is diagnostic
- Other cranial nerve schwannomas (cranial nerve V)
- Meningiomas (often multiple)

Spinal cord/canal
- Intradural, extramedullary meningiomas
- Schwannomas
- Intramedullary ependymoma

Pearls
- Presence of mass effect and contrast enhancement help to differentiate gliomas from hamartomas. Some hamartomas enhance; over time they should not change in size.
- Contrast-enhanced scans should be acquired in all patients to detect gliomas, small meningiomas, and neuromas.
- NF1 typically has lesions of neurons and astrocytes.
- NF2 typically has lesions of Schwann cells and meninges.

VON HIPPEL-LINDAU (VHL) DISEASE

VHL (cerebelloretinal hemangioblastomatosis; autosomal dominant with 100% penetrance) is characterized by the presence of hemangioblastomas and renal (renal cell carcinoma [RCC] and cysts), adrenal, pancreatic, and scrotal abnormalities. Associated with chromosome 3. Features:

Hemangioblastoma, 50%
- Cerebellum (most common location)
- Brainstem, spinal cord
- Retinal

Renal
- RCC, 50% (bilateral in 65%, multiple in 85%)
- Benign renal cysts, 60%

Adrenal glands
- Pheochromocytoma, 15%; bilateral in 40%

Pancreas
- Multiple cysts, 70%
- Cystadenocarcinoma
- Islet cell tumor

Scrotum
- Epididymal cysts, 10%

Other
- Hepatic cysts, 20%
- Splenic cysts, 10%

Radiographic features
- Hemangioblastomas: enhancing nodules in subpial location
- Multiple hemangioblastomas is diagnostic of VHL.
- MRI is the first study of choice.
- CT is often used to evaluate kidneys, adrenals, and pancreas.

Pearls
- Entire CNS must be imaged (brain and spinal cord).
- Most patients with solitary hemangioblastoma do not have VHL.
- Family screening is necessary.

TUBEROUS SCLEROSIS (BOURNEVILLE'S DISEASE)

Autosomal dominant (20%-50%) or sporadic (50%) or inherited (50%), neuroectodermal disorder. The clinical triad of adenoma sebacum, seizures, and mental retardation is found in a minority.

Radiographic features

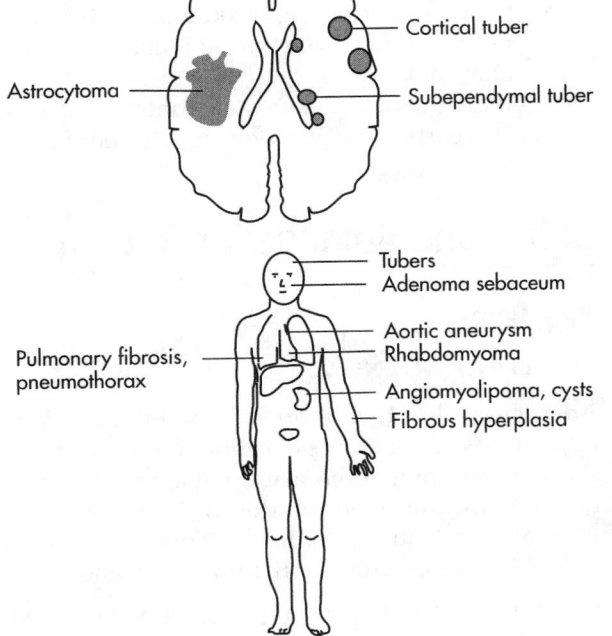

CNS (four major CNS lesions)
- Hamartoma containing abnormal neurons and astrocytes; typical locations:
    - Cortical (GM) tubers
    - Subependymal (candle drippings), hamartomas common near foramen of Monro
- Tubers:
    - Cortical location
    - Tubers may calcify (differential diagnosis: CMV, toxoplasmosis)
    - Noncalcified tubers: T1 hypointense, T2 hyperintense; do not enhance on CT but variable enhancement on MRI
- Subependymal giant cell astrocytoma
    - Located at foramen of Monro
    - Result in hydrocephalus
- Disorganized/dysplastic WM lesions:
    - Wedge-shaped tumefactive, and linear or curvilinear (radial bands) lesions in the cerebral hemisphere and multiple linear bands extending from a conglomerate focus near the fourth ventricle in to cerebellar hemispheres. Visualization of these radial bands are specific to tuberous sclerosis, and they are usually arranged perpendicular to the ventricles.

Kidney
- Angiomyolipoma, 50%, usually multiple and bilateral
- Multiple cysts

Bone, 50%
- Bone islands in multiple bones
- Periosteal thickening of long bones
- Bone cysts

Other
- Pulmonary lymphangioleiomyomatosis
- Spontaneous pneumothorax, 50%
- Chylothorax
- Cardiac rhabdomyomas, 5%
- Aortic aneurysm

STURGE-WEBER-DIMITRI SYNDROME (ENCEPHALOTRIGEMINAL ANGIOMATOSIS)

Capillary venous angiomas of the face and ipsilateral cerebral hemisphere. Clinical:
- Port-wine nevus of cutaneous distribution of cranial nerve V (V1 most frequent), unilateral
- Seizures, 90%
- Mental retardation
- Ipsilateral glaucoma
- Hemiparesis, 50%

Radiographic features

- Tramtrack cortical calcification (characteristic) that follow cortical convolutions; most common in parietal occipital lobes
- Atrophic cortex with enlarged adjacent subarachnoid space
- Ipsilateral thickening of skull and orbit
- Leptomeningeal venous angiomas: parietal > occipital > frontal lobes; enhancement
- Enlargement and increased contrast enhancement of ipsilateral choroid plexus
- MRI: cortical calcifications may be confused with flow voids because of their hypointensity

Sellar and Juxtasellar Region

Neoplasm

PITUITARY ADENOMA

Adenomas (10%-15% of primary brain neoplasms) originate from the anterior hypophysis. The old classification of pituitary adenomas is based on light microscopy staining (chromophobic, acidophilic, basophilic, mixed). The new classification is based on the hormones produced. Two types:

- Microadenomas (< 10 mm): often (75%) endocrinologically functional
- Macroadenomas (> 10 mm): often endocrinologically nonfunctional

FUNCTIONING PITUITARY MICROADENOMA

Tumor confined to the gland < 10 mm.

Types

- Prolactinoma (most common; galactorrhea, amenorrhea, decreased libido)
- Growth hormone (GH) (acromegaly, gigantism)
- Adrenocorticotropic hormone (ACTH) (Cushing's syndrome)
- Gonadotroph (infertility or menstrual problems in women, follicle-stimulating hormone).
- Mixed (prolactin, GH, thyroid-stimulating hormone least common)

Radiographic features

Sensitivity: MRI is the most sensitive imaging study to detect pituitary microadenomas

Technique

- Obtain coronal and sagital planes before and after administration of Gd-DTPA. Small abnormalities confirmed on both planes are real, whereas those seen on one view only are likely to be artifacts.
- Use high-resolution thin slices.

T1W noncontrast appearance

- Microadenomas are hypointense/isointense relative to pituitary
- Gland asymmetry
- Gland is convex superiorly (normal: flat or concave)
- Stalk deviation
- Depression of sella floor

Contrast enhancement: (Gd-DTPA)

- Dynamic imaging is required.
- Low dose (0.05 mmol Gd/kg): evaluation of microadenomas
- Normal dose (0.1 mmol Gd/kg): evaluation of macroadenomas
- Adenoma enhances less rapidly than normal pituitary.

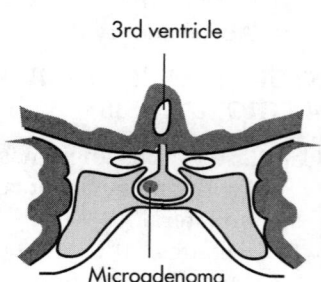

3rd ventricle

Microadenoma

Differentiation of adenoma type by enhancement pattern:
- ACTH adenomas usually enhance strongly (difficult to detect).
- 70% adenomas are hypointense relative to pituitary in dynamic phase.
- Adenoma may not be seen if only delayed images are acquired.
- Petrosal sinus sampling may be helpful if MRI is nondiagnostic.

NONFUNCTIONING PITUITARY MACROADENOMA

Unlike microadenomas, macroadenomas are symptomatic because of their mass effect (hypopituitarism, visual problems, etc.). Nevertheless, they may attain very large size before cranial nerves are affected. Macroadenomas secrete hormone subunits that are clinically silent. Current nomenclature is "null-cell adenoma" or "oncocytoma."

Radiographic features

Large tumor extends beyond the confines of the sella.

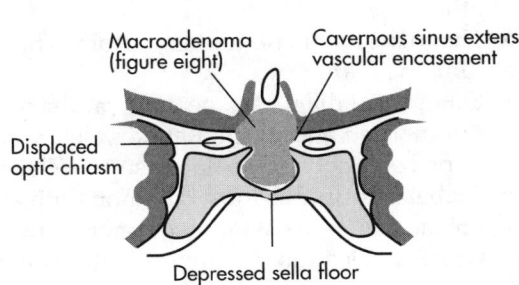

Macroadenoma (figure eight)
Cavernous sinus extension vascular encasement
Displaced optic chiasm
Depressed sella floor

- Intrasellar expansion (ballooning of sella)
- Extension into suprasellar cistern
     Figure-eight shape
     Thickening of cavernous sinus
     Encasement/narrowing of cavernous ICA flow void. Cavernous sinus involvement can be difficult to determine unless tumor surrounds the vessel/cavernous sinus.
     Compression of optic chiasm
     Upward displacement of third ventricle
     Obstruction of foramen of Monro with hydrocephalus, 10%
     Compression of frontal horn of lateral ventricles
     Splaying of cerebral peduncles

Morphologic features
- Calcification, uncommon (1%-8%)
- Intratumoral necrosis, hemorrhage (T1 hyperintense)
- Benign invasive adenoma cannot be distinguished from pituitary carcinoma, although malignant pituitary carcinoma is very rare (< 1% of adenomas).

Enhancement
- Intense but heterogenous

MRI features
- Heterogenous appearance because of solid and cystic components
- Use multiplanar MRI to define relationship of tumor to surrounding anatomy.

CRANIOPHARYNGIOMA

Craniopharyngiomas are benign tumors that arise from squamous epithelial remnants along Rathke's duct/pouch. Most common tumor of the suprasellar cistern. Age: 1st-2nd decade (> 50%). Location: 7% combined suprasellar/intrasellar; completely intrasellar craniopharyngiomas rare. Clinical findings:
- Growth retardation (compression of hypothalamus)
- Diabetes insipidus (pituitary compression)
- Bitemporal hemianopsia
- Headaches (most common)
- Cranial nerve palsies (cavernous sinus involvement)

Radiographic features

- Cystic mass (90%) with mural nodule in suprasellar location
- Calcification in 90% (children), less common in adults (50%)
- Enhancement of solid lesion rim, no enhancement of cystic lesion
- Variable signal intensity by MRI depending on cyst content: high protein content, blood, cholesterol. The most common MR appearance is T1W hypointensity and T2W hyperintensity).
- Obstruction of foramen of Monro with hydrocephalus, 60%
- Usually avascular by angiography

Pearls

- A suprasellar mass in a child or adolescent is a craniopharyngioma until proven otherwise.
- The majority of craniopharyngiomas have cystic components; purely solid tumors are rare.
- Differential diagnosis: necrotic pituitary adenoma, cystic optochiasmtic glioma, thrombosed aneurysm, Rathkes cleft cyst (no calcification, no enhancement)

Clinical presentations of pediatric suprasellar region lesions

- Diabetes insipidus most common with eosinophilic granuloma of stalk
- Precocious puberty most common with hypothalamic hamartoma
- Growth delay most common with craniopharyngioma

Other

EMPTY SELLA

Defect in sella diaphrgam with extension of CSF space into the sella. An empty sella is a common, anatomic variant. Incidence: 10% of adults. Clinical: incidental finding, asymptomatic, no clinical significance. Differentiate from:

- Cystic sella tumor
- Surgically removed pituitary gland
- Involuted pituitary (Sheehan's syndrome)

POSTSURGICAL SELLA

Small tumors are often removed via a transsphenoidal approach (anterior wall of sphenoid sinus → sella); typically sella and sphenoid sinus are packed with Gelfoam, muscle, fat; postsurgical fluid may be seen in the sphenoid sinus.

Radiographic features

- Image sella soon after surgery to establish baseline imaging appearance for further follow-up.
- Gd-DTPA fat-suppression MRI techniques are helpful to suppress bright signal from surgical fat plug in the sella and to enhance pituitary tissue.

ECTOPIC NEUROHYPOPHYSIS

The neurohypophysis (T1 hyperintense) is located in the hypothalamic region or in the sella; frequently associated with a small or absent pituitary gland (clinical: hypopituitarism).

PITUITARY APOPLEXY

Causes:

- Acute onset hemorrhage into pituitary adenoma with necrosis and infarction of the pituitary gland
- Sheehan's syndrome: postpartum infarction of anterior pituitary gland

Spine

Congenital

SPINAL DYSRAPHISM

A group of spinal anomalies involving incomplete midline closure of bone, neural, and soft tissues.

Classification

Open spinal dysraphism (spinal bifida aperta), 85%: posterior protrusion of spinal contents through the dorsal bone defect, neurological defects are common

- Myelomeningocele: protruding placode, almost 100% association with Chiari II
- Lipomyelomeningocele: protruding placode with fat
- Myelocele: neural placode flush with surface not covered by skin

Occult spinal dysraphism, 15%: no exposed neural tissue, covered by skin, neurological defects are uncommon

- Lipomyelomeningocele (not part of Chiari II)
- Meningocele
- Dorsal dermal sinus
- Spinal lipoma
- Tethered cord
- Split notochord syndromes

Open dysraphisms are nearly always diagnosed by prenatal US. CT and MRI are most commonly used to plan surgical repair.

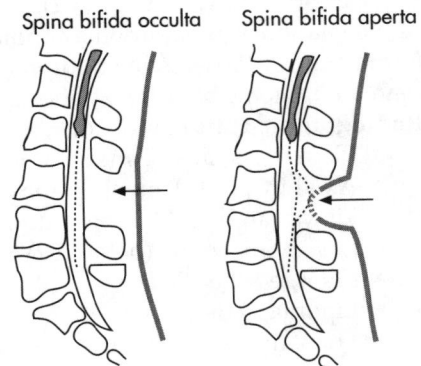

Spina bifida occulta   Spina bifida aperta

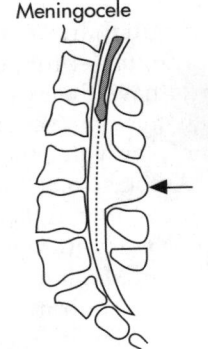

Meningocele

DORSAL DERMAL SINUS

Epithelialized sinus tract connecting the skin to the spinal canal/cord. May end in subcutaneous fat, meninges, or cord. 50% terminate in a dermoid/epidermoid. Location: lumbosacral > occipital. Clinical: infection, overlying hairy path or skin abnormality.

LIPOMYELOMENINGOCELE

Most common occult spinal dysraphism. Female > male. Presentation: usually in infancy, some into adulthood. Clinical: neurogenic bladder, orthopedic deformities, sensory problems. Not associated with Chiari II malformation.

Radiographic features

Plain film

- Incomplete posterior fusion (spina bifida)
- Widened spinal cord
- Segmentation anomalies

MRI

- Tethered cord
- Syringohydromelia, 25%
- Extradural lipoma contiguous with subcutaneous fat
- Nerve roots from placode

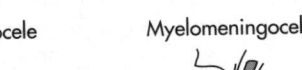

Lipomeningocele   Myelomeningocele

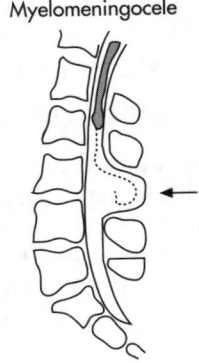

TETHERED SPINAL CORD

Neurological and orthopedic disorders associated with a short thick filum and an abnormally low (below L2) conus medullaris (normal location of cord at 16 weeks, L4/5; at birth, L2/3; later, L1/2). Commonly a component of other spinal malformations: spinal lipoma/lipomyelomeningocele, diastematomyelia, dermal sinus. Presents in children and young adults. Clinical: paresthesias, pain, neurogenic bladder, kyphoscoliosis, incontinence, spacticity.

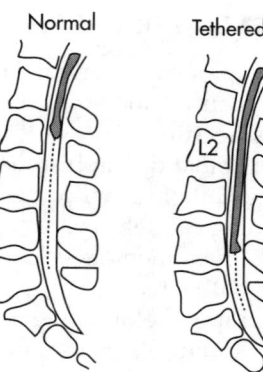

Radiographic features

- Plain films may or may not reveal osseous dysraphism.
- Axial MR or CT myelography are imaging studies of choice. Sagittal views can be difficult to interpret
- Low-lying conus (below L2)
- Enlarged thecal sac
- Lipoma, 50%
- Thick filum terminale > 1.5 mm

DIASTEMATOMYELIA (ONE OF THE "SPLIT NOTOCHORD SYNDROMES")

Sagittal division of spinal cord into two hemicords. The cords may be split by a fibrous septum or a bony spur. The two hemicords share a common thecal sac (50%) or have their own thecal sac (50%). Severe forms are associated with neurenteric cysts. Clinical presentation is similar to other occult spinal dysraphism. Do not confuse with diplomyelia, the true spinal cord duplication (very rare).

Associations

- Tethered cord
- Hydromyelia
- Meningocele, myelomeningocele, lipomyelomeningocele
- Abnormal vertebral bodies: hemivertebra, block vertebra, etc.
- Scoliosis, clubfoot, and cutaneous stigmata > 50%
- Chiari II

Other

- Most severe but rare dorsal enteric fistula

Radiographic features

- Usually thoracolumbar (85% below T9)
- MRI is the imaging study of choice.
- Osseous abnormalities are nearly always present.
    Segmentation anomalies (hemivertebra, block, butterfly, etc.)
    Incomplete posterior fusion
    Osseous spur, 50%
- Tethered cord, 75%

HYDROSYRINGOMYELIA

Term used to describe two entities that are often difficult to separate: abnormal dilatation of the central canal (hydromyelia) and short cord cavity (syrinx), which may or may not communicate with the central canal. Causes:

Congenital (usually results in hydromyelia)

- Chiari malformation
- Myelomeningocele

Acquired (usually results in syringomyelia)
- Posttraumatic
- Tumors

Infection

SPONDYLITIS AND DISKITIS

Spine infections may progress from spondylitis → diskitis → epidural abscess → cord abscess. Infective spondylitis usually involves extradural components of the spine such as posterior elements, disks (diskitis), vertebral body (osteomyelitis), paraspinous soft tissues. Cause:
- Pyogenic: *Staphylococcus aureus* > *Enterococcus*, > *E. coli*, *Salmonella*
- TB
- Fungal
- Parasitic

Radiographic findings
- Normal plain film findings for 8-10 days after infection
- T2 hyperintense disk
- Contrast enhancement
- Soft tissue mass (inflammation, abscess)

SPINAL TUBERCULOSIS (POTT'S DISEASE)

- Bone destruction is prominent, more indolent onset then pyogenic bone destruction
- Loss of disk height, 80%
- Gibbus deformity: anterior involvement with normal posterior vertebral bodies
- Involvement of several adjacent vertebral bodies with disk destruction
- Large paraspinous abscess
- Extension into psoas muscles (psoas abscess)

ARACHNOIDITIS

Causes
- Surgery ("failed back" syndrome)
- Subarachnoid hemorrhage
- Pantopaque myelography
- Infection

Radiographic features
- CT myelography is superior to MR for establishing the diagnosis. Never use ionic contrast material for myelography because it may cause a fatal arachnoiditis.
- Myelographic block is seen with severe adhesive arachnoiditis.
- Intradural scarring/loculation (limited enhancement)
- Clumping of nerve roots within the thecal sac (intrathecal pseudomass); blunting of caudal nerve root sleeves
- Intradural cysts (may be bright on T1W images)
- Irregular margins of thecal sac

6

Degenerative Abnormalities

DISK HERNIATION

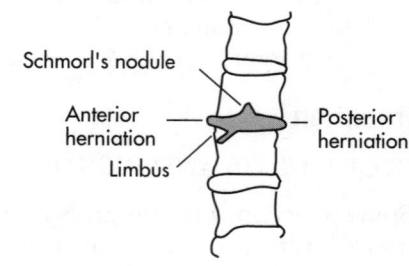

Spectrum of intervertebral disk herniation

Posterior disk herniation
- Intraspinal herniation (herniated disk)

Anterior disk herniation
- Elevation of the anterior longitudinal ligament
- May mimic anterior osteophytes

Schmorl's nodule
- Cephalocaudal extrusion of disk material
- Young adults (1-2 levels affected; Scheuermann's disease: > 3 levels affected)

Intravertebral disk herniation (limbus vertebra)
- Anterior herniation of disk material
- Triangular bone fragment

POSTERIOR DISK HERNIATION

The most important point in describing a disk herniation is the exact relationship of the disk to neural structures.
- Bulging disk: symmetrical perimeter expansion of a weakened disk; intact annulus
- Herniated disk: focal rather than diffuse bulge; annulus fibrosus is torn, disk material herniates through separation

Note that there is much controversy regarding these definitions and imaging findings; especially their clinical correlation to lower back pain and need for surgery. Imaging modalities are useful mainly to guide surgery.

Radiographic features

Techniques

Detection: MRI is the imaging study of choice

CT myelography
- Permits reliable visualization of nerve roots in the thecal sac
- Disadvantage: time-consuming, invasive

Plain films
- The diagnosis of herniation is not possible by plain film.
- All findings of degenerative joint disease (e.g., narrowing of disk space, spurring, eburnation, vacuum sign) may be found in patients with or without herniation.

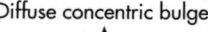
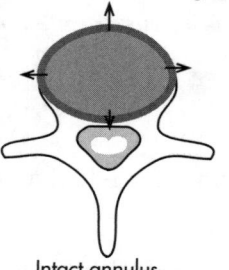

Diffuse concentric bulge — Intact annulus

Focal bulging disk — Intact annulus

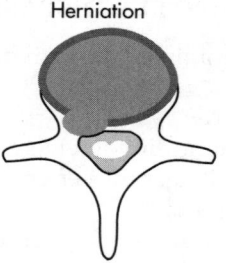

Herniation — Torn annulus

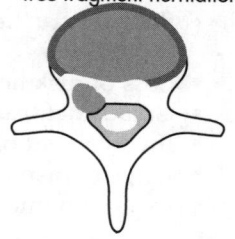

Extrusion, sequestration, free fragment herniation — Torn annulus

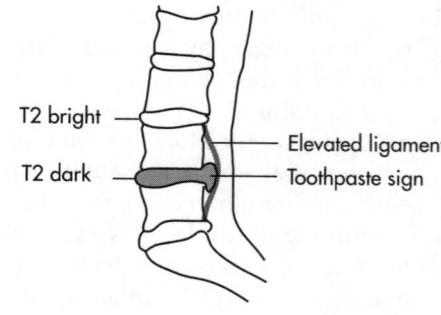

T2 bright — Elevated ligament

T2 dark — Toothpaste sign

MRI features

Techniques
- Sagittal T1W and T2W
- Axial T1W and/or FSE T2W (T1W at most institutions)
- Axial acquisitions should be angled to axis of disk space

Extruded disk material gives rise to the toothpaste sign (disk material is extruded from disk into the spinal canal like toothpaste); the material may be continuous with the disk (simple herniation) or be separated (free fragment herniation). Free fragments may have different MR signal characteristics from the native disk material.

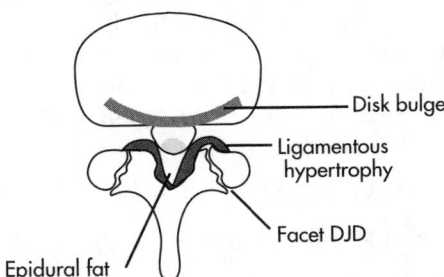

- Location of herniation
    - Paracentral (most common)
    - Posterolateral
    - Central (uncommon, ligament is strongest here)
    - Often missed by axial imaging:
        Lateral, extraforaminal extension
        Intraforaminal extension
- Role of contrast
    - Post operation: differentiate scar from residual/recurrent disk herniation
    - Helpful for confirming extruded fragments
    - Facilitates diagnosis of neuritis secondary to herniation
- Secondary degenerative abnormalities
    - Endplate marrow changes ("diskogenic" endplate disease)
        T1 dark/T2 bright: vascular granulation tissue *TYPE I*
        T1 bright/T2 isointense or bright: fatty marrow replacement *TYPE II*
        T1 dark/T2 dark: sclerosis *TYPE III*
    - Degenerated disks are T2 hypointense (loss of proteoglycans, H_2O). However, normally aging disks may also be hypointense.
    - Osteophytes, facet hypertrophy contribute to neural foraminal stenosis
    - Ligamentum flavum hypertrophy
- Location
    - Lumbar: L4/L5 or L5/S1, 95% (the first "freely mobile" nonsacralized disk level)
    - Thoracic: most common at the 4 lowest disk levels
    - Cervical: C5/C6 and C6/C7, 90%

SPINAL STENOSIS

Narrowing of the spinal canal with or without compression of the cord and/or CSF block.

Causes:

Acquired, most common
- Bulging or protruded disks
- Hypertrophy of ligamentum flavum
- Hypertrophy of facets
- Degenerative osteophytes
- Spondylolisthesis

Congenital:
- Short pedicles, thick laminae, large facets
- Morquio's syndrome
- Achondroplasia

Radiographic features

MRI is study of choice:
- T2W sequences best define the thecal sac.
- T1W sequences best define the lateral recesses (fat).
- Look for "trefoil" appearance of thecal sac, complete effacement of epidural fat.

CT myelogram useful in equivocal cases.

Associated spinal cord changes
- T2 hyperintensity: edema or gliosis
- Atrophy: chronic

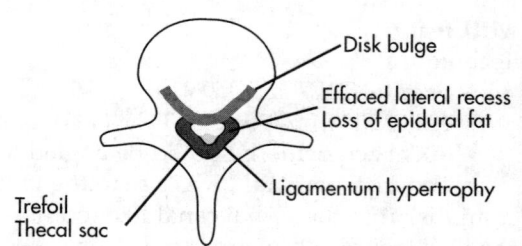

SPINAL BLOCK

Complete spinal stenosis with no communication of spinal fluid.

FORAMINAL STENOSIS

Stenosis of the intervertebral foramen that involves the exiting nerve as it passes under the pedicle. Causes:
- Degenerative osteophytes of the facets
- Spondylolisthesis
- Lateral herniated disks
- Fracture
- Postoperative scarring
- Lateral recess masses (extradural masses)

POSTOPERATIVE SPINE

Present clinically as "failed back" syndrome. Common problems:
- Recurrent disk herniation (operative site or another site)
- Scar formation
- Neural foramina stenosis
- Neuritis
- Arachnoiditis
- Lateral recess stenosis (simple laminectomy does not decompress the lateral recess)
- Dural bulge (pseudomeningocele)
- Diskitis
- Epidural hematoma or abscess

Radiographic features

Differentiation of recurrent disk herniation and epidural scar formation:
- Gd-DTPA–enhanced MRI is the study of choice.
- Scar tissue usually shows early homogeneous enhancement.
- Disk usually shows late peripheral enhancement (surrounding granulation tissue).

Detection of complications (see above)

ACUTE TRANSVERSE MYELOPATHY

Clinical syndrome with a variety of underlying causes:
- Acute infection
- Postinfection
    Vaccination
    Autoimmune
- Systemic malignancy
- Posttraumatic

Radiographic features
- MRI normal in 50% during acute phase
- T2W hyperintensity
- Focal cord enlargement
- Contrast enhancement may be present.

Tumors

APPROACH

- MRI is the imaging study of choice.
- CT indicated for osseous lesions; CT myelography is more useful than noncontrast CT.
- Classify lesions by their location in anatomical compartments:
    Intramedullary: within the spinal cord
    Intradural: within the dural sac, but outside cord
    Extradural: outside the thecal sac

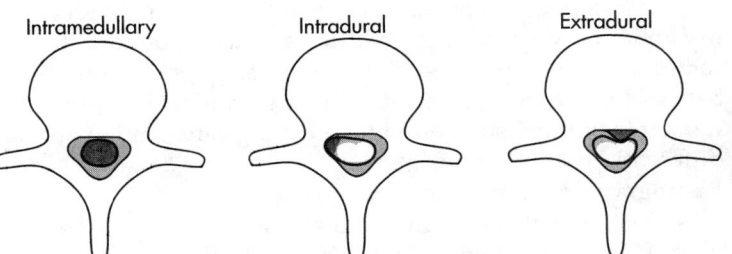

INTRAMEDULLARY TUMORS

Types
- Astrocytoma (most common)
- Ependymoma (second most common; lower spinal cord, conus medullaris and filum terminale)
- Hemangioblastoma
- Metastases (rare)

Radiographic features
- Expansion of cord
- Large cystic components, 50%
- Differentiation of different tumors is usually not possible by imaging methods.
- Describe the extent of the solid tumor and the extent of the cyst (during surgery the tumor will be removed while the cyst will be decompressed).

ASTROCYTOMA

Location: thoracic 65%, cervical 50%. Isolated conus medullaris involvement occurs in 3% of cases. Astrocytomas are rare in the filum terminale.

Radiographic features

- MR imaging: poorly defined margins and are isointense to hypointense relative to the spinal cord on T1W images and hyperintense on T2W images. The average length of involvement is seven vertebral segments. Cysts are a common feature, with both polar and intratumoral types being observed.
- Virtually all cord astrocytomas show at least some enhancement after the intravenous administration of contrast material.
- Widened interpedicular distance and bone erosion may be evident on conventional radiography and CT. Patients with holocord involvement tend to present with scoliosis and canal widening.

EPENDYMOMA

Location: cervical alone, 45%; cervicothroacic, 25%; thoracis alone, 25%; conus, 5%. Myxopapillary ependymoma is, in rare cases, found in the subcutaneous tissue of the sacrococcygeal region, usually without any connection with the spinal canal. It is believed that these arise from either heterotopic ependymal cell rests or vestigial remnants of the distal neural tube during canalization and retrogressive differentiation.

Radiographic features

- T1W: isointense or hypointense relative to the spinal cord
- T2W: hyperintense. About 20%-33% of ependymomas demonstrated the "cap sign," a rim of extreme hypointensity (hemosiderin) seen at the poles of the tumor on T2W images. Most cases (60%) also showed evidence of cord edema around the masses.
- Cysts in 80%, most of which are the nontumoral (polar) variety
- X-rays: scoliosis, 15%; canal widening, 10%; vertebral body scalloping, pedicle erosion, or laminar thinning
- CT: isoattenuated or slight hyperattenuated compared with the normal spinal cord. Intense enhancement with contrast. CT myelography shows nonspecific cord enlargement. Complete or partial block in the flow of contrast material.

HEMANGIOBLASTOMA

75% are intramedullary but can involve the intradural space or even the extradural space. Extramedullary hemangioblastomas are commonly attached to the dorsal cord pia or nerve roots. Location: thoracic, 50%; cervical cord, 40%. Most cord hemangioblastomas (80%) are solitary and occur in patients younger than 40 years. The presence of multiple lesions should should prompt work-up for VHL syndrome.

Radiographic features

- Diffuse cord expansion
- T1W: isointense, 50%; hyperintense 25%
- T2W: usually hyperintense with focal flow voids
- Cyst formation or syringohydromyelia is very common.
- Only 25% of hemangioblastomas are solid.

METASTASES

Intramedullary spinal metastases are relatively rare (1% of autopsied cancer patients). Location: cervical 45%, thoracic 35%, lumbar region 8%. Most metastases are solitary, with an average length of two to three vertebral segments. Routes of spread include hematogenous (via the arterial supply) and direct extension from the leptomeninges.
Primary tumors:

- Lung carcinoma, 40%-85%
- Breast carcinoma, 11%
- Melanoma, 5%
- Renal cell carcinoma, 4%
- Colorectal carcinoma, 3%
- Lymphoma, 3%

NERVE SHEATH TUMORS

Nerve sheath tumors are the most common intradural, extramedullary mass lesions.
Clinical: may mimic disk herniation.
Types

- Schwannoma
- Neurofibroma
- Ganglioneuroma
- Neurofibrosarcoma (rare)

Radiographic features
Location

- Intradural, extramedullary, 75%
- Extradural, 15%
- Intramedullary, < 1%
- Multiple in neurofibromatosis

Morphology

- Dumbbell shaped, 15%
- Enlargement of neural foramen
- Contrast enhancement, 100%
- T1W: isointense 75%, hyperintense 25%
- T2W: very hyperintense, target appearance common

NEOPLASMS OF THE FILUM TERMINALE

Common

- Ependymoma (especially myxopapillary)
- Astrocytoma (especially anaplastic and pilocytic)
- Hemangioblastoma

Less common

- Subependymoma
- Ganglioglioma
- Paraganglioma
- Metastasis
- Lymphoma
- PNET
- Neurocytoma
- Oligodendroglioma
- Mixed glioma
- Glioblastoma multiforme

Differential Diagnosis

Tumors

APPROACH TO INTRACRANIAL MASS LESION

(Mnemonic: "TEACH")
- **T**umor
    Primary
    Metastases
- **E**dema
- **A**bscess
- **C**yst, contusion
- **H**ematoma

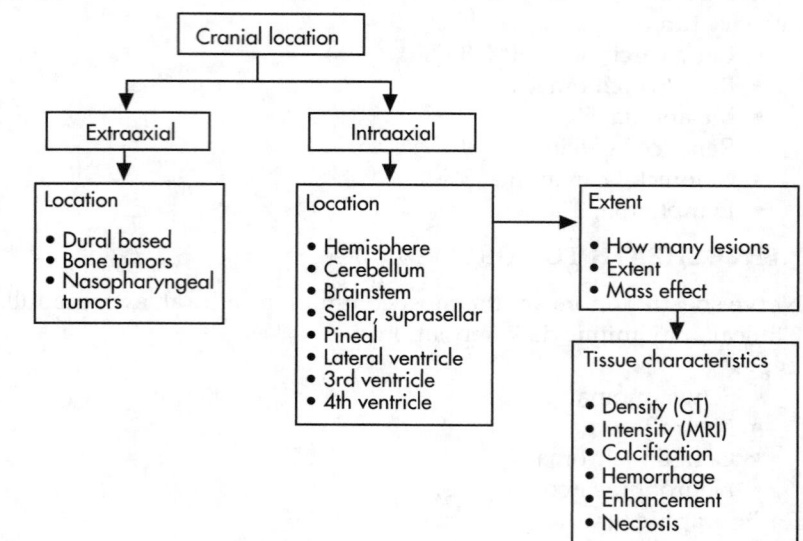

EXTRAAXIAL MASSES

Extraaxial, hemisphere
- Meningioma
- Metastases
- Lymphoma
- Arachnoid cyst
- Dermoid/epidermoid
- Other: hemorrhagic, infectious fluid collections

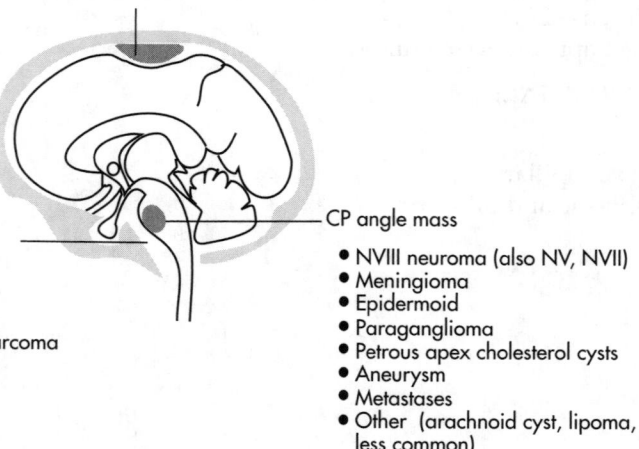

Clivus, prepontine cistern
- Metastases
- Meningioma
- Chordoma
- Chondroma, chondrosarcoma

CP angle mass
- NVIII neuroma (also NV, NVII)
- Meningioma
- Epidermoid
- Paraganglioma
- Petrous apex cholesterol cysts
- Aneurysm
- Metastases
- Other (arachnoid cyst, lipoma, dermoid less common)

INTRAAXIAL MASSES

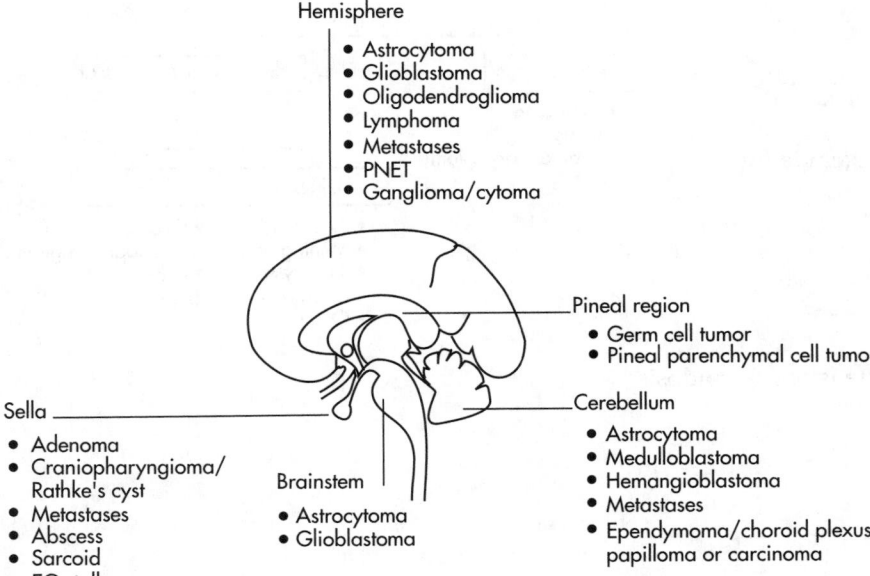

Hemisphere
- Astrocytoma
- Glioblastoma
- Oligodendroglioma
- Lymphoma
- Metastases
- PNET
- Ganglioma/cytoma

Pineal region
- Germ cell tumor
- Pineal parenchymal cell tumor

Sella
- Adenoma
- Craniopharyngioma/ Rathke's cyst
- Metastases
- Abscess
- Sarcoid
- EG stalk

Brainstem
- Astrocytoma
- Glioblastoma

Cerebellum
- Astrocytoma
- Medulloblastoma
- Hemangioblastoma
- Metastases
- Ependymoma/choroid plexus papilloma or carcinoma

MULTIPLE LESIONS

Tumor
- Metastases
- Multicentric glioma
- Lymphoma

Infection
- Abscess
- Fungus
- Cysticercosis
- Toxoplasmosis

Vascular
- Embolic infarctions
- Multifocal hemorrhage
- Diffuse axnal injury
- Contusions
- Cavernous hemangiomas
- Vasculitis

CORPUS CALLOSUM LESIONS

Tumors
- Astrocytoma (butterfly glioma)
- Lymphoma
- Lipoma (midline)

Demyelinating disease
- Multiple sclerosis
- Marchiafava-Bignami disease (alcoholics)
- Progressive multifocal leukoencephalopathy (rarely enhances)

Infarct (always also involves cingulate gyrus)

INTRASELLAR MASSES

- Pituitary adenoma
- Pituitary apoplexy
- Craniopharyngioma
- Cysts (Rathke's cleft, pars intermedia)
- Metastasis
- Aneurysm (radiologist must exclude for the surgeon preoperatively)
- Abscess

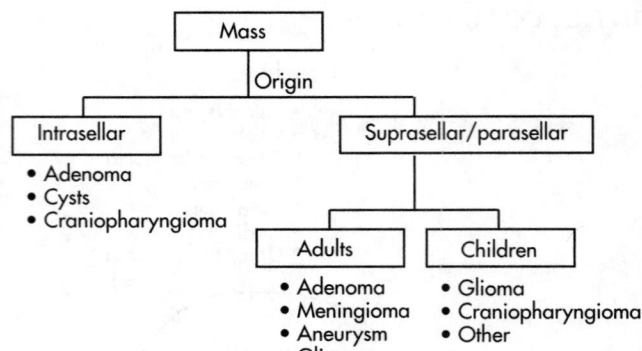

SUPRASELLAR MASSES

Mnemonic for suprasellar lesions:
"SATCHMOE"
- **S**ellar lesion with superior extension, sarcoidosis
- **A**neurysm, arachnoid cyst
- **T**eratoid lesions
    Germ cell tumors
    Epidermoid/dermoid
- **C**raniopharyngioma
- **H**ypothalamic glioma
- **M**etastases, meningioma
- **O**ptic nerve glioma
- **E**G

Adults
- Macroadenoma (most common)
- Meningioma
- Glioma
- Craniopharyngioma
- Aneurysm (rare, but important)

Children
- Craniopharyngioma (most common)
- Glioma (optic nerve, chiasm, hypothalamus)
- Germinoma
- Hypothalamic hamartoma
- EG

POSTERIOR FOSSA TUMORS

Approach
1. Intraaxial or extraaxial?
2. Location
    - Lateral (hemispheric): astrocytoma
    - Anterior: brainstem glioma
    - Posterior: medulloblastoma (midline)
    - 4th ventricle: ependymoma
3. Age
4. Spread
    - Through foramina of Luschka and Magendie: ependymoma

5. Cystic component
   - Pilocytic astrocytoma
   - Hemangioblastoma
6. Enhancement pattern
7. Dense cell packing
   - Medulloblastoma

Causes

Adults
- Metastases
- Hemangioblastoma
- Astrocytoma
- Extraaxial tumors (meningioma, schwannoma, epidermoid)

Children
- Cerebellar astrocytoma
- Medulloblastoma
- Brainstem glioma
- Ependymoma

BRAIN TUMORS IN INFANTS (≤ 2 YEARS)

- Teratoma (most common)
- PNET (primary cerebral neuroblastoma)
- Choroid plexus papilloma/carcinoma
- Anaplastic astrocytoma

INTRAVENTRICULAR TUMORS

Adults
- Gliomas
  - Astrocytoma (including giant cell type)
  - Subependymoma
- Meningioma
- Metastases
- Cysticercosis

Children
- Choroid plexus papilloma
- Ependymoma
- PNET (medulloblastoma)
- Teratoma
- Astrocytoma

CEREBELLOPONTINE ANGLE (CPA) MASS

- Acoustic neuroma, 90%
- Meningioma, 10%
- Epidermoid, 5%
- Arachnoid cyst
- Metastases
- Vertebrobasilar dolichoectasia
- Exophytic glioma
  - Ependymoma through Luschka
  - Brainstem astrocytoma
- Lipoma

Lateral ventricle
- 0-15 years
  - PNET
  - Choroid plexus papilloma
- 15-30 years
  - Glioma
  - Juvenile pilocystic astrocytoma
- > 30 years
  - Subependymoma
  - Astrocytoma
  - Metastases
  - Oligodendroglioma
  - Meningioma
  - Central neurocytoma

3rd ventricle
- 0-15 years
  - Astrocytoma
  - EG of stalk
  - Germinoma
  - Extrinsic craniopharyngioma
- 15-30 years
  - Colloid cyst
- > 30 years
  - Glioma
  - Metastases
  - Pituitary or pineal masses
  - Other (e.g., aneurysm, sarcoid)

4th ventricle
- 0-15 years
  - Ependyoma
  - Medulloblastoma
- 15-30 years
  - Choroid plexus papilloma
- > 30 years
  - Metastases/hemangioblastoma
  - Subependymoma

6

CYSTIC MASSES

Neoplastic
- Cystic astrocytoma/GBM
- Hemangioblastoma
- Metastases: squamous cell carcinoma

Benign (usually no peripheral enhancement)
- Dermoid/epidermoid
- Arachnoid cyst
- Colloid cyst
- Cavum variants
    - Cavum septum pellucidum
    - Cavum vergae
    - Cavum velum interpositum

TUMORS WITH CSF SEEDING

- Choroid plexus papilloma/carcinoma
- Ependymoma
- PNET tumors
    - Medulloblastoma
    - Pinealblastoma
    - Cerebral neuroblastoma
- Germinomas
- GBM

HYPERDENSE LESION (CT)

Tumors
- High-cell density
    - Lymphoma
    - PNETs (medulloblastoma)
    - Ependymoma
    - Germinoma
    - Other PNET
- Hemorrhagic tumors
    - GBM
    - Metastases: kidney, lung, melanoma, choriocarcinoma (mnemonic: CT/MR: choriocarcinoma, thyroid, melanoma, renal cell carcinoma)
- Calcified tumors (rare)
    - Mucinous metastases
    - All osteogenic tumors

Hemorrhage
- Hypertensive
- Trauma
- Vascular lesions

T2 HYPOINTENSE LESIONS (MRI)

Paramagnetic effects
- Ferritin, hemosiderin
- Deoxyhemoglobin
- Intracellular methemoglobin
- Melanin

Low spin density
- Calcification
- High nucleus/cytoplasm ratio (lymphoma, myeloma, neuroblastoma)
- Fibrous tissue (meningioma)

Other
- High protein concentration, > 35%
- Flow signal void

T1 HYPERINTENSE LESIONS (MRI)

Paramagnetic effects
- MRI contrast agent: Gd-DTPA
- Methemoglobin
- Melanin
- Ions: manganese, iron, copper, certain states of calcium

Other
- Fat: dermoid
- Very high protein concentration (i.e., colloid cyst)
- Slow flow

Abnormal Enhancement

LESIONS WITH NO ENHANCEMENT

- Cysts
- Tumors with intact blood-brain barrier (low-grade gliomas)

LESIONS WITH STRONG ENHANCEMENT

- Meningioma
- PNET (e.g., medulloblastoma)
- AVM
- Paraganglioma (very vascular)
- Aneurysm (nonthrombosed)
- HIV-associated lymphoma
- Glioblastoma multiforme

RING ENHANCEMENT

Tumor
- Primary brain tumors
- Metastases
- Lymphoma (AIDS)

Infection, inflammation
- Abscess
- Granuloma
- Multiple sclerosis
- Toxoplasmosis
- Cysticercosis
- Vascular

Vascular
- Resolving hematoma
- Infarct (nonacute)
- Thrombosed vascular malformation
- Thrombosed aneurysm
- Vasculitis

DIFFUSE MENINGEAL ENHANCEMENT

- Meningitis (viral, bacterial)
- Carcinomatosis
    Lymphoma
    Metastases
- Postoperative/postshunt
- SAH
- Intracranial hypotension
    CSF leak

BASILAR MENINGEAL ENHANCEMENT

Infection
- TB (most common)
- Fungal
- Pyogenic (more common on convexity)
- Cysticercosis

Tumor
- Lymphoma, leukemia
- Carcinomatosis

Inflammatory
- Sarcoid
- Rheumatoid pachymeningitis
- Whipple's disease

EPENDYMAL ENHANCEMENT

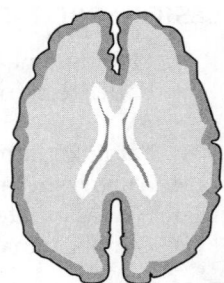

Tumor
- Lymphoma
- Metastases (lung, melanoma, breast)
- CSF seeding
    PNET
    GBM

Infection
- Spread of meningitis
- CMV (rare)

Inflammatory ventriculitis
- Postshunt/instrumentation
- Posthemorrhage

Basal Ganglia Signal Abnormalities

T2 HYPOINTENSE BASAL GANGLIA LESIONS

- Old age
- Any chronic degenerative disease
    MS
    Parkinsonian syndromes
- Childhood hypoxia

T2 HYPERINTENSE BASAL GANGLIA LESIONS

Mnemonic: "TINT"
- **T**umor
    - Lymphoma
- **I**schemia
    - Hypoxic encephalopathy
    - Venous infarction (internal cerebral vein thrombosis)
- **N**eurodegenerative diseases (uncommon)
    - Huntington's disease
    - Wilson's disease
    - Hallervorden-Spatz disease
    - Mitochondrial encephalopathies (e.g., Leigh/Kearns-Sayer syndrome)
    - Aminoacidopathies
- **T**oxin
    - CO, CN, H_2S poisoning
    - Hypoglycemia
    - Methanol

T1 HYPERINTENSE BASAL GANGLIA LESIONS

- Dystrophic calcifications (any cause)
- Hepatic failure
- Neurofibromatosis
- Manganese (used in formulas for TPN)

BASAL GANGLIA CALCIFICATION (INCREASED CT DENSITY)

Senescent/physiological/idiopathic calcification (most common)
Metabolic calcification
- Hypoparathyroidism (most common metabolic cause)
- Pseudohypoparathyroidism
- Pseudo-pseudohypoparathyroidism
- Hyperparathyroidism

Infection
- TORCH, AIDS
- Postinflammatory: TB, toxoplasmosis
- Cystercosis (common)

Toxic/postanoxic
- Lead
- CO
- Radiation therapy
- Chemotherapy

Other
- Fahr's disease
- Mitochondrial (common), encephalopathies (uncommon)
- Cockayne's syndrome

Congenital Abnormalities

SPECTRUM OF CYSTIC SUPRATENTORIAL CONGENITAL ABNORMALITIES

- Holoprosencephaly
- Hydranencephaly
- Aqueductal stenosis (severe obstruction hydrocephalus)
- Callosal dysgenesis (interhemispheric cyst)
- Other
    Porencephaly
    Arachnoid cyst
    Cystic teratoma
    Epidermoid/dermoid
    Vein of Galen AVM

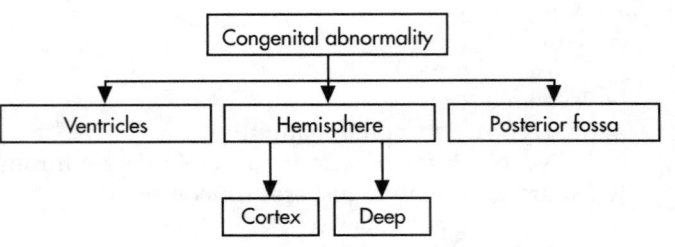

POSTERIOR FOSSA CYSTIC ABNORMALITIES

- DW malformation (vermian hypoplasia/aplasia and large posterior fossa)
- DW variant (normal size posterior fossa and vermian hypoplasia
- Mega cisterna magna (normal vermis)
- Retrocerebellar arachnoid cyst (must show mass effect)
- Chiari IV (near complete abscence of cerebellum)
- Other
    Epidermoid/dermoid
    Cystic tumor

Spine

SPINAL CORD COMPRESSION

Criteria
- No CSF seen around the cord (spinal block)
- Narrowed AP diameter of cord (< 7 mm)
- Deformity of cord

Causes
Infection (TB, pyogenic)
Compression fracture
- Malignancy
- Trauma

Spondylosis and disk disease
- Herniated nucleus, hypertrophy of ligaments
- Osteophyte, facet hypertrophy

Primary bone disorders (Paget's disease)
Other causes
- Benign tumors (e.g., angioma, cysts, lipoma)
- Epidural hematoma

INTRAMEDULLARY LESIONS

- Tumor
    Astrocytoma (most common)
    Ependymoma (second most common)
    Hemangioblastoma
    Metastases (rare)
- Demyelinating disease/myelitis
- Syringohydromyelia
    Tumor related
    Chiari malformation
- AVM
- Trauma (contusion)

INTRADURAL EXTRAMEDULLARY TUMORS

- Nerve sheath tumor (most common)
    Neurofibroma
    Schwannoma
- Meningioma (80% thoracic)
- Drop metastases
- Lipoma
- Teratomatous lesion
- Arachnoid cyst
- Arachnoiditis/meningitis
- AVM/AVF

EXTRADURAL LESIONS

- Disk
- Metastases
- Epidural abscess
- Hematoma
- Other
    Lipomatosis (thoracic)
    Synovial cyst

CYSTIC SPINAL LESION (SYRINGOHYDROMYELIA)

Criteria: Syringomyelia: cavity in spinal cord; may or may not communicate with central canal; for hydromyelia: dilatation of central canal. Cannot be differentiated with imaging. Cause:

Primary
- Chiari/malformations
- Spinal dysraphism
- DW
- Diastematomyelia

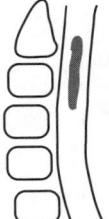

Acquired
- Tumor
  - Astrocytoma
  - Ependymoma
- Inflammatory
  - Arachnoiditis/meningitis
  - SAH
- Trauma
  - Spinal cord injury
  - Vascular insult

SUGGESTED READINGS

Atlas SW, editor: *Magnetic resonance imaging of the brain and spine,* Philadelphia, 2002, Lippincott Williams & Wilkins.

Brant-Zawadzki M, Norman D: *Magnetic resonance imaging of the central nervous system,* ed 1, Baltimore, 1987, Williams & Wilkins.

Edelmann RR, Hesselink JR: *Clinical magnetic resonance imaging,* Philadelphia, 1996, WB Saunders.

Grossman CB: *Magnetic resonance imaging and computed tomography of the head and spine,* Philadelphia, 1996, Lippincott Williams & Wilkins.

Latchaw RE: *MR and CT imaging of the head, neck, and spine,* ed 2, St Louis, 1991, Mosby.

Osborn AG: *Handbook of neuroradiology,* St Louis, 1996, Mosby.

Osborn AG: *Introduction to cerebral angiography,* Baltimore, 1980, Williams & Wilkins.

Osborn AG: *Diagnostic neuroradiology,* St Louis, 1994, Mosby.

Stark DD, Bradley W, editors: *Magnetic resonance imaging,* St Louis, 1998, Mosby.

Taveras JM, Ferrucci JT: *Radiology: diagnosis, imaging, intervention,* Philadelphia, 2002, Lippincott Williams & Wilkins.

Thrall J: *Current practice of radiology,* St Louis, 1993, Mosby.

Yock D: *MRI of CNS disease: a teaching file,* ed 2, St Louis, 1995, Mosby.

Chapter 7

Head and Neck Imaging

Chapter Outline

7

Temporal Bone

General

The temporal bone is divided into 5 portions:
- Mastoid (mastoid process: insertion for sternocleidomastoid muscle)
- Petrous portion (inner ear structures, skull base)
- Squamous portion (lateral inferior skull)
- Tympanic portion with tympanic cavity
- Styloid portion

EXTERNAL AUDITORY CANAL (EAC)

- Cartilaginous portion
- Bony portion

MIDDLE EAR

Composed of air-filled spaces that contain the ossicles and are divided into:
- Epitympanum
- Mesotympanum
- Hypotympanum

Boundaries of the middle ear are tympanic membrane laterally, the tegmen superiorly; and the inner ear (promontory) medially. The eustachian tube (pressure equalization) connects the middle ear with the nasopharynx. Three ossicles transmit sound waves from the tympanic membrane to the oval window in the vestibule:
- Malleus
- Incus
- Stapes (2 crura, 1 footplate)

INNER EAR

The inner ear (labyrinth) consists of:
- 3 semicircular canals, which connect to vestibule
- Vestibula with utricule and saccule
- Cochlea (sensorineural hearing), which connects to:
    Stapes → oval window
    Round window (allows for counterpulsation of fluid)

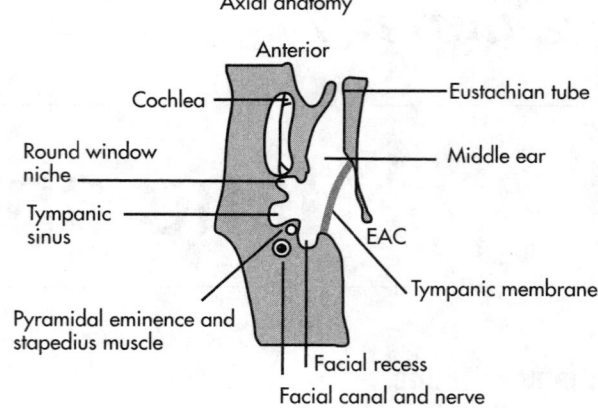

Axial anatomy

Anterior

Cochlea — Eustachian tube

Round window niche — Middle ear

Tympanic sinus — EAC

Pyramidal eminence and stapedius muscle — Tympanic membrane

Facial recess

Facial canal and nerve

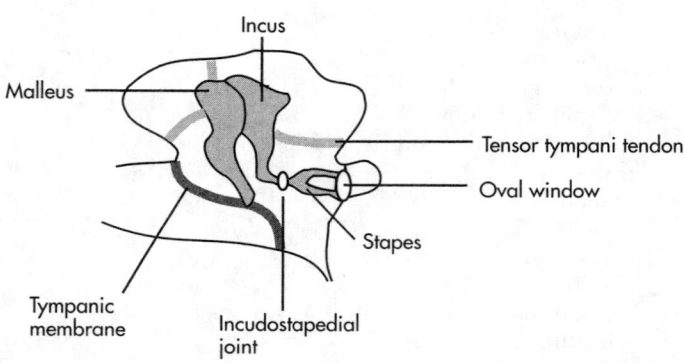

Coronal anatomy

Incus

Malleus — Tensor tympani tendon

Oval window

Stapes

Tympanic membrane — Incudostapedial joint

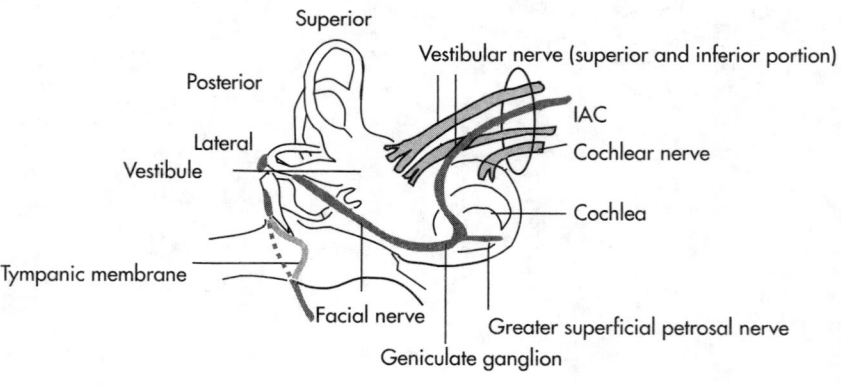

Superior

Posterior — Vestibular nerve (superior and inferior portion)

Lateral — IAC

Vestibule — Cochlear nerve

Cochlea

Tympanic membrane — Greater superficial petrosal nerve

Facial nerve

Geniculate ganglion

INTERNAL AUDITORY CANAL (IAC)

Left and right IAC should not differ > 2 mm in diameter.
Contents of IAC are divided by the falciform crest and "Bill's" bar:

- Facial nerve (anterior superior): NVII
- Superior vestibular nerve (posterior) with superior and inferior divisions: NVIII
- Inferior vestibular nerve (posterior): NVIII
- Cochlear part (anterior inferior): NVIII

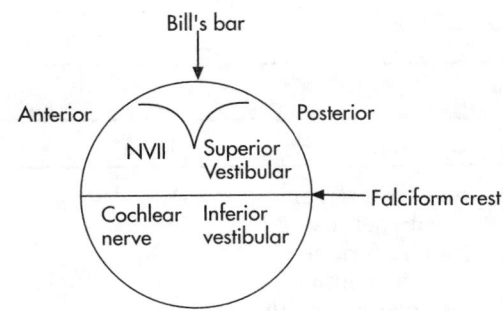

FACIAL NERVE

3 main portions of the facial nerve
- Intracranial (extracanalicular) portion
    Cerebellopontine angle (CPA) segment
    Meatal segment
- Intratemporal (intracanalicular) portion (30 mm)
    Labyrinth segment
    Tympanic (horizontal)
    Mastoid (vertical)
- Extracranial portion with 5 branches

The facial nerve gives rise to 4 branches
- Greater superficial petrosal nerve
- Stapedius nerve
- Chorda tympani
- Terminal branches (total of 5 extracranial branches)

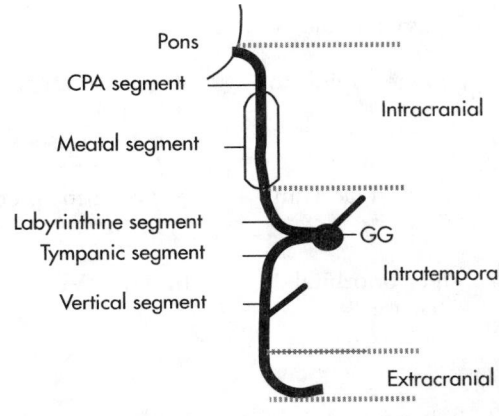

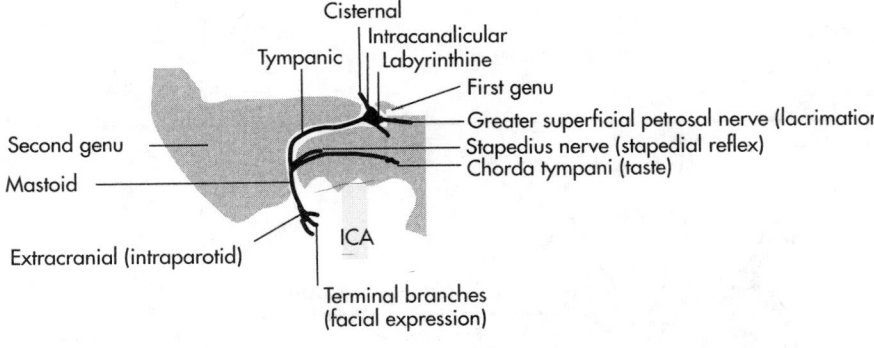

SKULL BASE

OVERVIEW OF FORAMINA			
Opening	Nerve	Artery	Vein
Jugular foramen pars nervosa	IX		Inferior petrosal sinus
Jugular foramen pars venosa	X, XI		Internal jugular vein
Foramen rotundum	V2	Artery of foramen rotundum	Emissary veins
Foramen ovale	V3	Accessory meningeal artery	Emissary veins
Foramen spinosum	Recurrent meningeal branch of mandibular nerve, lesser superficial petrosal nerve	Middle meningeal artery	Middle meningeal vein
Foramen lacerum	Nerve of the pterygoid canal	Meningeal branches of ascending pharyngeal artery	
Superior orbital fissure	III, IV, V, VI	Orbital branches of middle meningeal artery Recurrent meningeal branches of lacrimal artery	Ophthalmic veins
Stylomastoid foramen	VII		
Hypoglossal canal	XII		
Carotid canal	Sympathetics	ICA	
Vidian canal		Vidian artery	
Optic canal	II	Ophthalmic artery	

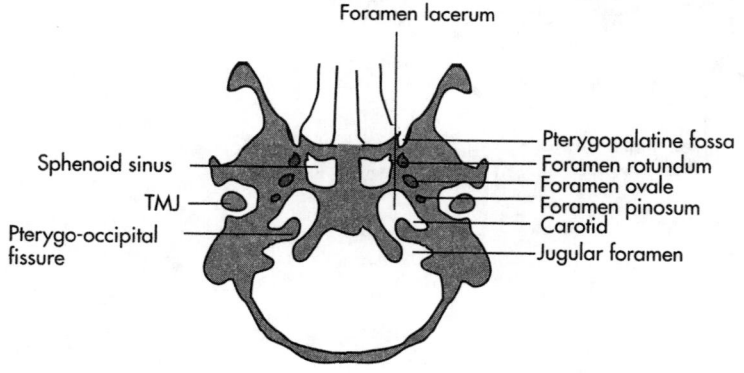

Foramen lacerum

Sphenoid sinus
TMJ
Pterygo-occipital fissure

Pterygopalatine fossa
Foramen rotundum
Foramen ovale
Foramen pinosum
Carotid
Jugular foramen

CRANIAL NERVES

- CNI: olfactory nerve
- CNII: optic nerve
- CNIII: oculomotor nerve
- CNIV: trochlear nerve
- CNV: trigeminal nerve
- CNVI: abducens nerve
- CNVII: facial nerve
- CNVIII: auditory nerve
- CNIX: glossopharyngeus nerve
- CNX: vagus nerve
- CNXI: spinal accessory nerve
- CNXII: hypoglossal nerve

Trauma

TEMPORAL BONE FRACTURES

Clinical findings
- Hearing loss
- Tinnitus
- Vertigo
- Bleeding into EAC
- Cerebrospinal fluid (CSF) leak
- Facial paresis

Radiographic features

TEMPORAL BONE FRACTURES		
Parameter	Longitudinal Fractures (Middle Ear Fracture)	Transverse Fractures (Inner Ear Fracture)
Frequency	80%	20%
Fracture line	Parallel to long axis	Perpendicular to long axis
Labyrinth	Spared	Involved: vertigo, sensori-neural hearing loss
Ossicles	Involved: conductive hearing loss	
Tympanic membrane	Involved	Spared
Facial paralysis	20%	50%

Fracture complications
- Ossicular fractures or dislocations
- Tympanic membrane perforation
- Hemotympanum
- NVII paralysis
- CSF otorrhea
- Meningitis, abscess
- Sinus thrombosis, rare
- Labyrinthitis ossificans (late)

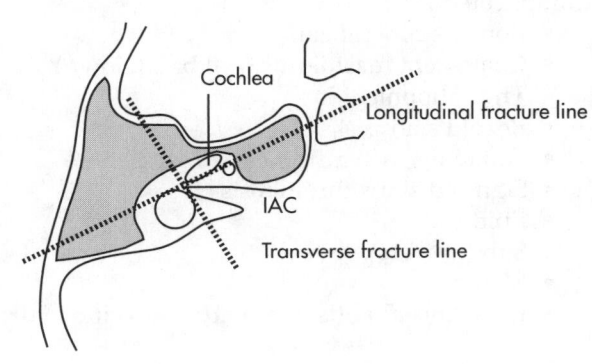

Indications for surgery in temporal bone fractures
- Ossicular fracture or dislocation
- Decompression of the facial nerve
- Labyrinthine fistulae
- CSF leaks

Inflammation

ACUTE INFLAMMATION

Acute inflammations of the middle and inner ear are rarely evaluated radiographically because they can be efficiently diagnosed and treated clinically. Types:
- Otitis media (edema fills middle ear cavity): acute, subacute, chronic forms
    Children: common
    Adults: less common; exclude nasopharyngeal carcinoma which causes serous otitis media
- Mastoiditis (bony destruction has to be present to make diagnosis, fluid-filled mastoid cells are also often present)
- Labyrinthitis
    Serous
    Toxic
    Suppurative

Complications
- Meningitis
- Sinus thrombosis
- Epidural abscess
- Petrositis (infection of petrous air cells)

BELL'S PALSY

Acute onset. Unilateral peripheral facial nerve palsy. Bell's palsy resolves in 6 weeks to 3 months. By MRI there is enhancement along facial nerve involving intracanalicular and labyrinthine segments that normally do not enhance in normal individuals. Facial nerve can normally enhance in its tympanic and mastoid segments due to right arterial supply. Facial nerve enhancement is nonspecific and can occur other inflammatory and neoplastic conditions. Perineural spread of tumor should also be considered.

MASTOIDITIS

Types
Uncomplicated forms:
- Edema and/or fluid only

Complicated form
- Bone demineralization
- Coalescent mastoiditis (cell breakdown)
- Thrombophlebitis
- Bezold's abscess
- Gradenigo's syndrome (petrositis)
- Sigmoid sinus thrombosis
- Epidural
- Subdural empyema
- Meningitis
- Focal encephalitis, brain abscess, otitic hydrocephalus

ACQUIRED CHOLESTEATOMA

Mass of keratin debris lined by squamous epithelium. Etiology: epithelial cells move into the middle ear via a perforation of the tympanic membrane. Secondary to eustachian tube dysfunction. Types:

- Acquired: chronic middle ear infection (common). Either in attic (Prussak's space or sinus location)
- Congenital (epidermoid): cholesteatoma arises from epithelial nests in middle ear, mastoid, or petrous bone including the labyrinth (uncommon)

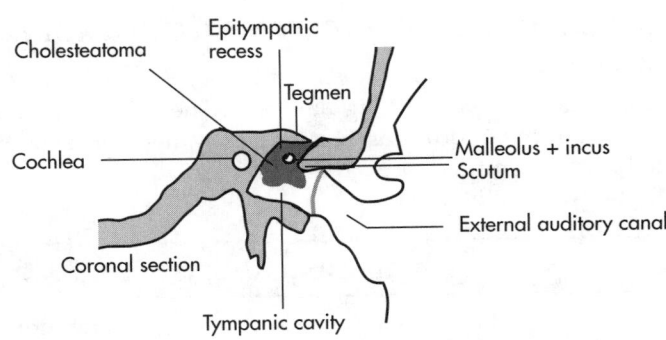

Radiographic features (acquired cholesteatoma)

- Soft tissue mass in middle ear
- Borders may be well- or ill-defined
- Erosion of incus and otic spur (scutum) common
- Bone resorption (collagenase) is typical and occurs most commonly in:
  - Ossicles
  - Lateral semicircular canal (fistula)
  - Tegmen tympani
  - Facial canal
- Mastoid air cells are typically underpneumatized and sclerotic
- Labyrinthine fistula formation in lateral semicircular canal, less common
- It is often impossible to distinguish chronic middle ear infection from cholesteatoma in cases with little bone destruction.

LOCATION OF ACQUIRED CHOLESTEATOMA		
	Attic Cholesteatoma	**Sinus Cholesteatoma**
TM perforation	Pars flaccida	Pars tensa
Location	Prussak's space	Sinus tymphani
Ossicles displaced	Medially	Laterally
Bone erosion	Lateral tymphanic wall (erosion of scutum is an early finding)	Initially subtle
Ossicle erosion	Head of malleus and long process of incus	Short process of incus and stapes

Complications of cholesteatoma

- Labyrinthine fistula (dehiscence of semicircular canals—most frequently lateral canal)
- Facial nerve paralysis (involvement of facial nerve canal)
- Sinus thrombosis
- Meningitis
- Encephalitis
- Abscess
- Petrous apex syndrome (Gradenigo's syndrome)

CONGENITAL CHOLESTEATOMA (EPIDERMOID)

Rare lesions that may occur in middle ear, mastoid, EAC, jugular fossa, labyrinth, petrous apex, CPA, and jugular fossa. The most common location is anterosuperior portion of the middle ear. Histologically, the cholesteatoma is made up of squamous cell lining, keratin debris, and cholesterol.

Radiographic features

SIGNAL CHARACTERISTICS RELATIVE TO BRAIN			
	Epidermoid (Congenital Cholesteatoma)	Cholesterol Granuloma (Cholesterol Cyst)	Mucocele
CT	≤	Isodense, no calcium, no enhancement	<
T1W	≤ (lamination)	> (cholesterol)	≤
T2W	>	> (methemoglobin)	>

CHOLESTEROL GRANULOMA (CHOLESTEROL CYSTS)

Subtype of granulation tissue that may be present anywhere in the middle ear, including the petrous apex. Clinical symptoms occur when the granuloma becomes expansile and causes bone erosion, such as in the petrous apex, leading to hearing loss, tinnitus, cranial nerve palsies. Histologically, cholesterol granulomas contain hemorrhage and cholesterol crystals.

Radiographic features

- Bone erosion of petrous apex
- Expansion of petrous apex
- CT: isodense relative to brain, no enhancement, no calcification
- MRI: hyperintense relative to brain on T1-weighted (T1W) images because of cholesterol content

MALIGNANT EXTERNAL OTITIS

Severe, life-threatening *Pseudomonas aeruginosa* infection in elderly diabetics. The aggressive infection spreads via cartilaginous fissures of Santorini and extends into:

- Middle ear
- Base of temporal bone
- Petrous apex (osteomyelitis)
- Parapharyngeal space
- Nasopharynx
- Meninges
- central nervous system
- Bone (osteomyelitis)

Radiographic features

- Mastoiditis
- Osteomyelitis of base of skull (jugular, sigmoid) and at bony/cartilaginous junction of EAC
- Sinus phelibitis, thrombosis
- Multiple cranial nerve paralyses

HEARING LOSS

Types of hearing loss:
    Conductive
- 3 main locations of abnormalities: tympanic membrane, ossicles, hyperostosis of oval window
- Common underlying causes: otitis, cholesteatoma, otosclerosis, trauma

    Sensorineural
- Evaluate inner ear, IAC
- Common underlying causes: idiopathic, hereditary, acoustic neuroma

PULSATILE TINNITUS

Causes of pulsatile tinnitus:
    Normal vascular variants
- Aberrant ICA
- Jugular bulb anomalies (high or dehiscent megabulb, diverticulum)
- Persistent stapedial artery

    Vascular tumors
- Glomus jugulare
- Glomus tympanicum

    Vascular abnormalities
- Arteriovenous malformation (AVM)
- Atherosclerosis
- ICA dissection or aneurysm at petrous apex
- Fibromuscular hyperplasia

    Other causes of tinnitus
- Paget's disease
- Otosclerosis
- Ménière's disease

Tumors

GLOMUS TUMORS

Glomus tumors (chemodectoma = nonchromaffin paraganglioma) arise from chemoreceptor cells in multiple sites in head and neck. Most tumors are benign, but 10% of glomus tumors are associated with malignant tumors elsewhere in the body. Ten percent are multiple, thus it is important to check other common locations in head and neck during imaging (glomus jugulare, vagale and carotid body tumor). Glomus tumors represent the most common middle ear tumor. Types:
- Glomus jugulare: origin at jugular bulb; more common
- Glomus tympanicum: origin at cochlear promontory; less common, rises from paraganglia along Jacobson's and Arnold's nerves within the tymphanic cavity

Clinical findings
- Pulsatile tinnitus (most common)
- Hearing loss
- Arrythmias
- Sudden blood pressure (BP) fluctuations

Radiographic features
- Glomus tympanicum typically presents as a small soft tissue mass centered over the cochlear promontory. Glomus tympanicum are usually indistinguishable from other soft tissue masses in the tympanic cavity.

- Glomus juglare are centered in the region of the jugular foramen and rarely extend below level of hyoid bone. They are accompanied by permeative bone changes in jugular foramen. Characteristic findings by MRI are multiple low signal intensity areas that represent flow voids in the tumor. This has a *salt and pepper* appearance.
- Intense contrast enhancement by CT, MRI, angiography
- Large tumors erode bone

BENIGN TEMPORAL BONE TUMORS

- Meningioma
- Facial neuroma, may arise anywhere along the course of NVII. In the IAC, the tumor is indistinguishable from an acoustic neuroma
- Osteoma
- Adenoma (ceruminoma = apocrine adenoma) in the EAC, benign but locally aggressive, rare
- Epidermoid (primary cholesteatoma)
- Petrous apex cholesterol granuloma

MALIGNANT TEMPORAL BONE TUMORS

- Carcinoma (most common tumors)
    Squamous cell carcinoma (SCC) arising from the EAC
    Adenocarcinoma
- Lymphoma
- Metastases: breast, lung, melanoma
- Chondrosarcoma, other primary bone tumors
- Rhabdomyosarcoma in children

Congenital Anomalies

OVERVIEW OF SYNDROMES

SYNDROMES ASSOCIATED WITH VARYING DEGREES OF DEAFNESS				
Syndrome	Inner Ear	Middle Ear	Outer Ear	Other Abnormalities
OTOCRANIOFACIAL				
Treacher Collins	+++	+++	0	Coloboma, mandibular hypoplasia ("fishmouth")
Crouzon's disease	+++	+++	0	Exophthalmos, craniosynostosis
OTOCERVICAL				
Klippel-Feil	++	++	+++	Cervical fusion, short neck
Cleidocranial dysostosis	+	+	++	Large head, underdeveloped facial bones, absent clavicles
OTOSKELETAL				
Osteogenesis	0	+	+++	Deformity, fractures, blue sclera
Osteopetrosis	++	++	+++	Increased bone density
OTHER				
Thalidomide	+++	+++	+++	Short limbs, cardiac, GI, hemangiomas

CONGENITAL ABNORMALITIES OF THE INNER EAR

- Cochlear malseptation (Mondini's deafness) results in < 2.5 cochlear turns and an "empty cochlea." Direct connection to CSF resulting in leaks and meningitis
- Single cochlear-vestibular cavity (Michel's deafness) results in < 2.5 cochlear turns. Hypoplastic petrous pyramid
- Small internal auditory canal
- Cochlear aplasia
- Large vestibule or aqueduct

PETROUS MALFORMATIONS ASSOCIATED WITH RECURRENT MENINGITIS

- Lamina cribrosa/spiralis defect at lateral end of IAC: perilymphatic hydrops develops with secondary displacement of stapes
- Dehiscence of tegmen tympani
- Wide cochlear aqueduct

Otodystrophies and Dysplasias

OTOSCLEROSIS

The osseous labyrinth (otic capsule) normally has a dense capsule. In otosclerosis, the capsule is replaced by vascular, irregular bony trabeculae and later sclerotic bone. Unknown etiology; inherited. Bilateral, 90%. Patients (female > male) present with hearing loss.

Types
- Fenestral otosclerosis: sclerosis around oval window including fixation of stapes. Clinical and audiometric diagnosis (conductive hearing loss). CT is rarely helpful.
- Cochlear otosclerosis: involves cochlea and otic capsule. CT findings:
  Deossification around cochlea (lucent halo)
  Sclerosis occurs later in disease

OTHER OTODYSTROPHIES AND DYSPLASIAS

- Paget's disease
- Fibrous dysplasia
- Osteogenesis imperfecta
- Osteopetrosis resulting in cupulolithiasis
- Craniometaphyseal dysplasia (Pyle's disease)
- Craniodiaphyseal dysplasia (Engelmann's disease)
- Cleidocranial dysostosis

7

Orbit

General

Orbital spaces

- Intraconal space: space inside the rectus muscle pyramid
- Extraconal space: space outside the rectus muscle pyramid
- Preseptal space
- Postseptal space
- Lacrimal fossa

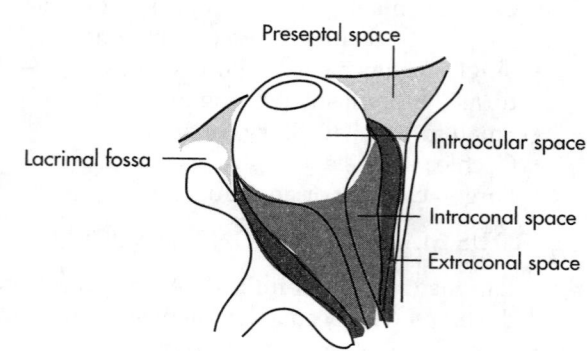

Orbital structures

- Globe (lens, anterior chamber, posterior chamber, vitreous, sclerouveal coat)
- Intraconal, extraconal fat
- Optic nerve and sheath
- Ophthalmic artery and vein
- Rectus muscles

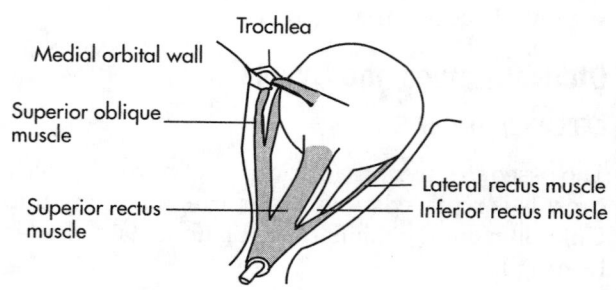

Orbital septum

- Represents condensed orbital rim periosteum
- Attaches to outer margins of bony orbit and deep tissues of lids
- Separates all the structures in the orbit from soft tissues in the face (preseptal vs. postseptal)

Globe

RETINOBLASTOMA

Malignant tumor that arises from neuroectodermal cells of retina. Clinical: leukocoria (white mass behind pupil). Age: < 3 years (70%)

- 30% bilateral, 30% multifocal within one eye
- 10% of patients have a familial history of retinoblastoma

Radiographic features

- Intraocular mass
- High density (calcification, hemorrhage)
- Dense vitreous, common
- Calcifications are common (90%); in absence of calcifications suspect other mass lesions:
    - Persistent hyperplastic primary vitreous
    - Retrolental fibroplasia
    - Toxocariasis
    - Coats' disease
- Primary role of imaging is to determine tumor spread:
    - Optic nerve extension, 25%
    - Scleral break-through
    - Metastases: meninges, liver, lymph nodes

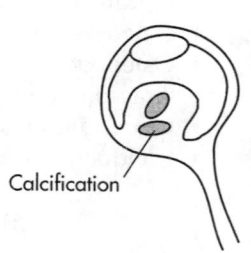

Pearls
- Tumors may occur bilaterally or trilaterally counting pineoblastoma
- Associated with other malignancies (osteosarcoma most common) later in life; postradiation sarcoma at 10 years: 20%, 20 years: 50%, 30 years: 90%

MELANOMA

Most common (75%) ocular malignancy in adults. Arises from pigmented choroidal layer; retinal detachment is common.

Radiographic features
- Thickening or irregularity of choroid (localized, polypoid or flat)
- Exophytic, biconvex mass lesion
- Usually unilateral, posterior location
- Retinal detachment, common
- Contrast enhancement
- MRI: T1 hyperintense, T2 hypointense
- Poor prognostic indicators:
    Large tumor size
    Heavy pigmentation
    Infiltration of the angles, optic nerve, sclera, ciliary body

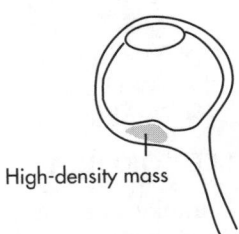

High-density mass

PERSISTENT HYPERPLASTIC PRIMARY VITREOUS (PHPV)

Caused by persistence of portions of the fetal hyaloid artery and primary vitreous. Associated with ocular dysplasias (e.g., Norrie's disease = PHPV, seizures, deafness, low IQ). Clinical: blindness, leukocoria, microphthalmia. Usually unilateral. Rare.

Radiographic features
- Small globe (microphthalmia)
- Vitreous body hyperdensity along the remnant of the hyaloid artery
- No calcification (in contrast to retinoblastoma)
- Complications:
    Retinal detachment
    Chronic retinal hemorrhage

RETROLENTAL FIBROPLASIA

Toxic retinopathy caused by oxygen treatment (e.g., for hyaline membrane disease). A retinal vasoconstriction leads to neovascularization of the posterior vitreous and retina. Hemorrhage with scarring, retraction, and exudate formation follows. Bilateral.

COATS' DISEASE

Primary vascular abnormality (exudative retinitis) causing lipoprotein accumulation in retina, telangiectasia, neovascularization, and retinal detachment (pseudoglioma). Age: 6-8 years, males. Rare.

Radiographic findings
- Dense vitreous with focal mass or calcium
- Unilateral

DRUSEN

Focal calcification in hyaline bodies in the optic nerve head. Usually bilateral and asymptomatic. Blurred disk margins may be mistaken for papilledema.

7

GLOBE SHAPE ABNORMALITIES

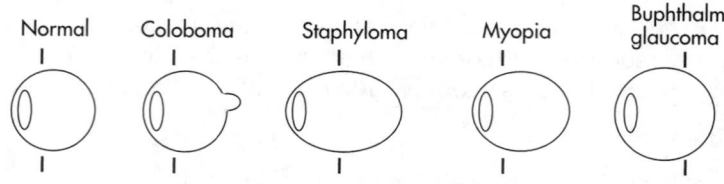

Normal   Coloboma   Staphyloma   Myopia   Buphthalmos glaucoma

- Coloboma: focal outpouching involving retina, choroid, iris; caused by deficient closure of fetal optic fissure; located in region of optic disk; associated with:
    - Morning glory anomaly
    - Microphthalmos with cyst
- Staphyloma: acquired defect of globe wall with protrusion of choroid or sclera
- Axial myopia: AP elongation but no protrusion
- Buphthalmos: congenital glaucoma; anterior ocular chamber drainage problem

LEUKOKORIA

Leukokoria refers to a white pupil. Clinical, not a radiologic finding. Underlying causes:
- Retinoblastoma
- PHPV
- Congenital cataract
- Toxocariasis
- Other
    - Sclerosing endophthalmitis
    - Coats' disease
    - Retrolental fibroplasia
    - Trauma
    - Chronic retinal detachment

Optic Nerve

OPTIC NERVE GLIOMA

Most common cause of diffuse optic nerve enlargement, especially in childhood. Pathology: usually well-differentiated, pilocytic astrocytoma. Clinical: loss of vision, proptosis (bulky tumors). 80% occur in first decade of life. In neurofibromatosis (NF) the disease may be bilateral.

Radiographic features
- Types of tumor growth: tubular, excrescent, fusiform widening of optic nerve
- Enlargement of optical canal; > 1 mm difference between left and right is abnormal
- Lower CT density than meningioma
- Contrast enhancement is variable
- Calcifications are rare (but are common in meningioma)
- Tumor extension best detected by MRI: chiasm → optic tracts → lateral geniculate body → optic radiation

OPTIC NERVE MENINGIOMA

Optic nerve sheath meningiomas arise from arachnoid rests in meninges covering the optic nerve. Age: 4th decade (80% female); younger patients typically have NF. Clinical: progressive loss of vision.

Radiographic features
Mass
- Tubular, 60%
- Fusiform, surrounding the optic nerve, 25%
- Eccentric, 15%
- Calcification (common)

Enhancement
- Intense contrast enhancement
- Linear bands of enhancement (nerve within tumor): "tram-track sign"

Other
- Sphenoid bone and/or optical canal hyperostosis

Extraocular Tumors

HEMANGIOMA

Common benign tumor of the intraconal space. Types:
Capillary hemangioma (children; strawberry nevus): no capsule
- Represent 10% of all pediatric orbital tumors
- Infiltrate conal and extraconal spaces
- Grow for < 1 year and then typically involute
- 90% are associated with cutaneous angioma

Cavernous hemangioma (adults): true capsule, benign
- Large dilated venous channels with fibrous capsule
    Dense enhancement with contrast
    Signal intensity similar to fluid (e.g., CSF) on T2W
- Well delineated, round
- Expansion of orbit
- Calcified phleboliths, rare
- Hemosiderin deposition
- No bone destruction but remodelling in large hemangiomas

DERMOID CYST

Common orbital tumor in childhood. Age: 1st decade.
Radiographic features
- Low CT attenuation and T1 hyperintensity (fat) is diagnostic
- Contiguous bone scalloping or sclerosis is common
- May contain debris (inhomogenous MRI signal)

LYMPHANGIOMA

2% of orbital childhood tumors. Age: 1st decade. Associated with other lymphangiomas in head and neck. Lymphangiomas of the orbit do not involute spontaneously.
Radiographic features
- Variable CT appearance because of different histological components (lymphangitic channels, vascular stroma)
- Multiloculated
- Rim enhancement
- Signal intensity similar to fluid (e.g., CSF) on T2W

7

LACRIMAL GLAND TUMORS

Lymphoid, 50%
- Benign reactive lymphoid hyperplasia
- Lymphoma

Epithelial tumors, 50%
- Benign mixed (pleomorphic) tumor (75% of epithelial tumors)
- Adenoid cystic carcinoma
- Mucoepidermoid carcinoma
- Malignant mixed tumor

RHABDOMYOSARCOMA

Most common malignant orbital tumor in childhood. Mean age: 7 years.

Radiographic features
- Large, aggressive soft tissue mass (intraconal or extraconal)
- Metastases to lung and cervical nodes

METASTASES

Children: Ewing's tumor, neuroblastoma, leukemia. Adults: breast, lung, renal cell, prostate carcinoma. Direct extension of SCC from paranasal sinus.

Inflammatory and Infiltrative Lesions

ORBITAL INFECTION

The orbital septum represents a barrier to infectious spread from anterior to posterior structures. Common causes of orbital infection include spread from infected sinus and trauma.

Radiographic features
- Periorbital cellulitis: soft tissue swelling
- Postseptal infection (true orbital cellulitis)
    - Subperiosteal infiltrate
    - Stranding of retrobulbar fat
    - Lateral displacement of enlarged medial rectus muscle
    - Proptosis

THYROID OPHTHALMOPATHY

Orbital pathology (deposition of glycoproteins and mucopolysaccharides in the orbit) caused by long-acting thyroid-stimulating factor (LATS) in Graves' disease. Clinical: painless proptosis, patients may be euthyroid, hypothyroid, or hyperthyroid. Grades:

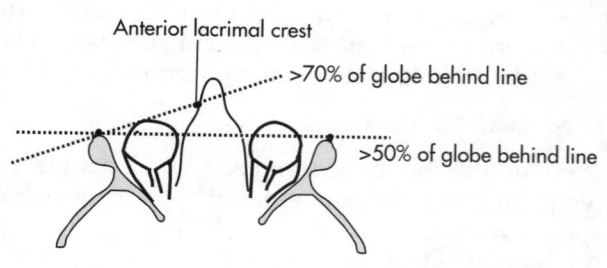

- Grade 1: lid retraction, stare, lid lag (spasm of upper lid due to thyrotoxicosis)
- Grade 2: soft tissue involvement
- Grade 3: proptosis as determined by exophthalmometer measurement
- Grade 4: extraocular muscle involvement; affects muscles at midpoint
- Grade 5: corneal involvement
- Grade 6: optic nerve involvement: vision loss

Treatment: prednisone → radiotherapy → surgical decompression; surgery or ^{131}I for thyroid.

Radiographic features

Exophthalmos

Muscle involvement
- Mnemonic for involvement: "**I'M SL**ow"

    Inferior (most common)

    Medial

    Superior

    Lateral
- Enlargement is maximum in the middle of the muscle and tapers toward the end (infiltrative, not inflammatory disease)
- Spares tendon insertions
- Often bilateral, symmetric

Other
- Optic nerve thickening
- Expansion of orbital fat

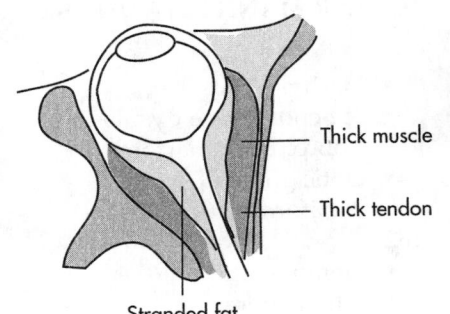

Exophthalmos

— Thick muscle

— Normal tendon

ORBITAL PSEUDOTUMOR

Inflammation of orbital soft tissues of unknown origin. Clinical: painful proptosis, unilateral, steroid responsive. Causes:
- Idiopathic
- Systemic disease: sarcoid, endocrine
- Unrecognized focal infections, foreign bodies

Radiographic features
- Infiltrating intraconal or extraconal inflammation presenting as ill-defined infiltrations or less commonly as a mass
- Typical features

    Unilateral

    Unlike thyroid opthalmopathy, pseudotumors involve tendons of muscles (because it is inflammatory disease)

    Muscle enlargement
- Stranding of orbital fat (inflammation)
- Enlarged lacrimal gland
- May involve orbital apex including superior orbital fissure (Tolosa-Hunt syndrome)

Thick muscle

Thick tendon

Stranded fat

DIFFERENTIATION		
	Pseudotumor	**Thyroid Opthalmopathy**
Involvement	Unilateral, 85%	Bilateral, 85%
Tendon	Involved	Normal
Muscle	Enlargement	Enlargement: I > M > S > L
Fat	Inflammation	Increased amount of fat
Lacrimal gland	Enlarged	
Steroids	Good response	Minimal response

7

ACUTE INFECTIONS

Bacterial infection (extraconal > intraconal) are often due to sinusitis, complicated by cavernous sinus thrombosis.

Trauma

Types:
- Blunt trauma with orbital blowout fractures, 50%
- Penetrating injury, 50%

Detection of ocular foreign bodies:
- Metal: objects > 0.06 mm^3
- Glass: objects > 1.8 mm^3
- Wood: difficult to detect because wood density is similar to that of soft tissue

Other

ERDHEIM-CHESTER DISEASE

Lipid granulomatosis with retroorbital deposition, xanthelasma of eyelids, skeletal manifestations (medullary sclerosis, cortical thickening) and cardiopulmonary manifestations due to cholesterol emboli. Rare.

OCULAR MANIFESTATIONS OF PHAKOMATOSES

NF1
- Lisch nodules
- Sphenoid bone dysplasia
- Choroidal hamartoma
- Optic glioma
- Plexiform neurofibroma

NF2
- Meningioma
- Schwannoma

Sturge-Weber
- Choroidal angioma
- Buphthalmos
- Glaucoma

Tuberous sclerosis
- Retinal astrocytic hamartoma

Von Hippel-Lindau (VHL)
- Retinal angioma

Pharynx, Larynx

General

ANATOMY

The upper aerodigestive tract consists of the pharynx and the larynx. The larynx connects pharynx and trachea. The pharynx is divided into:
- Nasopharynx: extends to inferior portion of soft palate
- Oropharynx: extends from soft palate to hyoid bone
- Hypopharynx (laryngeal part of pharynx): contains pyriform sinuses and posterior pharynx

The larynx contains:
- Laryngeal surface of epiglottis
- Aryepiglottic folds
- Arytenoid cartilage
- False cords
- True cords (glottis is the space between vocal cords)
- Subglottic larynx

AXIAL CT ANATOMY

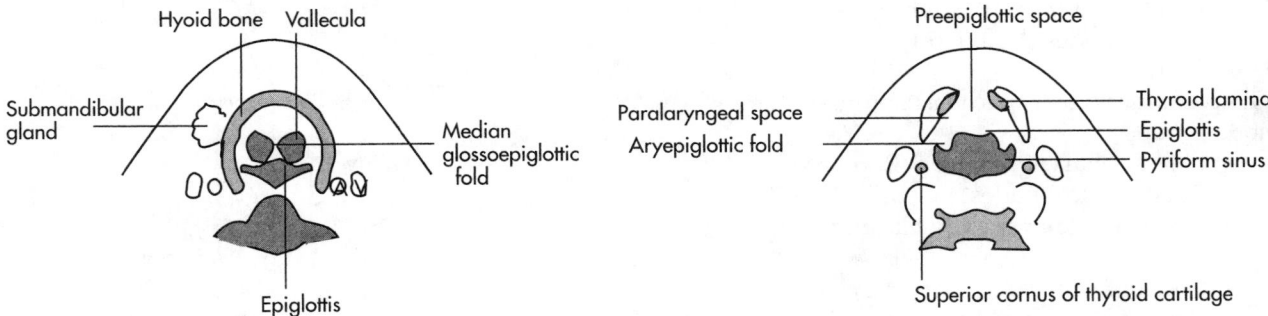

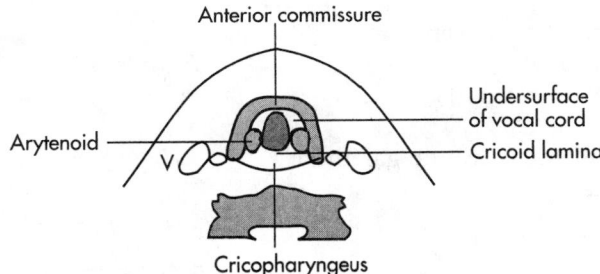

PARAPHARYNGEAL SPACE

Potential space filled with loose connective tissue. Space is pyramidal in shape with apex directed towards the lesser cornua of the hyoid bone and the base towards the skull base. Extends from skull base to mid-oropharynx. Borders:

- Lateral: mandible, medial pterygoid muscle
- Medial: superior constrictor muscles of pharynx, tensor and levator veli palatini
- Anterior: buccinator muscle, pterygoid, mandible
- Posterior: carotid sheath

Contents

Anterior (prestyloid) compartment
- Internal maxillary art.
- Interior alveolar, lingual, auriculotemporal nerves

Posterior (retrostyloid) compartment
- ICA, internal jugular vein (IJV)
- CN IX, X, XII,
- Cervical sympathetic chain lymph nodes

Medial (retropharyngeal) compartment
- Lymph nodes (Rouvière)

Lymphatics

The parapharyngeal space has abundant lymph node groups

- Lateral pharyngeal node (Rouvière)
- Deep cervical nodes
- Internal jugular chain including jugulodigastric node
- Chain of spinal accessory nerve
- Chain of transverse cervical artery

Paraganglia

Cells of neuroectodermal origin that are sensitive to changes in oxygen and CO_2. Types:

- Carotid body (at carotid bifurcation)
- Vagal bodies

Neoplastic transformation of the jugular bulb ganglion produces the glomus jugulare.

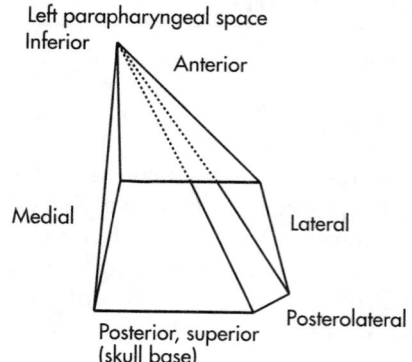

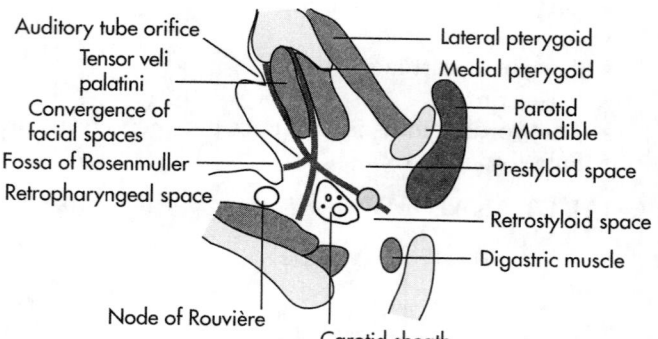

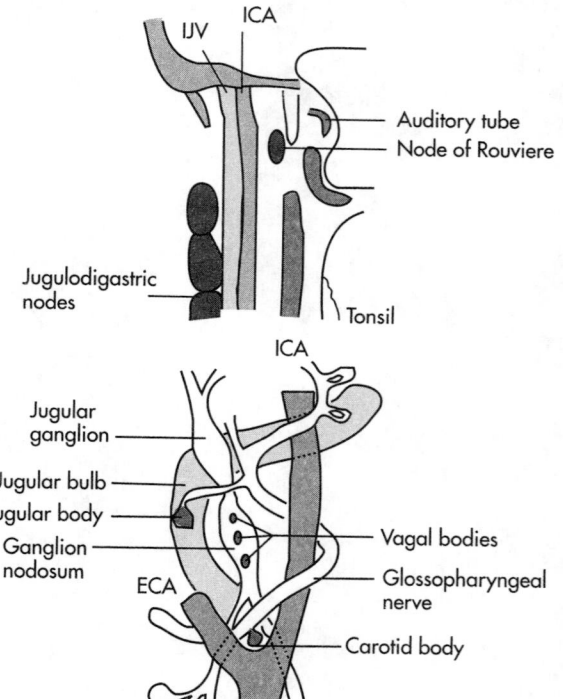

FLUOROSCOPIC VOCAL CORD EXAMINATION

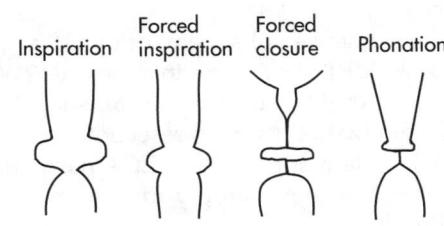

Inspiration   Forced inspiration   Forced closure   Phonation

Occasionally performed to evaluate the subglottic region (Valsalva maneuver), invisible by laryngoscopy.
- Phonation of "E" during expiration: adducts cords
- Phonation of "reversed E" during inspiration; distends laryngeal ventricles
- Puffed cheeks (modified Valsalva): distends pyriform
- Valsalva: distends subglottic region
- Inspiration: abducts cords

Nasooropharynx

THORNWALDT'S CYST

Cystic midline nasopharyngeal notochordal remnant (3% of population). May occasionally become infected. Age: 15-30

Radiographic features
- Hemispherical shaped soft tissue density seen on lateral plain films
- Typical cystic appearance by CT and MRI
- Location: midline; same level as adenoids

RETROPHARYNGEAL ABSCESS

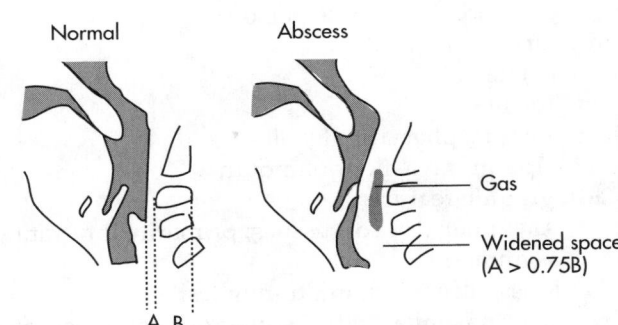

Normal   Abscess

Gas

Widened space (A > 0.75B)

A B

Cause: dental disease, pharyngitis, penetrating trauma, vertebral osteomyelitis. Organism: *Staphylococcus, Streptococcus*, anaerobes, tuberculosis (TB).

Radiographic features
- Widened retropharyngeal space
- May involve retropharyngeal, parapharyngeal, prevertebral, submandibular, masticator space, or spread to mediastinum
- CT apperance
  Gas
  Necrotic tissue and edema appears hypodense
  Stranding of fat
  Rim enhancement with contrast

JUVENILE ANGIOFIBROMA

Vascular tumor of mesenchymal origin. Most frequent benign nasopharyngeal tumor in adolescents (age: 10-20, males only). Clinical: epistaxis (very vascular tumor), mass in the pterygopalatine fossa; extension to infratemporal fossa, nasal cavity.

Radiographic features
Usually large soft tissue mass causing local bony remodeling
- Pterygopalatine fossa, 90%; with extension causing displacement of posterior wall of maxillary sinus
- Sphenoid sinus, 65%
- Pterygomaxillary fissure, infratemporal fossa, intracranial cavity via superior orbital fissure

Highly vascular:
- Intense enhancement by CT and MRI
- MRI: very hyperintense on T2W, flow voids
- Angiography: tumor blush

Embolization prior to resection
- Main supply from ECA particularly maxillary artery
- May have supply from ICA

Pearls
- Do not biopsy (hemorrhage)
- Recurrent if incompletely resected; recurrence rate today is low because of early diagnosis

SQUAMOUS CELL CARCINOMA (SCC)

SCC accounts for 80%-90% of malignant tumors in the nasooropharynx (lymphoma: 5%; rare tumors: adenocarcinoma, melanoma, sarcoma).

Location

Nasopharynx
- Tumors most commonly arise from lateral pharyngeal recess (fossa of Rosenmuller)
- Possibly associated with Epstein-Barr virus
- Common in Chinese persons

Oropharynx
- Palate
- Tonsil
- Tongue, pharyngeal wall
- Lips, gingiva, floor of mouth

Radiographic features
- Asymmetry of soft tissues; primarily infiltrating carcinomas produce only slight asymmetry
- Mass, ulceration, infiltrating lesion

Staging of nasopharyngeal squamous cell carcinoma

Primary tumor
- Tis: carcinoma in situ
- T1: tumor confined to 1 site of nasopharynx or no tumor visible
- T2: tumor involving 2 sites (both posterosuperior and lateral walls)
- T3: extension of tumor into nasal cavity or oropharynx
- T4: tumor invasion of skull, cranial nerve involvement, or both

Adenopathy
- No: clinically positive node
- N1: single clinically positive homolateral node ≤ 3 cm in diameter
- N2: single clinically positive homolateral node > 3 cm but not > 6 cm in diameter
- N3: node > 6 cm

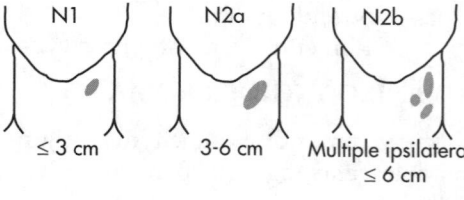
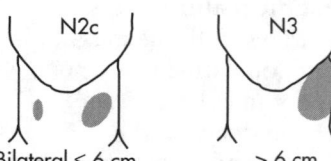

Distant metastasis
- M0: no evidence of metastasis
- M1: distant metastases present

Pearls
- Elderly patients with serous otitis media have nasopharyngeal carcinoma until proven otherwise
- 20% of tumors are submucosal and cannot be seen by the clinician
- Schmincke's tumor: undifferentiated cancer
- 80%-90% of patients with nasopharyngeal SCC have positive lymph nodes at presentation

OTHER NEOPLASMS

OVERVIEW OF OTHER HEAD AND NECK NEOPLASMS BY SITE			
Space	**Congenital**	**Benign**	**Malignant**
Prestyloid/ parapharyngeal	2nd branchial cleft cyst	Mixed tumor Neuroma	SCC of tonsil Salivary/parotid carcinoma Sarcoma Lymphoma
Poststyloid/ parapharyngeal		Paraganglioma Neuroma Chordoma	SCC Nodal metastases Lymphoma Neuroblastoma
Infratemporal fossa, masticator space	Lymphangioma Cystic hygroma	Odontogenic cyst Neural tumor Hemangioma	SCC Sarcoma (MFH, rhabdomyosarcoma) Lymphoma Salivary/parotid carcinoma
Floor of mouth, sublingual	Epidermoid, dermoid Teratoma Lymphangioma Cystic hygroma	Rannula Pleomorphic adenoma Neural tumor Hemangioma	Salivary/parotid SCC Sarcoma Lymphoma
Retropharyngeal	Meningocele	Chordoma Neural tumor Fibroma Teratoid	Sarcoma (muscle, neural, liposarcoma) Vertebral metastases Primary bone tumor Neuroblastoma

MFH, Malignant fibrous histiocytoma.

Hypopharynx, Larynx

VOCAL CORD PARALYSIS

Innervation of vocal cord muscles is through the recurrent laryngeal nerve of the vagus (NX). The left recurrent laryngeal nerve is more commonly injured. Causes of paralysis:
- Idiopathic
- Traumatic, surgery
- Tumor: mediastinum, left hilum, or lung apex
- Arthritis (degenerative changes of cricoarytenoid cartilage)

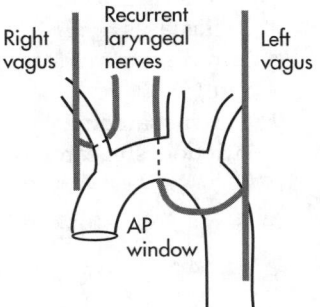

Radiographic features
- Abnormal movement of the involved cord
- Widening of laryngeal ventricle
- Expansion of pyriform sinus
- Flattening of false vocal cords
- Flattened subglottic angle

LARYNGOCELE

Dilatation of the laryngeal ventricle. Most commonly seen in glassblowers or patients with chronic obstructive pulmonary disease (COPD). May extend through the thyrohyoid membrane into the neck.

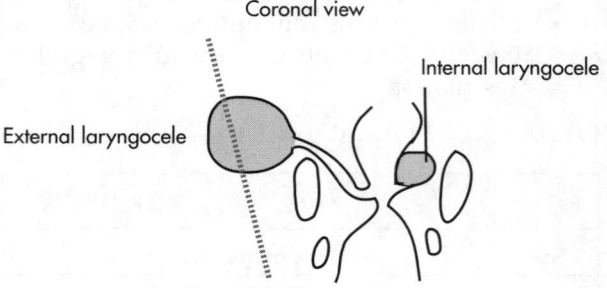

LARYNGEAL TRAUMA

Cause
Intubation: erosions, laryngomalacia, stenosis
Direct force: fractures. The main goal of CT is to demonstrate the presence of:
- Displaced fractures of thyroid or cricoid cartilage
- Arytenoid dislocation
- A false passage
- Displacement of epiglottis

Types
- Thyroid: longitudinal, paramedian, transverse, or comminuted fractures
- Cricoid: always breaks in 2 places, the posterior component is clinically often not recognized
- Epiglottis: may be avulsed posteriorly and superiorly
- Arytenoids: anterior and posterior dislocation

BENIGN LARYNGEAL TUMORS

- Papilloma and hemangioma are the most common tumors
- Less common tumors: chondroma, neurofibroma, fibroma, paraganglioma, rhabdomyoma, pleomorphic adenoma, lipoma
- Vocal cord polyps (not true tumors) are the most common benign lesion of the larynx

LARYNGEAL CARCINOMA

Histology
SCC, 90%
Others, 10%
- Adenocarcinoma
- Metastases
- Tumors arising from supporting tissues of larynx (chondrosarcoma, lymphoma, rare)
- Carcinosarcoma
- Adenocystic carcinoma

Types

Supraglottic, 30%
- Tumor arises from false cords, ventricles, laryngeal surface of epiglottis, arytenoids, aryepiglottic folds
- Usually large when discovered
- Treated by supraglottic laryngectomy or radiation

Glottic, 60%
- Tumor arises from true vocal cords including anterior commissure
- Usually small when discovered (hoarseness is an early finding)
- Early symptoms, good prognosis
- T1 tumors treated with cordectomy, hemilaryngectomy or radiation
- T3 tumors are treated with total laryngectomy

Subglottic, 10%
- Uncommon as an isolated lesion and usually seen as an extension of glottic tumors
- Poor prognosis because of early nodal metastases

Radiographic features

Common locations of mass lesions:
- Pyriform sinus (most common)
- Postcricoid
- Posterolateral wall

Determine mobility of cords (fluoroscopy); locate the cause of cord fixation:
- Cricoarytenoid joint arthritis
- Vocalis muscle invasion from tumor
- Paralaryngeal space tumor
- Recurrent laryngeal nerve paresis
- Idiopathic (? virus infection)

Invasion
- Fat spaces become obliterated; > 2 mm soft tissue indicates tumor spread to contralateral side of cord
- Thickening of anterior commissure
- Cartilage invasion: erosion, distortion (bowing, bulging, buckling), sclerosis (microinvasion)
- Adenopathy

Staging
- T1: confined to true vocal cords, normal mobility
- T2: confined to true vocal cords, limited mobility but no fixation of cords
- T3: fixation of cords

Pearls
- 25%-50% of supraglottic tumors have metastasized at time of surgery.
- Subglottic tumors metastasize most frequently.
- Glottic tumors confined to cords metastasize infrequently but spread locally to contralateral cord via anterior commissure or posterior interarytenoid area. Masses may also be due to hemorrhage, inflammation, edema, or fibrosis.

7

POSTSURGICAL LARYNX

Vertical hemilaryngectomy
- True vocal cord, laryngeal ventricle, false cord, ipsilateral thyroid lamina are removed
- Used to treat limited true vocal cord tumors or supraglottic tumors

Horizontal hemilaryngectomy (supraglottic)
- Epiglottis, aryepiglottic folds, false vocal cords, preepiglottic space, superior portion of thyroid cartilage, and portion of hyoid bone are removed.
- Used for selected tumors of epiglottis, aryepiglottic folds, and false vocal cord

Total laryngectomy
- Entire larynx and preepiglottic space, hyoid bone, strap muscles, and part of the thyroid gland are removed; permanent tracheostomy
- A neopharynx (extending from the base of the tongue to the esophagus) is created using muscular, mucosal, and connective tissue layers
- Used for extensive laryngeal tumors

Radical neck dissection
- Sternocleidomastoid muscle, IJV, lymph nodes, and submandibular salivary gland are removed
- Myocutaneous flaps are used for repair

Parapharyngeal Space

BRANCHIAL CLEFT CYST

Embryologic cysts derived from 1st or 2nd (most common) cervical pouch. Clinical: anterior triangle mass; may be infected.

Radiographic features
- Cyst location
     Type 1: EAC or parotid
     Type 2: anterior triangle, angle of mandible
- Signal intensity
     Water density (< 20 HU) unless infected (debris)
     Intense rim enhancement in infected cysts
- Cleft sinus passes between internal and external carotid artery

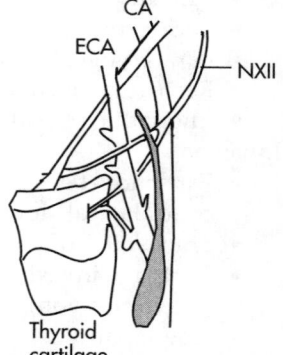

THYROGLOSSAL DUCT CYST

Extends from thyroid to foramen cecum. Clinical: palpable midline mass (80%). Represent 70% of congenital neck lesions.

Location
- Suprahyoid, 20%
- At hyoid bone 15%
- Infrahyoid, 65%

Radiographic features
- Thin-walled cystic structure
- Water density (< 20 HU)
- Thickening and enhancement of wall indicates infection

GLOMUS TUMORS (PARAGANGLIOMA, CHEMODECTOMA)

Benign tumors that arise from paraganglion cells of the sympathetic system. Tumors are very vascular and thus enhance extensively (CT, dense blush with angiography). Location:

- Skull base (glomus jugulare)
- Below skull base (glomus vagale)
- At carotid bifurcation (carotid body tumor)

GLASSCOCK-JACKSON GLOMUS TUMOR CLASSIFICATION	
Type	**Findings**
GLOMUS TYMPANICUM	
Type I	Tumor limited to promontory
Type II	Tumor completely filling middle ear space
Type III	Tumor filling middle ear, extending into mastoid or through tympanic membrane
Type IV	Tumor filling middle ear, extending into mastoid or through tympanic membrane to fill EAC; may extend anterior to internal carotid artery
GLOMUS JUGULARE	
Type I	Tumor involving jugulare bulb, middle ear, and mastoid
Type II	Tumor extending under internal auditory canal; may have intracranial extension
Type III	Tumor extending into petrous apex; may have intracranial extension
Type IV	Tumor extending beyond petrous apex into clivus or infratemporal fossa; may have intracranial extension

Sinuses, Nasal Cavity

General

SINUSES

- Frontal
- Ethmoid
- Sphenoid
- Maxillary

Osteomeatal complex (OMC)

- Control point for drainage from 3 sinuses: frontal, anterior ethmoid, maxillary
- Medial wall of OMC is formed by uncinate process
- Superolateral wall of OMC is formed by inferior orbital wall
- The infundibulum leads to the hiatus semilunaris
- The middle turbinate may contain an air cell (concha bullosa)
- Ostia for sinuses vary in size (depending on pO_2, mucus stasis)

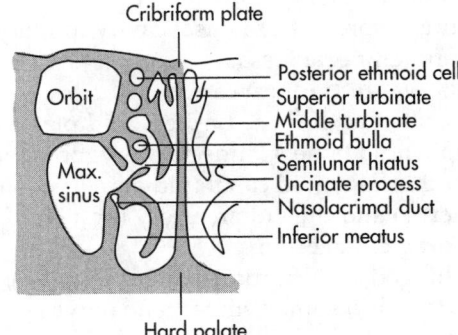

Labels: Cribriform plate, Orbit, Max. sinus, Hard palate, Posterior ethmoid cell, Superior turbinate, Middle turbinate, Ethmoid bulla, Semilunar hiatus, Uncinate process, Nasolacrimal duct, Inferior meatus

7

Cells

- Haller cells: ethmoidal cells extending along the medial floor of the orbit
- Onodi cells: most posterior ethmoidal cells that surround optic canal and optic nerve
- Agger nasi cells: ethmoid air cells frequently pneumatize adjacent bones such as frontal bone, maxilla, middle tubinate sphenoid, and/or lacrimal bone

Anatomic variation (may potentially lead to obstruction)

- Concha bullosa, 35%
- Septal deformity, 20%
- Paradox middle turbinate, 15%
- Reversed uncinate process
- Inferiorly migrated ethmoid bullae

Nasofrontal duct

- Frontal sinus drains directly into the frontal recess of the nasal cavity (85%)
- In 15% a nasofrontal duct drains frontal sinus into the ethmoid infundibulum

ANATOMICAL SPACES

Pterygopalatine fossa

Pyramidal space between upper pterygoid process and posterior wall of maxillary antrum. Fossa continues superiorly with the inferior orbital fissure and laterally with the infratemporal fossa. Pterygopalatine fossa is the crossroad of foramina and spread of pathology. Connections to other spaces:

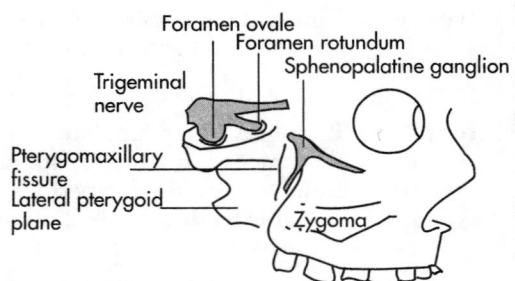

- Foramen rotundum leads to middle cranial fossa
- Sphenopalatine foramen connects to posterior nasal cavity
- Pterygoid (vidian) canal inferior and lateral to foramen rotundum (vessels and nerves)

Sphenopalatine foramen

The foramen extends from the pterygopalatine fossa to the posterior nasal cavity. Contains pterygopalatine vessels and nerves. Favored pathway of least resistance for tumor spread from nasal cavity to pterygopalatine fossa, inferior orbital fissure, and infratemporal fossa.

Pterygoid (vidian) canal

Located at the base of pterygoid plates below and lateral to foramen rotundum in the sphenoid bone. Connects pterygopalatine fossa and foramen lacerum. Contains nerve of the pterygoid canal (vidian nerve = continuation of greater superficial petrosal nerve) and the vidian artery (branch of the internal maxillary artery).

Foramen lacerum

Plugged with fibrocartilage during life; only branches of the ascending pharyngeal artery and some sympathetic nerves go through this foramen. Located at the base of the medial pterygoid plate. Favored site of nasopharyngeal carcinoma. Pathways to skull base:

- Fossa of Rosenmüller lies subjacent to foramen lacerum
- Prestyloid parapharyngeal space lies anterior
- Tensor and levator veli palatini take origin from this region
- Carotid artery rests on the foramen lacerum

Sinuses

ACUTE SINUSITIS

Frequency of involvement: maxillary > ethmoid, frontal > sphenoid sinus. Sinusitis is frequently associated with upper respiratory tract infections due to occlusion of draining ostia.

Types:
- Infectious sinusitis
    Acute
    Subacute
    Chronic
- Noninfectious (allergic)
- Dental infection and sinusitis (20% maxillary antrum)

Radiographic features
- Opacified sinus partial, complete
- Mucosal thickening
- Air-fluid levels
- Chronic sinusitis: mucosal hyperplasia, pseudopolyps, hyperostosis of bone
- Complications
    Mucous retention cyst
    Mucocele
    Osteomyelitis
    Cavernous sinus thrombosis
    Intracranial extension
        Empyema
        Cerebritis
        Abscess
    Orbital complications
- Recurrent sinusitis: hyperostosis, bone erosion (rare), mucosal hypertrophy

Pearls
- Plain film diagnosis of opaque sinus is nonspecific
- Obtain CT to assess bone detail and OMC anatomy for recurrent sinusitis
- Contrast-enhanced CT: tumors, polyps, and mucosa enhance, secretions do not enhance
- T2W: benign lesions are usually very bright; tumors have intermediate brightness

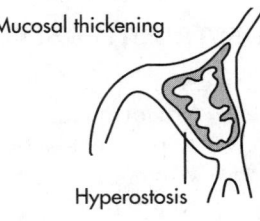

Mucosal thickening

Hyperostosis

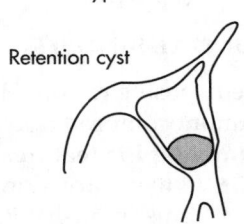

Retention cyst

MUCOUS RETENTION CYST

Incidence: 10% of population. Cysts occur from blockage of duct draining glands. Most commonly in maxillary sinus (floor).

Radiographic features
- Cysts adhere to sinus cavity wall without causing bony expansion (in contradistinction to mucocele)
- Rounded soft tissue mass T1W
- MRI signal intensity depends on pulse sequence used and protein content (see graph)

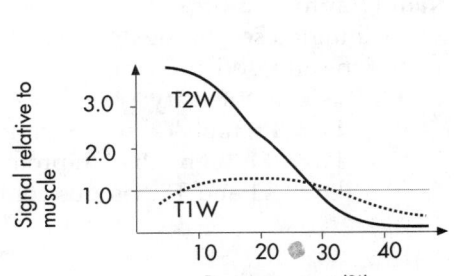

POLYPS

Most common tumors of sinonasal cavity. Diseases associated with sinonasal polyps:
- Polypoid rhinosinusitis (allergy)
- Infection
- Endocrine disorders
- Rhinitis medica (aspirin)

Radiographic features
- Location: ethmoid sinus > nose
- Soft tissue polyps are typically round
- Bony expansion and remodeling
- Very hyperintense on T2W
- Mucoceles may form as a result of blocked draining ostia

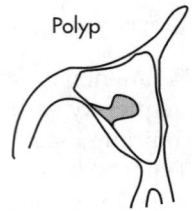

Polyp

DESTRUCTIVE SINUSITIS

Causes
- Mucormycosis
- Aspergillosis
- Wegener's granulomatosis
- Neoplasm

FUNGAL SINUSITIS

Predisposing factors: diabetes, prolonged antibiotic or steroid therapy, immunocompromised patient

Radiographic features
- Bony destruction and rapid extension into adjacent anatomic spaces
- Indistinguishable from tumor: biospy required
- Main role of CT/MRI is to determine extent of disease
- Aspergillosis may appear hyperdense on CT and hypointense on T1W
- If sphenoid sinus alone is involved, consider aspergillosis

MUCOCELE

True cystic lesion lined by sinus mucosa. Mucoceles occur as a result of complete obstruction of sinus ostium (inflammation, trauma, tumor). The bony walls of the sinus are remodelled as the pressure of secretions increases. In pediatric patients, consider cystic fibrosis. Location: frontal 65% > ethmoid 25% > maxillary > 10%. sphenoid (rare). Patients with polyposis may have multiple mucoceles.

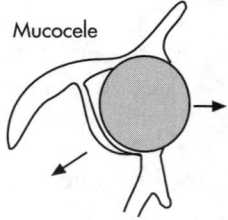

Mucocele

Radiographic features
- Rounded soft tissue density
- Typically isodense by CT
- MR signal intensity:
    Low T1, high T2: serous content
    High T1, high T2: high protein content
    Dark T1 and T2: viscous content

- Differential diagnosis signal voids within paranasal sinuses
  - Aerated sinus
  - Desiccated secretions
  - Calcifications
  - Fungal concretions (mycetoma)
  - Foreign body
  - Ectopic (undescended) tooth
  - Dentigerous cyst
  - Acute blood
- Distortion and expansion of bony sinus walls
- Nonenhancement unless infected (mucopyocele): rim enhancement
- Complication: breakthrough into orbit or anterior cranial fossa

BENIGN TUMORS

- Osteoma (most common paranasal sinus tumor)
- Papilloma
- Fibroosseous lesions
- Neurogenic tumors
- Giant cell granuloma

MALIGNANT TUMORS

Types

Squamous cell carcinoma, 90%
- Maxillary sinus, 80%
- Ethmoid sinus, 15%

Less common tumors, 10%
- Adenoid cystic carcinoma
- Esthesioneuroblastoma
  - Arises from olfactory epithelial cells
  - Commonly extends through cribriform plate
- Lymphoepithelioma
- Mucoepidermoid carcinoma
- Mesenchymal tumors: fibrosarcoma, rhabdomyosarcoma, osteosarcoma, chondrosarcoma
- Metastases from lung, kidney, breast

Tumor spread

Direct invasion
- Maxillary sinus:
  - Posterior extension: infratemporal fossa, pterygopalatine fossa
  - Superior extension: orbit
- Ethmoid or frontal sinus: frontal lobe

Lymph node metastases
- Submandibular, lateral pharyngeal, jugulodigastric nodes

Perineural spread
- Pterygopalatine fossa
- Connection to middle cranial fossa via foramen rotundum

ENDOSCOPIC SINUS SURGERY

The goal of endoscopic sinus surgery is to relieve obstructions of the sinus ostia. Endoscopic surgery replaces the more invasive procedures, such as Caldwell-Luc, for maxillary sinus access. Complications:
- Recurrent inflammatory disease due to adhesions, synechiae, incomplete removal, 10%
- Orbital complication, 5%
    Hematoma
    Abscess
    Optic nerve injury
- Intraoperative hemorrhage
- CSF leak, 1%
- Intracranial injury
- ICA dissection

Nose

COCAINE SEPTUM

Cocaine use can lead to nasal septal erosions and perforations because of its vasoconstrictive properties causing ischemia.

RHINOLITH

Calcification of foreign body or granuloma in nasal cavity. Clinical: nasal obstruction.

Glands and Periglandular Region

General

FLOOR OF MOUTH

- Formed by mylohyoid muscle
- Mylohyoid muscle extends from mandible to hyoid
- Above the mylohyoid muscle the floor is subdivided by different tongue muscles (genioglossus, geniohyoid)
- Sublingual space refers to the space between the mylohyoid and genioglossus-geniohyoid complex
- Submandibular space refers to space below mylohyoid. Not limited posteriorly; disease may spread to masticator or parapharyngeal space

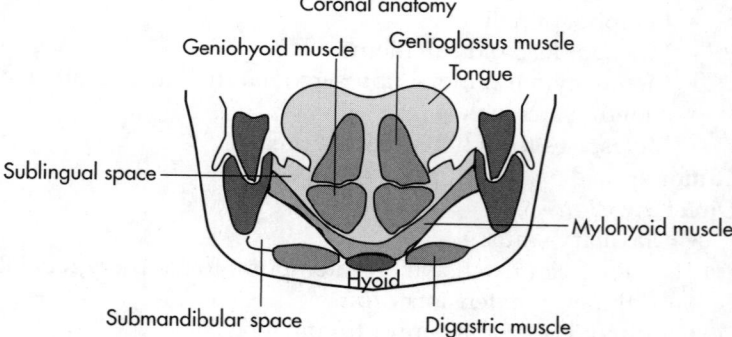

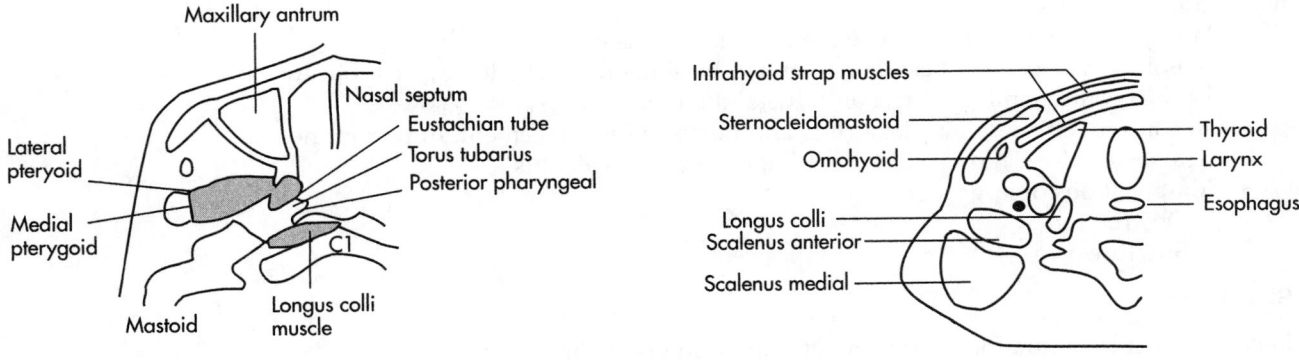

SUPERFICIAL NECK ANATOMY

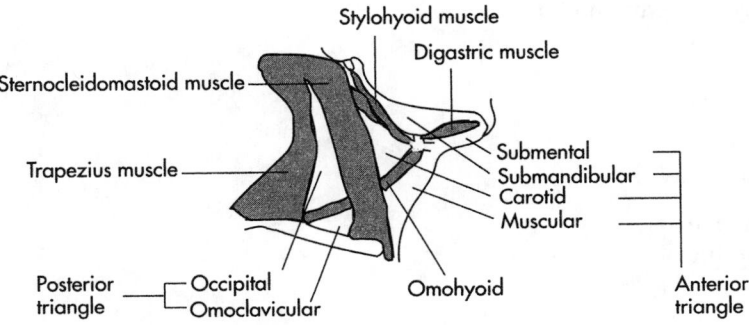

GLANDULAR STRUCTURES IN NECK

Salivary glands
- Parotid glands (inferior to external ear; Stenson's duct)
- Submandibular glands (medial to body of mandible; Wharton's duct)
- Sublingual glands (posterior to mandibular symphysis; Bartholin's duct)

Thyroid gland
Parathyroid gland

Salivary Glands

SIALOLITHIASIS (CALCULI)

Calculi are often composed of hydroxyapatite and multiple in 25% of patients. Total duct obstruction is usually due to calculi > 3 mm. Location:

Submandibular gland, 80%
- Most calculi are radiopaque (80%-90%). The higher incidence of submandibular calculi is due to (a) more alkaline pH of submandibular gland, which tends to precipitate salts; (b) thicker more mucousy submandibular saliva; (c) higher concentration of hydroxyapatite and phosphatase; (d) narrower Wharton's orifice compared with main lumen; (e) slight uphill course of salivary flow in Wharton's duct when patient is in upright position

Parotid, 20%
- 50% of calculi are radiopaque

Radiographic features

- Radiopaque calculi can often be seen on plain films or CT
- Radiolucent calculi are best demonstrated by sialography. Sialography typically shows a contrast filling defect and ductal dilatation
- On contract CT there may be strong and persistent enhancement. Important not to mistake calcification in stylohyoid ligament for a calculus
- Complications of large stones:
    Obstruction
    Strictures

SIALOSIS

Recurrent, noninflammatory enlargement of parotid gland (acinar hypertrophy, fatty replacement). Causes:

- Cirrhosis
- Malnutrition, alcoholics
- Drugs (thiourea, reserpine, phenylbutazone, heavy metal)

SIALOADENITIS

Acute sialoadenitis

- Bacterial, viral
- Abscess may form

Chronic, recurrent sialoadenitis

- Recurrent infection due to poor oral hygiene
- Sialography: multiple sites of peripheral ductal dilatation
- Small gland

Granulomatous inflammation

- Cause: sarcoid, TB, actinomycosis, cat-scratch disease, toxoplasmosis
- Produce intraglandular masses indistinguishable from tumors; biopsy is therefore required

SJÖGREN'S DISEASE

Autoimmune disease causing inflammation of secretory glands (e.g., lacrimal, parotid, submandibular, tracheobronchial tree). Male:Female = 1:9 (most common in menopausal women). Clinical features:

- Sicca complex: dry eyes (keratoconjuctivitis sicca), dry mouth, xerostomia (dry mouth)
- Systemic disease: rheumatoid arthritis

Radiographic features

Parotid gland enlargement (lymphoepithelial proliferation), 50%
Sialography patterns:

- Punctate: normal central and peripheral ductal system, punctate (1 mm) parenchymal contrast collections
- Globular: normal central system, peripheral duct system does not opacify, larger (> 2 mm) extraductal collections
- Cavitary: > 2 mm extraductal collections
- Destructive: ductal structures not opacified
- The MRI findings are similar to those seen by CT: parenchymal heterogeneity, cystic degeneration and fatty replacement

CYSTIC SALIVARY LESIONS

- Mucous retention cyst: true cyst with epithelial lining
- Ranula: retention cyst from sublingual glands in floor of mouth
- Mucocele (extravasation cyst): results from ductal rupture and mucous extravasation. Not a true cyst; composed of granulation tissue
- Benign lymphoepithelial cysts (BLC)
  - AIDS patients
  - Associated adenopathy and lymphoid hyperplasia may may be a clue to HIV seropositivity
  - Typically presents as bilateral parotid cysts, superficial in location
  - In absence of HIV infection, parotid cysts are rare
  - Warthin's tumor must be considered in the differential diagnosis
- Cystic tumors (Warthin's)
  - Bilateral in 10%
  - Accumulation of pertechnetate
  - Well-defined, lobulated, intermediate signal intensity mass with cystic areas

PAROTID TUMORS

Types

Benign, 80%

- Pleomorphic adenoma (most common), 70%
- Warthin's tumor (papillary cystadenoma lymphomatosum), 5% (of these 5%-20% are bilateral), male > female
- Rare: oncocytoma, hemangioma, adenoma

Malignant, 20%

- Mucoepidermoid carcinoma, 5%
- Carcinoma arising from pleomorphic adenoma, 5%
- Adenoid cystic carcinoma (cylindroma), 2%
- Adenocarcinoma, 4%
- Squamous cell carcinoma, 2%
- Oncocytic carcinoma, 1%

PLEOMORPHIC ADENOMA (MIXED TUMOR)

Most common (75%) benign salivary neoplasm. Clinical: unifocal mass, slow growing, well demarcated.

Radiographic features

- Well-circumscribed, encapsulated mass
- Superficial posterior glandular, location, 80%
- Lesions are hypoechoic by ultrasound (US)
- Moderate enhancement by CT
- Calcification in a parotid mass is very suggestive of pleomorphic adenoma
- Malignant transformation, 5%
- T1 hypointense, T2 hyperintense moderate enhancement
- MRI characteristics thay suggest malignancy include:
  - Irregular margins
  - Heterogeneous signal
  - Lymphadenopathy
  - Adjacent soft tissue or bone invasion
  - Facial perineural spread

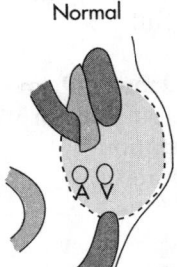

Normal

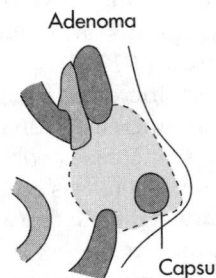

Adenoma

Capsule

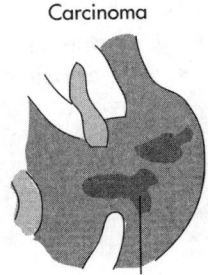

Carcinoma

Necrosis

7

- The deep lobe of the parotid gland extends between mandibular ramus and styloid process into the parapharyngeal space. For ideal surgical planning, masses arising from deep lobe (transparotid approach) must be differentiated from other parapharyngeal space masses (transcervical approach). In deep lobe masses there will be an absence of fatty tissue plane on some or all axial slices.. Normal parotid tissue partially wrapped around the mass or extension of mass laterally in to stylomandibular tunnel further suggests deep parotid lobe origin of mass.

MALIGNANT TUMORS

Radiographic features
- Areas of necrosis due to infarction (rapid growth)
- Locally invasive and agressive
- Lymph node metastases

Parathyroid

HYPERPARATHYROIDISM

Usually detected by increased serum calcium during routine biochemical screening. Incidence: 0.2% of the general population (female > male). Clinical manifestations of hyperparathyroidism: gastrointestinal complaints, musculoskeletal symptoms, and renal calculi. 3 types

Primary hyperparathyroidism:
- Adenoma, 80%
- Hyperplasia, 20%
- Parathyroid carcinoma, rare

Secondary hyperparathyroidism:
- Renal failure
- Ectopic parathormone (PTH) production by hormonally active tumors

Tertiary hyperparathyroidism: results from autonomous glandular function after long-standing renal failure

Clinical manifestations of hyperparathyroidism: GI complaints, musculoskeletal symptoms, and renal calculi.

Effect of PTH
- Increases vitamin D metabolism
- Increases renal calcium reabsorption (hypercalcemia)
- Increases bone resorption
- Decreases renal PO_4 resorption (hypophosphatemia)

Radiographic features

Parathyroid
- Single parathyroid adenoma, 80%
- Hyperplasia of all 4 glands, 20%

Bone
- Osteopenia
- Subperiosteal resorption (virtually pathognomonic)
- Brown tumors
- Soft tissue calcification

Renal
- Calculi (due to hypercalciuria)

PARATHYROID ADENOMA

Adenomas may consist of pure or mixed cell types, with the most common variant composed principally of chief cells. Some cases are associated with the multiple endocrine neoplasia (MEN) I syndrome. 80% single, 20% multiple.

Radiographic features

Detection

- US and scintigraphy are the best screening modalities
- Adenomas are hypoechoic by US
- If US is negative, further evaluation with CT or MRI may be helpful
- Angiography is reserved for patients with negative neck explorations and persistent symptoms
- Location:
    Adjacent to thyroid lobes
    Thoracic inlet
    Prevascular space in mediastinum (not in posterior mediastinum); the inferior glands follow the descent of the thymus (also a 3rd pouch derivative)

Angiography

- Adenomas are hypervascular
- Arteriography is most often performed following unsuccessful surgery and has a 60% success rate in that setting
- Venous sampling and venography: 80% success rate following unsuccessful neck explorations

HYPOPARATHYROIDISM

Cause

Idiopathic

- Rare; associated with cataracts, mental retardation, dental hypoplasia, obesity, dwarfism

Secondary

- Surgical removal (most common)
- Radiation
- Carcinoma
- Infection

TYPES OF HYPOPARATHYROIDISM				
Type	**Calcium**	**PO$_4$**	**PTH**	**Comments**
Hypoparathyroidism	↓	↑	↓	Surgical removal (most common cause)
Pseudohypoparathyroidism	↓	↑	∅↑	End-organ resistance to PTH (hereditary)
Pseudopseudohypoparathyroidism	∅	∅	∅	Only skeletal abnormalities (Albright's hereditary osteodystrophy)

Radiographic features
- Generalized increase in bone density, 10%
- Calcifications in basal ganglia
- Other calcifications: soft tissues, ligaments, tendon insertion sites

Thyroid

THYROID NODULE

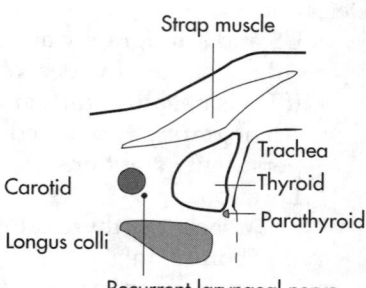

Thyroid US is usually performed with 5-10 MHz transducer. Images are obtained in transverse and longitudinal sections. Look for enlargement of lobes, cysts, hypoechoic or hyperechoic focal lesions and describe them as such.

Detection
- Allows precise localization of neck nodules (intrathyroid vs. extrathyroid)
- Detection of nonpalpable nodules in high risk groups (e.g., prior neck radiation, MEN II)
- Extent of disease (nodes, vessel invasion)
- Postsurgical follow-up

Differentiation
- US cannot reliably differentiate benign from malignant nodules
- US needle aspiration allows distinction of colloid cyst and adenoma
- Features suggestive of malignancy are:
  Solid mass
  Ill-defined margins
  Microcalcification rather than large or peripheral calcification

US guidelines for thyroid nodules:
- 80% of nodular disease is due to hyperplasia (pathologically they are referred to as hyperplastic, adenomatous, or colloid nodules).
- Malignant and benign nodules present simultaneously in 10%-20% cases, thus multiplicity is not a sign of benignity.
- Nodules with large cystic components are usually benign; however 20% of papillary cancers are cystic.
- Comet tail artifacts are seen in colloid cysts.
- In a solid hyperechoic nodule the incidence of malignancy is 5%.
- In a solid isoechoic nodule the incidence of malignancy is 25%.
- In a solid hypoechoic nodule the incidence of malignancy is 65%.
- A complete halo usually indicates a benign lesion; malignant lesions may be associated with incomplete halo.
- Haloes usually form around follicular lesions.

Types of Doppler color flow in thyroid nodules:
- Type 1: no flow
- Type 2: perinodular flow
- Type 3: intranodular flow (usually malignant)

Biopsy of focal nodules
- 25-G needle, US guidance
- Fine needle aspiration with little suction from 10-cc syringe
- Cytology interpretation
  Microfollicular: 5% malignant potential
  Macrofollicular: benign
  Mixed

Surgical removal
- High-risk group
- Cytologic findings are positive or equivocal
- Nodule grows despite suppressive T_4 therapy

THYROID FOLLICULAR ADENOMA

- Represent 5% of thyroid nodules
- Appear as solid masses with surrounding halo
- Difficult to differentiate from follicular cancer by cytology; thus these lesions need to be surgically resected

THYROIDITIS

OVERVIEW		
Type	Etiology	Clinical Manifestation
Subacute granulomatous thyroiditis (de Quervain's)	Postviral HLA-B35	Pain Hypothyroidism Systemic: fever, chills ESR > 50
Subacute lymphocytic thyroiditis	Autoimmune Postpartum	No pain Hypothyroidism
Hashimoto's thyroiditis*	Autoimmune HLA-DR3 HLA-B8	Early disease: hyperthyroidism 5% Late disease: hypothyroidism Antimicrosomal antibodies

*Hashimoto's thyroiditis is associated with pernicious anemia, SLE, Sjögren's, Addison's, Hashimoto's + Addison's = Schmidt's syndrome. Most thyroiditis shows Ga uptake.

Radiographic features
- Enlargement of thyroid
- Hypoechogenicity

GRAVES' DISEASE (DIFFUSE GOITER)

The etiology of Graves' disease is unknown but is associated with HLA-B8, DR3 (white patients), and HLA-Bw35, Bw46 (Asian patients). Pathogenetically it is an autoimmune disease in which T lymphocytes become sensitized to antigens within the thyroid gland and stimulate B lymphocytes to synthesize antibodies: thyroid-stimulating Ig (TSI). Graves' disease consists of one or more of the following:
- Thyrotoxicosis
- Goiter
- Ophthalmopathy
- Dermopathy: pretibial myxedema: accumulation of glycosaminoglycan in pretibial skin
- Rare findings:
    Subperiosteal bone formation (osteopathy of phalanges), rare
    Clubbing (thyroid acropathy)
    Onycholysis = separation of the nail from its bed
    Gynecomastia in males
    Splenomegaly, 10%
    Lymphadenopathy

Radiographic features

Scintigraphy

- Uniform distribution of increased activity by scintigraphy (Hashimoto thyroiditis can mimic this appearance, but Hashimoto patients are usually euthyroid)
- Elevated ^{131}I uptake: 50%-80%

US

- Enlarged thyroid
- Prominent pyramidal lobe

THYROID CANCER

Thyroid cancer is common (in 5% of all autopsies), but death due to thyroid cancer is uncommon (only 1200 deaths/year in the United States; the total of cancer deaths/year in the United States is > 500,000). Most common presentation of thyroid cancer is a solitary thyroid nodule. Incidence of thyroid cancer:

- In solitary nodule, 10%
- In hot nodule, very uncommon

Risk factors

- Male patient
- Young adult or child
- Palpable nodule
- Family history of goiter, thyroid cancer
- Prior head, neck irradiation

Poor prognostic factors

- Poor differentiation
- Male
- Advanced age
- Pain
- Lesion > 4 cm
- More than 4 adjacent structures involved

TYPES OF THYROID CANCER		
Type	Frequency	Comment
Papillary	60%	Metastases to cervical nodes, good prognosis
Follicular	25%	Aggressive, higher mortality (5-year survival is 50%)
Medullary	5%	Arises from C-cells (calcitonin); MEN association
Anaplastic	10%	Very aggressive, occur in older patients
Epidermoid	< 1%	
Other (lymphoma, metastases)	< 1%	

Staging

- T1:   nodule < 4 cm (= T1a) or > 4 cm (= T1b)
- T2:   nodule with partial fixation
- T3:   nodule with complete fixation
- N1:   regional nodes (ipsilateral 1a; contralateral 2b; bilateral 2c)
- N2:   fixed regional lymph nodes
- M1:   metastases

Radiographic features
- Cancers are most commonly detected during routine workup of nodules and multinodular goiter
- [131]I is used for detection of metastases
- Since normal hormone production can blunt TSH stimulation and prevent tumor detection, residual postsurgical thyroid tissue is usually ablated with [131]I
- Anaplastic and medullary cancers do not concentrate ^{131}I and are therefore not detectable by iodine scanning

Medullary thyroid cancer
- Thyroid mass
- Calcification, 10%
- Early spread to adjacent organs and chest
- Adenopathy
- Bullae formation, pulmonary fibrosis may occur as part of a desmoplastic reaction

Mandible and Maxilla

Cystic Masses

OVERVIEW

Odontogenic cysts
- Radicular cysts: caused by caries and infection; periapical lucency with sclerotic margins. Usually asymptomatic. No malignant potential.
- Dentigerous cyst
- Odontogenic keratocyst (basal cell nevus syndrome)
- Developmental lateral periodontal cyst (Botryoid cyst)

Nonodontogenic cysts
- Fissural cysts
    Nasopalatine duct cyst
    Globulomaxillary cyst
    Nasolabial cyst
- Solitary, simple hemorrhagic bone cyst
- Static bone cavity (Stafne cyst)

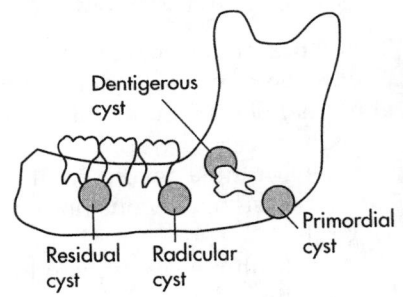

DENTIGEROUS CYST (FOLLICULAR CYST)

Most common pericoronal radiolucency. Formed by excessive accumulation of fluid between enamel and dental capsule. Most frequently seen in mandible (80%) with unerupted 3rd molars or maxilla (20%).

Radiographic features
- Well-corticated pericoronal radiolucency
- May become very large and occupy entire ramus
- Expansion of mandibular cortex
- May displace teeth
- Complications:
    Common: infection, pathologic fractures
    Rare: ameloblastoma, squamous cell carcinoma (SCC), mucoepidermoid carcinoma

ODONTOGENIC KERATOCYST

Aggressive cystic jaw lesion in mandible (70%) or maxilla (30%). Associated with basal cell nevus syndrome (Gorlin's) syndrome. High rate of recurrence.

Radiographic features

- Scalloped corticated border (typical)
- Large size, rapid growth
- Perforation of bone cortex
- Displacement of teeth

Benign Tumors

OVERVIEW

- Ameloblastoma
- Odontoma
- Fibromyxoma
- Cementoma

AMELOBLASTOMA (ADAMANTINOMA)

Multilocular expansile radiolucent lesion most commonly located in ramus area. Locally aggressive.

BASAL CELL NEVUS (GORLIN'S) SYNDROME

This syndrome, a phakomatosis, consists of multiple basal cell nevi of the skin, odontogenic jaw cysts (derived from odontogenic epithelium), and a variety of other abnormalities. Evolution of basal cell carcinoma at the age of 30 years.

Skin

- Multiple nevoid basal cell carcinoma, palmar plantar dyskeratosis, sebaceous cysts, cutaneous fibroma

Oral

- Multiple jaw cysts (odontogenic keratocysts), mandibular prognathism, cleft lip or palate, ameloblastoma, squamous cell carcinoma

Other

- CNS: agenesis of corpus callosum, congenital hydrocephalus, medulloblastoma, meningioma, cerebellar astrocytoma, craniopharyngioma, dural calcification
- Skeletal: rib anomalies, short 4th metacarpal (50%), vertebral anomalies, polydactyly, clavicular and scapular deformities
- Eyes: congenital blindness, cataracts, glaucoma, coloboma
- Genital: uterine and ovarian fibromas (often with calcification), hypogonadism, cryptorchism

Malignant Tumors

OVERVIEW

Primary odontogenic tumors, rare

- Odontogenic carcinoma
- Odontogenic sarcoma

Primary nonodontogenic primary tumors
- Osteosarcoma
- Chondrosarcoma
- Ewing's sarcoma
- Multiple myeloma
- Others

Metastases
- Carcinomas, 85% (breast, lung, renal)
- Sarcomas, 5%
- Other

PRIMARY ODONTOGENIC MALIGNANCIES

Extremely rare tumors. Always rule out primary nonodontogenic bone tumors which are more common. Classification:

Odontogenic carcinoma
- Malignant ameloblastoma
- Primary intraosseous carcinoma
- Other carcinomas arising from odontogenic epithelium

Odontogenic sarcoma
- Ameloblastic fibrosarcoma
- Ameloblastic odontosarcoma

Temporomandibular Joint (TMJ)

ANATOMY

Joint is composed of two synovial compartments separated by a fibrocartilage disk. Posterior capsular attachment is very elastic (bilaminar zone). In the open mouth position the condyle and disk translate anteriorly.

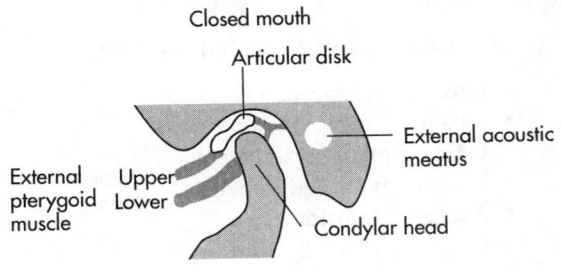

Closed mouth
Articular disk
External acoustic meatus
External pterygoid muscle
Upper
Lower
Condylar head

DISK DISPLACEMENT

Clinical: pain, clicking, locked jaw.

Types
- Anteromedial displacement with reduction (most common type); disk is displaced anteriorly in the open mouth view and recaptured in the closed mouth view
- Persistent anterior displacement; disk does not reduce closed lock
- Rotational displacement
- Medial displacement (uncommon)

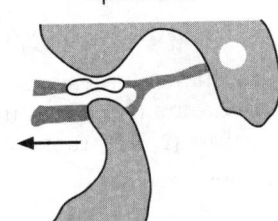

Open mouth

DEGENERATIVE CHANGES OF TMJ

Radiographic findings are similar to those of osteoarthritis in other joints:
- Joint space narrowing
- Subchondral sclerosis, spuring, pseudocyst formation
- Deformity
- Avascular necrosis

Differential Diagnosis

Temporal Bone

APPROACH

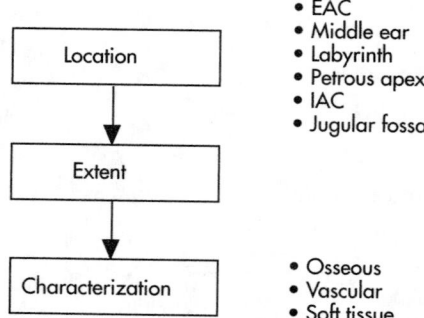

- EAC
- Middle ear
- Labyrinth
- Petrous apex
- IAC
- Jugular fossa

- Osseous
- Vascular
- Soft tissue

SOFT TISSUE MASS IN MIDDLE EAR

- Cholesteatoma
- Chronic otitis media
- Granulation tissue
- Cholesterol granuloma
- Glomus tympanicum tumor
- Aberrant internal carotid artery
- High or dehiscent jugular bulb

VASCULAR MASS IN MIDDLE EAR

- Glomus tympanicum
- Aberrant carotid artery
- Carotid artery aneurysm
- Persistent stapedial artery
- Exposed jugular bulb
- Exposed carotid artery
- Hemangioma
- Extensive glomus jugulare

INTRACANALICULAR INTERNAL AUDITORY CANAL MASSES

Exclusively intracanalicular lesions
- Acoustic neuroma (NVIII), common
- Facial neuroma (NVII), rare
- Hemangioma
- Lipoma

Not primarily intracanalicular
- Meningioma
- Epidermoid

JUGULAR FOSSA MASS

- Glomus jugular tumor, most common
- Neurofibroma, second most common
- Schwannoma
- Chondrosarcoma
- Metastases

MASTOID BONE DEFECT

- Neoplastic bone destruction
- Cholesteatoma
- Postoperative simple mastoidectomy
- Postoperative radical mastoidectomy
- Postraumatic deformity

Orbit

APPROACH TO ORBITAL MASSES

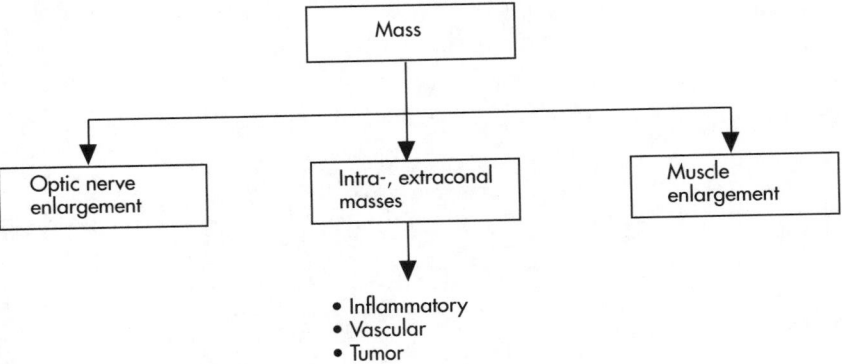

ORBITAL MASSES BY ETIOLOGY

Tumors
- Hemangioma (adults: cavernous; children: capillary)
- Lymphoma
- Metastases
- Lymphangioma
- Less common
    - Rhabdomyosarcoma
    - Hemangiopericytoma
    - Neurofibroma

Inflammatory
- Pseudotumor, common
- Thyroid ophthalmopathy, common
- Cellulitis, abscess
- Granulomatous: Wegener's disease

Vascular
- Carotid-cavernous fistula
- Venous varix
- Thrombosis of superior ophthalmic vein

Trauma
- Hematoma
- Foreign body

EXTRACONAL DISEASE

Nasal disease
- Infection
- Neoplasm

Orbital bone disease
- Subperiosteal abscess
- Osteomyelitis
- Fibrous dysplasia
- Tumors
- Trauma

Sinus disease
- Mucocele
- Invasive infections
- Neoplasm

Lacrimal gland disease
- Adenitis
- Lymphoma
- Pseudotumor
- Tumor

INTRACONAL DISEASE

Well-defined margins
- Hemangioma
- Schwannoma
- Orbital varix
- Meningioma

Ill-defined margins
- Pseudotumor
- Infection
- Lymphoma
- Metastases

Muscle enlargement
- Pseudotumor
- Graves' disease (thyroid ophthalmopathy)
- Myositis
- Carotid cavernous fistula

VASCULAR ORBITAL LESIONS

Tumor
- Hemangioma, hemangioendothelioma, hemangiopericytoma
- Lymphangioma
- Meningioma

Vascular (with enlarged superior ophthalmic vein)
- Carotid cavernous fistula
- Cavernous thrombosis
- Orbital varix
- Ophthalmic artery aneurysm

OPTIC NERVE SHEATH ENLARGEMENT

Tumor
- Optic nerve glioma
- Meningioma
- Meningeal carcinomatosis
- Metastases, lymphoma, leukemia

Inflammatory
- Optic neuritis
- Pseudotumor
- Sarcoid

Increased intracranial pressure

Trauma: hematoma

TRAMTRACK ENHANCEMENT OF ORBITAL NERVE

- Optic nerve meningioma
- Optic neuritis
- Idiopathic
- Pseudotumor
- Sarcoidosis
- Leukemia, lymphoma
- Perioptic hemorrhage
- Metastases
- Normal variant

OCULAR MUSCLE ENLARGEMENT

- Thyroid ophthalmopathy (most common cause); painless
- Pseudotumor; painful
- Infection from adjacent sinus
- Granulomatous: TB, sarcoid, cysticercosis
- Rare causes: high flow (dural AVM, carotid cavernous sinus fistula [CCF], lymphangioma), hemorrhage, tumor (lymphoma, rhabdomyosarcoma, leukemia, metastases), trauma, acromegaly, apical mass

ORBITAL MASSES

OVERVIEW		
	Children	Adults
Tumor	Retinoblastoma	Hemangioma
	Rhabdomyosarcoma	Schwannoma
	Optic nerve glioma	Melanoma
	Lymphoma	Meningioma
	Hemangioma	Lymphoma
Other	Dermoid cyst	Pseudotumor
		Trauma

Mnemonic for childhood orbital masses: "LO VISON"

- **L**eukemia
- **O**ptic nerve glioma
- **V**ascular malformation (hemangioma, lymphangioma)
- **I**nflammation
- **S**arcoma, rhabdomyosarcoma
- **O**phthalmopathy, orbital pseudotumor
- **N**euroblastoma

CYSTIC LESIONS OF THE ORBIT

- Dermoid
- Epidermoid
- Teratoma
- Aneurysmal bone cyst
- Cholesterol granuloma
- Colobomatous cyst

T1 HYPERINTENSE ORBITAL MASSES

Tumor
- Melanotic melanoma
- Retinoblastoma
- Choroidal metastases
- Hemangioma

Detachment
- Coats' disease
- Persistent hyperplastic primary vitreous
- Trauma

Other
- Hemorrhage
- Phthisis bulbi
- Intravitreal oil treatment for detachment

GLOBE CALCIFICATIONS

Tumor
- Retinoblastoma (95% are calcified, 35% are bilateral)
- Astrocytic hamartoma (associated with: tuberous sclerosis, NF)
- Choroidal osteoma

Infection (chorioretinitis)
- Toxoplasmosis
- Herpes
- CMV
- Rubella

Other
- Phthisis bulbi
    Calcification in endstage disease
    Shrunken bulb
- Optic nerve drusen
    Most common cause of calcifications in adults
    Bilateral

SUDDEN ONSET OF PROPTOSIS

- Orbital varix (worsened by Valsalva maneuver)
- Hemorrhage into cavernous hemangioma
- CCF
- Hemorrhage into lymphangioma
- Thrombosis of superior orbital vein

LACRIMAL GLAND ENLARGEMENT

Lymphoid lesions, 50%
- Benign lymphoid hyperplasia
- Pseudotumor
- Sjögren's syndrome
- Mikulicz's disease
- Lymphoma

Epithelial neoplasm
- Pleomorphic adenoma, 75%
- Adenoid cystic carcinoma

DIFFUSE BONE ABNORMALITY

Signs: bony enlargement (fibrous dysplasia), expansion, sclerosis.
- Fibrous dysplasia
- Paget's disease
- Thalassemia
- Congenital (rare): osteopetrosis, craniometa and diaphyseal dysplasia

7

Sinuses

RADIOOPAQUE SINUS

Normal variant
- Hypoplasia
- Unilateral thick bone

Sinusitis (acute: AFL; chronic: mucosal thickening, retention cysts)
- Allergic
- Fungal: aspergillosis, mucormycosis
- Granulomatous: sarcoid, Wegener's disease

Solid masses
- SCC
- Polyp, inverted papilloma
- Lymphoma
- Juvenile angiofibroma; most common tumor in children
- Mucocele: expansile, associated with cystic fibrosis in children

Postsurgical
- Caldwell-Luc operation

Nasooropharynx

MUCOSAL SPACE MASS

Tumors
- SCC
- Lymphoma
- Rhabdomyosarcoma
- Melanoma

Benign masses
- Adenoids
- Juvenile angiofibroma
- Thornwaldt's cyst

PARAPHARYNGEAL AND CAROTID SPACE MASSES

Tumor
- Salivary gland tumors, 80% are benign, 20% are malignant
- Neurogenic tumor (schwannomas, glomus vagale)
- Nasopharyngeal carcinoma
- Lymphadenopathy: benign, malignant

Abscess, cellulitis

PREVERTEBRAL MASS

- Metastases
- Chordoma
- Osteomyelitis, abscess
- Hematoma

Neck

CYSTIC EXTRATHYROID LESIONS

Neck
- Branchial cleft cyst (lateral to carotid artery)
- Thyroglossal duct cyst (midline mass)
- Ranula (retention cyst) of sublingual glands
- Retention cysts of mucous glands (parotid)
- Cystic hygroma (lymphangioma): most common < 2 years of age
- Rare lesions: cervical thymic cysts, dermoid, teratoma, hemangioma

Nasooropharynx
- Thornwaldt's cyst
- Mucous retention cyst (obstructed glands)
- Necrotic SCC (thick wall)

Larynx, paralaryngeal space
- Laryngocele
- Mucous retention cyst

CYSTIC THYROID LESIONS

- Colloid cysts
- Cystic degeneration
- Cystic tumor
    Papillary cancer
    Cystic metastases (papillary cancer)

SOLID NECK MASS

Tumor
- SCC of larynx or nasooropharynx (common)
- Lymphadenopathy
    Reactive hyperplasia
    Malignant
- Parotid tumors
- Neural tumors
    Neurilemoma
    Neurofibroma
    Glomus tumors
- Other rare tumors
    Mesenchymal, dermoid, teratoma

Inflammatory
- Infection (abscess, fungal, TB)
- Granulomatous inflammation (sarcoid, TB lymphadenitis = scrofula)

Congenital
- Ectopic thyroid

7

VASCULAR HEAD AND NECK MASSES

- Glomus tumor
    - Carotid body tumor
    - Glomus vagale
    - Glomus jugulare
    - Glomus tympanicum
- Hemangioma
- AVM
- Aneurysm (often ICA)
    - Pseudoaneurysm
    - Posttraumatic

AIDS

ENT complications occur in 50% of patients.

Parotid
- Multiple intraparotid cystic masses (benign lymphoepithelial lesion)
- Lymphadenopathy

Sinonasal
- Sinusitis (*Staphylococcus, Streptococcus, Pseudomonas > Legionella, Cryptococcus, Pneumocystis carinii,* CMV)
- Kaposi's sarcoma (uncommon)

Oral cavity
- *Candida*
- Periodontal and gingival infections

Pharynx/larynx
- Opportunistic infections
- Epiglottitis
- Lymphoma (tonsils)

Temporal bone (rare)
- Otitis media: *Pneumocystis carinii*
- Otitis externa: *Pseudomonas*

SUGGESTED READINGS

Bailey B (ed): *Head and neck surgery–Otolaryngology,* Philadelphia, 2001, Lippincott Williams & Wilkins.
Delbalso AM: *Maxillofacial imaging,* Philadelphia, 1990, WB Saunders.
Harnsberger HR: *Handbooks in radiology: head and neck imaging,* St Louis, 1994, Mosby.
Latchaw RE: *MR and CT imaging of the head, neck, and spine,* ed 2, St Louis, 1991, Mosby.
Mancuso A, Harnsberger HR, Dillon W: *Workbook for MRI and CT of the head and neck,* Baltimore, 1989, Williams & Wilkins.
Ramsey RG: *Neuroradiology,* Philadelphia, 1994, WB Saunders
Schnitzlein H, Murtagh F: *Imaging anatomy of the head and spine,* Baltimore, 1990, Urban & Schwarzenberg.
Som PM, Bergeron RT: *Head and neck imaging,* ed 2, St Louis, 1995, Mosby.
Valvassori GE: *Head and neck imaging,* New York, 1988, Thieme Medical Publishers.

Chapter 8

Vascular Imaging

Chapter Outline

8

Techniques

General

PREPROCEDURE EVALUATION

1. What is the indication for the procedure?
   - Diagnosis
   - Preoperative staging
   - Therapy
2. Define the problem
   - What is the diagnostic question that is to be answered?
   - What study can best answer the question (ultrasound [US], computed tomography [CT], magnetic resonance imaging [MRI], angiography)?
3. Patient history, interview, examination
   - Review chart
   - Key data: signs and symptoms
       Prior vascular surgery/interventions
       Prior studies
       Laboratory values
       Other medical illnesses
       Pulse examination
   - Explanation of the procedure to the patient
   - Obtain informed consent
4. Assess risk vs. benefit (there are no absolute contraindications to angiography)
   - Approach and access
   - Coagulopathy?
   - Renal insufficiency?
   - What are alternative options?
5. Preprocedural orders
   - Appropriate labs drawn (i.e., PT/PTT)?
   - Appropriate medication withheld (i.e., Coumadin)?
   - IV access present?
   - Hydration
   - Clear liquids only
   - Premedication if necessary

ACCESS

Types of arterial approaches
- Right femoral artery
- Left femoral artery
- Left axillary artery
- Right axillary artery
- Translumbar aorta
- Brachial arteries
- Antegrade femoral artery
- Through a surgical graft

Right femoral approach is the preferred route
- Easily accessible for manipulations and hemostasis
- Large caliber vessel
- Well-defined landmarks exist.
- Most angiographers are right-handed.
- Low complication rate compared to other approaches

Standard femoral approach: Seldinger technique
- Double wall technique is preferred.
- Advantages of "single wall" puncture are only theoretical.
- Use fluoroscopy to determine puncture level.
     Artery entry: midfemoral head
     Skin entry: inferior margin of femoral head
- Local anesthesia at skin entry site: 1%-2% lidocaine
- Palpate artery above site
- Advance 18-G Seldinger needle (45-60 degree angle) to bone.
- Remove central stylet and withdraw slowly.
- Advance guidewire through needle, while good pulsatile flow jets out the hub.
- Always fluoroscope when advancing a guidewire.
- Never advance guidewire against resistance.
- Exchange needle over wire for dilator or catheter.

Advantage of puncturing symptomatic extremity
- Inflow can be assessed by obtaining pull-down pressures.
- Should complications arise (i.e., emboli, thrombosis), they will affect the already compromised extremity.
- Conversion to antegrade approach is possible if necessary.

Disadvantage of puncturing symtomatic extremity
- May interfere with surgical procedure if complication develops (e.g., hematoma)
- If a severe stenosis is present, a catheter may obturate the vessel completely.

Axillary artery approach
- Main indication for this approach are nonpalpable femoral pulses (i.e., aortic occlusion)
- Left-side approach is preferred
     Easier to access descending aorta
     Left-sided approach crosses fewer CNS arteries
- 3J wire is preferred
- Disadvantages:
     Difficult to compress
     Relatively high incidence of complications (e.g., stroke, bleeding, thrombosis)
     Brachial plexus injury
- Always check for blood pressure differential to detect occult arterial disease.

Translumbar approach (TLA)
- Main indication for this approach are nonpalpable peripheral pulses
- High TLA is preferred: above abdominal aortic aneurysm, grafts, diseased distal aorta
- Disadvantages
     Patient must lie prone for entire study
     Higher incidence of bleeding (debatable)
     More difficult to manipulate catheters
- Use an 18-G needle/sheath system

8

Antegrade femoral approach
- The main indication for this approach is a distal extremity intervention (e.g., percutaneous transluminal angioplasty [PTA] of superficial femoral artery [SFA]).
- Retrograde catheterization may be converted to antegrade access with a Simmons 1 catheter and a 3J or angled glide wire.
- Difficult to manage in obese patients

ANGIOGRAPHY COMPLICATIONS

There are four types of complications:
- Puncture site complications (e.g., groin hematoma)
- Contrast agent complications (e.g., anaphylactoid reaction)
- Catheter-related complications (e.g., vessel dissection)
- Therapy-related complications (e.g., central nervous system [CNS] bleed during UK)

Puncture site and contrast media complications are the most frequent complications during angiography. Puncture site problems depend on coagulation status, size of catheter, patient body habitus, and compliance issues. The overall incidence of death related to angiography is very low (< 0.05%).

Puncture site complications
- Minor hematoma, > 5%
- Major hematoma that requires surgical therapy, < 0.5%
- Arteriovenous fistula (AVF), 0.05%
- Pseudoaneurysm, 0.01%
- Vessel thrombosis, 0.1%
- Neuritis
- Infection

Contrast complications (see also Chapter 19)
- Renal failure
- Cardiac failure
- Phlebitis (venography)
- Anaphylactoid reactions (rare with arteriography)

Catheter-related complications
- Cholesterol emboli
- Thromboembolism
- Cerebrovascular accident
- Arterial dissection

Pearls
- Complications can be limited by:
  Careful preangiography assessment (e.g., correct coagulopathies)
  Appropriate approach (e.g., history and pulse examination)
  Good technique (e.g., trained angiographer)
- Risk factors for development of AVF or pseudoaneurysm:
  Low puncture
  Heparinization
  Large catheters
- Most puncture site complications can be prevented by good manual compression and correction of coagulopathies prior to angiography.
- Always reassess patient after the procedure.

Hardware

CATHETERS

Generic types
Diagnostic catheters
- High-flow catheters with sideholes are used for central vessels (> 10 mL/sec)
- Low-flow catheters with endhole are used for selective arterial work

Therapeutic catheters
- Balloon catheters (PTA and occlusion balloon)
- Atherectomy catheters
- Coaxial infusion catheters
- Embolization catheters

Measurements
- Outer diameter (OD): catheter size is determined by the OD and given in "French" size. French (Fr) = the circumference in millimeters. Divide French size by 3 to obtain OD in mm.
- Inner diameter (ID): measured in 1/1000 of an inch
- Length: measured in centimeters. 65 cm is commonly used for abdominal studies. 100 cm is usually used for arch and carotid studies.

SPECIFIC CATHETERS		
Catheter Type	**Use**	
Pigtail	Aorta, pulmonary	
Cobra (C)	Mesenteric, renal, contralateral iliac	
Simmons (S)	Mesenteric, arch vessels	
Headhunter (H)	Carotid, arch vessels	
Berenstein	Carotid	
Davis	Arch, carotids, upper extremity	
Tracker	Coaxial subselection	

Cobra   Simmons   Pigtail

8

FLOW RATES OF INJECTIONS (MGH)			
	Catheter	Injection*	Comments
Abdominal aorta	Pigtail/tip occluded straight	20/40	Tip occluded straight catheter for iliac pressures
Celiac	C2, S2	6/60	Variations in anatomy are common
Renals	C2, S2	5/15	Multiple vessels in 25%
SMA	C2, S2	6/60	IA priscoline for venous phase
CT portography	In SMA	3/120	Helical CT
IMA	S2, CZ	2/20	Requires 2 runs to include entire vascular territory
Splenic	Variable	5/50	Good splenic vein opacification
Hepatic	Variable	5/50	Dual (artery, portal) blood supply; variable anatomy
Pelvis	Pigtail	10/40	Position above bifurcation
Internal iliac	C2, S2	5/25	
One leg runoff	Straight tip	4/48	In external iliac
Two leg runoff	Pigtail	6/72	Position above bifurcation
Arm	H1	variable	LOCA (reduces pain)
IVC	Pigtail	15/45	
Aortic arch	Pigtail	30/60	Higher injections in young patients
CCA	Davis A1	7/11	60% HOCA or LOCA
ICA	Davis A1	6/8	60% HOCA or LOCA
ECA	Davis A1	2/4	60% HOCA or LOCA
Vertebral	Davis A1	6/8	60% HOCA or LOCA
Coronary	Judkins	4/8	LOCA

*Flow rate (mL/sec)/total volume of injection (mL). For cut film.

Pearls

- Rate and volume of contrast are reduced for digital subtraction angiography (DSA).
- Rate and volume always depend on rate of blood flow and size of vessel observed under fluoroscopy.

Material

- Thermoplastics materials (polyurethane and polyethylene) are very commonly used for catheter manufacturing.
- Nylon: combined with polyurethane to manufacture high-flow, small French catheters
- Teflon: very stiff, low-friction material
- Braided catheters: internal wire mesh improves torquability

Pearls

- Shorter catheters allow for higher flow rates and easier exchangeability.
- The larger the ID, the better the flow dynamics.
- It is good practice to size catheters, sheaths, and wires prior to their use; considerable discrepancy of dimensions may occur (variable among manufacturers).
- Maximum flow rate and pressure tolerance of catheters is specified by manufacturer on package or insert.

GUIDEWIRES

All nonspecialty guidewires have a similar construction:
- Central stiff steel core with a distal taper
- Wire coilspring wound around core
- Thin filamentous safety wire holding the other two components together
- Most wires are coated with Teflon to decrease friction.

Measurements
- Length: 145 cm is the standard length and allows exchanges of 65 cm catheters. "Exchange length" wires are 220-250 cm in length and are used for long catheters.
- OD: guidewires are designated by OD in 1/1000 of an inch: 0.018-0.038 is the most common size range.
- J tip: refers to the radius of wire curvature in millimeters (i.e., a 3J wire has a 3-mm distal curvature)

SPECIFIC GUIDEWIRES	
Wire	**Major Use/Comments**
3J	Tortuous and diseased vessels, avoids selecting branch vessels
15J	Large vessels: femoral, aorta, IVC
Straight wire	Dissection is more common
Rosen	Exchanges/PTA
Amplatz stiff	Exchanges, tortuous iliac arteries
Bentson	Long flexible taper (floppy end)
Terumo	Slippery hydrophilic coating; glides well, torque guide

Pharmacological Manipulation

DRUGS COMMONLY USED			
	Dosage*	**Use**	**Comments**
VASODILATOR			
Papaverine	1 mg/min infusion	Mesenteric ischemia	Smooth muscle relaxant
Tolazoline (priscoline)	25 mg IA	Peripheral spasm	Direct muscle relaxant
Nitroglycerine	100 µg IA or IV	Peripheral spasm	Direct muscle relaxant
Nifedipine	10 mg SL	Peripheral spasm	Calcium channel blocker
VASOCONSTRICTOR			
Vasopressin (Pitressin)	0.2-0.4 U/min	GI bleeding	Contraindications: CAD, HTN, arrhythmias
Epinephrine	5 µg	Renal vasoconstriction	Differentiate tumor from normal renal vessels

IA, Intraarterial; *IV*, intravenous; *SL*, sublingual; *GI*, gastrointestinal; *CAD*, coronary artery disease; *HTN*, hypertension.
*See manufacturer's package insert for specific rates of administration.

Angiographic Interventions

EMBOLIZATION

Indication
Hemorrhage
- Gastrointestinal (GI) bleeding
- Varices
- Traumatic organ injury
- Bronchial artery hemorrhage
- Tumors
- Postoperative bleeding

Vascular lesions
- AVM or AVF
- Pseudoaneurysms

Preoperative devascularization
- Renal cell carcinoma
- AVM
- Vascular bone metastases

Other
- Hypersplenism
- Gonadal varices
- Hepatic chemoembolization

General principles
- Proximal occlusion is equivalent to surgical ligation. It does not compromise collateral flow. For this reason, it may be ineffective to control bleeding if collaterals continue to supply the bleeding site.
- Distal embolization usually infarcts tissue followed by necrosis.
- Temporary vs. permanent embolization: tumors, vascular lesions, varices, and preoperative embolizations are usually permanent occlusions. GI bleeding is best treated with Gelfoam at first (if vasopressin has failed).
- Be as selective as possible (i.e., use tracker catheter).
- Prevent reflux of embolic material into other vessels.
- Document preangiographic and postangiographic appearance.

Embolic agents
Temporary
- Surgical gelatin (Gelfoam): not FDA approved for embolization
- Pledgets are cut to size or occlude large vessels; Gelfoam powder occludes distal vessels and causes infarction.

Permanent
- Steel coils of variable: sizes are commercially available; coils obstruct proximal vessels
- Microcoils (platinum) are used to occlude more distal vessels.
- Detachable balloons are used for large vessel occlusion. FDA restricted. Useful for pulmonary AVF, carotid cavernous fistula.
- Polyvinyl alcohol (Ivalon): small particles for distal occlusion. 200-1000 μm. Suspend in albumin-contrast agent mixture.
- Absolute ethanol: causes tissue necrosis. Used with proximal balloon occlusion to minimize shunting and reflux. Useful for solid organ necrosis (i.e., malignant tumors).
- Plastic polymers: glue, tissue adhesives

EMBOLIZATION MATERIALS		
Material	Occlusion	Primary Use
TEMPORARY AGENTS		
Autologous blood clot	6-12 hrs	Rarely used nowadays
Gelfoam	Weeks	Upper GI bleed, pelvic trauma
PERMANENT AGENTS		
Ethyl alcohol (1 mL/kg)	Permanent	Tumors (causes coagulative necrosis)
Steel coils	Permanent	Large vessel, aneurysm, tumor
Polyvinyl alcohol (200-1000 μm)	Permanent	Tumors
Balloons	Permanent	High output AV fistulas
Cyanoacrylate	Permanent	AVM

Complications

- Postembolization syndrome (fever, elevated WBC), 40%
- Infection of embolized area (administer prophylactic antibiotics)
- Reflux of embolic material (nontarget embolization)
- Alcohol causes skin, nerve, and muscle infarction if used in the periphery; its use should be restricted to parenchymal organs.

HEPATIC CHEMOEMBOLIZATION

- Palliative only; prolonged survival or relief of endocrine symptoms
- Dual hepatic/portal supply allows for arterial embolotherapy
- Gelfoam or ethiodol mixed with chemotherapeutic agents is used
- Tumors: hepatocellular carcinoma, occular melanoma, metastatic endocrine tumors

Thrombolysis

Indication:
- Arterial graft thrombosis
- Native vessel acute thrombosis
- Before percutaneous intervention
- Hemodialysis AVF or graft
- Venous thrombosis
    - Axillosubclavian
    - Portal vein, SMV
    - IVC

General principles
- Always obtain a diagnostic angiogram prior to thrombolysis.
- Streptokinase is no longer used (antigenic side effects).
- rTPA is no more effective than UK but is much more expensive.

- Favorable prognostic factors for thrombolysis:
    Recent clot (< 3 months)
    Good inflow/outflow
    Positioned in thrombus
- Endpoints of thrombolysis therapy:
    No lysis present after 12 hours of infusion
    Major complication develops
    Severe reperfusion syndrome
    Progression to irreversible ischemia
- Successful thrombolysis is defined as:
    > 95% lysis of thrombus
    Clinical reperfusion
- Always treat underlying lesions.
- Overall success:
    Grafts, 90%
    Native arteries, 75%
- Heparinize concomitantly with UK infusion
- Monitor in ICU
- No good correlation between success, complications, and blood tests

THROMBOLYTIC AGENTS			
	SK	**UK**	**rTPA**
Source	*Streptococcus* culture	Renal cell culture	DNA technology
Dosage	5000 U/hr	100,000 U/hr	0.05 mg/kg/hr
Half-life	20 min	10 min	5 min
Treatment time	24-48 hr	24 hr	6 hr
Bleeding	20%	10%	10%
Cost	Cheap	Expensive	Very expensive

Techniques
Low-dose technique (constant)
- 100,000 U/hr of UK
- Repeat angiogram after 12 hours
High-dose technique (graded)
- 250,000 U/hr × 4 hours of UK
- Repeat angiogram then 125,000 U/hr
Pulse spray ultra-high dose
- 600,000 U/hr in 5000 U of UK bolus doses
- Aliquots every 30 seconds
Catheter placement
- Coaxial dual infusion is best
- 5 Fr catheter lodged in proximal thrombus
- T3 or infusion wire (Katzen) coaxially into distal thrombus
- Split infusion of UK into proximal and distal catheters
- Secure skin entry site

TPA infusion
- TPA (arterial): Infuse at 1 mg/hr total dose divided between infusion sites. Total maximum dose per patient is 100 mg. TPA has half-life of 6 minutes.
- TPA (venous): Same infusion rate as arterial, lower bleeding complication rate
- TPA (line clearance): 0.5 mg/hour × 3-4 hours

Contraindications
Absolute
- Active bleeding
- Intracranial lesion (stroke, tumor, recent surgery)
- Pregnancy
- Nonviable limb
- Revascularization of nonviable limb will cause acute renal failure and cardiovascular collapse due to lactic acid and myoglobin
- Infected thrombus

Relative
- Bleeding diathesis
- Cardiac thrombus
- Malignant hypertension
- Recent major surgery
- Postpartum

Complications
- Major hemorrhage, requiring termination of UK, surgery, or transfusion (e.g., intracranial bleed, massive puncture site bleed), 7%
- Minor hemorrhage, 7%
- Distal embolization
- Pericatheter thrombosis
- Overall, termination of therapy is required in 10%

Angioplasty

PTA is a method to fracture the vascular intima and to stretch the media of a vessel by a balloon. Atherosclerotic plaques are very firm and are fractured by PTA. Healing occurs by intimal hyperplasia.

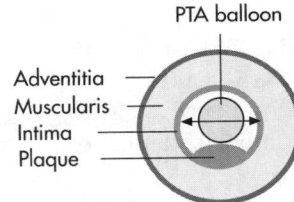
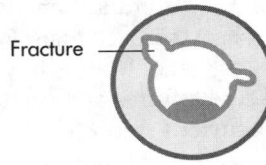

Indication
- Claudication or rest pain
- Tissue loss
- Nonhealing wound
- Establish inflow for a distal bypass graft
- Hemodialysis AVF or grafts

General principles
- Premedication with aspirin and 10 mg nifedipine
- Ipsilateral approach is preferred
- Heparinize (5000-10,000 U) after the lesion is crossed
- Diagnostic angiogram is obtained prior to PTA
- Measure pressure gradients with borderline lesions
- Significant gradient > 10 mm of Hg at rest; > 20 mm Hg after vasodilator; > 10% systolic blood pressure

- Pharmacological adjuncts
    - IA nitroglycerin or Priscoline for vasospasm and provoked pressure measurements
- Balloon size: sized to adjacent normal artery
    - Common iliac artery: 8-10 mm
    - External iliac artery: 6-8 mm
    - Superficial femoral artery: 4-6 mm
    - Renal artery: 4-6 mm
    - Popliteal artery: 3-4 mm
- Wire should always remain across lesion.
- Repeat angiogram and pressure measurements after angioplasty.
- Postprocedure heparin with "limited flow" results (dissection, thrombus)

Prognostic indicators

- Large vessels/proximal lesions respond better than small vessel/distal lesions.
- Stenoses respond better to PTA than occlusions.
- Short stenoses respond better to PTA than long stenoses.
- Isolated disease responds better to PTA than multifocal disease.
- Poor inflow or poor outflow decreases success.
- Limb salvage interventions have a poor prognosis.
- Diabetics have a poorer prognosis than nondiabetic patients.

PTA results

Iliac system
- 95% initial success
- 70%-80% 5-year patency

Femoral popliteal
- 90% initial success
- 70% 5-year patency

Renal artery
- 95% initial success
- Fibromuscular dysplasia: 95% 5-year patency
- Atherosclerosis: 70%-90% 5-year patency
- Ostial lesions have a poorer prognosis.

Acute failures are due to thrombosis, dissection, or inability to cross a lesion.

Recurrent stenosis
- Intimal hyperplasia (3 months to 1 year)
- Progression of disease elsewhere (> 1 year)

Complications

- Groin complications (same as diagnostic angiography)
- Distal embolism
- Arterial rupture (rare)
- Renal infarction or failure (with renal PTA)

INTRAVASCULAR STENTS

Metallic stents have an evolving role in interventional angiography. Current stents include:

Palmaz balloon expandable stent (Johnson and Johnson)
- Balloon mounted
- Placement is precise; shortens slightly
- Minimal elastic deformation due to hoop strength
- Should not be placed at sites where extrinsic forces could crush the stent
- Thoracic outlet veins
- Dialysis graft

Wallstent (Schneider)
- Bare
- Placement is less precise
- Considerable elastic deformity
- Useful in tortous vessels and tight curves

Gianturco zigzag stent (Cook)

Stent grafts (metallic stents combined with synthetic graft material) are currently investigational and used in aortic aneurysms and dissections.

Indications for metallic stents
- Unsuccessful PTA
- Recurrent stenosis
- Venous obstruction, thrombosis
- Transjugular intrahepatic portosystemic shunt

Indications for stents in revascularization procedures
- Long segment stenosis
- Total occlusion
- Ineffective or unsuccessful PTA:
    Residual stenosis > 30%
    Residual pressure gradient > 5 mm Hg
    Hard calcified plaque
    Large post-PTA dissection flap
- Recurrent stenosis after PTA
- Ulcerated plaque
- Renal ostial lesions

Stent results
- Iliac artery: over 90% 5-year patency (better than PTA)
- Renal artery and other vessels: limited long-term data

TRANSJUGULAR INTRAHEPATIC PORTOSYSTEMIC SHUNT (TIPS)

Established indications
- Portal hypertension with variceal bleeding that has failed endoscopic treatment
- Refractory ascites

Possible future indications
- Budd-Chiari syndrome
- Pretransplant

General principles
- Confirm portal vein patency prior to procedure (US, CT, or angiography).
- Preprocedure paracentesis may be helpful.
- Right internal jugular vein (IJV) is the preferred access vessel.
- Goal: portal-systemic gradient < 10 mm Hg, decompression of varices

Contraindications
- Polycystic liver disease
- Hepatic failure
- Severe right-sided failure
- Severe hepatic encephalopathy
- Portal vein thrombosis
- Active infection
- Large liver hypervascular tumor

8

Technique

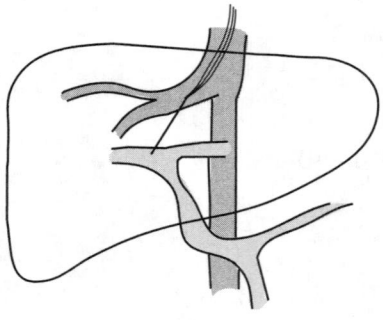 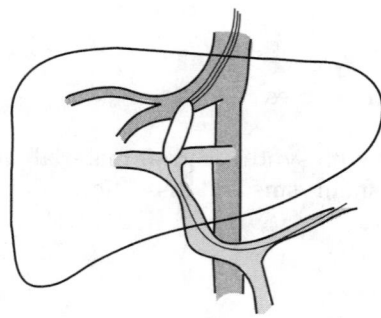 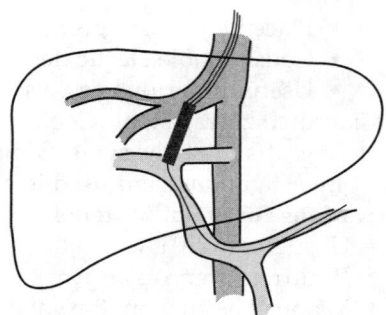

- Right IJV approach
- Obtain wedged hepatic pressure and venogram.
- Create tract from right hepatic vein to portal vein with 16-G needle.
- Advance catheter over wire into portal venous system.
- Obtain portal venogram.
- Measure portal pressures.
- Dilate tract with PTA balloon (8 mm).
- Deploy metallic stent (Palmaz or Wallstent).
- Dilate stent until gradient < 10 mm Hg.
- Coil embolization of varices is optional.

Results
- Patency: 50% at 1 year
- Recurrent bleeding in 10%

Complications
- Hepatic encephalopathy, 10%; more likely when residual gradient is less than 10 mm of Hg
- Bleeding
- Shunt thrombosis or stenosis
- Right heart failure
- Renal failure

Signs of malfunction
- No flow
- Low velocity flow (< 50-60 cm/sec) at portal venous end of shunt
- Reversal of flow in hepatic vein away from IVC
- Hepatopedal flow in intrahepatic portal vein
- Reaccumulation of ascites; varices; recanalized umbilical vein

TYPES OF VENOUS ACCESS	
Device	**Purpose/Situation**
External tunneled catheter (silicone or polyurethane)	Continuous use, multiple simultaneous uses
Implantable port	Intermittent use; immunocompromised patient
High flow catheter	Temporary hemodialysis; pheresis
PICC	Short-term use, usually < 2-3 months; infrequent blood drawing

PICC, Peripherally inserted central catheter.

Venous Access

CENTRAL VENOUS ACCESS CATHETERS

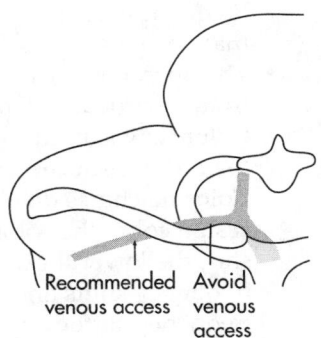

Recommended venous access | Avoid venous access

The catheters are typically inserted through axillary (subclavian), internal jugular, or arm vein. Pneumothorax, symptomatic vein stenosis, and thrombotic complications are less common with jugular than subclavian vein approaches. For the axillary vein puncture, the entry site should be lateral to the ribs in the subcoracoid region. This approach eliminates the possibility of pneumothorax and also ensures that the catheter is well within the subclavian vein as its passes through the costoclavicular space. If the catheter is extravascular at this site, chronic compression may occur and lead to catheter erosion and fracture—"pinch-off syndrome." For IJV puncture, a site on the mid-neck above the clavicle is selected. The vein is punctured under transverse US guidance, ensuring that the carotid artery is avoided.

COMPLICATIONS OF CENTRAL VENOUS CATHETER PLACEMENTS

- Pneumothorax
- Arterial puncture
- Hemorrhage or hematoma
- Occlusion
- Mechanical problems
- Air embolism
  This usually occurs when venous dilator is removed from peel away sheath to be replaced with the catheter.
  The embolism can be avoided by covering the opening with a gloved finger and removing the dilator with patient in suspended deep inspiration.
  If air does get sucked in, perform fluoroscopy of the chest. If there is air in the pulmonary artery, do the following:
  Place patient in left lateral decubitus position to keep air in the right chamber.
  Suck out air with Swan-Ganz balloon catheter.
  Administer supplemental O_2 and monitor patient.

Vascular Ultrasound

GENERAL

Frequency shift = 2 × transducer frequency × velocity of blood × cosine of angle × 1/speed of sound (1540 m/s). Cos of 90° = 0 and cos of 0° = 1. The optimal angle between the probe and the vessel is < 60°.

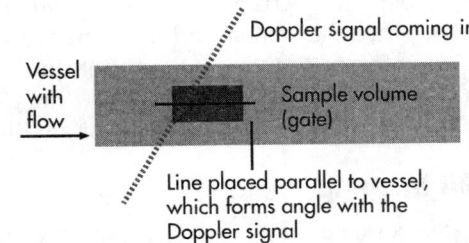

Doppler signal coming in

Vessel with flow

Sample volume (gate)

Line placed parallel to vessel, which forms angle with the Doppler signal

CONTINUOUS WAVE DOPPLER

- Performed with a pencil probe. No static image is produced, as the machine does not stop to listen. If one vessel is located behind the other, one cannot use continuous wave because it will reveal both waveforms.

8

PULSED WAVE DOPPLER

- Frequently used for interrogating arteries and veins; duplex refers to the fact that one gets gray scale and Doppler images.
- The operator can set the machine to listen only to those Doppler shifts coming from a particular depth. This is called *Doppler gate* or *sample volume*.
- Color flow is used to determine the direction of flow (by convention red is toward transducer and blue is away), as well as magnitude of shift.
- Color machines do not display velocity, since angle of insonation is not used to assign color; the color indicates magnitude of frequency shift. The greater the shift the lower the saturation of color. In simple terms: in a tortuous vessel, the frequency shifts and angle of insonation changes, thus change in color is due to frequency shift even though velocity is the same.
- It is important to remember that the color image is a display of average frequency shift and not peak frequency shift. Calculations of stenosis from Doppler data are based on peak frequency shift or peak velocities.

POWER DOPPLER US

- The signal is related to the number of moving targets (usually red blood cells). This technique ignores velocity and direction of flow. Used to detect flow and has high sensitivity.

ALIASING

Aliasing is the result of flow velocity exceeding the measuring ability of pulsed wave Doppler. By Doppler imaging, this is seen as a wraparound with high velocity below the bottom of the scale rather than on the top. By color imaging aliasing becomes evident by inversion of color (blue within an area of red and vice versa). Ways for reducing aliasing:

- Pulse repetition frequency (PRF) can be increased by raising the scale.
- The doppler shift can be reduced by manipulating variables of equation—thus either a greater angle (thus reduced cos 0 value) or a lower frequency can be used.
- Color aliasing refers to wrapping of signal displayed as areas of color reversal.
- Changes due to vessel tortousity can also change colors, but in that case color changes are marked by band of black, thus red to blue with black (no signal) in between. Artifacts due to 0 = 90 degrees.
- Since the ultrasound machine typically only displays either gray scale or color information, there is competition as to which signal is displayed. If gray scale gain setting is high, the color image is suppressed when flow is low, giving impression of absent flow or smaller lumen.

MR Imaging

NONCONTRAST IMAGING TECHNIQUES

Two main noncontrast MR angiography (MRA) techniques: time of flight (TOF) MRA and phase contrast (PC) MRA. Both techniques can be acquired in either two-dimensions (2D) or three-dimensions (3D).

TOF-MRA
- 3D has higher signal-to-noise ratio (SNR) and shorter imaging times than 2D.
- Works well for high flow arterial systems
- Limitations for imaging low flow venous systems

PC-MRA
- Less saturation effects
- Velocity flow information
- Longer imaging times

GD-ENHANCED MRA

A perfectly timed gadolinium contrast agent injection with 3D spoiled gradient-echo (SPGR) produces high SNR MRA covering extensive regions of vascular anatomy within a breath hold. Compared to noncontrast techniques, signal does not depend on inflow of blood, is not subject to problems of flow saturation, and reduces intravoxel dephasing. The IV-administered Gd shortens the T1 of blood to < 270 msec (T1 of fat) so that all bright signal essentially originates from vessels. Images are reconstructed as maximum intensity projections (MIP). Technique:
- Dose: Two or three bottles (20 mL each) of the gadolinium (about 0.3 mmol/kg Gd)
- Timing: Perfect contrast agent bolus timing is crucial to ensure that the maximum arterial Gd occurs during the middle of the acquisition, when central k-space data are acquired. Begin injecting Gd immediately after starting the scan. Finish the injection just after the midpoint of the MR acquisition. To ensure full use of the entire dose of contrast, flush the IV tubing with 20 mL of normal saline.

Other Techniques

DIGITAL SUBTRACTION ANGIOGRAPHY (DSA)

Venous DSA
- Catheter in central venous structure; a large volume and high concentration of contrast agent is given as a bolus.
- Adequate results in only 70% of patients
- Invasive study

Arterial DSA
- Advantages: lower iodine concentration required than for cut film, less pain, speedy
- Disadvantages: less resolution, motion, and bowel gas artifacts

PETROSAL VEIN SAMPLING

Venous blood is obtained from bilateral inferior petrosal veins (which drain the cavernous sinus) to detect for lateralization of hormones produced by pituitary tumors (very sensitive test). Simultaneous tracker catheters are advanced into the inferior petrosal veins. Simultaneous samples are obtained to distinguish paraneoplastic/endocrine production of hormones from pituitary sources and localize the abnormality to left or right.

LYMPHOGRAPHY

- 1 mL isosulfan blue injected between 1st-2nd and 4th-5th toes; wait 10 minutes for lymphatic uptake.
- Cutaneous cutdown to the fascia (dorsum of foot)
- Isolate a lymphatic; pass a silk suture above and below.
- Milk the blue dye into the vessel.
- Puncture lymphatic with a 30-G needle lymphography set.
- Hook-up needle to pump and inject oily contrast medium (Ethiodol)
- Obtain initial images of lymphatic vascular phase and later of the nodal phase.

Conscious Sedation

Form of sedation in which the patient is given sedation and pain medication but should remain easily arousable. The following parameters are continuously monitored:
- BP
- Oxygenation using a pulse oximeter
- ECG and heart rate

Conscious sedation is usually achieved by small aliquot dosing of midazolam and fentanyl.

COMMON MEDICATIONS AND DOSAGES*				
	IV Dosage	Total Dose	Duration (hr)	Comments
BENZODIAZEPINES				
Diazepam	1-5 mg	10-25 mg	6-24	Long acting
Lorazepam	0.5-2.0 mg	2-4 mg	6-16	
Midazolam	0.5-2.0 mg	< 0.15 mg/kg	1-2	Good amnesic effect; short-acting
NARCOTIC ANALGESICS				
Morphine	1-5 mg	< 0.2 mg/kg	3-4	Histamine release
Meperidine	12.5-25 mg	0.5-1 mg/kg	2-4	MAOI interaction
Fentanyl	15-75 µg	1-3 µg/kg	0.5-1	Immediate onset
Naloxone	0.4-0.8 mg	Repeated as needed	0.3-0.5	For narcotic overdose
ANTIEMETICS				
Metaclopramide	10 mg	0.5-1 mg/kg	1-2	Stimulates GI motility
Prochlorperazine	2.5-10 mg	10 mg	4-6	Adjust dosage for age
Promethazine	12.5-25 mg	25 mg	4-6	CNS depressant effects
Droperidol	0.625-1.25 mg	Higher dose: sedation	4-6	Potent antiemetic at low doses

MAOI, Monoamine oxidase inhibitor.
*See manufacturer's packet insert for specific rates of administration.

Coagulation

GENERAL

- Coumadin interferes with vitamin K-dependent synthesis of clotting factors.
- Heparin inactivates thrombin by combining with antithrombin III.
- Partial thromboplastin time (PTT) is the time required for 1 mL of recalcified whole blood to clot. It therefore reflects the intrinsic clotting axis.
- Prothrombin time (PT) is the time required for 1 mL of recalcified whole blood to clot in the presence of thromboplastin (phospholipid extract); it therefore reflects the extrinsic clotting axis.

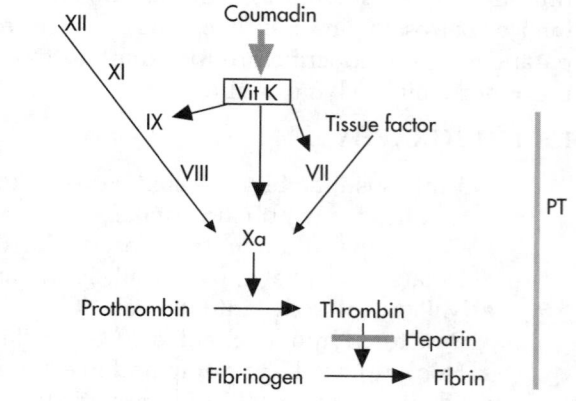

OVERVIEW		
Clotting Parameter	Normal Value	Causes of Abnormal Values
Prothrombin time (extrinsic coagulation system)	< 3 sec of control	Warfarin, heparin Liver disease Vitamin K deficiency (parenteral nutrition, biliary obstruction, malabsorption, antibiotics)
Coagulopathy (DIC, PTT thrombolytic therapy) PTT (intrinsic coagulation system)	< 6 sec of control	Lupus anticoagulant Hemophilia
Bleeding time		< 8 min platelet count < 50,000/mm^3 Qualitative: uremia, NSAIDs von Willebrand's disease

DIC, Disseminated intravascular coagulation.

NORMALIZATION OF PROLONGED COAGULATION TIMES

Interventions (biopsy, aspiration, drainage) should not be performed if coagulation times are markedly prolonged (i.e., beyond above values); correction of coagulopathies (see below) can often be achieved in several hours.

CORRECTING PROLONGED COAGULATION TIMES			
Anticoagulant	PT/PTT	Antidote	Normalization
Heparin	Both prolonged	Stop heparin IV protamine titration	3-6 hrs Minutes
Coumadin	Both prolonged	IV vitamin K for 3 doses Fresh frozen plasma	Days Minutes
Aspirin	Normal (platelet aggregation reduced)	Platelet concentrates Stop aspirin	Minutes Week

NEWER DRUGS FOR ANTICOAGULATION

Low molecular weight heparins
- Dalteparin: Dose: 15,000-18,000 U in 2 divided daily doses for deep vein thrombosis (DVT) treatment. No or minimal effect on PT and PTT. Effects are reversed with protamine: 1 mg/100 U of dalteparin.
- Enoxaparin: mechanism of action and antidote similar to dalteparin

Low molecular weight heparnoid (danaparoid)
- Indicated in patients who have developed heparin-induced thrombocytopenia (HIT). However, a 10%-20% cross-reactivity still occurs.
- Dose: 750 U subcutaneous BID in patients 50 to 90 kg
- No effects on PT or PTT
- Antidote same as dalteparin but only 30% reversal. Fresh frozen plasma (FFP) is given for reversal.

Recombinant hirudin (lepirudin)
- Indicated in patients who have developed HIT type II
- Dose: 0.4 mg/kg bolus followed by continuous infusion of 0.15 mg/kg/hr
- Half-life is 1.3 hours in normal individuals (longer in patients with renal failure)
- aPTT of 1.5 to 2.5 of patient's baseline is considered therapeutic
- No antidote known; treat overdose with blood products

Antiplatelet drugs
- Clopidogrel (Plavix). Prevents platelet aggregation. Dose: 75 mg once a day. The antiplatelet effect lasts for 7-10 days after discontinuation of drug. Prolongs bleeding time two times; no known antidote.

Thoracic Aorta and Great Vessels

General

ANATOMY

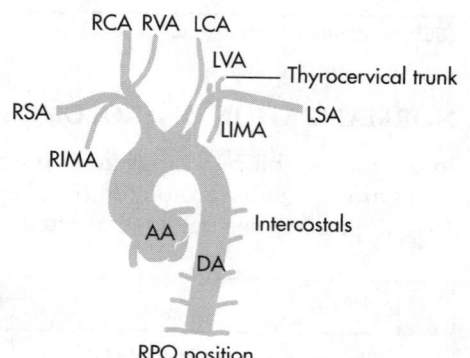

- The normal ascending aorta is always larger in diameter than the descending aorta.
- Branches:
    - Great vessels
    - Intercostal arteries
    - Bronchial arteries
- Normal great vessel configuration, 70% (see diagram). Variants occur in 30%:
    - Bovine arch 20%: common origin of brachiocephalic and left CCA
    - Left vertebral artery (LVA) comes off aortic arch between left CCA and subclavian artery (SA), 5%
    - Common carotid trunk 1%
    - Arteria thyroidea IMA to thyroid isthmus
- Intercostal arteries are usually paired from 3rd to 11th intercostal space; these arteries may give rise to spinal arteries.
- Bronchial artery configuration is quite variable. Most common configurations are:
    - Single right bronchial artery
    - Multiple left bronchial artery

IMAGING PRINCIPLES

CT
- Indications:
    - Diagnosis and surveillance of aneurysms
    - Aneurysm rupture
    - Aortic dissections
- Spiral CT is currently expanding CT indications
- CT is not yet validated as the sole evaluation of traumatic arch injuries.

MRI
- Indications:
    - Diagnosis and surveillance of aneurysms
    - Aortic dissection
- Allows evaluation of the aortic root better than CT
- MRA of great vessels is gaining in diagnostic importance.

Aortography
- Indications:
  - Preoperative aneurysm assessment
  - Traumatic arch injury
  - Equivocal CT or MRI
- Remains the gold standard diagnostic tool but is rarely the initial diagnostic examination for the thoracic aorta

Transesophageal echocardiography
- Indications:
  - Aortic dissection
  - Associated cardiac disease (AI, LV dysfunction)
- Not validated to evaluate traumatic aortic injury

Thoracic aortography technique
- Catheter: 7-8 Fr pigtail
- Contrast: Hypaque 76 or nonionic equivalent
- Rate: 30-40 mL/sec $\times$ 2 sec (total 60-80 mL)
- Fast filming: 3/sec $\times$ 3. Higher rate for DSA
- Always perform imaging in at least two orthogonal views.

Thoracic Aortic Aneurysm

GENERAL

True aneurysms contain all three major layers of an intact arterial wall. False aneurysms lack one or more layers of the vessel wall; false aneurysms are also called *pseudoaneurysms*. Most thoracic aortic aneurysms are asymptomatic and are detected incidentally. Clinical symptoms usually indicate large size, expansion, or contained rupture.

Causes
- Atherosclerosis (most common)
- Connective tissue diseases (Marfan, Ehler-Danlos)
- Syphilis
- Posttraumatic pseudoaneurysm
- Mycotic aneurysm
- Aortitis
  - Takayasu's disease
  - Giant cell aortitis
  - Collagen vascular diseases (rheumatoid arthritis, ankylosing spondylitis)

Pearls
- True aneurysms tend to be fusiform.
- False aneurysms tend to be saccular.
- Posttraumatic, mycotic, and postsurgical aneurysms are false aneurysms.

ATHEROSCLEROTIC ANEURYSM

90% of these aneurysms are fusiform because thoracic atherosclerosis is usually circumferential; 10% are saccular. A saccular shape should therefore raise the suspicion of a false aneurysm (pseudoaneurysm). Atherosclerotic thoracic aneurysm are more common in the descending aorta and have a high incidence of concomitant abdominal aortic aneurysm.

8

Complications

Expansion
- Pain
- Hoarseness, dysphagia
- Aortic insufficiency

Rupture (uncommon if < 5 cm)
- Rupture into pericardial or pleural space, trachea, mediastinum, esophagus
- Rupture into superior vena cava (SVC) (aortocaval fistula), pulmonary artery (aortopulmonary fistula)

Radiographic features

Angiography
- Most useful in preoperative assessment of asymptomatic patients
- Appearance
    Fusiform >> saccular
    Determine proximal and distal extent (often thoracoabdominal)
    Determine branch involvement
    Coexistent aneurysmal or occlusive disease?
- Not accurate in determining aneurysm size because of:
    Magnification
    Layering of contrast
    Thrombus in the lumen
- An indicator of an impending rupture is focal ectasia (so-called pointing aneurysm, or nipple of aneurysm).

CT
- Mural thrombus well seen
- Extraluminal extent and contained rupture better seen than by angiography

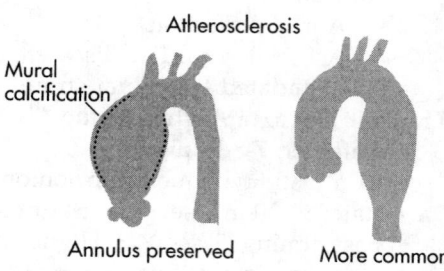

Atherosclerosis
Mural calcification
Annulus preserved   More common

CYSTIC MEDIAL NECROSIS

Degenerative process of the aortic muscular layer (media) causing aneurysms of the ascending aorta. Commonly involves aortic sinuses and sinotubular junction, resulting also in aortic insufficiency. Causes:
- Hypertension
- Marfan, Ehlers-Danlos, homocystinuria (structural collagen diseases)

Radiographic features
- Symmetrical sinus involvement (tulip bulb)
- Ascending aorta is most commonly involved.
- Dissection is a frequent complication.
- Calcifications are rare.

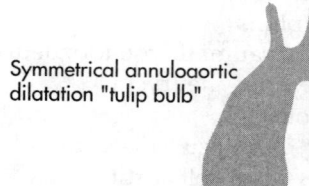

Medial degeneration
Symmetrical annuloaortic dilatation "tulip bulb"

SYPHILITIC ANEURYSMS

Syphilitic aneurysms are a delayed manifestation of tertiary synphilis 10-30 years after primary infection. Infectious aortitis occurs via vasa vasorum. 80% of cases involve the ascending aorta or the aortic arch.

Radiographic features
- Asymmetrical saccular sinus involvement
- Tree bark calcification is common.
- Dissections are rare.

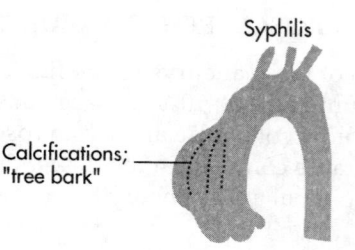

Syphilis
Calcifications; "tree bark"
Asymmetrical sinus dilatation

MYCOTIC ANEURYSMS

Mycotic aneurysms are saccular pseudoaneurysms located in ascending aorta or isthmus. Organisms: *Staphylococcus, Streptococcus, Salmonella*. CT often reveals perianeurysmal inflammation. Underlying diseases:
- Immunocompromised patients
- Intravenous drug abuse
- Endocarditis
- Postsurgical
- Idiopathic

Aortic Dissection

GENERAL

Aortic dissection represents a spectrum of processes in which blood enters the muscular layer (media) of the aortic wall and splits it in a longitudinal fashion. Most dissections are spontaneous and occur in the setting of acquired or inherited degeneration of the aortic media (medial necrosis). Medial necrosis occurs most commonly as an acquired lesion in mid-old age hypertensive patients. Dissections (spontaneous) almost exclusively originate in the thoracic aorta and secondarily involve the abdominal aorta by extension from above. Aortic dissection results in the separation of two lumens by an intimal flap. The false lumen represents the space created by the splitting of the aortic wall; the true lumen represents the native aortic lumen. "Dissecting aortic aneurysm" is somewhat of a misnomer because many dissections occur in normal caliber aortas. In chronic dissections the false channel may become aneurysmal.

Clinical
- Chest pain or back pain, 80%-90%
- Aortic insufficiency
- Blood pressure discrepancies between extremities
- Neurological deficits
- Ischemic extremity
- Pulse deficits
- Silent dissections are very rare.

Causes
Medial degeneration is a pathological finding associated with many diseases that predispose to dissection.
- Hypertension (most common)
- Structural collagen disorders
    Marfan syndrome
    Ehlers-Danlos syndrome
- Congenital
    Aortic coarctation
    Bicuspid or unicuspid valve
- Pregnancy
- Collagen vascular disease (very common)

Types

Classification is based on location because treatment and prognosis depends on the portion of aorta involved.

Stanford classification
- Type A, 60%: involves at least ascending aorta; surgical treatment
- Type B, 40%: limited to descending aorta; medical treatment

DeBakey classification
- Type I, 50%: involves ascending and descending aorta
- Type II, 10%: confined to ascending aorta
- Type III, 40%: same as a Stanford B

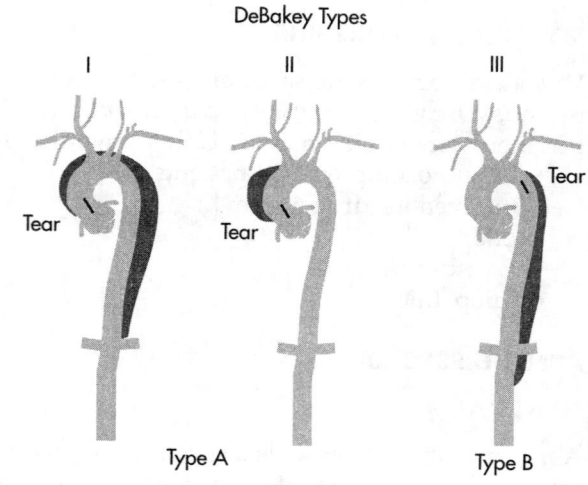

DeBakey Types

I   II   III

Tear   Tear   Tear

Type A   Type B

Stanford Types

Treatment

Stanford B: medical control of hypertension is the standard therapy. Surgery is indicated in complicated type B dissections:
- Ischemic extremity
- Mesenteric ischemia or renal artery compromise
- Rupture
- Aneurysmal enlargement of false lumen

Stanford A: require surgery because of involvement of aortic root
- Pericardial tamponade
- Coronary artery occlusion
- Aortic insufficiency

Indications for imaging
- Diagnosis
- Preoperative evaluation (angiography ± coronary angiography)
- Follow-up of postoperative and chronic dissections (CT or MRI)

```
                         ┌──────────────────┐
                         │ Clinical suspicion │
                         └──────────────────┘
        Clinical type A or              Stable
        complicated type B
              │                           │
              ▼                           ▼
     ┌──────────────────┐       ┌──────────────────────────────┐
     │   Aortography    │◄──────│ Trans-Esophageal Echocardiography │
     │ ± coronary       │ Type A│      (or contrast CT)         │
     │   angiography    │ or    └──────────────────────────────┘
     └──────────────────┘ complicated        │ Type B
                          type B             ▼
                                   ┌──────────────────┐
                                   │ Routine surveillance │
                                   │     CT or MRI      │
                                   └──────────────────┘
```

Goals of imaging studies
- Determine if ascending aorta is involved
- Determine origin and extent of dissection
- Define branch vessel involvement: coronary arteries, great vessels, mesenteric and renals, iliac arteries
- Determine if there is aortic regurgitation
- Find the intimal flap and entry/reentry points
- Evaluate patency of false lumen
- Determine if there is an extraaortic hematoma (pericardial, paraaortic, wall thickening)

Angiographic features
- Key diagnostic finding: intimal flap
- Intimal flap or false and true lumen are detectable in 85%-90%
- Delayed opacification of false lumen
- Compression of true lumen by false lumen
- Occlusion of branch vessels
- Soft tissue companion shadow adjacent aorta (hematoma, thrombosed false lumen)
- Abnormal catheter position
    Displaced from aortic wall by false lumen
    Inability to opacify true lumen (catheter in false lumen)
- Differentiation of true and false lumen
    Location: false lumen is anterolateral in ascending aorta and posterolateral in descending aorta
    Size: false lumen is larger and compresses true lumen
    Opacification: slower flow leads to delayed opacification of false lumen

CT features
- Same hallmark findings as angiography
    Intimal flap
    Two lumens (true and false)
- CT is more accurate in detection of:
    Thrombosed false channels
    Periaortic hematoma and pericardial/pleural blood
    Isolated aortic wall hematoma (hyperdense wall)
- CT is not accurate in evaluation of:
    Coronary arteries or great vessels
    Aortic valve
    Entry or exit sites
- Dynamic contrast-enhanced helical CT is the technique of choice.
    Precontrast scan (to detect wall hematoma)
    Dynamic contrast-enhanced helical CT (to detect intimal flap)
    Delayed contrast-enhanced helical CT (occasionally needed)
- Role of CT
    Triage patients with equivocal clinical findings
    Surveillance of chronic dissections

MRI features
- Conventional spin echo: excellent for detecting intimal flaps and wall hematoma
- Phase contrast gradient echo detects differential flow velocities in true and false lumens.
- Cine MR sequences allow detection of aortic insufficiency

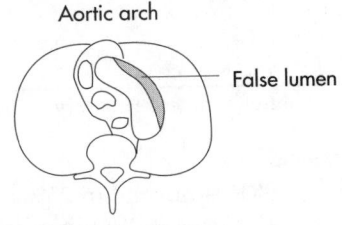

Aortic arch — False lumen

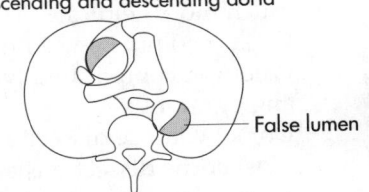

Ascending and descending aorta — False lumen

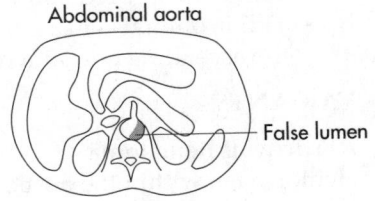

Abdominal aorta — False lumen

8

DIFFERENTIATION OF THROMBOSED ANEURYSM AND DISSECTION		
	Thrombosed Aneurysm	**Dissection**
Longitudinal extent	Usually focal	Extensive, > 6 cm
Calcification	Outside aortic shadow	Inside aortic shadow
Size of aorta	Large	Normal in acute phase, may become very large in chronic dissection
Aortic lumen	Large	Normal
Involved branches	Lumbar, IMA	Renal, SMA

IMA, Inferior mesenteric artery; SMA, superior mesenteric artery.

Pearls

- CXR is normal in 25% of aortic dissections.
- Abnormal CXRs in aortic dissection are nonspecific; clinical findings are usually much more helpful.
- CT should not be used to triage patients who are surgical candidates (suspected type A or complicated type B); a CT adds an unnecessary contrast burden before angiography.
- Do not confuse dissection with transection (traumatic aortic injury).
- Most aortic dissections are spontaneous; minor trauma may precipitate dissection in predisposed patients (Marfan syndrome) but this is the exception.
- TEE is often used as a first triage exam and answers the first critical question: Is the ascending aorta involved?

VARIANTS

Aortic wall hematoma

Hemorrhage within the aortic wall with no identifiable intimal flap or false lumen. This entry is caused by bleeding from vasa vasorum into the media. Not detected by angiography; noncontrast CT is the study of choice (hyperdense aortic wall).

Penetrating aortic ulcer

Found usually in association with an atherosclerotic aneurysm. An ulcer ruptures into the media and results in a contained rupture or focal dissection. Not a true dissection but has a similar presentation. High mortality because of rupture.

Chronic dissection

Type B or repaired dissections may persist with true and false lumens (double barrel aorta). These dissections are compatible with long survival. Surveillance imaging with CT or MRI is used to detect an enlarging false lumen (dissecting aortic aneurysm) or extension.

Traumatic Aortic Injury

GENERAL

Exact mechanism are unknown but shear forces of deceleration injury are postulated to be the main cause of traumatic aortic injury. Only 15%-20% of patients who sustain traumatic aortic injury survive and present for imaging evaluation. Aortic injury typically results in a false aneurysm involving disruption of either intima or intima and media, or all wall layers. Only 5% of untreated patients survive at 4 months.

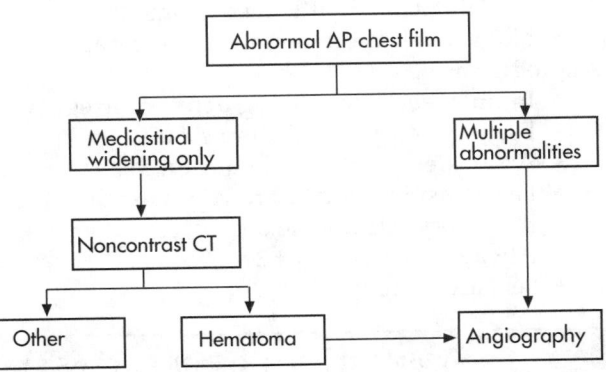

Location

- Aortic isthmus, 95%: between left subclavian artery and ligamentum arteriosum
- Proximal ascending aorta
- Descending aorta (at hiatus)
- Associated great vessel injury in 5%-10%

Approach

A history of appropriate mechanism of injury is a sufficient reason to evaluate a patient for aortic tear. The goal is to diagnose the injury as expeditiously as possible so that surgical repair can be undertaken. Angiography remains the most accurate imaging examination for the detection and preoperative staging and should therefore be the first-line examination in surgical candidates. CT may be used to accurately determine the absence or presence of mediastinal hematoma in low-risk patients with equivocal CXR and high-risk patients with normal chest radiograph.

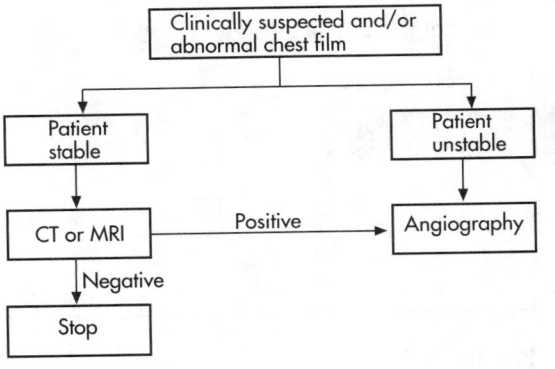

Chest radiograph

- Routinely obtained in all patients
- Look for signs of mediastinal hematoma:
    - Widened mediastinum or right paratracheal widening
    - Loss of aortic contour
    - Left apical cap
- Secondary signs are not specific:
    - Rightward displacement of nasogastric tube
    - Downward displacement of left bronchus
    - Fracture of first and second ribs
    - Hemothorax
- Only 15% of patients with mediastinal hematoma will have an aortic tear.
- Aortic injury occurs rarely in a normal mediastinum CXR.

CT

- Current role is to determine absence or presence of mediastinal hematoma.
- Patients with any appearance other than normal mediastinal fat should go straight to angiography.
- Pitfalls:
  Young patients with residual thymus
  Ventilated patients (motion artifact)
  Patients with little mediastinal fat
- Not yet validated to replace angiography

Angiography

- Intimal tear: linear filling defect or irregularity or aortic contour
- Pseudoaneurysm at isthmus, 80%
- Associated great vessel injuries, 5%
- False positive studies are very rare: ductus bump or diverticulum (remnant of the embryonic double arch)
- Always obtain at least 2 views
- Sensitivity, 100%

DIFFERENTIATION OF DUCTUS KNOB VS. AORTIC TEAR	
Ductus Knob	**Aortic Tear**
Smooth	Sharp
Round	Irregular
Broad neck	Narrow neck
No companion shadow	Companion shadow
Ductus diverticulum	Traumatic pseudoaneurysm

Pearls

- Some authors still consider the mechanism of injury alone (regardless of CXR findings) as an indication for aortography.
- CT and TEE have not been validated as adequate replacements for aortography.

Aortitis

TAKAYASU'S ARTERITIS (PULSELESS DISEASE)

Marked intimal proliferation and fibrosis lead to occlusion and narrowing of aorta and involved arteries; aneurysms may also be found. Age: 90% < 30 years (in contradistinction to all other arteritis). More common in females.

Types

- Type 1: aortic arch
- Type 2: abdominal aorta
- Type 3: entire aorta
- Type 4: pulmonary arteries

Radiographic features

- Stenoses of arch vessels (most common)
- Stenosis and occlusion of aorta (may mimic coarctation)
- Thickening of aortic wall
- Pulmonary artery involvement, 50%
- Abdominal coarctation and renal artery stenoses

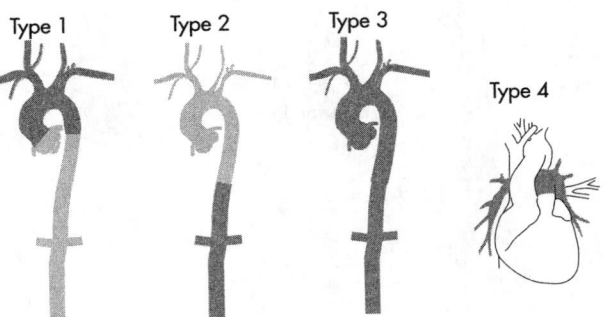

GIANT CELL ARTERITIS

- Older patients > 50 years
- Diagnosis: biopsy of temporal artery
- Most commonly involves medium size arteries
- Aorta is involved in 10%, most commonly ascending aorta
- Complications: aneurysm, dissection

SYPHILITIC AORTITIS

Syphilitic aortitis occurs 10-30 years after infection as the aorta becomes progressively weakened by inflammation and fibrosis (wrinkling of the intima) ultimately leading to aneurysm formation. Organism: *Treponema pallidum*. Diagnosis: postitive FTA-ABS, VDRL. Treatment: high-dose penicillin, resection of enlarging aneurysm.

Complications

- Aneurysm 10%
- Aortic valve disease
- Coronary artery narrowing at ostium 30%
- Gummatous myocarditis (rare)

Radiographic features

- Involvement: ascending aorta (60%) > aortic arch (30%) > descending thoracic aorta (10%)
- Tree bark appearance
- Saccular aneurysm of ascending aorta
- Heavy calcification of the ascending aorta is typical (but not common)

8

Abdomen and Pelvis

Abdominal Aorta

ANATOMY

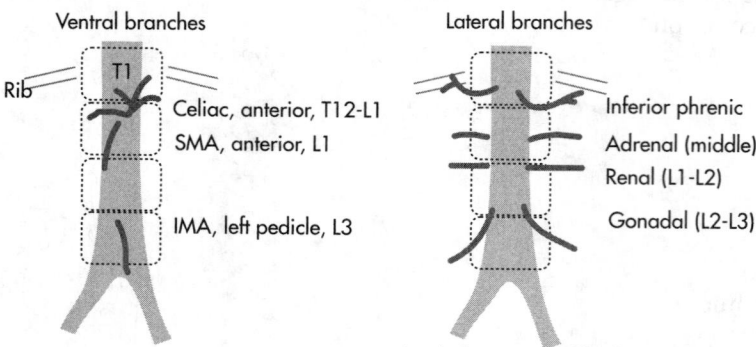

Ventral branches

Rib

T1

Celiac, anterior, T12-L1

SMA, anterior, L1

IMA, left pedicle, L3

Lateral branches

Inferior phrenic

Adrenal (middle)

Renal (L1-L2)

Gonadal (L2-L3)

(Excluding 4 paired lumbars)

ABDOMINAL AORTIC ANEURYSM (AAA)

Atherosclerotic aneurysms are most commonly located in the abdominal aorta. 90% of AAA are infrarenal. The major risk of an abdominal aneurysm is rupture but other complications occur:

- Expansion and/or leakage: pain
- Aortocaval fistula: congestive heart failure (CHF), leg swelling
- Distal embolization: blue toe syndrome
- Aortoenteric fistula
- Infection

The risk of rupture is small in aneurysm less than 5 cm but increases for aneurysms over 5 cm. Associated with other aneurysms, especially popliteal artery aneurysm.

Radiographic features

Plain film

- Determine size by atherosclerotic calcification
- Lateral projection is most helpful

CT

- AAA is defined as vessel diameter ≥ 3 cm
- Contrast-enhanced helical CT may provide preoperative assessment in simple cases.
- Most accurate imaging study to determine the size of aneurysm
- Best imaging study to detect a suspected rupture

Angiography

- Routinely used for preoperative staging
- Yields more accurate data regarding status of mesenteric and renal vessels than does CT
- Not reliable for size determination
- Allows mapping of pelvic and leg arterial anatomy
- Always define:
    Proximal and distal neck of aneurysm
    Patency of mesenteric vessels
    Presence of aberrant vessels

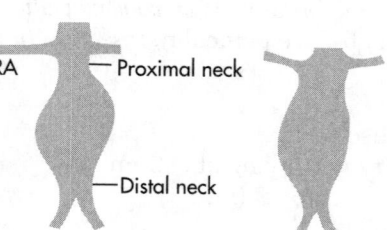

Infrarenal   Juxtarenal

RA

Proximal neck

Distal neck

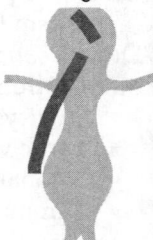

Hourglass

OTHER ABDOMINAL AORTIC ANEURYSMS

Inflammatory AAA

Represents 5% of all AAAs. The inflammatory mantle surrounding the AAA enhances on contrast CT. This entity must be differentiated from leaking or ruptured AAAs.

Mycotic AAA

The aorta is a common site for infected aneurysms. Mycotic aneurysms are typically eccentric saccular aneurysms in a location atypical for atherosclerotic AAAs. Organisms: *Salmonella, Staphylococcus*. Clinical: Fever of unknown origin (FUO).

Risk factors

- Arterial trauma
- Sepsis
- Immunosuppression
- Bacterial endocarditis
- IV drug abuse (IVDA)

AORTOILIAC OCCLUSIVE DISEASE

Multiple patterns exist:

- Infrarenal aortic occlusion: occlusion up to the level of renal arteries
- Distal aortoiliac disease: involves bifurcation and iliac arteries
- Small aorta syndrome: focal atherosclerotic stenosis of distal aorta; occurs most commonly in younger female smokers
- Multisegment disease: often associated with infrainguinal occlusive disease

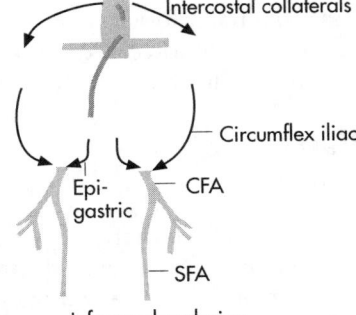
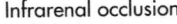

Infrarenal occlusion

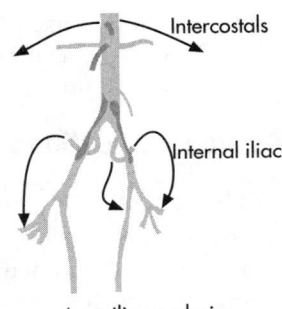

Aortoiliac occlusive

Common clinical symptoms include thigh, hip, and buttocks claudication, impotence, and diminished femoral pulses (Leriche's syndrome in men). In general, aortoiliac occlusive disease responds well to percutaneous interventions such as percutaneous transluminal angioplasty, endovascular metallic stents.

Radiographic features

- Arteriography is the imaging study of choice once the decision is made to intervene.
- Collateral arterial pathways:
    Internal mammary arteries → external iliac arteries via superior and inferior epigastric arteries
    IMA → internal iliac arteries via hemorrhoidal arteries
    Intercostal/lumbar arteries → external iliac arteries via deep circumflex iliac arteries
    Intercostals/lumbar arteries → internal iliac arteries via iliolumbar and gluteals
- Always measure pressure gradients across stenoses to determine their hemodynamic significance and to assess response to intervention.
- Role of MRA:
    2D TOF or Gd-DTPA 3D SPGR are commonly used techniques.
    Diagnostic study of choice in patients with high risk for contrast reactions or renal failure
    Good for visualizing distal "runoff" when aorta is occluded

ABDOMINAL AORTIC COARCTATION

Abdominal aortic coarctation may be congenital or acquired. Most commonly affects young adults or children. Clinical: renovascular hypertension (common), claudication, abdominal angina. Associations:

Congenital
- Thoracic aortic coarctation
- Idiopathic hypercalcemia syndrome (Williams syndrome)
- Congenital rubella
- Neurofibromatosis (NF)

Acquired
- Takayasu's arteritis
- Fibromuscular dysplasia
- Radiation therapy

Radiographic features
- Segmental coarctation is most common
- Coarctation usually involves the renal arteries
- IMA serves as major collateral vessel to lower extremities
- Diffuse hypoplasia is a less common form of presentation

Aortic Interventions and Surgery

ENDOVASCULAR STENT GRAFTS

Endovascular stent–graft implantation is an alternative to open surgery for the treatment of aortic aneurysm. Advantages of endovascular procedures are lower blood loss, shorter stay in intensive care and hospitalization, and quicker recovery. Common complications include that can be discerned by imaging include:
- Graft thrombosis
- Graft kinking
- Pseudoaneurysm caused by graft infection
- Graft occlusion
- Shower embolism
- Colonic necrosis
- Aortic dissection
- Hematoma at arteriotomy site
- Endoleak (see below for classification)

Endoleak classification (White)
- Type I endoleak is present when a persistent perigraft channel with blood flow develops. This can be due to inadequate or ineffective seal at the graft ends (either the proximal or distal graft) or attachment zones (synonyms: "perigraft endoleak" or "graft-related endoleak").
- Type II endoleak occurs when there is persistent collateral retrograde blood flow into the aneurysm sac (e.g., from lumbar arteries, the IMA, or other collateral vessels). There is a complete seal around the graft attachment zones so the complication is not directly related to the graft itself (synonyms: "retrograde endoleak"or "nongraft–related endoleak").
- Type III endoleak arises at the midgraft region and is due to leakage through a defect in the graft fabric or between the segments of a modular, multisegmental graft. This subgroup of endoleak is primarily due to mechanical failure of the graft (early component defect or late material fatigue). In some cases hemodynamic forces or aneurysm shrinkage may be contributory (synonyms: "fabric tear" or "modular disconnection").

- Type IV endoleak is detected by angiography or other contrast studies as any minor blush of contrast that is presumed to emanate from contrast diffusion across the pores of the highly porous graft fabric or perhaps through the small holes in the graft fabric caused by sutures or stent struts, etc. This is usually an intentional design feature, rather than a form of device failure. In practice, differentiation of type IV endoleak from type III can often be difficult, perhaps requiring postoperative, directed angiography (synonym: "graft porosity").
- Endoleak of undefined origin. In many cases, the precise source of endoleak will not be clear from routine follow-up imaging studies, and further investigation may be required. In this situation, it may be appropriate to classify the condition as "endoleak of undefined origin" until the type of endoleak is elucidated by further studies.
- Non-endoleak aneurysm sac pressurization (endopressure). In this situation, no endoleak is demonstrated on imaging studies, but pressure within the aneurysm sac is elevated and may be very close to systemic pressure (unpublished data). The seal is formed by semiliquid thrombus, and the pressure in the sac is similar to the pressures measured in the endoleak. The aneurysm is pulsatile; wall pulsatility also may be detected and monitored by specialized US techniques.

TYPE OF GRAFTS

- Bifurcation grafts are mainly used for AAA repair and aortoiliac occlusive disease.
  - End-to-side (used only for aortoiliac occlusive disease)
  - End-to-end
- Tube grafts are mainly used for AAA repair.
- Endarterectomy is usually used for aortoiliac occlusive disease.
- Aortofemoral bypass is mainly used in aortoiliac occlusive disease.
- Extraanatomical grafts
  - Axillofemoral
  - Axillobifemoral
  - Femoral-femoral

These grafts are preferred in patients with unilateral iliac disease, high surgical risk, severe scarring from prior vascular procedures, abdominal or groin infections, or chronic occlusion of one limb, and AFB.

AORTIC BIFURCATION GRAFTS (ONLAY GRAFTS, INVERTED Y GRAFTS)

Aortic onlay graft

The end of the graft is anastamosed to the ventral wall of the aorta. The distal lines are anastamosed to both CFA. Only used for occlusive disease. Features:

- Preserves flow to native pelvic arteries, especially internal iliac arteries
- Impotence is less common
- Higher incidence of graft occlusion

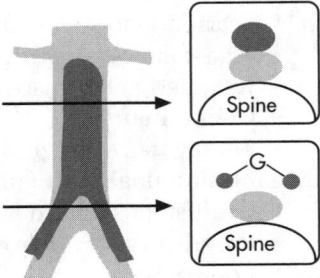

8

End-to-End Y Graft

Hemodynamically better than end-to-side anastomosis. Used for AAA and occlusive disease. May be bifurcated to iliac arteries or extended distally to CFAs. Advantages:
- More physiological flow at anastomosis
- Lower risk of aortoduodenal fistula
- Higher patency

WRAPPED GRAFT (TUBE GRAFT)

The graft is positioned within the aneurysm. The native aortic wall is sutured around the graft.

SURGICAL GRAFT COMPLICATIONS

CT is the study of choice for detecting:
- Perigraft infection
- Anastomotic pseudoaneurysm
- Hematoma, lymphocele
- Aortoenteric fistula

^{111}In-WBC may be helpful in detecting graft infection.

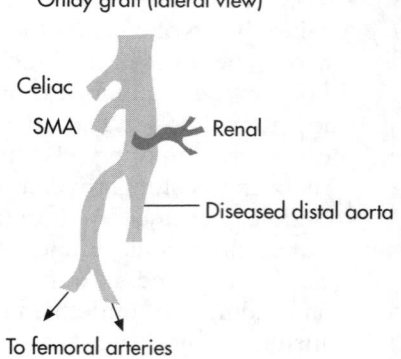

Onlay graft (lateral view)

Celiac
SMA
Renal
Diseased distal aorta
To femoral arteries

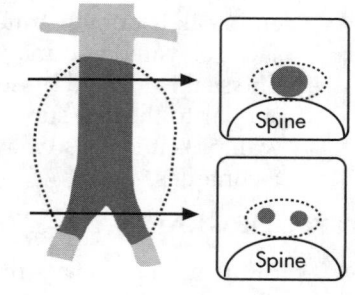

Spine

Spine

OVERVIEW	
Complication	Incidence (%)
Perigraft abscess	40
Groin infection	25
Pseudoaneurysm	20
Hematoma, lymphocele	10
Aortoenteric fistula	10
Other	10
Bowel infarction	
Abscess	

INFRAINGUINAL GRAFT FAILURE

Causes of early or subacute infrainguinal bypass graft failure
- Scarred vein segments
- Anastomotic stricture
- Retained valve cusps (in situ grafts)
- Clamp injury
- Nonligated vein graft tributaries that divert flow away from the graft

Late infrainguinal graft failure
- Graft stenosis from intimal hyperplasia
- Progression of atherosclerosis
- Poor runoff

Mesenteric Vessels

CELIAC AXIS

Arises at T12-L1. Branches:
- 1st branch: left gastric artery (LGA)
- 2nd branch: splenic artery
- 3rd branch: common hepatic artery (CHA)

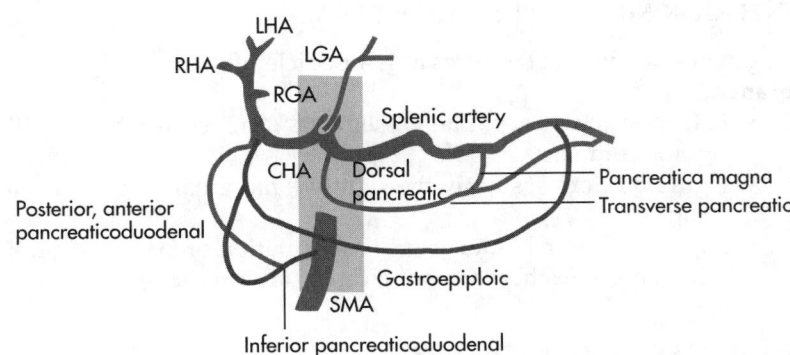

HEPATIC VASCULATURE

Hepatic arteries

The CHA represents the segment from the origin to take-off of GDA. The proper hepatic artery divides into LHA and RHA. Aberrations, 40%:
- RHA from SMA, 15%
- LHA from LGA, 10%
- Accessory LHA from LGA, 8%
- Accessory RHA from SMA, 5%
- RHA and LHA from SMA with no supply from celiac axis, 2%

Hepatic veins
- Hepatic venous drainage occurs via 3 hepatic veins that drain into the IVC.
- Hepatic veins define hepatic anatomical segments (8 segments, see Chaper 3).

SPLENIC ARTERY

Branches
- Dorsal pancreatic artery arises from splenic artery in 40%
- Pancreatica magna arises in midportion
- Short gastric arteries
- Left gastroepiploic artery
- Splenic polar branches

SUPERIOR MESENTERIC ARTERY (SMA)

The SMA arises at L1, 1-20 mm below the celiac axis. The first part lies immediately posterior to the body of the pancreas; it then passes ventral to the uncinate process (CT landmark).

Branches
- Inferior pancreaticoduodenal artery (1st branch)
- Middle colic artery (2nd branch)
- Jejunal and ileal arteries
- Right colic artery
- Ileocolic artery

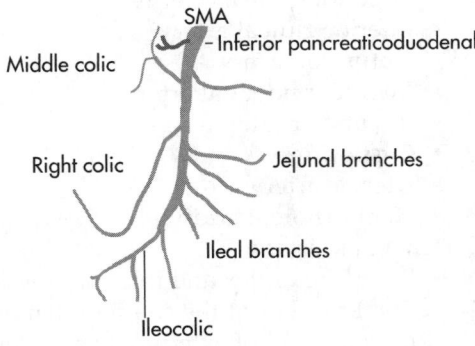

8

INFERIOR MESENTERIC ARTERY (IMA)

Originates below renal arteries at left pedicle of L3.

Branches

- Left colic artery: separate vessel in 40%; arises as a trunk with some sigmoid branches in 60%
- Sigmoid arteries: supply the sigmoid; marginal arteries (complex of arcades)
- Superior hemorrhoidal artery: continuation of IMA or sigmoid artery; becomes hemorrhoidal artery after passing over common iliac vessel

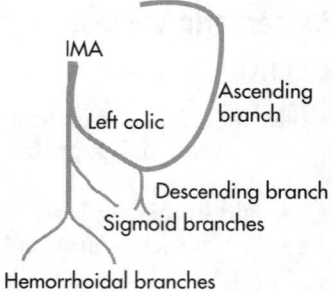

MESENTERIC COLLATERALS

Celiac artery to SMA

- Arc of Buehler: embryonic ventral communication of celiac artery to SMA
- Pancreaticoduodenal arcade

SMA to IMA

- Middle colic artery → left colic artery
- Arc of Riolan: short direct SMA-IMA communications
- Marginal arteries of Drummond: arcades along the mesenteric border of the colon

IMA to internal iliac artery

- Via superior hemorrhoidal artery

Rectal arcades

- Superior rectal artery from IMA
- Middle rectal artery from internal iliac artery
- Inferior rectal artery from pudendal artery

PELVIC ARTERIES

Internal iliac artery

- Superior gluteal artery
- Inferior gluteal artery
- Obturator artery
- Internal pudendal artery
- Iliolumbar artery
- Cystic artery
- Uterine artery
- Hemorrhoidal artery

External iliac artery

- Deep circumflex and inferior epigastric arteries are the first branches of the common femoral artery, thus marking end of external iliac vessels and the inguinal ligament

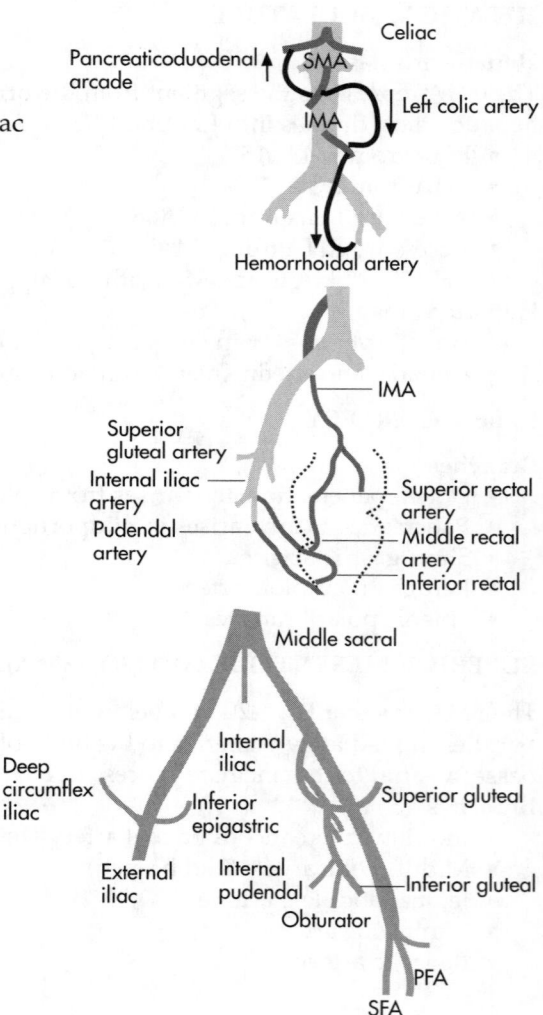

UPPER GI HEMORRHAGE

Endoscopy and conservative therapy are the primary forms of treatment. Angiography is used after failure of primary therapies. Rarely, massive upper GI bleeding can present as hematochezia. Causes:

- Gastritis (most common)
- Peptic ulcer disease
- Gastroesophageal varices
- Mallory-Weiss tear
- Other causes:
    Aortoduodenal fistula
    GI malignancy

Radiographic features

- Confirm active bleeding by a selective arteriogram
- The most common bleeding vessel in upper GI hemorrhage is the left gastric artery (LGA), 85%-90%.
- Extravascular contrast extravasation is the hallmark of active bleeding:
    Accumulation in bowel lumen
    Gastric "pseudovein" sign (contrast between rugal folds)
    Filling of pseudoaneurysm or pooling
- Normal variants of LGA origins:
    Celiac trunk (most common)
    Directly from aorta
    Common trunk with splenic artery from aorta
- Alternative sources for gastric bleeding:
    Right gastric artery (RGA)
    Left and right gastroepiploic arteries
    Short gastric arteries
- Common sources of duodenal bleeding:
    GDA and/or its branches
    Pancreaticoduodenal arcade

Bleeding scans are not usually helpful for evaluating upper GI bleeding.

Angiographic intervention

- Vasopressin
    Usually successful in gastritis, esophagogastric tears
    Proceed to embolization if no response after 30 minutes
- Embolization is more successful with tumors, peptic ulcer disease, and duodenal bleeds.
- Gelfoam embolization is used for self-limiting lesions (e.g., benign ulcers) because recanalization will occur after initial cessation of bleeding.
- Permanent embolization (polyvinyl alcohol, coils) is reserved for major arterial injury (e.g., tumor, duodenal ulcers, pseudoaneurysm).
- Embolization of upper GI does not result in ischemia because of rich collateral supply.

8

SUCCESS RATES OF TREATMENTS FOR UGI BLEEDING		
Type of Hemorrhage	Treatment	Success (%)
ESOPHAGOGASTRIC HEMORRHAGE		
Mallory-Weiss tear	Vasopressin	90
Diffuse gastric bleeding*	Vasopressin	80
Esophageal varices	IV (not IA) vasopressin	
	Endoscopic sclerosis	
	TIPS	
PYLORODUODENAL HEMORRHAGE		
Ulcer	Vasopressin	35
	Vasopressin and embolization	60

*Related to stress, trauma, surgery, burns, NSAIDs, etc.

LOWER GI HEMORRHAGE

Defined as bleeding distal to ligament of Treitz. 98% of hemorrhages are located in large bowel, 2% are located in small bowel. Endoscopy is performed to exclude rectal bleeding. Unlike with UGI hemorrhage, endoscopy is often technically not successful because bleeding obscures visualization. Causes:

Large bowel, 98%
- Diverticulosis (most common)
- Angiodysplasia
- Colon carcinoma
- Polyps
- Inflammatory bowel disease, other colitis
- Rectal disease
    Ulcer or tear
    Hemorrhoids
    Tumor

Small bowel, 2%
- Leiomyoma
- Arteriovenous malformation
- Ulcer (steroid therapy or transplant patients)
- Small bowel varices
- Other
    Inflammatory bowel disease (IBD)
    Diverticulosis, Meckel's diverticulum
    Small bowel tumors (e.g., metastases, Kaposi's sarcoma)

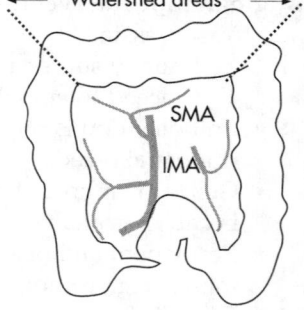

Radiographic features

Scintigraphic scans are sensitive and are often helpful.
- Threshold of detection is 0.1 mL/min.
- If scintigraphy is negative, the angiographic likelihood of a positive study is very low.
- Prolonged imaging can detect intermittent bleeding.

Selective SMA and IMA arteriogram
- Multiple runs should be obtained to cover entire vascular bed (colonic flexures, rectum).
- Anomalous arteries (e.g., middle colic) may require celiac arteriogram.

Angiographic intervention
- Intraarterial vasopressin is successful in 90%.
- Rebleed rate, 30%
- Unlike in the upper GI tract, embolization of the lower GI tract has a higher rate of complications because of less collateralization. Bowel ischemia and/or infarction occurs in 25%.

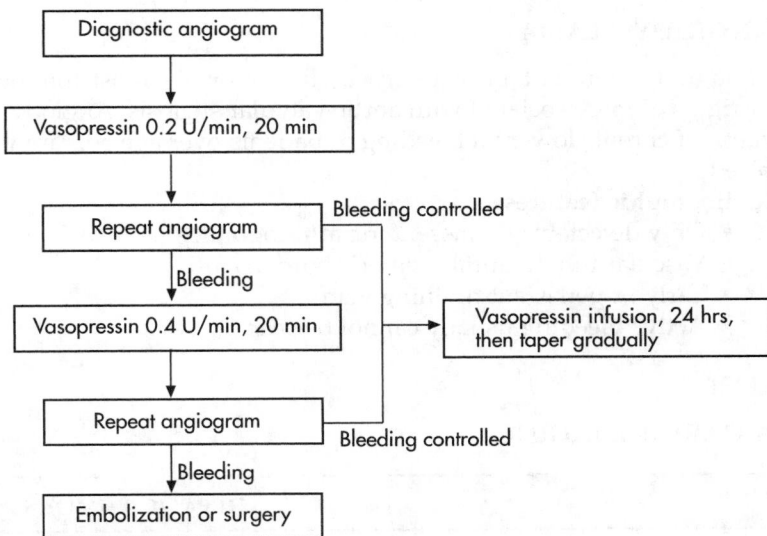

INTESTINAL ISCHEMIA

May be acute or chronic. Chronic ischemia occurs when progressive occlusive disease involves all three mesenteric arteries. Patients are usually not very ill and present with abdominal angina and weight loss. Patients with acute ischemia, in contradistinction, usually present with an acute abdomen and often have a deranged metabolic status and other concomitant medical conditions (e.g., shock, cardiac disease, sepsis).

Causes
Arterial occlusion
- Embolization
- In situ thrombosis
- Aortic dissection
- Primary mesenteric artery dissection (fibromuscular dysplasia [FMD], iatrogenic)
- Vasculitis

Nonocclusive arterial ischemia (most common)
- Atherosclerosis and low cardiac output/hypotension

Mesenteric venous thrombosis
Other
- Incarcerated hernia
- Volvulus
- Intussusception

Radiographic features
Angiography
- Helical CT often used for triage; angiography remains the study of choice.
- Filling defects or occlusions: thrombus, embolus
- In situ thrombosis occurs proximal (origin of SMA)
- Emboli tend to be peripheral and/or located at vascular branch points.
- Late phase: lack of veins, collaterals, filling defects (venous thrombosis)
- Diffuse vasospasm may accompany nonocclusive or occlusive etiology.

Angiographic interventions
- Intraarterial or venous thrombolysis
- Nonocclusive ischemia: IA papaverine, 30-50 mg/hr

ANGIODYSPLASIA

Thought to represent an acquired vascular anomaly, most commonly located in cecum or right colon. Associated with aortic valvular stenosis. Angiodysplasia is a common cause of chronic lower GI bleeding in patients over age 50; rarely presents as acute GI bleed.

Radiographic features
- Only detectable by mesenteric arteriography
- Vascular tuft on antimesenteric border
- Early or persistent draining vein
- Active bleeding usually cannot be seen.

Liver

ARTERIAL IMAGING

HEPATIC TUMORS		
Lesion	**Arterial Vascularity**	**Other Findings**
Hemangioma	Normal	Dense peripheral stain; small, multiple pools (cotton wool)
FNH	++	Spoke wheel appearance, 35%
Adenoma	+	Paradoxically not very vascular
Regenerating nodules	−	Often hypovascular, seen with cirrhosis
HCC	++, AV shunting	Portal vein invasion, 75%

VENOUS IMAGING

Indications
- Portal vein thrombosis
- Hepatic vein thrombosis (Budd-Chiari syndrome)
- Portal hypertension
- Evaluation of hepatic transplants
- TIPS evaluation
- Evaluation of portosystemic shunts

Imaging modalities

US
- Cannot reliably diagnose intrahepatic venoocclusive disease
- Useful for most other indications

Angiography
- Hepatic and wedged hepatic venography
- Portal venography
    - Arterial portography (late phase celiac/SMA arteriography)
    - Transhepatic direct portal venography
    - Transjugular direct portal venography
    - Percutaneous splenoportography
    - Umbilical vein catheterization

CT angiography and MRA
- Evolving roles

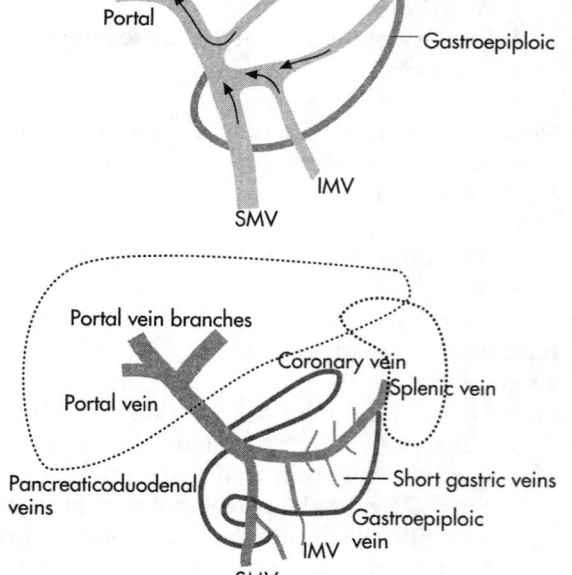

PORTAL HYPERTENSION

Defined as a portal pressure > 5-10 mm Hg. Most commonly caused by hepatic cirrhosis. Clinical manifestations occur because of altered flow dynamics; GI variceal bleeding is the most common presentation.

Causes

Presinusoidal
- Portal vein obstruction
    Thrombosis
    Tumor (pancreatic cancer, metastases)
- Schistosomiasis (most common cause worldwide)

Sinusoidal
- Cirrhosis

Postsinusoidal
- Budd-Chiari syndrome
- Hepatic vein or IVC occlusion

High flow states
- Traumatic AVF
- AVM (Osler-Weber-Rendu, HCC)

Physiology
- Elevated portal pressures
- Increased hepatic arterial flow to liver
- Biphasic or hepatofugal portal flow
- Decompression of portal venous system occurs via systemic collaterals:
    Coronary vein to azygous or hemiazygous veins: esophageal varices
    SMV/IMV to iliac veins: mesenteric varices, stomal varices
    IMV to inferior hemorrhoidal veins: hemorrhoids
    Umbilical vein to epigastric veins: caput medusa
    Splenic vein to azygous veins: gastric fundal varices
    Splenic vein to retroperitoneal veins: duodenal/retroperitoneal varices

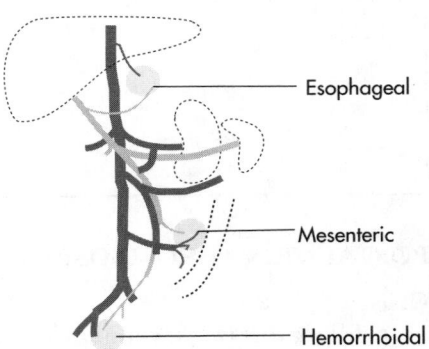

Esophageal

Mesenteric

Hemorrhoidal

Radiographic features

US
- Recanalized umbilical vein or hepatofugal flow is diagnostic
- Always demonstrate portal and splenic vein patency for determining treatment options.
- Portal collaterals
- Splenomegaly
- Ascites

Angiography
- Elevated portal pressure
    Corrected sinusoidal pressure (CSP) = hepatic wedge pressure − IVC pressure
    CSP < 5 mm Hg is normal
    Direct portal vein pressure < 5 mm Hg is normal.
- Portal flow away from liver
- Portosystemic collaterals or varices
- Corkscrew hepatic arteries
- Always exclude presinusoidal and postsinusoidal etiologies.

Treatment
- TIPS is the treatment of choice after conventional endoscopic techniques fail to control bleeding.
- Variceal embolization is adjunctive.
- Surgical portosystemic shunts

SURGICAL SHUNT TYPES		
Shunt Type	**Use**	
PORTACAVAL (Portal vein → IVC)	Performed for immediate decompression	Portacaval shunt Mesocaval shunt
SPLENORENAL (Splenic vein → renal vein) Warren (distal) Linton (proximal)	Common elsewhere Common at MGH	Splenorenal shunt: Warren Splenorenal shunt: Linton
MESOCAVAL (SMV → IVC)		

PORTAL VEIN THROMBOSIS

Causes
- Idiopathic (most common)
- Tumor (HCC, pancreatic cancer, metastases)
- Postoperative (splenectomy, transplant)
- Blood dyscrasias
- Coagulopathies
- Sepsis, pylephlebitis
- Pancreatitis
- Cirrhosis, portal hypertension

Complications: hepatic infarction, bleeding varices, mesenteric thrombosis, and presinusoidal portal hypertension.

Radiographic features

US
- Best screening imaging modality
- Thrombus appears echogenic
- Collaterals and varices

CT
- Hyperdense thrombus on noncontrast CT
- Low density filling defect on contrast CT
- Cavernous transformation: occurs in setting of subacute/chronic portal vein thrombosis: multiple portal tubular collaterals are present in porta hepatis

MRI
- T1 hyperintense portal vein thrombus
- Numerous portal flow voids (collaterals)

Angiography
- May be treated with intraarterial (SMA) or portal venous thrombolysis

Splenic vein occlusion (isolated)
- Segmental portal hypertension with gastric fundal varices
- Esophageal varices are absent
- Normal portal venous pressure
- Cannot be treated by TIPS

BUDD-CHIARI SYNDROME (BCS)

Obstruction of hepatic venous outflow resulting in hepatic enlargement, portal hypertension with varices, and ascites. Venous obstruction may be at the level of intrahepatic venules, the hepatic veins, or the IVC. Causes:

Hepatic vein thrombosis
- Hematologic disorders
- Coagulopathies
- Pregnancy
- Oral contraceptives
- Phlebitis
- Idiopathic

Tumor growth in hepatic veins and/or IVC
- Renal cell carcinoma
- HCC
- Adrenal carcinoma

Other
- IVC membrane or web (common in Asians)
- Constrictive pericarditis
- Right atrial tumor

Radiographic features
- Hepatic venography and inferior venacavography are diagnostic studies of choice.
- Spiderweb hepatic veins
- IVC narrowing or webs
- Stretched, straight hepatic arteries on arteriography

Kidneys

ANATOMY

Arteries
Single vessel 65%, multiple vessels 35% (aberrant vascular supply is common in malrotated or horseshoe kidneys). Branches of renal artery:
- Anterior and posterior division
- Segmental arteries (5 segments)
- Interlobar arteries (each supplies one renal column)
- Arcuate arteries → interlobular arteries → afferent glomerular arterioles

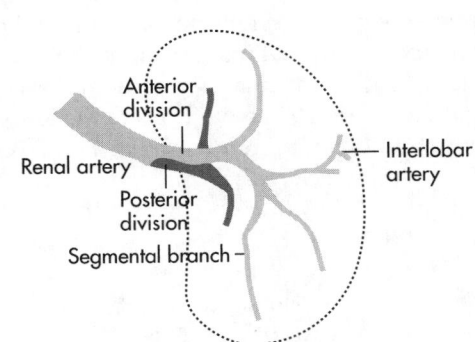

8

Variants
- Gonadal arteries arise from renal arteries in 20%.
- Inferior phrenic artery may occasionally arise from renal artery.
- Inferior adrenal arteries often arise from renal artery.

Veins
- Left renal vein is 3 times longer than the right; therefore the left kidney is used for transplants.
- Left renal vein passes anterior to the aorta (3% retroaortic) and under the SMA.
- Left renal vein receives left adrenal and gonadal veins.
- Multiple renal veins in 35%

INDICATIONS FOR RENAL ANGIOGRAPHY

Diagnostic renal arteriography
- Renovascular hypertension (detection of renal artery stenosis)
- Trauma
    AVF or pseudoaneurysm
    Traumatic bleeding, hematuria
    Devascularization injury
- Tumors (determine vascular supply)
- Transplant donors
    Number and location of renal arteries
    Complicating normal variants
    Detect unsuspected pathology

Renal venography
- Renin sampling in renovascular hypertension
- Diagnosis of renal vein thrombosis
- Evaluation for tumor extension into IVC or renal veins
- Unexplained hematuria (renal varices)

Angiographic interventions
- Renovascular hypertension: PTA or stents
- Embolization
    Preoperative tumor embolization to reduce blood loss
    Aneurysm
    Posttraumatic AVF
    Active bleeding (trauma, iatrogenic)

RENAL ARTERY STENOSIS (RAS)

Significant clinical entity because it is a potentially treatable cause of hypertension and, when advanced, of renal insufficiency. Renal artery stenosis may cause hyperreninemic HTN. Not all patients with RAS have HTN (thus RAS is not synonymous with renovascular HTN). Causes:
- Atherosclerosis, 70%
- FMD, 25%
- NF
- Arteritis:
    Takayasu's arteritis
    Polyarteritis nodosa
    Abdominal aortic coarctation

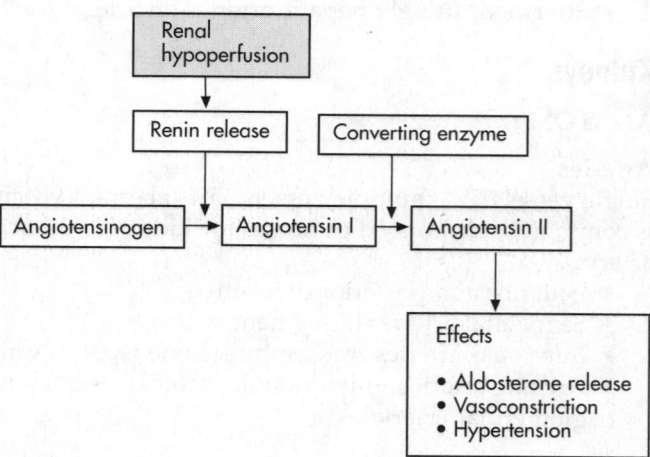

- Other
    - Radiation therapy
    - Aortic dissection
    - Pheochromocytoma

Radiographic features
- Radionuclide scan is often the first imaging study (see Chapter 6).
- RAS is hemodynamically significant if there is:
    - Lumen stenosis of $\geq$ 50%
    - Peak systolic pressure gradient > 15%
    - Poststenotic dilatation
    - Collaterals are present
- Renin vein sampling is helpful in some cases. Lateralizing renins (ratio > 1.5:1) indicate that revascularization will be beneficial.
- Pitfalls in angiographic diagnosis of RAS
    - Renal artery spasm (pseudostenosis)
    - Standing waves may simulate FMD.
    - Multiple views are usually required to unmask the entire renal artery.
- Accuracy of MRA
    - In comparison to angiography, MRA has sensitivity and specificity of greater than 90% for detecting renal artery stenosis (> 50%).
    - The protocol for imaging renal arteries includes: sagittal localizer, axial 2D T2-weighted sequence, 3D gadolium-enhanced MR angiography, and 3D phase contrast sequence.
    - 3D phase contrast imaging is used to evaluate the hemodynamic significance of renal artery stenosis.
    - With the combination of 3D PC imaging and 3D gadolium-enhanced imaging, the entire renal artery up to the first level of branching in the renal hilum can be evaluated.

RENAL ARTERY ATHEROSCLEROSIS

Most common cause of renovascular HTN. Occurs in older patients (over 50) and usually involves the proximal artery. Does not respond as well to percutaneous PTA as does FMD.

Radiographic features
- Ostial stenosis is usually associated with aortic plaque.
    - Poor PTA response, 30% patency
    - Metallic stents might improve patency rates.
- Main renal artery stenoses: 80% respond to PTA
- Distal and peripheral RAS may also occur.
- Frequently bilateral
- Two indications for revascularization:
    - Control HTN
    - Preserve renal function

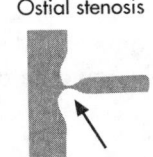

Ostial stenosis

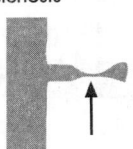

Mid–renal artery stenosis

FIBROMUSCULAR DYSPLASIA (FMD)

Proliferation of muscular and fibrous elements in middle- and large-sized arteries. Unknown etiology. 5 types exist and are classified by the layers of the arterial wall involved:

- Intimal fibroplasia (rare)
- Medial fibroplasia: most common type, 85%; causes classic stenoses alternating with aneurysms
- Perimedial fibroplasia; no aneurysms
- Medial hyperplasia (rare)
- Periadventitial fibroplasia (rare)

Distribution

- Renal arteries, 60%: most common site
- ICA or vertebral arteries, 35%
- Iliac arteries, 3%
- Visceral arteries, 2%

Radiographic features

- Most commonly located in mid and distal renal artery
- "String of beads" appearance is most common (85%).
- Smooth stenoses are less common (10%).
- Bilateral in 50%
- Excellent response to PTA (treatment of choice)

Pearls

- Most common cause of RAS in children
- Spontaneous renal artery dissection is due to FMD until proven otherwise.
- Always look for visceral vessel involvement and/or other aneurysms.
- Complications:
  - Spontaneous dissection
  - Aneurysm rupture, emboli
  - HTN
  - Renal insufficienty (rare)

RENAL ARTERIAL ANEURYSM

- FMD (common)
- Atherosclerosis (common)
- NF
- Angiomyolipoma
- Lymphangioleiomyomatosis
- Rare
  - Congenital
  - Inflammatory
  - Infectious
  - Posttraumatic

Intraparenchymal arterial aneurysm occur in:

- Polyarteritis nodosa
- Speed kidney (amphetamine abuse)

POLYARTERITIS NODOSA (PAN)

Vasculitis of small and medium-sized arteries. Autoimmune origin and associated with hepatitis B virus. Presents as systemic illness but renal manifestations are common: hematuria, hypertension, perinephric hematoma.

Radiographic features
- Aneurysm of interlobar and arcuate arteries
- Aneurysm tend to be smaller and more peripheral than in FMD.
- Renal infarctions
- Always evaluate visceral arteries.

RENAL VEIN THROMBOSIS

Most cases occur in children less than 2 years of age. Variable clinical presentation; many patients are asymptomatic.

Causes

Children
- Dehydration
- Sepsis
- Maternal diabetes

Adults
- Glomerulopathies (membranous type most common)
- Collagen vascular disease
- Diabetes
- Trauma
- Thrombophlebitis

Radiographic features

IVP
- Poor or absent nephrogram
- Enlarged kidney
- Ureteral notching

US
- Cannot accurately diagnose partial thrombosis
- More accurate in pediatric than in adult patients

CT/MRI
- Helpful to depict thrombus in main renal vein segment

Venography
- Protruding thrombus or lack of inflow on cavagram
- Selective renal venography is the most definitive study
- Left renal vein has more collaterals (gonadal, adrenal, ureterals)

Complications
- Pulmonary embolism
- Loss of renal function

8

Chest

General Anatomy

PULMONARY ARTERIES

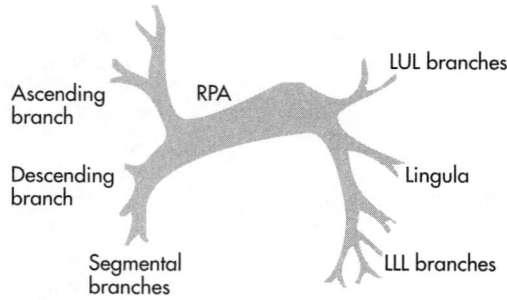

THORACIC VEINS

LIJV = left internal jugular vein
LEJV = left external jugular vein
LSCV = left subclavian vein
LTV = lateral thoracic vein
LSICV = left superior intercostal vein
LIMV = left internal mammary vein
HAZV = hemiazygos vein
AZV = azygos vein
RIJV = right internal jugular vein
REJV = right external jugular vein
RSCV = right subclavian vein
PICV = posterior intercostal vein
AICV = anterior intercostal vein
RTV = right thoracic vein
RIMV = right internal mammary vein
SVC = superior vena cava

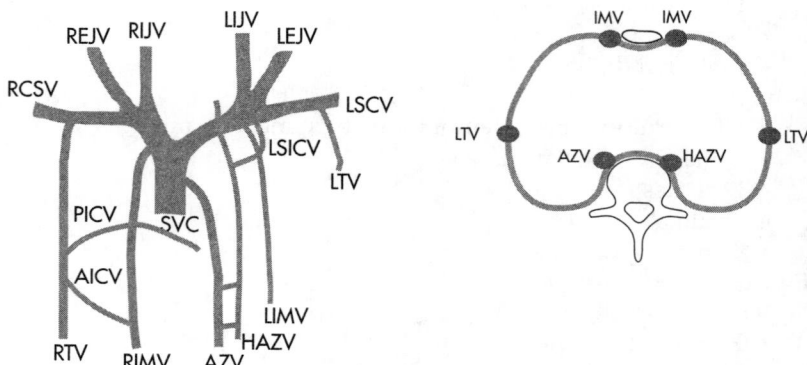

Angiographic Techniques

PULMONARY ANGIOGRAPHY

CATHETERS	
Type	**Comment**
Pigtail	Requires tip-deflecting device; maintains a stable position during high volume injections
Grollman	Secondary multipurpose curvature obviates need for tip-deflecting device
NIH catheter	Perforations possible
Balloon float catheter	Whips back with contrast injection because of floppiness

Indications
- Suspected pulmonary thromboembolism
- Diagnosis and treatment of pulmonary pseudoaneurysms and AVM
- Workup of pulmonary arterial hypertension

Technique
- Common femoral vein lies medial to artery
- Hand injection of inferior cava (cavogram) is performed to exclude IVC thrombus.
- Tip deflector directs catheter into right ventricle. Inability to advance the wire from RA into the RV can be due to primary placement in the coronary sinus.
- Ventricular ectopy is common when catheter is in RV.
- Tip deflector is needed to catheterize right PA but usually not left PA.
- Measure pulmonary arterial pressures
- Hand inject contrast agent to evaluate flow rate
- Views
     Right: PA and RPO magnified base
     Left: PA and LPO magnified base
     Additional views as needed
- Always pull catheter back through heart under fluroscopy.

PULMONARY PRESSURES			
Location	$P_{systolic}$	$P_{diastolic}$	P_{mean}
RA	—	—	0-5 mm Hg
RV	20-25 mm Hg	0-7 mm Hg	
PA	20-25 mm Hg	8-12 mm Hg	15 mm Hg
LA	—	—	5-10 mm Hg
LV	110-130 mm Hg	5-12 mm Hg	
Aorta	110-130 mm Hg	75-85 mm Hg	100 mm Hg

Pearls
- Transvenous pacer required if patient has preexisting LBBB
- Pulmonary hypertension: mean PA pressure > 15 mm Hg, systolic > 30 mm Hg
- All injections should be selective or subselective.
- Pulmonary pressures determine the type of contrast used at MGH (compromise between cost and risk):
     Normal pressures: HOCA
     Elevated pressures: LOCA
- Arterial flow with fluoroscopic hand injection determines rate of injection
     Normal flow: 22 mL/sec for 44 mL total
     Slow flow: reduce injection rate
     Fast flow: increase injection rate up to 30 mL/sec for 60 mL total
- No absolute contraindications
- Cut film is preferred over digital imaging:
     Better spatial resolution
     Less motion artifact
     Superior visualization of subsegmental and peripheral arteries

Complications
- Acute right heart failure (in pulmonary arterial hypertensives)
- Cardiac arrhythmias
- Death, < 0.3%

BRONCHIAL ARTERIOGRAPHY

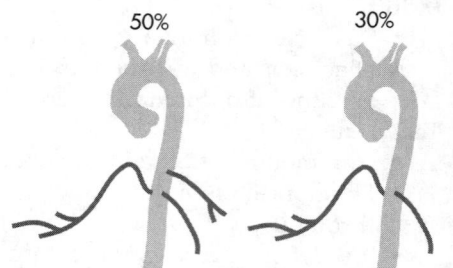

Indication: Hemoptysis, usually in patients with TB, cystic fibrosis, carcinoma.

Technique
- Descending thoracic aortogram is initially obtained as a road map.
- 90% of bronchial arteries originate from T4-T7 posterolaterally.
- Selective catheterization with Cobra or Simmons catheters
- DSA is preferable over cut-film.
- Embolization may be performed if active hemorrhage is present.

Complications
- Spinal cord injury
- Pain

BRONCHIAL ARTERY EMBOLIZATION

Indication: Hemoptysis

Technique
- Right femoral artery approach
- Descending aortogram to document takeoff of bronchial arteries
- Simmons, Cobra, or Berenstein for selective catheterization
- Use tracker to superselect bleeding vessel
- Use Polyvinyl alcohol, Gelfoam, or coils for embolization
- Systemic antibiotics are usually given.

Complications
- Reflux of embolization material
- Spinal artery injury, paralysis

Pulmonary Thromboembolism

Pulmonary embolism (PE) is a common complication of DVT. Despite the extrapolative and speculative nature of the medical literature concerning PE, a few generalizations apply:
- PE has high morbidity and mortality if not treated.
- Treatment significantly reduces morbidity and mortality.
- Subclinical PE is common and goes unrecognized.
- The clinical presentation of PE is most commonly nonspecific.
- Risk factors play an important role in the development of PE.
- Pulmonary arteriography is the gold standard for the detection of PE.

One or more preliminary diagnostic examinations are usually performed:
- Chest radiograph
    Exclude other causes of signs/symptoms (e.g., pneumonia)
    Triage to V/Q scan
    Required to optimally interpret V/Q scan
- V/Q scan (see Chapter 12)
    Useful with "clear" CXR
- Venous US
    Used to diagnose underlying DVT

Risk factors (same as for DVT)
- Postoperative patients, especially neurosurgical, orthopedic, and gynecological
- Trauma and burn patients
- Malignancy
- History of PE or DVT
- Immobility
- Obesity
- Congestive heart failure
- Neurological event
- Hormonal
    - Hormone therapy
    - Oral contraceptives
    - Pregnancy
- Coagulopathies, blood dyscrasias
    - Lupus anticoagulant
    - Protein C, S, or antithrombin III deficiencies
    - Polycythemia vera

INDICATIONS FOR PERFORMING PULMONARY ANGIOGRAPHY

Prior V/Q scan
- Intermediate or indeterminate V/Q scan
- Discrepancy between V/Q scan and clinical assessment (e.g., low probability scan and high clinical suspicion)

Without V/Q scan
- Complex therapeutic issues
- Hemodynamically unstable patient (may need embolectomy, lysis, etc.)
- Contraindication to anticoagulation
- A high likelihood of having a nondiagnostic V/Q scan

RADIOGRAPHIC FEATURES

Acute PE
- Embolus seen as intraluminal filling defect
- Tram tracking of contrast
- Abrupt cutoff of artery
- "Missing" vessels
- Angiographic findings do not always correlate with signs, symptoms, or V/Q scan findings.

Chronic PE
- Eccentric filling defects: "muralized" embolus
- Synechia or webs
- Smooth cutoffs
- "Missing" vessels
- Elevated pulmonary arterial pressures

Other Pulmonary Vascular Diseases

PULMONARY ARTERIOVENOUS MALFORMATION (AVM) OR FISTULA (AVF)

Most patients with pulmonary AVM/AVF are asymtomatic. Symptoms depend on size and number of lesions and when present include: dyspnea, cyanosis, clubbing. Paradoxical embolization: CVA, brain abscess.

Causes
Congenital
- Isolated, 50%
- Osler-Weber-Rendu syndrome, 50%

Acquired
- Trauma
- Infection
- Hepatogenic angiodysplasia

Radiographic features
CT, CXR
- Lung mass with feeding artery and draining vein

Angiography
- Most lesions are direct AVFS
- Lesions may be embolized with coils

Multiple in 35%
Most lesions occur in lower lobes
May be treated with transcatheter embolization

PULMONARY ARTERY PSEUDOANEURYSM

Cause: posttraumatic or iatrogenic pseudoaneurysms are most common. Clinical: hemoptysis. Treatment: transcatheter embolization (coils).

Extremities

Anatomy

LOWER EXTREMITY ARTERIES

Branches
Common femoral artery (CFA)
- SFA
- Profunda (PFA)
    Medial circumflex
    Lateral circumflex
    Descending branch

Popliteal artery
- Superior and inferior medial and lateral genicular arteries
- Anterior tibial artery: first trifurcation
- Posterior tibial artery
- Peroneal artery

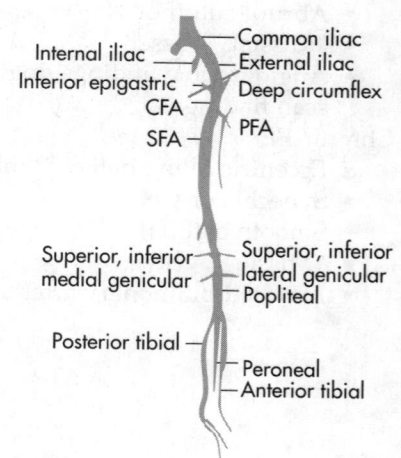

Foot
- Dorsal arteries (from anterior tibial artery): dorsalis pedis
  - Medial and lateral malleolar artery
  - Arcuate artery → metatarsal → digital arteries
- Plantar arteries (from posterior tibial)
  - Medial and lateral malleolar arteries
  - Medial and lateral plantar → plantar arch → metatarsal → digital arteries

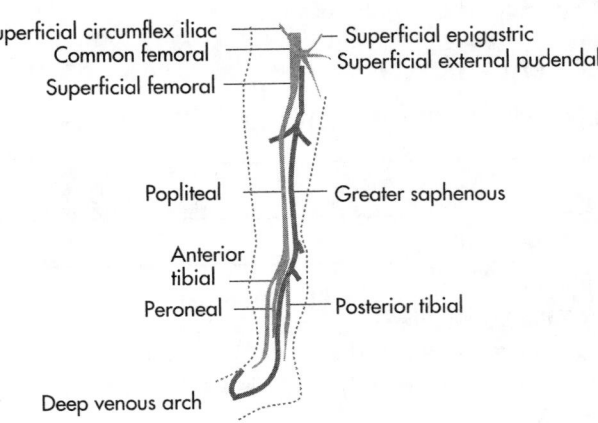

Collaterals

Collaterals develop in the setting of occlusive iliac and lower extremity disease.
- Internal mammary artery → inferior epigastric artery → CFA
- Lumbar/iliolumbar artery → circumflex iliac artery → CFA
- Lumbar/iliolumbar artery → lateral circumflex artery→ PFA
- Gluteal/obturator artery → lateral and medial circumflex artery → PFA
- PFA branches
- Geniculate branches

Persistent sciatic artery

- An embryonic sciatic artery remains the dominant flow inflow vessel to the leg; rare
- The aberrant vessel comes off the internal iliac artery, passes through the greater sciatic foramen, and runs deep to the gluteus maximus muscle.
- The aberrant artery joins the popliteal artery above the knee.
- The anomaly is usually bilateral.
- The artery is prone to intimal injury and aneurysm formation in the ischial region, due to its superficial location.

LOWER EXTREMITY VEINS

Calf veins are duplicated and follow the course of the arteries.

Common femoral vein
- Profunda vein
- Superficial femoral vein (receives blood from deep system via popliteal veins)

Deep calf system
- Anterior tibial veins (small)
- Peroneal veins
- Posterior tibial veins

Superficial calf system
- Greater saphenous vein (medial)
- Lesser saphenous veins (posterior calf)
- Many superficial collaterals connect the 2 saphenous veins.

8

UPPER EXTREMITY ARTERIES

Branches

Subclavian artery
- Vertebral artery
- Internal mammary artery
- Thyrocervical trunk
- Costocervical artery

Axillary artery
- Supreme thoracic artery
- Thoracoacromial artery
- Lateral thoracic artery
- Subscapular artery
- Humeral circumflex arteries

Brachial artery
- Profunda brachial artery
- Radial artery
- Ulnar artery
- Ulnar collaterals

Forearm
- Radial artery
    - Deep palmar arch
- Ulnar artery
    - Recurrent ulnar arteries
    - Common interosseous artery
    - Superficial palmar arch

Wrist, hand
- Deep palmar arch
- Superficial palmar arch

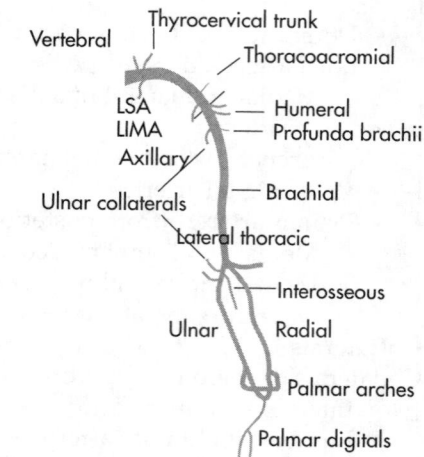

Lower Extremity

LOWER EXTREMITY OCCLUSIVE DISEASE

CAUSES	
Young Patients	**Old Patients**
Inflammatory Takayasu's disease Collagen vascular disease, autoimmune diseases, Buerger's disease	Atherosclerosis Embolism
DRUGS	
Ergotism (long, smooth narrowing) Amphetamine: speed kidney	
OTHER	
Spasm due to trauma (standing waves) Popliteal artery entrapment Radiation	

ATHEROSCLEROTIC OCCLUSIVE DISEASE

Intimal plaque formation leads to symptoms that depend on:
- Specific artery involved
- Severity of disease (degree of stenoses, multifocality)
- Superimposed complications:
  - Plaque ulceration or subintimal hemorrhage
  - Acute thrombosis
  - Distal embolization

Sudden changes in symptomatology usually indicate an acute complication. Clinical presentation is variable:
- Diminished pulses
- Claudication
- Hair loss, skin changes
- Tissue loss
- Rest pain
- "Cadaveric extremity": pale, paralyzed, pulseless, painful
- Gangrene

Risk factors for atherosclerosis of extremities are the same as for atherosclerosis elsewhere:
- Diabetes
- Hypertension
- Smoking
- Genetic predisposition, family history
- Hypercholesterolemia

Radiographic features
- Atherosclerotic disease is usually symmetrical and commonly affects arterial bifurcations.
- Location of involvement: SFA > iliac artery > tibial artery > popliteal artery > CFA
- Role of arteriography:
  - Preoperative staging
  - Percutaneous intervention: PTA, stent, atherectomy, lysis
- Assess hemodynamic significance of stenosis:
  - > 50% narrowing of luminal diameter
  - Presence of collaterals
  - Peak systolic pressure gradient across lesion > 10 mm Hg
- Role of MRA is still in evolution
- May perform limited DSA runoff using gadolinium chelate as contrast agent

Treatment
Angiographic (often used in conjunction with surgery)
- PTA
- Metallic stents
- Atherectomy (less commonly used)

8

Surgical
- In situ autologous saphenous vein graft
- Reversed vein graft
- Synthetic (polytetrafluoroethylene) grafts: usually not used below the knee
- Xenografts are no longer used
- Endarterectomy
- Amputation

ATHEROSCLEROTIC ANEURYSMAL DISEASE

Atherosclerosis in extremities may result in aneurysmal as well as occlusive disease. Location: popliteal artery (most common) > iliac artery > femoral artery. Frequently associated with AAA.

Clinical
- Popliteal aneurysm: Most common peripheral arterial aneurysm. 50% of aneurysms are bilateral, 80% are associated with aneurysm elsewhere. Commonly due to atherosclerotic disease or trauma. Angiography may show luminal dilatation or mural calcification. Remember that in 25% of cases popliteal artery aneurysms may not be associated with visible arterial dilatation by angiography. In these cases, secondary signs such as the "dog leg sign" (acute bend in lumen of the popliteal artery) may be helpful. The differential diagnosis associated with dog leg sign include (in addition to popliteal aneurysms) tortuous artery, popliteal artery entrapment syndrome, adventitital cystic disease, and Baker's cyst. Complications of aneurysm include distal embolization or thrombosis resulting in ischemia. Rupture is uncommon.
- Iliac aneurysms have a high incidence of rupture. Nearly all cases are associated with AAA.
- Common femoral aneurysm: distal embolization and/or thrombosis

ARTERIOMEGALY

- Diffusely enlarged vessels without focal aneurysms.
- Usually in aortoiliac and femoral-popliteal systems.
- Sluggish flow

ARTERIAL THROMBOEMBOLISM

Results in acute arterial occlusion and threatened limb. Clinical "5 Ps": pain, pallor, pulselessness, paresthesias, paralysis. Minimizing time from diagnosis to intervention is crucial to prevent limb loss.

Causes
- Cardiac: mural thrombus (most common)
    - Ventricular aneurysm
    - Myocardial infarction
    - Atrial fibrillation
- Aneurysms
- Iatrogenic
- Paradoxical embolus (DVT and right-to-left shunt)

Radiographic features
- Multiple lesions
- Emboli frequently lodge at bifurcations
- Lack of collateral vessels
- Severe vasospasm
- Filling defects with menisci
- Bilateral lesions

Treatment
- Surgical embolectomy
- Always differentiate arterial thrombembolism from in situ thrombosis secondary to atherosclerosis since therapy is different.

BUERGER'S DISEASE

Nonnecrotizing panarteritis of unknown etiology (thrombangitis obliterans); venous involvement occurs in 25%. Nearly all patients are smokers and 98% are male. Age: 20-40 years. Clinical: claudication is most common.

Location
- Calf and foot vessels (most common)
- Ulnar and radial arteries
- Palmar and digital arteries

Radiographic features
- Abrupt segmental arterial occlusions
- Intervening normal appearing arteries
- Multiple corkscrew collaterals
- Sparing of larger inflow arteries (e.g., iliac, femoral arteries)
- More than 1 limb affected. Lower extremity > upper extremity.

SMALL VESSEL ATHEROSCLEROSIS

Pattern of atherosclerosis in diabetics with preponderance of calf and foot involvement. High frequency of gangrene requiring amputation.

CHOLESTEROL OR ATHEROMA EMBOLI

Microemboli to distal small arteries result in painful ischemic digits, livido reticularis, "blue toe syndrome," and/or irreversible renal insufficiency. Source of emboli are most commonly atherosclerotic plaque from more proximal arteries. Emboli may occur spontaneously or after catheterization.

ERGOTISM

Bilateral, symmetrical, diffuse, and severe vasospasm. Primarily seen in young females on ergot medications for migraines. Reversible after discontinuation of medication.

POSTCATHETERIZATION GROIN COMPLICATIONS

Iatrogenic complications of femoral artery catheterization include most commonly:
- Hematoma
- Pseudoaneurysm
- AVF

8

Risk factors
- Anticoagulation
- Large catheters or sheaths
- Inadequate compression
- Poor access technique

Radiographic features
- US is the imaging study of choice to evaluate for complications.
- Hematoma: mass of variable echogenicity. No color flow within hematoma.
- Pseudoaneurysm:
    - Communicates with femoral artery
    - Swirling flow in pseudoaneurysm ("yin-yang") by color Doppler
    - To-and-fro flow at site of communication by pulse wave Doppler
    - Compression thrombosis with US transducer
- AVF:
    - More common with low entries (artery on top of vein)
    - Arterialized flow in the vein
    - Loss of high-resistance triphasic arterial waveform
    - Low-resistance diastolic flow in artery

DEEP VENOUS THROMBOSIS (DVT)

Lower extremity DVT is a medically important disease because it is the source of PE in 90% and because a high morbidity is associated with postphlebitic syndrome. Risk factors are related to Virchow's triad: stasis, hypercoagulability, and venous injury. Most DVT begin in the calf.

Locations
- Femoral-popliteal veins
- Pelvic veins
- Calf veins
- Intramuscular branches

Radiographic features
- US is the initial imaging study of choice for studying femoral-popliteal veins and has a high sensitivity (93%) and specificity (98%) for DVT.
- US is not nearly as accurate in calf or iliac veins.
- Dynamic compression US criteria:
    - Noncompressibility of vein
    - Echogenic lumen
    - Enlarged vein
- Color Doppler allows differentiation of occlusive and nonocclusive thrombi.
- Indirect iliac evaluation is possible by evaluating the pulse wave Doppler form. The waveform changes with respiration, augmentation, and Valsalva.

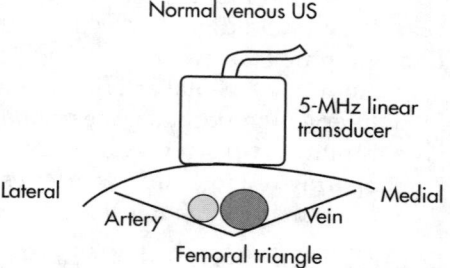

Normal venous US

5-MHz linear transducer

Lateral   Medial
Artery   Vein
Femoral triangle

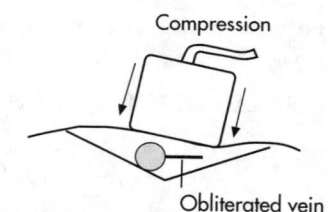

Compression

Obliterated vein

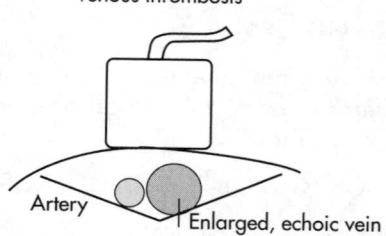

Venous thrombosis

Artery
Enlarged, echoic vein

- US "misses":
    DVT in small veins (e.g., calf)
    DVT of intramuscular veins
    Femoral profunda vein
    Iliac thrombus
    Acute DVT superimposed on chronic venous disease
- Venography is used when US is not definitive.
    Superior evaluation of calf veins
    Allows differentiation of acute from chronic thrombosis

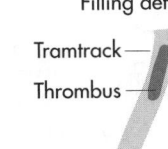

Compression

Noncompressible vein

Pearls

- Traditionally, infrapopliteal calf DVT is usually not treated medically. However, it is often followed serially with US to determine if there is proximal extension that would require treatment.
- More recently, there has been a trend to treat calf DVT to prevent postphlebitic syndrome; this concept, however, is evolving.

Filling defect

Tramtrack

Thrombus

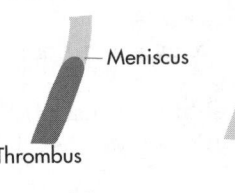

Occlusive thrombus

Meniscus

Thrombus

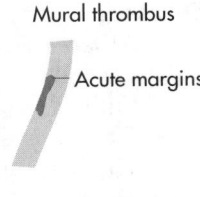

Mural thrombus

Acute margins

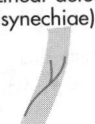

"Muralized" thrombus

Obtuse margin

Linear defects (synechiae)

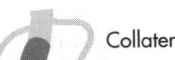

Chronic occlusion

Collaterals

IVC FILTERS

Indications: DVT and/or PE and one of the following:

- Contraindication to anticoagulation
- Failure of anticoagulation
- Complication of anticoagulation
- Prophylaxis
    Marginal cardiopulmonary reserve
    Preoperative protection
    Prophylactic filter placements are performed at some institutions; this indication is controversial, however.
- Documented DVT

Types

All filters have the same efficacy.

- Birdsnest (Cook) is only filter to accommodate a mega cava (< 28 mm diameter)
- Titaniumor Stainless Steel Greenfield (Medi-Tech)
- LGM filter (Vena-Tech)
- Simon nitinol filter (Bard) has the smallest delivery system. May be placed via brachial vein.

Technique

- Single wall aspiration technique for right femoral vein
- IVC venogram is performed to document patency at level of renal veins (usually at L1-2)
- Since caval thrombosis is a complication of filter placement, filters are usually below the renal veins and only suprarenally in selected cases.
- Large-bore left femoral vein introducer sheath

8

Complications
- Filter migration, <1%
- Filter failure (recurrent PE), 3%
- IVC thrombosis, 10%
- Groin complications

Upper Extremity

GENERAL

Diseases
- Atherosclerosis
- Vasculitis (Takayasu's, giant cell arteritis)
- Emboli
- Trauma (stabbing, gunshot), iatrogenic (cardiac catheterization)
- Thoracic outlet syndrome

Technique
- Transfemoral angiographic approach is preferred
    More flexibility
    Minimizes arterial spasm (also use spasmolytic drugs)
- Use LOCA to reduce pain and complications, especially to the carotid-vertebral system.
- Arch aortogram is obtained prior to selective work.
- Magnification, filtration, and subtractions are useful for hand arteriography.

THORACIC OUTLET SYNDROME

Compression of brachial plexus or subclavion vessels at the thoracic outlet. Three common sites of compression:
- Scalene triangle
- Costoclavicular space
- Pectoralis tunnel

Causes
- Brachial plexus compression (most common) causing neurological symptoms
- Subclavian artery: ischemia from distal emboli, claudication
- Subclavian vein thrombosis (any etiology)

PRIMARY SUBCLAVIAN VEIN THROMBOSIS

Primary thrombosis is also known as spontaneous or effort thrombosis or Paget-Schroetter disease. Thrombosis is caused by mechanical compression as the vein is impinged between the anterior scalene muscle, the first rib, and subclavius tendon or the costoclavicular ligament.

Radiographic features
- CXR may demonstrate cervical ribs, old fractures, etc.
- MRI is indicated if neurological symptoms are present.
- Arteriography:
    Subtle subclavian artery aneurysm (most common)
    Mural thrombus
    Distal emboli (forearm and hand)
    Arterial stenosis
    Arterial compression with hyperabduction

- Venography:
   - Dilatation or stenosis
   - Obstruction with hyperabduction

Treatment

For patients with thoracic outlet syndrome, an integrated approach that combines catheter directed therapy with delayed surgery is now the accepted treatment and includes the following:

- Thrombolysis as initial treatment
- A short course of anticoagulation with coumadin
- Conservative therapy when there is no extrinsic compression is detected after thrombolysis
- Surgical decompression for axillary or subclavian vein compression detected after thrombolysis
- Angioplasty or surgery for residual postoperative stenosis

HYPOTHENAR HAMMER SYNDROME

- Results from chronic repetitive trauma to the hand
- Trauma to distal ulnar artery as it crosses the hook of the hamate
- Aneurysm formation, occlusion, and distal embolization

AV FISTULAS FOR HEMODIALYSIS ACCESS

The ideal hemodialysis access is an endogenous arteriovenous fistula.

Types

Native fistula

- Brescia-Cimino fistula is side-to-side anastomosis of radial artery and cephalic vein at the wrist.
- Brachial artery and cephalic vein
- Brachial artery and basilic vein
- Femoral artery and saphenous vein

Synthetic bridge graft

- Manufactured out of PTFE
- Placed in forearm in straight configuration from radial artery to brachial vein or in looped configuration from brachial artery to brachial vein
- Can also be placed in upper arm brachial or axillary artery to high brachial vein
- Can be used earlier than native fistulas
- Generally do not have the longevity of the native grafts

Major disorders for AV fistulas

Failing dialysis graft

- Venous anastomotic stenosis; most likely to occur within first few centimeters of the anastomosis. Treated by dilatation by balloon angioplasty. Indications for stenting include restenosis, elastic recoil, and vein rupture.
- Arterial stenosis. Responsible for graft failure in < 15 % of cases.
- Intragraft stenosis is relatively uncommon.

Thrombosed dialysis graft

- In most cases, graft thrombosis occurs from progressive narrowing in the graft circuit (usually at the venous end). Treatment options: percutaneous therapy, pulse spray pharmacomechanical thrombolysis (PSPMT), mechanical thrombectomy.

Ischemia and steal syndrome

8

Trauma

INDICATIONS FOR ANGIOGRAPHY IN EXTREMITY TRAUMA

- Blunt trauma with pulsatile bleeding, expanding hematoma, pulse deficits, digital ischemia, or a bruit or thrill at trauma site
- High-velocity missile
- Low-velocity missile and clinical findings (expanding hematoma, loss of pulses)
- Crush injury
- Iatrogenic trauma
- Reconstructive surgery planned (e.g., free flaps, bone grafts)

TRAUMATIC INJURIES

Many possible injuries can occur:
- Intimal tear: linear defect in lumen; may progress to pseudoaneurysm
- Pseudoaneurysm: may be amenable to transcatheter embolization
- Mural hematoma
- Laceration
- Transection
- Dissection
- AVF early draining vein
- Distal embolization: may occur from proximal injuries
- Vasospasm

Pearls
- All patients with posterior knee dislocations should undergo arteriography because:
    - High incidence of popliteal artery injury and thrombosis
    - High rate of limb loss
- Hemorrhage secondary to pelvic fractures rarely requires arteriography.
- Vasospasm and compartment syndrome cannot be distinguished by arteriography in many instances.

Differential Diagnosis

General

ANEURYSM

Atherosclerosis
- Aorta
    - Abdominal aorta (most common)
    - Descending thoracic aorta
- Peripheral vasculature (popliteal > iliac > femoral)

Infection (mycotic)
- Bacterial (*Staphylococcus, Salmonella*)
- Syphilis

Inflammation
- Takayasu's disease
- Giant cell arteritis
- Collagen vascular diseases
    Polyarteritis nodosa

Congenital
- Structural collagen diseases
    Marfan syndrome
    Homocystinuria
    Ehlers-Danlos syndrome
- Fibromuscular dysplasia
- Neurofibromatosis
- Pseudoxanthoma elasticum
    Trauma

ISCHEMIA

Arterial
- Dissection
- Embolus
- Thrombosis, thrombosed aneurysm
- Vasculitis
- Drugs

Venous
- Thrombosis (phlegmasia cerulea dolens)

Low flow
- Hypovolemia, shock
- Hypoperfusion

PERIPHERAL VASCULAR DISEASE

- Occlusive atherosclerosis
- Aneurysmal atherosclerosis
- Small vessel atherosclerosis (diabetics)
- Embolic disease
    Thromboembolic
    Cholesterol emboli
    Plaque emboli
- Vasculitis
- Other
    Buerger's disease
    Medication

EMBOLI

Cardiac emboli
- Atrial fibrillation
- Recent acute myocardial infarction
- Ventricular aneurysm
- Bacterial endocarditis
- Cardiac tumor (myxoma)

8

Atherosclerotic emboli
- Aortoiliac plaque
- Aneurysm (AAA, popliteal)

Paradoxical emboli; (R-L shunt)
- DVT

ANGIOGRAPHIC TUMOR FEATURES

Mnemonic: "BEDPAN"
- **B**lush
- **E**ncasement of arteries
- **D**isplacement of arteries
- **P**uddling of contrast
- **A**rteriovenous shunting
- **N**eovascularity

"MANY VESSELS"

DIFFERENTIATION OF HYPERVASCULAR LESIONS		
	Early Draining Vein	Mass Effect
Arteriovenous malformation	Yes	No (only in brain)
Extensive collaterals	No	No
Tumor neovascularity	Yes in AV shunting	Yes from tumor

Thorax

AORTIC ENLARGEMENT

- Aneurysm
- Dissection
- Poststenotic dilatation due to turbulence:
    Coarctation
    Aortic valvular disease
    Sinus of Valsalva aneurysm

AORTIC STENOSIS

Congenital
- Coarctation
- Pseudocoarctation
- Williams syndrome (supravalvular aortic stenosis)
- Rubella syndrome

Aortitis
- Takayasu's disease (most common arteritis to cause stenosis)

Other
- Neurofibromatosis
- Radiation

PULMONARY ARTERY STENOSIS

- Williams syndrome (infantile hypercalcemia)
- Rubella syndrome
- Takayasu's disease
- Associated with congenital heart disease (especially tetralogy of Fallot)

Abdomen

HYPERRENINEMIC HYPERTENSION

Decreased renal perfusion
- Atherosclerosis
- Fibromuscular dysplasia

Renin-secreting tumors

Renal compression
- Large intrarenal masses (cysts, tumors)
- Subcapsular hemorrhage (Page kidney)

RENAL TUMORS

Renal cell carcinoma
- 80% hypervascular
- Neovascularity
- AV shunting
- Parasitization

Angiomyolipoma
- Aneurysms
- Fat content

Oncocytoma
- Spoke wheel, 30%
- Most hypovascular

RENAL ARTERIAL ANEURYSM

Main artery aneurysm
- FMD (common)
- Atherosclerosis (common)
- Neurofibromatosis
- Mycotic
- Trauma
- Congenital

Distal intrarenal aneurysms
- Polyarteritis nodosa
- IVDA (septic)
- Other vasculitides (Wegener's, collagen vascular disease)
- Traumatic pseudoaneurysm
- RT
- Amphetamine abuse (speed kidney)

8

SUGGESTED READINGS

Abrams HL, editor: *Abrams angiography: vascular and interventional radiology,* Boston, 1997, Little, Brown.

Castaneda-Zuniga WR: *Interventional radiology,* Philadelphia, 1997, Lippincott Williams & Wilkins.

Cope C et al: *Atlas of interventional radiology,* New York, 1990, Gower Medical Publishers.

Dyer R, editor: *Handbook of basic vascular and interventional radiology,* London, 1993, Churchill Livingstone.

Gedgaudas E, Moller JH, Castaneda-Zuniga WR, et al: *Cardiovascular radiology,* Philadelphia, 1985, WB Saunders.

Johnsrude IS et al: *A practical approach to angiography,* Baltimore, 1987, Williams & Wilkins.

Kadir S: *Atlas of normal and variant angiographic anatomy,* Philadelphia, 1990, WB Saunders.

Kadir S: *Current practice of interventional radiology,* New York, 1991, BC Decker.

Kadir S: *Diagnostic angiography,* Philadelphia, 1986, WB Saunders.

Kadir S: *Teaching atlas of interventional radiology: diagnostic and therapeutic angiography,* New York, 1999, Thieme.

LaBerge JM: *Interventional radiology essentials,* Philadelphia, 2000, Lippincott Williams & Wilkins.

Wojtowycz MM: *Handbook of interventional radiology and angiography,* St Louis, 1995, Mosby.

Chapter 9

Breast Imaging

Chapter Outline

Breast Imaging

Mammography Techniques

Mammography is primarily a screening not a diagnostic tool. The mediolateral oblique and craniocaudal views are standard screening views, while additional views described below are mainly used for further evaluation of lesions.

MAMMOGRAPHIC VIEWS

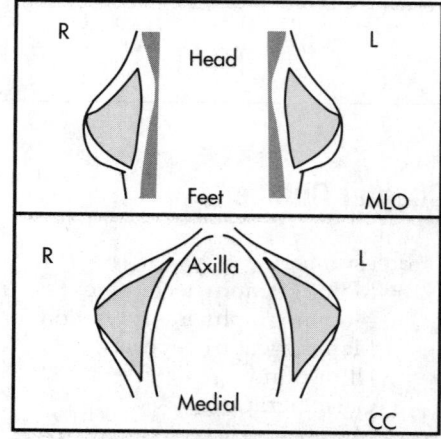

Mediolateral oblique (MLO) view
This standard view is a projection parallel to the pectoralis major muscle (C-arm of mammographic unit is 40°-60°). The pectoralis should be seen to the level or below of the axis of the nipple and appear convex (never concave towards the nipple).

Craniocaudal (CC) view
Projection with slight rotation toward the sternum to detect posteromedial tumors that may be missed on the MLO view. In general, better breast compression is achieved with the CC view than with the MLO view.

Straight lateral view
This view is a true mediolateral projection (x-ray beam parallel to floor). Used commonly to evaluate calcifications.

Axillary tail view (Cleopatra view)
This view allows imaging of the axillary tail of the breast. It resembles the mediolateral view but allows evaluation of breast tissue more laterally oriented.

Cleavage valley view
Modified CC view that improves visualization of area between breasts. Both breasts are positioned on the detector.

Spot compression views
With or without microfocus magnification. For evaluation of margins and morphology of lesions. Spreads structures, useful to determine if densities are real or not.

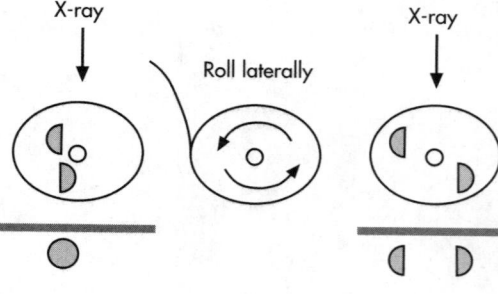

Rolled views
- Roll breast laterally: superior lesion moves laterally
- Roll breast medially: superior lesion moves medially

Proper positioning
Proper positioning is crucial for lesion detection. A cancer not imaged will not be detected. For both the CC and MLO views, the mobile border of the breast (CC: inferior border, MLO: lateral border) should be moved as far as possible toward the fixed border before placing the breast on the bucky. Check for correct positioning on CC and MLO views:
- Pectoralis muscle: On the MLO view, the pectoralis major should be convex anteriorly (never concave) and be seen to or below the level of the axis of the nipple. On the CC view, the muscle is seen approximately 35% of the time. The perpendicular distance from the nipple to the pectoralis on the MLO is used as a reference for adequacy of the CC view. The measurement on the CC view (taken as the distance from the nipple to the pectoralis or the back of the image) should be within 1 cm of the MLO measurement.

- The nipple should be in profile on at least one view. This may require an extra view in addition to the screening CC and MLO views.
- Retroglandular fat should usually be seen behind all fibroglandular tissue.
- Improper positioning on the MLO results in sagging, which is manifested by low nipple position and skin folds near the inframammary fold. The breast should be pulled up and out.
- Skin folds are usually not problematic in the axilla but can obscure lesions elsewhere. Repeat such views.
- Although the CC view is taken to include all of the medial breast tissue, exaggerated positioning is not desired. To check for this, make sure the nipple is near midline and not off to one side.
- On the MLO view, check for "cutoff" of inferior breast or axillary tissue resulting from placing the breast too low or too high on the bucky.
- Problems with compression or cutoff may be related to the image receptor size. Both 18 × 24 cm and 24 × 30 cm sizes are available. Too small a size results in cutoff. Too large can impair compression by impinging on other body parts.
- Motion is best detected by checking the septations located inferiorly and/or posteriorly or calcifications which will be blurred by motion.

COMPRESSION

Compression should always be symmetrical. Breast compression is used to reduce patient dose and improve image quality:
- Reduction of motion artifacts by immobilization of breast
- Reduction of geometric blur
- Reduction in change of radiographic density (achieve uniform breast thickness)
- Reduction of scattered radiation by decreasing breast thickness

PATIENT INTERACTION

The comparable radiation risk of mammography (~200 mR/breast per view with grid) is very low; in a population of 1 million, one would expect 800 occult, naturally occurring cancers and only 1-3 cancers (absolute risk model) induced by mammography. This risk is similar to:
- Breathing Boston air for 2 days
- Riding a bicycle for 10 miles
- Driving a car for 300 miles
- Eating 40 tablespoons of peanut butter

OBTAIN HISTORY

- Family history
- Risk factors for breast cancer
- Complaints
  - Mass, thickening
  - Pain
  - Nipple discharge

Mammography Interpretation

VIEWING CONDITIONS

Ideally, dedicated mammography viewing equipment is used. Minimal requirements include:
- Adequate view box luminescence
- Low ambient light
- Masking of mammograms to exclude peripheral viewbox light
- Magnifying glass: each film should be reviewed with a magnifying glass following initial inspection

IMAGE LABELLING

American College of Radiology (ACR) requirements:
- Markers identifying the view and side are required and are to be placed near the axilla to guide orientation
- An identification label must include the patient name (first and last), ID number, facility name and location, and technologist's initials if not included elsewhere on the film
- Cassette number (Arabic numeral)

Optional
- Technical factors
- Mammography unit number (Roman numeral)

DOUBLE READING

While it is not the standard of practice, institutions performing double reading of screening mammograms report increases in cancers detected ranging from 6.4% - 15%. Massachusetts General Hospital (MGH): 7.7%.

EVALUATION OF THE MAMMOGRAM

Each mammogram should be systematically evaluated for:
- Adequate quality of study, additonal views required?
- Adequate penetration of fibroglandular breast tissue
- Skin, nipple, trabecular changes
- Masses present?
- Calcifications
- Axillary nodes
- Asymmetry (usually a variant of normal)
- Architectural distortion

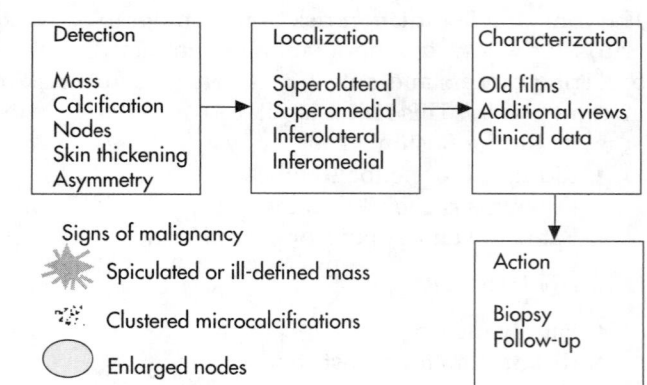

Comparison with prior films is mandatory. Breast cancers can grow slowly, and minimal progressive changes need to be documented. All masses and calcifications need to be further characterized. If the initial views are not adequate, additional views have to be obtained.

QUALITY CONTROL

ACR requirements:
- Daily: processor, darkroom cleanliness
- Weekly: screen cleanliness, viewbox
- Monthly: replenishment rates, phantom, visual checklist. Some mammographers advocate more frequent evaluation of phantom images since such phantom images evaluate the entire imaging system
- Quarterly: fixer retention, repeat/reject, light x-ray field alignment analysis
- Semiannually: darkroom fog, screen-film contact, compression, viewbox luminance

Mammography Reporting (Bi-Rads)

MASS

Breast masses vary in appearance and are usually classified according to their border: a potential mass seen on a single view only is called a "density."

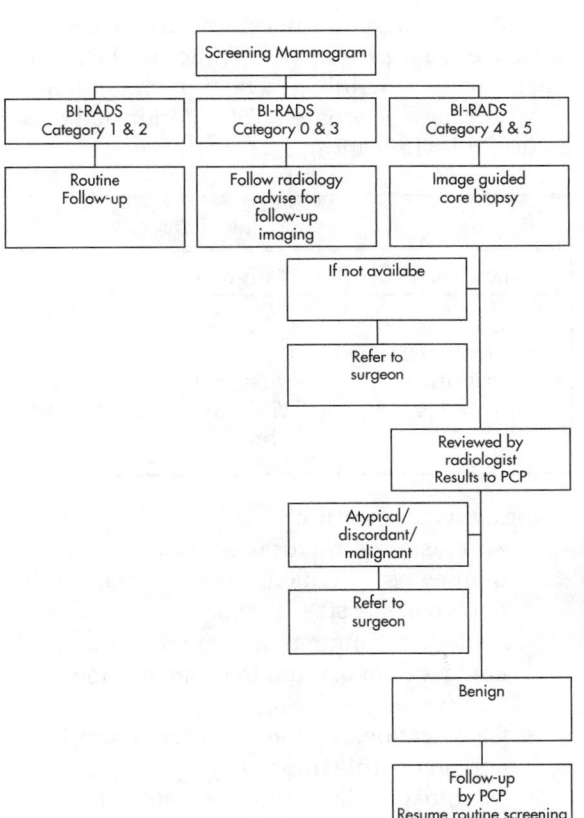

- Spiculated: a spiculated tumor margin is the only specific sign of malignancy; however, not all spiculated masses are cancers. Spiculated masses are the easiest masses to diagnose, although they may be obscured by fibroglandular tissue. Spiculations are also seen in:

  Scar tissue (usually resolve in 1 year if a surgical scar and in 3 years if a postradiation scar)

  Desmoid tumors
- Indistinct borders: rapidly growing tumors that do not elicit significant fibrous tissue reaction. Some benign lesions may also have indistinct or fuzzy margins:

  Fat necrosis

  Elastosis refers to radial scar, indurative mastopathy or sclerosing duct hyperplasia; elastosis is probably a form of sclerosing adenosis

  Infection/abscess
- Microlobulated: small lobulations are more worrisome for malignancy than larger lobulations
- Obscured: margin cannot be seen or evaluated because of overlying normal tissue
- Circumscribed masses with well-defined borders: uncommon sign of malignancy; only 2% of solitary masses with smooth margins are malignant

Other features of mass lesions are less useful:
- Size: the larger the tumor the worse the prognosis. Malignant tumors larger than 1 cm are twice as likely to have spread to axillary nodes. A biopsy should be considered in any solitary, noncystic lesion larger than 8 mm. If spiculated, any size lesion should be biopsied. The size of a mass does not correlate with likelihood of malignancy.

- Shape: the more irregular the mass, the greater the likelihood of malignancy. Shapes are classified as round, oval, lobular, or irregular.
- Density: malignant lesions are usually very dense for their size; lucent, fat-containing lesions, on the contrary, are benign (posttrauma oil cyst, lipoma, galactocele). Lesions are described as high, equal, or low density or as fat-containing.
- Location: distinguish parenchymal mass from skin lesion. Small lesions in the periphery of the upper outer quadrant are most likely lymph nodes.
- Multiplicity: multiple, well-circumscribed masses are commonly benign fibroadenomas (younger patients), cysts after 35 years of age. In older patients, metastases from other primaries should be excluded.

CALCIFICATIONS

50% of all malignant tumors are discovered by mammography because of the presence of suspicious calcifications. Once detected, calcifications should be categorized as definitively benign, malignant, or suspicious (i.e., biopsy is necessary). In asymptomatic women, 75% of biopsied clustered calcifications are benign, 25% are associated with cancer.

EVALUATION OF CALCIFICATIONS		
Parameter	Malignant	Benign
Size	< 1 mm	> 1 mm
Number per cm^3	> 5	< 5
Distribution	Clustered	Scattered (not clustered)
Morphology	Wild, unordered, fine linear branching	Round, lucent center, solid rods

Malignant calcifications
- A "cluster of microcalcifications" is usually defined as > 5 calcifications per cm^3 of tissue.
- Each particle size is invariably < 2 mm (except comedocarcinoma); most malignant calcifications are less than 0.5 mm in diameter; lower limit of detectability is 0.2-0.3 mm.
- Calcifications within a cluster typically vary in size and shape (pleomorphis).
- Malignant calcifications are almost always located in ducts (intraductal component), even when the tumor is not.
- Dot-dash branching pattern and irregular shapes are typical of malignant calcification.
- The use of microfocal spot magnification improves the diagnostic accuracy in the evaluation of calcification.
- Always biopsy suspicious calcifications.

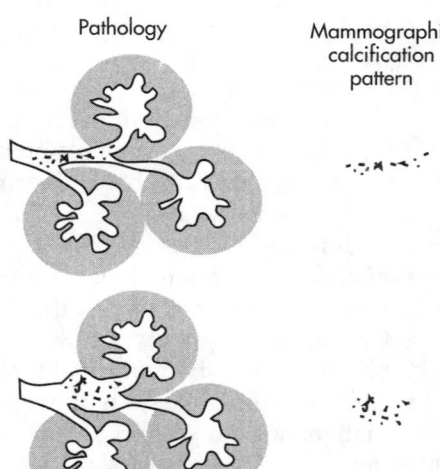

Pathology

Mammographic calcification pattern

Benign calcifications

Calcifications, when multiple, are described as clustered, linear, segmental (distributed along multiple branches of a duct system), regional (occupy a large volume but not in a ductal distribution) or diffuse. Types:

Round
- May vary in size; classified as punctate if < 0.5 mm
- Probably clustered benign; 6-month follow-up for 2-year interval

Dystrophic
- Irregular, > 0.5 mm, often lucent centers

Large rodlike calcification
- > 1 mm continuous rods, may branch
- Benign secretory disease (plasma cell mastitis) or duct ectasia

Skin calcifications
- Polyhedral shape with lucent centers
- Appearance is usually typical so that no further workup is required; occasionally a "skin localization" with tangential views will be useful

Vascular calcifications
- Parallel tracks

Coarse
- Involuting fibroadenoma

Rim calcification
- Cyst
- Fat necrosis

Milk of calcium
- Layering calcification in microcysts
- Fuzzy, amorphous on CC view
- Semilunar on linear or MLO view

Suture calcification
- Linear or tubular with shape of knot

Others
- Round, dystrophic: follow-up for 6 months for 2 years
- Pleomorphic calcifications: biopsy
- Unsure: follow-up or biopsy

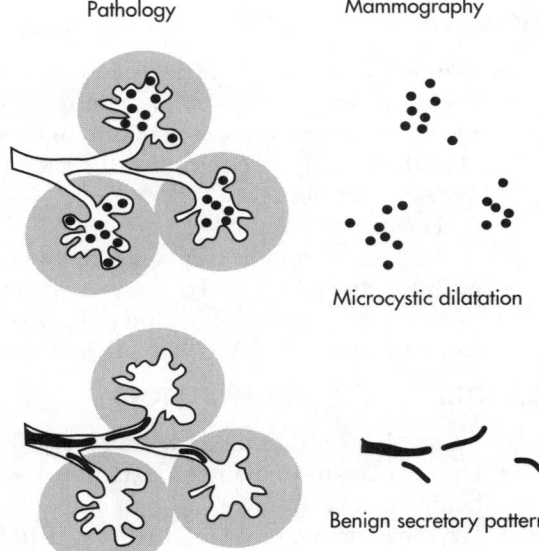

Pathology   Mammography

Microcystic dilatation

Benign secretory pattern

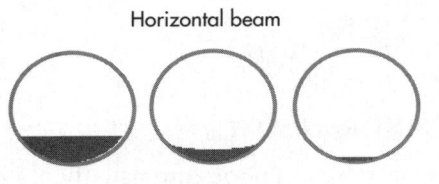

Horizontal beam

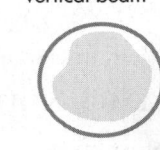

Vertical beam

ARCHITECTURAL DISTORTION

Architectural distortion refers to a tumor-associated desmoplastic response that results in a focal change of breast parenchyma. Architectural distortion should always be seen on at least 2 views. Mammographic signs of a desmoplastic response include:
- Abnormal arrangement of Cooper's ligaments
- Ducts and periductal fibrosis
- "Pulling in" of superficial structures

9

SKIN, NIPPLE, TRABECULAR CHANGES

- Skin retraction due to fibrosis and shortening of Cooper's ligaments (skin becomes flat or concave); the tumor itself is almost always palpable if skin retraction is present on the mammogram
- Skin thickening (> 3 mm) may be a sign of malignancy or benign conditions. Types:
   Focal: local tumor
   Diffuse: sign of edema; may be due to inflammatory cancer
- Nipple retraction is worrisome when acute and unilateral
- Fine linear nipple calcification obliges one to rule out Paget's disease (other causes of nipple calcification are benign)

ABNORMAL DUCTAL PATTERNS

Cancer may cause shortening, dilatation, or distortion of ducts. Mammography:
- Ducts > 2 mm in diameter extending > 2 cm into the breast are usually due to benign duct ectasia.
- Asymmetrical-appearing ducts are usually a normal variation, although this can be a very rare indication of malignancy.
- Symmetrical ductal ectasia is a benign condition.

BREAST LESIONS THAT ARISE IN MAIN SEGMENTAL DUCTS

- Papillomas
- Papillary cancer

BREAST LESIONS ARISING IN TERMINAL DUCTS

- Peripheral papillomas
- Epithelial hyperplasia
- Ductal carcinoma in situ (DCIS)
- Invasive ductal carcinoma

LYMPH NODE ABNORMALITIES

Normal intramammary lymph nodes are usually only visible in the upper outer quadrant. Nodes may occasionally be seen below the medial plane. There have been rare reports of lymph nodes in the medial breast. An increase in size, number, or density of axillary lymph nodes is abnormal: axillary nodes > 2 cm or intramammary nodes > 1 cm without lucency or hilar notch are suspicious (if lucent fat center is present, even larger nodes may be benign); nodes that contain tumor lose the radiolucent hilum and appear dense, although benign hyperplasia may appear similar. Nodal calcification implies:
- Metastases (most common)
- Lymphoma
- Rheumatoid arthritis and previous gold injections

ASYMMETRY OF BREAST TISSUE

Asymmetrical dense tissue is seen in 3% of breasts, usually upper outer quadrant, and is considered a normal variant (caused by fibrosis). The mammographic finding of asymmetrical breast tissue is suspicious only if it is *palpable* or if there are associated abnormalities (mass, calcifications, architectural distortion, or if asymmetry has developed over time). The following are the criteria that an opacity has to fulfill to be called asymmetrical tissue:

- Not a mass (i.e., changes morphology on different views)
- Contains fat
- No calcifications
- No architectural distortion
- If asymmetrical tissue is palpable, ultrasound may be useful for further workup

SKIN CALCIFICATIONS

- Suspect skin calcification, if superficial in location
- Periaerolar, axillary, or medial location
- Tiny hollow spherical calcifications
- Plaquelike on one view and linear on another view

Mammography Reporting

DICTATION

Reports are organized by a short description of breast composition, description, and location of significant findings, as well as any interval changes, and an overall impression. The ACR categorizes reports into 6 categories:

0 = Needs additional mammographic or other imaging evaluation. This includes interpretations awaiting old films for comparison.
1 = Negative: breasts are symmetrical and normal, return to annual screening
2 = Benign finding: includes typical nodes, calcified fibroadenomas, lucent lesions (implants), and scattered benign calcifications, return to annual screening
3 = Probably benign, follow-up suggested: multiple, rounded densities, borderline calcifications → 6 month follow-up
4 = Suspicious and should be biopsied: indicates 20%-30% chance of malignancy → biopsy
5 = Cancer with 99% certainty: spiculated lesions → biopsy/excision

Pearls
- Short-term follow-up less than 6 months is almost never useful because most processes will not change over such a short interval. The rare exception is a suspected hematoma, which would be expected to show signs of regression at 3 months.
- Heterogeneously dense and extremely dense parenchymal patterns lower the sensitivity of mammography, and a short statement to this effect may be included in the report.

REASONS FOR MISSING BREAST CANCER

- Failure to detect lesions
- Faulty technique
    Underexposure on mammogram
    Patient motion
    Poor film screen contact
    Dense or nodular parenchymal pattern
    Subthreshhold size
- Misdiagnosis of lesions

COMMONLY MISSED LESIONS

- Invasive lobular carcinoma. Mammographically this lesion appears as architectural distortion and asymmetrical density. Lack of a discrete mass or clustered microcalcifications can make this lesion difficult to detect.
- Invasive ductal carcinoma
- DCIS coexistent with atypical ductal hyperplasia on core needle biopsy.
- Palpable mass: palpable masses not seen on mammography must be investigated further. Spot films or tangential films over the palpable mass may disclose a mass that is otherwise occult.

Ultrasound (US)

Indications
- Women under age 28 (MGH threshold) with a palpable lump should be evaluated with US because the palpable lesion most likely represents a fibroadenoma. The decision to biopsy a solid mass in a young woman must be made by the patient and her physician since the risk of malignancy is very low.
- Differentiation of cyst from solid structure (use 7.5 or 10 MHz transducer): no internal echoes; through transmission; thin imperceptible wall. Abscess and hematoma may mimic a solid mass. If there are low-level echoes, a mass lesion has to be excluded by biopsy/aspiration.

Interpretation
- Ultrasound cannot detect most small calcifications.
- Fibroadenomas are usually hypoechoic and well circumscribed.
- Lymphomas are usually hypoechoic.
- Lipomas are difficult to differentiate from surrounding tissue.
- Oil cysts are hypoechoic and have poor through transmission.
- Benign lymph nodes may have a characteristic central echogenic center due to fat in the lymph node hilum.
- Cysts and solid lesions often cannot be differentiated from one another on mammograms, particularly well-circumscribed mammographic densities.

Galactography

Indications
- Workup of solitary and spontaneous duct discharge
- Identify deep lesions that might be missed by surgery
- May be used to identify proximal lesions, since papilloma and cancer have a similar appearance

Technique

1. Patient sitting or lying down
2. Express secretions to identify duct origins
3. Prep breast
4. Blunt pediatric sialogram needle
5. Inject 0.1-2 mL of water-soluble contrast agent
6. Avoid air bubbles
7. Obtain mammogram. Look for filling defects, distorted ducts, extravasation.

MR Imaging (MRI)

Advantages

- Images breast implants and ruptures
- Highly sensitive to small abnormalities
- Used effectively in dense breasts
- Evaluation of inverted nipples for cancer
- Determines the extent of breast cancer
- Determines what type of surgery is indicated (lumpectomy or mastectomy)
- Evaluation of breast cancer recurrence and residual tumors after lumpectomy
- Evaluation of axillary lymph nodes
- Can be useful in cutaneous disorders such as neurofibromatosis
- Characterization of small abnormalities
- May be useful in screening women at high risk for breast cancer, according to recent studies

Limitations

- MRI takes 30-60 min compared to 10-20 min for screening mammography.
- The cost of MRI is several times the cost of mammography.
- MRI requires the use of a contrast agent.
- MRI can be nonspecific; often it cannot distinguish between cancerous and noncancerous tumors.
- Minimally invasive breast biopsy techniques need to be further developed to evaluate abnormalities detected with MRI.
- Advanced MRI techniques may not be available at many outpatient centers.

Technique

- Prone position
- Dedicated bilateral surface coils are usually receive-only coils but can be transmit/receive coils
- 1.5 T for optimum MRI

Contrast enhancement by MRI

- Cancer
- Benign masses
- Regional enhancement: usually implies benign etiology
- Patchy enhancement (i.e., enhancement in one part of the breast that seems to be confined to one ductal system): reasonable likelihood of underlying obstructing malignancy
- Diffuse enhancement is felt to be a benign pattern (fibrocystic or proliferative changes)

9

Evaluation of implants (see section on implants in this chapter)
- Silicone has long T1 and long T2.
- Proton signal is from methyl groups in the dimethyl polysiloxane polymer.
- The silicone shell is of lower signal than the silicone within the implant because of greater cross-linking of methyl groups.
- Fast-spin echo T2W, as well as orthogonal silicone-sensitive (fat-suppressed) inversion recovery sequences, are obtained. Chemical H_2O supression will yield a silicone-only image.
- MRI of implant rupture: 94% sensitivity, 97% specificity (compare to US: 70% sensitivity, 92% specificity)

Evaluation of malignancy
- MRI is useful in patients with dense breasts not well evaluated with mammography or with known multicentric lesions (i.e., in different quadrants).
- Most protocols use dynamic contrast enhancement pattern of breast lesion on fat-suppressed images, usually a volume acquisition.
- Cancer enhances more rapidly than benign lesions, and the critical period is in the first 3 min.
- For lesions 1 cm or greater: 88%-100% sensitivity, 30%-97% specificity
- DCIS generally enhances more slowly than invasive cancers and findings overlap significantly with hyperplasia. May not enhance. MRI should not be used to evaluate malignant character of microcalcification.
- The use of MRI for monitoring postsurgical or postradiation patients for recurrence or for screening of patients with implants is questionable since a trend toward a more advanced stage at diagnosis is known (although the risk of malignancy is the same as in patients without implants).

Biopsy

MGH statistics: between 1978 and 1988, 3000 biopsies were performed. Of those, 25% proved to be malignant (25% positive predictive value). Breast biopsies do not seed tumors in the needle tract.

NEEDLE LOCALIZATION FOR SURGICAL BIOPSY/EXCISION

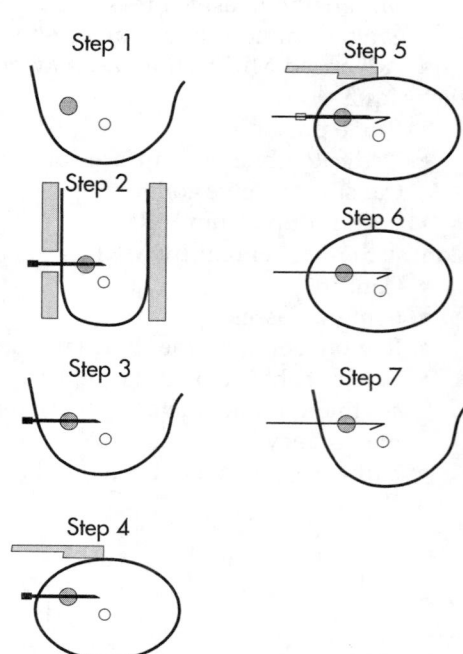

1. Identify lesion (use 90° angle films to direct needle parallel to chest wall); choose shortest distance to lesion
2. Obtain view with breast in compression device; clean skin with iodine 3 times, then once with alcohol; pass needle tip in direction of x-ray beam past lesion
3. Obtain a second film; if the needle is in good position take a 90° opposed film
4. If needle is in appropriate location (tip 1 cm beyond lesion), pass hook wire through needle. Pull needle back to engage hook; the wire may back out somewhat when patient stands up
5. Take a third mammogram perpendicular to wire with wire in place
6. A mammogram of the postbiopsy specimen should be obtained to ensure that the lesion is included in the specimen.

TECHNIQUE OF LOCALIZING LESION SEEN ONLY ON A SINGLE VIEW (TRIANGULATION)

Same as above technique with the following modifications:

1. Place the breast in compression in the position in which the lesion is seen.
2. Pass the needle tip deep to the lesion (TLN: true length of needle; PLN: projected length of needle; TLPN: true length to pull back needle; PLPN: projected length to pull back needle; TDL: true depth of lesion).
3. With slight repositioning to oblique the needle, its projection allows use of similar triangles to calculate the distance of pull back.
4. The needle is adjusted accordingly and the wire deployed after confirming needle position.
5. Take a mammogram with the wire in place in the orthogonal position.

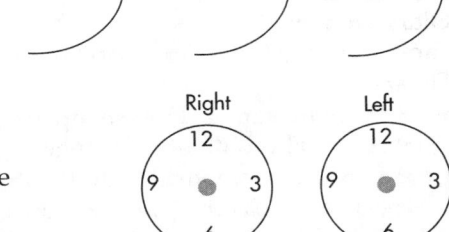

$$TLPN = (TLN \times PLPN) / PLN$$

Alternative technique

This technique allows localization of an unseen lesion on the CC view if it is only visible on the straight lateral and MLO view.

1. Align straight lateral, oblique, and CC views from left to right.
2. Nipple should be on a horizontal line.
3. Connect the lesion on any two views by a straight line.
4. Lesion should be located along path of the line on the 3rd view.
5. When describing the location of a lesion, the breast is seen as the face of a clock, and the location in this plane is given as clock position. Depth is then indicated as anterior, middle, or posterior.
6. Additional descriptions are subareolar, central, or axillary tail area.

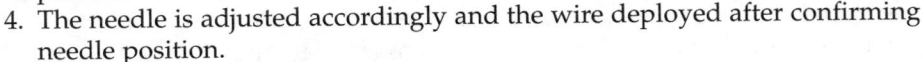

LESION SEEN ON CT BUT NOT EASILY SEEN MAMMOGRAPHICALLY

These are usually lesions near the chest wall.

1. Place a linear marker or localization grid over the lesion and scan.
2. Once the lesion is scanned determine the percutaneous puncture site with the linear marker or grid.
3. Because of breast mobility, the patient is left in the gantry and the needle is advanced. Caution is necessary not to advance through the chest wall.
4. Confirm needle position with CT and deploy wire.

CORE BIOPSY

Indications

- Solid mass lesion in young patient that is most likely benign (i.e., core biopsy thus avoids an excisional biopsy)
- Solid mass lesion that is most likely malignant (i.e., patients would go directly to radical mastectomy avoiding an excisional biopsy)
- Some mammographers also biopsy suspicious calcifications; however, this is not universally accepted.

Technique
- US guidance or stereotactic mammographic unit
- In general, a 14-G needle is used.

Breast Cancer

General

INCIDENCE

11% of women age 20 in the United States will develop breast cancer if they live to age 85 (4%, if the high-risk groups are excluded). Breast cancer is the second leading cause of cancer death (lung is first) in women. There are approximately 45,000 deaths/year from breast cancer in the United States and over 185,000 new cases each year. The presumed etiology of breast cancer is DNA damage, with estrogen playing a key role. 25% have p53 mutations (tumor-suppressor gene located on chromosome 17). 40% of inherited breast cancers (5%-10% of all breast cancers) have BRCA1 mutations (tumor-suppressor gene located on chromosome 17); 40% have BRCA2 mutations (chromosome 13). 75% of breast cancers occur in women with no risk factors.

Risk factors

Older women

Family history (1st degree: mother or sister)

Other
- Early menarche, late menopause, late first pregnancy, nulliparity
- Atypical proliferative changes
- Lobular carcinoma in situ (LCIS) is not in itself considered malignant, but carries a 30% risk of breast cancer (15% in each breast)
- Prior history of breast cancer (in situ or invasive) increases the risk for a second cancer by 1% per year.

SCREENING

General
- Early screening campaigns have led to the detection of 75% of malignancies in stage 0 (in situ) or stage 1.
- All palpable lesions should be referred for a mammogram in appropriately aged women; the mammogram aids in detection of multifocal disease and bilateral disease (4% of cancers are bilateral).
- Screening has led to nearly a 30% reduction in mortality compared with unscreened group.
- More than 40% of cancers are detected by mammography only.
- Approximately 10% of cancers are palpable but not seen on mammography.
- There is decreased lead time in finding cancers in females under 50 (lead time 2 years), such that yearly screening is more important at this age than in patients over 50 (lead time 3-4 years).
- Radiation risk of screening is higher in young females (teens to early 20s), but is negligible after 35-40 years of age.

Health Insurance Plan (HIP) study, New York

A total of 62,000 patients were offered screening: 31,000 by mammography and physical examination and 31,000 by physical examination only; patients were then followed for the development of breast cancer. After 18 years of follow-up, there was a 23% lower mortality rate from breast cancer in patients who had a mammogram.

Breast Cancer Detection Demonstration Program (BCDDP)
- 88% of cancers are detected by mammogram.
- 42% of cancers are detected by mammogram only.
- 20% of cancers were not detected by mammogram or physical examination within 1 year.
- 9% of cancers are detected by physical examination only.

It was concluded from this study that physical examination and mammography are two complementary studies that do not replace each other, although mammography is the more sensitive study for detection of small lesions.

SCREENING RECOMMENDATIONS

Asymptomatic women
- MGH follows ACR recommendations of yearly screening after age 40.
- Monthly breast self-examination to begin at age 20
- Medical examination every 3 years between 20 and 40 years (yearly after 40)
- No mammography screening before the age of 35 unless inherited risk suspected

Mammography at any age over 28-30 for the following
- Palpable mass (if not a simple cyst by US)
- Bloody discharge
- Planned breast surgery (unless under 25 years of age)

PROGNOSIS

Annual incidence of breast cancer has increased 1% per year since 1940. A recent larger increase may be due to earlier detection. Mortality may be decreasing. Survival rates decrease with positive nodal involvement. The involvement of nodes correlates with primary tumor size (cancers > 1 cm have nodal involvement in 30%; cancers < 1 cm have nodal involvement in only 15%). Doubling time of breast cancer is 100-180 days.

BREAST CANCER SURVIVAL RATE

OVERVIEW		
Stage	**5-Year Survival (%)**	**10-Year Survival (%)**
DCIS or < 5 mm	98	95
Negative nodes	85	75
Positive nodes	55	40
Metastases	10	2

STAGING

Lymph nodes
Axillary lymph nodes are divided into 3 levels
- Level I: low axilla
- Level II: more medial under pectoralis minor
- Level III: most medial under clavicle

Positive supraclavicular and internal mammary nodes are considered distant metastases.

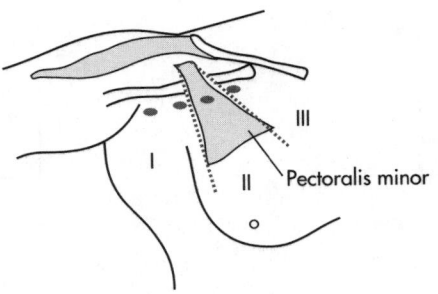

9

Staging system
- Stage 0 ductal carcinoma in situ (DCIS)
- Stage 1 small cancers
    Cancers < 2 cm in diameter
    No axillary or distant disease
- Stage 2 large cancers
    Cancers 2-5 cm in diameter, or
    Axillary node involvement
    No distant metastases
- Stage 3 extensive local/regional spread
    Cancers > 5 cm, or
    Cancers fixed to pectoralis, or
    Cancers with lymph nodes fixed together in a matted axillary mass
- Stage 4 distant metastases

Metastatic spread
- Axillary lymph nodes
- Bones
- Lungs
- Liver
- Opposite breast
- Skin

SENSITIVITY OF DETECTION

- 20% of cancers appear within 1 year of a negative screen are missed by the combination of mammography and physical exam.
- 10% of cancers missed on initial mammography may be seen with additional views.
    50% of mammography misses are unavoidable due to truly normal findings.
    30% of mammography misses are due to observer oversight or poor positioning.

Specific Neoplasm

PATHOLOGY

99% of all malignant breast tumors are epithelial tumors (adenocarcinomas) that have their origin in the terminal duct lobular unit (TDLU). Of these, 90% are ductal and 10% are lobular in origin.

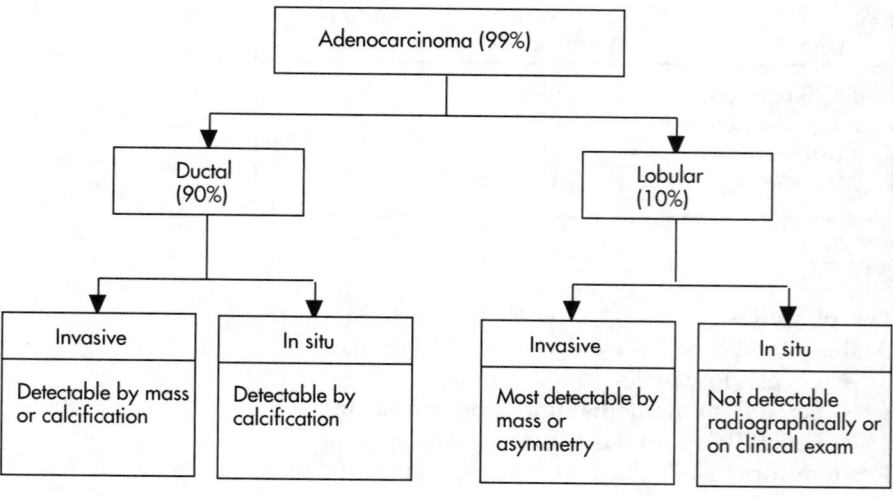

Classification

1. Tumors of ductal epithelial origin
   Carcinoma in situ (DCIS)
   Invasive carcinoma:
   - Not otherwise specified (NOS)
   - Medullary carcinoma (extensive lymphocytic infiltrate; good prognosis)
   - Mucinous or colloid carcinoma (extensive mucin production; well differentiated)
   - Papillary carcinoma (related to small duct papillomas; low lethality, can be intracystic)
   - Tubular carcinoma (attempts to form ducts, well differentiated; most benign and slow growing of all breast carcinomas)
   - Inflammatory carcinoma (aggressive with early dermal lymphatic invasion)
   - Paget's disease (tumor cells involve the nipple)
2. Tumors of lobular origin
   Lobular carcinoma
   - Carcinoma in situ (LCIS)
   - Invasive lobular carcinoma
3. Tumors of stromal origin
   Sarcoma: fibrosarcoma, liposarcoma
   Lymphoma
4. Rare tumors
   Phylloides tumor
   Carcinosarcoma
5. Metastases to breast
   Melanoma (most common)
   Lymphoma
   Lung, renal, primary tumor

Pearls

- Tubular, mucinous, and medullary carcinoma are the three tumors with the best prognosis.
- Phylloides tumors and cysts are the two fastest growing breast lesions.
- Most of the tumors cannot be differentiated by mammography; the tissue-specific diagnosis is usually made by histology.

OVERVIEW OF INFILTRATING TYPE BREAST CANCERS			
Type	Frequency (%)	Positive Node (%)	5-Year Survival (%)
Ductal (NOS)	80	60	55
Lobular	8	60	50
Medullary	4	40	65
Colloid	3	30	75
Comedo	5	30	75
Papillary	1	20	85

9

DCIS (COMEDOCARCINOMA, CRIBRIFORM)

Noninfiltrating, intraductal carcinoma is confined to ducts, which it fills and plugs up. The centers of the tumor may undergo necrosis, and cheesy material can usually be expressed (hence the term *comedocarcinoma*). Typically, exuberant calcification (heterogeneous and irregular) are produced in the necrotic debris.

INVASIVE DUCTAL CARCINOMA (NOS)

Most common form of breast cancer (80%). Probably arises from DCIS and typically measure about 2 cm at diagnosis (in the absence of screening). Microscopically the tumor has extensive collagen. Calcifications are common. Infiltration of tumor occurs into:

- Dermal lymphatics that leads to inflammation and skin thickening
- Perivascular and perineural spaces
- Desmoplastic response of breast tissue causes radiographically visible spiculations

MEDULLARY CARCINOMA

Uncommon (4%), well-differentiated tumor that may get very large (5-10 cm) before discovery. Histologically the tumor is highly cellular with little stroma. Typically, there is a striking lymphocytic infiltration. Tumor has high thymidine labeling. Soft to palpation due to lack of desmoplastic reaction. Mammographically the tumor presents as a mass as opposed to calcifications (typically absent). By US the tumors may show posterior enhancement rather than shadowing.

PAPILLARY CARCINOMA

Uncommon (1%) tumor that usually occurs near menopause. Tumors are usually not palpable but rather present with bloody discharge. At the time of diagnosis, tumors are usually large (> 5 cm). Slower growth rate and better prognosis than infiltrative ductal carcinoma (NOS).

TUBULAR CARCINOMA

Rare, well-differentiated, most benign of all breast carcinomas. Histologically characterized by tubule formation. Mammographically the tumor is indistinguishable from other malignant tumors (spiculated margins, etc.), although tumors tend to be small (1-2 cm) due to slow growth.

INFLAMMATORY CARCINOMA

Uncommon (< 1%), aggressive tumor with early dermal lymphatic invasion. The diagnosis is based on clinical findings of inflammation (usually there is no mass seen by mammography):

- Increased warmth (inflammation)
- Diffuse brawny induration of breast skin
- Erysipeloid edge (peau d'orange)
- Nipple usually retracted and crusted
- Axillary lymphadenopathy is commonly present
- Mammographically there is typical skin thickening (due to carcinomatosis of dermal lymphatics)

PAGET'S DISEASE

Represents 5% of mammary carcinomas and typically occurs in older patients. Paget's disease is a lesion of the nipple that is caused by epidermal infiltration of a ductal carcinoma. Clinically, there are eczematoid nipple changes and occasionally serous or bloody nipple discharge. Because of the early clinical signs this cancer leads to early detection and thus has a good prognosis.

LOBULAR CARCINOMA IN SITU (LCIS)

Does not produce gross morphological changes on clinical or mammographic examination (LCIS is a histological diagnosis). This tumor tends to occur in younger women. 30% risk of eventually developing breast cancer (15% each breast), which may be ductal or lobular.

INFILTRATING LOBULAR CARCINOMA

80% have additional foci of LCIS.

PHYLLODES TUMOR

Rare fibroepithelial tumor that is usually benign; however, 25% will recur and 10% metastasize. Tumor is partially or completely encapsulated. Histologically the tumor resembles a giant fibroadenoma. Age 40-50 years.

METASTASES

- Melanoma is most common metastasis to breast followed by sarcomas, lymphoma, lung cancer, gastric cancer.
- Usually round, multiple, well-defined lesions
- Calcifications are not a typical feature of metastases (in contradistinction to primary breast tumors).

LYMPHOMA

- Secondary lymphoma (non-Hodgkin's > Hodgkin's) of the breast is more common than primary lymphoma, although both are rare (0.3% of all breast malignancies).
- Presents as palpable mass or diffuse thickening with large axillary nodes.

Mammographic Signs of Malignancy

Primary signs (due to the tumor itself; most reliable signs). 20%-30% with these findings will have breast cancer:
- Mass with spiculated or ill-fined margin
- Malignant calcifications

Secondary signs (occur as a result of the tumor; less specific signs)
- Architectural distortion
- Skin, nipple, trabecular changes (thickening, retraction)
- Abnormal ductal patterns
- Lymphadenopathy
- Asymmetry of breast tissue

9

Noncancerous Lesions

Normal Breast

ANATOMY

The mammary gland overlies the fascia of the pectoralis major and is attached to the overlying skin by bands of connective tissue (Cooper's ligament). Lymphatic drainage:

- Axillary nodes, 75%
- Internal mammary nodes, 25%
- Posterior intercostal nodes (rare)
- Contralateral nodes (uncommon unless ipsilateral obstruction present)

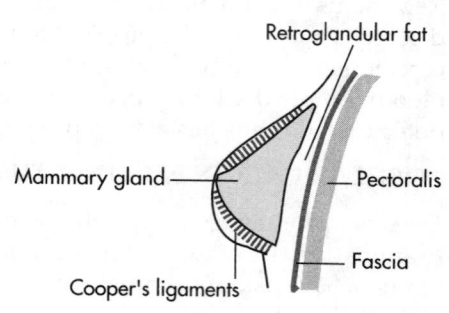

The gland is divided into 15-20 lobes, that are arranged in a radial pattern. Each lobe drains separately into the nipple via a lactiferous duct; however some ducts may join prior to ending in the nipple: usually there are 5-10 openings.

The collecting ducts terminate proximally in TDLUs, which are composed of an extralobular terminal duct, intralobular terminal duct, and ductules. The ductules are the most peripheral structures. The lobule (500 μm) is the smallest structural unit of the breast.

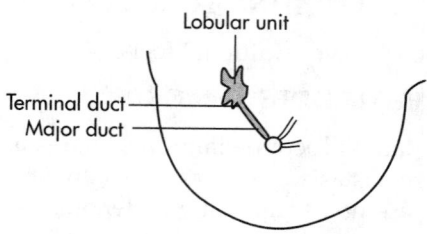

Ducts are surrounded by cellular connective tissue including lymphatics. The epithelium of the TDLU comprises two layers:

- Luminal true epithelial layer
- Deep myoepithelial layer

Most malignant tumors and fibrocystic changes arise from the TDLU (i.e., are epithelial in origin), but some arise from supporting stroma.

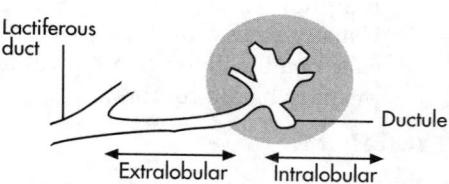

DENSENESS OF BREAST TISSUE

After the age of 30, the parenchymal pattern of the breast does not vary much except for changes in body habitus and/or estrogen levels (which cause parenchyma to become denser). Menopause does not change the breast pattern. Most commonly the density of breast tissue is categorized as:

- Mostly fat
- Fat with some fibroglandular tissue
- Extensive heterogeneously dense with fibroglandular tissue
- Extremely dense breast tissue

Benign Processes

FIBROCYSTIC CHANGES

Fibrocystic changes refer to cellular proliferation in terminal ducts, lobules, and connective tissue with development of fibrosis. Within this spectrum are changes that are symptomatic or asymptomatic, are or are not associated with increased risk for developing cancer (see list), and can be (fibrosis) or cannot be (epithelial proliferation) seen by mammography.

Risk

Increased risk for developing cancer (5 times)
- Atypical hyperplasia (lobular or ductal)

Increase risk for developing cancer (2 times)
- Hyperplasia, moderate or florid, solid or papillary
- Sclerosing adenoma

No increased risk
- Cysts
- Fibroadenoma
- Fibrosis
- Adenosis
- Duct ectasia
- Mild hyperplasia (< 4 cell layers in depth)
- Mastitis
- Metaplasia (squamous, apocrine)

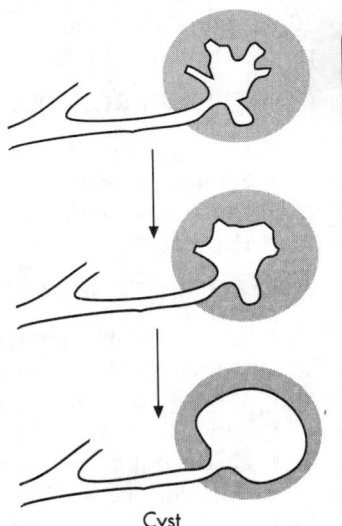

Terminal duct lobular unit

Benign lesions → Cystic disease / Epitheliosis / Epithelial hyperplasia / Adenosis / Duct ectasia / Intraductal papilloma / Fibroadenoma

Malignant lesions → Normal epithelium → Atypical duct hyperplasia → Duct carcinoma in situ → Infiltrating carcinoma

CYSTIC DISEASE

Cysts arise from terminal acini and enlarge because of obstruction or secretion imbalance. Cysts are classified according to their size.
- Microcyst (< 3 mm), believed to be a normal finding
- Macrocyst (> 3 mm), present in up to 50% of adult population

Histologically, cysts have an epithelial lining. Spectrum of clinical presentations:
- Asymptomatic
- Palpable mass
- Pain from enlargement or rupture

Radiographic features

Mammography
- Multiple, rounded densities may be lobulated.
- Cysts may leak and cause inflammation and pericystic fibrosis.
- Cyst wall may calcify or the cysts may contain precipitated milk of calcium. In the medial-lateral views the x-ray beam is horizontal, allowing visualization of calcium fluid level within the cyst.
- Some cysts recur and should be re-aspirated; if recurrent after 2nd aspiration, many surgeons prefer to biopsy the cyst (although the data supporting this approach are obscure).
- Tumor within a cyst is very rare but if seen usually represents a papilloma (papillary carcinoma would be the most common intracystic malignancy).
- The presence of cysts does not exclude cancer elsewhere in the breast.

Lobule

9

Cyst

US

- Cyst appearance:
  - Anechoic with enhanced through-transmission
  - Sharply defined anterior and posterior margin
  - Round or oval
- A cyst with classic US appearance does not require aspiration
- Thinly septated cysts are not worrisome

FIBROADENOMA

Fibroadenomas are the most common benign solid breast lesion. They are characterized by the presence of glandular and fibrous components (focal glandular hypersensitivity to estrogen?) and proliferation of connective tissue of the lobule. Commonly found from adolescence to age 40.

Clinical spectrum

- Palpable mass during reproductive age
- Sensitive to hormonal influences, therefore often enlarge during pregnancy and usually involute at menopause
- Malignancy reported to occur within fibroadenomas since they contain epithelium; however, this is very rare

Radiographic features

- Well-defined, often lobulated masses
- Halo often surrounds the mass (Mach effect)
- Often contain typical popcorn calcification, a result of myxoid degeneration
- Multiple, 20%
- Rarely, fibroadenomas contain microcalcifications and are then indistinguishable from malignancy
- Well-circumscribed and relatively hypoechoic by US

Circumscribed mass

Partially circumscribed

Popcorn calcification

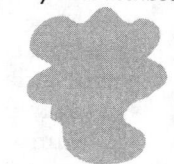

Multilobulated mass

Giant fibroadenoma

Giant fibroadenoma or juvenile fibroadenoma is a more cellular variant that occurs at 10-20 years. Most commonly solitary. Giant fibroadenoma is indistinguishable from a phyllodes tumor by imaging.

COMPLEX FIBROADENOMA

- Cysts greater than 3 mm
- Sclerosing adenosis
- Epihelial calcification
- Papillary apocrine changes

PHYLLODES TUMOR

- Similar to fibroadenoma
- Large rapidly growing breast mass
- Majority of lesions are benign. 10%-15 % are malignant with lung metastases
- Patients are typically older than those with fibroadenomas
- Large round or oval masses, with smooth borders
- US: solid mass with low level internal echoes
- Small fluid filled spaces or cysts may be present
- Biopsy required for definite diagnosis

FIBROSIS

Dense fibrosis (focal, diffuse) arises from unknown etiology. Focal forms can mimic cancer and are diagnosed by biopsy.

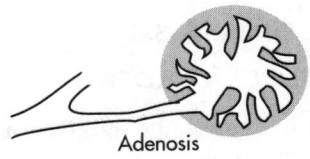
Adenosis

ADENOSIS

Benign entity characterized by a proliferation of glandular structures:
- Formation of new ductules and lobules
- Terminal intralobular ducts accompanied by proliferation of epithelium
- Overgrowth of myoepithelial cells
- May be combined with sclerosis (sclerosing adenosis); this entitiy may be palpable and may contain diffuse calcifications
- Cystic lobular hyperplasia refers to a process similar to adenosis but which typically has cystic dilatation of lobules. calcium within these cystic spaces often appears as milk of calcium (tea-cup configuration).

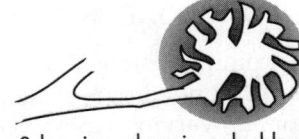
Sclerosing adenosis, palpable

Radiographic features
- Adenosis rarely forms a visible mass.
- May contain round, diffuse, segmental, or malignant-appearing clustered microcalcifications

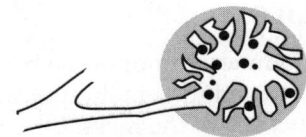
Pearl-type calcification

DUCTAL ECTASIA

Benign entity that represents accumulation of cellular debris in enlarged subareolar ducts. Patients typically present with nonsanguinous discharge and/or pain (inflammatory response). Plasma cell mastitis refers to an inflammatory component associated with extensive secretory calcifications.

Radiographic features
- Enlarged ducts can occasionally be seen by mammography.
- Often associated with extensive benign secretory calcifications

PAPILLOMA WITH FIBROVASCULAR CORE

Solitary intraductal papillomas
Benign lesions (hyperplastic epithelium on a stalk) usually found in an ectatic subareolar major duct. A papilloma is the most common cause of bloody or serous nipple discharge (duct ectasia is the second most common cause). Mammographic appearance:
- Occasionally seen as small mass lesion (subareolar)
- May be detected because of dilated duct
- Rarely contains benign calcifications (raspberry type)
- Galactography confirms diagnosis
- Unlike papillomatosis, there is no increased risk of cancer

Papillomatosis
Refers to multiple peripheral papillomas that are located in the duct lumen just proximal to the lobule. Increased risk for malignancy.

RADIAL SCAR

Idiopathic scarring process, not related to a surgical scar. Pathologically, there is sclerosing ductal hyperplasia. Has the same mammographic findings as a spiculated tumor or postsurgical scar. Usually does not have a central mass. Usually not palpable.

9

Benign Masses

TUBULAR ADENOMA

Uncommon, benign tumor consisting of tubular structures. The lactating adenoma is a variant.

LIPOFIBROADENOMA (HAMARTOMA)

Uncommon, large (3-5 cm) breast tumor that is palpable in 75%. Typically the tumor is surrounded by a pseudocapsule (displaced surrounding trabeculae). Tumors contain varying amounts of fat which may occasionally be difficult to differentiate from fat in the remainder of the gland.

LIPOMA

Common tumor of the breast. Usually slow growing and seen in older patients. Easily detected mammographically because of the thin capsule (may be calcified) and lucency of the mass. Lipomas are most common in women over 40 years of age.

TENSION CYSTS

Develop as a result of an obstructed apocrine cyst. The obstruction may be caused by epithelial hyperplasia, fibrosis, kinking of duct, cancer, etc.

GALACTOCELE

Milk-containing cysts caused by inspissated milk obstructing a duct. Galactoceles typically occur in 20- to 30-year-old patients postlactation. Since milk contains fat, these lesions may be entirely lucent. A horizontal beam may show a fat-fluid level.

DESMOID

Extraabdominal desmoids are very rare breast lesions. Desmoids are usually in close proximity to the pectoralis muscle. May have spiculated borders, thus mimicking cancer. Never contain microcalcifications.

Inflammation

MASTITIS

Types
- Acute mastitis (puerperal mastitis): staphylococcal infection related to lactation (pain, erythema, clinical diagnosis)
- Mastitis in older patients (nonpuerperal mastitis): secondary to infection of sebaceous glands; may proceed to abscess
- Plasma cell mastitis: rare aseptic inflammation of subareolar region; elderly women, often bilateral and symmetrical; thought to result from extravasation of intraductal secretions with subsequent reactive inflammation
- Granulomatous mastitis (rare): TB, sarcoid

Radiographic features

Density
- Areas of diffusely increased density
- May mimic inflammatory cancer (especially in older patients)
- Abscess appears as focal mass

Nodes
- Axillary adenopathy is common

Skin
- Skin thickening
- Nipple retraction

FAT NECROSIS

Results from blunt trauma, surgery, or radiotherapy. Lipocytes necrose, fat liquefies (oil cysts), and fibrosis develops before healing.

Radiographic features
- Poorly defined mass with ill-defined hazy borders (may mimic cancer)
- Unlike cancer, fat necrosis decreases in size over time
- May form a lucent oil cyst
- Rim calcifications are common
- Coarse calcifications
- Microcalcifications indistinguishable from breast cancer (rare)

IMPLANTS

Implants used for breast augmentation include most commonly silastic bags filled with silicone or saline. Implant leakage occurs in 1%-2%. Old silicone injections (no longer used) present as multiple curvilinear calcifications near the skin surface (0.5-2 cm; differential diagnosis: scleroderma). There are 2 locations for surgical implants (without clear-cut evidence of which one is superior):
- Subpectoral implants
- Retroglandular implants

There are many types of implants:
- Single lumen: silicone or saline
- Double lumen: inner silicone/outer saline
- Reverse double-lumen: inner saline/outer silicone
- Other: e.g., expander, foam
- Multiple stacked implants

To diagnose breast cancer in patients with implants, the entire remaining glandular tissue has to be imaged. The screening mammographic examination for patients with implants consists of four views:
- Routine CC and MLO
- Implant displaced CC and MLO (Ecklund)

If the implant is not freely movable so that adequate displacement is not possible, a straight lateral view is added to image the posterior tissue above and below the implant.

9

Radiographic evaluation

Contour abnormalities

- Breast forms a fibrous capsule around the implant.
- Rupture can be intracapsular (implant shell only) or extracapsular (implant shell and fibrous capsule).
- Gel bleed: microscopic silicone leaks through intact shell. A gel bleed can usually not be detected by imaging.
- Flaps ("linguini sign" by MRI) may represent intracapsular rupture.
- Radiating folds: normal findings not to be confused with rupture.
- Crenulated margins indicate capsular contracture.
- Focal bulges: may represent a rupture or a herniation though the fibrous capsule
- Inverted teardrop: nonspecific sign seen with extensive gel bleed or focal intracapsular rupture; occurs when silicone enters radial fold and then leaks between internal and external capsules

Calcifications

- Silcone-induced tissue calcifications may have a variety of sizes and shapes
- Capsular calcification is due to an inflammatory response

US

- Implants are normally hypoechoic
- Echogenic implants are abnormal ("snowstorm" or "stepladder" appearance of ruptured implants)

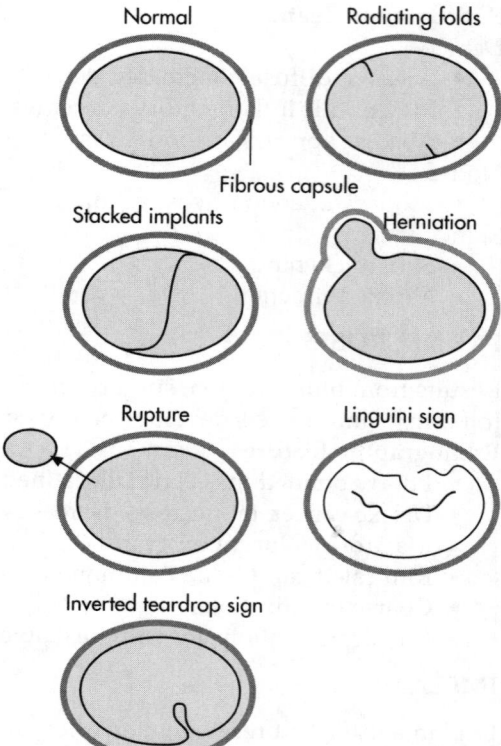

POSTSURGICAL BREAST

IMAGING FINDINGS IN THE POSTSURGICAL BREAST			
Finding	0-6 Months (%)	7-24 Months (%)	> 2 Years (%)
Skin changes	95	55	25
Architectural distortion	85	35	15
Loss of tissue	10	10	5
Parenchymal scar	30	5	3
Calcification	5	5	5
Fat necrosis	5	1	1
Foreign body	1	1	1

Postsurgical scars and spiculated tumors have the same mammographic appearance and can usually not be separated reliably without knowledge of the clinical findings. Findings suggestive of scars:

- Involution with time (should be gone by 1 year)
- Long curvilinear spicules extending to skin

Post-reduction mammography

Mammograms may show any of the findings listed above as well as a swirling appearance of the parenchyma in the inferior breast. The retroareolar ducts may be interrupted.

POSTRADIATION BREAST

Typical radiation dose is 50 Gy to the breast and boosting 60-75 Gy at lumpectomy site. The postradiation mammograms should be performed 6 months after initiation of therapy and followed annually. Women with diffuse intraductal disease may be at increased risk of recurrence following radiotherapy.

Radiographic features

- Diffuse density of entire breast, unilateral (edema); most pronounced at 6 months, nearly gone at 24 months
- Thickening of skin and of trabecula usually resolves within months, but may progress to permanent fibrosis. Persistent distortion or scar after 1 year is difficult to differentiate from tumor
- Calcifications following radiation therapy may represent:
    - Residual tumor calcifications (although all should have been removed by surgery)
    - Benign dystrophic calcifications, which arise 2-4 years after radiation (usually large with central lucency)

Male Breast

The normal male breast is predominantly composed of fat that has no lobules and only rudimentary ducts. Therefore, male breasts do not develop fibroadenomas.

GYNECOMASTIA

Gynecomastia refers to an enlargement of the male breast (most common male breast abnormality). Gynecomastia occurs most commonly in adolescent boys and men > 50 years. Gynecomastia is usually asymmetric. Two types:

- Florid type (usually pubertal type): predominantly epithelial proliferation, edema, and cellular stroma
- Fibrous type (usually older men): predominantly fibrosis

Causes

Drugs
- Reserpine
- Spironolactone
- Cimetidine
- Marijuana
- Estrogens

Secreting testicular tumors (increased estrogen production)
- Seminoma
- Embryonal cell carcinoma
- Choriocarcinoma

Hepatic cirrhosis
- Inadequate estrogen degradation

Radiographic features
- Subareolar increased density, which is typically flame-shaped (the normal male breast is predominantly fatty)
- Unilateral or bilateral, symmetrical or asymmetrical
- Secretions may be present especially in gynecomastia secondary to estrogens

9

MALE BREAST CANCER

Very rare tumor (0.2% of male malignancies). Mean age: 70 years. Risk factors include exposure to ionizing radiation, occupational exposure to electromagnetic field radiation, cryptorchidism, testicular injury, Klinefelter's syndrome, liver dysfunction, family history of breast cancer, previous chest trauma, and advanced age. Mammographic findings in male breast cancer are similar to those in female cancer. For mammography of the male breast, bilateral studies are performed routinely, even if the symptoms are only unilateral. Histology: infiltrating ductal carcinoma or ductal carcinoma in situ (even in men with gynecomastia, lobule formation is rare). Gynecomastia does not increase a man's risk of developing breast carcinoma.

Male breast cancer usually occurs in a subareolar location or are positioned eccentric to the nipple. The lesions can have any shape but are frequently lobulated. Calcifications are fewer in number, coarser, and less frequently rod-shaped than those seen in female breast cancer. Secondary features include skin thickening, nipple retraction, and axillary lymphadenopathy.

Differential Diagnosis

Mass Lesions

SPICULATED MASSES

All spiculated masses are suspicious for neoplasm and should be biopsied. Causes:
- Malignancy
- Radial scar (benign sclerosing adenosis)
- Fat necrosis
- Postsurgical scar
- Superimposed tissue mimicking a lesion
- Desmoid

MASS WITH MICROLOBULATION

- Cancer

MASS WITH MACROLOBULATION

- Phyllodes tumor
- Fibroadenoma
- Simple cyst
- Intramammary lymph node

WELL-CIRCUMSCRIBED MASSES (ROUNDED DENSITIES)

- Cysts (common lesion < 40 years; less common in postmenopausal women)
- Fibroadenoma (most common lesion in the 10-40 year age group)
- Hematoma (seat belt injury, biopsy)
- Lymph nodes are common in upper outer quadrant. However, they are suspicious if:
    >1 cm without fat
    No lucent center or hilar notch

- Skin
    - Seborrheic keratosis is most common skin lesion seen by mammography
    - Nipple imaged out of profile
- Malignant tumors
    - Primary tumors rarely present as well-circumscribed mass lesions; however, the following types can occur:
    - Invasive (NOS)
    - Papillary cancer
    - Medullary cancer
    - Colloid cancer
    - Metastases (rare)
- Other
    - Fibrosis (may be isolated, dense, and sharply marginated; never distorts architecture)
    - Trauma (hematoma): usually resolves weeks after trauma; scars can persist
    - Phyllodes tumor: rare lesion, usually benign (15% malignant), variant of fibroadenoma (benign giant fibroadenoma, very dense)

Approach

- Lesions < 8 mm: follow-up in 6 months (US is less accurate in these small lesions)
- Lesions > 8 mm: US to determine whether the lesion is a cyst

DEVELOPING DENSITY ON MAMMOGRAM

- Carcinoma
- Hematoma
- Cysts
- Hormonal changes in fibroglandular tissue

LUCENT LESIONS (FATTY LESIONS)

- Hamartoma (lipofibroadenomas; usually large)
- Lipoma
- Traumatic oil cysts
- Galactocele (rare, may have fat-fluid level, lactating breasts)

GIANT MASSES (> 5 CM)

Tumors
- Hamartoma (in older patients)
- Cystosarcoma phylloides
- Giant fibroadenoma (young patients: 10-20 years)

Abscess

Other

NIPPLE RETRACTION

- Acquired with age (usually bilateral and symmetric)
- Hamartoma or seroma
- Congenital
- Tumor
- Inflammatory

NIPPLE DISCHARGE

- Papilloma (most common cause)
- Duct ectasia (2nd most common cause)
- Only 5% of cancers (especially intraductal carcinoma) present with nipple discharge as a solitary finding
- Others
    Papillomatosis
    Fibrocystic changes

PROMINENT DUCTS

- Duct ectasia (bilateral)
- Intraductal papilloma (unilateral)
- Intraductal carcinoma (unilateral)
- Vascular structures mimicking ducts

TRABECULAR THICKENING

- Mastitis (always obtain a follow-up view to exclude an underlying mass)
- Inflammatory carcinoma
- Postradiation
- Postreduction mammoplasty
- Lymphatic or SVC obstruction, including metastases to local lymph nodes
- Metastases

MALE BREAST ENLARGEMENT

- Gynecomastia (most common cause)
- Abscess
- Lipoma
- Sebaceous cysts
- Breast cancer (uncommon)

Skin

DIFFUSE SKIN THICKENING (> 2.5 mm)

Tumor
- Inflammatory breast cancer
- Lymphoma
- Leukemia

Inflammation
- Acute mastitis
- Abscess
- Radiation
- Postsurgical

Lymphatic obstruction
- Lymphatic spread of tumor to axilla (breast, lung)

Generalized edema
- Right heart failure
- Central venous obstruction
- Nephrotic syndrome

RINGLIKE PERIPHERAL CALCIFICATION IN MASS

- Fibroadenoma
- Calcified cyst
- Oil cyst
- Fat necrosis

FOCAL SKIN THICKENING

Tumor
- Carcinoma
- Intradermal metastases
- Skin lesions (usually have radiolucent rim around them): seborrheic keratitis, moles, warts

Inflammation
- Plasma cell mastitis
- Dermatitis
- Prior trauma, biopsy
- Fat necrosis
- Mondor's disease (thrombosis of superficial veins)

SUGGESTED READINGS

Breast imaging reporting and data system (BI-Rads), ed 2, Reston, Va, 1995, American College of Radiology.

Egan RL: *Breast imaging: diagnosis and morphology of breast diseases*, Philadelphia, 1988, WB Saunders.

Homer MJ: *Mammographic interpretations: a practical approach*, Philadelphia, 2000, WB Saunders.

Kopans D: *Breast imaging*, Philadelphia, 1997, Lippincott Williams & Wilkins.

Peters ME, Voegeli CM: *Breast imaging*, London, 1989, Churchill Livingstone.

Sickles EA, Destouet JM, Eklund GW, et al: *Breast disease (test and syllabus)*, ed 2, Reston, Va, 1993, American College of Radiology.

9

Chapter 10

Obstetric Imaging

Chapter Outline

First Trimester

General

REFERENCE

All ages in this section refer to the menstrual age or gestational age based on the last menstrual period (LMP) and not the embryonic age based on day of conception. A 4-week pregnancy by the LMP method thus corresponds to a 2-week pregnancy by the conception method. All measurements given in this section are for transvaginal sonography (TVS) unless otherwise stated.

ROLE OF IMAGING

1st trimester
1. Confirm an intrauterine pregnancy (IUP)
2. Date an IUP (confirm gestational age)
3. Determine fetal number and placentation
4. Evaluation for an ectopic pregnancy
5. Evaluation of 1st trimester bleeding: assess viability
    - Normal IUP
    - Abortion: impending, in progress, incomplete, missed
    - Ectopic pregnancy
    - Subchorionic hemorrhage

2nd trimester
1. Determine fetal number and viability
2. Placental evaluation and location
3. Estimate amount of amniotic fluid
4. Assess gestational age and growth
5. Fetal survey
6. Evaluate adnexa and cervix

3rd trimester
1. Fetal presentation (vertex, breech)
2. Type of placenta
3. Membranes
4. Cervical os
5. Biophysical profile, growth

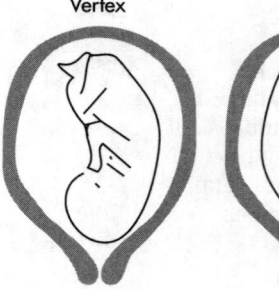

Vertex   Breech

PRENATAL SCREENING

Screening tests
- Ultrasound (US)
- Alpha-fetoprotein (AFP)
- β-Human chorionic gonadotropin (βHCG)
- Amniocentesis
- Chorionic villous sampling (CVS)
- Fetal blood sampling

Reasons for prenatal screening
- Advanced maternal age (most common) (≥ age 35 years)
- Prior children with chromosomal abnormalities or structural defects
- Family history of genetic or metabolic disorder
- Exposure to teratogens (drugs, infections)

ALPHA-FETOPROTEIN (AFP)

- AFP is formed by the fetal liver, yolk sac, and gut and is found at different concentrations in fetal serum, amniotic fluid, and maternal serum (MSAFP).
- In the normal fetus, AFP originates from fetal serum and enters amniotic fluid through fetal urination, fetal GI secretions, and transudation from membranes (amnion and placenta).
- Elevated MSAFP levels occur if there is transudation of AFP into the maternal serum such as in open neural tube defects (AFP screening has an 80%-90% sensitivity for detection) or in fetal swallowing problems (abdominal wall defect).
- MSAFP is best measured at 16 weeks
- False positive causes of elevated AFP:
  - Gestational age ≥ 2 weeks than estimated clinically
  - Multiple gestations
  - Fetal death
- In case of elevated AFP, test for acetycholinesterase in amniotic fluid, which is present in neural tube defects.

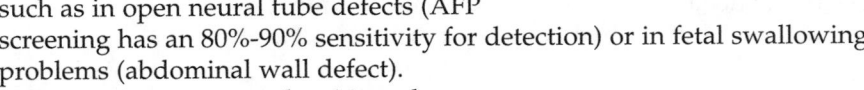

βHCG

Normal βHCG levels correlate with size of gestational sac until 8th to 10th week. Thereafter βHCG levels decline. Initially, the doubling time for the βHCG is approximately 2-3 days. Third International Reference Preparation = 1.84 × Second International Reference Preparation.

FOUR PATTERNS OF βHCG IN PREGNANCY		
βHCG (mIU/mL)*	**US**	**Outcome**
< 1000	Gestational sac present	Abortion likely
< 1000	Gestational sac absent	Not diagnostic, repeat
> 1000-2000	Gestational sac present	Normal pregnancy
> 2000	Gestational sac absent	Ectopic likely

*Second International Standard.

TRIPLE SCREEN MARKERS			
Risk Category	**AFP**	**HCG**	**Estriol**
NTD/abdominal wall defect	Increased	Not applicable	Not applicable
Trisomy 21	Reduced	Increased	Low
Trisomy 18	Reduced	Increased	Increased

NTD, Neural tube defect.

AMNIOCENTESIS

Performed at 15-16 weeks using an US-guided transabdominal approach. Desquamated cells of amniotic fluid are cultured and then karyotyped 2-3 weeks later. In twin pregnancies, indigo carmine is injected into the amniotic cavity punctured first to assure sampling of both cavities. The main complication is fetal loss (0.5%).

Indications for amniocentesis

- Advanced maternal age ≥ 35 years
- Abnormal MSAFP
- History of genetic or chromosomal disorders
- Fetal anomalies: central nervous system (CNS) lesions, large choroid plexus cyst (controversial), cystic hygroma, nuchal thickening, heart defects, congenital dislocation of the hip (CDH), duodenal atresia, omphalocele, cystic kidneys, hydrops, pleural effusions, ascites, clubfoot, two vessel umbilical cord, facial anomalies, short femur

CHORIONIC VILLOUS SAMPLING (CVS)

- Performed earlier than amniocentesis: 10-12 weeks
- Transcervical or transabdominal approach under US guidance

FETAL BLOOD SAMPLING

- Allows rapid chromosomal analysis within 2-3 days
- Percutaneous US-guided sampling of umbilical vessels

First Trimester Imaging

APPROACH TO FIRST TRIMESTER SONOGRAM

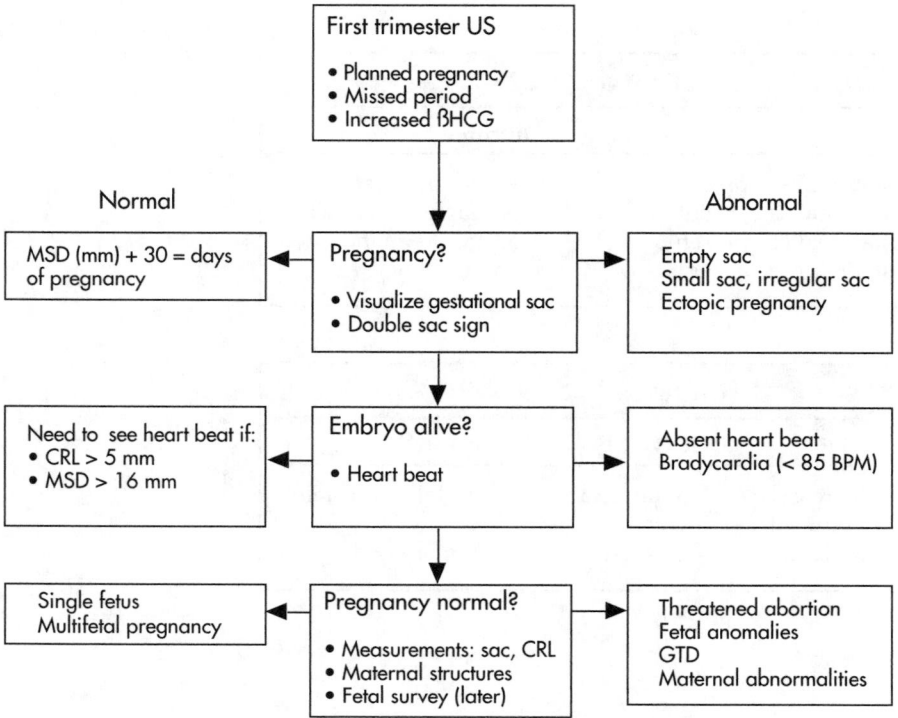

Normal Pregnancy

EARLY DEVELOPMENT

- Fertilization occurs in fallopian tubes
- Oocyte + sperm cell = zygote
- Cleavage occurs in fallopian tube
- Morula enters uterine cavity
- Blastocyst implants into endometrial wall
- Corpus luteum develops from ruptured graafian follicle (usually < 2 cm). Corpus luteum regresses at 10 weeks when its function is taken over by placenta
- Corpus luteum secretes progesterone and induces decidual reaction

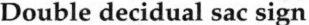

AMNIOTIC AND CHORIONIC MEMBRANES

- Amniotic cavity is initially small
- Embryo lies within the amniotic cavity
- Amniotic cavity enlarges and ultimately fuses with the chorion (14-16 weeks)
- Yolk sac is located outside the amniotic cavity but within the chorionic cavity; it is connected to primitive gut by the omphalomesenteric duct

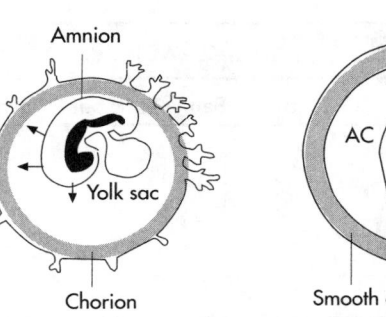
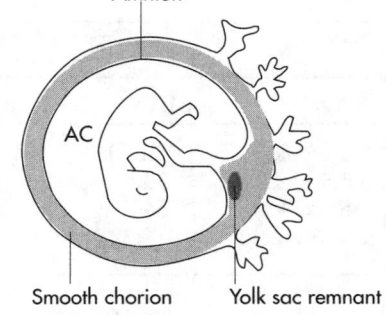

Double decidual sac sign

The double decidual sac sign is a useful early sign of IUP. It is based on the demonstration of three layers of different echogenicity:

- Decidua parietalis (hyperechoic)
- Fluid in the uterine cavity (hypoechoic)
- Decidua capsularis (hyperechoic)

The double bleb sign refers to the presence of an amnion and yolk sac at 5-6 weeks. The embryo lies between these two structures.

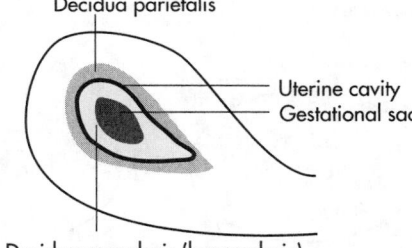

YOLK SAC

- Provides nutrients to the embryo until placental circulation is established.
- Angiogenesis and hematopoiesis occur in the wall of the yolk sac.
- Dorsal part is later incorporated into the primitive gut and remains connected by the omphalomesenteric (vitelline) duct.

FETAL HEART

A fetal heart beat should always be detectable if the crown-rump length (CRL) is ≥ 5 mm by TVS. Absence of cardiac activity in embryos > 5 mm is indicative of fetal demise.

Pearls

- Occasionally embryonic cardiac activity may be seen before a distinct embryo is visualized.
- In patients with threatened abortion, demonstration of cardiac activity is the single most important role of US.

Gestational Sac

NORMAL GESTATIONAL SAC

The gestational sac is the implantation product that occurs in the uterus on approximately day 21. At that time the blastocyst is approximately 0.1 mm in size and cannot be seen by US. Normal sacs become visible when they reach 2-3 mm. Measurements:

$$\text{Mean sac diameter (MSD)} = \frac{(\text{length} + \text{width} + \text{height})}{3}$$

$$\text{Normal MSD (mm)} + 30 = \text{days of pregnancy}$$

After the gestational sac has developed, a yolk sac, the fetal heartbeat, and the embryo will become visible.

TVS LANDMARKS (ACCURACY ± 0.5 WEEK)					
Age	βHCG	Gestational Sac	Yolk Sac	Heart Beat	Embryo (Fetal Pole)
5 weeks	500-1000	+	−	−	−
5.5 weeks	> 3600	+	+	−	−
5 weeks	> 5400	+	+	+	−
> 6 weeks		+	+	+	+

Order of appearance of structures: gestational sac → yolk sac → embryo (fetal pole) → amnion.

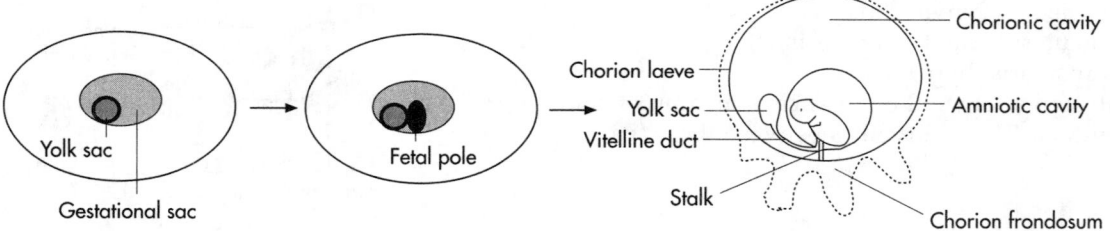

CORRELATION OF MSD AND βHCG LEVELS

- βHCG and MSD increase proportionally until the 8th week (25 mm MSD)
- βHCG doubles every 2-3 days
- βHCG levels decline after 8 weeks
- Normal MSD growth: 1.1 mm/day
- Discordance between MSD and βHCG indicates an increased probability of demise

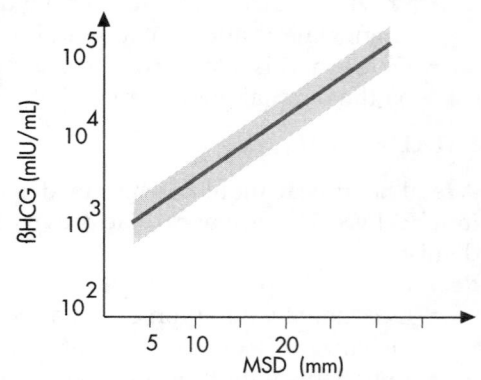

CRITERIA FOR THE DIAGNOSIS OF ABNORMAL GESTATIONAL SACS

MAJOR CRITERIA (POSITIVE PREDICTIVE VALUE 100%)	
Finding*	MSD
ABNORMAL FINDING BY TVS	
No yolk sac	$\geq$ 8 mm
No heart beat	$\geq$ 16 mm
ABNORMAL FINDING BY TAS	
No yolk sac	$\geq$ 20 mm
No heart beat	> 25 mm
Low βHCG for a given MSD†	

*For example, a yolk sac should always be seen by TAS if the MSD is > 20 mm or by TVS if the MSD is > 8 mm.
†Consult a normogram.

Minor criteria
- Irregular contour of sac
- Decidual reaction < 2 mm
- Choriodecidual reaction not echogenic
- Absent double decidual sac
- Low position

SMALL GESTATIONAL SAC

Patients with small sac size have a high likelihood (> 90%) of pregnancy loss. Rule of thumb:

$$\text{MSD (in mm)} - \text{CRL (in mm)} < 5 \text{ mm indicates loss of pregnancy}$$

EMPTY GESTATIONAL SAC

Refers to a gestational sac that does not contain a yolk sac or embryo. An empty gestational sac may represent:
- An early normal IUP (if MSD < 8 mm)
- An anembryonic pregnancy: blighted ovum (if MSD > 8 mm)
- Pseudogestational sac of ectopic pregnancy

Blighted ovum refers to an abnormal IUP with developmental arrest occurring before formation of the embryo.

PSEUDOGESTATIONAL SAC

20% of patients with ectopic pregnancies have an intrauterine pseudogestational sac (i.e., intrauterine fluid collection rimmed by endometrium). Differentiation from gestational sac:
- Pseudogestational sacs are located centrally in uterine cavity not ecentric like true sac.
- Pseudogestational sacs do not have a yolk sac.
- Pseudogestational sacs have an absent double decidual sign.

10

Threatened Abortion

Threatened abortion is a clinical term encompassing a broad spectrum of disease that occurs in 25% of pregnancies and results in true abortion in 50%. Threatened abortion includes:

- Blighted ovum
- Ectopic pregnancy
- Inevitable abortion
- Incomplete abortion
- Missed abortion

Signs and symptoms of threatened abortion include bleeding, pain, contractions, open cervix. If a live embryo is identified, predictors of poor outcome are:

- Bradycardia (< 85 bpm)
- Small gestational sac size (if MSD − CRL < 5 mm)
- Subchorionic hemorrhage (large)

TERMINOLOGY OF ABORTION

Threatened abortion
- Vaginal bleeding with closed cervical os during the first 20 weeks of pregnancy
- Occurs in 25% of first trimester pregnancies
- 50% survival

Inevitable abortion
- Vaginal bleeding with open cervical os; an abortion in progress

Incomplete abortion
- Retained products of conception causing continued bleeding

Spontaneous abortion
- Vaginal bleeding, passage of tissue
- Most common in 1st trimester
- No US evidence of viable IUP; ectopic pregnancy must be excluded
- High percentage have chromosomal abnormalities

Missed abortion
- Retention of a dead pregnancy for at least 2 months

EMBRYONIC DEMISE (DEAD EMBRYO)

The most common cause for embryonic death is a chromosomal abnormality that leads to arrested development. Any of the following indicate embryonic demise:

- CRL > 5 mm and no cardiac activity
- MSD ≥ 8 mm and no yolk sac
- MSD ≥ 16 mm and no embryo
- Absent yolk sac in presence of an embryo
- Absent cardiac activity in embryo seen by transabdominal ultrasound (TAS). If early, need to confirm with TVS.

BRADYCARDIA

If the heart rate is ≤ 85 bpm at 5-8 weeks, spontaneous abortion will nearly always occur. Follow-up US is recommended to assess for viability.

NORMAL FETAL HEART RATES	
Time	Mean (bpm)
5-6 weeks	101
8-9 weeks	143
> 10 weeks	140

The presence of cardiac activity indicates a good but not a 100% chance that a pregnancy will progress to term. There is still a 20% chance of pregnancy loss during the first 8 weeks even if a positive heartbeat is present. During the 9th-12th weeks, the chance of fetal loss decreases to 1%-2% in the presence of a positive heart beat.

SUBCHORIONIC HEMORRHAGE

Venous bleeding causing marginal abruption with separation of the chorion from the endometrial lining extending to the margin of the placenta. Usually (80%) occurs in the late 1st trimester and presents as vaginal bleeding. Prognosis: generally good if there is a fetal heartbeat and bleeding is minimal.

PERCENTAGE OF PREGNANCY LOSS IN FIRST TRIMESTER WITH AND WITHOUT VAGINAL BLEEDING		
Week	Bleeding (%)	No Bleeding (%)
< 6	35	20
7-8	20	5
9-11	5	1-2

Ultrasound features
- Associated with marginal separation of placenta
- Hypoechoic or hyperechoic blood separates chorion from endometrium
- Distinguish from retroplacental bleed and abruption by location and extent of placental involvement

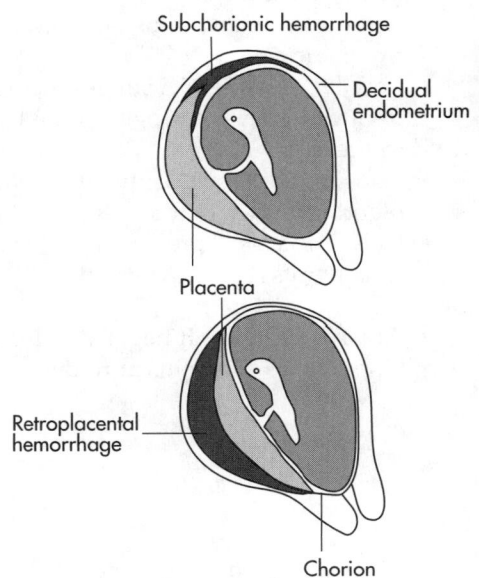

Subchorionic hemorrhage

Decidual endometrium

Placenta

Retroplacental hemorrhage

Chorion

10

Ectopic Pregnancy

General

LOCATION OF ECTOPIC PREGNANCY

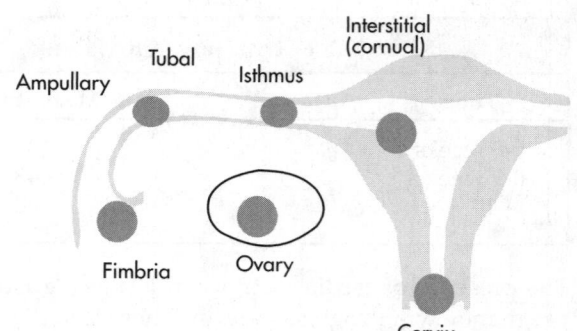

- Tubal, 97%
    Ampullary (most common)
    Isthmus
- Interstitial (cornual) 3%
- Ovarian, 1%
- Cervical (very rare)
- Fimbria (very rare)

CLINICAL

Incidence: 0.5%-1% of all pregnancies. Triad:
- Pain, 95%
- Hemorrhage, 85%
- Palpable adnexal mass, 40%

RISK FACTORS

- Prior ectopic pregnancy
- IUD
- History of pelvic inflammatory disease
- Tubal surgery or other tubal abnormalities
- In vitro fertilization

Diagnosis

DIAGNOSTIC TESTS

Serum markers
- Normal βHCG doubling time depends on the age of the pregnancy but on average is 2 days.
- Ectopic pregnancies usually have a slower increase in βHCG than normal pregnancies.
- Low levels of βHCG suggest ectopic pregnancy.
- Reduced levels of progesterone P4 suggest ectopic pregnancy.

Culdocentesis
- Considered to be positive if > 5 ml of nonclotted blood is aspirated; clotted blood indicates that a vessel has been entered; dry tap is nondiagnostic.
- Culdocentesis is preferred to detect ectopic pregnancy of < 6 weeks; at later time points, US is preferred.

US
- Always use TVS. If negative, also perform TAS.
- Doppler US can be used to detect peritrophoblastic flow.

US FEATURES OF ECTOPIC PREGNANCY

Uterus
- May be normal
- Thick decidual cast with no gestational sac
- Pseudogestational sac
  Fills endometrial cavity symmetrically
  May be large
- No double decidual sign but rather a single rim of echoes around pseudogestational sac

Extrauterine structures
- Free fluid in cul de sac (bleeding). May be anechoic or echogenic
- Simple adnexal cyst (10% chance of pregnancy)
- Complex adnexal mass (95% chance of ectopic)
- Tubal ring sign (95% chance of ectopic): echogenic rim surrounding an unruptured ectopic
- Live embryo outside uterus; 100% specific but only seen in 25%

Pearls
- A normal TVS does not exclude an ectopic pregnancy
- A normal IUP virtually excludes the presence of an ectopic pregnancy. The likelihood of a coexistent ectopic pregnancy is 1:7000 in pregnancies with risk factors or 1:30,000 in pregnancies with no risk factor.
- Cornual ectopic pregnancy
  Symptoms occur later than with ectopic pregnancies in other locations
  Hemorrhage is more severe (uterus more hypervascular, erosion of uterine artery).
  Higher morbidity and mortality. Look for complete rim of myometrium around gestational sac.
- Cervical ectopic pregnancy
  Requires evacuation

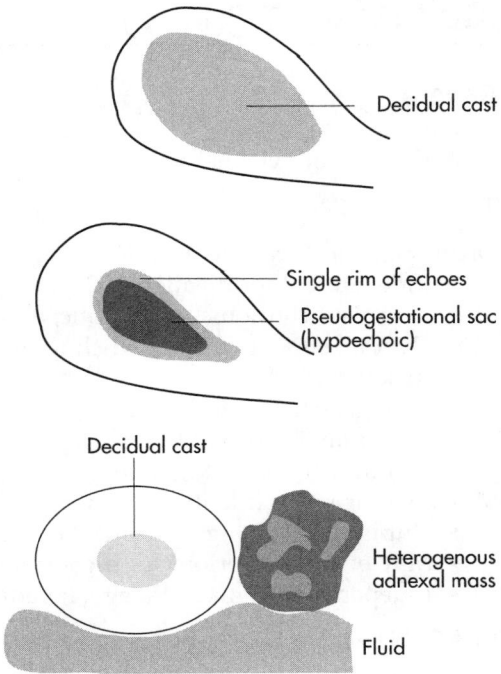

Decidual cast

Single rim of echoes
Pseudogestational sac (hypoechoic)

Decidual cast

Heterogenous adnexal mass

Fluid

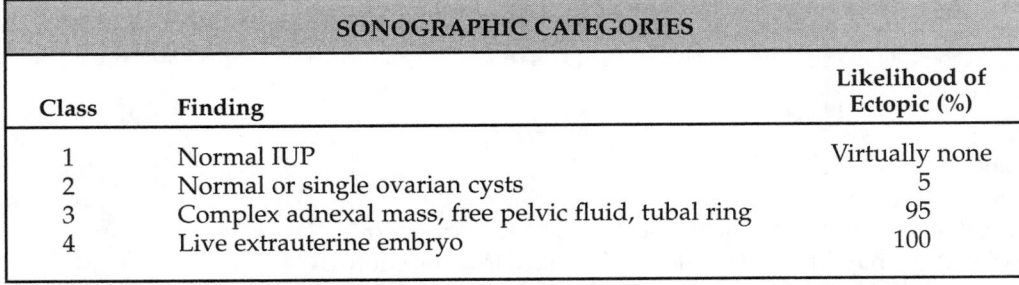

SONOGRAPHIC CATEGORIES		
Class	Finding	Likelihood of Ectopic (%)
1	Normal IUP	Virtually none
2	Normal or single ovarian cysts	5
3	Complex adnexal mass, free pelvic fluid, tubal ring	95
4	Live extrauterine embryo	100

*Likelihood of a coexistent ectopic pregnancy is 1/7000 pregnancies; more common with ovulatory induction and in vitro fertilization.

10

Multifetal Pregnancy

General

Incidence: 1% of live births

TYPES

Dizygotic twins (fraternal), 70%
- Independent fertilization of 2 ova
- Always dichorionic, diamniotic; each ovum has its own placenta and amnion. Overall, 80% of twins are dichorionic, diamniotic.
- Risk factors:
    Advanced maternal age
    Family history of twins
    Ethnicity (e.g., Nigerian)

Monozygotic twins (identical), 30%
- Duplication of single fertilized ovum
- May be monochorionic or dichorionic
- Independent of maternal age, heredity, and race

PLACENTAL UNIT

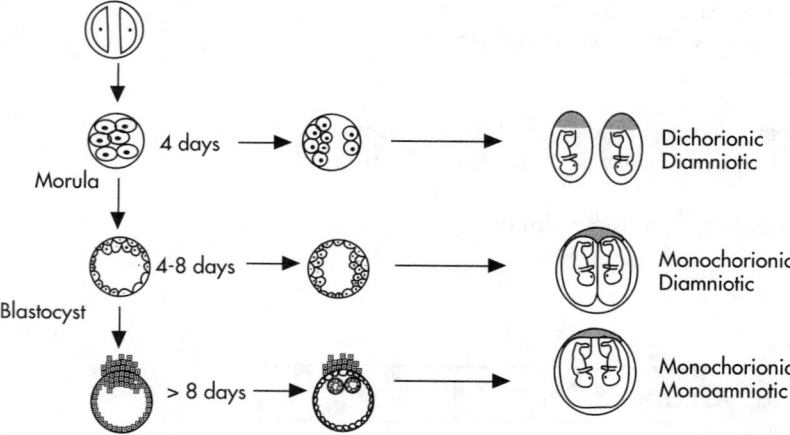

- Amnionicity: number of amniotic sacs
- Chorionicity: number of placentas
- Dizygotic twins are always diamniotic, dichorionic (i.e., have 2 sacs and 2 placentas). The 2 placentas may fuse but do not have vascular connections.
- Monozygotic twins have different amnionicity and chorionicity depending on the stage of cleavage of the single fertilized ovum.
- The amnionicity/chorionicity determines the risk of complications:
    Monoamniotic > Monochorionic, diamniotic > dichorionic
    Monoamniotic: cord entanglement
    Monochorionic: intraplacental vascular communication

US IMAGING

Approach
1. Define presence and number of twins
2. Determine amnionicity and chorionicity
3. Growth estimation: determine fetal weight for each twin
4. Are there complications or anomalies?

US features
Findings definitely indicating dichorionicity
- Separate placentas
- Different fetal sex
- Thick membrane separating twins in 1st trimester
- Chorionic peak: chorion extending into intertwin membrane

Findings indicative of diamnionicity
- Thin membrane in 1st trimester
- 2 yolk sacs

In the 2nd trimester, the sensitivity for finding an amnion is only 30%. In 70% of cases, an amnion is present but not visible.

Pearls
- Dichorionicity is easiest to establish in 1st trimester
- Different genders of fetuses always indicates dichorionicity
- Failure to identify a separating amnion is not a reliable sign to diagnose monoamnionicity
- Twin peak sign

Complications

OVERVIEW OF COMPLICATIONS IN TWIN PREGNANCIES

All twins
- Increased incidence of premature labor
- Fetal mortality 3 times higher than for single pregnancy
- Neonatal mortality 7 times higher than for single pregnancy

Dichorionic, diamniotic twins
- Perinatal mortality, 10%

Monochorionic, diamniotic twins (MD twins)
- Perinatal mortality, 20%
- Twin-twin transfusion
- Acardia
- Demise of co-twin
- Twin embolization syndrome
- Structural abnormalities

Monoamniotic, monochorionic (MM) twins
- Perinatal mortality, 50%
- Entangled cords
- Conjoined twins
- All the MD complications as well

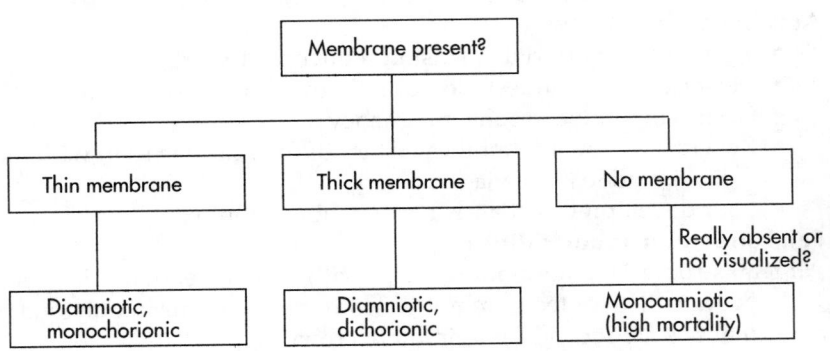

TWIN-TWIN TRANSFUSION SYNDROME

Only occurs in monochorionic twins (25%). Results from AV communications in placenta. Very poor prognosis.

US features

Recipient twin

- Large twin (increased estimated fetal weight [EFW])
- Polyhydramnios
- Polycythemia
- Fetal hydrops

Donor twin (pump twin)

- Small twin pinned to side of gestational sac (decreased EFW) "stuck twin"
- Oligohydramanios

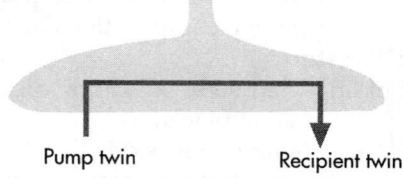

Monochorionic placenta

Pump twin   Recipient twin

CONDITIONS ASSOCIATED WITH DEMISE OF A TWIN

Vanishing twin ("blighted twin")

Demise of a twin in the early 1st trimester (<15 weeks) and subsequent resorption of the dead fetus. Risk to the surviving twin is minimal, especially if dichorionic.

Fetus papyraceus

Demise of a twin in the 2nd or 3rd trimester and persistence of the dead fetus as an amorphous mass or flattened structure along the uterine margin. Complications: premature labor, obstruction at labor, embolization.

Twin-twin embolization syndrome

Occurs only in monochorionic twins because they share a common placenta. Demise of one twin leads to passage of thromboplastic material into the circulation of the live twin. Results in thrombosis and multiorgan failure in the live twin and maternal disseminated intravascular coagulation (DIC).

Acardiac parabiotic twin

- Twin reversal arterial perfusion sequence (TRAPS)
- Most extreme manifestation of twin transfusion syndrome
- Occurs in monochorionic pregnancy
- Reversal of flow in umbilical artery of the acardiac twin with blood entering via the vein and leaving via the artery
- Poor development of acardiac twin above thorax

Fetal structural abnormalities

All fetal structural abnormalities occur with higher frequency in twins (monozygotic > dizygotic). Most defects are not concordant and occur in only one twin. Some abnormalities are secondary to in utero crowding.

Conjoined twins

Only occurs in MM twins. 75% are females. Prognosis is related to degree of joining and associated anomalies:

- Thoracopagus (most common, 70%): thorax is fused
- Omphalopagus, xiphopagus: anterior abdomen is fused
- Pygopagus: sacrococcygeal fusion
- Craniopagus: cranium is fused

Ectopic twin pregnancy

There may be an increase in this condition because of more widespread use of ovulation induction and in vitro fertilization techniques. Incidence: 1/7000; consider if the patient has previously mentioned risk factors.

Second and Third Trimester

General

Some pathological entities in this section are described in more detail in Chapter 11.

FETAL SURVEY		
Organ/Views	**Normal Appearance**	**Common Anomalies**

Supratentorium
  Ventricular view
  Thalamic view
		Hydrocephalus
		Holoprosencephaly
		Hydranencephaly
		Agenesis corpus callosum
		Anencephaly (lethal)
		Encephalocele
		Spina bifida
		Abnormal contour
		Scalp edema
		Cystic hygroma
		Cystic masses
		Hemorrhage

Posterior fossa Cerebellar view		Large cisterna magna Dandy-Walker malformation Banana sign (spina bifida)

Orbits
  Axial view
		Anophthalmia
		Proptosis
		Hypertelorism, hypotelorism (orbital
		  spacing)

Nose and lip
  Sagittal profile
  Coronal view
  Axial view
		Facial cleft
		Proboscis
		Micrognathia
		Facial mass

Spine
  Longitudinal view
    (coronal and sagittal)
  Axial view (posterior
    and lateral)
		Spina bifida
		Scoliosis
		Sacral agenesis
		Sacrococcygeal teratoma

10

	FETAL SURVEY—cont'd	
Organ/ Views	**Normal Appearance**	**Common Anomalies**

Heart, lungs
  4-chamber view
  Short-axis view
  Outflow tract view
	Ventricles / Atria / Patent foramen / Aorta	CHD: VSD, TA, TGA, DORV,
		  tetralogy of Fallot
		Dextroposition
		Cardiac masses
		Lung masses
		Effusion

Gastrointestinal	Stomach / Spine	Esophageal atresia Duodenal atresia Small bowel atresia Ascites Meconium peritonitis Situs
Kidneys	Spine / RK / LK / Pelvis	Renal agenesis Hydronephrosis MCDK APCKD Hydroureter Ectopic kidney
Bladder		Outlet obstruction Exstrophy
Cord, abdominal wall	Liver / Spine / Vein / Arteries	Gastroschisis Omphalocele Limb–body wall complex 2-vessel cord
Extremities		Dwarfism Clubfoot Hands, fingers Polydactyly

CHD, Congenital heart disease; *VSD,* ventricular septal defect; *TA,* truncus arterious; *TGA,* transposition of great arteries; *DORV,* double outlet right ventricle; *MCDK,* multicystic dysplastic kidney; *ARPCKD,* autosomal-recessive polycystic kidney disease.

Pearls

- A normal cavum septum pellucidum, ventricular atrium (< 10 mm), and cisterna magna virtually exclude all neural axis abnormalities
- The 2 most common forms of neural tube defects are:
    - Anencephaly (missing cranial vault)
    - Myelomeningocele (most are associated with Chiari malformation). A normal cisterna magna excludes nearly all cases of myelomeningocele.
- Always obtain a 4-chamber view and 2 views of cardiac outflow tracts (LV → aorta, RV → PA)
- Bladder and stomach should be visualized by 14 weeks. If they are not seen, rescan the patient in 2 hours: bladder should fill within this time frame
- Any structure or mass that touches the fetal spine most likely originates from the genitourinary (GU) tract

Fetal Neural Axis

ANATOMY

Normal CNS structures

- Ventricles: < 10 mm at atrium
  Choroid plexus in atria of lateral ventricles should fill atrium
  Choroid absent in anterior or occipital horns
- Cisterna magna: 4-10 mm
- Thalami are in midline
- Cavum septum pellucidum

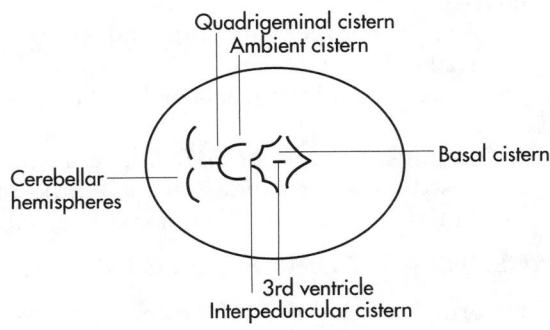

Signal intensities

Hyperechoic structures
- Choroid plexus
- Pia-arachnoid
- Dura
- Cerebellar vermis
- Specular reflections from ventricles

Hypoechoic structures
- Brain white matter
- Cerebral spinal fluid (CSF)

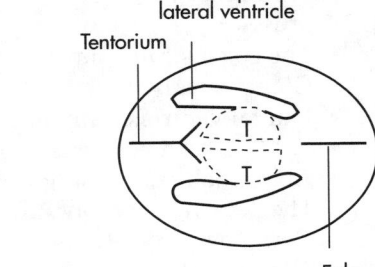

Spine

- 3 hyperechoic ossification centers
  Posterior ossification centers: 2 neural arches
  Anterior ossification center: vertebral body
- Spinal cord is hypoechoic

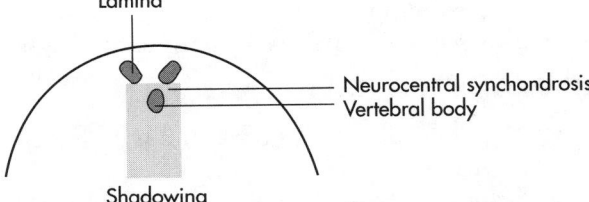

HOLOPROSENCEPHALY

Failure of midline cleavage of the forebrain:
- Alobar form: no cleavage
- Semilobar form: partial cleavage
- Lobar form: almost complete cleavage

US features

Alobar holoprosencephaly
- Monoventricle communicates with dorsal cyst
- Thin anterior mantle of brain tissue: "horseshoe" or "boomerang"
- Fused thalami
- No falx, corpus callosum, or septum pellucidum
- No brain tissue around dorsal cyst

Semilobar holoprosencephaly
- Monoventricle with rudimentary occipital horns
- Posterior brain tissue is present (no dorsal cyst)
- Fused thalami
- Partial falx posteriorly
- No corpus callosum or septum pellucidum

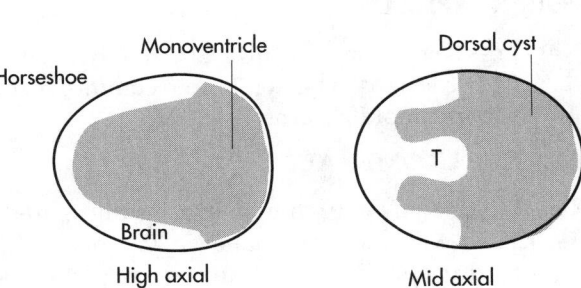

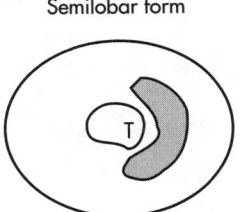

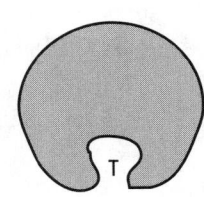

Coronal

10

Lobar holoprosencephaly
- Very difficult to make specific diagnosis

All types have:
- Absent septum pellucidum and corpus callosum
- Thalamic fusion
- Associated midline facial anomalies: clefts, cyclopia, hypotelorism

Pearls
- Identification of septum pellucidum excludes all types of holoprosencephaly
- Fused thalami excludes severe hydrocephalus
- Anterior cerebral mantle (horseshoe) excludes hydranencephaly

AGENESIS OF CORPUS CALLOSUM (ACC)

The normal development of the corpus callosum begins anterior (genu) and progresses to posterior (splenium). Agenesis may be partial (affects dysgenesis posterior aspects) or complete.

US features
- The corpus callosum is not visible in complete agenesis
- Colpocephaly
- Lateral ventricles are displaced laterally
- Enlarged 3rd ventricle expands superiorly
- Abnormal (sunburst) gyral pattern in interhemispheric fissure is a late feature
- The presence of a cavum septum pellucidum excludes complete ACC
- Common associations:
    Dandy-Walker (DW) syndrome
    Holoprosencephaly
    Heterotopias
- TVS scanning often helpful for early diagnosis

HYDRANENCEPHALY

- Near total absence of cerebrum with intact cranial vault, thalamus, and brainstem
- Secondary to occlusion of supraclinoid arteries

PORENCEPHALY

- Less severe vascular insult than in hydranencephaly
- Cystic lesions are often in free communication with the ventricle or subarachnoid cisterns

VENTRICULOMEGALY

Refers to dilated (> 10 mm) ventricles (measured at level of atrium). Associated with other anomalies in 75% of cases. Types:
- Hydrocephalus (noncommunicating, obstructive > communicating)
- Brain atrophy (enough brain tissue developed which regresses later)
- Colpocephaly (not enough brain tissue developed)

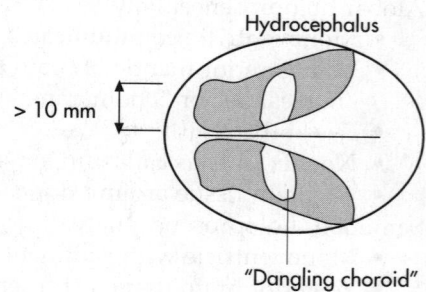

Hydrocephalus

> 10 mm

"Dangling choroid"

Hydrocephalus is the most common CNS abnormality. Causes:
Obstructive (common)
- Spina bifida is the most common cause of hydrocephalus
- Aqueductal stenosis
- DW syndrome
- Encephalocele
- Arnold-Chiari malformation

Nonobstructive (uncommon)
- Hemorrhage
- Infection: cytomegalovirus (CMV), *Toxoplasma* (calcification)

US features
- Enlarged ventricles (> 10 mm)
- Dangling choroid plexus in the lateral ventricle
- The presence of colpocephaly should prompt search for possible callosal agenesis

CYSTIC STRUCTURES

Cystic teratoma
- Most common congenital intracranial tumor
- Solid and cystic components

Choroid plexus cysts
- Very common between 12-24 weeks (2nd trimester); most resolve by 3rd trimester
- Usually multilocular, 5-20 mm; may be bilateral
- Most cysts < 10 mm are of no consequence
- Cysts > 10 mm may indicate trisomy 18, and amniocentesis is often performed, although controversial. Look for other findings of trisomy 18.

Arachnoid cysts
- Cystic space within the pia-arachnoid has a ball valve communication with the subarachnoid space.
- Congenital or acquired (after hemorrhage, infection)
- No communication with ventricle
- Must differentiate from cystic teratoma, porencephaly, arteriovenous malformation (AVM)

HEMORRHAGE

Similar imaging features and classification (Papile grades 1-4) to germinal matrix hemorrhage in prematures but different etiology. In utero hemorrhage is very common. Causes:
- Maternal hypertension, eclampsia
- Isoimmune thrombocytopenia
- Maternal hemorrhage
- Nonimmune hydrops

10

DANDY-WALKER SYNDROME

Abnormal development of posterior fossa structures characterized by:

- Posterior fossa cyst that communicates with the 4th ventricle
- Hypoplasia of the cerebellar vermis
- Variable hydrocephalus

US features

- Posterior fossa cyst separates the cerebellar hemispheres and connects to the 4th ventricle
- Absence or hypoplasia of vermis
- Other associations
    - Hydrocephalus
    - ACC
    - CHD

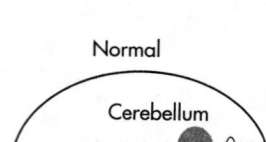
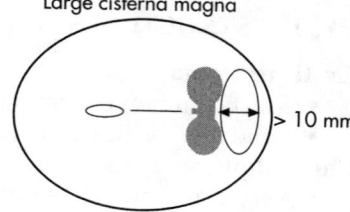

LARGE CISTERNA MAGNA

Diagnosis of exclusion; must exlude DW complex.

US features

- AP diameter > 10 mm
- No communication with 4th ventricle

NEURAL TUBE DEFECT (NTD)

Incidence: 1:600 births in the United States. Increased risk (3%) in parents with prior NTD child. Screening: amniotic and MSAFP are increased because of transudation of fetal serum AFP across the NTD. Spectrum of disease:

- Anencephaly (most common)
- Spina bifida and meningomyelocele
- Face and orbits usually intact
- Encephalocele (least common)

ANENCEPHALY

- Complete absence of cranial vault (acrania) and cerebral hemispheres; should be symmetrical. Asymmetrical absence should raise the suspicion of amniotic band syndrome (ABS).
- Angiomatous tissue covers base of the skull.
- Some functioning neural tissue is nearly always present.
- Polyhydramnios, 50%
- Should not be diagnosed before 14 weeks of age (skull is not ossified)

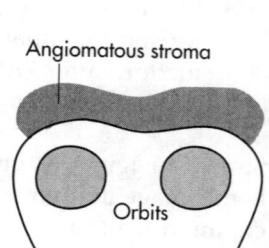

ENCEPHALOCELE

Herniation of intracranial structures through a cranial defect. Most defects are covered by skin and MSAFP levels thus are normal. Location: occipital 70%, frontal 10%. Lesions are typically midline. Asymmetric lesions should raise the suspicion of ABS. Prognosis depends on the amount of herniated brain. Mortality 50%, intellectual impairment 50%-90%.

Associations
- Other intracranial anomalies
- ABS
- Meckel's syndrome

US features
- Extracranial mass lesion (sac)
- The sac may contain solid (brain tissue), cystic (CSF space), or both components; absence of brain tissue in the sac is a favorable prognostic indicator.
- Bony defect
- Lemon sign (skull deformity)

SPINA BIFIDA AND MYELOMENINGOCELE

Location: lumbosacral > thoracic, cervical spine. MSAFP is elevated unless the myelomeningocele is covered with skin. Incidence: 0.1% of pregnancies.
Associations (due to imbalanced muscular activity):
- Clubfoot
- Hip dislocations

US features
Spine
- Complex mass outside spinal canal
- Sac is best seen when surrounded by amniotic fluid
- Sac may be obscured if oligohydramnios is present
- Separation of posterior lamina

Indirect signs
- Lemon sign: bifrontal indentation. In 90% of fetuses with spina bifida < 24 weeks. In older fetuses (24-37 weeks), lemon sign disappears. Lemon sign rarely seen in a normal fetus.
- Banana sign: represents the cerebellum wrapped around the posterior brain stem secondary to downward traction of the spinal cord as part of Arnold-Chiari malformation.
- Hydrocephalus, 90%

Pearls
- Most spina bifida are suspected because of head abnormalities (e.g., banana sign).
- Spina bifida is almost always associated with a Chiari malformation.
- A normal cisterna magna exludes spina bifida.
- Spina bifida is the most common cause of ventriculomegaly.

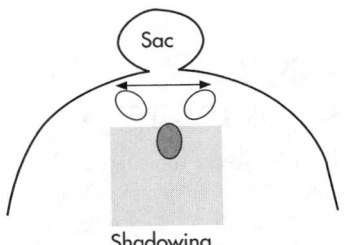

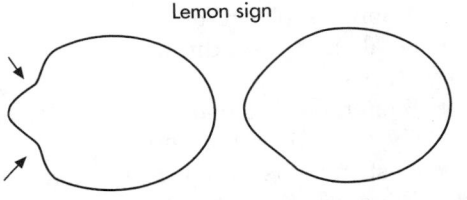

Lemon sign

Concave frontal contour   Flattened frontal contour

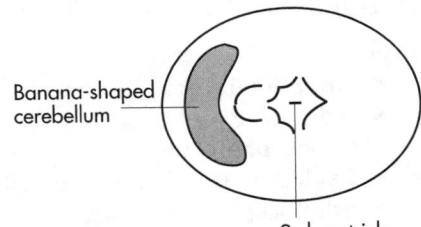

Banana-shaped cerebellum

3rd ventricle

10

ALGORITHM FOR INTRACRANIAL MALFORMATIONS

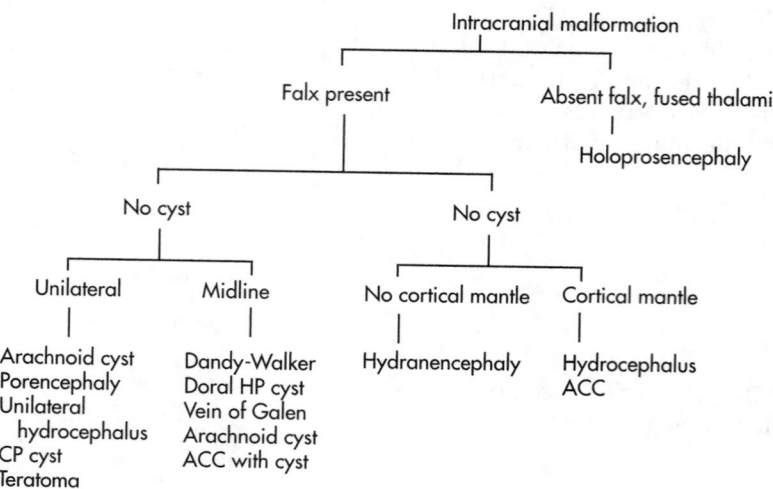

Face, Neck

CYSTIC HYGROMA

Fluid-filled structures caused by lymphatic malformation (? obstructed). Location: neck, upper thorax. Prognosis depends on size: high incidence of hydrops and in utero death in large lesions. Cystic hygromas in noncervical location do not carry a significant risk of chromosomal anomalies and have a favorable outcome. Amniocentesis is performed in cervical cystic hygromas because of frequently associated syndromes:

- Turner's, 45XO (most common)
- Trisomies (21, 18, 13)
- Noonan's syndrome
- Fetal alcohol syndrome

US features

- Bilateral, posterolateral cystic head and neck masses
- Cysts are usually multiple
- Cysts may become very large and extend to thorax
- Generalized lymphedema (nonimmune hydrops)
- Cyst multiplicity and intact skull exclude encephalocele

OTHER ANOMALIES OF THE FACE AND NECK

Types

- Anophthalmia: no orbits
- Arhinia: absent nose
- Cebocephaly: hypotelorism and rudimentary nose
- Cyclopia: usually one eye, with supraorbital proboscis
- Ethmocephaly: hypotelorism and proboscis
- Facial clefts (lip, palate, or face)
- Flattened nose
- Hypotelorism: distance between eyes is decreased
- Hypertelorism: distance between eyes is increased

- Macroglossia: large tongue
- Micrognathia: small mandible
- Nuchal thickening (> 5 mm)
- Proptosis: eye protrudes from skull
- Proboscis: cylindrical appendage near the orbits
- Single nostril

Associations

- Holoprosencephaly: cyclopia, ethmocephaly, cebocephaly, clefts, hypotelorism
- Cloverleaf skull: proptosis
- Craniosynostoses: hypertelorism
- Frontal encephalocele: hypertelorism
- Median cleft face syndrome: hypertelorism and clefts
- Beckwith-Wiedemann: large tongue
- Trisomy 21: nuchal thickening

Heart

DETECTION

Cardiac abnormalities are often difficult to detect because of small heart size, complex anatomy, and rapid heart rate. Since cardiac abnormalities may be associated with a chromosomal abnormalities (15%-40%), amniocentesis is indicated in all patients with cardiac defects.

Cardiac abnormalities best detected on 4-chamber view:

- Septal defect—ventricular septal defect (VSD), AV canal
- Endocardial cushion defect
- Hypoplastic left heart: absent or small LV
- Ebstein's anomaly: large RA and small RV; tricuspid valve within RV
- Critical aortic stenosis: RV < LV. Coarctation: LV < RV

Cardiac abnormalities best detected on outflow tract views:

- Tetralogy of Fallot: large aorta overriding a small PA
- Transposition of great arteries: large vessels run in a parallel plane
- Truncus arteriosis: single truncal vessel overriding the septum
- Pentalogy of Cantrell
    - Omphalocele
    - Sternal cleft
    - Cardiac exstrophy
    - CVS malformations
    - Anterior diaphragmatic hernia

Cardiac abnormalities often missed:

- Isolated atrial septal defect (ASD)
- Isolated VSD
- Aortic or pulmonic stenosis
- Coarctation of the aorta
- Total anomalous pulmonary venous connection (TAPVC)

Other detectable abnormalities:

- Rhabdomyoma: most common prenatal and neonatal cardiac tumor (commonly associated with tuberous sclerosis)
- Endocardial fibroelastosis: markedly echogenic myocardium
- Ectopia cordis: heart is located outside of thoracic cavity
- Cardiomyopathy: dilated heart, poor contractility

10

MATERNAL RISK FACTORS FOR CHD

- Diabetes
- Infection: rubella, CMV
- Collagen vascular disease: systemic lupus erythematosus (SLE)
- Drugs: alcohol, trimethadione, phenytoin, lithium
- Family history of heart disease

FETAL ARRHYTHMIAS (USE M-MODE OR DOPPLER US FOR EVALUATION)

- Premature atrial contractions (PAC) are the most common fetal arrhythmia
- PACs and premature ventricular contractions (PVCs) are benign (most disappear in utero)
- Supraventricular tachycardia (HR ≥ 180) is the most common tachyarrhythmia:
    10% incidence in CHD: structural abnormalities uncommon
    May lead to hydrops. Treatment: digoxin, verapamil
- Fetal bradycardia (HR < 100 for > 10 seconds) usually indicates fetal hypoxia distress
- Fetal heart block: 40%-50% have structural abnormality
    40% incidence in CHD
    Associated with maternal SLE

Thorax

PULMONARY HYPOPLASIA

Types
- Primary pulmonary hypoplasia (idiopathic)
- Secondary hypoplasia:
    Bilateral
        Oligohydramnios (Potter's sequence)
        Restricted chest cage (skeletal dysplasias)
    Unilateral
        Congenital cystic adenoid malformation (CCAM)
        Congenital diaphragmatic hernia (CDH)
        Hydrothorax

US features
- Small thorax
- Low thoracic circumference (below 2 standard deviations of normal) is suggestive but not diagnostic of pulmonary hypoplasia
- Fetal lung maturity is most accurately determined by the lecithin:sphingomyelin ratio in amniotic fluid samples (normal ratio > 2). The echogenicity pattern of lung is an unreliable indicator of lung maturity

CONGENITAL CYSTIC ADENOID MALFORMATION

Hamartomatous malformation of the lung. Usually unilateral, involving one lobe.
Types
Macroscopic types: includes type I and II; cysts > 5 mm
- Hydrops is uncommon
- Overall good pronosis

Microscopic type: smalls cysts with solid US appearance
- Hydrops is common
- Very poor prognosis

US features

Solid or cystic pulmonary mass
- Macroscopic type appears cystic
- Microscopic type appear solid

Mass effect on normal lung determines prognosis:
- Pulmonary hypoplasia
- Mediastinal shift: impaired swallowing → polyhydramnios
- Cardiac compromise

BRONCHOPULMONARY SEQUESTRATION

Only the extralobar type is usually detected prenatally.

Types
- Intralobar: pulmonary venous drainage
- Extralobar: systemic venous drainage

Associations (extralobar form 65%, intralobar 10%)
- Congenital diaphragmatic hernia (most common)
- Foregut abnormalities
- Sternal abnormalities

US features
- Well-defined, homogenous, echogenic mass
- Most common location (90%) is left lung base
- May mimic microcystic CCAM
- Complications (mass effect on esophagus → impaired swallowing)
    Polyhydramnios
    Fetal hydrops

CONGENITAL DIAPHRAGMATIC HERNIA (BOCHDALEK HERNIA)

90% are on the left side, 95% unilateral. Mortality: 50%-70% (because of pulmonary hypoplasia). Because of commonly associated anomalies, all patients with CDH should have an amniocentesis.

US features

Chest
- Stomach and/or bowel adjacent to heart (key finding) on 4-chamber view
- Herniation into chest may occur intermittently
- Peristaltic movements in chest
- Shift of heart and mediastinum

Abdomen
- Absent stomach in abdomen
- Small abdominal circumference (because of herniation of organs into chest)

Other
- Polyhydramnios (impaired swallowing)
- Always look for associated anomalies (anencephaly is most common)

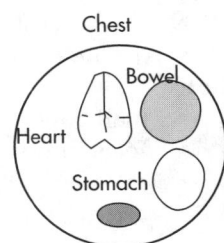

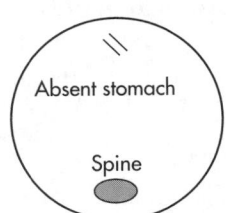

10

MEDIASTINAL MASSES

Mediastinal masses
  Anterior and middle mediastinum
  - Teratoma
  - Cystic hygroma
  - Normal thymus
  Posterior mediastinum
  - Neurogenic tumors
  - Enteric cysts

PLEURAL EFFUSION

Causes
- Fetal hydrops
- Underlying chest mass (CCAM, CDH, sequestration)
- Chromosomal anomalies
- Infection
- Idiopathic

US features
- Crescentic fluid around lung ("bat wing appearance")

Abdomen

NORMAL ANATOMY

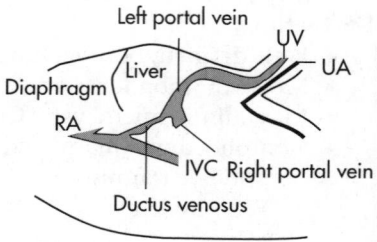

Umbilical vessels
- 1 umbilical vein (UV) connects to either portal system:
  UV → left portal vein → ductus venosus → IVC
  UV → left portal vein → right portal vein → liver
- 2 umbilical arteries (UAs) connect to internal iliac arteries

Stomach
- Always visible by 14 weeks
- Anechoic because it contains swallowed amniotic fluid

Bowel
- Small bowel is meconium filled and appears echogenic (pseudomass)
- Meconium is passed only during fetal distress
- 95% of infants born with meconium-stained amniotic fluid are older than 37 weeks
- Large bowel is fluid filled and appears hypoechoic

Adrenal glands
- Usually well seen because they initially are 20 times their adult size relative to the kidney
- Adrenal glands can be mistaken for kidneys (hypoechoic rim, echogenic center: Oreo cookie sign)

Other
The gallbladder is seen in nearly all fetuses by 20 weeks. The spleen is seen from 18 weeks on; it appears isoechoic to kidneys and hypoechoic relative to liver. The pancreas is not routinely seen.

GASTRIC ABNORMALITIES

Echogenic material in the stomach (gastric pseudomass)
- Debris
- Blood clot
- Vernix

Failure to visualize stomach
- Oligohydramnios (not enough fluid to swallow; most common cause)
- Esophageal atresia (always look for other VACTERL associations)
- Diaphragmatic hernia
- Swallowing abnormality (cranial defect)
- Situs abnormality: look on both sides

DUODENAL ATRESIA

Associated anomalies occur in 50% of patients with duodenal atresia. Therefore a chromosomal analysis and detailed fetal survey are indicated:
- Down syndrome, 30%
- Malrotation, 20%
- Heart disease, 20%
- Other: renal anomalies, tracheoesophageal fistula, VACTERL

Radiographic features
- Double-bubble sign (can be seen as early as 24th week of gestation)
- Polyhydramnios

MECONIUM

Echogenic material within the bowel may represent:
- A normal finding if present in 2nd trimester
- Cystic fibrosis (carrier testing of parents performed)

There are 3 meconium-associated problems during pregnancy:

Meconium peritonitis (10% have cystic fibrosis)
- Sterile chemical peritonitis develops after bowel perforation
- Calcification, 85%
- Ascites, 55%
- Polyhydramnios
- Causes (can be determined in only 50% of cases)
    - Volvulus
    - Atresia
    - Intussusception
    - Meconium ileus

Pseudocyst
- Inflammatory response around walled-off peritoneal meconium

Ileus (100% have cystic fibrosis)
- Inspissation of thick meconium in distal ileum
- Bowel dilatation, 25%
- Polyhydramnios, 65%

10

ASCITES

Ascites is always an abnormal finding.
Causes
Isolated ascites

- Urinary ascites
- Meconium peritonitis, bowel rupture
- Ruptured ovarian cyst

Hydrops
Pseudoascites: the hypoechoic anterior abdominal wall musculature may be mistaken for ascites

Adrenal Gland

Neuroblastoma

- Most common antenatal tumor (arises from adrenal gland)
- Usually unilateral
- Hyperechoic
- Often metastasizes to placenta, liver, subcutaneous tissues
- Often associated with hydrops

Abdominal Wall

ANATOMY

- Midgut elongation and umbilical herniation: 8 weeks
- Rotation and peritoneal fixation: 12 weeks

Pearls

- 20% of normal pregnancies may show herniated bowel at 12 weeks
- Bowel outside of fetal abdomen beyond 14 weeks is always abnormal

ANTERIOR WALL DEFECTS

OVERVIEW			
	Gastroschisis	**Omphalocele**	**LBWC**
Location	Right-sided defect	Midline defect	Lateral
Size of defect	Small (2-4 cm)	Large (2-10 cm)	Large
Umbilical cord insertion	Anterior abdominal wall	On omphalocele	Variable
Membrane	No	Yes (3 layers)	Contiguous with placenta
Liver involved	No	Yes	Yes
Bowel involved	Common	Uncommon	Uncommon
Ascites	No	Yes	Yes
Other anomalies	Rare	Common (50%-70%)	Always

ALGORITHM FOR ANTERIOR ABDOMINAL WALL DEFECTS

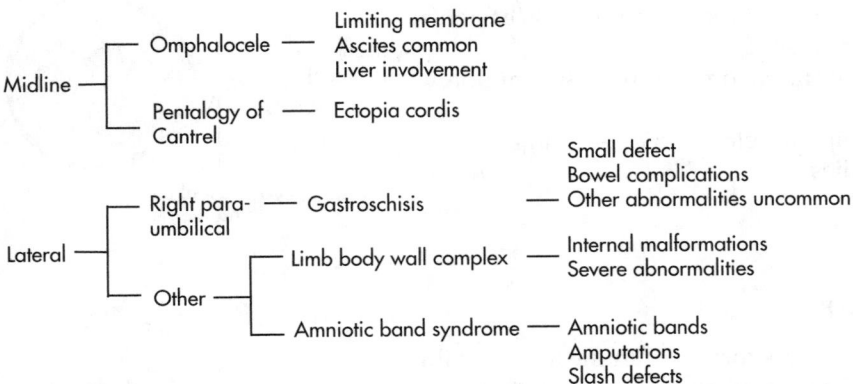

GASTROSCHISIS

Gastroschisis is a defect involving all 3 layers of the abdominal wall. MSAFP is elevated. Incidence 1:3000. Mortality 10%. Gastroschisis has a better prognosis than omphalocele because of the lower incidence of associated anomalies. Associated anomalies are usually limited to the GI tract and result from bowel ischemia:

- Intestinal atresia or stenosis
- Bowel perforation
- Meconium peritonitis

US features

- Wall defect is usually small, < 2 cm
- Defect located to the right side of the umbilical cord, 90%
- Bowel outside abdominal cavity. By definition, the bowel is nonrotated
- Externalized structures appear disproportionately large relative to abdominal wall defect
- Bowel wall thickening, dilatation may indicate ischemia and potential for perforation

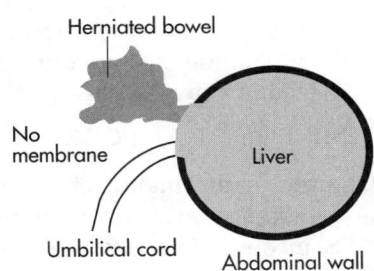

OMPHALOCELE

A large midline abdominal wall defect is covered by a membrane consisting of peritoneum (inside layer), amnion (outside layer), and Wharton's jelly (between the 2 layers). Rupture of the membrane occurs in 10%-20%. Mortality is 80%-100% depending on severity of concurrent abnormalities. In contrast to gastroschisis, MSAFP levels are normal if the membrane is intact. Unlike gastroschisis, omphaloceles are frequently (50%-70%) associated with other severe malformations:

- GU, GI, CNS, cardiac anomalies
- Pentalogy of Cantrell: omphalocele, CDH, sternal cleft, ectopia cordis, CHD
- Beckwith-Wiedemann: omphalocele, macroglossia, gigantism, pancreatic hyperplasia with hypoglycemia
- Trisomies (13 > 18 > 21)
- Turner's syndrome

10

US features

- Umbilical cord enters centrally into herniated sac
- Layers of the covering membrane (peritoneum, amnion, Wharton's jelly) may occasionally be distinguished
- Defect may contain any intraabdominal organ but most commonly liver with or without bowel
- If bowel loops lie within the omphalocele it indicates a higher incidence of karyotypic anomalies
- Allantois cyst is often present
- Ascites
- Associated cardiac anomalies, 40%

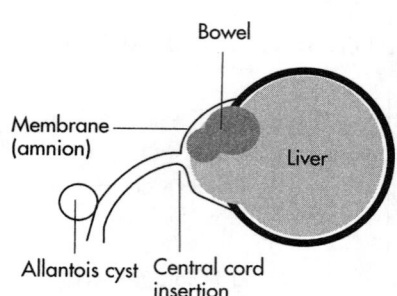

AMNIOTIC BAND SYNDROME (ABS)

The amnion is ruptured and multiple bands form within the amniotic fluid. Amniotic bands result in amputation defects of abdominal wall, trunk, and extremities.

US features

- Limb entrapment in bands
- Multiple asymmetrical limb amputations or facial defects
- Asymmetric encephalocele (adherence of fetus to "sticky" chorion)
- Gastropleural schisis
- Abdominal wall defects similar in appearance to gastroschisis
- Bands are occasionally visualized
- Associated anomalies: syndactyly, clubfoot
- Amniotic band syndrome must be differentiated from chorioamniotic separation, normal unfused amnion in first trimester, uterine synechiae (also called amniotic sheets), and from fibrin strands that occur after amniocentesis.

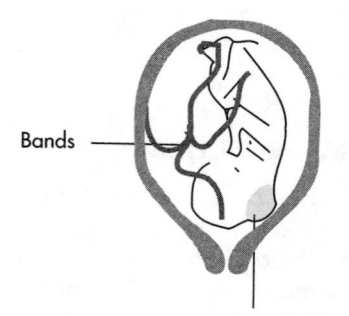

LIMB-BODY WALL COMPLEX (LBWC)

Complex malformation characterized by eccentric body wall defect involving thorax and abdomen, extremities, cranium, and face. Thought to represent a severe form of ABS; incompatible with life.

US features

Thoracoabdominal defect

- Defects are usually large
- Fetal membranes are contiguous with defect

Neurologic abnormalities

- NTD common: encephaloceles, meningomyeloceles
- Scoliosis (common)
- Anencephaly

Other abnormalities

- Cardiovascular anomalies
- Single umbilical artery
- The constellation of omphalocele and scoliosis suggests presence of LBWC

Urinary Tract

NORMAL DEVELOPMENT

Renal morphology
- Kidneys are routinely seen at 16 weeks of age.
- Pyramids and medulla can be differentiated at 23-26 weeks of age.
- Normal renal pelvis is normally < 10 mm in diameter. Measurement is a function of gestational age.
- Ratio of renal to abdominal area on cross-section is constant (0.3 ± 0.03).
- Ratio of renal pelvis to kidney in cross-section is normally < 0.5.

Renal function can be estimated by evaluation of:
- Urine in bladder: routinely seen at 16 weeks; the normal urinary bladder fills and empties every 30-45 minutes. Fetal urine becomes major source of amniotic fluid by 16 weeks.
- A normal amniotic fluid volume is an indicator of good prognosis.
- Oligohydramnios is an indicator of bad prognosis.

Amniotic fluid
- Fetal urine accounts for almost all amniotic fluid in 2nd half of pregnancy.

POTTER'S SYNDROME

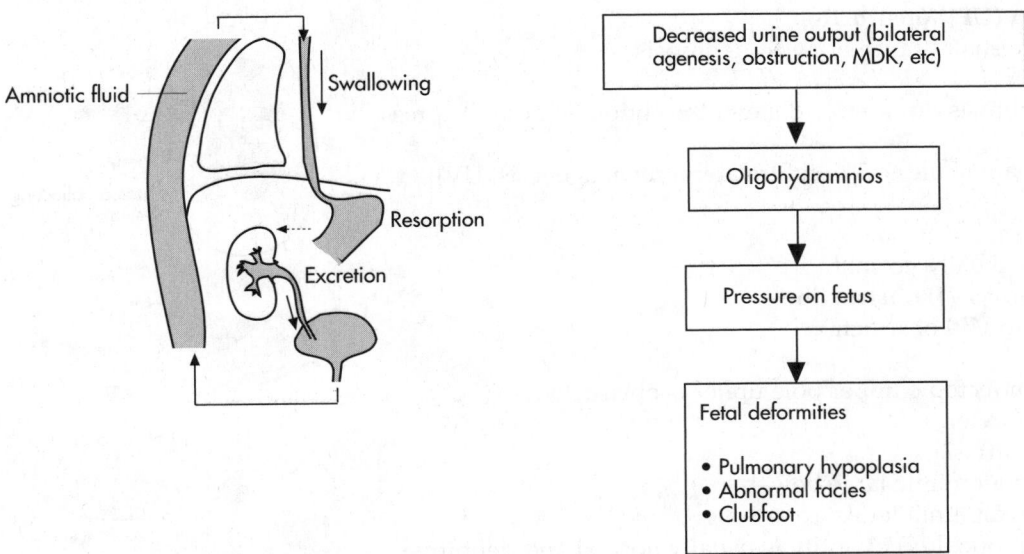

Also referred to as Potter's sequence. Renal failure causes decreased urine output, which results in oligohydramnios. Pulmonary hypoplasia, contractures, and Potter facies result. Underlying renal causes:
- Bilateral renal agenesis
- Posterior urethral valves
- Infantile polycystic dysplastic kidney (PCDK)
- Multicystic dysplastic kidney (MCDK)

10

RENAL AGENESIS

Unilateral renal agenesis is 4 times more common than bilateral agenesis. Bilateral agenesis is always fatal at birth because of associated pulmonary hypoplasia.

US features
- Kidney are not visualized; do not mistake adrenal glands or bowel loops for kidneys
- Fetal bladder does not fill during a 2-hour US examination
- Severe oligohydramnios
- Small fetal thorax (pulmonary hypoplasia)
- Potter facies and limb deformity

URINARY TRACT OBSTRUCTION

Approach
1. Upper or lower obstruction?
2. Renal function impaired (oligohydramnios?)
3. Associated anomalies?
4. Surgical decompression required to improve prognosis?
   - Normal amniotic fluid indicates excellent prognosis.
   - Oligohydramnios indicates poor outcome.
   - Renal dysplasia indicates poor outcome.

Ureteropelvic junction (UPJ) obstruction
- Most common antenatal cause of hydronephrosis
- Bilateral UPJ, 20%
- Severe hydronephrosis can greatly distend the abdomen and compress the thorax
- Associated renal anomalies, 25%: contralateral renal agenesis, UVJ obstruction
- Paranephric urinoma
- Amniotic fluid is usually normal

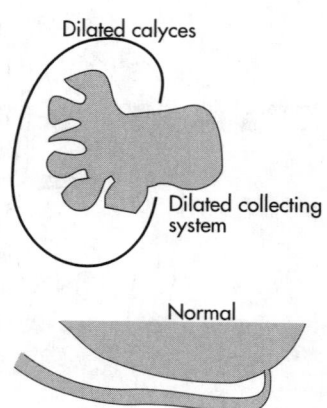

Dilated calyces

Dilated collecting system

Ureterovesical junction (UVJ) obstruction
- Less common than UPJ obstruction
- Common causes
  - Duplex system (ectopic upper pole ureter is obstructed)
  - Primary megaureter
  - Distal ureteral atresia
- A dilated ureter may mimic large bowel
- Most obstructions are unilateral
- As with UPJ, amniotic fluid quantity is usually normal and definitive diagnosis can be made in neonatal period
- Associated renal anomalies: UPJ obstruction, MCDK

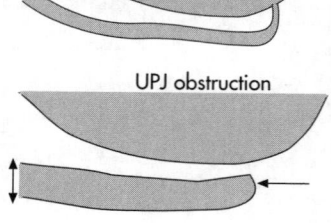

Normal

UPJ obstruction

Bladder outlet obstruction
- Most common cause: posterior urethral valves in males (much less common: caudal regression syndrome, megacystis-microcolon-intestinal hypoperistalsis, which is very rare)
- Dilated bladder and posterior urethra ("key-hole" appearance)
- Thickened bladder wall (> 2 mm)
- Dystrophic bladder wall calcification
- Pyelocaliectasis, 40%
- Urine ascites
- Oligohydramnios, 50%

ANTENATAL PREDICTORS OF POOR POSTNATAL RENAL FUNCTION

Ultrasound
- Severe oligohydraminos
- Increased renal echogenecity
- Renal cortical cysts
- Slow bladder refilling after emptying

Fetal urine
- Increased Na, Ca, and osmolality

Fetal blood
- Increased b2 microglobulin

RENAL CYSTIC DISEASE

Multicystic dysplastic kidney (MCDK) disease
Cystic dysplasia secondary to in utero obstruction. Severity related to degree of obstruction and time of occurrence. Most common neonatal renal mass. Usually unilateral; incompatible with life if bilateral.

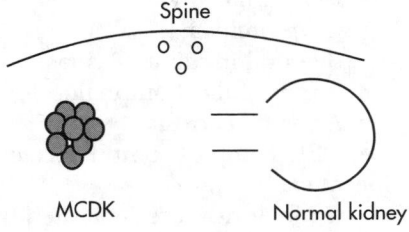

US features
- Paraspinal mass with numerous macroscopic cysts
- Cysts are usually noncommunicating (differentiation from hydronephrosis is thuse possible)
- Ureter and renal pelvis are atretic and not visualized
- Contralateral renal anomalies, 40%:
    UPJ obstruction common
    Agenesis (lethal)
    MCDK (lethal if bilateral)

Autosomal-recessive polycystic kidney disease (ARPCKD) (infantile polycystic kidney disease)
A heterogeneous spectrum of renal and liver disease. Renal disease predominates in the severe perinatal form; inverse relationship between hepatic and renal disease.

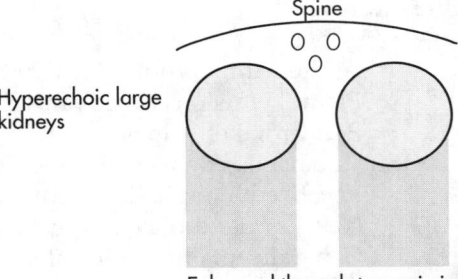

US features
- Bilaterally enlarged, hyperechoic kidneys
- Enhanced renal through-transmission
- Individual cysts cannot be visualized by US
- Liver fibrosis
- Potter sequence: absent bladder, oligohydramnios, small thorax

Cystic renal dysplasia
Nonspecific dysplasia secondary to collecting system obstruction.
- Small bilateral renal cortical cysts
- Prognosis depends on residual renal function
- Search for oligohydramnios and cause of obstruction (e.g., UPJ, UVJ obstruction)

Meckel-Gruber syndrome
- Characteristic features (need 2 of the 3 features for diagnosis):
    Bilateral MCDK, 95%
    Occipital encephalocele, 80%
    Polydactyly, 75%
- Fatal at birth because of pulmonary hypoplasia
- Autosomal recessive; 25% recurrence risk in subsequent pregnancies

10

Megacystis-microcolon-intestinal-hypoperistalsis syndrome
Rare nonobstructive cause of megacystis. Female preponderance.
- Normal or increased amniotic fluid
- Dilated small bowel may be present but is rare

EXSTROPHY

Difficult to detect prenatally. Most cases are suspected because of failure to visualize a normal bladder. Some are suspected because of associated infraumbilical omphaloceles.

Bladder exstrophy
Defect of lower abdominal and anterior bladder wall. Associated findings:
- Epispadia, always
- Cryptorchism
- Bilateral inguinal hernias
- Infraumbilical omphalocele
- Anorectal atresia
- OEIS complex (omphalocele, exstrophy, imperforate anus, spinal anomalies)

Cloacal exstrophy
Two hemibladders are separated by intestinal mucosa. Each hemibladder has its own ureters. Associated with mulitple GI and GU anomalies.

Hydrops Fetalis

GENERAL

Hydrops refers to excessive accumulation of serous fluid within body cavities and fetal soft tissues. Incidence: 1:700-1000.

US features
- Effusions
  - Ascites (fluid around urinary bladder) is the first and most reliable sign
  - Pleural effusions (in advanced disease)
  - Pericardial effusions
- Subcutaneous edema (skin thickening > 5 mm)
  - Localized: lymphatic obstruction, vascular abnormalities
  - Neck, upper thorax: suspect Down syndrome, Turner's syndrome
  - Generalized: often associated with cardiovascular anomalies
- Placental edema (placenta is > 4 cm thick)
- Polyhydramnios (75%) is more common than oligohydramnios

Types
- Immune hydrops fetalis, 10%
- Nonimmune hydrops fetalis, 90%

Approach
Hydrops is a fetal emergency. Immediate steps to be taken:
1. Determine maternal immune status.
2. Prepare for fetal transfusion.
3. Search for structural abnormalities and determine cause of hydrops.
4. Biophysical profile.

IMMUNE HYDROPS FETALIS (IHF)

Pathophysiology

- Rh-negative mother develops immunoglobulin G (IgG) antibodies to fetal Rh-antigen after first exposure (e.g., delivery, abruption). Production of maternal antibodies can be tested with the indirect Coombs' test.
- In second fetus, Ag-Ab interaction causes anemia → extramedullary hematopoiesis → hepatomegaly → portal-venous hypertension → hydrops
- Prophylaxis: administer anti-Rh antigen immunoglobin (Rhogam) to all Rh-negative mothers at 28 weeks. This effectively blocks maternal sensitization.
- Good prognosis

Role of prenatal US

Establish and monitor severity of IHF

- Effusions, anasarca, placental edema, polyhydramnios

US-guided therapeutic interventions

- Blood transfusions via the umbilical cord
- Fetal blood sampling through umbilical vessel puncture

NONIMMUNE HYDROPS FETALIS (NIHF)

NIHF represent 90% of fetal hydrops. The overall prognosis is poor because of the frequent inability to treat underlying causes or even the failure to identify an underlying cause. Mortality: 50%-90%. Concomitant oligohydramnios indicates very poor prognosis. In many instances, the pathophysiology of NIHF is poorly understood.

Etiologies

- Cardiac, 25%
    Tachyarrhythmias (most common; most treatable)
    Structural defects
- Idiopathic, 20%
- Chromosomal anomalies, 10%
    Turner's syndrome
    Trisomy 21
- Twin-twin transfusion, 10%
- Anemias
- Infections (CMV, toxoplasmosis, parvovirus)
- Other, 25%
    Chest masses: CCAM, CDH, sequestration
    Skeletal dysplasia: dwarfism, osteogenesis imperfecta, arthrogryposis
    GU anomalies
    Lymphatic anomalies: cystic hygroma, lymphangiectasial, lymphedema
    Placental chorioangioma
    GI anomalies: meconium peritonitis

Complications of fetal hydrops

- Neonatal death from pulmonary hypoplasia or structural anomalies
- Maternal hypertension, 30%
- Maternal anemia, 20%
- Maternal hydrops (Mirror syndrome)

10

Extremities

SKELETAL DYSPLASIAS (DWARFISM)

Approach (see also Chapter 11)

1. Measure long bones and place the abnormality in one of the following categories:
   - Rhizomelic: disproportionate shortening of proximal limb (humerus, femur)
   - Mesomelic: disproportionate shortening of distal long bones (tibia, radius, ulna)
   - Micromelia: entire limb shortened. Subclassify:
     Mild
     Severe
     Bowed
2. Look for associated findings: bowing, fractures, ossification, skull shape
3. Obtain family history
4. Consult nomograms and reference texts

Thanatophoric dwarf

Most common lethal dysplasia. Sporadic:
- Cloverleaf skull (trilobed) is the key finding, 15%
- Severe micromelia
- Polyhydramnios, 75%
- Nonimmune hydrops
- Small thorax

Homozygous achondroplasia

Autosomal dominant lethal dysplasia that resembles thanatophoric dwarf. Both parents are achondroplasts (key observation). Similar US features as in thanatophoric dwarfs.

Achondrogenesis (type I)

Autosomal recessive lethal dysplasia.
- Severe micromelia
- Absent vertebral body ossification
- Ossified calvarium (feature distinguishing from hypophosphatasia)

Osteogenesis imperfecta (type II)

Autosomal recessive lethal condition with severe hypomineralization.
- Unossified skull
- Multiple fractures and long bone angulation/thickening

Congenital lethal hypophosphatasia

Autosomal recessive lethal condition with imaging features similar to osteogenesis imperfecta type II.
- Fractures are less common
- Long bones are thin and delicate

Short rib–polydactyly syndromes

Spectrum of inherited disorders.
- Severe micromelia differentiates this condition from Jeune's and Ellis-van Creveld syndrome
- Short ribs and narrow thorax
- Polydactyly

Camptomelic dysplasia

Lethal dysplasia with mild micromelia and anterior bowing of long bones.

Chondrodysplasia punctata

Lethal autosomal recessive dysplasia that is not frequently diagnosed in utero.

- Stippled epiphyses (only specific feature)

Heterozygous achondroplasia

- Decreased femur after 27 weeks is sensitive indicator of this dysplasia
- Narrow lumbosacral interpedicular distance

Asphyxiating thoracic dysplasia (Jeune's syndrome)

Autosomal recessive dysplasia which is usually lethal.

- Small thorax
- Polydactyly
- May be indistinguishable from Ellis-van Creveld syndrome

Chondroectodermal dysplasia (Ellis-van Creveld syndrome)

Appears similar to Jeune's syndrome except that 50% of fetuses have ASD and usually nonlethal.

Diastrophic dysplasia

Nonlethal autosomal recessive dwarfism.

- Hitchhikers thumb: abducted thumb
- Flexion contractures
- Clubfoot

CLUBFOOT (TALIPES)

Types

Idiopathic (good prognosis, more common)
Secondary (worse prognosis)

- Trisomy 18
- Amniotic band syndrome
- Meningocele

US features

- Foot is at right angle to tibia
- Abnormal position of a foot has to persist (i.e., a permanent flexion has to be differentiated from temporary flexion)
- Metatarsal bones seen in same plane as tibia-fibula plane

EXTREMITY ABNORMALITIES

Short radial ray (radial hypoplasia)

Radius and ulna normally end at the same level. In radial hypoplasia the radius is shorter. Associations:

- Fanconi's anemia
- Thrombocytopenia-absent radius syndrome (TAR) syndrome
- Holt-Oram syndrome
- VACTERL
- Klippel-Feil syndrome
- Mental retardation (Cornelia de Lange syndrome)

Limb anomalies

- Acromelia: shortening of distal extremity
- Adactyly: absence of digits
- Amelia: absence of extremity
- Camptomelia: bent limb
- Hemimelia: absence of distal limb
- Mesomelia: shortening of middle segments (forearm)
- Polydactyly: supernumerary digits

10

Sirenomelia

Severe manifestation of caudal regression syndrome (mermaid syndrome).
- Fusion of lower extremities
- Oligohydramnios
- Bilateral renal agenesis or MCDK

ARTHROGRYPOSIS MULTIPLEX

Neural motor unit defect that results in deformities and disability. Rare. Diseases with similar imaging appearance:
- Oligohydramnios
- Fetal akinesia syndrome
- Pena-Shokeir syndrome

US features
- Fetus presents as "buddha" (no movement)
- Hydrops
- Clubfoot, 75%
- Flexion deformities, 50%
- CDH, 40%

SYNDROMES

Trisomy 21 (Down syndrome)

13%-50% may not have any sonographically detectable abnormalities. Most common anomaly is CHD (40%-50%); AV canal defect is usually mentioned but ASD and VSD are most common. Other anomalies:
- Duodenal atresia (rarely identified before 25 weeks)
- Hydrothorax
- Hydrops
- Omphalocele
- Increased nucal thickness—40 % ($\geq$ 6 mm at 14-21 weeks; $\geq$ 3 mm at 10-12 weeks); measure at level of cerebellum and thalami arrow
- Echogenic bowel: other causes of echogenic bowel (similar or increased echogenecity compared to adjacent bone):

    Trisomy 21

    Cystic fibrosis

    CMV

    Intrauterine growth retardation (IUGR)

    Intramniotic bleeding normal
- Short femur length
- Shorter humeral length
- Pyelactasis

    > 4 mm before 33 weeks

    > 7 mm after 33 weeks
- Echogenic intracardiac focus

    Most commonly in LV

    But can also be seen in RV
- Small frontal lobes
- Separation of great toe from second toe
- Hypoplasia of fifth digit and clinodactly (incurving of fifth digit to fourth)

Trisomy 18 (Edward's syndrome)
- CHD, 90%
- IUGR, 60%
- Single umbilical artery, 80%
- Choroid plexus cysts, 30%
- Polyhydramnios
- Characteristic face:
     Dolichocephaly, strawberry skull
     Micrognathia
     Low ears
- Skeletal abnormalities
     Clenched hand with overlap of 2nd and 3rd digit, 80%
     Rockerbottom feet
- GI anomalies (hernia, omphalocele, atresias)

Trisomy 13 (Patau's syndrome)
- CHD, 80%
- CNS abnormalities, 70%
     Holoprosencephaly
- IUGR
- Abnormal face
     Cleft defects
     Microphthalmia/hypotelorism
- Skeletal abnormalities
     Polydactyly, 70%
     Rockerbottom feet
- GU anomalies

Meckel-Gruber syndrome
- Bilateral MCDK, 95%
- Occipital encephalocele, 80%
- Postaxial polydactyly, 75%

Measurements and Growth

Measurements

RECOMMENDATIONS

Fetal measurements become less accurate as a pregnancy progresses. Therefore the gestational age assigned at the initial scan should be considered a baseline and later age determinations should be based on the initial scan. Best measurements:

First trimester
- MSD
- CRL

2nd, 3rd trimester
- Biparietal diameter (BPD) and occipitofrontal diameter (OFD)
- Head circumference (HC)
- Femur length (FL)
- Abdominal diameter (AD)
- Abdominal circumfeence (AC)
- Composite (BPD, HC, AC, FL)

CONFIDENCE LIMITS OF MEASUREMENTS		
Time	US Finding/Measurement	Confidence Limits
TVS		
5 weeks	MSD	
5.5 weeks	MSD + yolk sac	± 1
6 weeks	MSD + yolk sac, fetal heart, CRL	± 0.5
TAS		
6-13 weeks	CRL	± 0.5
2nd trimester	Corrected BPD	± 1.5
3rd trimester	Corrected BPD or composite	± 3.2

ESTIMATED GESTATIONAL AGE (EGA)

- EGA in days (± 1 week) = MSD + 30
- EGA in weeks = CRL + 6.5

GESTATIONAL SAC

- Accurate size measurements are possible up to 5-6 weeks
- Sac measurements are made from inside to inside border of hypoechoic sac
- In ovoid sacs determine 3 diameters:

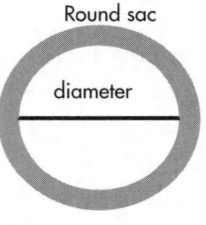
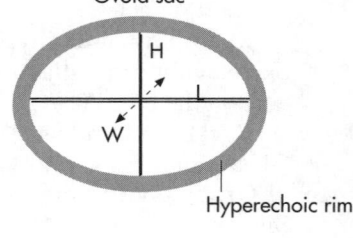

$$MSD = \frac{(L + W + H)}{3}$$

- Only need to measure 1 diameter in perfectly round sacs

CROWN-RUMP LENGTH (CRL)

- Accurate size measurements are possible from 6-12 weeks (1st trimester)
- The CRL is the most accurate estimation of fetal age (± 0.5 week)
- Measure longest longitudinal diameter of fetal axis, excluding yolk sac
- After 13 weeks, CRL measurements are not reliable because of fetal flexion

HEAD MEASUREMENTS

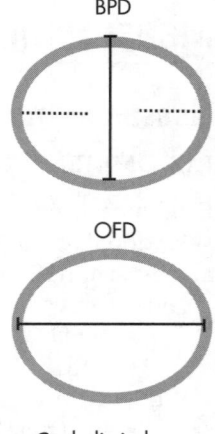

Biparietal diameter (BPD)
- BPD = inner-to-outer wall measurement)
- OFD = mid-to-mid wall measurement)
- BFD and OFD are measured at the widest portion of the skull at the level of the thalami

Cephalic index
- Used to determine whether head shape is normal or whether it needs correction
- Cephalic index: (A/B) × 100
- Normal index: 70-86
- Note that A and B are outer-to-outer wall measurements

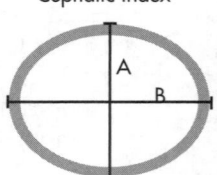

Corrected biparietal diameter
- Most accurate predictor of age in 2nd trimester
- Corrects for shape abnormalities of the head
- Corrected BPD = $\dfrac{\text{BPD} \times \text{OFD}}{\sqrt{1.265}}$
- Rough estimation of age:

  BPD (cm) $\times$ 4 + 2 weeks = age in weeks

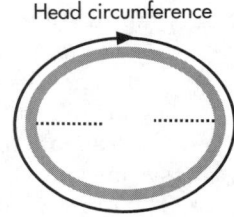
Head circumference

Head circumference
- Same accuracy as BPD measurements
- HC = 1.57 $\times$ (outer BPD + outer OFD)

ABDOMINAL MEASUREMENTS

- Measurements are performed at level of liver
- Intrahepatic umbilical vein serves as a landmark and should be equidistant from lateral abdominal walls
- All measurements are outer edge measurements
- Types of measurements
  Abdominal diameter (AD)
  Abdominal circumference (AC) = 1.57 $\times$ (AD$_1$ + AD$_2$)

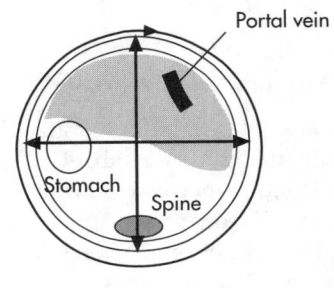
Portal vein
Stomach   Spine

FEMUR LENGTH MEASUREMENT

- Only the hyperechoic diaphysis is included in the measurement
- The epiphyseal cartilage is not calcified and therefore appears hypoechoic

ESTIMATED FETAL WEIGHT (EFW)

- Use 3 body measurements (head, abdomen, femur length) to compute EFW
- Correlate EFW to gestational age; 95% confidence interval is ± 15% (2 standard deviations) of the determined value (approximately ± 15-20%)

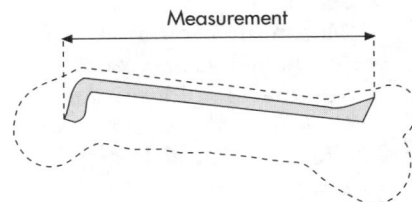
Measurement

Growth Abnormalities

ABNORMALLY SMALL FETUS (IUGR)

Small for gestational age (SGA) = IUGR. Definition: EFW is present if weight is < 10th percentile of normal. Best time for screening is 34 ± 1 week.

Maternal causes
- Primary placental insufficiency
- Secondary placental insufficiency
  Hypertension
  Collagen vascular disease, vasculitis
- Nutrition or toxin related
  Alcohol or drug abuse
  Smoking
  Starvation
  Teratogenic medications

10

Fetal causes

- Chromosomal anomaly
- Infection (TORCH)
- Normal small infant

Sonographic determination

- No single parameter best defines IUGR
- Different criteria (BPD, EFW, AD, FL) and clinical signs (e.g., placental grade, alcohol abuse, hypertension) have varying prognostic value.
- HC/AC ratio detects 70% of all IUGR but misses 30% of IUGR that appear symmetrical.
- The most reliable criteria to determine the presence of IUGR is the combination of EFW + amniotic fluid volume (AFV) + presence of maternal hypertension. Doppler of umbilical cord s/d ratio elevated.

ABNORMALLY LARGE FETUS

Large for gestational age (LGA): EFW is present if weight is > 90th percentile. Macrosomia is a subset of LGA defined as fetal weight > 4000 g at birth. Important to recognize because a large fetus has increased morbidity and mortality.

Risk factors

- Maternal diabetes (most common)
- Maternal obesity
- Prior LGA infant
- Prolonged pregnancy

Complications

- Asphyxia
- Meconium aspiration
- Neonatal hypoglycemia
- Trauma (shoulder dystocia, brachial plexus palsy)

Biophysical Profile (BPP)

Method for assessing antepartum risk of fetal asphyxia. Goal of the BPP is to identify a fetus at risk for perinatal death or complications thus directing obstetric management and altering perinatal outcome. More sensitive and specific than a non-stress test alone.

MANNING CRITERIA FOR FETAL VIABILITY		
Parameters	**Criterion of Normal**	**Indicator of**
1. Fetal heart acceleration	≥ 2 episodes of ≥15 bpm in 20 min	Acute hypoxia
2. Breathing movements	≥ 1 episode ≥ 30 sec in 30 min	Acute hypoxia
3. Gross body movements	≥ 3 movements in 30 min	Acute hypoxia
4. Muscular tone	≥ 1 flexion and extension of extremity	Acute hypoxia
5. Amniotic fluid volume	≥ 2 cm in perpendicular plane	Chronicity

Binary assignment: 2 points for normal, 0 points for abnormal. The score is the sum of all points.

Clinical relevance
- Score 8-10: retest after periodic interval
- Score 4-6:
    Mature lung: deliver now
    Immature lung: close monitoring
- Score 0-2: delivery indicated

Mortality
- Score 8-10: 0.1%
- Score 6: 1%
- Score 4: 3%
- Score 2: 10%
- Score 0: 30%

Fetomaternal Structures

General

APPROACH

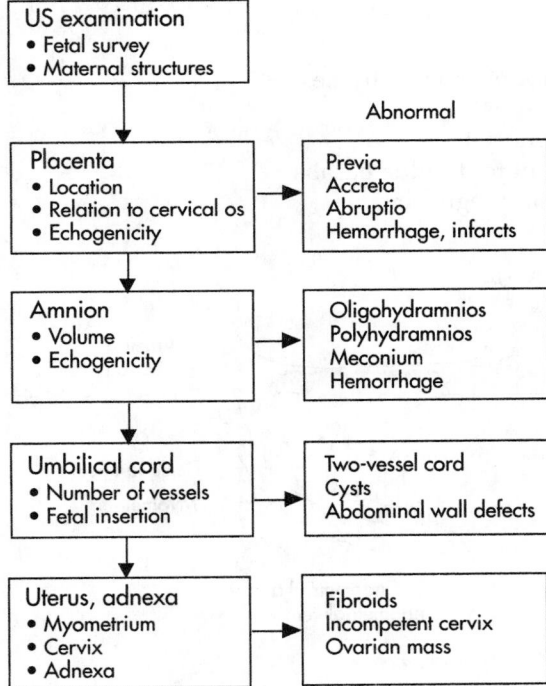

Placenta

NORMAL DEVELOPMENT

Placenta is derived from 2 units:
- Maternal decidua basalis
- Fetal chorion frondosum

Decidua (maternal endometrium)
- Decidua capsularis: layer that covers implanted embryo
- Decidua parietalis: layer lining the uterine cavity
- Decidua basalis: layer between embryo and myometrium

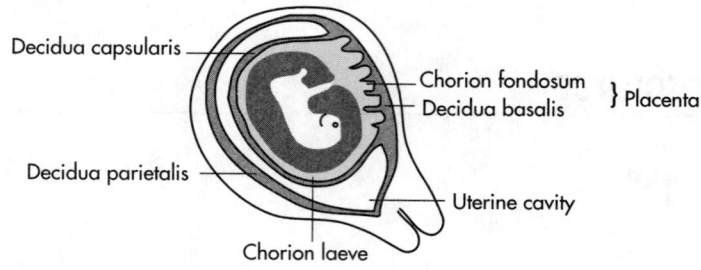

Chorion (fetal component)
- Chorion results from fusion of trophoblast and extraembryonic mesenchyme
- Layers
    Chorion laeve: smooth portion of chorion surrounds embryo
    Chorion frondosum: forms primordial placenta, adjacent to decidua basalis
- *Chorion* and *placenta* are terms used interchangeably later in pregnancy

Placental unit
- First, the trophoblast differentiates into 2 layers: an inner layer of cytotrophoblasts and an outer layer of syncytiotrophoblasts
- Syncytiotrophoblasts erode endometrium and a lacunar network of maternal blood develops around the syncitiotrophoblast
- Villi form from columns of syncitiotrophoblast and proliferate
- The functional unit of the placenta is the cotyledon; the entire placenta consists of 10-30 cotyledons
- Measurements of final placenta:
    Diameter: 15-20 cm
    Weight: 600 g
    Thickness < 4 cm

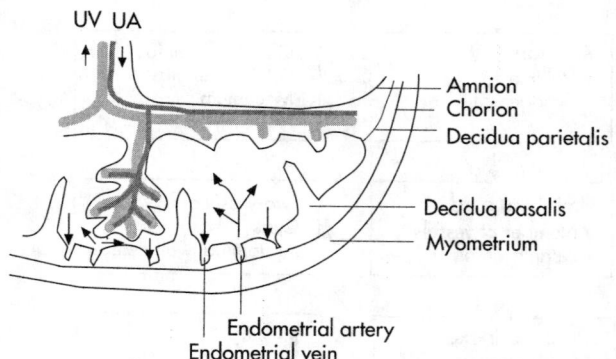

US FEATURES

Normal placenta
- Appears hyperechoic relative to adjacent myometrium
- Draining veins can be seen in the basal plate
- Spiral arterioles are too small to be seen by US
- Placental calcifications are physiological and have no clinical significance; calcifications occur primarily along basal plate and septa
- Normal hypoechoic or anechoic foci in placenta may represent fibrin, thrombus, maternal lakes, cysts

Placental variants

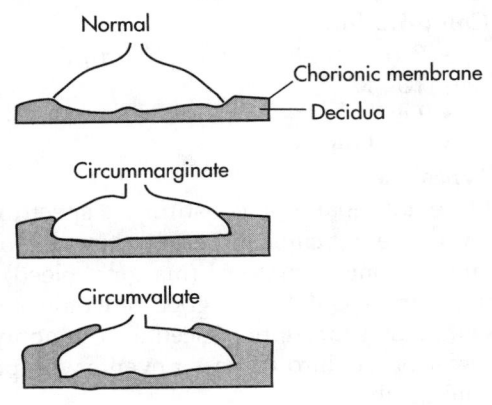

Normal

Chorionic membrane
Decidua

- Succenturiate lobe: an accessory placental lobe.
  Complication: hemorrhage from connecting vessels
- Extrachorial placenta: fetal membranes do not extend to the edge of the placenta. Types:
    Circummarginate: no clinical significance
    Circumvallate: predisposes to hemorrhage

Circummarginate

Circumvallate

Placental grading

Grading system originally described by Grannum to reflect the normal maturation of the placenta. Grade 3 placentas are most mature and usually indicate term. Classification is generally of no clinical use.

- Grade 0: smooth surface, homogenous
- Grade 1: scattered calcification
- Grade 2: calcification in chorionic plate and basal plate
- Grade 3: calcification extend continuously from chorionic plate to basal surface, dividing placenta into cotyledons; posterior shadowing

PLACENTA PREVIA

A placenta previa covers the internal cervical os. Incidence 1:200. Incidence increases with age, multiparity, prior C-sections, and smoking. A pregnancy with placenta previa should be delivered by C-section. Complications:

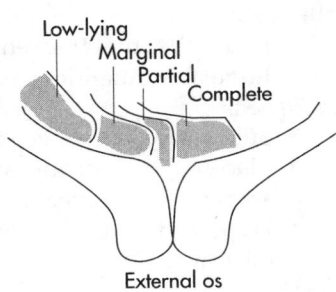

Low-lying
Marginal
Partial
Complete

External os

- 3rd trimester bleeding, 90%
- Premature delivery
- Perinatal death
- Maternal death

Types

- Marginal: placenta extends to os
- Complete: complete coverage of os
- Low-lying placenta: placental edge within 2 cm of os

US features

- Transperineal or endovaginal US often useful to establish diagnosis
- Determine the subtype of placenta previa
- Placental position can change during pregnancy (regressing placenta previa) because of differential growth of lower uterine segment; 60%-90% of patients with 2nd trimester placenta previa will have a normal placenta at term
- Placenta previa can be mimicked by (false positive):
    Overdistended bladder (rescan with empty bladder after 20-30 minutes)
    Focal myometrial contractions

PLACENTAL SEPARATION

Premature separation of a normal placenta from the myometrium results in hemorrhage and hematomas. Incidence: 1% (may be as high as 4% because a separation often goes undiagnosed). Recurrence rate 5%-10%. Increased risk of abruptio with:

- Parity
- Age
- Preeclampsia, eclampsia
- Trauma
- Uterine anomalies
- Cocaine abuse

10

Complications
- 3rd trimester bleeding (abruptio)
- IUGR
- DIC
- Fetal death

Types

Placental separation constitutes a spectrum of abnormalities with different clinical presentations and outcomes. Subchorionic hematoma (marginal bleed) usually occurs early in pregnancy and has a good outcome. Large retroplacental hematomas (abruptio placenta) commonly present as catastrophic third trimester events with pain, bleeding, and fetal death.

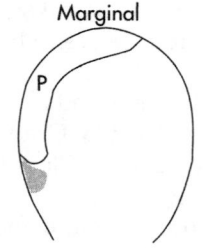
Marginal

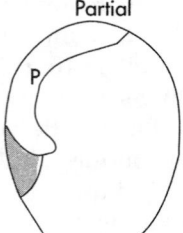
Partial

US features

Specific
- Retroplacental hematoma
- Elevation of fetal membranes (subchorionic hematoma)

Suggestive
- Focal placental thickening
- Edge abnormalities

Nonspecific
- Subchorionic hypoechoic areas
- Placental hypoechoic areas

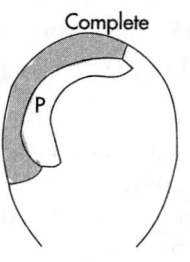
Complete

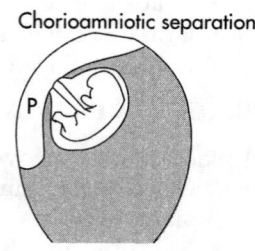
Chorioamniotic separation

Appearance of hemorrhage
- Hyperechoic acute hemorrhage may mimic an echogenic placenta (false negative)

CLINICAL SIGNS OF PLACENTAL SEPARATION		
	Retroplacental Hematoma	**Marginal Separation**
Time	Late, > 20 weeks	Early, < 20 weeks
Type of hemorrhage	Arterial (spiral arteries)	Venous
Vaginal bleeding	Occasionally	Yes
Symptoms	Major	Minor
Prognosis	Worse	Better
Common terminology	Abruptio placenta	Subchorionic hemorrhage

PLACENTA ACCRETA

The normal decidua forms a barrier to deep invasion of chorionic villi into the uterus. In placenta accreta there is loss of the normal placenta/myometrium border. The risk of placenta accreta is higher in patients with prior C-section.

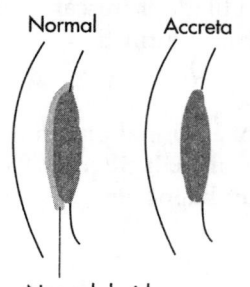
Normal   Accreta

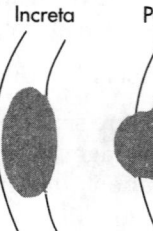
Increta   Percreta

Normal decidua

Types
- Placenta accreta, 80%: chorionic villi adhere to myometrium
- Placenta increta, 15%: villi invade myometrium
- Placenta percreta, 5%: villi completely penetrate myometrium (usually into bladder)

Complications
- Maternal hemorrhage after delivery
- Postpartum infection (retained placenta)

Imaging features
- Very difficult to diagnose by US
- MRI may prove helpful

NORMAL INTRAPLACENTAL LESIONS

All of the following lesions except infarcts appear as anechoic or hypoechoic foci within the placenta and have no pathological significance:
- Fibrin depositions in 25% of pregnancies
- Intervillous thrombosis
- Maternal lakes
- Septal cysts
- Small infarcts are of no clinical significance (if the infarct area is > 10% of placental area, IUGR commonly results from hypoxia). Infarcts are usually not detected unless they hemorrhage.

CHORIOANGIOMA

Benign vascular malformation of the placenta. Most chorioangiomas are small and are of no significance. Complications of large lesions are related to shunting:
- Polyhydramnios
- Hydrops
- IUGR
- Premature labor
- Fetal death

US features
- Chorioangioma may appear as a mixed hyperechoic/hypoechoic solid mass
- Flow in lesions can be demonstrated by Doppler US (in contrast to hemorrhage)
- Polyhydramnios

Gestational Trophoblastic Disease

CLASSIFICATION

Gestational trophoblastic disease (GTD) is a proliferative disease of the trophoblast that may present as:
- Hydatidiform mole (partial or complete)
- Invasive mole
- Choriocarcinoma

Modified NIH classification
Nonmetastatic trophoblastic disease
- Hydatidiform mole
- Persistent mole (> 8 weeks)
- Invasive mole or choriocarcinoma confined to uterus

10

Metastatic trophoblastic disease
- Low risk
    - < 4 months
    - βHCG < 100,000 mIU/ml
    - Lung or vaginal metastases
- Intermediate risk
    - > 4 months
    - βHCG > 100,000 mIU/mls
    - Lung or vaginal metastases
- High risk
    - CNS or liver metastases

KAROTYPES			
Type	Malignant Potential	Karyotype*	Fetal Tissue
Complete mole	Yes (20%)†	46 XX > 46 XY	No
Partial mole	No	69 (triploidy)	Yes

*DNA in all hydatidiform moles is paternal in origin.
†15% invasive mole, 5% choriocarcinoma.

HYDATIDIFORM MOLE

Most benign and most common form of GTD. Incidence 1:1,500 (geographic variation). Risk factors: increased age, prior GTD, Asian. Clinical:
- Uterus too large for dates
- Elevated βHCG (levels can be used to monitor treatment and regression of disease)
- Molar vesicles passed per vagina
- Hemorrhage (common)
- Hyperemesis gravidarum

US features
- Hyperechoic soft tissue mass fills uterine cavity
- Cystic degeneration of mole (vesicular appearance)
- Large, usually multiseptated theca lutein adnexal cysts, 50%
- Absence of fetal parts

Prognosis of hydatidiform mole
- Resolution after evacuation, 80%
- Locally invasive mole, 15%
- Metastatic choriocarcinoma, 5%

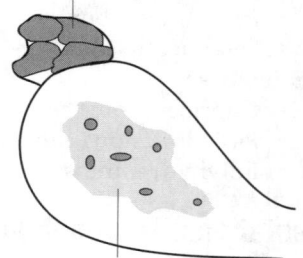

Theca lutein cyst

Echogenic contents with cystic structure

VARIANTS

Incomplete or partial mole
A pregnancy with a formed but abnormal placenta (cystic spaces) and an abnormal dysmorphic fetus. Genetic triploidy (69 chromosomes). May develop persistent GTD but has no malignant potential.

Coexistent trophoblastic disease and a living fetus
Very rare. May be seen in a twin pregnancy with GTD of one placenta.

Hydropic degeneration of the placenta
Hydropic degeneration of the placenta does not represent GTD. There is enlargement of chorionic villi but βHCG is low. Most frequently seen with a missed abortion.

CHORIOCARCINOMA

Malignant form of GTD. Incidence 1:40,000 pregnancies; only 5% of moles progress to choriocarcinoma. Choriocarcinoma is preceded by:
- Mole, 50%
- Abortion, 25%
- Normal pregnancy, 20%
- Ectopic pregnancy, 5%

Metastases
- Lung
- Brain
- Liver
- Bone
- GI tract

Amnion

NORMAL AMNIOTIC FLUID

Volume

Several methods are used for assessment of fluid; there is no evidence that any method is better than the other:
- Subjective assessment (recommended by most sonographers)
    Anterior uterine wall displaced away from fetal body (good sign)
    Fetal extremities readily visible because of excessive fluid
    Umbilical cord readily visible
- Single deepest pocket measurement, > 7 cm
- 4-quadrant amniotic fluid index

Echogenicity

Normal amnion is anechoic

Low-level echoes may be due to:
- Vernix
- Hemorrhage
- Meconium

Pearls
- Amniotic fluid volume is dynamic because of constant production (fetal urination) and consumption (fetal swallowing and lung absorption).
- The greater the degree of polyhydramnios, the greater the likelihood that a major malformation and a chromosomal abnormality are present.

POLYHYDRAMNIOS

Amniotic fluid volume more than expected for gestational age and defined as:
(1) amniotic fluid index > 20-24; (2) largest fluid pocket greater than 8 cms, or
(3) fluid volume larger than 1500-2000 cm^3. Causes:

Idiopathic, 40%

Maternal, 40%
- Diabetes
- Hypertension

10

Fetal, 20%
- CNS lesions (neural tube defect)
- Proximal GI obstruction
- Chest masses
- Twin-twin transfusion
- Nonimmune hydrops

OLIGOHYDRAMNIOS

Amniotic fluid volume less than expected for gestational age. First trimester oligohyramnios results in failure of pregnancy in 95% (pulmonary, hypoplasia, limb contractures). Criteria:
- 4-quadrant amniotic fluid index < 5
- Largest pocket method: < 1 × 1 cm

Causes
Mnemonic: DRIPPC
- **D**emise
- **R**enal abnormalities (decreased urine output)
- **I**UGR, 80%
- **P**remature rupture of membranes
- **P**ost dates
- **C**hromosomal anomalies

Umbilical Cord

CORD ANATOMY

The normal umbilical cord measures 1-2 cm in diameter. The cord contains 2 arteries and 1 vein. Placental insertion:
- Central insertion, 90%
- Marginal insertion, 5% (no clinical significance)
- Insertion on membranes at distance from placenta (velamentous insertion); may cause bleeding in antenatal period, 5%

VASA PREVIA

Velamentous insertion of the umbilical cord with vessels traversing the internal cervical os. Use Doppler US to confirm vessels at the os. Complication: hemorrhage at delivery.

TWO-VESSEL CORD

Umbilical cord containing only 1 artery and 1 vein. Incidence 1%. Associated with structural and chromosomal abnormalities in 50%.

STRAIGHT CORD

A normal cord appears twisted by US (coiled cord), a result of fetal movement. Straight cords are commonly associated with other anomalies. Mortality 10%.

Uterus and Adnexa

INCOMPETENT CERVIX

Premature dilatation of cervical canal before start of labor. Clinical: painless cervical dilatation, prolapse of membranes into vagina, recurrent 2nd trimester abortions.

Causes
Prior injury (most common)
- Abortion, ectopic
- Prior pregnancy
- Curettage, conization, dilatation
- Fetal anatomic variants

Congenital
- Prior diethystilbestrol (DES) exposure in utero
- Inadequacy of lower uterine segment?

US features
Technique
- TAS: bladder should not be fully distended
- TVS: insert probe 3-4 cm into vagina to visualize cervix
- Translabial US

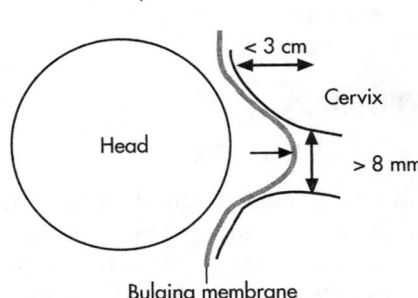

Criteria
- Shortening of cervix < 3 cm
- Cervical canal width > 8 mm
- Prolapse of:
  Membrane
  Cord
  Fetal parts

Management issues
- Serial imaging should be performed if incompetent cervix is suspected but not shown by the first US; an incompetent cervix is a dynamic process
- Serial assessment of the efficacy of surgical cerclage should be monitored by US; sutures usually appear as hyperechoic structures with posterior shadowing
- Main complication of incompetent cervix: 2nd trimester abortion

UTERINE FIBROIDS

Most common uterine mass identified during pregnancy. Most fibroids do not change size during pregnancy, however, some may enlarge due to elevated estrogen levels. Focal myometrial contractions (FMC) may be mistaken for fibroids. FMC are transient and usually disappear within 10 minutes.

DIFFERENTIATION OF FIBROID VS. FMC		
	Fibroid	**FMC**
Echogenicity	Hypoechoic	Isoechoic
Attenuation of beam	Yes	No
Heterogenous	Yes	No
Persistence	Yes	Resolves

ADNEXAL MASSES

Corpus luteum cyst (CLC)
Most common adnexal mass during 1st trimester. CLC secretes progesterone to support the pregnancy until placental progesterone secretion is established.

10

US features

- Most masses are < 5 cm and unilocular
- May contain septations and/or debris
- Typically resolve by 16 weeks
- CLCs are physiological structures. Do not mention them in report unless:
    - Very big
    - Symptomatic
    - Hemorrhagic

Other adnexal masses

- Benign cystic teratoma
- Cystadenoma
- Endometriosis
- Appendicitis

Pelvimetry

MEASUREMENTS

Can be obtained from plain films, CT, or MRI. MRI is now the modality of choice for pelvimetric measurements. Pelvimetry isused to determine pelvic dimensions in breech presentations.

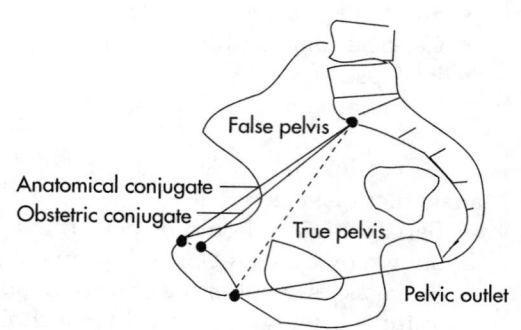

- Obstetric conjugate (> 10 cm), sacral promontory to superior symphysis pubis
- Anatomical conjugate, sacral promontary to superior symphysis pubis
- Diagonal conjugate (> 11.5 cm), sacral promontory to subpubic angle
- Bispinous diameter (> 10.5 cm), distance between ischial spines

Differential Diagnosis

First Trimester

FIRST TRIMESTER BLEEDING

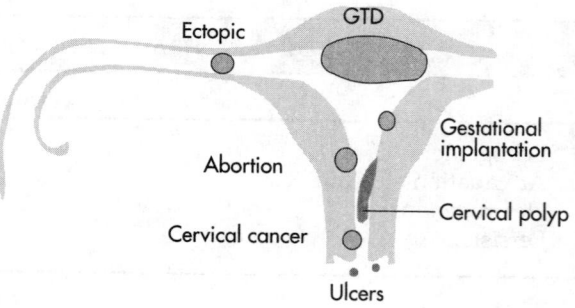

Pregnancy related (common)

- Normal intrauterine pregnancy (implantation bleed)
- Abortion (impending, in progress, incomplete)
- Ectopic pregnancy
- GTD
- Subchorionic hemorrhage

Unrelated to pregnancy (rare)

- Polyp
- Cancer
- Vaginal ulcers

EMPTY SAC

- Normal early IUP
- Blighted ovum (anembryonic gestation)
- Ectopic pregnancy (pseudogestational sac)

ECHOGENIC CENTRAL CAVITY

Normal pregnancy
- Decidua in early, not yet visible IUP
- Hemorrhage

Ectopic pregnancy
- Decidual reaction

Abortion
- Retained products after an incomplete abortion

COMPLEX INTRAUTERINE MASS

- Missed abortion with placental hydropic degeneration
- Fetal demise with retained tissue
- Molar pregnancy
- Degenerated uterine fibroid
- Endometrial carcinoma

AFP ABNORMALITIES

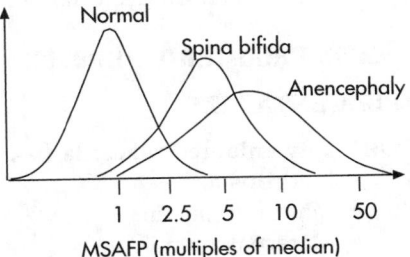

Elevated MSAFP (> 2 mutiples of median)

- Fetal abnormalities, 60%
    NTD
    Abdominal wall defects
    Cystic hygroma
    Gastrointestinal obstruction, atresia
    Liver disease: hepatitis
    Renal disease: congenital nephrosis
- Incorrect dates, 20%
- Multiple gestation, 15%
- Fetal demise, 5%
- Low birth weight
- Placental abnormalities (abruption, mole)

Low MSAFP (< 0.5 multiples of median)

- Down syndrome
- Trisomy 18 (T18)
- Incorrect dates

10

PREDICTORS OF POOR OUTCOME

- Fetal heartbeat not seen with CRL > 5 mm
- MSD ≥ 8 mm and no yolk sac (TVS)
- MSD ≥ 16 mm and no fetal pole (TVS)
- βHCG > 1000 mIU/ml and no gestational sac
- βHCG > 3600 and no yolk sac
- Heart rate < 90 bpm
- MSD—CRL < 5 mm
- Irregular gestational sac
- Abnormal yolk sac (> 6 mm, calcified, irregular)
- Absent double decidual sign with MSD > 10 mm
- Empty sac, large sac
- Large subchorionic hematoma
- < 2 mm choriodecidual reaction

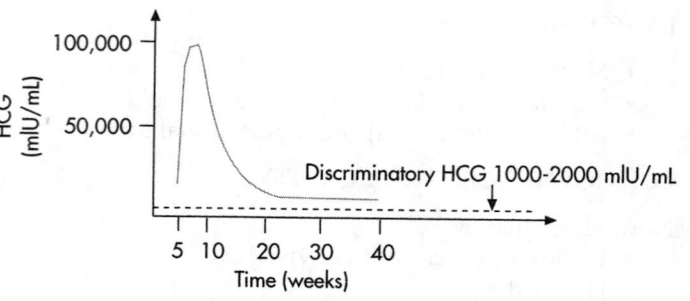

Second and Third Trimester

PLACENTA SIZE

Diffusely enlarged placenta (> 4 cm thick)
- Hydrops fetalis
- Maternal diabetes
- Maternal anemia
- Congenital infection (TORCH)
- Intraplacental hematoma

Small placenta (hypoperfusion)
- Maternal hypertension
- Toxemia
- Severe diabetes
- IUGR

ABNORMAL PLACENTAL ECHOTEXTURE

- Partial mole
- Hydropic placenta
- Hemorrhage or abruption
- Common but insignificant findings (venous lakes, fibrin, intervillous thrombosis, septal cysts, infarcts)

UMBILICAL CORD ABNORMALITIES

Solitary umbilical artery
- Trisomies 13, 18
- Structural anomalies

Enlargement of umbilical cord
- Edema
- Hematoma
- Cysts (allantoic, omphalomesenteric)
- Mucoid degeneration of Wharton's jelly

Other
- Knots
- Varices

RISK FACTORS FOR PRETERM DELIVERY

- Prior preterm delivery
- Multiple gestation (triplets > twins)
- Uterine anomaly, 25%
- DES exposure of mother in utero, 25%
- Incompetent cervix, 25%
- Large fibroid, 20%
- Polyhydramnios, 20%

ABNORMAL LOWER UTERINE SEGMENT

- Prolapse of cord (emergency; put patient in Trendelenburg position and call obstetrician)
- Incompetent cervix
- Placenta previa
- Cerclage
- Low fibroid

THIRD TRIMESTER BLEEEDING

- Placenta previa, 10%
- Abruptio placentae
- Cervical lesions
- Idiopathic (occult abruptio)

MASSES DURING PREGNANCY

Uterus
- Fibroid
- Focal myometral contractions
- GTD
- Hemorrhage

Adnexal
- Corpus luteum cyst
- Dermoid (fat)
- Theca lutein cysts
- Other ovarian neoplasms

Other
- Pelvic inflammatory disease
- Other organs: appendiceal abscess, diverticulitis

FREQUENTLY MISSED LESIONS

- NTD
- Facial anomalies
- Head anomalies in near field
- Heart defects
- Limb anomalies
- Difficulties with imaging in oligohydramnios

10

FETAL DEATH

- No fetal heart beat
- Absent fetal movement
- Occasional findings:
    Overlapping skull bones (Spalding's sign)
    Gross distortion of fetal anatomy (maceration)
    Soft tissue edema: skin > 5 mm
- Uncommon findings:
    Thrombus in fetal heart
    Gas in fetal heart

Fetal Head and Spine

CYSTIC CNS STRUCTURES

Supratentorial
- Choroid plexus cysts
- Ventriculomegaly, hydrocephalus
- Hydranencephaly
- Porencephaly
- Holoprosencephaly
- Arachnoid cyst
- Teratoma

Posterior fossa
- DW complex
- Arachnoid cyst
- Mega cisterna magna

Midline cysts
- Cavum septum pellucidum
- Dorsal cyst in ACC
- Vein of Galen AVM

HYDROCEPHALUS

Noncommunicating
- NTD: Chiari II malformation, meningocele, meningomyelocele, encephalocele, spina bifida
- Dandy-Walker complex
- Aqueduct stenosis
- ACC (colpocephaly)

Communicating (rare prenatally)
- Hemorrhage
- Infection

CYSTIC HEAD AND/OR NECK MASSES

- Cystic hygroma
- Encephalocele (bony calvarial defect)
- Hemangioma
- Teratoma (solid elements)
- Branchial cleft cyst (anterolateral) or thyroglossal (midline) duct cyst
- Umbilical cord tangled around neck

CYSTIC BACK MASSES

- NTD
- Cystic teratoma

HYPERECHOIC BRAIN MASS

- Hemorrhage
- Teratoma
- Lipoma of corpus callosum

INCOMPLETE MINERALIZATION OF THE SKULL

- Osteogenesis imperfecta
- Achondrogenesis, type 1 (skull usually partially ossified)
- Hypophosphatasia

SKULL DEFORMITIES

Lemon sign
- Myelomeningocele
- Encephalocele

Cloverleaf skull
- Craniosynostosis
- Thanatophoric dwarfism
- Other rare skeletal dysplasias

KYPHOSCOLIOSIS

Isolated finding: hemivertebra, butterfly vertebra
Complex anomalies
- VACTERL complex
- Limb-body wall complex
- Any skeletal dysplasia

Fetal Chest

CYSTIC THORACIC MASSES

- Diaphragmatic hernia (stomach adjacent to heart)
- CCAM, type 1, 2
- Cysts: bronchogenic, enteric duplication, pericardial
- Cystic hygroma

SOLID (ECHOGENIC) MASSES

- Diaphragmatic hernia
- CCAM, type 3
- Pulmonary sequestration
- Tumors
    Teratoma
    Rhabdomyoma of the heart

PLEURAL EFFUSION

Unilateral usually due to lung masses
- CHD
- Sequestration
- CCAM

Bilateral
- Fetal hydrops (any cause)
- Pulmonary lymphangiectasia (rare)

Unilateral or bilateral
- Idiopathic
- Infection
- Chromosomal anomalies

Fetal Abdomen

ABNORMAL STOMACH

Absent stomach bubble
- Oligohydramnios
- Swallowing abnormality (CNS defect)
- Esophageal atresia
- Congenital diaphragmatic hernia
- Situs abnormality
- Risk of chromasomal abnormalities (trisomy 18)

Double-bubble (associated with polyhydramnios)
Mnemonic: LADS
- **L**adds's bands
- **A**nnular pancreas
- **D**uodenal atresia
- **S**tenosis of the duodenum

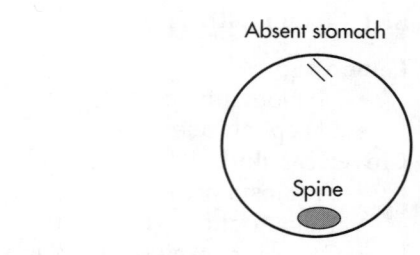

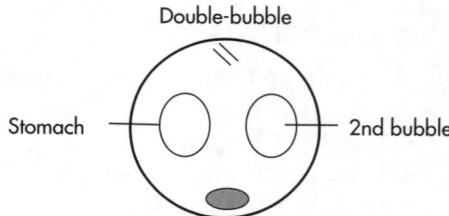

DILATED BOWEL

- Atresia
- Stenosis
- Volvulus
- Meconium ileus
- Enteric duplication
- Hirschsprung's disease

Pearls
- Proximal obstructions are usually associated with polyhydramnios
- Distal obstructions are usually associated with normal amniotic fluid volume (colon absorbs fluid)

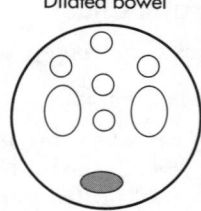

ECHOGENIC BOWEL CONTENT

Criteria: bowel content as bright as iliac bone.
- Normal variant during 2nd trimester (transient inspissation)
- Cystic fibrosis (most common cause)
- Down syndrome (rare but has been reported)
- IUGR
- CMV infection

ABDOMINAL CALCIFICATION

Bowel related (usually occurs with obstruction)
- Meconium peritonitis (most common cause)
- Meconium ileus
- Atresias
- Volvulus

Related to other organs
- Renal
- Liver: infections (TORCH)
- Neuroblastoma
- Teratoma
- Fetal gallstones (usually resolve without consequences)

HYDRONEPHROSIS

The most common causes are:
- UPJ obstruction
- UVJ obstruction (primary megaureter)
- Duplicated collecting system with obstruction of upper pole
- Bladder outlet obstruction
    Male
        PUV (thick bladder wall)
        Prune-belly syndrome (normal bladder wall)
    Females and males
        Caudal regression syndrome
        Megacystis-microcolon-intestinal hypoperistalsis
        Ureteral agenesis
        Maternal drugs
        Ectopic ureterocele

COMMON RENAL ANOMALIES

- Agenesis
- Ectopic kidney
- Hydronephrosis
- Cystic disease
    ARPCKD (infantile form): enlarged hyperechoic kidneys
    Multicystic dysplastic kidneu: large, noncommunicating hypoechoic cysts

CYSTIC ABDOMINAL STRUCTURES

- Hydronephrosis, bladder outlet obstruction
- Fluid-filled dilated bowel
- Ascites
- Meconium pseudocyst
- Fetus in fetu
- Cysts
    Mesenteric cysts
    Urachal cysts
    Duplication cysts
    Ovarian cysts
    Choledochal cysts

10

LIVER

Hepatic calcifications
- Infection: TORCH

Hepatic cysts
- Simple cyst
- Polycystic disease
- Choledochal cyst, Caroli's disease
- Hamartoma

Hepatic masses
- Teratoma
- Hepatoblastoma
- Hemangioma, hemangioendothelioma
- Hamartoma

SPLENOMEGALY

- Rh immune hydrops
- Premature rupture of membranes
- TORCH infection

ASCITES

- Hydrops (any cause)
- Urine ascites
- Meconium peritonitis
- Infection
- Pseudoascites

ANTERIOR WALL DEFECTS

Midline
- Omphalocele
- Pentalogy of Cantrell

Lateral
- Gastroschisis
- Limb-body wall complex
- Amniotic band syndrome

Infraumbilical
- Bladder or cloacal exstrophy

ANOMALIES IN SACRAL REGION

- Teratoma
- Meningocele (anterior or posterior)
- Caudal regression syndrome (e.g., sacral agenesis, sirenomelia)

Fetal Extremities

FRACTURES

- Osteogenesis imperfecta
- Hypophosphatasia

POLYDACTYLY

- Familial
- Trisomy 18, trisomy 13
- Meckel-Gruber syndrome
- Jeune's syndrome
- Short-rib polydactyly syndromes

SUGGESTED READINGS

Callen PW: *Ultrasonography in obstetrics and gynecology,* Philadelphia, 2000, WB Saunders.

Fleischer AC, Kepple DM: *Transvaginal sonography,* Philadelphia, 1995, JB Lippincott.

Hegge FN: *A practical guide to ultrasound of fetal anomalies,* Philadelphia, 1992, Lippincott Williams & Wilkins.

Mittlestaedt CA: *General ultrasound,* New York, 1992, Churchill Livingstone.

Nyberg DA, Hill LM, Böhm-Véler M, et al: *Transvaginal ultrasound,* St Louis, 1992, Mosby.

Nyberg DA, Mahony B, Pretorius D: *Diagnostic ultrasound of fetal anomalies: text and atlas,* Chicago, 1990, Year Book Medical Publishers.

Rumack CM: *Diagnostic ultrasound,* St Louis, 1998, Mosby.

Sauerbrei EE, Nguyen KT, Nolan RL: *A practical guide to ultrasound in obstetrics and gynecology,* Philadelphia, 1998, Lippincott Williams & Wilkins.

Tessler F, Perrella R, Grant E, et al: *Handbook of endovaginal sonography,* New York, 1992, Thieme Medical Publishers.

10

Chapter 11

Pediatric Imaging

Chapter Outline

Respiratory Tract
    Upper airway
    Congenital pulmonary abnormalities
    Pneumonia
    Neonatal respiratory distress
    Mediastinum
Gastrointestinal Tract
    General
    Esophagus
    Stomach
    Duodenum, small bowel
    Colon
    Liver, biliary
Genitourinary Tract
    General
    Congenital anomalies
    Renal cystic disease
    Inflammation
    Tumors
    Ovarian masses
    Other

Musculoskeletal System
    Trauma
    Infection
    Degenerative and chronic traumatic disease
    Metabolic abnormalities
    Congenital anomalies
    Arthritis
    Other disorders
Pediatric Neuroimaging
    Cranial ultrasound
    Skull
    Spine
Differential Diagnosis
    Chest
    Abdomen
    Genitourinary system
    Central nervous system
    Musculoskeletal
    Other

Respiratory Tract

Upper Airway

APPROACH

Inspiratory stridor is the most common indication for radiographic upper airway evaluation. The main role of imaging is to identify conditions that need to be treated emergently and/or surgically (e.g., epiglottitis, foreign bodies). Technique:

1. Physician capable of emergency airway intervention should accompany child
2. Obtain 3 films:
   - Lateral neck-full inspiration, neck extended
   - AP and lateral chest-full inspiration, include upper airway
3. Fluoroscope the neck if radiographs are suboptimal or equivocal
4. Primary diagnostic considerations
   - Infection (epiglottitis, croup, abscess)
   - Foreign body (airway or pharyngoesophageal)
   - Masses (lymphadenopathy, neoplasms)
   - Congenital abnormalities (webs, malacia)
5. If upper airway is normal consider:
   - Pulmonary causes (foreign body, bronchiolitis)
   - Mediastinal causes (vascular rings, slings)
   - Congenital heart disease (CHD)

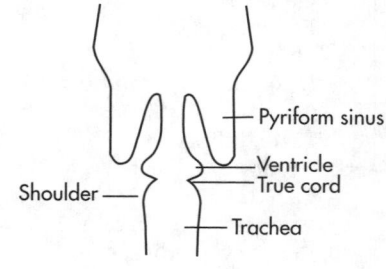

NORMAL APPEARANCE

- 3 anatomical regions
    Supraglottic region
    Glottic region: ventricle and true cords
    Subglottic region
- Epiglottis and aryepiglottic folds are thin structures
- Glottic shoulders are seen on AP view
- Adenoids are visible at 3-6 months after birth
- Normal retropharyngeal soft tissue thickness (C1-C4) = ¾ vertebral body width

LARYNGOMALACIA

Common cause of stridor in the 1st year of life. Immature laryngeal cartilage leads to supraglottic collapse during inspiration. Stridor improves with activity and is relieved by prone positioning or neck extension. Self-limited course. Diagnosis is established by fluoroscopy (laryngeal collapse with inspiration).

TRACHEOMALACIA

Collapse of trachea with expiration. May be focal or diffuse; focal type is usually secondary to congenital anomalies that impress on the trachea such as a vascular ring.

WEBS

Most common in larynx.

TRACHEAL STENOSIS

- Diffuse hypoplasia, 30%
- Focal ringlike stenosis, 50%
- Funnel-like stenosis, 20%

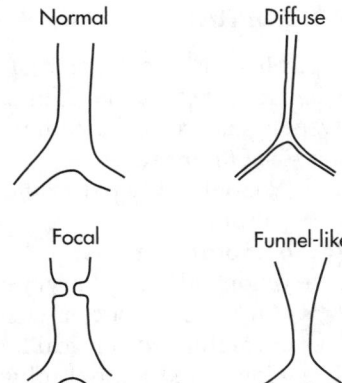

Normal   Diffuse

Focal   Funnel-like

SUBGLOTTIC STENOSIS

Fixed narrowing at level of cricoid. Failure of laryngeal recanalization in utero.

EPIGLOTTITIS

Life-threatening bacterial infection of the upper airway. Most commonly caused by *Haemophilus influenzae*. Age: 3-6 years (older age group than with croup). Clinical: fever, dysphagia, drooling, sore throat. Treatment: prophylatic intubation for 24-48 hours, antibiotics.

Radiographic features
- Thickened aryepiglottic folds (hall mark)
- Key radiographic view: lateral neck
- Thickened epiglottis
- Subglottic narrowing due to edema, 25%: indistinguishable from croup on AP view
- Distention of hypopharynx

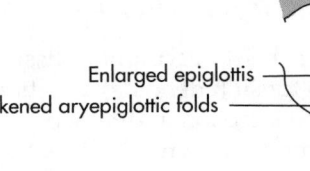

Enlarged epiglottis
Thickened aryepiglottic folds

Pearls
Other causes of enlarged epiglottis or aryepiglottic folds:
- Caustic ingestion
- Hereditary angioneurotic edema
- Omega-shaped epiglottis (normal variant with normal aryepiglottic folds)
- Stevens-Johnson syndrome

CROUP

Subglottic laryngotracheobronchitis. Most commonly caused by parainfluenza virus. Age: 6 months–3 years (younger age group than epiglottitis). Clinical: barking cough, upper respiratory tract infection. Self-limited illness.

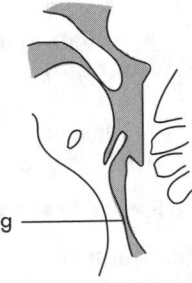

Subglottic narrowing

Radiographic features
- Subglottic narrowing (inverted "V" or "steeple sign")
- Key view: AP view
- Lateral view should be obtained to exclude epiglottitis
- Steeple sign: loss of subglottic shoulders

Pearls
- Membranous croup: uncommon infection of bacterial origin (*Staphylococcus aureus*). Purulent membranes in subglottic trachea
- Epiglottitis may mimic croup on AP view

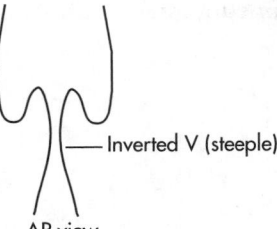

Inverted V (steeple)

AP view

11

RETROPHARYNGEAL ABSCESS

Typically due to extension of a suppurative bacterial lymphadenitis, most commonly *S. aureus, Streptococcus B,* oral flora. Age: < 1 year. Clinical: fever, stiff neck, dysphagia, stridor (uncommon). Most cases present with cellulitis rather than true abscess. Other causes:

- Foreign body perforation
- Trauma

Radiographic features

- Widened retropharyngeal space (most common finding)
- Air in soft tissues is specific for abscess
- Straightened cervical lordosis
- Computed tomography (CT) is helpful to define superior and (inferior mediastinal) extent
- Plain film findings are usually nonspecific
- Main differential diagnosis:
    Retropharyngeal hematoma
    Neoplasm (i.e., rhabdomyosarcoma)
    Lymphadenopathy

TONSILLAR HYPERTROPHY

The tonsils consist of lymphoid tissue that encircle the pharynx. Three groups: pharyngeal tonsil (adenoids), palatine tonsil, and lingual tonsil. Tonsils enlarge secondary to infection and may obstruct nasopharynx and/or eustachian tubes. Rarely, bacterial pharyngitis can lead to a tonsillar abscess (Quinsy abscess), which requires drainage. Specific etiologies:

- Mononucleosis (Epstein-Barr virus)
- Coxsackie virus (herpangina, hand-foot-mouth disease)
- Adenovirus (pharyngoconjunctival fever)
- Measles prodrome (rubeola)
- β-hemolytic streptococcus (Quinsy abscess)

Radiographic features

- Mass in posterior nasopharynx (enlarged adenoids)
- Mass near end of uvula (palatine tonsils)
- CT is useful to determine the presence of a tonsillar abscess

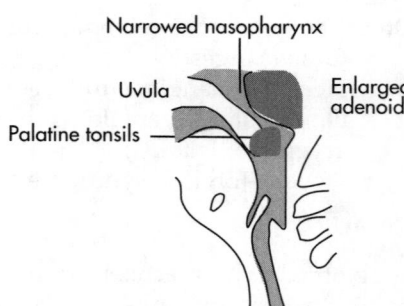

AIRWAY FOREIGN BODY

Common cause of respiratory distress. Age: 6 months-4 years. Acute aspiration results in cough, stridor, wheezing; chronic foreign body causes hemoptysis or recurrent pneumonia. Location: right bronchi > left bronchi > larynx, trachea

Radiographic features

Bronchial foreign body

- Unilateral air trapping causing hyperlucent lung, 90%
- Expiratory film or lateral decubitus make air trapping more apparent
- Atelectasis is uncommon, 10%
- Only 10% of foreign bodies are radioopaque
- Chest fluoroscopy or CT should be performed if plain films are equivocal

Tracheal foreign body

- Foreign body usually lodges in sagittal plane
- CXR is usually normal

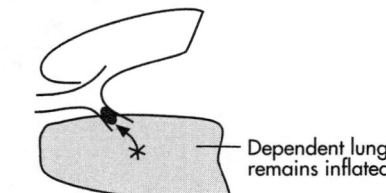

Congenital Pulmonary Abnormalities

BRONCHOPULMONARY FOREGUT MALFORMATION

Bronchopulmonary foregut malformations arise from a supernumerary lung bud that develops below the normal lung bud. Location and communication with gastrointestinal (GI) tract depend on when in embryonic life the bud develops. Most malformations present clinically when they become infected (communication with GI tract). Spectrum:

OVERVIEW OF BRONCHOPULMONARY MALFORMATIONS	
Malformation	**Location**
Sequestration	
Intralobar	60% basilar, left
Sequestration	80% left or below diaphragm
Bronchogenic cyst	Mediastinum, 85%; lung, 15%
CCAM	All lobes
Congenital lobar emphysema	LUL, 40%; RML, 35%; RUL, 20%

PULMONARY SEQUESTRATION

Clinical: recurrent infection, lung abscess, bronchiectasis, and hemoptysis during childhood. Pathology:

- Nonfunctioning pulmonary tissue (nearly always posteromedial segments of lower lobes)
- Systemic arterial supply: anomalous arteries from the aorta (less commonly branch of the celiac artery)
- No connection to bronchial tree

11

TYPES OF PULMONARY SEQUESTRATION*		
Feature	**Intralobar Sequestration**	**Extralobar Sequestration**
Age	Older children, adults	Neonates
Pleura	Inside lung (intralobar)	Outside lung (extralobar, own pleura)
Forms	Airless (consolidation) and air-containing, cystic type	Always airless (pleural envelope) unless communication with GI tract
Venous return	Pulmonary vein	Systemic: IVC, azygos, portal
Arterial supply	Thoracic aorta > abdominal aorta	Thoracic aorta > abdominal aorta

Associations	In 10% of patients:
	    Skeletal anomalies, 5%
	    Foregut anomalies, 5%
	    Diaphragmatic anomalies
	    Rare other associations
		In 65% of patients:
		    Diaphragmatic defect, 20%
		    Pulmonary hypoplasia, 25%
		    Bronchogenic cysts
		    Cardiac anomalies

IVC, Inferior vena cava.
*Location of all sequestrations: posterobasal, L > R.

Radiographic features

- Large (> 5 cm) mass near diaphragm
- Air-fluid levels if infected
- Surrounding pulmonary consolidation
- Sequestration may communicate with GI tract

BRONCHOGENIC CYST

Result from abnormal budding of the tracheobronchial tree. Cysts contain respiratory epithelium. Location:

- Mediastinum, 85% (posterior > middle > anterior mediastinum)
- Lung, 15%

Radiographic features

- Well-defined round mass in subcarinal/parahilar region
- Pulmonary cysts commonly located in medial ⅓ of lung
- Initially no communication with tracheobronchial tree
- Cysts are thin walled
- Cysts can be fluid or air filled

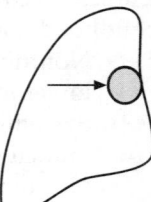

CONGENITAL CYSTIC ADENOID MALFORMATION (CCAM)

CCAM refers to a proliferation of polypoid glandular lung tissue without normal
alveolar differentiation. Clinical: respiratory distress during first days of life.
Treatment: surgical resection (sarcomatous degeneration has been described). Types:

- Macrocystic (Stocker types 1 and 2): single cyst or multiple cysts > 5 mm
  confined to one hemithorax; better prognosis; common
- Microcystic (Stocker type 3): homogenous echogenic mass without discernible
  individual cysts; closely resembles pulmonary sequestration or intrathoracic
  bowel from a diaphragmatic hernia; less common

Radiographic features

- Multiple cystic pulmonary lesions of variable size
- Air-fluid levels in cysts
- Variable thickness of cyst wall

CONGENITAL LOBAR EMPHYSEMA

Progressive overdistention of one or more pulmonary lobes but usually not the entire
lung. 10% of patients have congenital heart disease (patent ductus arteriousus [PDA]
and ventricular septal defect [VSD]).

Causes:

Idiopathic, 50%
Obstruction of airway with valve mechanism, 50%

- Bronchial cartilage deficiency or immaturity
- Mucus
- Web, stenosis
- Extrinsic compression

Radiographic features

- Hyperlucent lobe (hallmark)
- First few days of life: alveolar opacification because there is
  no clearance of lung fluid through bronchi
- May be asymptomatic in neonate but becomes symptomatic
  later in life
- Use CT to differentiate from bronchial obstruction
- Distribution

  LUL, 40%
  RML, 35%
  RUL, 20%
  2 lobes affected, 5%

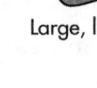

Shifted
thymus

Large, lucent hemithorax

PULMONARY HYPOPLASIA

Types of pulmonary underdevelopment

- Agenesis: complete absence of one or both lungs (airways, alveoli, and vessels)
- Aplasia: absence of lung except for a rudimentary bronchus which ends in a
  blind pouch
- Hypoplasia: decrease in number and size of airways and alveoli; hypoplastic PA

Scimitar syndrome (hypogenetic lung syndrome, pulmonary venolobar syndrome)
Special form of hypoplastic lung in which the hypoplastic lung is perfused from the aorta and drained by the IVC or portal vein. The anomalous vein has a resemblance to a Turkish scimitar (sword). Associations:

- Accessory diaphragm, diaphragmatic hernia
- Bony abnormalities: hemivertebrae, rib notching, rib hypoplasia
- CHD: atrial septal defect (ASD), VSD, PDA, tetralogy of Fallot

Radiographic features

- Small lung (most commonly the right lung)
- Retrosternal soft tissue density (hypoplastic collapsed lung)
- Anomalous vein resembles a scimitar
- Systemic arterial supply from aorta
- Dextroposition of the heart (shift because of hypoplastic lung)

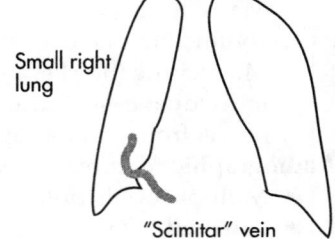

Small right lung

"Scimitar" vein

CONGENITAL DIAPHRAGMATIC HERNIA (CDH)

Incidence: 1 in 2,000-3,000 births. Mortality rate of isolated hernias is 60% (with postnatal surgery) and higher when other abnormalities are present. Clinical: respiratory distress in neonatal period. Associated abnormalities:

- Pulmonary hypoplasia (common)
- CNS abnormalities
    Neural tube defects: spina bifida, encephalocele
    Anencephaly

Types
Bochdalek's hernias (90% of CDH): posterior

- 75% are on the left, 25% on right
- Right sided hernias are more difficult to detect because of similar echogenicity of liver and lung
- Contents of hernia: stomach, 60%; colon, 55%; small intestine, 90%; spleen, 45%; liver, 50%; pancreas, 25%; kidney, 20%
- Malrotation of herniated bowel is very common

Morgagni hernias (10% of CDH): anterior

- Most occur on right (heart prevents development on the left)
- Most common hernia contents: omentum, colon
- Accompanying anomalies common

Eventration

- Due to relative absence of muscle in dome of diaphragm
- Associated with:
    Trisomies 13, 18
    Congenital CMV, rubella
    Arthrogryposis multiplex
    Pulmonary hypoplasia

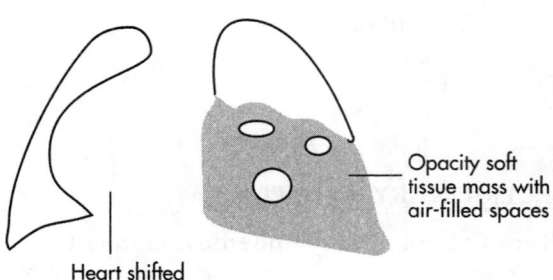

Heart shifted

Opacity soft tissue mass with air-filled spaces

Radiographic features

- Hemidiaphragm not visualized
- Multicystic mass in chest
- Mass effect

KARTAGENER'S SYNDROME

Kartagener's syndrome (immotile cilia syndrome) is due to the deficiency of the dynein arms of cilia causing immotility of respiratory, auditory, and sperm cilia.

Radiographic features
- Complete thoracic and abdominal situs inversus
- Bronchiectasis
- Sinus hypoplasia and mucosal thickening

Pneumonia

Childhood pneumonias are commonly caused by:
- Mycoplasma, 30% (lower in age group < 3 years)
- Viral, 65% (higher in age group < 3 years)
- Bacterial 5%

VIRAL PNEUMONIA

Causes: respiratory syncytial virus (RSV), parainfluenza

RADIOGRAPHIC PATTERNS OF PNEUMONIA			
Pattern		**Frequency**	**Description**
Bronchiolitis		Common	Normal CXR Overaeration is only diagnostic clue Commonly due to RSV
Bronchiolitis + parahilar, peribronchial opacities		Most common	Dirty parahilar regions caused by: Peribronchial cuffing (inflammation) Hilar adenopathy
Bronchiolitis + atelectasis		Common	Disordered pattern with: Atelectasis Areas of hyperaeration Parahilar + peribronchial opacities
Reticulonodular interstitial		Rare	Interstitial pattern
Hazy lungs		Rare	Diffuse increase in density

11

Pearls
- All types of bronchiolitis and bronchitis cause air-trapping (overaeration) with flattening of hemidiaphragms
- RSV, mycoplasma, and parainfluenza are the most common viruses that cause radiographic abnormalities (in 10%-30% of infected children)
- Any virus may result in any of the 5 different radiographic patterns

BACTERIAL PNEUMONIA

The following 3 pathogens are the most common:
- Pneumococcus (age 1-3)
- *S. aureus* (infancy)
- *H. influenzae* (late infancy)

Radiographic features

Consolidation
- Alveolar exsudate
- Segmental consolidation
- Lobar consolidation

Other findings
- Effusions
- Pneumatocele

Complications
- Pneumothorax
- Bronchiectasis (reversible)
- Swyer-James syndrome (acquired pulmonary hypoplasia), radiographically characterized by small, hyperlucent lungs with diminished vessels (focal emphysema)
- Bronchiolitis obliterans

Round pneumonia
- Pneumococcal pneumonia in early consolidative phase
- Pneumonia appears round because of poorly developed collateral pathways (pores of Kohn and channels of Lambert)
- With time the initially round pneumonia develops into a more typical consolidation

Recurrent infections
- Cystic fibrosis
- Recurrent aspirations
- Rare causes of recurrent infection
  - Hypogammaglobulinemia (Bruton's disease; differential diagnosis clue: no adenoids or hilar lymph nodes)
  - Hyperimmunoglobulinemia E (Buckley's syndrome)
  - Immotile cilia syndrome (Kartagener's)
  - Other immunodeficiencies
  - Bronchopulmonary foregut malformation

ASPIRATION PNEUMONIA

Aspiration pneumonia results from inhalation of swallowed materials or gastric content. Gastric acid damages capillaries causing acute pulmonary edema. Secondary infection or acquired respiratory distress syndrome (ARDS) may ensue.

Causes

Aspiration due to swallowing dysfunction (most common cause)
- Anoxic birth injury (common)
- Coma, anesthesia

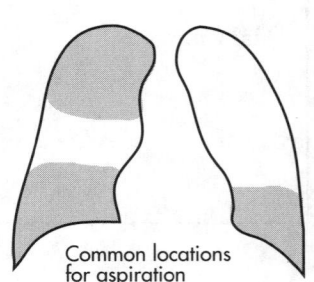

Common locations for aspiration

Aspiration due to obstruction
- Esophageal atresia or stenosis
- Esophageal obstruction
- Gastroesophageal reflux, hiatal hernia
- Gastric or duodenal obstruction

Fistula
- Tracheoesophageal fistula

Radiographic features
- Recurrent pneumonias; distribution:
    Aspiration in supine position: upper lobes, superior segments
        of lower lobes
    Aspiration in upright position: both lower lobes
- Segmental and subsegmental atelectasis
- Interstitial fibrosis
- Inflammatory thickening of bronchial walls

Neonatal Respiratory Distress

Respiratory distress in the newborn is usually due to one of 4 disease entities:
- Hyaline membrane disease (HMD)
- Transient tachypnea of the newborn (TTN)
- Meconium aspiration
- Neonatal pneumonia

NEONATAL RESPIRATORY DISTRESS				
Disease	**Lung Volume**	**Opacities**	**Time Course**	**Complication**
Hyaline membrane disease	Low	Granular	4-6 days	PIE, BPD, PDA
Transient tachypnea	High or normal	Linear, streaky*	< 48 hours	None
Meconium aspiration	Hyperinflation	Coarse, patchy	At birth	PFC, ECMO
Neonatal pneumonia	Anything	Granular	Variable	

*Ground glass opacity at birth.

The most common complications of HMD are:
- Pulmonary interstitial emphysema (PIE)
- Persistent PDA
- Bronchopulmonary dysplasia (BPD)

HYALINE MEMBRANE DISEASE (HMD)

HMD is caused by surfactant deficiency. Surfactant diminishes surface tension of expanding alveoli. As a result, acinar atelectasis and interstitial edema occur. Hyaline membranes are formed by proteinaceous exudate. Symptoms occur within 2 hours of life. The incidence of HMD depends on the gestational age at birth.

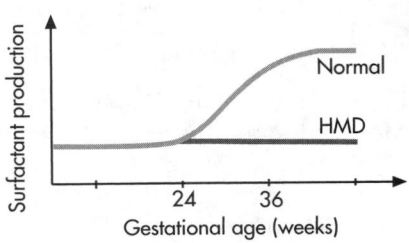

11

INCIDENCE OF HYALINE MEMBRANE DISEASE	
Birth at Gestational Age (Weeks)	Incidence (%)
27	50
31	16
34	5
36	1

Radiographic features

- Any opacity in a premature infant should be regarded as HMD until proven otherwise
- Lungs are opaque (ground glass) or reticulogranular (hallmark)
- Hypoaeration (atelectasis) leads to low lung volumes: bell-shaped thorax (if not intubated)
- Bronchograms are often present
- Absence of consolidation or pleural effusions
- In contrast to other causes of respiratory distress syndrome in neonates, pleural effusions are uncommon
- CXR signs of premature infants:
    No subcutaneous fat
    No humeral ossification center
    Endotracheal tube present

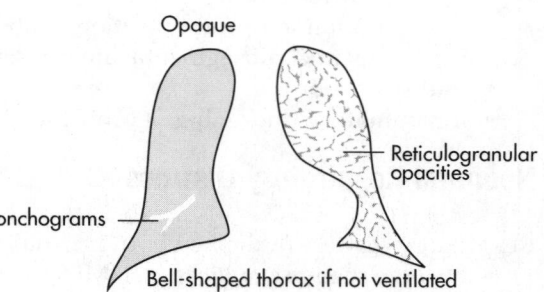

In most cases of HMD the diagnosis is made clinically but may initially be made radiographically. The role of the radiologist is to assess serial chest films. Treatment complication of HMD:

- Persistent PDA (signs of congestive heart failure [CHF]); the ductus usually closes within 1-2 days after birth in response to the high Po_2 content
- Air-trapping: PIE and acquired lobar emphysema
- Diffuse opacities (whiteout) may be due to a variety of causes:
    Atelectasis
    Progression of HMD
    Aspiration
    Pulmonary hemorrhage
    CHF
    Superimposed pneumonia

PULMONARY INTERSTITIAL EMPHYSEMA (PIE)

PIE refers to accumulation of interstitial air in peribronchial and perivascular spaces. Most common cause: positive pressure ventilation. Complications:

- Pneumothorax
- Pneumomediastinum
- Pneumopericardium

Radiographic features

- Tortuous linear lucencies radiate outward from the hilar regions
- The lucencies extend all the way to the periphery of the lung
- Lucencies do not change with respiration

BRONCHOPULMONARY DYSPLASIA (BPD)

Caused by oxygen toxicity and barotrauma of respiratory therapy. There are 4 stages in the development; the progression of BPD through all 4 stages is now rarely seen because of the awareness of this disease entity.

STAGES OF BRONCHOPULMONARY DYSPLASIA			
Stage	Time	Pathology	Imaging
1	< 4 days	Mucosal necrosis	Similar to HMD
2	1 week	Necrosis, edema, exudate	Diffuse opacities
3	2 weeks	Bronchial metaplasia	Bubbly lungs*
4	1 month	Fibrosis	Bubbly lungs*

*Bubbly lungs (honeycombing): rounded lucencies surrounded by linear densities; hyperaeration.

Prognosis of stage 4
- Mortality, 40%
- Minor handicaps, 30%
- Abnormal pulmonary function tests in almost all in later life
- Clinically normal by 3 years, 30%

MECONIUM ASPIRATION SYNDROME

Meconium (mucus, epithelial cells, bile, debris) is the first stool that is evacuated within 12 hours after delivery. In fetal distress, evacuation may occur into the amniotic fluid (up to 10% of deliveries). However, in only 1% does this aspiration cause respiratory symptoms. Only meconium aspirated to below the vocal cords is clinically significant. Meconium aspiration sometimes clears in 3-5 days. CXR nearly always returns to normal by 1 year of age.

Radiographic features
- Patchy, bilateral opacities
- Atelectasis
- Hyperinflated lungs
- Pneumothorax, pneumomediastinum, 25%

Complication
- Mortality (25%) from persistent fetal circulation

NEONATAL PNEUMONIA (NP)

Pathogenesis
Transplacental infection
- TORCH
- Pulmonary manifestation of TORCH is usually less severe than other manifestations

Perineal flora (group B streptococcus, enterococcus, *Escherichia coli*)
- Ascending infection
- Premature rupture of membranes
- Infection while passing through birth canal

Radiographic features
- Patchy asymmetrical opacities in a term baby represent neonatal pneumonia until proven otherwise
- Hyperinflation

11

TRANSIENT TACHYPNEA OF THE NEWBORN (TTN)

TTN (wet lung syndrome) is a clinical diagnosis. It is caused by a delayed resorption of intrauterine pulmonary liquids. Normally, pulmonary fluids are cleared by:
- Bronchial squeezing during delivery, 30%
- Absorption, 30%: lymphatics, capillaries
- Suction, 30%

Causes
- Cesarean section, premature delivery, maternal sedation (no thoracic squeezing)
- Hypoproteinemia, hypervolemia, erythrocythemia

Radiographic features
- Fluid overload (similar appearance as noncardiogenic pulmonary edema)
    Prominent vascular markings
    Pleural effusion
    Fluid in fissure
    Alveolar edema
- Lungs clear in 24-48 hours

EXTRACORPOREAL MEMBRANE OXYGENATION (ECMO)

Technique of providing prolonged extracorporeal gas exchange. Indications: any severe respiratory failure with predicted mortality rates of > 80%. Exclusion criteria for ECMO:
- < 34 weeks of age
- > 10 days of age
- Serious intracranial hemorrhage
- Patients that require epinephrine

Complications
- Late neurological sequela; developmental delay, 50%
- Intracranial hemorrhage, 10%
- Pneumothorax, pneumomediastinum
- Pulmonary hemorrhage (common)
- Pleural effusions (common)
- Catheter complications

Mediastinum

THYMUS

The ratio of thymus:body weight decreases with age. Thymus is routinely identified on CXR from birth to 2 years of age. Size and shape of the thymus are highly variable from person to person.

COMMON MEDIASTINAL TUMORS

Anterior
- Thymic hyperplasia and thymic variations in shape and size (most common)
- Teratoma
- T-cell lymphoma
- Cystic hygroma
- Thymomas are extremely rare

Middle
- Adenopathy (leukemia, lymphoma, TB)
- Bronchopulmonary foregut malformation

Posterior
- Neuroblastoma
- Ganglioneuroma
- Neurofibromatosis
- Neurenteric cysts
- Meningoceles

Pearls
- Any pediatric anterior mediastinal mass is thymus until proven otherwise
- Posterior mediastinal masses are the most common abnormal chest masses in infants

Gastrointestinal Tract

General

EMBRYOLOGY

The GI tract develops from three embryological precursors, each of which have a separate vascular supply: foregut, midgut, hindgut.

EMBRYONIC PRECURSORS OF GI TRACT		
Origin	**Vascular Supply**	**Derivatives**
Foregut	Celiac artery	Pharynx, lower respiratory tract, esophagus, stomach, liver, pancreas, biliary tree, duodenum
Midgut	SMA	Distal duodenum, small bowel, ascending colon
Hindgut	IMA	Transverse colon, rectum, bladder, urethra

SMA, Superior mesenteric artery; *IMA,* inferior mesenteric artery.

Bowel is formed in 3 steps:
- Rotation
- Fixation
- Canalization

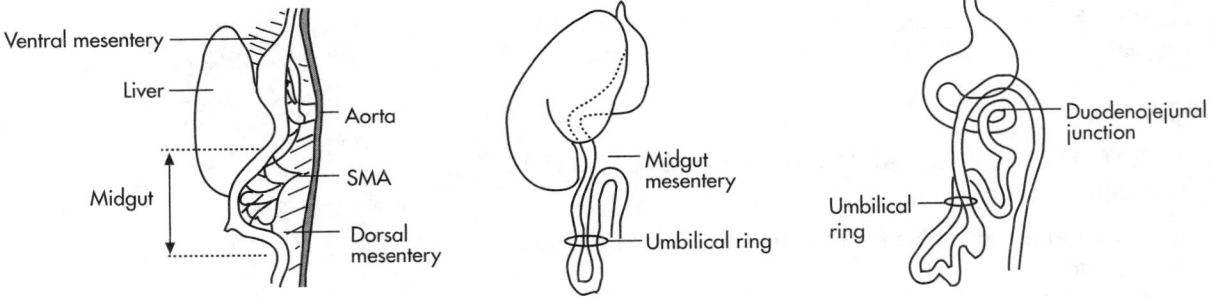

Rotation

- Duodenojejunal loop (first 270° loop) brings stomach into horizontal axis and puts liver into right and spleen into left abdomen. The common bile duct (CBD) is associated with the ventral pancreas and becomes located dorsally because of the rotation. Before the rotation, the 1st loop rotation results in the duodenojejunal junction being located to the left.
- Cecocolic loop (second 270° loop). The small bowel develops from the dorsal mesentery, and then rotates 270° so that the cecum lies near the right upper quadrant (RUQ). It later descends to the right lower quadrant (RLQ).

Fixation

Fixation is incomplete at birth. Abnormal fixation of the colonic mesentery to the posterior abdominal wall results in potential spaces into which bowel may herniate (paraduodenal hernias). Abnormalities of fixation include:
- Increased mobility (cecal bascule)
- Internal hernia (paraduodenal, paracecal)

Canalization

After forming a primitive tube, the bowel lumen solidifies and then recanalizes to form the viable lumen. Anomalies in this step may result in atresia or duplication.
- Atresia
  - Duodenal atresia results from failure of recanalization of the foregut (10 weeks); frequently associated with other abnormalities (malrotation 50%, Down syndrome 30%, esophageal atresia)
  - Jejunoileal atresia results from an ischemic insult, not a failure of recanalization; occurs later and is usually an isolated phenomenon
- Duplication
  - Abnormal recanalization: small intramural duplication cysts may develop
  - Notochordal adhesion: a portion of bowel remains adherent to the notochord and a diverticulum may develop

UMBILICAL ARTERY (UA) LINE

Traverses the UA, the internal iliac artery, and the infrarenal aorta. The tip of the line should be located above the renal arteries between levels T8 and T12. An alternative location of the catheter tip is below the renal arteries between levels L3 and L4.

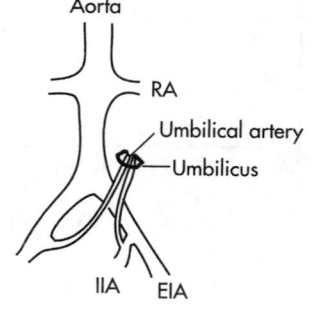

UMBILICAL VEIN (UV) LINE

The UV line should traverse the UV, portal sinus (junction of left and right portal vein), ductus venosus (which closes at 96 hours of life), and IVC and end in the right atrium. The line can easily be misplaced in a portal or hepatic branch (the tip then projects over the liver).

Esophagus

ESOPHAGEAL ATRESIA (EA) AND TRACHEOESOPHAGEAL FISTULA (TEF)

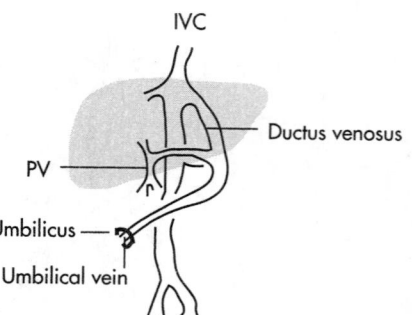

Spectrum of anomalies involving esophagus and trachea. There are two clinical presentations:
- Early presentation in EA with a pouch (N-type, 85%): vomiting, choking, difficulty with secretions
- Late presentation of recurrent pneumonias if there is a fistula between esophagus and trachea (H-type, 5%)

Types
- TEF, N-type fistula, 85%
- Pure EA without fistula, 10%
- TEF, H-type fistula (no atresia), 1%
- Other forms

Associations
VACTERL
- **Vertebral** anomalies
- **Anorectal** anomalies
- **Cardiovascular** anomalies
- **Tracheal** anomalies
- **Esophageal** fistula
- **Renal** anomalies: renal agenesis
- **Limb** anomalies: radial ray

Cardiac anomalies
- VSD
- Ductus arteriosus
- Right aortic arch

EA is associated with other atresias and/or stenosis
- Duodenal atresia
- Imperforate anus

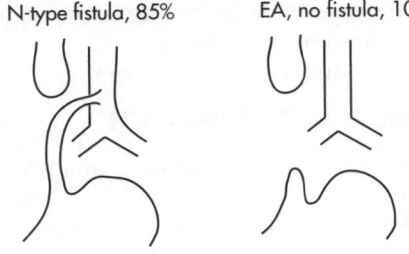

N-type fistula, 85%   EA, no fistula, 10%

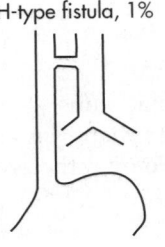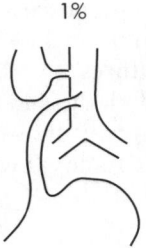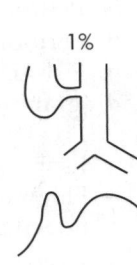

H-type fistula, 1%   1%   1%

Radiographic features
Plain film findings
- Gas-filled dilated proximal esophageal segment (pouch)
- Gasless abdomen (EA-type)
- Excessive air in stomach (H-type)
- Aspiration pneumonia

Procedures
- Pass 8 Fr feeding tube through nose to the level of atresia; distal end of tube marks level of atresia; inject air if necessary
- Definite diagnosis is established by injection of 1-2 mL of liquid barium; this, however, should be done only at a large referral institution
- Videotape the injection

Main differential diagnosis
- Traumatic perforation of posterior pharynx
- Pharyngeal pseudodiverticulum

GASTROESOPHAGEAL REFLUX

Causes
- Immaturity of lower esophageal sphincter during first 3 months of life (usually resolves spontaneously)
- Congenital short esophagus
- Hiatal hernia
- Chalasia (lower esophageal sphincter fails to contract in resting phase; differentiate from achalasia in adults)
- Gastric outlet obstruction

11

Radiographic features

Barium swallow

- Determine presence of reflux
- Exclude organic abnormalities

Gastroesophageal scintigraphy

- Most sensitive technique to determine reflux and gastroesophageal emptying
- Semiquantitative method
- Anatomy only poorly visualized

ESOPHAGEAL FOREIGN BODY

Foreign bodies in the esophagus may cause airway symptoms by:

- Direct mechanical compression of airway
- Periesophageal inflammation
- Perforation and abscess
- Fistulization to trachea

Radiographic features

- Foreign body lodges in coronal plane
- Esophagram may show inflammatory mass
- Fluoroscopic removal with Foley catheter in select instances (e.g., nonembedded)

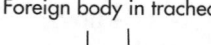
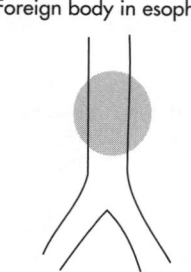
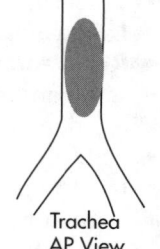

Foreign body in esophagus   Foreign body in trachea

Trachea
AP View

Stomach

HYPERTROPHIC PYLORIC STENOSIS (HPS)

Caused by hypertrophy of the circular musculature of the pylorus. Incidence: 1:1000 births. Male:female = 4:1. Unknown etiology. Treatment: pyloromyotomy. Clinical: projectile nonbilious vomiting after each feeding; peaks at 3-6 weeks after birth; never occurs after 3 months; palpable antral mass (olive sized), weight loss, dehydration, jaundice, alkalosis. Associations:

- EA, TEF, hiatal hernia
- Renal abnormalities
- Other: Turner's syndrome, trisomy 18, rubella

Radiographic features

Plain film

- Gastric distention (> 7 cm)
- Peristaltic waves result in a "caterpillar" appearance to the distended stomach
- Decreased air in distal bowel
- Thick antral folds

US

- HPS appears as target lesion (anechoic mass in RUQ with central echoes due to gas)
- Scan in RPO projection (move fluid into antrum)
- Size criteria are used to establishthe diagnosis of HPS:
     Pyloric muscle thickness > 3.5-4 mm
     Pyloric length > 15-18 mm
- Useful as first imaging modality

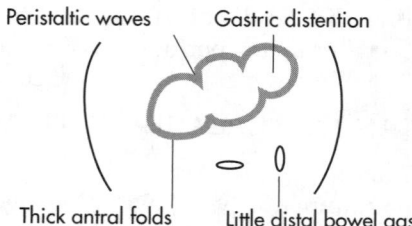

Peristaltic waves   Gastric distention

Thick antral folds   Little distal bowel gas

Upper GI technique:

1. Insert an 8 Fr feeding tube to (a) decompress the stomach and (b) drain gastric contents before administration of contrast agent
2. Patient in RAO (to visualize the pylorus)
3. Instill 10-20 mL of barium
4. Wait for pylorus to open, obtain spot views
5. Get air contrast view by turning patient supine
6. If there is no pyloric stenosis, get a lateral and AP view to exclude malrotation
7. UGI findings of HPS:
   - Indented gastric antrum (shoulder sign)
   - Compression of duodenal bulb
   - Narrow and elongated pylorus: string sign

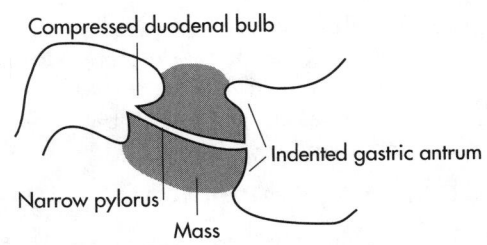

PYLOROSPASM

Intermittent findings of pyloric stenosis. Treatment: antispasmodic drugs.
Associations:
- Adrenogenital syndrome
- Dehydration
- Sepsis

Radiographic features
- Pyloric musculature is of normal thickness
- Prominent mucosa (echogenic)
- Exclude secondary causes of pylorospasm (e.g., ulcer)

VOLVULUS

Mesenteroaxial volvulus. Pylorus lies above gastroesophageal (GE) junction
- Occurs with eventration of left diaphragm or diaphragmatic hernia
- Acute syndrome: obstruction, ischemia

Organoaxial volvulus: rotation around long axis of stomach
- Rare in children
- Associated with large hiatus hernia
- Lesser curvature is inferior and greater curvature lies superior
- Associated gastric outlet obstruction

Duodenum, Small Bowel

CONGENITAL DUODENAL ATRESIA, STENOSIS

Results from failure of recanalization (around 10 weeks). Incidence: 1:3500 live births. Atresia:stenosis = 2:1. Clinical: common cause of bowel obstruction, bilious vomiting within 24 hours after birth. Treatment: duodenojejunostomy or duodenoduodenostomy.

Associations
- 30% have Down syndrome
- 40% have polyhydramnios and are premature
- Malrotation, EA, biliary atresia, renal anomalies, imperforate anus with or without sacral anomalies, CHD

11

Radiographic features

- Enlarged duodenal bulb and stomach (double-bubble sign)
- Small amount of air in distal small bowel does not exclude diagnosis of duodenal atresia (hepatopancreatic duct may bifurcate in Y shape and insert above and below atresia)

DUODENAL DIAPHRAGM

Variant of duodenal stenosis caused by an obstructive duodenal membrane. The pressure gradient through the diaphragm causes the formation of a diverticulum ("wind sock" appearance).

ANNULAR PANCREAS

Uncommon congenital ringlike position of pancreas surrounding the second portion of duodenum. Results from abnormal rotation of embryonic pancreatic tissue. The annular pancreas usually causes duodenal narrowing. Diagnosis made by ERCP and MRCP.

MALROTATION AND MIDGUT VOLVULUS

Normally, the rotations place the ligament of Treitz to the left of the spine at level of duodenal bulb. Distal end of mesentary is in RLQ. In malrotation the mesenteric attachment is short, allowing bowel to twist around the superior mesenteric vessels. SMV compression (edematous bowel) is followed by SMA compression (gangrene).

Associations

- Gastroschisis
- Omphalocele
- Diaphragmatic hernia
- Duodenal or jejunal atresia

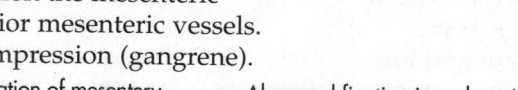

Normal fixation of mesentery · Abnormal fixation in malrotation

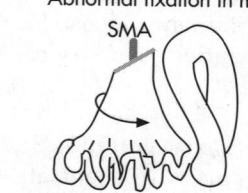

Radiographic features

Plain film

- Suspect diagnosis in the setting of bowel obstruction and abnormally positioned bowel loops
- A normal position of the cecum does not exclude malrotation, but makes it much less likely

US

- Reversal of SMA (right) and SMV (left) location may occasionally be diagnosed by color Doppler
- Distended proximal duodenum
- Usually not useful

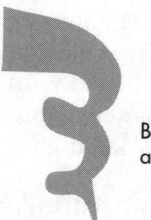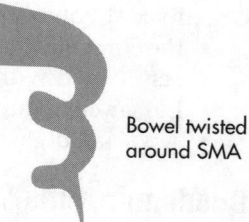

Bowel twisted around SMA

UGI

- Abnormal position of duodenojejunal junction because of absence of ligament of Treitz
- Beaking at site of obstruction
- Spiraling of small bowel as it twists around SMA (corkscrew)
- Edema of bowel wall
- Early diagnosis is essential to prevent bowel necrosis

Barium enema

- A normal barium enema will rule out 97% of malrotation
- Can determine if there is a concomitant cecal volvulus

CT

- SMA to right of SMV
- Gastric outlet obstruction
- Spiraling of decodenum and jejunum around SMA axis

LADD'S BANDS

Peritoneal bands in patients with malrotation. The bands extend from malplaced cecum to porta hepatis and may cause duodenal obstruction.

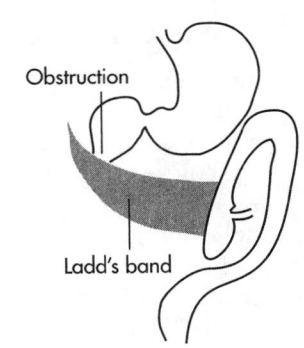

SMALL BOWEL ATRESIA

Due to in utero ischemia rather than recanalization failure. Ileum is most commonly affected followed by jejunum and duodenum; may involve multiple sites. Association:
- Polyhydramnios, 20%-40%

Radiographic features
- Dilated small bowel
- Microcolon

MECONIUM ILEUS

Occurs in 10% of patients with cystic fibrosis, meconium ileus is the presenting symptom. Thick, tenacious meconium adheres to the small bowel and causes obstruction, usually at the level of the ileocecal valve. Meconium ileus can be uncomplicated (i.e., no other abnormalities) or complicated (50%) by other abnormalities such as:
- Ileal atresia
- Perforation, peritonitis
- Stenosis
- Volvulus

Radiographic features
Plain film
- "Soap bubble" appearance (air mixed with meconium)
- Small bowel obstruction
- Calcification due to meconium peritonitis, 15%

Enema with water-soluble contrast medium
- Microcolon is typical: small unused colon
- Distal 10-30 cm of ileum is larger than colon
- Inspissated meconium in terminal ileum
- Hyperosmolar contrast may stimulate passage of meconium

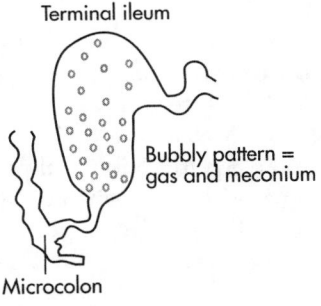

OTHER MECONIUM PROBLEMS

Meconium plug syndrome
Neonatal intestinal obstruction due to colonic inertia (in contradistinction to meconium ileus where there is accumulation of meconium in small bowel). Because of the inertia the colon usually requires an enema to stimulate peristalsis. Usually occurs in full-term babies. In the spectrum with small left colon syndrome. No association with cystic fibrosis.

Meconium peritonitis
Due to antenatal perforation of bowel. The inflammatory response may cause peritoneal calcification as early as 12 hours after perforation.

Meconium ileus equivalent
Occurs in older patients with cystic fibrosis, usually patients who do not excrete bile salts. The inspissated fecal material causes intestinal obstruction.

11

INTUSSUSCEPTION

Invagination of a segment of bowel into more distal bowel. Types:
- Ileocolic
- Ileoileocolic
- Ileoileal
- Colocolic

Ileocolic and ileoileocolic intussusception make up 90% of all intussusceptions. 90% of all pediatric intussusceptions have no pathological lead point; in the remaining 10% the lead point is due to:
- Meckel's diverticulum
- Polyp or other tumors
- Cysts

Symptoms
- Usually in the first 2 years of life (40% from 3-6 months), rarely in neonates
- Pain, 90%
- Vomiting, 90%
- Mass, 60%
- Blood per rectum, 60%

Radiographic features
Plain film
- Frequently normal (50%)
- Intraluminal convex filling defect in partially air-filled bowel loop (commonly at hepatic flexure)

Ultrasound (US)
- Target or doughnut sign

Intussusception reduction (80% success rate)
1. Dilute contrast (e.g., Cystoconray 17%) in bag placed 3 feet above table top. Alternatively, air reduction is commonly used.
2. Avoid abdominal palpation.
3. Maintain constant hydrostatic pressure. If patient evacuates around tube, repeat filling may be performed up to 3 tries before surgery is contemplated.
4. Successful reduction is marked by free flow of contrast into the terminal ileum. Fluoroscopy is used to evaluate for a pathological lead point. A postevacuation and a 24-hour film are obtained.
5. Contraindications to reduction:
   - Perforation
   - Peritonitis
6. Complications
   - Recurrence in 6%-10% (half within 48 hours after initial reduction)
   - Perforation during radiographic reduction is rare (incidence: 1:300 cases)

DUPLICATION CYSTS

Location: small bowel (terminal ileum) > esophagus > duodenum > jejunum > stomach (incidence decreases from distal to proximal, skips the stomach). Duplication cysts typically present as an abdominal mass. Small bowel duplications are most commonly located on the mesenteric side; esophageal duplications are commonly located within the lumen.

RADIOGRAPHIC FEATURES

- Round fluid-filled mass displacing adjacent bowel
- May contain ectopic gastric mucosa (hemorrhage)
- Calcifications are rare
- Communicating vertebral anomalies (neurenteric cysts; most common in esophagus)

OMPHALOMESENTERIC DUCT ANOMALIES

Omphalomesenteric duct anomalies are due to persistence of the vitelline duct, which connects the yolk sac with the bowel lumen through the umbilicus. Spectrum:

- Meckel's diverticulum
- Patent omphalomesenteric duct (umbilicoileal fistula)
- Omphalomesenteric cyst (vitelline cyst)
- Omphalomesenteric sinus (umbilical sinus)

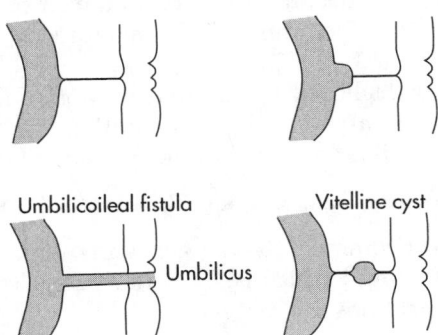

Meckel's diverticulum

Persistence of the omphalomesenteric duct at its junction with the ileum. Rule of 2s:

- Occurs in 2% of population (most common congenital GI abnormality)
- Complications usually occur before 2 years of age
- The diverticulum is located within 2 feet of the ileocecal valve
- 20% of patients have complications
  - Hemorrhage from peptic ulceration when gastric mucosa is present within lesion
  - Inflammation and ulcer
  - Obstruction

Radiographic features

- Difficult to detect because diverticuli usually do not fill with barium
- Pertechnetate scan is the diagnostic imaging modality of choice to detect ectopic gastric mucosa; sensitivity 95%
- False positive pertechnetate studies may occur in:
  - Crohn's disease
  - Appendicitis
  - Intussusception
  - Abscess

Colon

APPENDICITIS

Age: > 4 years (most common cause of small bowel obstruction) (see also Chapter 3).

Radiographic features

Plain film

- Mass in RLQ
- Obliterated properitoneal fat line
- Sentinel loop
- Fecalith

US
- May be useful in children
- Thickened appendiceal wall shadowing appendicolith, RLQ abscess

Barium enema (rarely done)
- A completely filled appendix excludes the diagnosis of appendicitis
- 15% of normal appendices do not fill with contrast
- Signs suggestive of appendicitis
    Beak of barium at base of appendix (mucosal edema)
    Irregularity of barium near tip of cecum
    Deformity of cecum (abscess, mass effect)

CT
- Helical CT with opacification of the gastrointestinal tract achieved through the oral or rectal administration of 3% diatrizoate meglumine solution is useful to diagnose or exclude appendicitis and to establish an alternative diagnosis

NECROTIZING ENTEROCOLITIS (NEC)

Most common GI emergency in premature infants. Precise etiology unknown (ischemia? antigens? bacteria?). Develops most commonly within 2-6 days after birth. Indications for surgery:
- Pneumoperitoneum

Increased incidence in neonates with:
- Premature infants
- Neonates with bowel obstruction (e.g., atresia)
- Neonates with CHD

Radiographic features
- Small bowel dilatation: adynamic ileus (first finding)
- Pneumatosis intestinalis, 80% (second most common sign)
- Gas in portal vein may be seen transiently; this finding does not imply as bad an outcome as it does in adults
- Pneumoperitoneum (20%) indicates bowel perforation: football sign (floating air and ascites give the appearance of a large elliptical lucency in supine position)
- Barium is contraindicated; use water-soluble contrast if a bowel obstruction or Hirschsprung's disease needs to be ruled out.

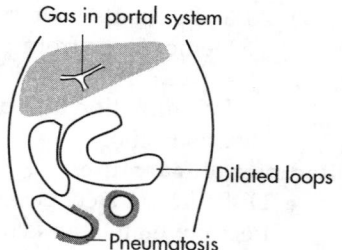

Complications
Acute
- Perforation

Later in life
- Bowel stricture
- Complications of surgery: short small bowel syndrome, dumping, malabsorption
- Complications of associated diseases common in premature infants:
    Hyaline membrane disease
    Germinal matrix hemorrhage
    Periventricular leukomalacia

HIRSCHSPRUNG'S DISEASE

Absence of the myenteric plexus cells (agangliosis, incomplete craniocaudal migration of embryonic neuroblasts) in distal segment of the colon causes hypertonicity and obstruction. Clinical: 80% (male:female = 6:1) present in the first 6 weeks of life with obstruction, intermittent diarrhea or constipation. Diagnosis: rectal biopsy. Treatment: colostomy (Swenson, Duhamel, Soave operations), myomectomy. Association: Down syndrome.

Complications

- Intestinal obstruction (in neonates)
- Perforation
- Enterocolitis 15%, etiology uncertain

Radiographic features

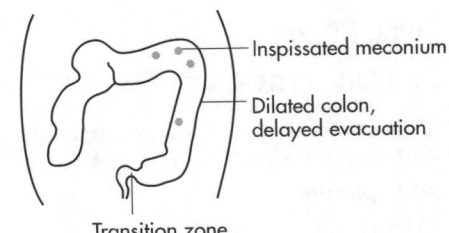

- Bowel gas pattern of distal colonic obstruction on plain film
- Barium enema is normal in 30%
- Transition zone between normal and stenotic colonic segment
- Rectum: sigmoid diameter ratio (normal 1:0) is abnormal (< 1.0) because of the narrowed segment
- Significant barium retention on the 24-hour barium enema film may be helpful
- Transition zone in rectosigmoid, 80%

CONGENITAL ANORECTAL ANOMALIES

Failure of descent and separation of hindgut and genitourinary (GU) system in second trimester.

High (supralevator) malformations

- Rectum ends above levator sling
- High association with GU (50%) and cardiac anomalies

Low (infralevator malformations)

- Rectum ends below levator sling
- Low association with GU anomalies (25%)

OVERVIEW		
	Male	**Female**
High malformation	Fistula to urethra or less commonly to the bladder	Rectovaginal fistula, hydrometrocolpos
Low malformation (bowel passes through levator sling)	Anoperineal fistula	Fistula to lower portion of urethra, vagina perineum

Associated anomalies are very common:

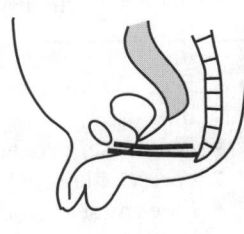
High malformation

- Sacral anomalies, 30% (tethered cord)
- Currarino's triad: anorectal anomaly, sacral bone abnormality, and presacral mass
- Genitourinary anomalies, 30%
- VACTERL
- GI anomalies: duodenal atresia, EA

Radiographic features

Plain film

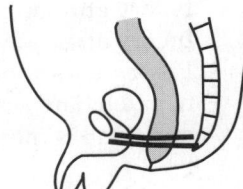
Low malformation

- Low colonic obstruction
- Gas bubbles in bladder or vagina
- Determine location of the gas-filled rectal pouch to the M-line (line drawn through junction of upper ⅔ and lower ⅓ of ischia; line indicates level of levator sling)
- Upside-down views can be obtained to distend distal rectal pouch

Magnetic resonance imaging (MRI)
- Determine location of rectal pouch with respect to levator and to determine if the malformation is supralevator or infralevator type
- Facilitates the detection of associated spinal anomalies

Liver, Biliary

BILIARY ATRESIA

Unknown etiology (severe hepatitis, sclerosing cholangitis with vascular component?). Associated with trisomy 18 and polysplenia.

Types
- Correctable: portoenterostomy (Kasai procedure)
- Noncorrectable

Imaging features

US
- Normal gallbladder in 20%

HIDA scan
- No visualization of bowel at 24 hours
- Good hepatic visualization within 5 minutes
- Increased renal excretion
- Main differential diagnosis is neonatal hepatitis. Findings of neonatal hepatitis include:

    Bowel activity present at 24 hours
    Decreased and slow hepatic accumulation of tracer
    GB may not be seen

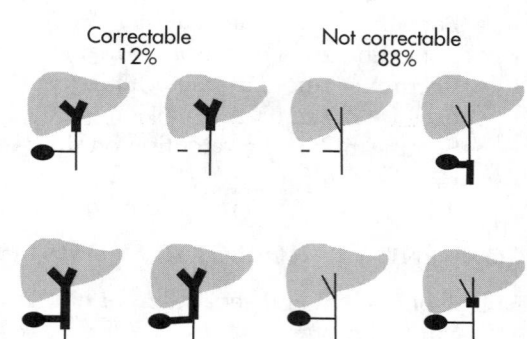

Correctable 12%   Not correctable 88%

NEONATAL HEPATITIS VS. BILIARY ATRESIA	
Neonatal Hepatitis	**Biliary Atresia**
Male premature newborns	Females
TORCH	Polysplenia
Skeletal abnormality	Choledochal cyst

- Both diseases present with conjugated hyperbilirubinemia during first week of life.
- The Kasai procedure for treatment of biliary atresia is often successful if the correct diagnosis is made by 40 days of age.
- One must exclude the presence of cystic fibrosis in patients thought to have biliary atresia. Inspissated bile in cystic fibrosis can be indistinguishable from biliary atresia by US or nuclear scan.
- Preprocedural phenobarbitol (5 mg/kg/day × 5 days) improves sensitivity of hepatobiliary scans. The finding of normal (1.5 cm or more) or enlarged (3 cm or more) GB is more supportive of diagnosis of hepatitis.

HEMANGIOENDOTHELIOMA

Most common benign pediatric liver tumor. 85% present at < 6 months. Associated cutaneous hemangiomas in 50%.

Complications
- CHF because of AV shunt, 15%
- Intraperitoneal bleed
- Disseminated intravascular coagulopathy
- Thrombocytopenia (platelet trapping)

Radiographic features
- Complex, hypoechoic mass by US
- Similar signal intensity/contrast characteristics as adult hemangioma

MESENCHYMAL HAMARTOMA

- Occurs during first 10 years of life
- Large multiloculated cystic lesion
- Large cysts > 10 cm may be seen
- 10% are exophytic

HEPATOBLASTOMA

Most common primary malignant liver tumor in children. Age: < 2 years.

Associations:
- Beckwith-Wiedeman syndrome
- Hemihypertrophy

Radiographic features
- Large hepatic mass
- Mixed echogenicity (US)
- Calcification, 50%
- Metastases: lungs > lymph nodes, brain

HEPATOCELLULAR CARCINOMA (HCC)

Second most common malignant primary liver tumor in children. Age: > 3 years.

Associations:
- Glycogen storage disease (von Gierke's)
- Galactosemia
- Tyrosinemia
- Biliary atresia

Radiographic features
- Difficult to distinguish from hepatoblastoma other than by clinical picture
- Lower incidence of calcification than hepatoblastoma

HYPOVOLEMIC SHOCK

- Small hyperdense spleen
- Marked enhancement of bowel wall, kidneys, and pancreas
- Dilated fluid-filled bowel
- Small caliber aorta and IVC

11

Genitourinary Tract

General

RENAL DEVELOPMENT

The kidney develops in 3 stages:

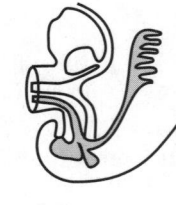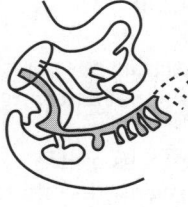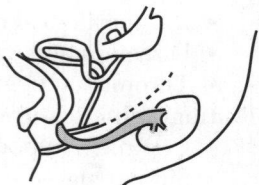

- Pronephros (3rd week): tubules drain into an excretory duct that terminates in the cloaca
- Mesonephros (4th week): serves as precursor for:
  - Male: vas deferens, seminal vesicles, ejaculatory duct
  - Female: vestigial
- Metanephros (5th week): ureteral bud develops from mesonephric duct; the ureteral bud elongates, undergoes divisions, and forms renal tubules while ascending along the posterior coelomic wall; at 12 weeks, there are 7 anterior and 7 posterior renal lobes separated by a fibrous groove; at 28 weeks the boundaries between renal lobes become indistinct; persistence of fibrous groove is evident after birth.

GENITALIA

Wolffian duct

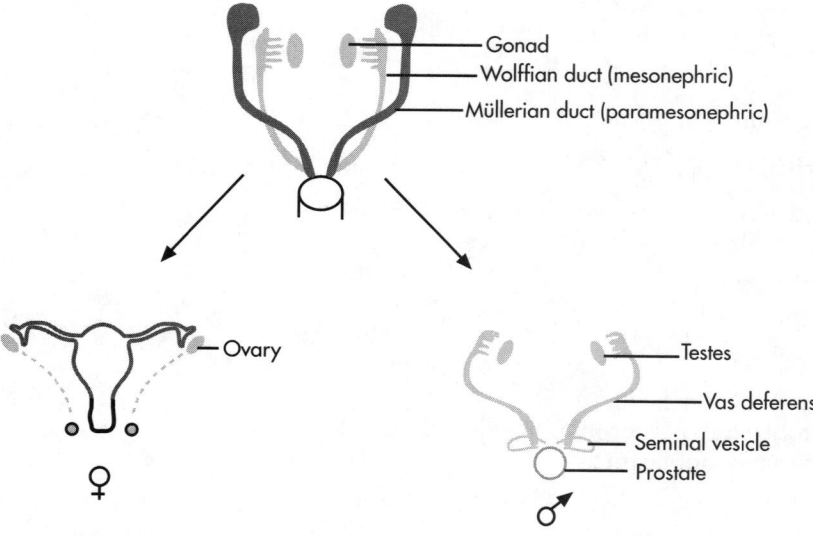

- Anlage for vas deferens, seminal vesicles, epididymis
- Guides ureteric migration to bladder
- Induces kidney development and ascent
- Induces Müllerian duct development in females

Müllerian duct
- Forms entire female genitalia except distal third of vagina

CLOACA

Divided by the cloacal (urorectal) septum into:
- Dorsal portion → rectum
- Ventral portion → allantois (atrophies as umbilical ligament), bladder, urogenital sinus (pelvic, phallic portions)

Wolffian and Müllerian ducts drain into the ventral portion of cloaca.

URACHUS

The umbilical attachment of the bladder (initially allantois then urachus) usually atrophies (umbilical ligament) as the bladder descends into the pelvis. Persistent canalization of the urachus may lead to urine flow from the bladder to the umbilicus.

Patent urachus

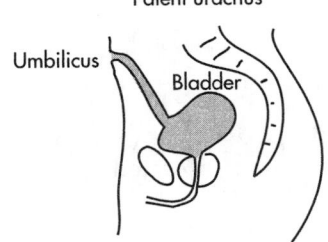

Urachal cyst

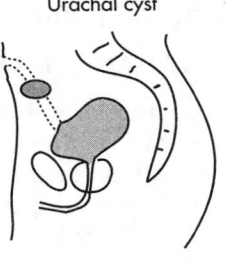

Urachal sinus

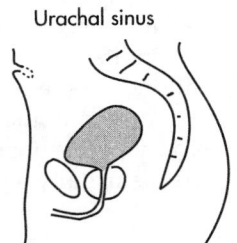

Vesicourachal diverticulum

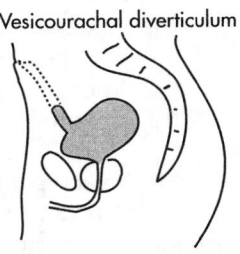

UTERUS

- The prepubertal uterus has a tubular configuration (anteroposterior cervix equal to anteroposterior fundus) or sometimes a spade shape (anteroposterior cervix larger than anteroposterior fundus)
- The endometrium is normally not apparent; however, high-frequency transducers can demonstrate the central lining
- The length is 2.5-4 cm; the thickness does not exceed 10 mm

OVARIES

- Ovarian volume: $V = \frac{1}{2}$ length × width × depth.
- The mean ovarian volume in girls less than 6 years of age is less than or equal to 1 cm^3.
- The ovarian volume increases after 6 years of age.
- In prepubertal girls (6-10 years old), ovarian volumes range from 1.2 to 2.3 cm^3. In premenarchal girls (11-12 years old), ovarian volumes range from 2 to 4 cm^3. In postmenarchal girls, the ovarian volume averages 8 cm^3 (range, 2.5-20 cm^3).

VOIDING CYSTURETHROGRAM (VCUG)

1. Pediatric VCUGs are performed by the radiologist, with attempts to minimize fluoroscopy time (optimally less than 15 second total).
2. Catheterize with an 8 Fr feeding tube (5 Fr in neonate).
3. AP spot films of the renal fossae and bladder.
4. Contrast instilled by gravity drip (bottle positioned 40 cm above table).
5. When patient indicates urge to urinate or signs of imminent voiding are seen, obtain bilateral oblique spots of bladder to include urethral catheter.
6. When voiding commences, catheter is removed. In female, 2 camera spots of distended urethra are obtained with slightly obliqued positioning. In the male, 2 camera high oblique spots are obtained during voiding.
7. Quickly fluoroscope the renal fossae during voiding; if reflux is observed, obtain spot film.
8. After completion of urination, obtain AP spots of bladder and renal fossae.

11

Congenital Anomalies

RENAL ANOMALIES

Anomalies of position
- Malrotation around vertical axis (most common)
- All malpositioned kidneys are malrotated
- Ectopic kidney
    Usually located in pelvis
    Most ectopic kidneys are asymptomatic, but pelvic kidneys are more susceptible to trauma and infection. Pelvic kidneys may complicate natural childbirth later in life.
    When a single orthopic kidney is seen on IVP, a careful search for the contralateral collecting system in the pelvis is mandated since the kidney itself may be obscured by pelvic bones.
    An ectopic thoracic kidney is usually an acquired duplication through the foramen of Bochdalek.

Anomalies of form
- Horseshoe kidney
- Pancake kidney. Results from fusion of both kidneys in the pelvis, usually near the aortic bifurcation
- Cross-fused ectopia
- Renal hypoplasia
    Incomplete development resulting in a smaller (< 50%) kidney with fewer calyces and papillae (< 5) but normal function
    Not to be confused with dysplasia, which results from collecting system obstruction and creates a bizarre appearance of the kidney. Hypoplastic kidneys are smooth with short infundibulae and sometimes have clubbed calyces.
    Segmental hypoplasia (Ask-Upmark kidney): usually upper pole with deep transverse groove. Associated with severe hypertension. Etiology is controversial (congenital vs. sequelae of pyelonephritis).

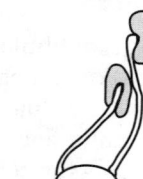

Crossed ectopia, fusion   Crossed ectopia

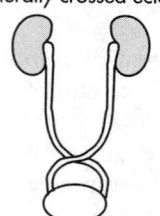

Bilaterally crossed ectopia

Anomalies of number
- Unilateral renal agenesis (1:1000 births); associated with hypoplasia or aplasia of testicle or vas deferens, cornuate uterus; hypertrophy of contralateral kidney
- Bilateral renal agenesis
- Supernumerary kidney (very rare)

Complications of renal congenital anomalies
- Infection
- Obstruction
- Calculus
- Trauma

HORSESHOE KIDNEY

Most common anomaly of renal form. In horseshoe kidneys the lower poles are fused across the midline. Incidence: 1:400 births. Associated anomalies, 50%:
- Ureteropelvic junction (UPJ) obstruction, 30%
- Ureteral duplication, 10%
- Genital anomalies
- Turner syndrome
- Other anomalies (GI, cardiac, skeletal), 30%

Radiographic features
- Inferior fusion (isthmus)
- Abnormal axis of each kidney (bilateral malrotation)
- Variable blood supply

RENAL ECTOPIA

Crossed ectopia refers to a kidney on the opposite side from ureteral bladder insertion. The lower kidney is the one that is usually ectopic. Abnormal rotation is common, and renal pelvices may face opposite directions. In 90% there is fusion of both kidneys. Incidence: 1:1000 births. Incidence of associated anomalies is low. Slightly increased incidence of calculi.

URETERAL DUPLICATION

2 ureters drain one kidney (incidence 1:150). Duplications may be incomplete (Y ureter) or complete:
- Orthotopic ureter: drains lower pole and enters bladder near trigone
- Ectopic ureter: drains upper pole and enters bladder inferiorly and medially (Weigert-Meyer rule); the ectopic ureter may be stenotic and obstructed

Complications
- Reflux in orthotopic ureter, causing urinary tract infection (UTI)
- Obstruction of ectopic ureter
- Ureterocele

Radiographic features (Lebowitz)
- Increased distance from top of nephrogram to collecting system: hydronephrotic upper pole moiety causes mass effect (1)
- Abnormal axis of collecting system (2)
- Concave upper border of renal pelvis (3)
- Diminished number of calyces compared to normal side; drooping lily sign (4)
- Lateral displacement of kidney and ureter (5)
- Spiral course of ureter (6)
- Filling defect in the bladder (ureterocele)

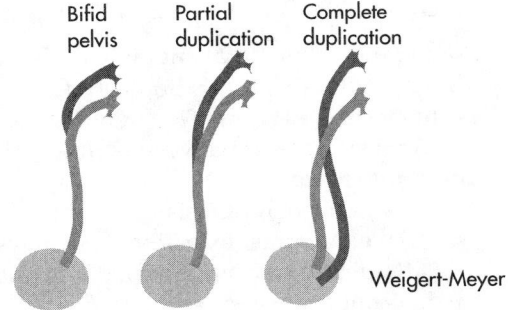

Bifid pelvis   Partial duplication   Complete duplication

Weigert-Meyer

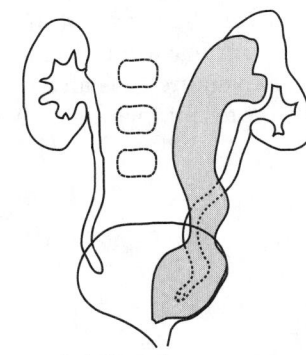

Pathological appearance

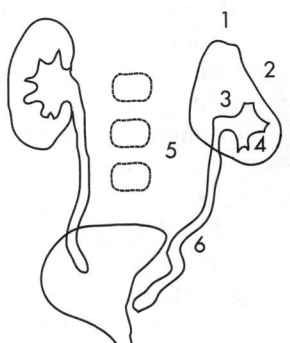

IVP appearance

11

URETEROCELE

A ureterocele refers to a herniation of the distal ureter into the bladder. Two types:

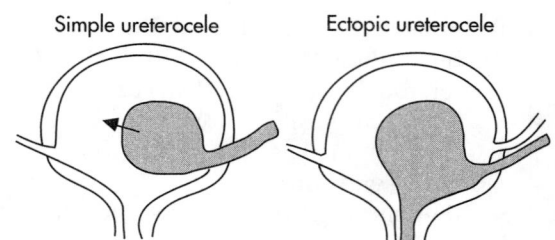

Simple (normal location of ureter), 25%
- Almost always occurs in adults
- Usually also symptomatic in children

Ectopic (abnormal location of ureter), 75%
- Almost always associated with duplication
- Unilateral, 80%
- May obstruct entire urinary tract
- Female incontinence (wetting) is seen with an ectopic ureter without ureterocele but not with an ectopic ureter alone

Radiographic features
- Ureterocele causes filling defect in bladder on IVP
- Typical appearance of a cystic structure by US
- Ureterocele may be distended, collapsed or everted to represent a diverticulum
- Complications

      Ureteroceles may contain calculi

      May be very large (bladder outlet obstruction)

CONGENITAL URETEROPELVIC JUNCTION (UPJ) OBSTRUCTION

Most common congenital anomaly of the GU tract in neonates. 20% of obstructions are bilateral. Treatment: pyeloplasty. Causes:
- Intrinsic, 80%: defect in circular muscle bundle of renal pelvis
- Extrinsic, 20%: renal vessels (lower pole artery or vein)

Radiographic features
- Caliectasis, pelviectasis
- Delayed contrast excretion of kidneys; poor opacification of renal parenchyma
- Differentiation from prominent extrarenal pelvis may require Whitaker test to determine presence and degree of obstruction

MEGAURETER

Congenital dilatation of distal ureter due to functional (not mechanical) obstruction (abnormal development of muscle layers, achalasia of ureter). 20% are bilateral. Most commonly diagnosed prenatally. Symptoms: asymptomatic (most common), pain, UTI, mass. Most commonly (95%), a megaureter is an isolated finding; associated disorders are uncommon (5%), but if present include:

Ipsilateral
- Calyceal diverticulum
- Papillary necrosis

Contralateral
- Reflux
- Ureterocele
- Ureteral duplication
- Renal ectopia or agenesis
- UPJ obstruction

Radiographic features
- Ureter dilated above dysfunctional distal ureteral segment
- Nonpropulsive motion in dilated ureteral segment

CIRCUMCAVAL URETER

Congenital abnormality of the IVC (not the ureter). Normally the IVC is derived from supracardinal vein, which is posterior to ureter. If the IVC is derived from the right subcardinal (most common) or postcardinal veins (both of which lie anterior to ureter), a portion of lumbar ureter becomes trapped behind the cava. Mostly in males.

Radiographic features
- Ureter passes behind IVC and emerges medial to the IVC on its course to pelvis.
- The anomaly is on the right unless patient has situs inversus.
- The anomaly can be bilateral if the IVC is duplicated.
- Types:
    Low loop (more common)
        Fish hook or reverse J course
        Ureter is obstructed
        Ureter emerges between cava and aorta and descends into the pelvis
    High loop (less common)
        Obstruction is mild
        Retrocaval segment runs obliquely at level of UPJ
        May simulate UPJ obstruction

BLADDER EXSTROPHY-EPISPADIA COMPLEX

Defect in lower abdominal wall, pubic area anterior wall of bladder and dorsal aspect of urethra; the defect causes the bladder to be open and the mucosa to be continuous with skin. Most common congenital bladder abnormality; overall rare (1:50,000). Always associated with epispadia (male: urethra ends on dorsal aspect of penis, female: cleft of entire dorsal urethra). Simple episadias without exstrophy are uncommon.

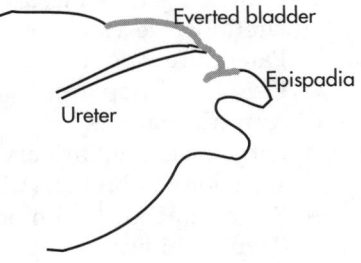

Radiographic features
- Diastasis of symphysis (width correlates with severity of exstrophy
- Omphalocele confluent with exstrophic bladder
- Cryptorchism
- Inguinal hernia
- Acquired ureterovesical junction (UVJ) obstruction in untreated cases
- Findings afetr surgical repair:
    Small bladder
    Reflux
- Other associated anomalies
    Rectal prolapse
    Bifid, unicornuate uterus
    Spinal anomalies

11

CLOACAL EXSTROPHY

More severe defect than isolated bladder exstrophy. Occurs earlier in embryogenesis.
Findings:
  Bone
  - Spina bifida aperta
  - Lipomyelomeningocele
  - Diastasis of symphysis
  Bladder
  - Exstrophy
  Colon
  - Exstrophy

PRUNE BELLY SYNDROME (TRIAD SYNDROME)

Nonhereditary disorders (1:50,000) characterized by triad:
- Widely separated abdominal rectus muscles (wrinkled appearance of skin looks like a prune)
- Hydroureteronephrosis (giant nonobstructed ureters)
- Cryptorchidism (bladder distention interferes with descent of testicles)

Prognosis: lethal in most severe cases, renal failure is common in milder cases.
Severe cases are associated with other anomalies:
- Dysplastic kidneys
- Oligohydraminos
- Pulmonary hypoplasia
- Urethral atresia
- Patent uruchus
- Prostatic hypoplasia

Radiographic features
- Large distended urinary bladder is the hallmark
- Vesicoureteral reflux (VUR) is common
- Patent urachus (common)
- Cryptorchidism

POSTERIOR URETHRAL VALVES (PUV)

PUV represent congenital folds (thick folds > thin folds) located in the posterior urethra near the distal end of the veru. Nowadays commonly discovered on prenatal US. Treatment: electrode fulguration.

Clinical findings
- PUV are the most common cause (35%) of obstructive symptoms (hesitancy, dribbling, enuresis)
- UTI, 35%
- Palpable bladder or kidney in neonates, 20%
- Hematuria, 5%

Types
- Type I (most common): derive from plica colliculi (normal tissue folds that extend inferiorly from verumontanum). Distal leafletsare thickened and fused at the level of membranous urethra
- Type III: represents a diaphragm

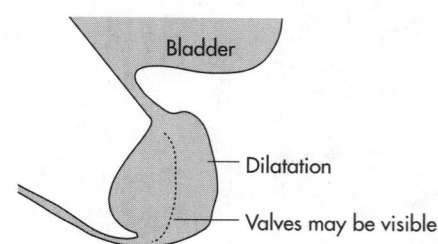

Radiographic features
- Verumontanum is enlarged in type I but not type III.
- Type I causes crescentic filling defect that bulges into contrast column (spinnaker sail appearance).
- Windsock appearance may be seen with type III.
- Posterior urethra above valves is dilated and elongated.
- Bladder trabeculation, saccules, and small diverticuli
- VUR
- Hydroureter and hydronephrosis
- In utero complications:
    Oligohydramnios
    Urine leak, 15%: urinoma, urine ascites
    Hydronephrosis
    Prune belly

MALE HYPOSPADIA

Ectopic ending of the urethra on the ventral aspect of the penis, scrotum, or perineum. Hyposadia is the result of a defective midline fusion of the genital folds. Incidence: 1:300 births. Associations:
- Cryptorchidism, 30%
- Inguinal hernias, 10%
- Urinary tract abnormalities (slightly higher incidence than in general population)

Radiographic features
- VCUG is performed in more severe cases, in patients with symptoms or other anomalies
- Enlarged urticle, 20%

CAUDAL REGRESSION

Insult to the caudal mesoderm results in spectrum of abnormalities:
- Agenesis of sacrum (20% occur in infants of diabetic mothers)
- Partial absence or underdevelopment of lower extremities
- GU and GI anomalies

Types of sacral agenesis
- Type 1: unilateral agenesis
- Type 2: bilateral agenesis with normal sacroiliac joint articulation
- Types 3-4: total absence of sacrum, variable fusions of vertebral bodies with ilia

Renal Cystic Disease

AUTOSOMAL RECESSIVE KIDNEY DISEASE (ARKD)

ARKD = infantile polycystic kidney disease (IPKD) = Potter type 1 = polycystic disease of childhood. 1:10,000-50,000 births.

Types

Antenatal form: 90% of tubules show ectasia
- Oligohydramnios in utero
- Death from renal failure, respiratory insufficiency after birth (75% within 24 hours)

11

Neonatal form: 60% of tubules show ectasia, minimal hepatic fibrosis
- Renal failure within 1st month of life
- Infants usually die within 1 year

Infantile form: 20% of tubules show ectasia, moderate hepatic fibrosis
- Symptoms appear at 3-6 months
- Death from renal failure, portal hypertension, arterial hypertension

Juvenile form: 10% of tubules show ectasia, severe hepatic fibrosis
- Disease appears at 1-5 years of age
- Death from portal hypertension

The less severe the renal findings, the more severe hepatic periportal cirrhosis. Hepatic fibrosis is also associated with:
- Adult polycystic kidney disease
- Multicystic dysplastic kidneys
- Caroli's disease
- Choledochocele

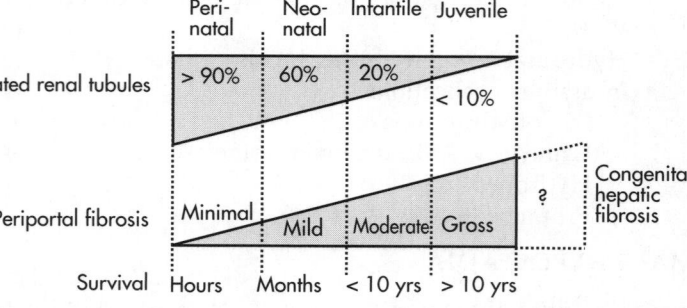

Autosomal recessive polycystic disease (Blythe Ockendon classification)

Radiographic features

Kidneys
- Enlarged hyperechoic kidneys (hallmark)
- Cysts 1-2 mm are only seen with high-resolution US equipment
- Faint, striated nephrogram due to tubular ectasia (similar appearance as in medullary sponge kidney; IVP seldom performed today)

US findings (in utero)
- Nonvisualization of urine in bladder
- Enlarged, hyperechoic kidneys
- Oligohydramnios (nonfunctioning kidneys)

Lung
- Pulmonary hypoplasia (because of external compression)
- Pneumothorax

Liver
- Hepatic fibrosis
- Portal venous hypertension

MULTICYSTIC DYSPLASTIC KIDNEYS (MCDK)

Collection of large, noncommunicating cysts separated by fibrous tissue; there is no functioning renal parenchyma. Results from occlusion (severe UPJ obstruction) of fetal ureters before 10 weeks of gestation. Absent or atretic renal vessels and collecting system. Because MCDK is involute, serial US follow-up is usually performed until disappearance. Associations:
- UPJ obstruction in contralateral kidney
- Horseshoe kidney

Radiographic features
- Cystic renal mass with no excretory function
- Hypertrophy of contralateral kidney
- Thick fibrous septae between cysts
- Calcification of cyst wall in adults
- Atretic ureter
- Absence of renal artery

MULTILOCULAR CYSTIC NEPHROMA (MLCN)

Congenital renal lesion characterized by large (> 10 cm) cystic spaces. Cysts are lined by cuboidal epithelium. The lesion has biphasic age and sex distribution. It occurs in children ages 2 months to 4 years with 75% *male* predilection, and in adults over 40 years of age with 95% *female* predilection. May present with hematuria due to prolapse of mass into the renal pelvis. Two distinct histological entities: cystic nephroma without blastema elements within septa and cystic, partially differentiated nephroblastoma, which has blastema elements in the septa. The two entities are indistinguishable by imaging.

Radiographic features

- Contrast-enhanced CT scans demonstrate a well-defined intrarenal, multilocular mass that compresses or displaces the adjacent renal parenchyma. The septations enhance, but the cysts do not.
- Calcifications are uncommon.
- MLCN are surgically removed because distinction from cystic Wilms' tumor is not possible by imaging modalities.

Inflammation

URINARY TRACT INFECTION (UTI)

UTI is defined as > 100,000 organisms/mL in a properly collected urine specimen; any bacterial growth in urine obtained by suprapubic puncture or catheterization is also abnormal. Any of the urinary structures may be involved (e.g., bladder: cystitis; prostate: prostatitis, renal tubules: pyelonephritis, urethra: urethritis). Pathogenetically, UTI are most commonly ascending infections (especially in females: short urethra). Most common organism: *E. coli* (70%).

Modalities for imaging of the UTI/VUR complex

1. Is there a structural abnormality of the urinary tract causing stasis that predisposes to infection?
   - US the imaging modality of first choice.
   - Structural abnormalities are frequently detected prenatally.
   - In case of abnormality, further imaging studies are usually required.
   - US should be obtained in all children after the first UTI.
2. Is there primary VUR?
   - VCUG or radionuclide cystography are imaging modalities of first choice.
   - VCUG should be obtained in:
        All children with UTI < 4 years old
        All older children with abnormal US, bladder dysfunction, or repeated UTI
3. Is there acute pyelonephritis?
   - Renal cortical scintigraphy has the highest sensitivity and specificity of imaging modalities and should be obtained if results would affect management.
   - US and IVP have a low sensitivity and specificity.
4. Is there parenchymal scarring ?
   - Small scars are best detected with renal cortical scintigraphy.
   - Larger scars can be detected by US or IVP.
   - Wait at least 4 months after UTI to assess for scarring; earlier on, many patients have abnormalities that are not permanent.

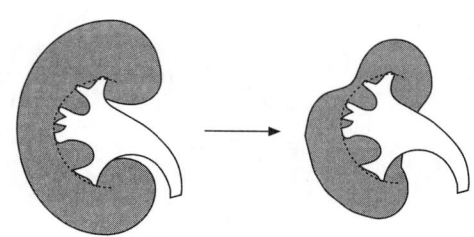

11

VESICOURETERAL REFLUX (VUR)

Primary VUR is due to immaturity or maldevelopment of the UVJ with incompetence of the antireflux flap valve action:

Immaturity is due to unerdeveloped longitudinal muscle of the submucosal ureter; with growth, the submucosal ureter elongates and the valve mechanism becomes competent (children with VUR often outgrow the reflux by 10 years of age, depending on grade of reflux and type)

Other causes of reflux (secondary reflux)
- Periureteral diverticulum
- Ureterocele
- Ureteral duplication
- Bladder outlet obstruction

Complications
- Cystitis
- Pyelonephritis
- Renal scarring occurs with intrarenal reflux of infected urine
- Hypertension and end-stage renal disease (in 10%-20% of renal scarring)

Incidence

Reflux seen in 30%-50% of children with UTI, in 20% of siblings (higher in younger children, lower in older children)

Radiographic features

Grading of reflux (international grading system)
- Grade I: reflux to ureter but not to kidney
- Grade II: reflux into ureter, pelvic and calices without dilations
- Grade III: reflux to calices with mild dilatation, blunted formices
- Grade IV: to calices with moderate dilatation, obliteration of formices
- Grade V: gross dilatation, tortuous urteres

Tumor

Most renal masses are benign in infants < 2 months of age; the frequency of malignancy increases with age. Approximately 87% of solid renal neoplasms in children are Wilms' tumors; other tumors include clear cell sarcoma (6%); mesoblastic nephroma (2%); rhabdoid tumor (2%); lymphoma (< 0.5%); renal cell carcinoma (< 0.5%).

MOST COMMON AGE AT PRESENTATION FOR SOLID RENAL MALIGNANCIES		
Renal Neoplasm	Age Range	Peak Age
Wilms' tumor		
Unilateral form	1-11 yrs	3½ yrs
Bilateral form	2 mon-2 yrs	15 mon
Nephroblastomatosis	Any age	6-18 mon
Renal cell carcinoma	6 mon-60 yrs	10-20 yrs*
Mesoblastic nephroma	0-1 yrs	1-3 mon
Multilocular cystic renal tumor		
Cystic nephroma	Adult female	Adult female
Cystic partially differentiated nephroblastoma	3 mon-4 yrs	1-2 yrs
Clear cell sarcoma	1-4 yrs	2 yrs
Rhabdoid tumor	6 mon-9 yrs	6-12 mon
Angiomyolipoma	6-41 yrs	10 yrs†
Renal medullary carcinoma	10-39 yrs	20 yrs
Ossifying renal tumor of infancy	6 days-14 mon	1-3 mon
Metanephric adenoma	15 mon-83 yrs	None
Lymphoma		
Hodgkin's	> 10 yrs	Late teens
Non-Hodgkin's	Any age child	<10 yrs

*von Hippel-Lindau disease.
†Tuberous sclerosis, neurofibromatosis, von Hippel-Lindau disease.

WILMS' TUMOR

Arises from metanephric blastema. Most common solid renal tumor of childhood. Third most common malignancy in children after leukemia and brain tumors and third most common cause of all renal masses after hydronephrosis and multicystic dysplastic kidney. 50% < 2 years, 75% < 5 years, extremely rare in the newborn. Wilms' tumors are bilateral in 5%-10% and multifocal in 10%. Nephroblastomatosis is a precursor of Wilms' tumor. Two loci on chromosome 11 have been implicated in the genesis of a minority of Wilms' tumors. Locus 11p13 is known as the *WT1* gene, and locus 11p15 is known as the *WT2* gene. An abnormal *WT1* gene is present in patients with WAGR syndrome (Wilms' tumor, aniridia, genitourinary abnormalities, mental retardation) or Drash syndrome (male pseudohermaphroditism, progressive glomerulonephritis); an abnormal *WT2* gene is present in patients with Beckwith-Wiedemann syndrome or hemihypertrophy.

Clinical
- Palpable abdominal mass, 90% (12 cm mean diameter at diagnosis!)
- Hypertension, 50%
- Pain, 35%
- Uncommon presentations: hematuria (5%), fever (15%), anorexia (15%)
- Wilms' tumor manifests as a solid intrarenal mass with a pseudocapsule and distortion of the renal parenchyma and collecting system. The tumor typically spreads by direct extension and displaces adjacent structures but does not typically encase or elevate the aorta; such encasement or elevation is a distinguishing characteristic of neuroblastoma

11

Associations
- Sporadic aniridia (35% will get Wilms' tumor)
- Hemihypertrophy
- Drash syndrome: pseudohermaphroditism, glomerulonephritis and Wilms' tumor
- Beckwith-Wiedemann syndrome: macroglossia, omphalocele, visceromegaly

Radiographic features

Tumor
- Large (mean 12 cm) mass arising from cortex of kidney
- Usually exophytic growth; pseudocapsule
- Cystic areas in tumor: hemorrhage, necrosis
- <15% have calcifications
- Intrarenal mass effect causes distortion of the pyelocalyceal system
- Less contrast enhancement than residual renal parenchyma
- Vascular invasion in 5%-10% (renal vein, IVC, right atrium)

Staging (similar to that of adenocarcinoma in adults)
- Stage I confined to kidney, 95% 2-year survival
- Stage II extension into perinephric space, 90%
- Stage III lymph node involvement
- Stage IV metastases to lung, liver, 50%
- Stage V bilateral renal involvement
- By MRI, Wilms' tumors demonstrate low signal intensity on T1W images and high signal intensity on T2W images. MRI also permits assessment of caval patency and multifocal disease.
- MRI has been reported to be the most sensitive modality for determination of caval patency, but it requires sedation.

Current screening recommendations for patients at risk with Wilms' include: US every 4 months for a year; followed by repeat imaging every 8 months for 2 years and then every 12 months until the child is 10 years of age and CT scanning every 6 months for a year followed by every 12 months for 4 years and again at 10 years of age.

NEPHROBLASTOMATOSIS

Nephrogenic rests are foci of metanephric blastema that persist beyond 36 weeks gestation and have the potential for malignant transformation into Wilms' tumor.

Present in 30% of bilateral Wilms' tumors
Present in 100% of bilateral Wilms' tumors

Radiographic features
- Multiple solid, subcapsular mass lesions are virtually diagnostic.
- Lesions are hypovascular (little enhancement by CT) and hypoechoic (US). By CT, macroscopic nephrogenic rests appear as low-attenuation peripheral nodules with poor enhancement relative to that of adjacent normal renal parenchyma. By MRI, the nodules demonstrate low-signal-intensity foci on both T1W and T2W images.
- Requires close follow-up to 7 years of age to screen for Wilms' tumor.

RENAL CELL CARCINOMA (RCC)

- RCC has been reported in patients less than 6 months of age. However, the tumor is rare in children, accounting for less than 7% of all primary renal tumors manifesting in the first 2 decades of life.

- RCC is associated with von Hippel-Lindau disease. The tumors tend to be multiple and manifests at a young age. This disease must be ruled out in pediatric patients diagnosed with RCC, especially when the tumor is bilateral.

CLEAR CELL SARCOMA

Represents 6% of all pediatric renal tumors. Highly malignant with worse prognosis than Wilms' tumor. High propensity for skeletal metastases. Cannot be distinguished from Wilms' by imaging studies alone.

RHABDOID TUMOR

Tumor originating in renal sinus (unlike Wilms', which arises from renal cortex) representing 2% of all renal cell tumors (early childhood). Poor prognosis and common metastases to lung, liver and brain. Associated with primary brain tumors of neuroectodermal origin including medulloblastoma, ependymoma, glioma and PNET.

Radiographic features

- Difficult to distinguish from Wilms' tumor by imaging alone
- A centrally located renal mass with subcapsular fluid collection and posterior fossa mass will suggest correct diagnosis
- Peripheral subcapsular fluid collection adjacent to solid tumor lobules is present in 70% of malignant rhabdoid tumors

NEUROBLASTOMA

Most common abdominal malignancy in the newborn; rare tumor (incidence 1:30,000). Arises in neural crest tissue (adrenal medulla, sympathetic neural system, Zuckerkandl). Age: 2 years, better prognosis under 1 year. Clinical: elevated VMA and HVA; may cause paraneoplastic syndrome.

Neuroblastoma

Organ of Zuckerkandl — Aortic bifurcation
Adrenal — 35% adrenal
Sympathetic chain — Neck, thorax, abdomen, pelvis

Radiographic features

- Solid tumor
- Hyperechoic by US
- Calcification in 85%
- Readily extends across midline
- Frequently encases vessels
- 65% are metastatic at initial presentation; common extensions:
    Bone
    Neural foramina (evaluate)
    Lymph nodes
    Liver, lung (uncommon)

11

FEATURES DISTINGUISHING BETWEEN WILMS' TUMOR AND NEUROBLASTOMA		
Feature	Wilms' Tumor	Neuroblastoma
Age	2-3 years	< 2 years
Origin	Kidney	Retroperitoneal neural crest
Renal mass effect	Intrinsic mass effect	External compression
Laterality	10% bilateral	Almost always
Calcification	< 15%	85%-95%
Vessel involvement	Renal vein invasion in 5%-10%	Frequent encasement

STAGING

- Stage 1: confined to organ of origin
- Stage 2: does not cross midline; homolateral lymph nodes
- Stage 3: crosses midline
- Stage 4: metastases to skeleton, lymph nodes
- Stage 4S: skin liver marrow; less than 1 year of age; good prognosis

MESOBLASTIC NEPHROMA (HAMARTOMA)

Most common solid renal mass in the neonate; uncommon in children and rare in adults. The tumor is benign (hamartoma) and is composed primarily of mesenchymal, connective tissue (cut surface looks like leiomyoma of the uterus). Treatment: surgical resection because of uncertainty that it may contain sarcomatous degeneration.

Radiographic features

- Solid, very large intrarenal mass in neonate. Imaging studies demonstrate a large solid intrarenal mass that typically involves the renal sinus. The mass replaces a large portion of renal parenchyma and may contain cystic, hemorrhagic, and necrotic regions. Local infiltration of the perinephric tissues is common.
- Often evenly hypoechoic (cystic) regions

ANGIOMYOLIPOMA

- These tumors most often occur sporadically. However, they may occur in 40%-80% of patients with tuberous sclerosis. Angiomyolipoma is also associated with neurofibromatosis and von Hippel-Lindau disease.
- In children, angiomyolipomas are rare in the absence of tuberous sclerosis.
- Lesions smaller than 4 cm in diameter are typically asymptomatic; those larger than 4 cm in diameter are more likely to spontaneously hemorrhage. Severe retroperitoneal hemorrhage has been termed *Wunderlich syndrome.*

OSSIFYING RENAL TUMOR OF INFANCY

- Ossifying renal tumor of infancy is a rare benign renal mass.
- Patients have ranged in age from 6 days to 14 months, with 10 of 11 having hematuria as the presenting symptom.
- Boys > girls
- The mass is believed to arise from urothelium and is attached to the renal medulla, specifically the papillary region of the renal pyramids. From this location, it extends in a polypoid fashion into the collecting system.
- At imaging, the renal outline is usually maintained; however, filling defects with partial obstruction of the collecting system are often seen. Because of its location within the collecting system and its characteristic ossification, ossifying renal tumor of infancy may mimic a staghorn calculus, which would be exceedingly rare in the age group in which this lesion occurs.

METANEPHRIC ADENOMA

- Metanephric adenoma, also known as nephrogenic adenofibroma or embryonal adenoma, is a benign renal tumor.
- Presenting features include pain, hypertension, hematoma, a flank mass, hypercalcemia, and polycythemia.
- No age prediction
- By US, the mass is well defined and solid. It can be hypoechoic or hyperechoic, or even cystic with a mural nodule.
- By CT performed before IV administration of contrast material, the mass may be isoattenuating or hyperattenuating and small calcifications may be present. The lesion enhances less-than-normal renal parenchyma.

Ovarian Masses

Cyst
- Fairly common
- May cause large abdominal mass
- If > 3 cm, need to follow up with US

Teratoma
- Most common ovarian neoplasm in children
- Most occur in adolescents
- Imaging
  Plain film: abdominal or pelvic mass; calcification, 65%
  US: mixed echogenicity
  CT: soft tissue, calcific, and fatty components in tumor

Amputated ovary
- Secondary to torsion with subsequent infarction
- Produces stippled calcification in atrophied ovary

Other

NEONATAL ADRENAL HEMORRHAGE

Common disorder in the perinatal or occasionally prenatal period. Right 70%, left 20%, bilateral 10%. Predisposing conditions:
- Traumatic delivery
- Hypoxia
- Sepsis
- Maternal diabetes mellitus

Radiographic features
- Initially appears as solid mass, increased density by CT early
- Liquification occurs within 10 days to produce a cystlike appearance
- Wall calcification
- Main differential diagnosis: neuroblastoma

11

RENAL ARTERY STENOSIS

- Fibromuscular hyperplasia (most common)
- Other less common causes:
  Neurofibromatosis
  Williams syndrome (idiopathic hypercalcemia of infancy)
  Middle aortic syndrome
  Takayasu's
  Posttransplant

RENAL VEIN THROMBOSIS

Enlarged echogenic kidneys with loss of corticomedullary differentiation. Causes:
- Nephrotic syndrome
- Protein c or S deficiency
- Dehydration
- Polycythemia
- Burns
- Left adrenal hemorrhage
- Posttransplant

Musculoskeletal System

Trauma

GENERAL

The immature skeleton has growth plates, cartilaginous epiphysis, and a thick, strong periosteum. Pediatric bone is more elastic than adult bone: bowing and bending injuries are therefore more common than breaking and splintering. Overall, childhood fractures are less common than adult fractures.

Types of fractures
- Elastic deformation (momentary)
- Bowing (permanent)
- Torus (buckle) fractures: buckling of cortex
- Greenstick fracture: incomplete transverse fracture with intact periosteum on the concave side and ruptured periosteum on the convex side. Occurs in patients of elementary school age.
- Complete fracture

Fracture healing
Fracture healing is rapid in children.
- Periosteal new bone: 1 week
- Loss of fracture line: 2-3 weeks
- Hard callus: 2-4 weeks
- Remodeling of bone: 12 months

Pearls
- Hyperemia from fracture healing may lead to overgrowth of an extremity

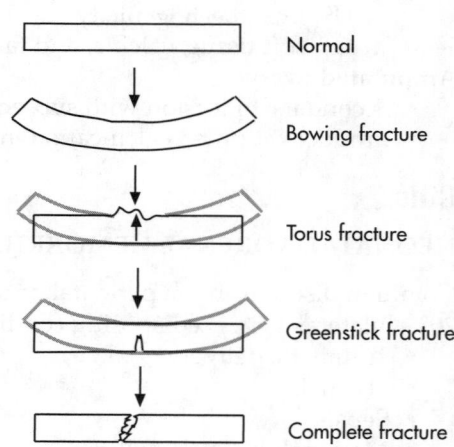

Normal

Bowing fracture

Torus fracture

Greenstick fracture

Complete fracture

NORMAL VARIANTS FREQUENTLY CONFUSED WITH DISEASE

- Nutrient foramina: lucencies extending through cortex with straight parallel margins. Usually extend away from joint central to periphery.
- Scalloping of medial distal fibula: this finding may be confused with a buckle fracture or superficial bone destruction.
- Serpentine physes may appear as lucencies suggesting fracture
- Distal femoral cortical irregularity: posteromeidal metaphysis
- Apophyses of the inferior pubic ramus: theses apophyses often ossify asymmetrically
- Dense metaphyseal bands affecting zone of provisional calcification; most common 2-6 years of age
- Calcaneal apophysess: normally denser than adjacent bone; frequently fragmented
- Calcaneal pseudocyst

SALTER-HARRIS FRACTURES

Epiphyseal plate fractures are analogues to ligamentous injuries in the adult. Growth plate injuries represent 35% of all skeletal injuries in children. Age: 10-15 years (75%). The most common sites for injury are wrist (50%) and ankle (30%). Because the physis is injured in Salter-Harris fractures permanent deformities may occur. Mnemonic: "SALTR." Increasing grade correlates with increasing risk of deformity; risk of deformity also varies with joint—distal femur > distal radius

Slipped (type 1)
Above (type 2)
Lower (type 3)
Together (type 4)
Ruined (type 5)

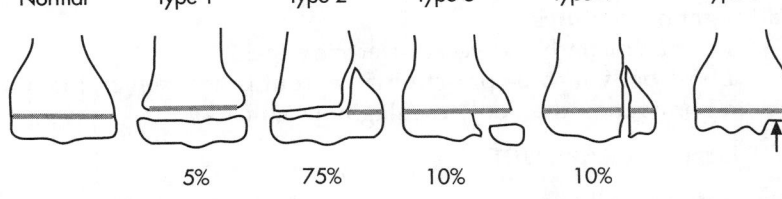

ELBOW INJURIES

The distal humeral shaft has 4 ossification centers. Ossification sequence (mnemonic: "CRITOE"):

- **C**apitellum, 1 year
- **R**adial head, 5 years
- **I**nternal (medial) epicondyle, 7 years
- **T**rochlea, 10 years
- **O**lecranon, 10 years
- **E**xternal (lateral) epicondyle, 11 years

In females, ossification centers appear 1-2 years earlier than in males.

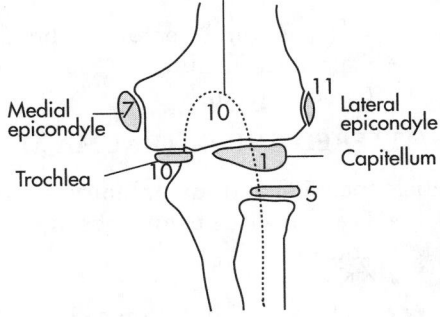

Several radiological lines and signs are important in evaluating elbow injuries:

- Anterior humeral line passes through the middle ⅓ of the capitellum
- Radiocapitellar line passes through the capitellum on all views and confirms the articulation between radial head and the capitellum
- Coronoid line projects anterior to the developing capitellum
- Fat pad sign (posterior pad is normally absent, anterior fat pad is usually present); absence of the posterior fat pad sign virtually excludes a fracture (90% of patients with fat pad sign have a fracture)

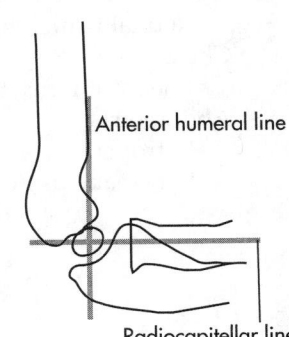

11

Common types
- Supracondylar fracture, 60%
- Lateral condylar fracture, 15%
- Medial epicondylar fractures, 10%

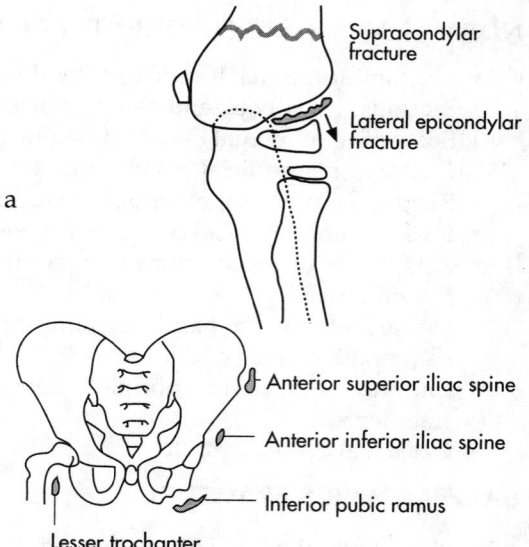

Supracondylar fracture

Lateral epicondylar fracture

LITTLE LEAGUE ELBOW

Inflammatory reaction (epiphysitis) of the medial epicondyle as a response to trauma (avulsion tear).

AVULSION FRACTURES

Abnormal stress on ligaments and tendons. Common sites:
- Iliac spine
    Superior: sartorius
    Inferior: rectus femoris
- Pubic ramus: adductors, gracilis
- Lesser trochanter: iliopsoas

Anterior superior iliac spine

Anterior inferior iliac spine

Inferior pubic ramus

Lesser trochanter

OSTEOCHONDROSIS DISSECANS

Marginal fracture of subchondral bone, adjacent cartilage, or both near a joint surface. Male:female = 3:1. Bilateral in 35%. 50% of patients have a history of trauma. In osteochrondrosis dissecans of the knee, the medial epicondyle is affected in 90%.

Radiographic features
- Lucent epicondyle defects, sclerotic edges
- Loose body may be present in joint (but is not seen on plain film unless it is a bony rather than only cartilaginous chip)

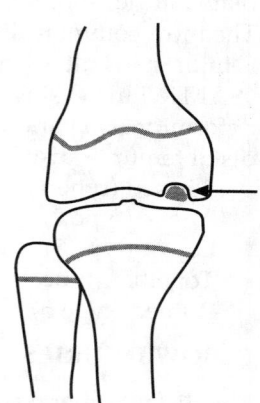

TODDLER'S FRACTURE

Stress fracture in lower extremity commonly due to fall. Most common fracture sites:
- Isolated spiral fracture of the tibial shaft
- Calcaneal fracture
- Cuboid fracture

BATTERED CHILD (TRAUMA X)

Incidence: 1% of trauma. Injuries:
- Fractures (see below; absence of fractures does not imply absence of abuse)
- CNS
    Subdural hematoma
    Retinal hemorrhage
- Chest
    Pneumothorax, pneumoperitoneum
- Abdomen
    Retroperitoneal hematoma
    Pancreatic pseudocysts

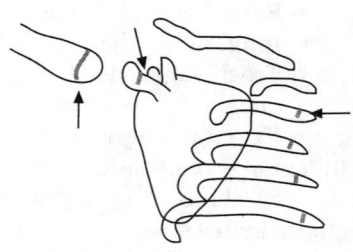

Radiographic features

Typical for battered child:

- Most common child abuse fracture is the diaphyseal fracture, which is indistinguishable from an innocent fracture
- Highly specific fractures are less common, and include metaphyseal fractures of long bones
- Posterior rib fractures

The 3 "S"s:

- Scapular fractures, uncommon
- Spinous process fractures, uncommon
- Sternal fractures, uncommon

Common fractures also often seen in other types of trauma

- Multiple, bilateral fractures
- Skull fractures
- Fractures of long bones

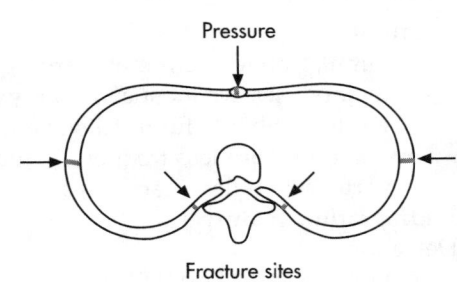

Pressure

Fracture sites

X-RAY VS. SCINTIGRAPHY FOR DETECTION OF CHILD ABUSE		
	Skeletal Survey	**Bone Scan**
Sensitivity	Moderate	High
Specificity	High	Low
Sedation required	Rare	Common
Radiation dose	Very low	Low
Need for additional studies	Occasionally	Always
Cost	Low	High
Utility	Screening	Equivocal cases

Infection

HEMATOGENOUS OSTEOMYELITIS

Common hematogenous bacterial osteomyelitis pathogens in children:

- Children (unifocal): *Staphylococcus* (85%), *Streptococcus* (10%)
- Neonates (multifocal): *Streptococcus* > *Staphylococcus*
- Immunocompromised adults: short bones of hand and feet: *Staphylococcus*
- Drug addicts: *Pseudomonas*, 85%, *Klebsiella, Enterobacter*
- Sickle cell disease: *Salmonella*

In otherwise healthy adults, hematogenous osteomyelitis is very rare; osteomyelitis in adults usually follows direct implantation after surgery or trauma.

Pathogenesis

Bacteria pass through nutrient vessels to metaphyses, where organism proliferate. Metaphyseal inflammatory reaction progresses to edema, pus, necrosis, thrombosis.

In older children, the cartilaginous growth plate becomes avascular and acts as a barrier to epiphyseal extension.

11

Location

- Tubular bones with most rapid growth and largest metaphyses are most commonly affected, 75%: femur > tibia > fibula; distal end > proximal end
- Flat bones are less frequently infected, 30%: vertebral bodies, iliac bones

Radiographic features

Detection

- Bone scan (^{99m}Tc-MDP > ^{67}Ga imaging) becomes positive within 24 hours after onset of symptoms (90% accuracy)
- Hyperemia on blood pool images
- Hot spot on delayed images
- Plain film
    Soft tissue swelling, obliteration of fat planes: 3 days
    Bone destruction, periosteal reaction: 5-7 days (children), 10-14 days (adults)

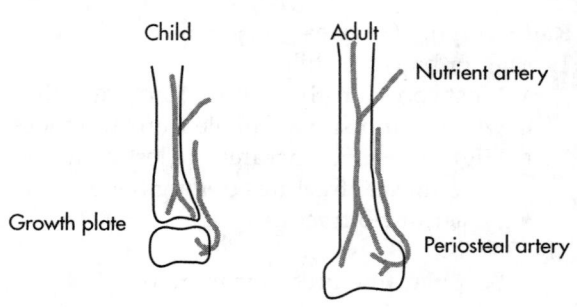

Child   Adult

Nutrient artery

Growth plate   Periosteal artery

Plain film

- Soft tissue swelling (earliest sign; often in metaphyseal region), blurring of fat planes, sinus tract formation, soft tissue abscess
- Cortical loss (5-7 days after infection), bone destruction
- Involucrum: shell of periosteum around infected bone (20 days after infection)
- Sequestrum: segmented or necrotic cortical bone separated from living bone by granulation tissue; may be extruded (30 days after infection)
- Periosteal bone formation
- Separation of epiphysis/metaphysis

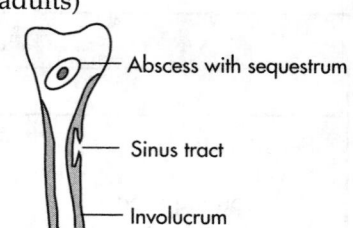

Abscess with sequestrum

Sinus tract

Involucrum

CHRONIC OSTEOMYELITIS

Chronic osteomyelitis may follow acute osteomyelitis. Often caused by less virulent organism, increased resistance, or partial treatment.

Radiographic features

- Brodie's abscess:
    Lucent well-defined lesion with thick sclerotic rim
    Typically in metaphysis or diaphysis of long bones
- Thick and dense cortex
- Sinus tracts to skin

Degenerative and Chronic Traumatic Disease

OVERVIEW

Three distinct conditions of the hip occur in children, each of which affects a different age group:

- Neonates, infants: congenital dislocation of the hip (CDH)
- School age: Legg-Calvé-Perthes (LCP) disease
- Adolescents: slipped capital femoral epiphysis (SCFE)

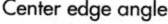

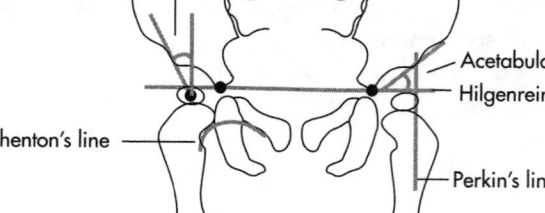

Center edge angle

Acetabular angle 15°-35°

Hilgenreiner line

Shenton's line

Perkin's line

OVERVIEW			
	CDH	LCP	SCFE
Age	Neonate	5-8 years	Puberty
Sex	Females (estrogen)	Males	Overweight males
Cause	Joint laxity: femoral head falls out of acetabulum	Osteonecrosis	Salter-Harris 1 fracture
Imaging	Putti's triad	Subchondral fissure	Posterior slippage
	US diagnostic	Fragmented epiphysis	Irregular growth plate

DEVELOPMENTAL DYSPLASIA OF HIP (CONGENITAL DISLOCATION OF THE HIP)

An abnormally lax joint capsule allows the femoral head to fall out of the acetabulum, leading to deformation. Predisposing factors for the development of CDH are:
- Abnormal ligamentous laxity (effect of estrogen; female:male = 6:1)
- Acetabular dysplasia (there are 2 components to the acetabular dysplasia: increased acetabular angle and shallow acetabular fossae)

CDH occurs most commonly (70%) in the left hip. Bilateral involvement is seen in 5%.
Treatment:
- Cast: flexion + abduction + external rotation
- Salter osteotomy if chronic

Clinical findings
- Ortolani's jerk or click sign
- Barlow's sign
- Limited abduction of flexed hip
- Shortening of one leg
- Waddling gait

Radiographic features
US (commonly used today)
- Normal femoral head is covered at least 50% by acetabulum
- In CDH, < 50% of femoral head is covered by acetabulum

Plain film (rarely used today)
- Putti's triad
    Superolateral displacement of proximal femur
    Increase in acetabular angle
    Small capital femoral epiphysis
- Femoral head is located lateral to Perkin's line
- Other features that are sometimes present
    Abnormal sclerosis of the acetabulum
    Formation of a false acetabulum
    Shallow acetabulum and other deformities
    Delayed ossification of femoral head

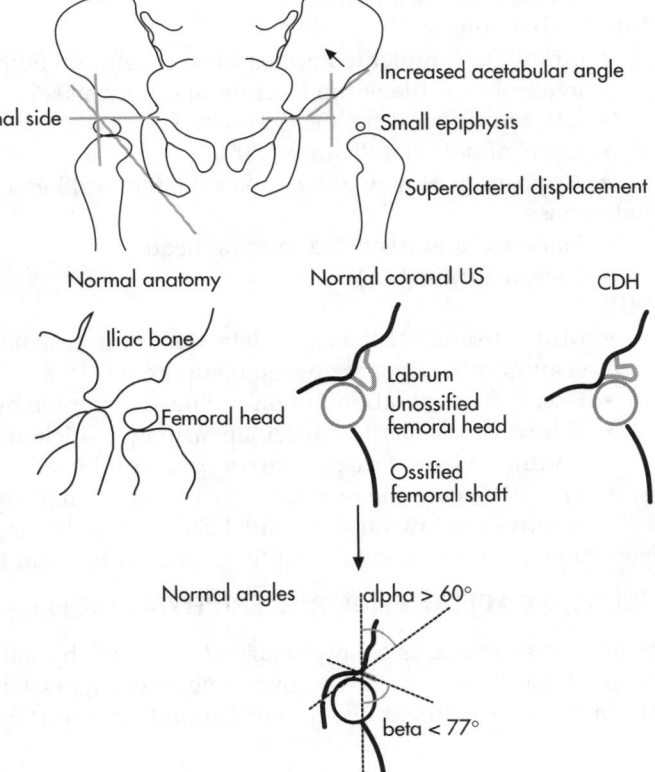

11

Pearls
- In the neonate, radiographic evaluation of hip dislocation is unreliable because of paucity of skeletal ossification; diagnosis becomes more reliable at 1-2 months of age
- AP is the best view to demonstrate abnormalities; the frogleg view is useless because the hip is reduced in this position

LEGG-CALVÉ-PERTHES (LCP) DISEASE

Avascular necrosis of the femoral head. Age: white males, 5-8 years. Bilateral in 15%. Treatment: the femoral head or acetabular component has to be remodeled to achieve acetabular coverage and thus prevent lateral subluxation:
- Abduction bracing (cast)
- Varus derotation osteotomy

Radiographic features

Early phase
- Widened joint: may be due to increased cartilage or joint effusion (earliest sign)
- Subchondral fissure fracture, best seen on frogleg view (tangential view of cartilage)
- Increase in bone density

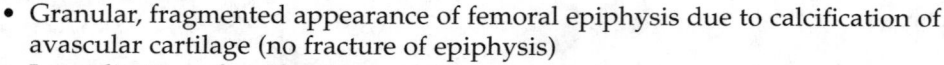

Intermediate phase
- Granular, fragmented appearance of femoral epiphysis due to calcification of avascular cartilage (no fracture of epiphysis)
- Lateralization of ossification center
- Cysts of demineralization (30%)
- Apposition of new bone makes the femoral head appear dense

Late phase
- Flattened and distorted femoral head
- Osteoarthritis (OA)

MRI
- MRI is useful for the early detection of disease before radiographic or scintigraphic findings become apparent
- Useful for evaluation of femoral head coverage by acetabulum
- Allows assessment of articular cartilage. Thickening of the hyaline cartilage leading to lateral displacement of femoral head
- In LCP disease the normal high T2 signal intensity of the femoral head epiphysis is low on T1W and T2W images. During repair phase, fat containing marrow returns to the epiphysis and high signal intensity appears.

SLIPPED CAPITAL FEMORAL EPIPHYSIS (SCFE)

Similar appearance as a Salter-Harris type 1 epiphyseal plate fracture of the proximal femur. Cause: unknown. Age: overweight teenagers. Clinical: pain 90%, history of trauma 50%. Treatment: fixation of femoral epiphysis (pins, bone pegs).

Radiographic features
- 15%-25% are bilateral, subtle changes are difficult to detect
- Always obtain AP and lateral view
- Malalignment of epiphysis–femoral neck line (Salter-Harris type 1 fracture)
- Widened growth plate
- Decreased height of epiphysis (slips posterior)
- Decreased angle of femoral neck anteversion by CT

Complications
- Osteonecrosis
- Chondrolysis (cartilage necrosis) from pins
- Varus deformity
- Degenerative OA

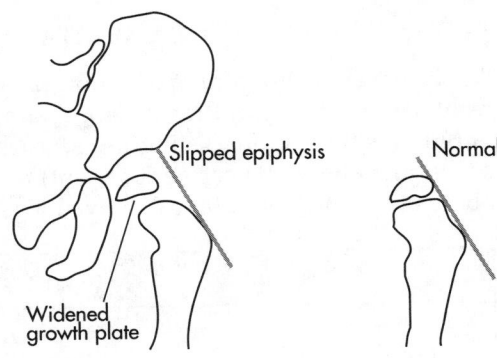

OSTEOCHONDROSIS

Osteochondrosis refers to abnormal bone and cartilage at the end of bone. The term is a catch-all term referring to a spectrum of diseases:
Abnormal endochondral ossification secondary to repeated stress without
osteonecrosis
- Scheuermann's disease: spine
- Blount's disease: tibial epiphysis
- Osgood-Schlatter disease: tibial tubercle

Osteonecrosis disease, probably not, old news
- Kienböck disease: lunate
- Freiberg's disease: metatarsals
- LCP

SCHEUERMANN'S DISEASE (ADOLESCENT KYPHOSIS)

Vertebral osteochondrosis refers to the kyphotic deformity of the thoracic (75%) or thoracolumbar (25%) spine in teenagers (13-17 years). Diagnostic criteria:
- Kyphosis must be > 35°
- Anterior wedging of at least one vertebral body of > 5°
- Usually 3-5 vertebral bodies are involved

Schmorl's theory: all pathological changes in the spine result from herniation of disk material through congenital defects into the vertebral endplates during time of excessive growth in adolescence.

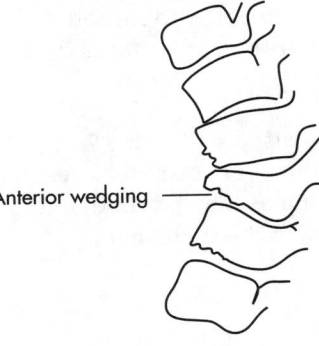

Radiographic features
- Progressive narrowing of disk spaces
- Wedging of the anterior portion of vertebral bodies (posterior portion protected by posterior articulation)
- Irregularity of endplates
- Changes seen in > 3 vertebral bodies
- Multiple Schmorl's nodes

11

BLOUNT'S DISEASE (CONGENITAL TIBIA VARA)

Abnormal endochondral ossification caused by stress and compression. The disease results in deformity of the medial proximal tibial metaphysis and epiphysis. 2 forms of Blount's disease are distinguished: early onset (infantile, onset 1-3 years) and late onset (juvenile, 4-10 years; adolescent) forms. Both forms occur more commonly in obese black children. Clinical: bowed legs, pain.

BLOUNT'S DISEASE		
Clinical	Early Onset (Infantile)	Late Onset (Juvenile, Adolescent)
Onset	1-3 years	> 4 years
Frequency	Common	Infrequent
Site	Bilateral (80%)	Unilateral (90%)
Recurrence after surgery	Low	High
Course	Progressive deformity	Less deformity

Radiographic features

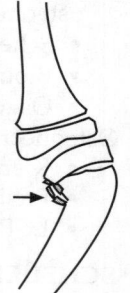

- Fragmentation of medial tibial epiphysis
- Irregular medial physeal line
- Beaking of proximal medial tibial metaphysis
- Bone bridge across the medial physis while the lateral growth plate remains open
- Metaphyseal-diaphyseal angle (MDA) > 11°
- Tibiofemoral angle (TFA) > 15°, i.e., tibia vara; this finding alone, however, is not diagnostic for Blount's disease

OSGOOD-SCHLATTER DISEASE

Painful irregularity of tibial tuberosity secondary to repeated trauma to deep fibers of patellar tendon. Male:female = 5:1; 25% are bilateral.

Radiographic features

- Irregular tibial tuberosity
- Thickening of patellar tendon; soft tissue swelling around patellar ligament
- Obliteration of infrapatellar fat pad

FREIBERG'S DISEASE

Osteonecrosis of the distal end of the 2nd (75%) or 3rd (25%) metatarsal. Bilateral in 10% of patients. Occurs between 11-15 years. Freiberg's disease the only osteonecrosis more frequent in females (75%) than in males (25%). Commonly associated with hallux valgus and short 1st metatarsal.

FOOT ANGLES

Diagnosis of foot abnormalities requires measurement of angles between talus and calcaneus and between forefoot and hindfoot. Films should be obtained while weight bearing.

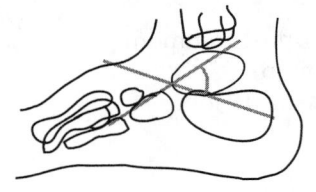

CLUBFOOT (TALIPES EQUINOVARUS)

Common abnormality (1:1,000); bilateral 50%. The typical clubfoot contains 4 separate components (always need an AP and lateral view):

- Hindfoot varus is the key radiological finding: AP talocalcaneal angle < 20°
- Equinus deformity of the heel: lateral talocalcaneal angle < 35°
- Adduction and varus deformity of the forefoot (metatarsus adductus): 1st metatarsal bone is displaced medially with respect to the the long axis of the talus
- Talonavicular subluxation: medial subluxation of the navicular bone; the subluxation is infrequently diagnosed because ossification has not occurred at the time of clubfoot diagnosis

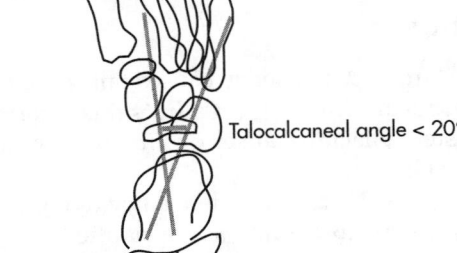

CONGENITAL VERTICAL TALUS

Rare deformity characterized by dorsal dislocation of the navicular bone on the talus. Axis of the talus is steep, and a convex plantar surface of the foot may result (rockerbottom feet). Associations:

- Meningomyelocele
- Arthrogryposis
- Trisomies 13-18

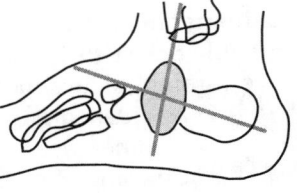

11

TARSAL COALITION

Fusion of 2 or more tarsal bones. Union may be complete, partial, bony, cartilaginous, or fibrous. Present at birth but usually asymptomatic until early adulthood. Location:
- Calcaneonavicular (most common)
- Talocalcaneal (common)

Commonly results in spastic flatfoot. Bilateral.

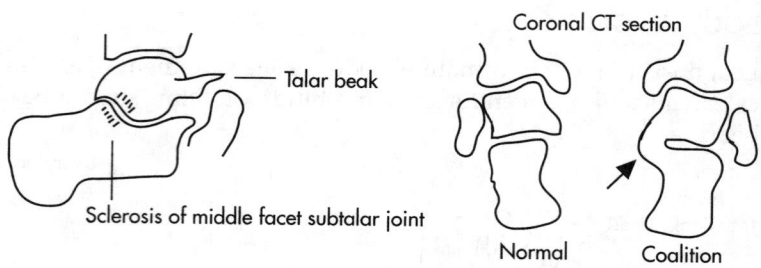

VARUS AND VALGUS

Varus and valgus refer to the relationship of a distal part of an extremity to a proximal part (e.g., femur/tibia). Varus referes to an angulation of the distal bone toward the midline. Valgus refers to an angulation of the distal bone away from the midline.

Metabolic Abnormalities

RICKETS

Vitamin D deficiency causes failure of mineralization of bone and cartilage (in adults this is termed osteomalacia). Causes of Vitamin D deficiency:

GI tract
- Nutritional deficiency (common)
- Absorption abnormalities

Skin disease

Liver disease

Renal
- Renal tubular acidosis
- Renal failure (loss of calcium)

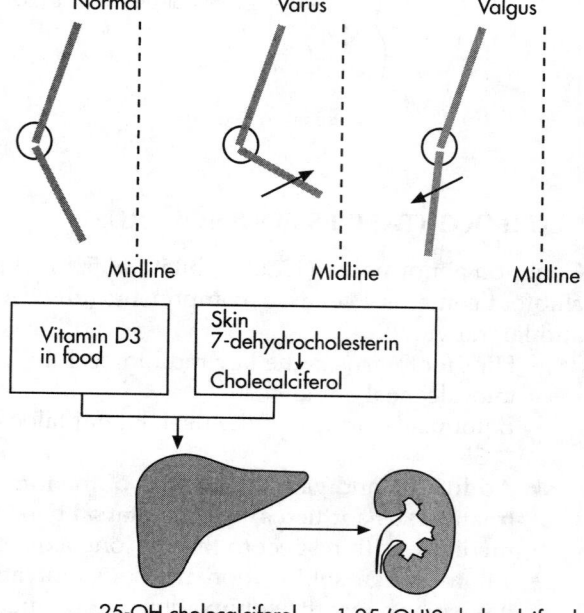

Radiographic features

Infantile rickets (6-18 months of age)
- Growth plate abnormalities (especially long bones)
    A widened growth plate is due to rickets until proved
        otherwise
    Cupping of metaphysis
    Disorganized (frayed) metaphysis
- Bowing deformities of bones
- Delayed closing of fontanelles
- Softening of cranial vault (craniotabes)
- Rachitic rosary: enlargement of cartilage at costochondral junction

Vitamin D–resistant rickets (> 2 years of age)
- Bowing of extremities is marked
- Bones may appear sclerotic occasionally

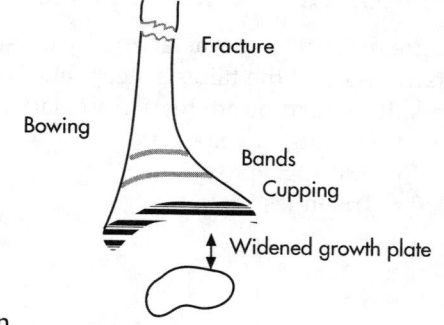

Congenital Anomalies

Radiological parameters used in the description of dysplasias:
- Size of bones
- Pattern of distribution of abnormal bones
- Bone density and structure
- Shape of bones
- Time of onset of abnormality

DWARFISM

Skeletal dysplasias can be categorized according to the relative shortening of humerus or femur in relation to radius or tibia:
- Rhizomelic dysplasia: shortening of proximal limb (humerus or femur) in relation to distal limb (radius or tibia)
- Mesomelic dysplasia: shortening of distal limb (radius or tibia) in relation to proximal limb (humerus or femur)
- Micromelic dysplasia: shortening of proximal and distal limbs

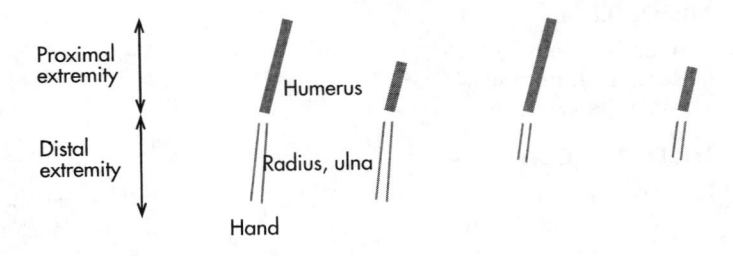

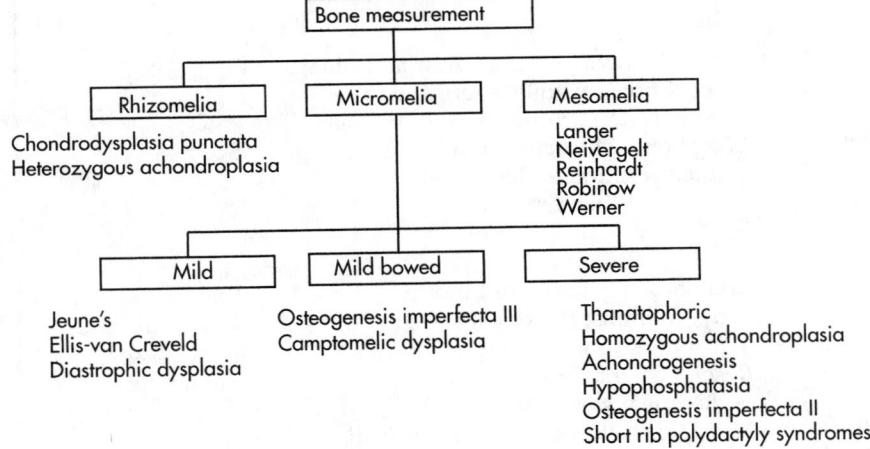

OVERVIEW OF SYNDROMES			
Syndrome	Lethal	In Utero Features (US)	Other Features
RHIZOMELIA			
Chondrodysplasia punctata	Yes	Hypertelorism, metaphyseal splaying, coronal clefts in vertebra bodies	
Achondroplasia (heterozygous form)	No	Femur length normal until 20 wk; below 95% confidence limits of mean by 27 wk	See p. 857
MESOMELIA			
Langer, Nievergelt, Reinhardt, Robinow's, Werner's syndrome	No	Mesomelic shortening	
MILD MICROMELIA			
Jeune's syndrome (asphyxiating thoracic dysplasia)	Yes	Small thorax; squared iliac wings; polydactyly; ± renal anomalies	Similar to Ellis-van Creveld syndrome
Ellis-van Creveld syndrome	Yes	Similar to Jeune's syndrome; ASD 50%	
Diastrophic dysplasia		Clubfoot; hitchhiker thumb; scoliosis; joint flexion contractures	
MILD BOWED MICROMELIA			
Camptomelic dysplasia	Yes	Anterior bowing of the femur and tibia; short fibulae; limbs short due to bowing; ± scoliosis; absent scapulae	
Osteogenesis imperfecta type III	No	Long bones shortened; bowed; ± fractures; humeri less severely involved than femurs	See p. 857
SEVERE MICROMELIA			
Thanatophoric dysplasia	Yes	Limb bowing; narrowed thorax; hydramnios; cloverleaf skull (15%); ± ascites or nonimmune hydrops	Both parents of normal stature
Achondroplasia, dysplasia homozygous form	Yes	Resembles thanatophoric with cloverleaf skull	Rib fractures
Osteogenesis imperfecta type II	Yes	Multiple fractures; hypomineralization; thick long bones	
Hypophosphatasia (congenital lethal)	Yes	Similar to osteogenesis imperfecta; poor mineralization	No rib fracture
Achondrogenesis	Yes	Absent vertebral ossification	
Short rib polydactyly syndromes	Yes	Short ribs; narrow thorax; polydactyly	

Pearls
- The diagnosis of a specific skeletal dysplasia is based on the best fit of clinical, biochemical, and radiological data.
- A specific diagnosis is often of no help in management except for determining prognosis and genetic counseling.

OSTEOGENESIS IMPERFECTA (OI)

Inadequate osteoid formation but normal mineralization (thin, osteoporotic fragile bones) causes severe bowing and fractures. Autosomal dominant, 1:40,000 births. Classification:

Type 1: tarda form (OIT, Ekman-Lobstein syndrome), 90%: more benign form with normal life expectancy. Findings:
- Blue sclera, 90%
- Laxity of ligaments
- Dental abnormalities (dentin dysplasia), 30%
- Deafness (otosclerosis), 20%
- Osseous abnormalities

Type 2: congenita (OIC, Vrolik type), 10%: death in utero or neonatal period; detected by prenatal US

Type 3: fractures at birth, progressive limb deformity, occasional fractures, normal sclerae and hearing

Type 4: bone fragility, normal sclerae, normal hearing, discolored teeth

Radiographic features

General
- Bowing deformities: genu valgum, coxa vara
- Thinning of cortex
- Frequent fractures

Skull
- Wormian bones

Spine
- Vertebral scalloping
- Severe kyphoscoliosis

Pelvis
- Acetabular protrusion is common

ACHONDROPLASIA

Common dysplasia characterized by abnormal bone formation at growth plate. Autosomal dominant (homozygous forms fatal, patients with heterozygous form have normal life span).

Radiographic features
- Rhizomelic dwarfism: short limbs (particularly proximal segments of femurs, humerus)
- Short and stubby fingers
- Spine
  Short interpedicular distance (typical)
  The interpedicular distance narrows distally
  Spinal stenosis is due to short pedicles
- Ping-pong paddle pelvis
  Iliac bones are rounded
  Horizontal acetabular roofs
- Skull
  Small skull base (enchondral ossification) and small foramen magnum
  Normal-sized calvarium (membranous ossification): frontal bossing

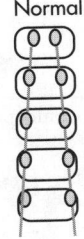
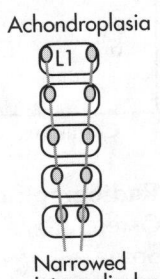

Normal   Achondroplasia

L1

Narrowed interpedicular distance

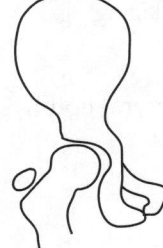
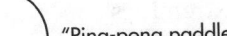

Normal   Achondroplasia

"Ping-pong paddle"

11

CHONDROECTODERMAL DYSPLASIA

Ellis-van Creveld syndrome is characterized by distal (acromelic) limb shortening.
Radiographic features
- Polydactyly (always present)
- Proximal phalanges longer than distal phalanges
- Shortened tubular bones with coned-shaped epiphysis
- Short ribs
- ASD, 50%

MUCOPOLYSACCHARIDOSIS

Excess of mucopolysaccharide accumulation secondary to enzyme deficiencies. The specific diagnosis is made according to:
- Age
- IQ
- Corneal clouding
- Urinary excretion of heparan, keratin, dermatan
- Other clinical findings

		MUCOPOLYSACCHARIDOSIS SYNDROMES		
Type	**Name**	**Inheritance**	**Deficient Enzyme**	**Prominent Features**
1H	Hurler's	AR	a-L-iduronidase	CC, LIQ, HS
1S	Scheie's	AR	a-L-iduronidase	CC, aortic valve disease
2	Hunter's	Male recessive	a-L-iduronate-2-sulfatase	LIQ
3	Sanfilippo's	AR	Heparan N-sulfatase	LIQ, coarse facial features
4	Morquio's	AR	Galactosamine-6-sulfate sulfatase	CC, HS, dwarfism
6	Maroteaux-Lamy	AR	Arylsulfatase B	Short stature, HS
7	Sly's	AR	Glucuronidase	LIQ, HS, pneumonias
8	DiFerrante	Genetic trait	Glucosamine-6-sulfate sulfatase	Short stature

CC, Corneal clouding; HS, hepatosplenomegaly; LIQ, low IQ.

Radiographic features
Osteoporosis
Spine
- Oval, hook-shaped vertebral bodies
- Severe hyperlordosis, scoliosis
Pelvis
- Hypoplastic with some flaring
Extremities
- Shortened bones
- Dysplastic changes at femoral epiphysis
- Short thick finger bones

CLEIDOCRANIAL DYSOSTOSIS

Defect in ossification of enchondral and intramembranous bones
- Wormian bones
- Clavicle deformity (either absent, partially absent, or unfused)
- Failure of midline ossification (delayed closure of symphisis pubis, fontanelles, mandible, neural arches, sternum, vertebral bodies)
- Supernumerary epiphysis

OSTEOPETROSIS

Osteoclast failure (bone remodels incompletely). Types:
- Autosomal recessive: lethal (anemia, thrombocytopenia, cranial foramina too small → hydrocephalus)
- Autosominal dominant: Albers-Schönberg disease, marble bones

Radiographic features
- Generalized osteosclerosis
- Erlenmeyer flask deformity of distal femur
- Bone-within-bone appearance
- Alternating dense and lucent metaphyseal lines

Complications
- Frequent fractures
- Anemia (bone marrow replacement)
- Cranial nerve palsies

Arthritis

JUVENILE RHEUMATOID ARTHRITIS (JRA)

RA with onset at < 16 years. 70% of JRA is seronegative. Still's disease = JRA + lymphadenopathy + splenomegaly.

Radiographic features
- Spinal involvement is very common (70%) and typically precedes peripheral arthritis:
    Diffuse ankylosis of posterior articular joints (diagnostic)
    C2 subluxation (due to destruction of posterior ligament)
    Odontoid fracture
- Monoarticular in early course in 25%
- Periosteal new bone formation is common (uncommon in adults)
- Soft tissue swelling edema, synovial congestion
- Growth retardation secondary to premature closure of growth plates: short metacarpals
- Overgrowth of epiphyses (increased perfusion)

Other Disorders

CAFFEY'S DISEASE (INFANTILE CORTICAL HYPEROSTOSIS)

Cortical periostitis at multiple sites. The etiology is unknown (viral?). Self-limited and benign condition. Occurs before 6 months of age.

Radiographic features
- New bone (periostitis) formation along tibia, ulna, mandible

11

SHORT STATURE

Dwarfism: height is > 4 standard deviations below the mean. Human growth hormone (HGH) deficiency: at least two different HGH stimulation tests (hypoglycemia, dopamine, exercise, arginine) have to be abnormal (< 5 mg/mL) to establish the diagnosis.

Classification

HGH deficiency (pituitary dwarfism)
- Isolated HGH deficiency
- Craniopharyngioma, infections

Peripheral tissue nonresponsive to HGH
- African pygmies
- Turner's syndrome
- Constitutional short stature

Systemic diseases (most common)
- Hypothyroidism (cretinism)
- Cyanotic CHF
- Chronic pulmonary disease

Approach
- Rule out chronic systemic disease (most common cause of short stature)
- Rule out osseous defects
- If HGH stimulation is normal: measure somatomedins

KLIPPEL-TRÉNAUNAY SYNDROME

Consists of enlarged extremity, cutaneous vascular lesions, and diffuse venous and lymphatic malformations. Generally involves only one of the lower extremities, although bilateral involvement, upper extremity involvement, or extension into the trunk may occur. Klippel-Trénaunay syndrome must be distinguished from Parkes Weber syndrome (enlarged extremity is due to underlying AVM). The cutaneous vascular lesion is generally a capillary malformation and usually involves the enlarged limb, although involvement of the whole side of the body or of the contralateral limb may be seen. In over two thirds of patients, a characteristic incompetent lateral venous channel arises near the ankle and extends a variable distance up the extremity to the infrainguinal or pelvic deep venous system. Clinical findings: lymphangitis, cutaneous lymphatic vesicles, lymphorrhea, or mass effect from macrocystic portions of lymphatic malformations. Extension of venous malformation into the pelvis may result in recurrent rectal bleeding or hematuria.

Radiographic findings
- Bone elongation causing leg length discrepancy, soft-tissue thickening, or calcified phleboliths
- Venography usually demonstrates extensive dilation of superficial veins and enlarged perforating veins. In some patients, segmental absence or hypoplasia of the deep venous system is seen and must be distinguished from incomplete filling with contrast material at venography.
- MRI demonstrates a lack of enlarged high-flow arterial structures. T2W imaging shows malformed venous and lymphatic lesions as areas of high signal intensity. MRI depicts deep extension of low-flow vascular malformations into muscular compartments and the pelvis and their relationship to adjacent organs, as well as bone or soft tissue hypertrophy.

Pediatric Neuroimaging

Cranial Ultrasound

CORONAL VIEWS (6 SECTIONS)

1. Frontal lobe view, interhemispheric fissure
2. Circle of Willis view (5-pointed star or bull's head appearance: MCA = horns, sphenoid sinus = bull's head; thalami = within bull's horns); germinal matrix (echolucent area adjacent to the ventricles), internal capsule, corpus callosum, interhemispheric fissure
3. Basilar artery view (pulsating structure within interpeduncular cistern): 3rd ventricle
4. Glomus view: glomus of choroid plexus is very echogenic
5. Tentorium cerebelli view: cerebellar vermis gives the appearance of a Christmas tree, quadrigeminal plate
6. Occipital lobe view: decussation of fibers of optic tract

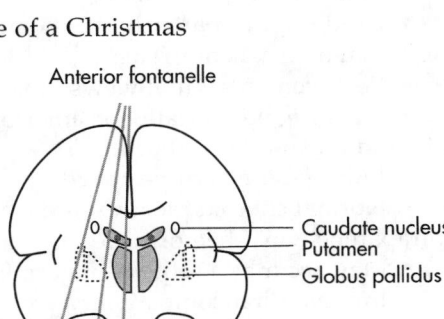

SAGITTAL VIEWS (6 SECTIONS)

1. 2 views are taken in the midline; bring into alignment the echogenic vermis of the cerebellum and the corpus callosum; 3rd ventricle and corpus callosum represent the best reference points
2. Parasagittal view of thalamus, choroid plexus
3. Parasagittal view slightly more lateral to first parasagittal view

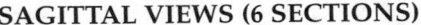

INDICATIONS FOR CRANIAL US

Screening for ventricular dilatation and hemorrhage
- Extracorporeal membrane oxygenation (ECMO) patients (ligation of ipsilateral carotid artery; anticoagulation)
- Premature infants (5%-50% incidence of hemorrhage); screen all neonates < 1500 g or < 32 weeks
- Low Apgar score

Diagnostic cranial US
- Neurological changes
- Cranial dysmorphism (Down syndrome, trisomy 18, meningomyelocele)
- Seizures

Follow-up of hemorrhage

GERMINAL MATRIX HEMORRHAGE

Germinal matrix represents highly vascular tissue located near the caudothalamic groove (inferior to lateral ventricles). Germinal matrix exists only during 24th-32nd week of gestation and the matrix is highly vulnerable to hypoxemia and ischemia. Later in pregnancy, the mature neuroectodermal cells of the germinal matrix migrate to the cerebral cortex.

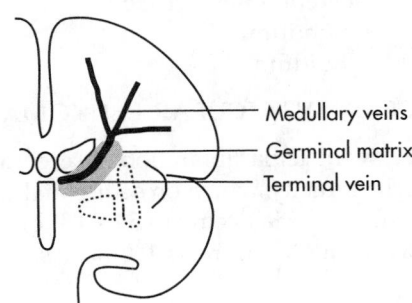

11

Causes of hemorrhage
- Trauma: birth
- Coagulopathies: e.g., ECMO, Rh incompatibility, drugs

Radiographic features

General US appearance of hemorrhage
- Acute hemorrhage (< 7 days): very hyperechoic, no shadowing
- Aging hemorrhage
  Echogenicity decreases within 2-3 weeks
  Abnormal area decreases in size

Grading of hemorrhage
- Grade 1: subependymal hemorrhage; no long-term abnormality
- Grade 2: intraventricular hemorrhage without ventricular dilatation; 10% mortality
- Grade 3: intraventricular hemorrhage with ventricular dilatation; 20% mortality
- Grade 4: intraparenchymal hemorrhage; > 50% mortality

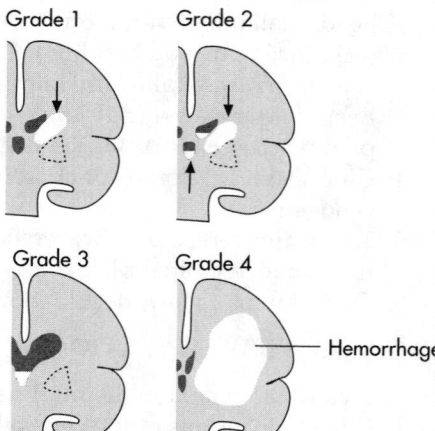

Germinal matrix hemorrhage
- Best seen on sagittal views
- Most frequent location is anterior to caudothalamic groove

Choroid plexus hemorrhage
- Lumpy-bumpy appearance
- Normal choroid plexus pulsates; a blood clot does not

Intraparenchymal hemorrhage
- May occur as a sequela of germinal matrix hemorrhage, birth trauma, Rh incompatibility, etc.
- Intraparenchymal hemorrhage ultimately results in porencephaly
- Hematoma becomes hypoechoic within a few days to weeks

Ventricular dilatation occurs in 75% after hemorrhage
- Ventricles on the coronal scan should not occupy more than ⅓ of the entire hemisphere
- Serial qualitative assessment of ventricular size is more useful in practice than quantitative determination of ventricular size
- Rounding of superolateral angles of frontal horns, dilatation of occipital horns

OTHER TYPES OF HEMORRHAGE (SEE ALSO CHAPTER 6)

Cortical hemorrhage
- AV malformations
- Inflammation
- Trauma
- Tumor

Extracerebral hemorrhage
- Subdural
- Epidural

PERIVENTRICULAR LEUKOMALACIA

Periventricular infarction of cerebral tissue is initially characterized by an increased echogenicity, which on sequential US may transform into cystic areas. Periventricular leukomalacia occurs in 5%-10% of premature infants. Pathogenesis: hypoxemia causes white matter necrosis. Clinical: spastic diplegia and intellectual deficits.

Location (in watershed areas of arterial blood flow)
- Adjacent to trigone of the lateral ventricles
- At level of foramen of Monro

Imaging features

Acute phase
- Broad zone of increased periventricular echogenicity
- May be symmetrical
- Differential diagnosis:
    Periventricular echogenic halo from normally dense venous plexus
    Germinal matrix hemorrhage

Chronic phase (> 2 weeks)
- Small cyst formation ("Swiss cheese" appearance)

Differential diagnosis of porencephaly and cysts of periventricular leukomalacia
- Porencephaly seldom disappears over time
- Porencephaly most often represents an extension of ipsilateral ventricle or subarachnoid space
- Porencephaly is almost always asymmetrical

CHOROID PLEXUS CYST

Cysts arise from choroid plexus and occur in 2%-4% of neonates.
- Small cysts (< 10 mm) usually disappear by 28 weeks
- Large cysts (> 10 mm) are frequently associated with trisomy 18; amniocentesis is usually performed once a large cyst is diagnosed

VP SHUNT COMPLICATIONS

- CSFoma: accumulation of fluid collection near intraabdominal catheter tip. Common in patients with abdominal adhesions due to prior surgery.
- Occlusion
- Infection
- Overshunting (collapsed ventricles)
- Disconnection

Skull

SUTURES

See diagram.

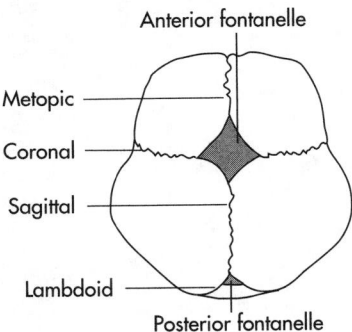

CRANIOSYNOSTOSIS

Premature closure of sutures (sagittal suture, 60%; coronal suture, 20%) results in skull shape abnormalities. Treatment: craniectomy. Causes:

Primary closure
Secondary closure
- Skeletal dysplasia
- Metabolic
- Ventricular shunting
- Hematologic disorders

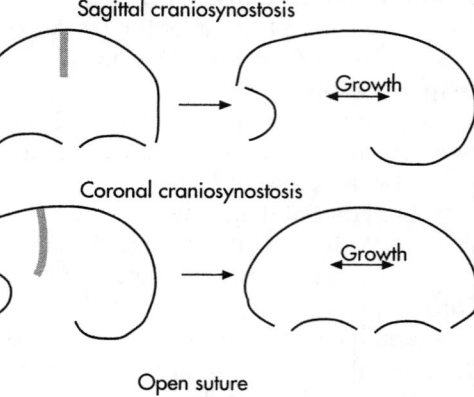

Sagittal craniosynostosis

Growth

Coronal craniosynostosis

Growth

MULTIPLE LACUNAE

Criteria: prominent depressions in inner table of skull.
Causes:
- Physiological up to 6 months
- Increased intracranial pressure
- Mesenchymal dysplasia (lacunar skull, Lückenschädel)
    Meningoceles
    Myelomeningoceles
    Encephaloceles

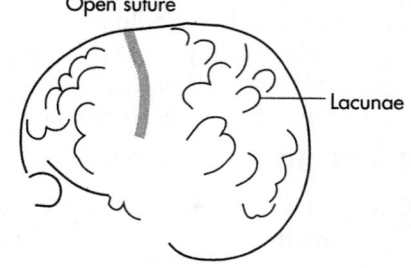

Open suture

Lacunae

WORMIAN BONES

Intrasutural bones (named after Worms, a Danish anatomist), most commonly located in lambdoid suture. Common causes:
- Normal finding until 1 year of age
- Osteogenesis imperfecta
- Cleidocranial dysplasia
- Hypothyroidism

Mnemonic for Wormian bones: PORKCHOPS
- **P**yknodysostosis
- **O**steogenesis imperfecta
- **R**ickets in healing
- **K**inky hair syndrome
- **C**leidocranial dysplasia
- **H**ypothyroidism
- **O**topalatodigital syndrome
- **P**achydermoperiostosis
- **S**yndrome of Down

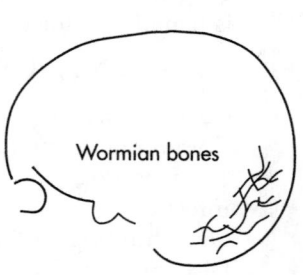

Wormian bones

SKULL FRACTURES

Neonatal skull fractures with torn dura rarely develop into:
- Growing skull fractures
- Leptomeningeal cysts
    Widely separated skull bone
    Meninges herniate through torn dura

Spine

DEVELOPMENT

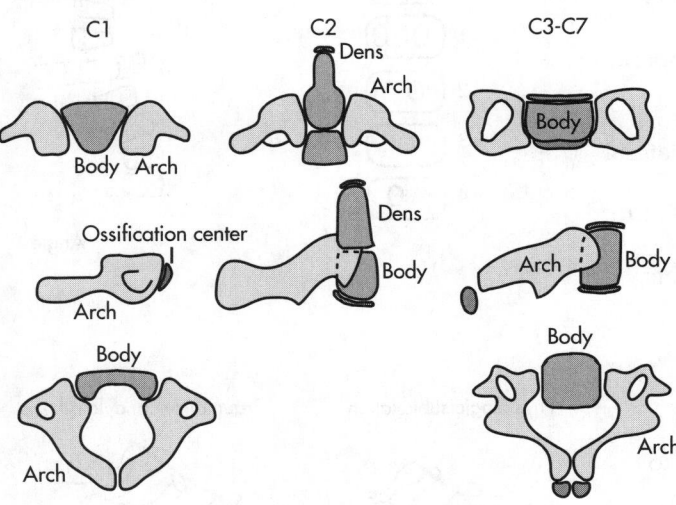

SCOLIOSIS

Scoliosis refers to lateral curving of the spine with varying degrees of rotation of the vertebral bodies around a vertical axis. Types:

Idiopathic, 90%
- Mild form: 3% prevalence
- Severe form: 0.1% prevalence

Secondary
- Congenital
    Hemivertebra
    Trapezoidal vertebra
    Unilateral neural arch fusions
- Growth asymmetry due to trauma, infection, radiation, neurofibromatosis
- Leg length discrepancy

Preoperative radiographic features
- Determine type of scoliosis and degree of flexibility of spine
- Measure the scoliotic curve (Cobb method)
- Determine the degree of rotation: semiquantitate the midline shift of one of the pedicles toward the midline and score 0 to +4; rotation determines the extent of required bone fusion and the rigidity of the curve

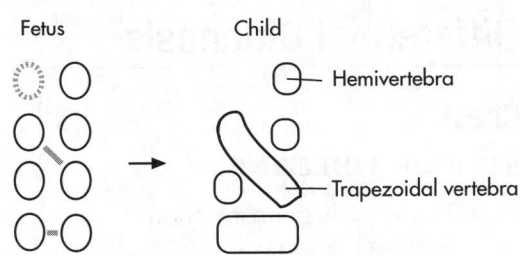

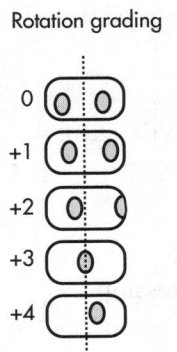

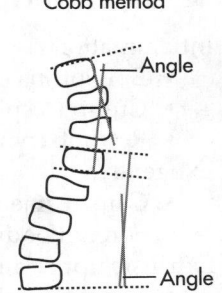

11

Postoperative radiographic features
- Correction of scoliosis: the general goal is to achieve 50% correction of the scoliotic curve and to maintain normal lung function because scoliosis causes respiratory compromise
- Bony fusion is complete within 9 months postoperative; best seen on 60° supine/oblique projections
- Types of surgery
  - Anterior approach: Dwyer cable; screws in lateral vertebral bodies are fastened with cable
  - Posterior approach: Harrington rod placement to achieve fusion of vertebrae
- Evaluate hardware: slippage or fracture of brackets, Harrington rod, or Dwyer cable

Rotation grading

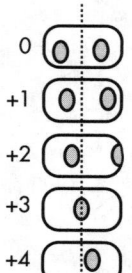

Cobb method

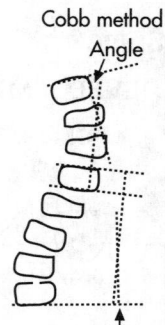

CERVICAL SPINE INJURIES

Cervical spine injuries are uncommon in children.
Pseudosubluxation
Physiological anterior displacement of C2 or C3 due to normal laxity of ligaments of the cervical spine:
- C2/C3 (25% of children < 8 years): normal up to 3 mm (posterior line maintains alignment)
- C3/C4: 15% of children < 8 years

Physiologic subluxation

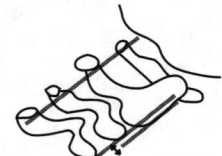

Traumatic spondylolisthesis

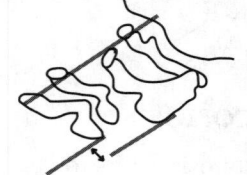

Differential Diagnosis

Chest

STRIDOR, WHEEZING

- Upper airway obstruction
- Tracheal lesions
- Rings and slings
- Foreign bodies
- Asthma

UPPER AIRWAY OBSTRUCTION

Inflammation
- Epiglottitis (*H. influenzae*)
- Croup (respiratory syncytial virus)
- Retropharyngeal abscess

Exogenous
- Caustic injection
- Foreign body

Extrinsic upper airway compression
- Thyroglossal duct cysts
- Branchial cleft cysts
- Other masses

BUBBLY LUNGS IN NEONATES

- Bronchopulmonary dysplasia (most common)
- Pulmonary interstitial emphysema
- Cystic fibrosis
- Wilson-Mikity syndrome (form of bronchopulmonary dysplasia)

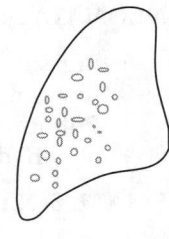

MASS LESIONS IN THE AIRWAYS

Lymphangioma and hemangioma may occur in any of the 3 locations
  Nasal cavity, nasopharynx
- Antrochoanal polyp
- Meningoencephalocele
- Angiofibroma
- Lymphadenopathy
- Neuroblastoma
- Rhabdomyosarcoma

Oropharynx
- Lymphadenopathy
- Ectopic thyroid tissue

Hypopharynx, larynx, or trachea
- Retention cysts
- Papillomas

NEONATAL LUNG MASSES

Lung bases; costophrenic angle obliterated
- Sequestration
- Congenital diaphragmatic hernia
- CCAM (first few hours of life)
- Hypoplastic lung (scimitar syndrome)
- Phrenic nerve paralysis: elevation of hemidiaphragm

Other lung zones
- Pulmonary tumor
    Neuroblastoma
    Pulmonary blastoma
    PNET (Askin tumor)
- Congenital lobar emphysema (only early in disease, later lobar emphysema will be partially aerated)

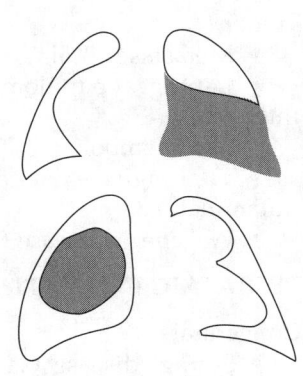

HYPERLUCENT LUNG

- Large anterior pneumothorax (common)
- Congenital lobar emphysema
- Congenital lung cyst
- Bronchiolitis obliterans (Swyer-James syndrome, not until > 7 years)
- Obstructive emphysema
    Obstruction at bronchiolar level: cystic fibrosis, asthma, pneumonia
    Foreign body
    Extrinsic compression: rings and slings, adenopathy, bronchogenic cyst
- CCAM

11

NEONATAL PNEUMOTHORAX

- Pressure ventilation
- Interstitial pulmonary emphysema
- Pulmonary hypoplasia (fetal anuria syndrome, Potter sequence, oligohydramnios)

SMALL SOLITARY PULMONARY NODULE

Congenital
- Bronchogenic cyst (common); 65% arise in lung, 35% from tracheobronchial tree
- Sequestration
- AVM, varix
- Bronchial atresia

Infection
- Round pneumonia, most common
- Granuloma
- Abscess cavity

Tumor
- Primary: PNET, pulmonary blastoma
- Neuroblastoma, Wilms' tumor metastases

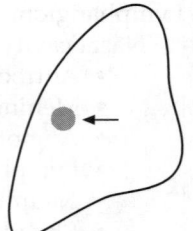

MULTIPLE PULMONARY NODULES

Tumor
- Metastases: Wilms' tumor, teratoma, rhabdomyosarcoma, osteosarcoma (OSA)
- Laryngeal papillomatosis (pulmonary lesions are rare)

Infection
- Septic emboli
- TB, fungus

Inflammatory
- Wegener's disease (sinuses also involved)

PEDIATRIC INTERSTITIAL PATTERN

Congenital
- Storage disease: Gaucher's, Nieman-Pick
- Lymphangiectasia (severe disease, usually fatal by 1-2 years)

Other common causes
- Viral pneumonia
- Bronchopulmonary dysplasia
- Hyaline membrane disease
- Histiocytosis X

PEDIATRIC CHEST WALL TUMORS

Common signs: pleural effusion, rib destruction, soft tissue density
- Eosinophilic granuloma (EG)
- Askin tumor (PNET)
- Neuroblastoma
- Metastases
- Ewing's sarcoma

Abdomen

DILATED STOMACH

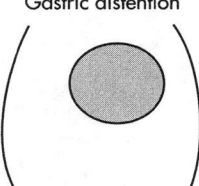

Gastric distention

A dilated air-filled stomach may be due to gastric outlet obstruction (no or little distal gas, permanent dilated stomach, contractile waves) but is most commonly due to air-swallowing during crying (normal distal gas, temporary distention occurs, no contractile waves). Causes of gastric outlet obstruction:
- Hypertrophic pyloric stenosis
- Pylorospasm
- Antral web
- Antral gastritis
- Rare
    Duplication cysts
    Ectopic pancreatic tissue
    Polyps, neoplasm

DOUBLE BUBBLE

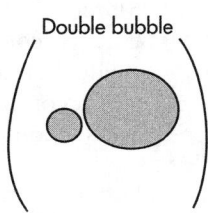

Double bubble

Gas in stomach and duodenal bulb with no or little gas distally is indicative of duodenal obstruction:
- Duodenal atresia (associated with Down syndrome) or stenosis, most common
- Annular pancreas, 2nd most common
- Duodenal diaphragm, bands
- Midgut volvulus, most important entity to diagnose because of high mortality if undiagnosed). Clinical: bilious vomiting.
- Vascular
    Preduodenal vein
    SMA syndrome
- Rare
    Duplication cysts
    Adhesions

PROXIMAL BOWEL OBSTRUCTION

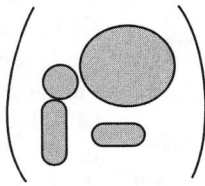

Neonates (congenital causes)
- Atresia/stenosis of small bowel
- Midgut volvulus
- Ladd's bands

Children (> 1 year)
- Intussusception (most common)
- Incarcerated inguinal hernia (6-24 months)
- Perforated appendicitis

11

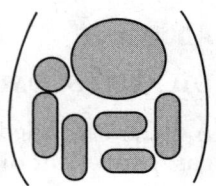

DISTAL BOWEL OBSTRUCTION

- Hirschsprung's disease
- Meconium plug syndrome
- Colonic atresia/stenosis
- Imperforate anus
- Meconium ileus
- Rare causes:
    Volvulus
    Presacral tumors
    Post-NEC strictures

MICROCOLON

Criteria: narrowed (unused) colon. The diagnosis is usually established by barium enema. Causes:

- Diabetic mothers
- Maternal $MgSO_4$ use
- Unused colon (no fecal material or succus has passed through the colon)
    Ileal atresia
    Meconium ileus
- Total colonic Hirschsprung's disease

Pearls

- Differentiation of small and large bowel in infants is not possible; refer to proximal and distal bowel
- In patients with low obstructions proceed to enema (water-soluble isoosmolar agents preferred over barium)
- Patients with meconium ileus almost always (98%) have cystic fibrosis. 10%-20% of patients with cystic fibrosis have meconium ileus.

PEDIATRIC PNEUMATOSIS INTESTINALIS

- Necrotizing enterocolitis
- Less common causes (benign pneumatosis; pathogenesis unclear)
    Cystic fibrosis
    Collagen vascular disease
    Leukemia
    Milk intolerance
    Immunodeficiency
- Obstruction
- Steroid use

GASLESS ABDOMEN

After birth, air appears normally in the GI tract: stomach, 2 hours; small bowel, 6 hours; rectum, 24 hours. Causes of gasless abdomen:

Severe vomiting, most common
- Gastroenteritis
- Appendicitis

Impaired swallowing
- Esophageal atresia
- Neurologic impairment
- Mechanical ventilation (paralyzed bowel)

Displaced bowel loops
- Bowel not in abdomen (e.g., hernia, omphalocele)
- Masses
- Ascites

ABDOMINAL CALCIFICATIONS

- Intraabdominal: meconium peritonitis (most common)
- Renal
     Neuroblastoma, Wilms' tumor
     Nephrocalcinosis
     Renal cysts
     Urinary tract calculus
- Bowel: fecalith of appendix, Meckel's diverticulum
- Bladder: hemorrhagic cystitis (Cytoxan therapy)
- Adrenal: hemorrhage, Wolman's disease (very rare)
- Cholelithiasis (sickle cell anemia)
- Liver: hepatoblastoma, granuloma

COMMON ABDOMINAL MASS LESIONS

OVERVIEW	
Neonates (< 1 month)	**Older Infants and Children**
RENAL, 55%	**RENAL, 55%**
Hydronephrosis	Wilms' tumor
MCDK	Hydronephrosis
GASTROINTESTINAL, 15%	**GASTROINTESTINAL, 15%**
Duplication	Appendiceal abscess
Meconium pseudocyst	Intussusception
Pseudocyst proximal to atresia	Neoplasm
RETROPERITONEAL, 10%	**RETROPERITONEAL, 25%**
Adrenal hemorrhage	Neuroblastoma
GENITAL, 15%	**GENITAL, 5%**
Ovarian cyst	Ovarian cyst
Hydrometrocolpos	Hydrometrocolpos
HEPATOBILIARY, 5%	**HEPATOBILIARY, 5%**
Hemangioendothelioma	Hepatoblastoma
Choledochal cyst	

11

GASTRIC FILLING DEFECT

- Foreign bodies, most common
- Lactobezoar (improperly prepared milk), phytobezoars, trichobezoars
- Congenital anomalies
    Duplications
    Ectopic pancreatic tissue
- Inflammation, rare
    Crohn's disease
    Chronic granulomatous diseases (immunodeficiency of the phagocytosis
        type)
- Tumors, rare
    Hamartoma
    Peutz-Jeghers disease

THICK FOLDS

Submucosal edema
- Enteritis

Submucosal tumor
- Lymphoma, leukemia

Submucosal hemorrhage
- Henoch-Schönlein purpura
- Hemolytic uremic syndrome
- Coagulopathies (e.g., hemophilia, vitamin K, anticoagulants)

GI HEMORRHAGE

- Meckel diverticulum
- Juvenile polyps
- Inflammatory bowel disease
- Portal hypertension

PEDIATRIC LIVER LESIONS

Benign
- Cysts
- Hemangioendothelioma
- Mesenchymal hamartoma

Malignant
- Hepatoblastoma
- Hemangioendothelioma (neonate)
- Hepatocellular carcinoma, if there is underlying liver disease (glycogen storage disorders, portal venous hypertension)
- Metastases from Wilms' tumor or neuroblastoma

FATTY LIVER

- Chronic protein malnutrition (most common cause)
- Congenital
    Cystic fibrosis
    Glycogen storage disease
    Wilson's disease
    Galactosemia
    Fructose intolerance
    Reye's syndrome
- Hepatitis
- Drugs: chemotherapy, steroids, hyperalimentation

PEDIATRIC CHOLELITHIASIS

Hemolysis
- Sickle cell anemia (small spleen)
- Thalassemia (large spleen)
- Spherocystosis
Other
- Cystic fibrosis
- Drugs: furosemide
- Metabolic disorders: hyperparathyroidism (HPT)
- Premature infants with hyaline membrane disease

HYDROPS OF GALLBLADDER

- Sepsis
- Burns
- Leptospirosis
- Kawasaki disease

CHOLECYSTITIS

- Sickle cell
- Hemolytic anemia

BILARY STRICTURES

- Pancreatitis
- Gallstones
- Ascending cholangitis
- Post-Kasai procedure
- Liver transplant

FATTY REPLACEMENT OF PANCREAS

- Cystic fibrosis
- Schwachman: Diamond syndrome:
    Metaphyseal dysplasia
    Cyclic neutropenia
    Pancreatic fatty replacement
    Flaring of ribs

11

PEDIATRIC PANCREATITIS

- Trauma
- Viral infection
- Sepsis
- Idiopathic
- Anomaly
- Drugs (steroids, etc.)
- Metabolic
    Cystic fibrosis
    Hyperlipidemia

Genitourinary System

CYSTIC RENAL MASSES

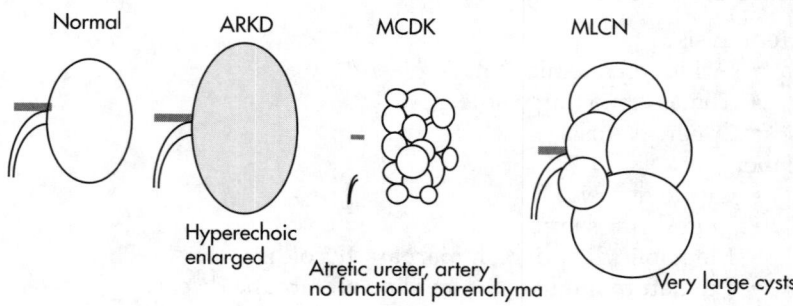

Cystic disease (differentiate from
  hydronephrosis)
- Autosomal recessive kidney
  disease (infantile polycystic
  kidney disease)
- Multicystic dysplastic kidney
- Multilocular nephroma
- Cysts associated with
  phakomatoses
    von Hippel-Lindau disease
    Tuberous sclerosis
- Other cystic diseases (see Chapter 4)
Tumors
- Cystic Wilms' tumor
- Cystic adenocarcinoma

HYDRONEPHROSIS

Most common abdominal mass in neonates. Causes (in decreasing order of
frequency):
- Reflux
- UVJ obstruction
- Ureterovesical obstruction
- Ectopic ureterocele
- Posterior urethral valves
- Prune belly

SOLID RENAL MASSES

- Wilms' tumor: most common solid tumor in children; rare in newborn
- Mesoblastic nephroma: the only solid renal mass lesion in newborns
- Nephroblastomatosis: subcortical masses; associated with Wilms' tumor
- Angiomyolipoma: fatty mass; associated with tuberous sclerosis
- Secondary tumors
    Lymphoma
    Neuroblastoma
    Leukemia: diffuse, bilateral enlargement
- Rare renal tumors
    Clear cell sarcoma
    Malignant rhabdoid
    Renal cell carcinoma

DIFFUSELY HYPERECHOIC RENAL KIDNEY IN NEWBORN

Increased size
- ARPCKD (bladder is usually empty)
- CMV glomerulonephritis (bladder may have some urine)
- Glomerular cystic disease
- Diffuse cystic dysplasia

Decreased size
- Renal dysplasia from obstructive uropathy or necrosis

ECHOGENIC KIDNEY (CORTEX SIMILAR TO SPLEEN OR LIVER WITH PRESERVED CORTICOMEDULLARY DIFFERENTIATION)

- ATN
- Glomerulonephritis
- Renal infiltration
- Glycogen storage disease
- Diabetes
- Renal vein thrombosis
- Leukemia is the only malignancy causing this appearance
- HIV
- Kawasaki disease

LOSS OF NORMAL CORTICOMEDULLARY DIFFERENTIATION

- Pyelonephritis; focal nephronia
- Infantile polycystic kidney
- Adult polycystic kidney
- Medullary cystic kidney
- Late renal vein thrombosis

11

MEDULLARY NEPHROCALCINOSIS

- Furosemide therapy
- Hyperparathyroidism
- RTA (distal tubular defect)
- Hypercalcemia or hypercalciuria
    Milk alkali
    Idiopathic hypercalciuria
    Sarcoidosis
    Hypervitaminosis D
- Oxalosis
- Medullary sponge

CONGENITAL URETERIC OBSTRUCTION

- Primary megaureter
- Ureterocele (ectopic or orthotopic)
- Distal ureteral stenosis
- Ureteral atresia
- Circumcaval ureter
- Bladder diverticulum

ADRENAL MASS

- Neonatal hemorrhage, common
- Neuroblastoma
- Rare adrenal pediatric tumors
    Teratoma
    Adenoma
    Carcinoma
    Pheochromocytoma
- Other retroperitoneal masses
    Wilms' tumor
    Hydronephrotic upper pole
    Retroperitoneal adenopathy
    Hepatoblastoma
    Splenic mass

CYSTIC STRUCTURE IN OR NEAR BLADDER WALL (US)

Bladder
- Hutch diverticulum
- Urachal remnant (dome of the bladder)
- Normal "bladder ears" (incompletely filled bladder extends into femoral/inguinal canal)

Ureter
- Ectopic insertion of ureter
- Ureterocele
- Megaureter

Other
- Ovarian cyst
- Mesenteric, omental cyst

LARGE ABDOMINAL CYSTIC MASS

- Lymphangioma (multiseptated noncalcified)
- Enteric duplication cyst (unilocular non calcified with bowel signature)
- Meconium pseudocyst (unilocular containing echoes and debris)
- Choledochal cyst
- Adrenal hemorrhage
- Ovarian cyst

PRESACRAL MASS

- Rectal duplication
- Anterior meningocele
- Teratoma
- Neuroblastoma

INTERLABIAL MASS

- Ectopic ureterocele
- Periurethral cysts
- Rhabdomyosarcoma of vagina
- Prolapsed urethra
- Imperforate hymen

Central Nervous System

ENLARGED HEAD (MACROCEPHALY)

Hydrocephalus (most common cause of enlargement before closure of sutures)
- Communicating (more common)
- Noncommunicating (less common)

Rare causes
- Subdural hematoma
- Calvarial abnormalities
    Benign macrocrania
    Chondrodystrophies
- Brain abnormalities
    Beckwith-Wiedemann syndrome
    Hemiatrophy
    Cerebral gigantism

SMALL HEAD (MICROCEPHALY)

- Absent or atrophic brain (congenital infection, fetal alcohol syndrome)
- Craniosynostosis
- Shunt placement

THICK SKULL

Metabolic/systemic
- Healing stage of renal osteodystrophy
- Hyperparathyroidism (salt and pepper skull)
- Anemias (compensatory hematopoiesis): sickle cell disease, thalassemia

11

Tumor
- Leukemia, lymphoma

Other
- Chronic decreased intracranial pressure (shunts; most common cause of calvarial thickening)
- Dilantin therapy
- Dysplasia
   Fibrous dysplasia
   Engelmann's disease

LYTIC SKULL LESIONS

- EG
- Leukemia, lymphoma
- Fibrous dysplasia
- Dermoid, epidermoid
- Hyperparathyroidism

INTRACRANIAL CALCIFICATION

Differentiate abnormal from physiological intracranial calcifications. The latter include:
- Choroid plexus calcification
- Habenula calcification
- Pineal gland calcification
- Falx: dura, pacchionian bodies calcification
- Hemangioblastoma calcification

Abnormal calcifications have a wide differential (mnemonic: "TIC MTV"):

Tumor
- Children: craniopharyngioma > oligodendroglioma > gliomas > other tumors
- Adults: meningioma > oligodendroglioma > ependymoma

Infection
- Children: TORCH
- Adults: cysticerosis, TB

Congenital, degenerative, atrophic lesions
- Congenital atrophy or hypoplasia
- Tuberous sclerosis (75% have calcifications)
- Sturge-Weber syndrome (tramtrack gyral calcifications)

Metabolic
- Idiopathic hypercalcemia
- Lead poisoning (rare today)
- Hypoparathyroidism
- Fahr's disease (familial)

Trauma

Vascular lesions
- AVMs (vein of Galen aneurysm)
- Hematoma
- Aneurysms

ENLARGED SELLA TURCICA

- Tumor (most common cause)
  - Craniopharyngioma, most common
  - Optic chiasm, hypothalamic glioma, 2nd most common
  - Less common: germ cell tumors, meningioma, pituitary adenoma
- Increased intracranial pressure
- Empty sella
- Nelson's disease

Musculoskeletal

COMMON PEDIATRIC BONE TUMORS

Primary
- EG
- Ewing's sarcoma
- OSA
- Bone cysts
  - UBC: (single cavity, fallen fragment sign)
  - ABC: eccentric

Secondary
- Neuroblastoma metastases
- Lymphoma
- Leukemia

Tumors with fluid-fluid level
- ABC
- Telangiectatic OSA
- Giant cell tumor
- Single cysts with pathological fracture

WIDENED JOINT SPACE

Widened joint spaces in pediatric patients are most commonly seen in hip joint or shoulders; other joints have strong capsules. Causes of widened joint space:

Joint effusion
- Septic arthritis
- Hemarthrosis (intraarticular fracture, hemophiliac)
- Transient toxic synovitis (viral)
- JRA

Synovial thickening without articular cartilage destruction
- JRA
- Hemophiliac arthropathy

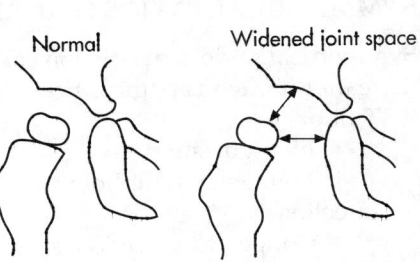

BOWED BONES

Anterior and posterior bowing (fetal malposition) is always abnormal. Anterior bowing may be associated with medial and lateral bowing. Isolated medial bowing is usually idiopathic. Common causes of anterior bowing:

Metabolic
- Rickets (most common)

Dysplasia
- Neurofibromatosis (primary bone dysplasia)
- Osteogenesis imperfecta
- Fibrous dysplasia

DIFFUSE PEDIATRIC OSTEOPENIA

- Rickets
- Hyperparathyroidism (secondary to renal disease = renal rickets)
- Immobilization
- JRA
- Uncommon causes
    Infiltrative disease: gangliosidosis, mucolipidosis
    Same causes as in adults (see previous sections)

DIFFUSELY DENSE BONES IN CHILDREN

Congenital
- Osteopetrosis
- Pyknodysostosis
- Melorheostosis
- Progressive diaphyseal dysplasia (Engelmann's disease)
- Infantile cortical hyperostosis
- Idiopathic hypercalcemia of infancy (Williams syndrome)
- Generalized cortical hyperostosis (van Buchem's disease)
- Pachydermoperiostosis

Other
- Hypothyroidism
- Congenital syphilis
- Hypervitaminosis D

SYMMETRICAL PERIOSTEAL REACTION IN CHILDREN

Symmetrical periosteal reaction can be physiological during first 6 months of life; thereafter it often is pathological. Wide differential (mnemonic: "TIC MTV").

Symmetrical periosteal reaction

Tumor
- Neuroblastoma
- Leukemia, lymphoma

Infection
- Congenital infection: syphilis, rubella

Congenital
- Caffey's disease (infantile cortical hyperostosis)
- Osteogenesis imperfecta

Metabolic
- Hypervitaminosis A, D
- Prostaglandin E therapy
- Scurvy

Trauma
- Battered child syndrome (subperiosteal hematoma)

Vascular
- Bone infarctions (sickle cell disease)

Mnemonic for periosteal reaction: "SCALP"
- **S**curvy
- **C**affey's disease
- **A**ccident, hypervitaminosis A
- **L**eukemia, lues
- **P**hysiological, prostaglandin inhibitors

DEFORMED EPIPHYSIS

Epiphyseal defect may be solitary (e.g., osteochondritis dissecans), cause complete fragmentation of epiphysis, or affect multiple epiphyses (syndromes).

Acquired (single epiphysis)
- Avascular necrosis:
    LCP disease (most common)
    Steroids
- Trauma (osteochondritis dissecans)
- Infection
- Hypothyroidism

Congenital dysplasia (multiple epiphysis, all rare)
- Multiple epiphyseal dysplasia
- Myer's dysplasia
- Morquio's syndrome

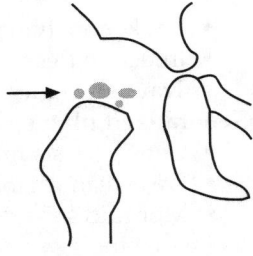

ENLARGED EPIPHYSIS

Most commonly caused by hyperemia associated with chronic arthritis.
- Hemophiliac joints
- JRA
- Chronic infectious arthritis
- Healed LCP disease
- Epiphyseal dysplasia hemimelia (Trevor's)

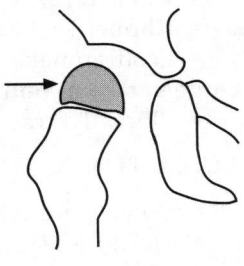

TRANSVERSE METAPHYSEAL LINES

Transverse metaphyseal bands are the result of abnormal enchondral bone growth; undermineralization leads to lucent lines and repair leads to dense metaphyseal lines. In some diseases, dense and lucent lines coexist.

Lucent lines
- Neonates: stress lines (hypoperfusion of rapidly growing metaphyses of long bones) due to fever, congenital heart disease, any severe disease
- > 2 years of age consider tumors:
    Neuroblastoma metastases
    Lymphoma, leukemia

Dense lines
- Neonates: growth recovery lines
- > 2 years of age:
    Heavy metal poisoning (lead bands)
    Healing rickets

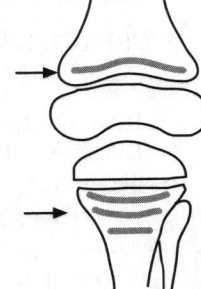

WIDENED GROWTH PLATE

Widened growth plate: > 1 mm.
- Rickets (most common)
- Salter-Harris fracture, type 1
- Tumor: lymphoma, leukemia, neuroblastoma
- Infection: osteomyelitis

11

METAPHYSEAL FRAGMENTS

- Battered child (corner fractures)
- Trauma
- Blount's disease
- Osteomyelitis

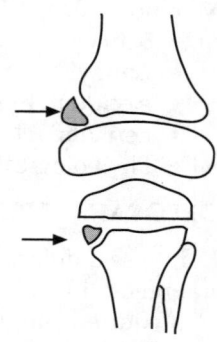

VERTEBRAL ABNORMALITIES

Vertebra plana (localized platyspondyly)
- Metastases (neuroblastoma most common)
- EG
- Leukemia, lymphoma
- Infection (less common)
- Trauma

Generalized platyspondyly (decreased height of vertebral body)
- Osteogenesis imperfecta
- Dwarfism (thanatophoric, metatropic)
- Morquio's syndrome
- Cushing's syndrome

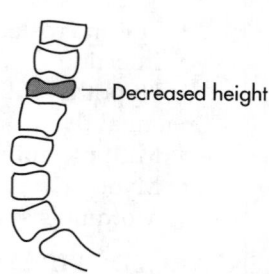

Fused vertebrae
- Isolated fusion of vertebral bodies
- Klippel-Feil syndrome (C2-C3 fusion, torticollis, short neck)
- Posttraumatic

Large vertebral body, or other abnormal shapes
- Blood dyscrasia (expansion of red marrow): sickle cell, thalassemia

ALTLANTOAXIAL SUBLUXATION

- Down syndrome
- Morquio's syndrome
- JRA
- Trauma

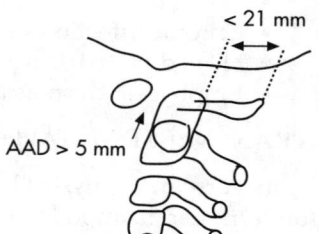

DISK SPACE NARROWING

Common
- Infection (pyogenic, tuberculous, brucella, typhoid)
- Block vertebra: congenital or acquired
- Scheuermann's disease
- Severe kyphosis or scoliosis

Uncommon
- Congenital
- Cockayne
- Kniest dysplasia
- Morquio's syndrome
- Spondyloepiphyseal dysplasia

Acquired
- Inflammatory arthritis (rheumatoid, anklylosing spondylitis)
- Herniated disk
- Neuropathic arthropathy (syrinx)
- Trauma

Enlarged disk space
- Osteoporosis
- Biconcave vertebra due to several causes
- Gaucher's disease
- Platyspondyly
- Sickle cell anemia
- Trauma

Intervertebral disk space calcification

Common
- Idiopathic (transient in children)
- Posttraumatic

Uncommon
- Spinal fusion
- Ochronosis
- Aarskog syndrome
- Ankylosing spondylitis
- Cockayne's syndrome
- Homocystinuria
- Hypercalcemia
- Hyperparathyroidism
- Hypervitaminosis D
- Infection
- Paraplegia
- Juvenile chronic arthritis

PEDIATRIC SACRAL ABNORMALITIES

- Meningocele
- Neurofibromatosis
- Presacral teratoma
- Agenesis

RADIAL RAY DEFICIENCY

Absence of 1st and/or 2nd digits of hand; often involves radius.
- Holt-Oram syndrome (cardiac, chest wall anomalies)
- Poland's syndrome
- Fanconi's anemia
- Thrombocytopenia–absent radius syndrome

POLYDACTYLY

- Familial polydactyly
- Chondroectodermal dysplasia (Ellis-van Creveld syndrome)
- Trisomies 13-15
- Laurence-Moon-Bardet-Biedel syndrome

ABNORMAL 4TH METACARPAL

Short metacarpal
- Turner's syndrome
- Growth arrest: sickle cell disease, infections

Long metacarpal
- Macrodystrophia lipomatosa
- Neurofibromatosis

11

DELAYED BONE AGE

Systemic diseases (most common)
- Hypothyroidism (cretinism; typical: hypoplastic T12 and L1)
- Cyanotic congenital heart failure
- Chronic pulmonary disease

HGH deficiency (pituitary dwarfism)
- Isolated HGH deficiency
- Craniopharyngioma, infections

Peripheral tissue nonresponsive to HGH
- African pygmies
- Turner's syndrome
- Constitutional short stature

HEMIHYPERTROPHY

Enlargement of an extremity (rare).
- Intraabdominal tumors (frequently Wilms')
- Arteriovenous fistula
- Lymphangioma
- Isolated anomaly (idiopathic)

Other

DOWN SYNDROME

- Duodenal atresia
- Tracheoesophageal fistula, esophageal atresia
- Endocardial cushion defect
- Hirschsprung's disease
- Multiple sternal ossification centers
- 11 ribs

WILLIAMS SYNDROME (INFANTILE IDIOPATHIC HYPERCALCEMIA)

- Aortic stenosis (supravalvular)
- Peripheral pulmonic stenosis
- Diffuse coarctation of abdominal aorta and stenosis of visceral branches
- Multisystem abnormalities
      Retardation
      Dentation abnormalities
      Elfin facies

BECKWITH-WIEDEMANN SYNDROME

- Macroglossia
- Visceromegaly (e.g., liver, kidneys , pancreas, etc.)
- Gigantism
- Omphalocele
- Wilms' tumor

PREMATURE INFANTS

- Hyaline membrane disease
- Necrotizing enterocolitis
- Germinal matrix hemorrhage
- Periventricular leukoencephalopathy
- PDA

SUGGESTED READINGS

Barr L, editor: *Handbook of pediatric imaging,* New York, 1991, Churchill Livingstone.

Blickman JG: *Pediatric radiology: the requisites,* St Louis, 1998, Mosby.

Donnelly LF: *Fundamentals of pediatric radiology,* Philadelphia, 2001, WB Saunders.

Kirks DR: *Practical pediatric imaging: diagnostic radiology of infants and children,* Philadelphia, 1997, Lippincott Williams & Wilkins.

Kleinman PK: *Diagnostic imaging of child abuse,* Baltimore, 1987, Williams & Wilkins.

Seibert JJ, James CA: *Pediatric radiology casebase: the baby minnie of pediatric radiology,* New York, 1998, Thieme Medical Publishers.

Silverman FN, Kuhn JP: *Caffey's pediatric x-ray diagnosis: an integrated imaging approach,* St Louis, 1993, Mosby.

Stringer DA: *Pediatric gastrointestinal imaging,* Toronto, 2000, BC Decker.

Swischuk LE: *Emergency radiology of the acutely ill of injured child,* Philadelphia, 2000, Lippincott Williams & Wilkins.

Swischuk LE: *Imaging of the newborn, infant, and young child,* Philadelphia, 1997, Lippincott Williams & Wilkins.

11

Chapter 12

Nuclear Imaging

Chapter Outline

Pulmonary Imaging

Radiopharmaceuticals

Pulmonary scintigraphy uses ventilation agents and/or perfusion agents, depending on the specific imaging task.

OVERVIEW				
Agent	**Half-Life**	**Main Energy**	**Collimator**	**Comments**
VENTILATION				
^{133}Xe	5.2 days	81	Low	Cheap; washout images helpful
^{127}Xe	36.4 days	203	Medium	Postperfusion imaging possible (high energy)
^{81m}Kr	13 sec	191	Medium	Postperfusion imaging possible; limited availability
^{99m}Tc DTPA aerosol	6 hr	140 keV	Low	Delivery not as good as with gases; multiple projections possible
PERFUSION				
^{99m}Tc MAA	6 hr	140 keV	Low	

If both ventilation (V) and perfusion (Q) imaging are performed (V/Q scan), the ventilation imaging part is usually performed first because the 81-keV ^{133}Xe photon energy lies in the range of significant Compton downscatter of the 140 keV ^{99m}Tc photon. Examination rooms must have negative internal pressure so that escaped Xe is not recirculated to other areas. Exhaled Xe can be vented to the outside atmosphere.

^{133}XENON

^{133}Xe is the most commonly used ventilation agent. It is relatively cheap and has a physical half-life of 5.2 days. Xe is a inert gas that distributes to lung spaces through normally ventilated areas. 3 phases of distribution are usually distinguishable although the biological half-life is less than 1 minute:

- Inspiration (15-20 seconds)
- Equilibrium (patient breathes Xe/O_2 mixture in a closed system for 3-5 minutes)
- Washout (patient breathes room air and exhales into charcoal trap)

Less than 15% of inhaled gas is absorbed in the body. Since Xe is highly soluble in fat, it localizes to liver and fatty tissues once absorbed. Xe also adsorbs onto plastic syringes (10% at 24 hours), for which reason glass syringes are used for handling. Cannot perform xenon ventilation on portable basis, as negative pressure is required to remove gas. Technetium aerosol can be used for portable scans.

^{127}XENON

^{127}Xe has a similar pharmacological behavior to ^{133}Xe. However, its physical half-life is longer (36.4 days vs. 5.2 days), it is more expensive, and its main photon energy is higher (203 vs. 81 keV). Because of the higher photon energy, ventilation imaging can be performed after the ^{99m}Tc MAA scan (140 keV main energy). Thus the best projection for ventilation imaging can be selected based on the perfusion scan. The high energy of the nuclide requires a medium-energy collimator so that collimators have to be changed between perfusion and ventilation study.

^{81m}KRYPTON

The availability of ^{81m}Kr/⁸¹Rb generators is the major limitation of using this nuclide. Because of the short physical half-life (13.4 seconds), washout images cannot be obtained, limiting the sensitivity for detection of obstructive lung disease. As with ¹²⁷Xe, ventilation imaging can be performed after the ^{99m}Tc MAA scan. A high main photon energy of 191 keV requires the use of a medium-energy collimator (lower resolution, collimators have to be changed during the study). The short half-life of ^{81m}Kr results in images comparable to xenon washin images, even though the images are obtained with continuous breathing of krypton. The higher energy of krypton permits ventilation imaging either before or after perfusion imaging. Because the krypton ventilation images are performed with continuous breathing, it is normal to see some tracer activity in the trachea on the anterior view.

^{99m}Tc DTPA AEROSOL

A large amount (1110-1850 MBq) of activity is loaded into a specially shielded nebulizer that produces droplets containing the radionuclide. Approximately 18 to 28 MBq of activity reaches the lungs during the 3-5 minutes of breathing. Once in the lungs, droplets diffuse through interstitium into capillaries and ^{99m}Tc DTPA is finally excreted renally. Pulmonary clearance usually takes > 1 hour (much faster in smokers, IPF, ARDS), for which reason the aerosol can not be used for single breath or washout phase imaging. Slow pulmonary clearance allows multiple projection images to be obtained typically in the same views as in the perfusion study. Because the aerosol delivers only a small amount of activity (20% of activity used for perfusion imaging), ventilation imaging is performed before perfusion imaging. Alternatively, a reduced dose of MAA (1 mCi) can be given first for perfusion imaging. Particle deposition in large central airways occurs in obstructive lung disease.

^{99m}Tc MACROAGGREGATED ALBUMIN

The theoretical basis for using macroaggregated albumin particles (MAA) in perfusion imaging is that particles become physically trapped in arterioles, thus allowing one to measure regional perfusion. MAA is prepared by heat and pH denaturation of human serum albumin (HSA). For quality assurance purposes, the size of at least 100 particles has to be determined (optimum from 10-90 μm; particles should not be < 10 μm or > 150 μm). 200,000-700,000 MAA particles are injected IV, to occlude precapillary arterioles (20-30 μm) and capillaries (8 μm). Injection of less than 70,000 particles leads to a statistically inaccurate exam (because of quantum mottle). The number of injected particles should be reduced in:
- Pulmonary hypertension
- Neonates, pediatric patients
- Right-to-left shunts

Pharmacokinetics
- > 90% of particles are trapped in lung capillaries during 1st pass (particles < 10 μm are phagocytosed by liver and spleen).
- Approximately 100,000 of the 280 billion capillaries are occluded during a normal lung perfusion scan.
- Particles are cleared from lungs by enzymatic hydrolysis (biological half-life: 2-10 hours).
- Renal clearance of ^{99m}Tc MAA is 30%-40% at 24 hours.
- Because the particle number/dose must be known at time of administration, all doses must be given within 6 hours of preparation.

12

Technique

INDICATIONS

Common indications for pulmonary imaging include:
- Pulmonary embolism (PE)
    - Elective V/Q scan
        - Clinical suspicion of PE (symptomatic patient and risk factors)
        - Baseline posttreatment scan
    - Emergency V/Q scan (e.g., at night)
        - Symptomatic patient and risk factor and normal or abnormal CXR
- Surgical applications
    - Preoperative evaluation of lung function (quantitative)
    - Postsurgical bronchial stump leaks (Xe may show air leak)
    - Transplant rejection (decreased MAA perfusion)
- R-L shunts

CONTRAINDICATIONS

No absolute contraindications exist. Relative contraindications include:
- Pulmonary arterial hypertension (PAH)
- R-L shunts (particles end up in systemic circulation)
- Hypersensitivity to HSA

PROTOCOL

1. Obtain history and risk factors
2. Ventilate patient with ^{133}Xe (370-740 MBq) and image in posterior projection: The gamma energy of xenon is 81 keV and will be attenuated by 10 cm of inflated lung and overlying breast tissue.
    - Initial breath: single image
    - Equilibrium: 2×90-second images
    - Washout: 3×45-second images
    - Retention: LPO, posterior, RPO images of 45 seconds each
3. Injection of ^{99m}Tc MAA (150 MBq) in supine position and image:
    - 6-standard views: posterior, RPO, LPO, anterior, RAO, LAO
    - Lateral views (usually not helpful)

Information that should be obtained in all patients:

CXR (within 12 hours of assessment)
- Normal or minimal lung abnormality on CXR is typical in PE.
- Normal CXR does not exclude PE but facilitates interpretation of a V/Q· scan (i.e., absence of matched hypoventilated/hypoperfused consolidations)

Arterial blood gases
- $Po_2 < 80\%$ is seen in 80% of patients with PE.
- An Aa gradient of > 14 mm Hg is seen in only 90% of patients

Lower extremity US (optional)
- Sensitivity for detecting femoropopliteal deep venous thrombosis (DVT), 95%
- Only approximately 30% of patients with PE have documented DVT

Imaging

NORMAL IMAGES

Xenon ventilation

Homogenous distribution of activity occurs in the 3 phases:

- Washin
- Equilibrium
- Washout; complete clearing should occur within 2-3 minutes

Trapping of Xe on washout is indicative of airway obstruction (e.g., bullae, COPD). Hallmarks of obstructive disease are decreased washin, slow equilibration, and delayed washout.

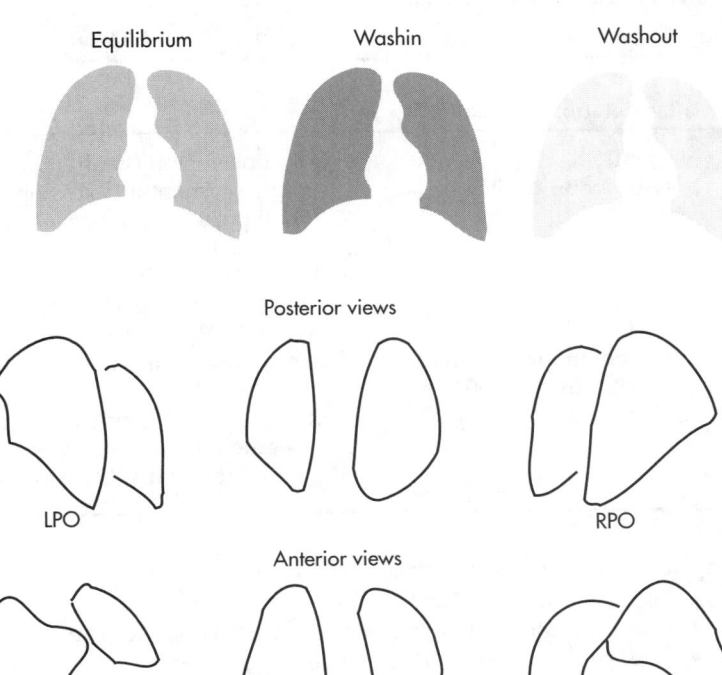

Perfusion

- Normal identifiable structures: heart, aortic arch, fissures
- Anterior indentation on lung on LPO represents the heart
- Slight gradient of activity from posterior to anterior reflects greater perfusion to dependent portions of lung in supine patient
- Activity at apex is usually less than at bases (less parenchymal volume at apex)
- Subsegmental perfusion defects occur in 7% of normal population

PULMONARY EMBOLISM

V/Q imaging requires the use of two sequential tracers: a ventilation (i.e., breathing) agent and a perfusion (i.e., intravascular) agent. Two tracers are used rather than one because altered pulmonary perfusion alone is a nonspecific finding that occurs in many pulmonary diseases, but V/Q mismatches are fairly specific for PE. V/Q mismatch refers to regions of decreased perfusion ("cold") that have normal ventilation. If the perfusion part of the study is normal, PE is excluded and ventilation imaging is not required.

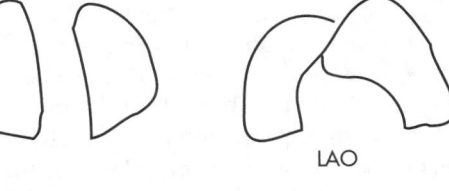

V/Q mismatch (PE)

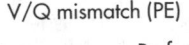

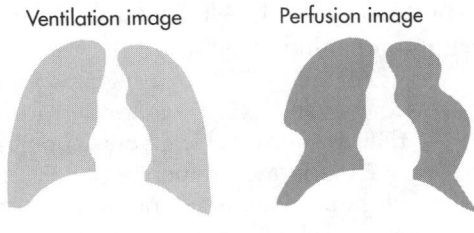

V/Q match (many pulmonary diseases)

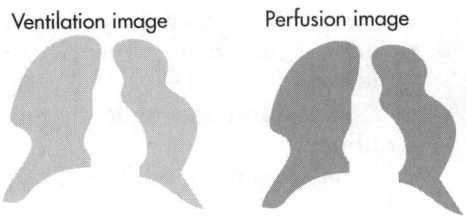

Scheme for interpretation (Prospective Investigation of Pulmonary Embolism Diagnosis, PIOPED)

1. Classify perfusion defects by size and segmental anatomy
   - Small segmental defect: < 25% of pulmonary segment affected
   - Moderate segmental defect: 25%-75% of a pulmonary segment affected
   - Large segmental defect: 75% of pulmonary segment affected
   - Lobar defect
   - Nonsegmental defect
2. Correlate perfusion and ventilation images
3. Cannot interpret study if >75% of a lung zone has obstructive disease

12

INTERPRETATION OF SCAN RESULTS		
Interpretation/Frequency	**Pattern**	**Probability of PE (%)**
Normal, 5%	Normal perfusion (ventilation and CXR may be abnormal)	0-5
Low probability, 55%	1. Single segmental perfusion defect (subsegmental)	10-15
	2. Small perfusion defect	
	3. Any perfusion defect with larger corresponding CXR abnormality	
	4. Nonsegmental perfusion abnormalities	
	5. Matched V/Q abnormalities	
Intermediate probability (indeterminate), 30%	Any scan not falling into high or low probability group	30-40
High probability, 10%	1. 2 segmental V/Q mismatches	90-95
	2. 1 segmental and > 2 subsegmental V/Q defects	
	3. 4 subsegmental V/Q mismatches	

Implications of scan results
- High probability: treat for PE
- Intermediate/indeterminate: pulmonary angiogram
- Low probability: unlikely to be PE. Consider other diagnoses. Obtain pulmonary angiogram if clinical suspicion remains very high
- Normal perfusion study excludes PE

V/Q scan to monitor sequelae/resolution of PE
- Most PE perfusion abnormalities resolve within 3 months. Thus a baseline posttreatment scan should be obtained several months after initial diagnosis.
- Baseline scans are helpful to diagnose recurrent PE.
- Acute perfusion defects tend to be sharply defined; old or resolving perfusion defects tend to be less well-defined.

Modified PIOPED criteria for scan interpretation
High probability > 80%
- > 2 large (> 75% of a segment) segmental perfusion defects without corresponding ventilation or radiographic abnormalities, or substantially larger than either matching ventilation or chest roentgenogram abnormalities
- > 2 moderate segmental (> 25% and < 75% of a segment) perfusion defects without matching ventilation or chest roentgenogram abnormalities and 1 large mismatched segmental defect
- > 4 moderate segmental perfusion defects without ventilation or chest roentgenogram abnormalities

Intermediate (indeterminate) probability, 20%-80%
- Single moderate mismatched segmental perfusion defect with normal chest radiograph
- One large and one moderate mismatched segmental defect with a normal radiograph
- Not falling into normal/very low, low, or high probability categories

Low probability, < 20%
- Any perfusion defect with a substantially larger chest roentgenogram abnormality
- Large or moderate segmental perfusion defects involving no more than 50% of the combined lung fields with matching ventilation defects either equal to or larger in size, and chest roentgenogram either normal or with abnormalities substantially larger than perfusion defects
- Any number of small segmental perfusion defects with a normal chest roentgenogram

Pearls
- Small perfusion defects (rat bites) almost never represent PE
- If ventilation abnormalities occupy > 75% of lung, PIOPED criteria classify the abnormality as indeterminate or nondiagnostic for PE
- If etiology of a matched V/Q abnormalities and CXR abnormality is unknown then scan is classified as indeterminate
- Intermediate and indeterminate scans have the same diagnostic significance (i.e., a PE has not been ruled in or ruled out). Some radiologists use the terms interchangeably

OTHER PATTERNS

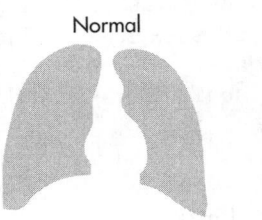
Normal

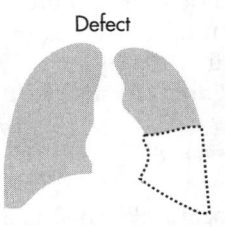
Defect

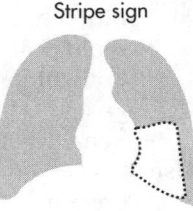
Stripe sign

Stripe sign
This sign refers to a perfusion abnormality with a zone of preserved peripheral perfusion. Because PE is pleural based, presence of this sign makes PE unlikely.

Reverse mismatch
Normal perfusion with abnormal ventilation. Most commonly due to atelectasis

Pulmonary edema
- Redistribution of blood away from dependent portions of the lung
- Pleural effusions, fissural "highlighting"

Bullae, emphysema, COPD
- Delayed washout on ventilation images: air trapping
- Matched V/Q defects

Pulmonary arterial hypertension
Diffusely heterogeneous perfusion with many small perfusion abnormalities

Transplant
- Poor perfusion to lung apices may be normal after lung transplant

EVALUATION OF LUNG FUNCTION

Commonly performed in patients undergoing lung resection. Using a computer program, the overall ventilation and perfusion of each lung is determined.

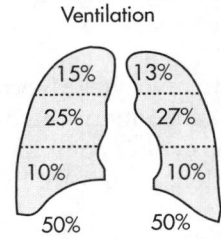
Ventilation

15%	13%
25%	27%
10%	10%
50%	50%

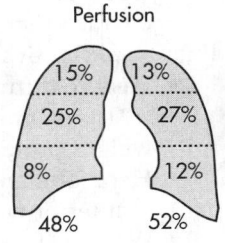
Perfusion

15%	13%
25%	27%
8%	12%
48%	52%

12

Cardiac Imaging

Radiopharmaceuticals

^{201}THALLIUM CHLORIDE

^{201}Tl ("perfusion marker") is cyclotron produced. It distributes proportionally to cardiac output in all tissues except brain (because of intact blood-brain barrier) and fat. Cellular uptake occurs in any tissue if the cellular Na^+/K^+ pump is intact.

Pharmacokinetics

- Myocardial extraction: 3%-4% of total dose (at rest). Localization in myocardium occurs in 2 phases:

    Intial distribution and cellular extraction based on blood flow, which is close to 90%

    Delayed "redistribution" based on continued extraction of thallium from blood and ongoing washout of previously extracted thallium

    Unlike the reextraction of thallium by myocardium the washout component of redistribution strongly depends on coronary perfusion, with ischemic areas demonstrating much slower washout than normal regions

- Blood half-life: ranges from 0.5 minutes (exercise) to 3 minutes (rest)
- Biological half-life: 10 days ± 2.5 days
- Long biological and physical half-life (73 hours) limit dose (1-2 mCi) that can be given
- Renal clearance 4%-8%

Use

- Imaging of myocardial ischemia and infarctions
- Parathyroid adenoma localization

^{99m}Tc SESTAMIBI

^{99m}Tc sestamibi is an isonitrile (hexakis 2 methoxy-isobutyl isomitrile) containing 6 isonitrile components. Sestamibi has a high 1st pass extraction, a distribution proportional to blood flow, and few or no metabolic side effects. Advantages over ^{201}Tl:

$$\left[\begin{array}{ccc} & R & R \\ R - & Tc & - R \\ & R & R \end{array} \right]^{-} \qquad R = -C \equiv N - \overset{\displaystyle CH_3}{\underset{\displaystyle CH_3}{C}} - CO - CH_3$$

- Better dosimetry: higher dose can be given resulting in higher photon flux
- Preferred agent for SPECT imaging (more photons)
- Higher energy than ^{99m}Tc photons: less tissue attenuation
- Preferred for obese patients
- Good correlation between ^{201}Tl and ^{99m}Tc MIBI in terms of imaging characteristics

Pharmacokinetics

- Passive diffusion into myocyte. Myocardial uptake is proportional to diffusion.
- ^{99m}Tc sestamibi is retained in myocardium because of binding to a low molecular weight protein in the cytosol complex.
- Hepatobiliary excretion: prominent liver activity (may interfere with evaluation of inferior wall).
- Wait 30-60 min before imaging to allow some hepatic clearance.
- There is no myocaridal redistribution, thus imaging can be performed 1-2 hours after injection.

^{99m}Tc TEBOROXIME

^{99m}Tc teboroxime is a neutral lipophilic boronic acid dioxine for cardiac imaging. Avidly extracted from blood by myocardium. Myocardial uptake has a linear correlation with blood flow so that regional uptake is a suitable marker of myocardial perfusion. The main disadvantage is rapid myocardial clearance that necessitates imaging immediately after injection and limits its versatility.

Pharmacokinetics
- Cardiac extraction: 3.5% (higher than isonitriles)
- Hepatobiliary excretion (may interfere with inferior wall evaluation)
- Biological half-life: 10-20 min
- Very rapid myocardial clearance
- No redistribution

COMPARISON OF AGENTS			
	^{201}Thallium	^{99m}Tc Sestamibi	^{99m}Tc Teboroxime
Dose	74-111 MBq	740-1850 MBq	740-850 MBq
Imaging time	Immediate	60 min	1-2 min
Cardiac half-life	3-5 hrs	5 hrs	5-10 min
Cardiac uptake	3%-4%	2%	3%-4%
Redistribution	Yes	Slight	No

^{99m}Tc RBC LABELING

Autologous RBC labeling is best performed by one of 3 methods of pertechnetate incorporation into RBC. RBC labeling is based on the principle that (+ 7) TcO_4 crosses the RBC membrane but reduced (+ 4) Tc does not. TcO_4 can be reduced intracellularly to (+ 4) Tc with tin (Sn^{2+}); reduced Tc binds to the beta chain of hemoglobin.

Uses
- Cardiac-gated blood-pool studies
- Bleeding studies
- Hemangioma characterization
- Spleen imaging (alternative to sulfur colloid)

Methods of labeling autologous RBCs

In vivo labeling
- 1 mg of stannous pyrophosphate injected IV
- After 20 minutes 740 MBq of ^{99m}TcO$_4^-$ is injected
- Disadvantage: labeling efficiency < 85%; low target-to-background ratio

Modified in vivo labeling
- 1 mg of stannous pyrophosphate injected IV
- After 20 minutes, 5 mL of blood is withdrawn and incubated in a syringe with 740 MBq of ^{99m}TcO$_4$ for 10 minutes
- Incubated RBC are reinjected
- Advantage of this method is a higher labeling efficiency: 30 minutes after injection 90% of administered radioactivity remains in the intravascular space

In vitro labeling
- Entire labeling procedure is performed outside patient
- Requires 30 minutes

12

Causes of poor RBC labeling
- Drug interactions (e.g., heparin, doxorubicin, contrast agents)
- Antibodies: transfusions, transplantation
- Short incubation time
- Too much or too little stannous ion

Pearls
- In vivo methods suffice in clinical practice
- Heat-damaged RBCs are used for selective spleen imaging
- ^{99m}Tc labeled human serum albumin (HAS) is an alternative agent for blood pool imaging but provides less target-to-background due to extracellular diffusion.
- New long circulating polymers are currently being developed that may obviate the need for RBC labeling.

Myocardial Perfusion Scintigraphy

GENERAL

Myocardial ischemia is only demonstrated if ^{201}Tl is in circulation while there is myocardial ischemia. For this reason, patients have to be exercised for a few minutes after IV injection of ^{201}Tl ("initial images"). The sensitivity of ^{201}Tl imaging depends directly on the degree of exercise achieved. A coronary stenosis must exceed 90% of normal diameter before resting blood flow is impaired; with maximum exercise, however, stenosis of > 50% is hemodynamically significant.

Images acquired several hours after initial IV injection show a different pattern; areas of initially high activity washout faster so areas of initially low activity may have relatively higher activity ("redistribution image"). To obtain good quality redistribution images, a 2nd dose of ^{201}Tl is injected 3-4 hours after initial imaging. Reinjection improves differentiation of defects and improves the sensitivity for ischemia as compared to simple redistribution imaging.

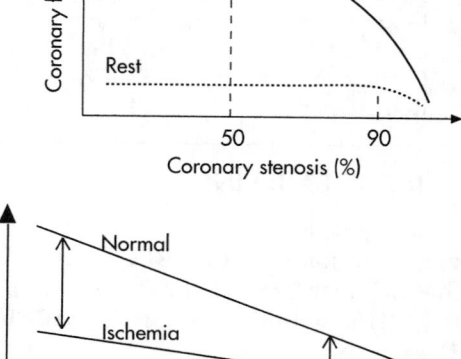

TECHNIQUES

There are 3 techniques of nuclear cardiac perfusion imaging:
Physical exercise test (significant increase in myocardial workload). This is the preferred technique:
- Treadmill test (Bruce protocol or modified protocol)
- Bicycling

Pharmacological "stress" test (no significant increase in myocardial workload)
- Coronary flow increases after administration of vasodilators; stenotic vessels do not respond as much and areas of hypoperfusion are accentuated
- Workload is not increased, ischemia seldomly occurs
- Agents used: dipyridamole (acts indirectly by reducing the degradation of endogenous adenosine)
- Adenosine (Adenocard): direct vasodilator with short duration
- Dobutamine

Rest study
- Use: patients for whom exercise or dipyridamole is contraindicated (intraaortic balloon pump, coronary artery bypass graft)
- Not sensitive for detecting ischemia
- Used mainly to determine myocardial viability

Treadmill test
1. Patient NPO to decrease splanchnic activity
2. Patient is exercised on treadmill to maximum stress (i.e., completion of protocol) or other endpoint
   - $\geq$ 85% predicted maximum heart rate (PMHR = 220 − age in years)
   - Unable to continue secondary to fatigue or dyspnea
   - Cardiovascular signs/symptoms: severe angina, hypotension, arrhythmias, ischemic electrocardiogram (ECG) changes
3. First dose of ^{201}Tl injected at peak exercise (75 MBq). Continue exercise for 1 minute
4. Image immediately
5. Second dose of ^{201}Tl (37 MBq) injected at rest after 3-4 hours to obtain redistribution images

Factors that limit exercise stress test:
- Inadequate stress decreases diagnostic sensitivity
- Heart rate should increase to at least 85% of PMHR
- Drugs that limit heart rate response decrease sensitivity of the stress test (beta-blockers, calcium channel blockers, digoxin)
- Nondiagnostic ECG: left ventricle hypertrophy, left bundle branch block, baseline ST-T abnormalities

Dipyridamole test
1. Patient NPO (no coffee, caffeine, or other xanthine products for 24 hours)
2. Dipyridamole IV infusion (0.6 mg/kg over 4 minutes): HR increases 20%, BP decreases 10 mm Hg
3. ^{201}Tl (74 MBq) is given 10 minutes after the dipyridamole is started (peak blood dipyridamole level)
4. Image immediately
5. Administer aminophylline (50-100 mg) to reverse side effects of dipyridamole
6. Reinject ^{201}Tl (30 MBq) for redistribution images

Rest and redistribution study
1. Injection of 1st dose of ^{201}Tl (74 MBq)
2. Image immediately
3. No reinjection of 2nd dose

12

NORMAL IMAGES AND VARIANTS

Uniform distribution of activity should be present in the myocardium.

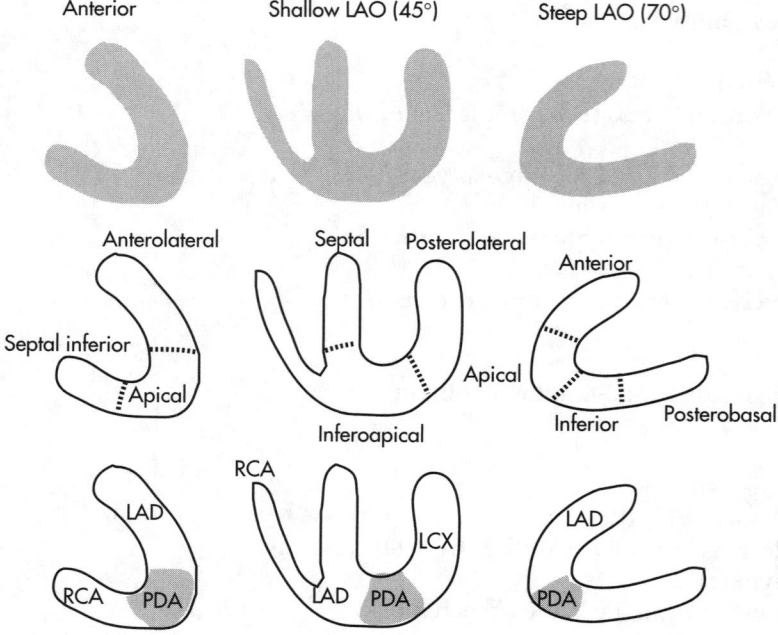

Variations

- Diaphragmatic attenuation: inferior myocardial wall especially on anterior and steep LAO views, may be attenuated.
- Thin basal myocardium: decreased activity along the most superior aspect of images (cardiac valve plane)
- Nonuniform activity may be seen in the proximal septum.
- Lung uptake is normal if lung:heart ratio is < 50%. A ratio of > 0.5% pulmonary activity indicates left ventricular (LV) dysfunction with or without pulmonary edema. Increased lung activity correlates with elevated pulmonary capillary wedge pressure.
- Splanchnic uptake may be seen after recent meal, inadequate exercise, and in dipyridamole and in MIBI studies.
- Right ventricular (RV) activity at rest (i.e., on redistribution images but not on stress images) indicates hypertrophy.
- "Hot" papillary muscles may make adjacent myocardium appear hypoperfused.
- Apical thinning refers to decreased activity in the cardiac apex (common in dilated hearts).

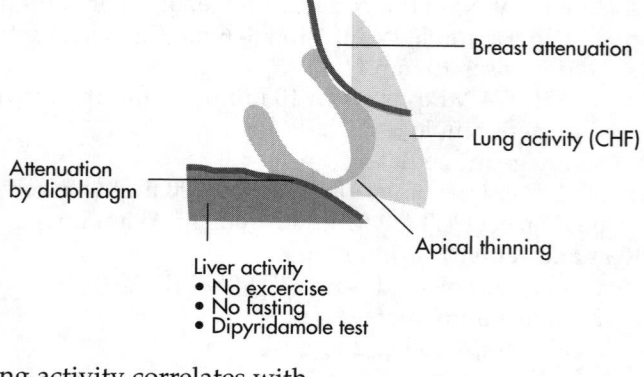

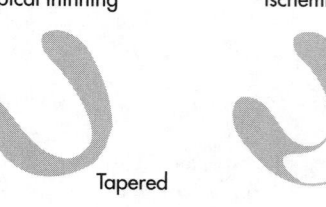

Image interpretation
1. Adequacy of study
   - Did patient achieve 85% PMHR?
   - Splanchic uptake (minimal exercise, not NPO)
2. Lung uptake
   - Lung/heart ratio > 0.5 indicates exercise-induced LV dysfunction
3. Heart size and wall thickness
   - Subjective assessment
   - Transient cavitary dilatation (dilated cavity on initial but not delayed images) is a sign of LV dysfunction
4. Distribution defects
   - Full-thickness defect
   - Partial-thickness defects
   - Reversible vs. irreversible defects

ABNORMAL PLANAR SCAN PATTERNS

Three patterns:

Reversible perfusion pattern
- Perfusion defect is present in the stress image with partial or complete fill-in on redistribution images
- Indicative of ischemia
- Rare conditions with this pattern causing false positives for ischemia: Chagas' disease, sarcoid, hypertrophic cardiomyopathy

Irreversible, fixed perfusion pattern
- Perfusion defect persists
- Much less specific for ischemia than reversible defects
- Often seen with scars (old myocardial infarction), cardiomyopathies, idiopathic hypertrophic subaortic stenosis, coronary spasm, infiltrative or metastatic lesions

Rapid washout pattern
- Stress view is normal and redistribution images demonstrate defects
- Least specific pattern
- May occur in coronary artery disease (CAD), cardiomyopathy, or normal patients

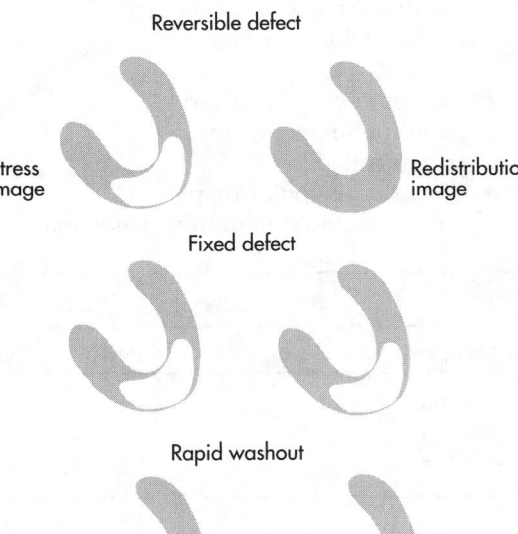

Reversible defect

Stress image / Redistribution image

Fixed defect

Rapid washout

SENSITIVITY AND SPECIFICITY			
	Exercise ECG (%)	201Tl Stress Test (%)	SPECT
Sensitivity	60	85	Marginal improvement over 201Tl
Specificity	85	85	Possibly lower

Sensitivity of 201Tl varies with extent of disease:
- 80% sensitivity for single vessel disease
- 95% sensitivity for triple vessel disease

Dipyridamole 201Tl scan appears to have similar sensitivity/specificity as exercise 201Tl.

12

SPECT IMAGING

Advantages of SPECT:
- Improved sensitivity for detection of moderate CAD
- More accurate anatomical localization (especially LCX territory)

Technique
- Best performed with multidetector camera
- Images are obtained over a 180° arc at 6° intervals: 45° RAO to 45° LPO
- The slice thickness is approximately 1 cm
- Total imaging time: single detector 20-30 minutes; multidetector 10-15 minutes
- Anterior planar images needed to assess lung activity

Interpretation
- 3 standard image reconstruction planes (cardiac axes: short, horixontal long and vertical)
- Compare initial and redistribution images as in planar imaging
- Quantitative polar maps are adjunct to qualitative visual analysis

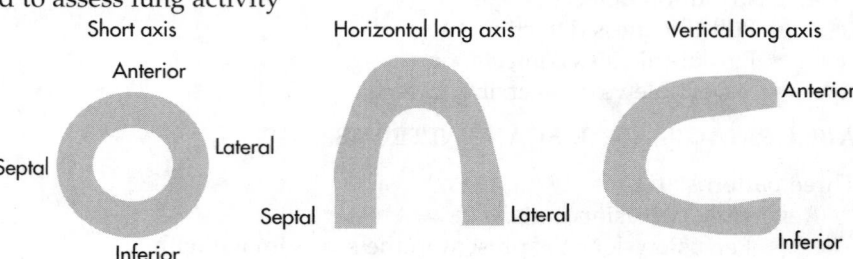

PET IMAGING		
Myocardium	**Perfusion (NH$_3$)**	**Metabolism (FDG)**
Normal	+	+
Ischemia	− or decreased	+
Necrosis	−	−

HIBERNATING MYOCARDIUM

Refers to chronic ischemia: poorly perfused heart at rest with loss of functional wall motion but which is still viable
- Fixed defects on 4-hour thallium images
- Diminished wall motion seen
- Requires revascularization procedure
- Re-image at 24 hour after second injection

STUNNED MYOCARDIUM

- Acute event that results from ischemic injury
- Normal or near normal perfusion with decreased contractility
- Acute coronary artery occlusion

Acute Myocardial Infarct (AMI) Imaging

^{99m}Tc PYROPHOSPHATE IMAGING

Limited indications because AMI is more diagnosed by ECG and elevated enzymes.

Technique

- ^{99m}Tc pyrophosphate (370-550 MBq) is injected at rest. Pyrophosphate binds to denatured proteins and parallels calcium metabolism.
- Imaging is performed 2-4 hours after injection.

Interpretation

- Scans become increasingly positive for 72 hours after infarct. Insensitive within the first 24 hours and 10 days after the MI.
- Focal myocardial activity represents accumulation in damaged myocardium. The severity of uptake may be graded:
  - Grade 0: no uptake, normal
  - Grade 1: less uptake than rib
  - Grade 2: more uptake than rib
  - Grade 3: more uptake than sternum
- A cardiac doughnut pattern may be present: absence of flow to central region of the infarct

Differential diagnosis of thoracic soft tissue uptake of ^{99m}Tc pyrophosphate:

- Infarction
- Direct myocardial injuries (contusion/trauma, cardioversion, myocarditis, cardiac surgery)
- All cardiomyopathies
- Pericarditis, endocarditis
- Unstable angina
- Calcification (dystrophic, valvular, costal cartilage)
- Breast tumors
- Blood pool activity

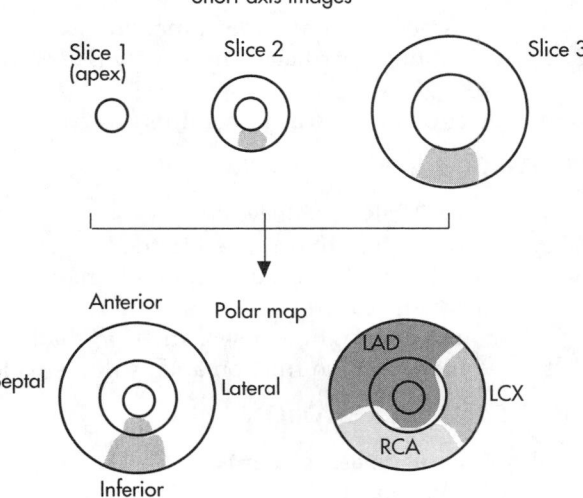

RESTING ^{201}THALLIUM SCAN

^{201}Tl is injected at rest. The distribution reflects coronary artery perfusion. Very reliable if performed within 12-24 hours after Q-wave infarcts (sensitivity 90%). Sensitivity decreases with time following the infarct, possibly related to the resolution of the associated ischemia. The sensitivity is also lower for non–Q-wave infarcts.

Ventricular Function Imaging

GENERAL

Two different approaches exist to studying ventricular function:

1st pass studies

- Immediately after IV injection of a radiotracer (e.g., ^{99m}Tc DTPA) the bolus is imaged as it passes through heart, lungs, and great vessels. The acquisition ends before the agent recirculates.
- A multidetector camera (multiple crystals and photomultiplier tube) for rapid data aquisition is required
- Advantages: fast, determination of transit time, intracardiac shunts detectable, RV ejection fraction (RVEF) can be obtained
- Disadvantages: imaging time and count density limited

Equilibrium studies (gated-blood pool study, GBPS)

- The blood pool is currently best imaged with ^{99m}Tc-labeled RBC
- Gating to the cardiac cycle (frame mode, list mode)
- Allows evaluation of segmental wall motion

12

Indications

- Assessment of ventricular function in CAD and cardiomyopathies
- Evaluation of cardiac drug toxicity (Adriamycin is often discontinued if EF < 45%)
- Detection of intracardiac shunts

PROTOCOL

1. Inject ^{99m}Tc RBC (740 MBq)
2. Gated images are triggered to the R-wave. Arrhythmias have R-R interval variability and cause distortion of images. Arrhythmia filtering should therefore be performed.
3. Acquire images in 3 views: anterior, shallow LAO (45°), steep LPO (30°)
5. Calculate ejection fraction and evaluate wall motion

IMAGE INTERPRETATION

Qualitative image assessment

1. Adequacy of study
   - Determine if labeling of RBC is adequate (free TcO_4 uptake in stomach, thyroid, cardiac-to-background activity)
   - Determine if gating is adequate (jumps, count drop-off at end of cycle)
2. Heart
   - Size of cardiac chambers
   - Thickness of myocardial walls and septum
   - Ventricular wall motion is graded segmentally. Segments should contract simultaneously; anterior, posterior, lateral walls move to a greater extent than septum or inferior wall; septum should move toward the LV. Atypical motion:
     - Hypokinesis: minimal wall movement (e.g., injured myocardium)
     - Akinesis: no wall movement (e.g., scarred myocardium)
     - Dyskinesis: paradoxical wall movement (e.g., aneurysm)
3. Lung
   - Lung activity should be similar to liver activity
   - Evaluate for areas of oligemia
4. Great vessels
   - Determine course and caliber
   - Aorta should be ⅔ of diameter of PA

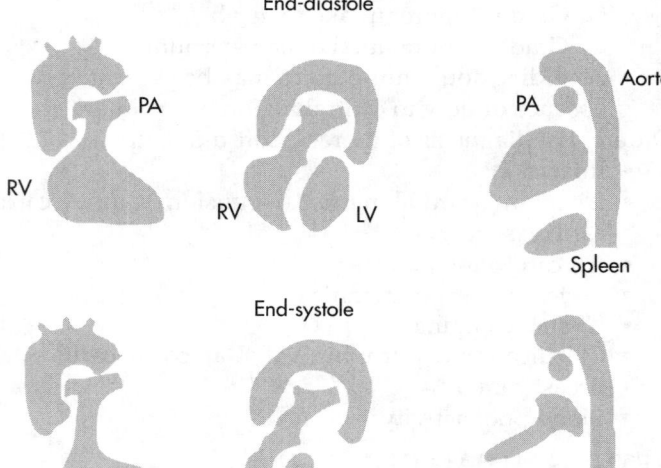

Quantitative image assessment

The LV volume is graphed over time by edge tracing algorithms. The most common quantitative parameters are EF and peak filling rate. Stroke volume or index and cardiac index can also be obtained. Quantitative data are obtained from shallow LAO (45°) projection:

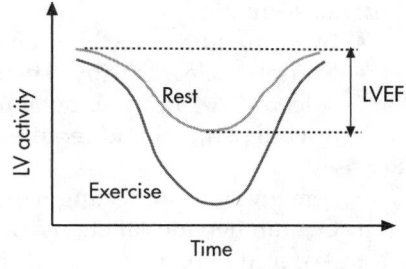

EF (systolic function)

- $LVEF = \dfrac{\text{end-diastolic volume (EDV)} - \text{end-systolic volume (ESV)}}{EDV}$

- Normal values: LVEF 50%-65%
- Normal variability: 5%

Peak filling rate (Diastolic function)

- Index of early ventricular filling
- Abnormalities in peak filling rates may precede EF changes (diastolic dysfunction may be present with normal LV systolic function)

Pearls

- GBPS is the preferred and most accurate imaging technique for LVEF determination.
- LVEF calculations by echocardiography are often less accurate than by nuclear imaging because:
   Cardiac visualization is incomplete, making quantitation difficult.
   Sampling error is related to operator differences.
- LVEF determination by contrast ventriculography is limited by geometric inaccuracy.

Gastrointestinal Imaging

Radiopharmaceuticals

GENERAL

OVERVIEW		
Radiopharmaceutical	**Target**	**Main Use**
^{99m}Tc sulfur colloid	RES distribution	Atypical splenic tissue, liver lesion
^{99m}Tc HIDA	Biliary excretion	Acute cholecystitis
^{99m}Tc RBC	Blood pool	Hemangioma, bleeding
$^{99m}TcO_4$	Mucosal secretion	Meckel scan

^{99m}TECHNETIUM SULFUR COLLOID

Sodium thiosulfate reacts with acid to form sulfur, which reacts to form a colloid. Tc is contained within the colloid in the (+7) valence state. Gelatin stabilizes the colloid sulfide.

$$S_2O_3^{-2} + 2H^+ \rightarrow S + SO_2 + H_2O$$
$$7S_2O_3^{-2} + {}^{99m}TcO_4^- + 4H^+ \rightarrow {}^{99m}Tc_2S_7 + 5SO_4^{-2} + 2HSO_4^- + 2H_2O$$

EDTA is added to bind free TcO_4^-.

12

Pharmacokinetics

- Blood half-life is 2-3 minutes. 90% extraction during first pass.
- Complete clearance by reticuloendothelial system (RES) of liver (80%-90%), spleen (5%-10%), and bone marrow. Localization of the agent in these tissues is flow dependent and requires functional integrity of RES cells.

Pearls

- Sensitivity for detecting hepatic metastases is lower than with CT.
- Overall hepatic function can be assessed by the pattern of uptake.
- Accumulation of ^{99m}Tc sulfur colloid in renal transplants indicates rejection.
- In severe liver dysfunction an increase in activity can be seen in marrow, spleen, lungs, and even kidneys ("colloid shift").

^{99m}Tc HEPATOBILIARY AGENTS

All newer hepatobiliary agents are Tc-labeled iminodiacetic acid derivatives, (abbreviated HIDA where *H* stands for hepatic). Commonly used compounds are the diisopropyl derivative (disofenin, DISIDA), which has the highest biliary excretion, and mebrofenin (BROMIDA), which has the fastest hepatobiliary extraction.

Pharmacokinetics

- Blood half-life is short (10-20 minutes depending on compound)
- 95%-99% biliary excretion into small bowel
- Urinary excretion may be higher in patients with impaired liver function or CBD obstruction

RES Colloid Imaging

INDICATIONS

- Define functioning splenic tissue
- Determine if a primary liver mass has RES activity
- Bone marrow imaging (rare)

IMAGE INTERPRETATION

- Normal liver uptake >> spleen uptake
- Colloid shift occurs in cirrhosis: spleen, bone marrow uptake >> liver uptake. Other causes:
  - Hepatic cirrhosis
  - Alcoholic liver disease
  - Portal hypertension
  - Diffuse metastases with severly impaired liver function
  - Fatty infiltration of liver
  - Diffuse hepatitis
  - Hemochromatosis
  - Amyloidosis
  - Lymphoma
  - Leukemia
  - Sarcoidosis
- All hepatic mass lesions are cold except for FNH, which may have RES activity

- Causes of pulmonary uptake of ^{99m}Tc colloid
    - Hepatic cirrhosis
    - COPD with superimposed infection
    - Estrogen therapy
    - Neoplasms (primary and mets, including hepatoma)
    - DIC
    - Histiocytosis X
    - Faulty colloid preparation → excessive aluminum
    - Transplant recipient
    - Pulmonary trauma
- Nonvisualization of spleen on colloid scan
    - Splenectomy
    - Sickle cell disease
    - Congenital absence of spleen (Ivemark's syndrome)
    - Tumor replacement
    - Infarction
    - Traumatic avulsion or volulus
    - Functional asplenia
        - Postsurgical hypoxia
        - GVHD
        - Chronic hepatitis
        - SLE

Hepatobiliary Imaging

NORMAL SCAN

Protocol
1. Inject 185-300 MBq of ^{99m}Tc-labeled IDA (higher dose if bilirubin elevated)
2. Static images every 5 minutes until the GB and small bowel are identified (usually at < 1 hour); when GB and intestines are visualized, the study is completed
3. Delayed imaging is necessary if GB is not visualized (up to 4 hours)
4. Administer morphine if GB is still not seen

Interpretation

Immediate	10 minutes	1 hour
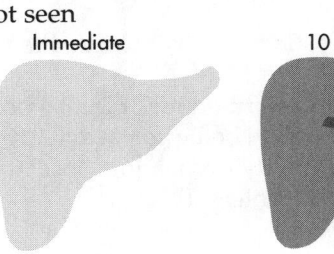	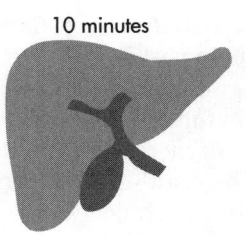	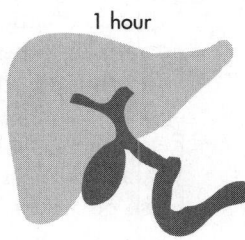

1. Hepatic activity can be
    - Normal
    - Delayed (reduced hepatic extraction in hepatocellular disease). With bilirubin levels > 20 mg/dL, study results are usually equivocal
2. GB activity
    - Present (normal)
    - Nondemonstration of GB at 1 hour after injection may be due to:
        - Prolonged fasting (> 24 hours, GB is filled with bile)
        - Recent meal (GB is contracted)
        - Acute cholecystitis
3. Bowel activity
    - Present (normal)
    - Absent (abnormal)

12

Pharmacological intervention if GB is not visualized

There are two pharmacological maneuvers that can be performed in an attempt to visualize the GB if it has not become apparent after 1 hour of imaging:

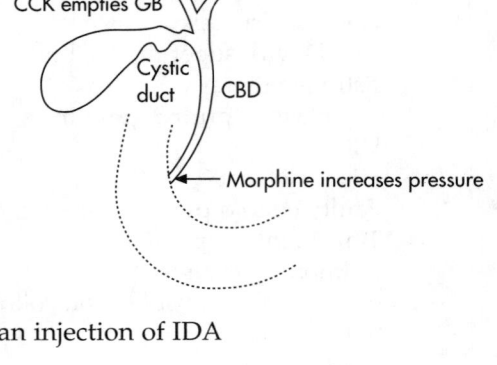

- Sincalide (CCK-8)
    Used to contract the GB to avoid false positive results
    Dose is 0.02-0.04 μg/kg in 10 ml of saline; given slow to avoid discomfort and spasm of GB neck
    This drug may obscure the diagnosis of chronic cholecystitis by speeding up the visualization of the GB. One way around this it to give CCK only if the GB is not visualized at 30-60 minutes; CCK is followed by an injection of IDA 15-30 minutes later.
- Morphine is often given before 4 hours to make the diagnosis of acute cholecystitis
    Dose is 0.04 mg/kg given slowly
    Causes spasm of sphincter of Oddi
    Can convert true positive in case of cystic duct sign to false negative

ACUTE CHOLECYSTITIS

Acute cholecystitis usually results from acute obstruction of the cystic duct. This is commonly due to:

- Cystic duct calculus (most common)
- Other causes (acalculous cholecystitis) usually related to inspissated bile in cystic duct
- Trauma
- Burn
- Diabetes

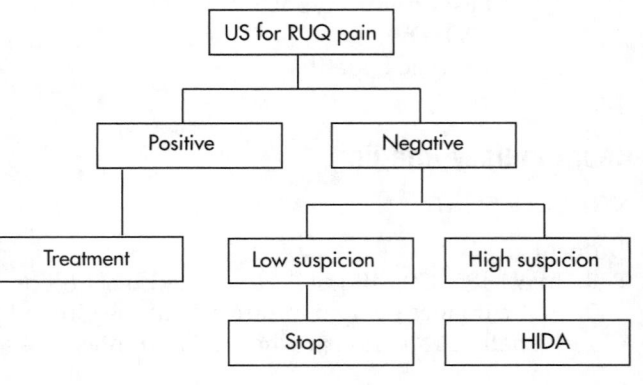

Indication for scintigraphic imaging

- Normal US but high clinical suspicion for cystic duct calculus
- Normal US and suspicion for acalculous cholecystitis

Imaging findings

- Nonvisualization of GB due to cystic duct obstruction. Prerequisites for establishing the diagnosis:
    Prolonged imaging (has to be performed for at least 4 hours)
    Pharmacological intervention has to be performed: CCK or morphine
- Pericholecystic rim of increased activity (hyperemia, local inflammation) in 60%
- Visualization of GB excludes acute cholecystitis
- False positives for acute cholecystitis
    Recent meal within 4 hours of imaging
    Prolonged fasting for 24 hours of hyperalimentation
    Alcoholism
    Pancreatitis
    Chronic cholecystitis
    Hepatocellular dysfunction
    Cholangiocarcinoma of cystic duct
- False negatives
    Acalculous cholecystits
    Duodenal diverticulam simulating GB
    Accesory cystic duct
    Biliary duplication cyst

CHRONIC CHOLECYSTITIS

- Delayed visualization of GB (can occur with acute cholecystitis)
- GB showing a blunted response to CCK is more likely to be chronically inflamed
- Delayed biliary to bowel time in presence of normal GB

LIVER TUMORS

HIDA IMAGING OF PRIMARY HEPATIC TUMORS			
	Flow	Uptake	Clearance
FNH	↑	Immediate	Delayed
Adenoma	Nl	None	—

Bowel Imaging

HEMORRHAGE

Protocol
1. Tracers:
   - ^{99m}Tc RBC, long half-life, low lesion/background ratio
   - ^{99m}Tc sulfur colloid, short half-life, high lesion/background ratio
2. Sequential imaging for 1 hour
3. Additional delayed or spot images depending on findings

Imaging findings
Scintigraphic evaluation usually limited to lower gastrointestinal bleeders. Three patterns:
- Uptake conforming to bowel with no change over time: inflammatory bowel disease, faulty labeling (TcO_4^- excreted into bowel)
- Uptake conforming to bowel with progressive accumulation over time: hemorrhage. Criteria for active bleeding:
    - Activity appears and confirms to bowel anatomy
    - Activity usually increases with time
    - Activity must move antegrade or retrograde in bowel
- False positive
    - Free pertechnetate
    - Activity in bladder or urinary tract
    - Uterine or penile flush
    - Accessory spleen
    - Hemangioma of liver
    - Varices
    - Aneurysm, other vascular structures
- False negative
    - Bleeding too slow
    - Intermittent bleeding

12

HEMANGIOMA IMAGING

^{99m}Tc RBC imaging is occasionally performed to diagnose hepatic hemangiomas although helical CT with contrast and MRI are now used more commonly. The sensitivity of RBC imaging for detection of hemangiomas depends on lesion size: < 1 cm 25%, 1-2 cm 65%, > 2 cm 100%.

MECKEL SCAN

Meckel's diverticulum (incidence 2% of general population) is a remnant of the omphalomesenteric duct. 50% of Meckel's diverticula contain ectopic gastric mucosa, which secretes ^{99m}TcO$_4^-$. Meckel's diverticula that do not contain gastric mucosa are not detectable. Most diverticula are asymptomatic, but complications may occur:

- Bleeding (95% of bleeding Meckel's diverticula have gastric mucosa)
- Intestinal obstruction
- Inflammation

Technique

1. Patient NPO
2. H$_2$ blockers (cimetidine) block secretion of ^{99m}TcO$_4^-$ into the bowel lumen and improve the target/background ratio of Meckel's diverticula (300 mg qid for 1-3 days before the study)
3. 370 MBq ^{99m}TcO$_4^-$ IV
4. Sequential imaging for 1 hour
5. Drugs to enhance the sensitivity detecting Meckel's diverticulum
   Cimetidine to block release of pertechnate from mucosa. Dose: 300 mg 4 times a day; 20 mg/kg body/day for 2 days before
   Pentagastrin to enhance uptake of ^{99m}TcO$_4^-$. Note that pentagastrin must be administered before the ^{99m}TcO$_4^-$ dose
   Glucagon to decrease small bowel or diverticular motility. Administer IV 10 minutes before study.

Imaging findings

- Activity in a Meckel's diverticulum increases over time, just like gastric activity. Other causes of increased RLQ activity (e.g., inflammation, tumor) show an initial increase of activity with virtually no changes later on (related to hyperemia and expansion of extracellular space).
- Normal gastric activity quickly enters the lumen and is transported into small bowel; once the activity reaches the small bowel, it can be confused with a Meckel's diverticulum.
- False positives
   Urinary tract activity
   Other ectopic gastric mucosa,
   Hyperemic inflammatory lesions
   AV malformations, hemangioma, aneursym
   Neoplasms
   Intussusception
- False negatives
   Minimal amount of gastric mucosa
   Rapid washout of pertechnetate
   Meckel's diverticulum with impaired blood supply

GASTRIC EMPTYING

Indications
- Children with gastroesophageal (GE) reflux
- Adults with diabetic gastroparesis

The stomach handles liquids and solids differently: liquids empty faster and show a monophasic exponential clearance. Solids empty after an initial delay, but emptying is nearly linear.

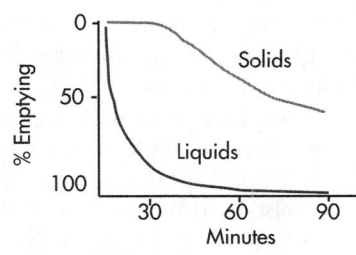

Liquid phase emptying (usually in children, "milk-scan")
- 3.7-37 MBq of ^{99m}Tc sulfur colloid or ^{111}In DTPA added to formula or milk
- Need to image long enough to determine the emptying half-time (image acquisition at 0, 10, 30, 60, 90 minutes)
- Emptying half-time is usually 30 minutes
- Usually performed in conjunction with a GE reflux study while increasing abdominal pressure with a binder (in adults only)

Solid phase emptying (usually for adults)
- 3.7-37 MBq of ^{99m}Tc sulfur colloid is added to raw eggs before scrambling them. ^{99m}Tc-labeled resins or iodinated fibers are alternatives.
- Emptying half-time is usually 1-2 hours.

Genitourinary Imaging

Radiopharmaceuticals

OVERVIEW		
	Radiopharmaceutical	**Comment**
IMAGING OF RENAL FUNCTION		
Glomerular filtration rate	^{99m}Tc DTPA	Inexpensive
Effective renal plasma flow	^{99m}Tc MAG$_3$	Good in renal failure
IMAGING OF RENAL MASS		
Tubular mass	^{99m}Tc DMSA	40% cortical binding
	^{99m}Tc glucoheptonate	20% cortical binding

The only 2 agents routinely used for renal imaging today are ^{99m}Tc DTPA and ^{99m}Tc MAG$_3$. The choice of agent depends on the type of information required:
- Quantification of split renal function: DTPA or MAG$_3$
- Renovascular hypertension: DTPA or MAG$_3$
- Renal failure, follow-up studies: MAG$_3$ preferred
- Obstructive uropathy: MAG$_3$ preferred

DMSA (imaging of renal cortex for scarring in children) and ^{99m}Tc glucoheptonate have limited use. Agents filtered through kidney deliver greatest radiation dose to bladder, whereas tracers bound to renal cortex result in higher renal radiation (i.e., ^{99m}Tc-DMSA)

12

^{99m}Tc DTPA

^{99m}Tc DTPA is an inexpensive chelate used primarily for dynamic renal and brain imaging. It has the same biodistribution as gadolium DTPA used in MRI.

Pharmacokinetics
- Rapid extravascular, extracellular distribution
- Cleared by glomerular filtration (glomerular filtration rate [GFR] agent)
- 5%-10% plasma protein binding, thus calculated GFR is lower than that obtained by inulin
- Immediate images provide information about renal perfusion
- Delayed images provide information about renal function (GFR) and collecting system
- Target organ: bladder (2.7 rads/370 MBq)
- Hydration and frequent voiding reduces patient radiation dose

^{99m}Tc MAG$_3$

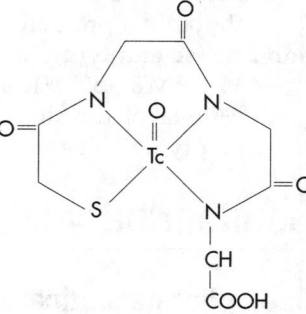

MAG$_3$ is a chelate for ^{99m}Tc. It is physiologically analagous to ^{131}I-ortho iodo-hippuran but has more favorable dosimetry and results in better images. Administered dose: 185-370 MBq. More expensive than DTPA.

Pharmacokinetics
- Cleared mostly by tubular secretion: effective renal plasma flow (ERPF) agent
- Minimal glomerular filtration
- Agent of choice in patients with renal insufficiency. Provides better images because it is not GFR dependent.
- Target organ: bladder (4.8 rads/370 MBq)

Renal Imaging

INDICATIONS

Renovascular hypertension
- Screening of hypertensive patients with high risk
- Renal flow assessment after revascularization procedure (PTA or surgical)

Renal transplant
- Acute tubular necrosis vs. acute rejection
- Other: cyclosporine toxicity, arterial occlusion, urinary obstruction or urinary leak

Determination of split function
- Prior to nephrectomy
- Radiation therapy planning
- Functional determination prior to surgical repair (e.g., obstructed kidney)

PROTOCOL

1. Bolus injection of tracer
2. Immediate imaging of sequential flow images: 1-3 second frames up to 1 minute to measure perfusion
3. Delayed images obtained at 60 sec/frame for 30 minutes. These images may be summed to obtain 5-minute static images.

NORMAL IMAGES

Perfusion images (rapid sequential imaging for 1st minute)
- Aorta is seen first
- Prompt renal activity within 6 seconds of peak aortic activity
- Kidney perfusion should be symmetrical

Static images (1-30 minutes)
- Symmetrical renal uptake, normal renal size
- Peak cortical activity at 3-5 minutes
- Peak renal uptake should be higher than spleen uptake
- Collecting system and ureters begin to fill after 4-5 minutes
- Cortical activity decreases with time

Quantitative split renal function
- Determined by ROI over each kidney with background correction. Measure activity of both kidneys 2-3 minutes after injection (before collecting system fills).
- Split renal function should be 50% on either side.

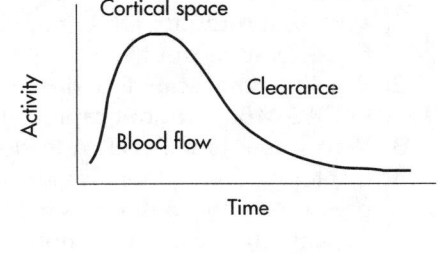

Interpretation
1. Perfusion images (symmetrical or asymmetrical perfusion? prompt or delayed excretion?)
2. Static images
   - Size and shape of kidney
   - Clearance of tracer through ureters into bladder
3. Quantitative data
   - Determine split renal function in %
   - Transit time: clearance of half of maximum activity

RENOVASCULAR HYPERTENSION

5% of hypertensive patients have treatable renal artery stenosis. ^{99m}Tc DTPA and ^{99m}Tc MAG$_3$ studies in these patients may show a unilateral reduction in flow, whereas function is often normal. Captopril (ACE inhibitor) can be used to differentiate normal and dysfunctional stenotic renal arteries. Captopril dilates the efferent arteriole, thus decreasing the GFR of the stenotic kidney.

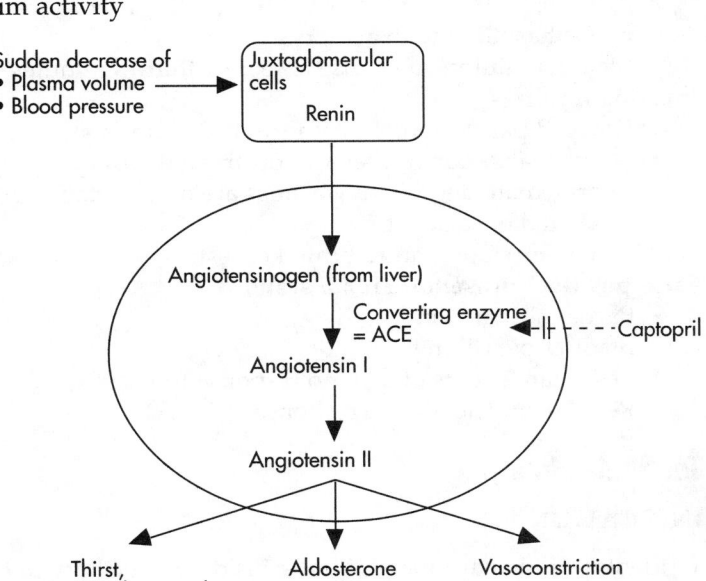

12

Technique

1. Withhold diuretics for 48 hours and ACE inhibitors for 1 week; hydrate patient to decrease risk of hypotension
2. Baseline renal scan: low-dose ^{99m}Tc DTPA (37-185 MBq) without captopril
3. Wait 4 hours for Tc DTPA to clear
4. Captopril, 50 mg PO; measure blood pressure every 15 minutes for 1 hour
5. Repeat renal scan after 1 hour

Interpretation

- Bilateral disease is difficult to diagnose
- A variety of patterns have been described:
  - Decreased flow in stenotic kidney (perfusion images)
  - Decreased excretion and prolonged cortical transit time (static image)
  - Prolonged washout in stenotic kidney (static images)

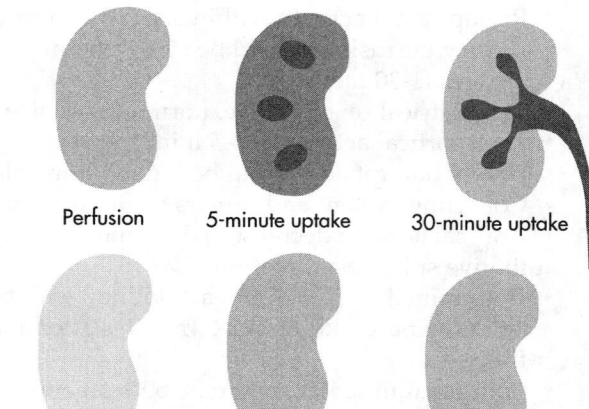
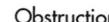
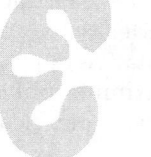
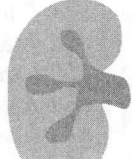

Normal — Perfusion — 5-minute uptake — 30-minute uptake

Stenosis

Obstruction

OBSTRUCTION

If delayed images and attempts at postural drainage fail, furosemide should be given to differentiate nonobstructive dilated collecting systems from obstructed collecting systems ("diuretic renogram").

Technique

- Proceed with the standard renal scan
- Administer furosemide IV 0.3-0.5 mg/kg after dilated pelvis has filled with activity
- Maximal diuretic response is seen within 15 minutes

Imaging findings

- Delayed parenchymal clearance (> 20 minutes) in obstructed kidney
- Nonvisualization of ureter in obstructed kidney
- Intermediate degrees of washout are of uncertain significance:
  - Partial obstruction?
  - Patient may require Whitaker test.

False positive furosemide renal scans

- Partial obstruction
- Bladder overfilling
- Less than 2 years of age (no response to Lasix)
- Renal insufficiency (no response to Lasix)

Testicular Imaging

INDICATION

To identify testicular torsion. Now considered ancillary to testicular US, which can be performed more promptly and is more specific.

PROTOCOL

- Positioning: scrotum on sling, penis taped to anterior abdominal wall
- Inject TcO_4 intravenously
- Flow images acquired over 1 minute
- Delayed static images: mark scrotal raphe for accurate anatomic localization

NORMAL IMAGES

- Slight uptake of tracer in both testes
- Testes can not be separated from scrotum
- Bladder activity is usually seen superior to testes

Interpretation

Flow images
- Increased (hyperemia) or not increased (no hyperemia)
- Decreased flow cannot be detect

Static images
- Cold testes
- Ring sign
- Hot testes

TORSION

Imaging findings

- Photopenic ("cold") testis indicates torsion
- "Ring sign" or "bull's eye": peripheral rim of increased activity with central zone of photopenia may represent inflammation of dartos and infarcted/necrotic testicle
- "Ring sign": delayed/missed torsion (the more pronounced the rim, the later the torsion or scrotal abscess)
- "Nubbin sign" area of increased activity that extends from the iliac arteries and ends at the torsion. Indicates increased perfusion to the scrotum via the pudendal arteries.
- Torsion of appendix testis cannot be diagnosed (too small).
- Testes in children < 2 years are usually too small to be imaged.

OVERVIEW OF TESTICULAR ABNORMALITIES		
Disease	**Flow Images**	**Static Images**
Early torsion (<6 hr)	Normal	Cold testis
Late torsion	Variable	Cold testis, hyperemic scrotum (ring sign)
Epididymitis, orchitis	Increased	Increased uptake
Abscess	Increased	Ring sign
Tumor	Variable	Variable
Trauma	Normal or increased	Normal or increased

12

Adrenal Imaging

METAIODOBENZYLGUANIDINE (MIBG)

Adrenal medullary imaging agent MIBG is recognized as a neurotransmitter precursor in:

- Any neuroectodermal tumor: carcinoid (even metastatic), neuroblastoma, pheochromocytoma, paraganglioma (extraadrenal pheochromocytoma)
- Normal activity is also seen in liver, spleen, salivary glands, myocardium

Technique

- Block uptake of free iodine into thyroid by administering Lugol's solution
- 18 MBq MIBG IV
- Imaging at 1, 2, 3 days after administration

Interpretation

- Absent or faint uptake is normal.
- Bilateral increased uptake indicates hyperplasia.
- Unilateral increased adrenal uptake is suspicious for a neuroectodermal tumor.
- Distant metastases are also detectable.

Bone Imaging

Radiopharmaceuticals

^{99m}Tc PHOSPHONATES

Agents are classified according to the phosphate linkage:

- P-C-P: phosphonates
- P-O-P: polyphosphates
- P-N-P: imidophosphates
- P-P: pyrophosphates

Methylene diphosphonate (MDP) and hydroxymethylene diphosphonate (HMDP) are the most commonly used agents; both agents resist in vivo hydrolysis by alkaline phosphatase.

Pharmacokinetics

- 50% of injected MDP localizes to bone.
- 70% of dose is excreted renally within 24 hours.
- Biodistribution may be considerably altered by abnormal cardiac output, renal function, and medications.
- MDP is chemiabsorbed onto hydroxyapatite (exact mechanism unknown). 80% of tracer that ultimately localizes in skeleton does so within 5-10 min. However, one typically waits for 2-3 hrs for imaging to minimize ECF and blood activity.
- Bone uptake depends on 2 factors:
    Osteoblastic activity (most important)
    Blood flow (less important)
- ^{99m}Tc MDP also reacts with mitochondrial calcium crystals. Uptake thus occurs in various types of cell injury:
    Tissue infarction: myocardial, splenic, cerebral
    Cardiac contusion, cardiac surgery, unstable angina pectoris, myopathies
- Critical organ is the bladder. Minimize radiation exposure by hydration and frequent voiding (this also helps to detect pelvic lesions).

BONE MARROW AGENTS

^{99m}Tc sulfur colloid is most commonly used for bone marrow imaging. InCl$_2$ is an alternative agent but is not available for clinical use at present. Bone marrow scintigraphy is not important in current practice and has a few limited indications.

Indications
- Determine viability of red marrow
- Localization of marrow prior to bone marrow aspiration

Bone Imaging

Indications
- Detection of metastases
- Staging of malignancies
- Detection of osteomyelitis
- Detection of radiographically occult fractures
- Determine multiplicity of lesions (e.g., fibrous dysplasia, Paget's)
- Diagnosis of reflex sympathetic dystrophy

TECHNIQUE

1. Inject 740 mBq ^{99m}Tc MDP IV
2. Image 2-4 hours later
3. May have to wait longer before imaging patients with renal insufficiency to allow for soft tissue clearance
4. Have patient urinate immediately before imaging to decrease bladder activity
5. 2 image acquisition formats:
   - Whole body single pass (lower resolution)
   - Spot-views (longer time of acquisition, better resolution)

NORMAL IMAGES

Adults
- Locally increased activity may be a normal variant:
  - Patchy uptake in the skull may be normal
  - Common location for degenerative changes (usually at both sides of a joint)
    - Sternoclavicular joint, manubriosternal joint
    - Lower cervical and lumbar spine (usually at concavity of scoliosis)
    - Knees, ankle, wrists, 1st carpometacarpal joint
  - Tendon insertions
  - Regions of constant stress
  - Geometric overlap of bones (ribs)
- Normal, secondary uptake of the label:
  - Nasopharynx
  - Kidneys
  - Soft tissues
- Findings that are always abnormal
  - Strikingly asymmetrical changes
  - Very hot spots
- The older the patient, the higher the proportion of poor quality scans

Children
- Intensive accumulation in growth plates

12

TUMORS

Indications for obtaining a bone scan
- Diagnosis
- Initial staging
- Follow therapeutic response

Imaging features
- The majority of bone tumors are "hot" lesions
- Cold lesion (purely osteolytic tumors with no blastic activity): renal cell carcinoma, thyroid cancer, anaplastic tumors, neuroblastoma (uncommon)
- Superscan: diffusely increased bone activity with little to no renal activity. Most commonly due to diffuse osseous metastases: (prostate carcinoma)
- Normal distribution: marrow tumors such as lymphoma, leukemia, multiple myeloma
- Soft tissue lesions (tracer uptake in tumor)
- Normal (false negative)

SPECIFIC METASTASES	
Tumor	Comment
Prostate cancer	PSA may be more specific for follow-up*
RCC	Osteolytic metastases usually well seen by plain film
Bronchogenic carcinoma	Usually associated with bone pain (especially squamous cell)
Lymphoma	Often false negative (inapparent lesions)
Myeloma	Often false negative (inapparent lesions)
Neuroblastoma	Metastases to metaphyses may mimic normal growth plate

PSA, Prostate-specific antigen; RCC, renal cell carcinoma.

Tumors that commonly metastasize to bone:
- Breast
- Prostate
- Lung
- Renal
- Thyroid

Metastases preferentially localize in bones with red marrow:
- Ribs   35%
- Spine   25%
- Pelvis   5%
- Extremities 15%
- Skull   5%

Increased uptake can also be observed in the in the following conditions:
- Brain infarcts
- Splenic infarcts
- Intramuscular injection sites
- Adrenal neuroblastoma
- Meningioma
- Malignant ascites
- Paget's disease of the breast

Bony lesions commonly missed on scan:
- RCC metastases
- Thyroid metastases
- Multiple myeloma
- Neuroblastoma
- Highly anaplastic tumors

OSTEOMYELITIS

Osteomyelitis is commonly evaluated with a 3-phase bone scan: flow ("flow images"), immediate static ("blood pool image"), and delayed static images (metabolic image). Increased activity on flow images suggests hyperemia, often present in inflammation and stress fractures.

3-PHASE BONE SCAN			
Disease Process	Flow Images	Blood Pool Images	Delayed Images
Cellulitis	+	+	–
Osteomyelitis	+	+	+
Fracture	+	+	+
Noninflammatory	–	–	+

Pearl
- Bone scan allows detection of osteomyelitis much earlier (24-72 hours after onset) than plain radiographs (7-14 days).
- Bone scan is sensitive but nonspecific for osteomyelitis.
- Combined ^{99m}Tc-MDP/^{111}In WBC scanning maximizes sensitivity and specificity and is the preferred technique for the diagnosis of osteomyelitis.
- ^{67}Ga uptake that focally exceeds ^{99m}Tc MDP uptake or differs in distribution increases specificity for diagnosis of infection.
- Sensitivity (95%) and specificity (70%-90%) for detection of osteomyelitis by 3-phase bone scan and MRI are similar.
- Lesions hot on all 3 phases of the bone scan:
    Osteomyelitis
    Trauma
    Hypervascular tumor
    RDS
    Neuropathic joint

FRACTURES

Indications for bone scans
- Stress fractures
- Avulsion injuries
- Radiographically occult fractures
- Shin splints
- Osteochondritis dissecans
- Osteonecrosis
- Hip replacement (loosening)
- Child abuse

12

Scintigraphic features

- Time after fracture at which bone scan becomes positive correlates with age of patient:

    Adult: 24 hours

    Older patients: 72 hours (i.e., need delayed images if initial images are negative)

- Bone uptake returns to normal within 1 (ribs) to 3 years (elderly patients, long bones)

REFLEX SYMPATHETIC DYSTROPHY (RSD)

- Bone scan is imaging study of choice for RSD
- Interpretation requires knowledge of duration of symptomatology

FINDINGS		
	Perfusion/Blood Pool Images	Delayed Images
Very early	Increased	Increased
Within 1 year	Increased/normal	Increased
Late	Decreased	Decreased
Children	Normal/increased	Any appearance

PROSTHESIS

DIFFERENTIATION BETWEEN PROSTHESIS LOOSENING AND INFECTION		
	Loosening	Infection
MDP flow image	Normal	Increased
MDP static image	Slight focal increase	Very hot
Ga imaging	Normal	Increased uptake
WBC imaging	Normal	Increased uptake

Total hip replacement (THR)

- More accurate in evaluation of femoral component
- Cemented THR MDP scan should be negative within 6 months after THR unless infected or loosened
- Noncemented THR: may remain hot for up to 24 months
- [111]In WBC or ^{67}Ga may help to differentiate infection from loosening

Bone scan is of little use for evaluating loosening of knee replacements because increased activity is a normal finding

Marrow Imaging

TECHNIQUE

1. Inject 370 MBq ^{99m}Tc colloid IV (higher dose than liver/spleen scan)
2. Image entire skeleton

IMAGING FEATURES

Distribution of activity parallels hematopoietic distribution.
Normal appearance
- Diffuse skeletal activity up to age 8 (diffuse hematopoietic marrow)
- Activity limited to axial skeleton by age 25 (hematopoietic marrow limited to axial skeleton)
- Lower thoracic spine and ribs obscured by intense liver/spleen activity
Abnormal appearance
- Chronic anemias: peripheral marrow expansion with activity in distal extremities
- Lymphoproliferative disorders: bone scan may be useful to localize marrow site for biopsy
- Acute bone infarction (e.g., sickle cell disease): diminished activity, heterogeneous

Thyroid Imaging

Radiopharmaceuticals

OVERVIEW

- ^{123}I: used for routine imaging. Expensive (cyclotron produced). Imaging should be performed after 24 hours. Organification
- ^{99m}TcO$_4^-$ used if imaging has to be performed within 1 hour, if patients receives PTU (unlike I, TcO$_4$ is not organified) or if patient is not able to ingest I orally. Disadvantage: 5% trapped, no organification.
- ^{131}I: now used only for therapeutic purposes (cancer) because of high energy (364 KeV), long half-life (8 days), and beta and gamma decay.

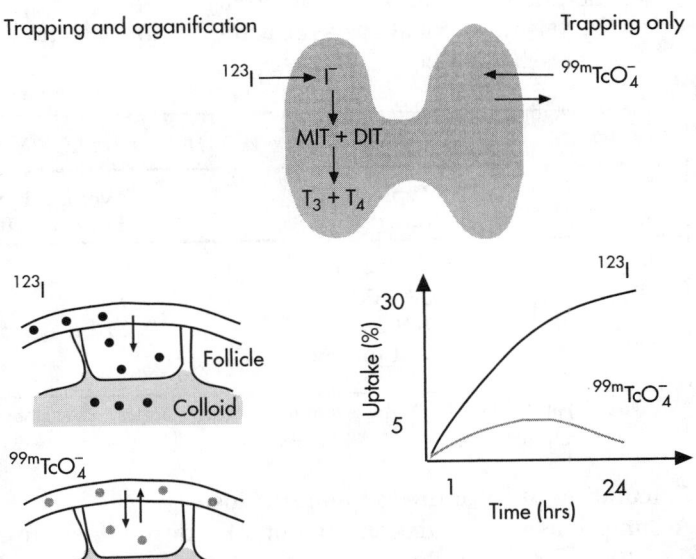

^{123}IODINE

^{123}I is the diagnostic agent of choice for thyroid imaging because of lower patient radiation exposure and higher counting efficiency when compared to ^{131}I. Dose 4-7 MBq sodium iodide PO. Image 24 hours after administration.

Pharmacokinetics

- Readily absorbed from GI tract; primary distribution in extracellular fluid
- Sodium iodide is trapped and organified by the thyroid; there is also trapping by stomach and salivary glands (but no organification)
- Physical half-life: 13 hours
- 35%-70% renal excretion within 24 hours
- Tissue localization:
    Thyroid and thyroid metastases
    Nasopharynx
    Salivary glands
    Stomach
    Colon
    Bladder
    Rarely in lactating breasts

^{131}IODINE

Indications

- Not for general thyroid imaging because of unfavorable dosimetry
- Detection of thyroid metastases
- Therapeutic thyroid radioablation
- There is no rational basis for using ^{131}I for detection of substernal goiters as suggested in older textbooks

TYPICAL DOSAGES OF RADIOACTIVE IODINE			
Agent*	Typical Dose (mCi)	Average Thyroid Exposure (Rad)	Dosage Rate (Rad/MCi)
^{123}I	0.1-0.4 PO	8	11-22
^{131}I	2-10 PO	9.6	1100-1600
^{99m}TcO$_4^-$	1-10 IV	2 (lowest of all)	0.12-0.2
^{125}I	Not for imaging†		

*Tc (140 keV) and ^{123}I (159 keV) have similar photon energies. ^{127}I is stable, nonradioactive iodine.
†^{125}I is a contaminant.

Calculation of ^{131}Iodine therapeutic dose

Assumptions for calculation: 80% uptake, desired glandular dose 8,000-10,000 rads (i.e., 100 µCi/g), gland weight 60 g. To calculate required dose:

$$\text{Dose (µCi)} = (60 \text{ g} \times 100 \text{ µCi/g})/0.8 \times 1000 = 7.5 \text{ µEQ}$$

Complications of ^{131}Iodine treatment

- Bone marrow depression
- Sterility if pelvic metastases present
- Leukemia

PERTECHNETATE

$^{99m}TcO_4^-$ distributes similarly to ^{111}In but is not organified when trapped in the thyroid. Also accumulates in salivary glands, stomach, and choroid plexus.

Applications
- Thyroid imaging
- Blood pool imaging (testicular torsion)
- Ectopic gastric mucosa (Meckel's scan)
- Dacryoscintigraphy (nasolacrimal drainage system)
- Brain imaging (passes into brain if there is a blood-brain barrier defect; rarely used)

Pharmacokinetics
- Rapid (30-minute) extraction of $^{99m}TcO_4^-$ by thyroid.
- Thyroid releases $^{99m}TcO_4^-$ over a period of several hours; at 24 hours there is virtually no $^{99m}TcO_4^-$ left in the thyroid

^{123}I	$^{99m}TcO_4^-$
Oral	IV
Organified	Not organified
Image late; 24 hrs	Image early; 20 minutes
Maximum uptake at about 24 hrs	Maximum uptake at about 20 min
Can be incorporated into thyroid hormone	Cannot be incorporated into thyroid hormone

Thyroid Imaging

IODINE UPTAKE TEST

This test determines how much of orally ingested ^{123}I is accumulated in the thyroid at 24 hours. It is thus a measure of I trapping and organification. The test cannot be used as a marker of thyroid function (this is done by measurements of T_3/T_4). Uptake values are classified as hyperthyroid, euthyroid, and hypothyroid states.

Technique
- Measure the dose of ^{123}I to be ingested (8 MBq, 1-2 capsules)
- Imaging of thyroid 24 hours after oral administration of capsules; as spatial resolution is not crucial, imaging is performed at 20 cm for 5 minutes without the pinhole insert
- Thyroid uptake calculation:
    $$Uptake = (Counts\ in\ neck - Background/Ingested\ dose) \times Decay\ factor$$
- Normal values: 10%-30% or orally ingested dose in thyroid

Increased uptake
- Hyperthyroidism
- Iodine starvation
- Thyroiditis
- Hypoalbuminemia
- Lithium use

12

Decreased uptake

- Hypothyroidism
- Thyroid hormone therapy, Lugol's solution, PTU
- Medications
    Iodinated contrast agents
    Certain vitamin preparations
- Thyroiditis

NORMAL IMAGING

Patient examination

Short medical history

- Hypothyroidism (edema, dry skin, bradycardia, decreased reflexes, hypothermia, loss of lateral eyebrows)
- Hyperthyroidism (diarrhea, sweating, tachycardia, warm and moist skin, ophthalmopathy)
- Enlargement of gland (goiter, nodule)

Current drug history including exposure to iodine contrast agents

Palpation of thyroid

Appearance of normal thyroid scans

Homogenous uptake

Each lobe measures 2-5 cm; slight asymmetry is common

Variants:

- Thin pyramidal lobe arising superiorly from isthmus; accentuated in:
    Graves' disease
    Postsurgical patients
- Lactating breast
- Ectopic thyroid (sublingual, substernal), congenital absence of a lobe (rare)
- $^{99m}TcO_4^-$ scans:
    Uptake of TcO_4^- in salivary glands
    Thin, linear band of superimposed activity often represents swallowed $^{99m}TcO_4^-$ activity in the esophagus (have patient drink water)

Interpretation

1. Uptake
   - Homogenous, heterogenous
   - Decreased, increased, normal
2. Size, shape
   - Enlarged, normal
   - External compression
3. Nodules
   - Hot, cold
   - Extrathyroid nodules (e.g., metastases)

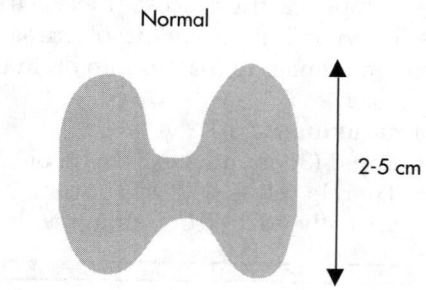

Normal

2-5 cm

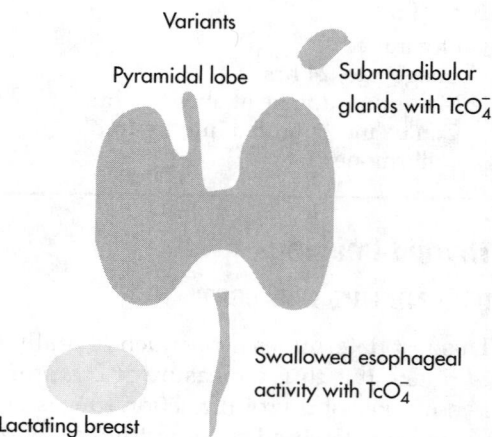

Variants

Pyramidal lobe

Submandibular glands with TcO_4^-

Swallowed esophageal activity with TcO_4^-

Lactating breast

COLD NODULE

Of all palpable nodules, 90% are cold, and of these 90% are benign. A cold nodule is nonfunctioning and has to be further worked up to exclude cancer. Cold nodes may represent:

- Adenoma/colloid cyst, 85%
- Carcinoma, 10%
- Focal thyroiditis
- Hemorrhage
- Lymph node
- Abscess
- Parathyroid adenoma

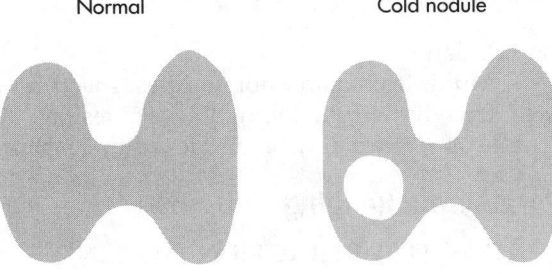

Normal   Cold nodule

MALIGNANT VS. BENIGN COLD NODULES	
Benign	**Malignant**
Older patients	Younger patients
Female	Male
Sudden onset	History of radiation, positive family history
Soft, tender lesion	Hard lesion
Multiple nodules	Other masses in neck
Response to suppression	No response to suppression therapy or iodine therapy

HOT NODULE

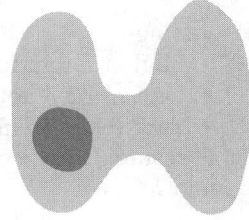

Cold nodule

The vast majority of hot nodules represent hyperfunctioning adenomas, half of which are autonomous (i.e., grow without stimulus of thyroid stimulating hormone, TSH). Autonomous nodules should be suppressed for 5 weeks with T_4 to turn off TSH. If the nodule stays hot, it is a true autonomous nodule that should be treated by surgery, ^{131}I, or alcohol ablation if clinically symptomatic.

Discordant nodules

Refers to hot nodule by $^{99m}TcO_4^-$ imaging and a cold nodule by ^{123}I imaging (i.e., a nonfunctiong nodule). Knowing whether a nodule is discordant is usually of little value per se.

HYPERTHYROIDISM

Graves' disease

- Diffuse toxic goiter (Graves' disease): most common form of hyperthyroidism
- Nodular toxic goiter (Plummer's disease)
- Functioning adenoma
- Struma ovarii (ovarian teratoma that contains functional thyroid tissue)

12

MULTINODULAR GOITER

Goiter

- Enlarged gland
- Multiple cold and hot nodules: spectrum of thyroid adenomas ranging from hyperfunctioning to cystic lesions
- Appearance may be mimicked by Hashimoto thyroiditis

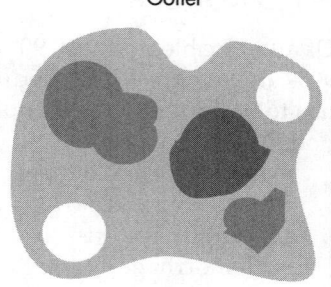

Parathyroid Imaging

$^{99m}TcO_4^-/^{201}Tl$ SUBTRACTION IMAGING

Technique
1. IV injection of 74-111 MBq of ^{201}Tl. Imaging for 15 minutes with pinhole collimator. ^{201}Tl localizes in normal thyroid and enlarged parathyroid gland
2. IV injection of 185-370 MBq of $^{99m}TcO_4^-$. Imaging for 15 minutes. $^{99m}TcO_4^-$ localizes in thyroid but not parathyroid
3. Electronic subtraction of images

Interpretation
- Sensitivity for detecting parathryoid adenomas by scintigraphy: 70%
- Specificity for lesion characterization is only 40% because ^{201}Tl accumulation may also occur in:
   - Benign thyroid adenomas
   - Lymph nodes
   - Carcinomas
- Most authors believe that ^{99m}Tc MIBI is superior to $^{99m}TcO_4^-/^{201}Tl$ subtraction imaging. In ^{99m}Tc MIBI imaging early and late images are compared. Parathyroid adenomas retain ^{99m}Tc MIBI and persist as focal hot spots on delayed images.

^{99m}Tc SESTAMIBI IMAGING OF PARA THYROID

Advantages:
- Higher target to background ratios rather than with thallium
- Delayed 2-3 hours increases the sensitivity of this technique
- Parathyroid activity persists while thyroid fades away

^{99m}Tc sestamibi is also used for imaging of thryoid tumors, as well as brain, lung, and bone tumors.

Miscellaneous Imaging Techniques

^{18}FDG-PET Imaging

RATIONALE FOR ^{18}FDG

- Malignancies often have increased glycolysis.
- Glucose and ^{18}FDG uptake into malignant cells is facilitated by increased expression of the glucose transporter in tumor cells.
- FDG uptake by neoplastic tumors in vivo depends on numerous physiological factors such as tissue oxygenation, regional blood flow, peritumoral inflammatory reactions, etc. FDG uptake is not specific for tumors.

PRACTICAL ASPECTS OF PET TUMOR IMAGING

- Most scanner utilize bismuth germanate (BGO) or NaI crystals.
- Resolution typically varies between 4-6 mm FWHM.
- Field of view (FOV) varies between 10-16 cms in most scanners with largest FOV for single acquisition around 55 cms.
- Patients fast for several hours before the study because elevated serum glucose can decrease cellular FDG uptake. Water is permitted to promote diuresis.
- In diabetics, insulin is adjusted so that fasting blood glucose level is below the preferred level of 130 mg/dL.
- FDG is injected intravenously, 100-400 MBq.
- Multiple emission images are obtained 30-60 minutes after FDG injection.
- Abdominal scanning starts from the inguinal region to minimize bladder activity.
- Data is reviewed in different planes.
- Image fusion: anatomical CT image is fused with PET scan, providing concomitant analysis of metabolic and structural information.
- Standardized uptake value (SUV) is a simple semiquantitative value that relates the concentration of FDG in the tumor to the average concentration in the body. Higher values indicate likely tumors.

NORMAL FDG-PET SCAN

- Normal FDG uptake predominates in brain where gray matter avidly concentrates.
- Myocardial uptake is variable depending on the availability of substrate. About 40% of fasting patients show considerable myocardial uptake.
- FDG is concentrated and eliminated by kidney. Activity seen in the kidney and bladder.
- Activity in GI tract varies. Stomach, colon (flexures and sigmoid colon) can be seen.
- Resting muscle does not show high uptake, but uptake may vary in tensed muscles or with recent muscular activity.

EVOLVING INDICATIONS FOR FDG-PET SCAN

- Differential diagnosis of solitary pulmonary nodules
- Preoperative staging of cancer
- Differentiation of postsurgical changes and residual disease
- Demonstration of suspected recurrence
- Follow-up therapy

PET IN LUNG CANCER

- Used in the diagnosis/workup for solitary pulmonary nodules. The negative predictive value is high. In patients with negative results, follow-up at 3-6 month intervals for at least 2 years is recommended.
- Used in hilar and mediastinal staging. One recommended strategy is to operate on patients with negative PET; patients with positive results should have confirmatory transbronchial biopsy or mediastinoscopy.
- Used for follow-up in patients with small cell carcinoma.

12

MELANOMA

- PET can be useful in detecting lymph node and visceral metastases.
- Small subcutaneous lesions can be easily missed.
- PET combined with CT scanning is very useful in detection of recurrence and follow-up staging in colorectal carcinoma.
- PET has been shown to be effective in detecting local and regional recurrence.
- PET can be used in staging patients with suspected or demonstrated recurrence.

PANCREATIC CARCINOMA

- Differentiation of pancreatic carcinoma from pancreatitis
- Staging of extent of tumor preoperatively

LYMPHOMA

- PET has been demonstrated in some studies to reveal more lesions than CT and clinical examination. Main value in staging is to provide a baseline for subsequent evaluation of therapy.

BREAST CANCER

- Accurate in detecting primary lesions > 0.5 cm. Useful in patients with previous implant surgery or in patients with dense breasts.
- Useful for nodal extension of disease
- Suspected recurrence
- Therapy and follow-up

Gallium Imaging

ISOTOPE

^{67}Ga citrate is most commonly used for imaging of tumors and inflammation.

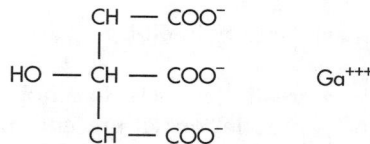

Pharmacokinetics

- Physical half-life: 78 hours
- Blood half-life: 12 hours
- ^{67}Ga is bound to iron transport proteins such as transferrin, ferritin, lactoferritin
- ^{67}Ga localizes in infections and tumors because of:
    Uptake in leukocytes
    Transferrin and lactoferrin binding at site of infection
    Abnormal vascular permeability at sites of inflammation and tumors
- Renal and fecal excretion

Radiation

Major radiation is to bone marrow (9 rad), bowel (9 rad), spleen and liver (7 rad).

Technique

- Usual dosage is 185-300 MBq. Higher doses increases lesion detectability
- Imaging 48-72 hours after IV administration
- All 3 major photopeaks (93, 185, 300 keV) are used for imaging to increase signal-to-noise ratio (SNR).

NORMAL IMAGES

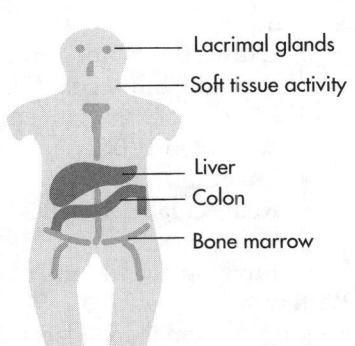

Lacrimal glands
Soft tissue activity
Liver
Colon
Bone marrow

- Low-quality images because:
    Relatively low dosage
    Residual blood activity
    Delayed imaging (days after injection)
    Need a medium energy collimator that has a lower spatial
      resolution
- Liver has the most intense uptake
- Colonic excretion becomes prominent after 48 hours and limits the
  utility of the technique for abdominal imaging
- Uptake in salivary glands, lacrimal glands, breast
- Epiphyseal plates are prominent in children
- Lung activity is minimal
- Renal activity is normal early only; activity after 72 hours is always abnormal

APPLICATIONS

Chest
Uptake occurs in a wide variety of inflammatory diseases and can be used to
determine whether an interstitial process is active or inactive (e.g., interstitial fibrosis
is not Ga avid). Most common indications:
- Sarcoid activity
- Detection of early *Pneumocystis carinii* pneumonia
- Lymphoma imaging (residual disease vs. inactive fibrosis)
- Ga-avid tumors: lymphoma > hepatocellular carcinoma > others

Other applications
- Osteomyelitis imaging
- Cardiac amyloidosis
- Increased parotid or lacrimal uptake
    Sarcoid
    Sjögren's syndrome
    Radiation

Leukocyte Imaging

PREPARATION

WBC labeling can be used as a marker of acute inflammation. WBC labeling is
performed with ^{111}In oxine, a lipophilic compound that diffuses through cell
membranes. Once inside the cell, In and oxine dissociate and In binds to intracellular
proteins; oxine diffuses out of cells. Tc HMPAO labeling of WBC is also used. Chronic
infection may cause false negative scans.

Indications
- All infectious processes in abdomen (^{67}Ga is less suited because of its bowel
  excretion)
- Osteomyelitis
- Vascular graft infections

12

Technique

1. Draw 50 mL blood from patient (anticoagulated with heparin).
2. Separate buffy coat (Ficoll).
3. 37 MBq of ^{111}In oxine or ^{111}In tropolone is incubated (30 minutes) with the separated WBC.
4. Wash cells.
5. Reinject labeled WBC (usually 7.4-18 MBq). Labeling procedures takes about 2 hours.
6. Imaging at 24 hours after injection.

Radiation

Major radiation is to spleen (20 rad), liver (3 rad), and bone marrow (2 rad). Radiation to other organs is low.

OTHER INFECTION IMAGING AGENTS

OPTIMAL IMAGING TIME	
Agent	Time (Hrs)
^{67}Ga	48
^{111}In-oxine WBC	24
^{111}In-IgG	12-24
^{99m}Tc HMPAO WBC	2
Chemotactic peptides	1
Long circulating polymers	1-12

NORMAL IMAGING

- Images have low SNR
- Spleen very hot (in contrast to Ga images where liver is very hot)
- No bowel activity
- No activity in lacrimal glands

Brain Imaging

^{99m}Tc HMPAO

Hexamethylpropyleneamine oxime (HMPAO) is a lipophilic agent that passes through the intact blood-brain barrier, is trapped within neurons, and remains there for several hours after IV administration. The compound is only stable for about 30 minutes after preparation and should therefore be administered immediately. Quality control is necessary to determine the amount of a less lipophilic complex of DL, HMPAO, which does not accumulate in the brain.

Pharmacokinetics

- Brain activity maximum at 1 minute, plateau at 2 minutes (88% peak activity)
- Brain activity remains constant for 8 hours
- Organ uptake
    Brain, 4%
    Liver, 11%
    Kidneys, 4%
    Bladder, urine, 3%
- Gray matter activity > white matter activity

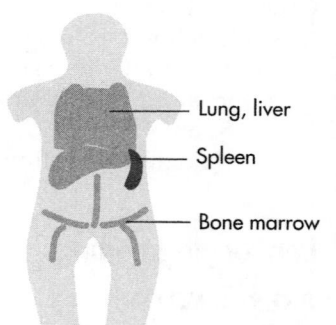

Lung, liver

Spleen

Bone marrow

BRAIN DEATH STUDY

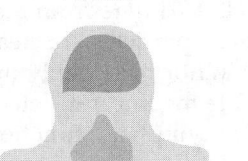
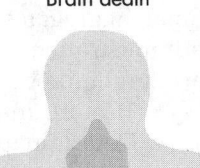

Normal   Brain death

Brain death is defined as absent cerebral blood flow despite maintained cardiac and respiratory function. Brain scans are useful to confirm the presence of brain death particularly in barbiturate intoxication and hypothermia (EEG less reliable). There are 2 types of studies:

- ^{99m}Tc DTPA flow study to demonstrate absence of flow
- ^{99m}Tc HMPAO study (preferred method)

Technique

1. Freshly prepare ^{99m}Tc HMPAO
2. Inject 555-740 MBq (high dose)
3. Scalp tourniquet to diminish activity from external carotid circulation (only needed for ^{99m}Tc DTPA but not for ^{99m}Tc HMPAO)
4. Obtain flow images (optional)
5. Obtain delayed images 5-15 minutes after injection

Imaging findings

- No flow
    - Absent ICA
    - Absent sinuses
- Absent cerebral uptake of HMPAO
- Slight perfusion of scalp veins may be present

HMPAO SPECT IMAGING

Indications

Dementia

- Alzheimer's disease: bilateral perfusion defects in temporoparietal regions
- Multiinfarct dementia: asymmetric perfusion defects

Movement disorders

- Parkinson's disease: increased perfusion in basal ganglia
- Huntington's disease: decreased striatal metabolism

Tumor

- Residual/recurrent tumor vs. radiation necrosis

Technique

1. Freshly prepare ^{99m}Tc HMPAO
2. Inject 555-740 MBq
3. Imaging 20 minutes after injection
4. 30-40 second acquisitions per view
5. Reconstructions in 3 orthogonal planes

Lymphoscintigraphy

AGENTS

Sulfide colloid

^{99m}Tc sulfide colloid (particle size 3-12 nm) differs from ^{99m}Tc sulfur colloid (particle size 500-1000 nm) used for liver spleen imaging. Sulfide colloid used for lymphoscintigraphy is prepared by reacting hydrogen sulfide with antimony potassium tartrate to provide Sb_2S_3. Polyvinylpyrrolidone stabilizes the colloid sulfide and limits particle growth.

12

Human serum albumin (HSA) nanocolloid

Small aggregates of HSA (differs from macroaggregated albumin in size). After SC administration (0.2 mL), particles are cleared by lymphatic vessels (30% at 3 hours); accumulation occurs in normal local lymph nodes. Indications:

- Tumor (unreliable method for detecting lymph node metastases)
- Determination of lymphatic function in lymphedema

Tumor Imaging

AGENTS

OVERVIEW	
Agent	Targets/Tumor Localization
NONSPECIFIC AGENTS	
^{67}Ga	Multiple mechanism
^{201}Tl	Multiple mechanism
^{99m}Tc sestamibi	Perfusion imaging
^{18}FDG-PET	Glucose metabolism
^{99m}Tc polymers	Neovascularity capillary permeability
SPECIFIC AGENTS	
^{99m}Tc MDP	Bone mineral
^{131}I	Thyroid cancer
^{131}MIBG	Adrenal tumors
Monoclonal antibodies	Tumor surface antigens
Somatostatin analogues	Somatostatin receptors

ONCOSCINT (^{111}IN DTPA LABELED B72.3 MONOCLONAL ANTIBODY)

Murine immunoglobulin G monoclonal antibody directed against a high molecular weight glycoprotein (TAG-72) expressed in the majority of colorectal and ovarian tumors. Properties:

- Biological half-life: 56 ± 14 hours
- Urine excretion (72 hours): 10%
- Used at 185 MBq; imaging at 48-72 hours
- Normal distribution: liver > spleen > bone marrow > other

Somatostatin Analog Imaging

SOMATOSTATIN

Human somatostatin (cyclic 14 amino acid peptide) has broad action, usually inhibitory in nature. A large variety of neuroendocrine cells have somatostatin receptors and imaging may be useful in these cases:

- Paraganglioma
- Pituitary adenoma
- Islet cell tumors
- Pheochromocytoma
- Adrenal neuroblastoma

- Pulmonary oat cell tumors
- Lymphoma
- Medullary thyroid carcinoma
- GI, chest carcinoids

OCTREOTIDE IMAGING

Octreotide (phe-cys-phe-trp-lys-thr-cys-thr), a synthetic cyclic octapeptide is used for clinical imaging. This agent has similar pharmacologic action to somatostatin and can be labeled with either ^{123}I or ^{111}In after certain molecular modification. Blood half-life: 6 hours. Urine excretion 50% at 6 hours. In abscence of tumors, the main distribution is to spleen, kidneys, and liver.

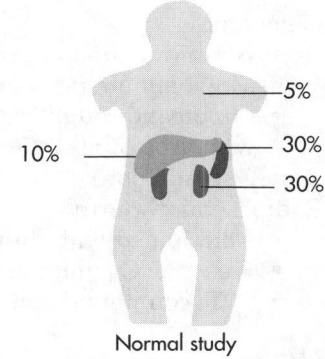

5%
10%
30%
30%

Normal study

Differential Diagnosis

Radiopharmaceuticals

OVERVIEW					
Organ	Pharmaceutical	Dose (mCi)*	Mode of Decay	Excretion	Critical Organ (rad/dose)
Bone	^{99m}Tc MDP	20	IT	Renal	2-3/bladder
Lung	^{99m}Tc MAA	4	IT	Renal	1.0/lung
	^{133}Xe	10	β-	Lungs	0.3/lung
Heart	^{201}Tl	2-4	EC	Minimal renal	2.2/kidney
	^{99m}Tc RBC	20	IT	Renal	0.4/body
Thyroid	^{123}I	0.2	EC	GI, renal	5/thyroid
	^{131}I	5-10	β-	GI, renal	500-1000 thyroid
Renal	^{99m}TC DTPA	10	IT	Renal	2-5/bladder
	^{99m}MAG$_3$	10	IT	Renal	2-5/bladder
Liver-spleen	^{99m}Tc sulfur colloid	5-8	IT	None	1-2/liver
Hepatobiliary	^{99m}Tc DISIDA	5-8	IT	Biliary	1.6/bowel
Brain	^{99m}Tc DTPA	20	IT	Renal	2-5/bladder
	^{99m}Tc HMPAO	20	IT	Renal, GI	5/Lacrimal gland
Infection-tumor	^{67}Ga citrate	5-10	EC	GI, renal	4.5/Colon
	^{111}In WBC	0.2-0.5	EC	None	20/Spleen
GI bleed	^{99m}Tc RBC	20	IT	Renal	0.4/body
Meckel's diverticulum	^{99m}Tc O4	15	IT	GI	2/Stomach
LeVeen shunt	^{99m}Tc MAA	3	IT	Renal	Lung/peritoneum
Gastric emptying	^{99m}Tc sulfur colloid	0.5	IT	GI	Colon
Ureteral reflux	^{99m}Tc sulfur colloid	0.5	IT	Urinary	Bladder

*1.0 MBq = 27mCi; 740 MBq = 20 mCi; 1.0 mCi = 37 MBq.

12

QUALITY ASSURANCE FOR RADIOPHARMACEUTICALS

Generator
- Aluminum breakthrough: $< 10\ \mu g/ml$
- Molybdenum (Mo) breakthrough: $< 0.15\ \mu Ci/1\ mCi$ of ^{99m}Tc
- Mo breakthrough is determined by counting the eluate in a well counter without (counts $^{99m}Tc + {}^{99}Mo$) and with a lead shield (count only 600 keV beta ($-$) radiation)

Radiochemical purity
- Determined with thin layer chromatography
- Free $^{99m}TcO_4^-$ migrates in saline and methanol
- ^{99m}Tc compounds migrate in saline only

Lung

V/Q MISMATCH

- Pulmonary embolism
- Vasculitis radiation therapy, Wegener's, autoimmune
- Tumor compression of PA
- Pleural effusion
- Radiation therapy
- Hypoplastic PA

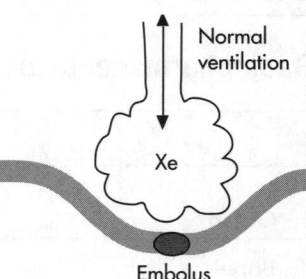

CAUSES OF PULMONARY EMBOLISM

- Venous thrombus (most common cause)
- Fat embolism; although present in most skeletal trauma, only 1% manifest clinical syndrome
- Tumor embolism
- Amniotic fluid embolism
- Parasites, especially schistosomiasis
- Talc embolism in intravenous drug abuser (widespread micronodular disease of the lungs)
- Oil embolism from Ethiodol following lymphangiogram
- Mercury embolism: thermometer accidents (metallic densities)
- Air embolism: rarely has plain film manifestations

MATCHED V/Q DEFECTS

Any primary pulmonary parenchymal abnormality may result in secondary arteriolar constriction thus causing a matched V/Q defect.
- Consolidation: pneumonia, edema
- COPD
- Atelectasis
- Tumor
- Bullous disease
- Pneumonectomy, surgery
- Pneumonia
- Enlarged hilar nodes
- Edema
- Firbosis
- Pulmonary infarction

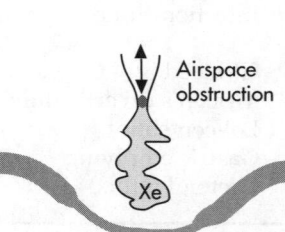

DECREASED PERFUSION IN ONE LUNG

- Embolus
- Pneumothroax
- Massive effusion
- Tumor
- Pulmonary agenesis or hypoplasia
- Swyer-James syndrome

Cardiovascular

FALSE NEGATIVE THALLIUM STUDIES

- Submaximal exercise (high splanchnic uptake)
- Noncritical stenosis ($< 40\%$)
- Small ischemic area
- Coronary collaterals
- Multivessel disease
- Medications:
    Blunted cardiac response to exercise (beta blockers, clacium channel blockers, digoxin)
    Altered myocardial extraction (furosemide, lidocaine, dipyridamole, dexamethasone, isoproteranol)

FALSE POSITIVE THALLIUM STUDY

- Any cardiomyopathy
- Aortic valve stenosis
- Mitral valve prolapse
- Left bundle branch block (LBBB)
- Infiltrative cardiac disease (sarcoidosis, Chagas' disease, amyloidosis)

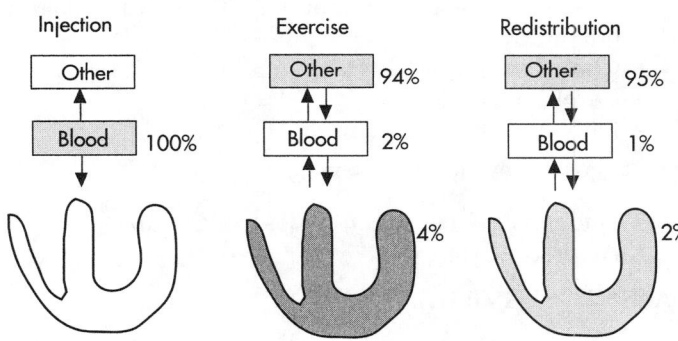

PARADOXICAL SEPTAL MOVEMENT

- Septal ischemia
- Previous cardiac surgery
- RV overload
- LBBB or pacer placement

PYROPHOSPHATE UPTAKE

- MI
- Unstable angina
- LV aneurysm
- Cardiomyopathy
- Valvular calcification
- Any cause of myocardial injury
    Contusion or surgery
    Cardioversion
    Myocarditis
    Pericarditis

12

Gastrointestinal

PATTERNS IN HIDA STUDIES

GB not visualized
Give morphine to increase pressure or cholecystokinin to contract GB. Causes:
- Acute cholecystitis
- Prolonged fasting
- Recent meal

Biliary system not visualized
- Biliary atresia
- Long-standing bile duct obstruction

Low hepatic activity, renal activity
- Severe hepatocellular disease
- Neonatal hepatitis; to improve the excretion of tracer in neonatal hepatitis, patients can be pretreated with phenobarbital (5 mg/kg for 5 days)

Bowel not visualized
- Choledocholithiasis
- Ampullary stenosis

Abnormal tracer collections
- Bile leak (postsurgical, trauma); do delayed imaging to differentiate leak from GB or bowel
- Choledochal cyst
- Caroli's disease
- Duodenal diverticulum

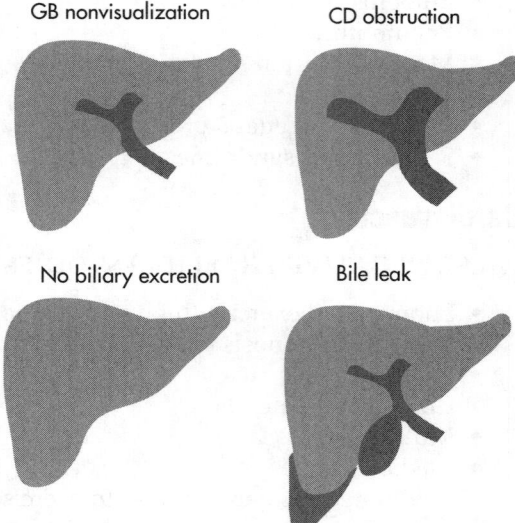

GB nonvisualization

CD obstruction

No biliary excretion

Bile leak

FALSE NEGATIVE HIDA STUDY

- Duodenal diverticulum may simulate GB
- Accessory cystic duct

FALSE POSITIVE HIDA STUDY

- Recent meal (within 4 hours)
- Prolonged fasting, ICU patients, parenteral nutrition
- Pancreatitis
- Hepatocellular dysfunction
- Right lower lobe pneumonia
- Cholangiocarcinoma involving cystic duct

FOCAL LIVER UPTAKE WITH ^{99m}Tc SULFUR COLLOID

- Focal nodular hyperplasia
- Regenerating nodule
- Budd-Chiari syndrome (hot caudate lobe)
- Vena cave obstruction (umbilical vein delivery to segment 1)

BLEEDING STUDIES

- Uptake conforming to bowel with no change over time: inflammatory bowel disease, faulty labeling (^{99m}TcO$_4^-$ excreted into bowel)
- Uptake conforming to bowel with progressive accumulation over time: hemorrhage
- Uptake not conforming to bowel: aneurysm

RLQ ACTIVITY ON MECKEL SCAN

- Meckel's diverticulum or other duplication cysts with ectopic gastric mucosa
- Renal (ectopic kidney, ureteral stenosis)
- Very active bleeding sites
- Tumors
- Inflammatory bowel disease

RAPID GASTRIC EMPTYING

- Postoperative: BI, BII
- Peptic ulcer disease, Zollinger-Ellison syndrome
- Drugs: erythromycin, metoclpromide, domperidone
- Sprue
- Vagotomy with distal partial gastrectomy

DELAYED GASTRIC EMPTYING

- Diabetes
- Hyperglycemia
- Acidosis
- Ileus
- Chronic gastritis
- Chronic ulcer disease
- Drugs—opiates, antacids, gastrin

Genitourinary

PATTERNS

Focal renal defects
- Tumor: solid, cystic
- Infection: abscess, cortical scarring
- Congenital: duplex system
- Trauma
- Vascular: complete stenosis

Focal hot renal lesions
- Collecting system
- Urinary leak
- Cross-fused ectopia
- Horseshoe kidney

Dilated ureter or collecting system
- Reflux (most common)
- Obstructed ureter

Delayed uptake and excretion (renal failure)
Prerenal: poor flow and uptake, unilateral
- Arterial stenosis
- Venous thrombosis

Renal (bilateral)
- Acute tubular necrosis: normal flow, poor uptake
- Glomerulonephritis: poor flow and poor uptake
- Chronic renal failure

Postrenal
- Obstruction: dilated calyces

Nonvisualized kidney
- Nephrectomy
- Ectopic kidney pelvis, fused ectopia
- Renal artery embolus
- Renal artery occlusion

Testicular Anomalies

Decreased uptake
- Torsion
- Orchiectomy

Increased uptake
- Orchioepididymitis

Ring sign
- Late torsion
- Tumor
- Abscess
- Trauma

Bone

FOCAL HOT LESIONS

Mnemonic: TIC MTV
- **T**umor
- **I**nflammation
  - Osteomyelitis
  - Infectious, inflammatory, metabolic arthritis
- **C**ongenital
  - Osteogenesis imperfecta
  - TORCH infections
- **M**etabolic (usually diffuse, multifocal lesions)
  - Marrow hyperplasia
  - Paget's disease
  - Fibrous dysplasia
- **T**rauma
  - Stress fracture, avulsion injuries
  - Osteonecrosis
  - Sudeck's dystrophy
  - Total hip replacement
  - Child abuse
- **V**ascular
  - Sickle cell (infection vs. infarcts)

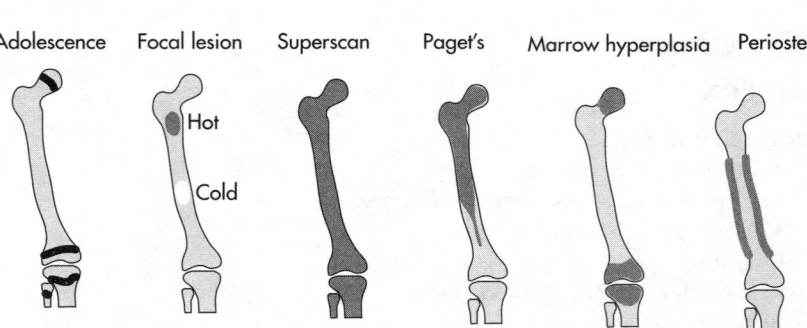

Adolescence   Focal lesion   Superscan   Paget's   Marrow hyperplasia   Periosteal

Hot

Cold

FOCAL COLD BONE LESIONS

Metastases most common cause (80%)
- Multiple myeloma, lymphoma
- Renal
- Thyroid
- Neuroblastoma

Primary bone lesions
- Unicameral bone cyst, ABC, EG

Vascular
- Infarction (acute)
- Aseptic necrosis (early)
- Radiation therapy (endarteritis obliterans)

Artifact
- Overlying pacemaker, barium, jewelry

SUPERSCAN

Criteria: diffuse high bone uptake, diminshed soft tissue and renal activity, high sternal uptake (tie sign), increased uptake at costochondral junction (beading).

Metastases (usually also causes focal abnormalities)
- Prostate metastases (most common)
- Lung cancer
- Breast cancer

Metabolic
- Hyperparathyroidism
- Renal osteodystrophy
- Osteomalacia
- Paget's disease (hot and cold lesions are typically combined)

Myeloproliferative disease
- Myelofibrosis (large spleen)

DIFFUSE PERIOSTEAL UPTAKE (TRAMTRACK SIGN)

Criteria: bilateral, diffuse periosteal uptake
- Hypertrophic osteoarthropathy (lower extremity > upper extremity)
- Child abuse
- Thyroid acropachy

EXTRAOSSEOUS ACTIVITY

Normally, the kidneys and bladder are the only organs apparent on a bone scan.
Causes of increased soft tissue activity:

Soft tissues
- Renal failure
- Radiotherapy ports
- Myositis
  Myositis ossificans
  Dermatomyositis
  Rhabdomyolysis (e.g., ethylene glycol poisoning, alcohol)
- Tumors with calcifications

Kidney
- Focal
    Obstruction
    Calcifying metatases
    Radiation to kidney
    RCC
- Diffuse
    Obstruction
    Dehydration
    Metastases
    RCC
    Chemotherapy
    Thalassemia
    Iron overload
    Pyelonephritis

Breast
- Pregnancy, lactation
- Inflammatory breast lesions
- Steroids

Stomach, GI
- Free $^{99m}TcO_4^-$
- Hyperparathyroidism
- Bowel infarction

Liver
- Metastases
- Simultaenous/prior administration of sulfur colloid
- Diffuse hepatic necrosis
- Elevated serum aluminum levels
- Colloid formation
- Hepatoma
- Amyloidosis

Spleen
- Blood dyscrasia (sickle cell, thalassemia: increased intracellular calcium)

Chest
- Cardiac infarction
- Lung tumors

Other
- Urine contamination

Thyroid

DIFFUSELY INCREASED THYROID UPTAKE

Criteria: > 30% uptake, enlarged gland, pyramidal lobe
- Graves' disease (usually hyperthyroid)
- Early Hashimoto's thyroiditis (usually euthyroid)
- Rare causes:
    Iodine starvation
    Thyroid metabolism anomalies

DIFFUSELY DECREASED THYROID UPTAKE

Criteria: nonvisualized gland or low uptake, salivary glands may show high uptake because of adjusted windowing. Causes:

Thyroiditis
- Painful (subacute granulomatous: de Quervain's disease)
- Painless (subacute lymphocytic)
- Late Hashimoto's disease

Medications
- Thyroid hormone therapy
- Iodine
    Iodinated contrast agents
    Vitamin preparations
    Lugol's solution
- PTU
- Tapazole

Thyroid ablation
- Surgery
- ^{131}I

HETEROGENOUS THYROID UPTAKE

Criteria: enlarged gland (goiter), hot and cold areas
- Multinodular goiter
- Multiple autonomous nodules
- Hashimoto's thyroiditis
- Cancer

SUGGESTED READING

Delbeke D, Martin WH, Patton JA, et al: *Practical FDG imaging*, New York, 2002, Springer Verlag.

Habibian RM: *Nuclear medicine imaging: a teaching file*, Philadelphia, 1999, Lippincott Williams & Wilkins.

Mettler F, Guiberteau M: *Essentials of nuclear medicine imaging*, Philadelphia, 1998, WB Saunders.

Palmer E, Scott J, Strauss H: *Practical nuclear medicine*, Philadelphia, 1992, WB Saunders.

Thrall J, Ziessman H: *Nuclear medicine: the requisites*, St Louis, 2000, Mosby.

Wieler HJ, Coleman RE, editors: *PET in clinical oncology*, New York, 2000, Springer Verlag.

12

Chapter 13

Contrast Agents

Chapter Outline

13

X-ray Contrast Agents

General

COST OF CONTRAST AGENTS

Average cost estimates per patient dose
- Ionic iodinated IV agent $ 10
- Nonionic iodinated agent $ 100
- Gastrografin for CT $ 1
- Barium $ 10
- Gadolinium chelate for MRI $ 100

Iodinated Contrast Agents

CLASSIFICATION

A variety of iodinated contrast agents have been developed and are distributed by different manufacturers. The agents all consist of iodinated benzene ring derivatives and ionic agents are typically formulated as sodium and/or meglumine salts. 2 genetic classes of agents:
- High osmolar contrast agents (HOCAs, "ionics")
- Low osmolar contrast agents (LOCAs, "nonionics" and "ionic-LOCAs")

OVERVIEW OF COMMERCIAL AGENTS IN UNITED STATES			
Manufacturer	**HOCA**	**LOCA**	**Ionic LOCA**
Berlex (Schering)	Urovist Angiovist	Ultravist	
Mallinckrodt	Conray Vascoray	Optiray	Hexabrix
Squibb (Bracco)	Renovue Renografin Renovist	Isovue	
Nycomed/Sanofi/Winthrop	Hypaque	Omnipaque Visipaque	
Cook Imaging		Oxilan	

Iodine content

For nonionic agents, the iodine (I) content is easy to determine because it is written on the label. For example, Omnipaque 300 contains 300 mg I/mL of solution. For ionic agents, the I content has to be calculated because contrast concentrations are expressed as salt weight basis. For example, Conray 60 contains 60% meglumine iothalamate = 600 mg salt/mL = 282 mg I/mL. Because meglumine and sodium have different molecular weights, a 60% (weight/volume) solution of contrast contains different amounts of I, depending on the accompanying cation:
- 60% meglumine diatrizoate: 282 mg I/mL
- 60% sodium diatrizoate: 358 mg I/mL

Meglumine vs. sodium salts

- All HOCA are ionic. They are organic acids consisting of an amion (radiodense iodinated benzoic acid derivative) and cation (sodium or meglumine).
- Sodium salts result in better renal opacification than meglumine salts (therefore sodium salts are used in Urovist).
- Sodium/meglumine diatrizoate mixtures have a lower incidence of ventricular fibrillation than pure meglumine solutions.

HOCA

There are 2 major ionic agents on the market, differing in the R-group:
- Diatrizoate (i.e., Hypaque)
- Iothalamate (i.e., Conray)

The osmolarity of ionic agents depends on the concentration, which typically ranges from 30% (550 mOsm/kg H_2O) to 76% (~ 2000 mOsm/kg H_2O). The ionic agents have been in clinical use since the 1950s.

Radiodense anion   Cation

Meglumine$^+$

NONIONIC LOCA

Nonionic agents have a lower incidence of adverse reactions (by a factor of 6 for all reactions and a factor of 9 for severe reactions) and are equally effective as imaging agents. They are much higher in cost when compared to HOCA. There are 4 nonionic agents on the market, differing in the R-groups:
- Iopamidol (Isovue)
- Iohexol (Omnipaque)
- Ioversol (Optiray)
- Iopromide (Ultravist)

Nonionic agents do not require an accompanying cation and therefore have lower osmolality. The osmolality depends on the concentration, which typically ranges from 300 mg I/mL (= 670 mOsm/kg H_2O) to 370 mgI/mL (= 800 mOsm/kg H_2O). Ionic agents have been in use since 1986. Iodixanol is a new nonionic dimer that is iso-osmolar to blood at all concentrations.

IONIC LOCA

There is only one agent on the market in the United States: ioxaglate (Hexabrix). It is a monoacid dimer that is available at a concentration of 320 mg I/mL (600 mOsm/kg H_2O).

Na$^+$ or meglumine$^+$

13

PHARMACOLOGY

Plasma levels of iodinated agents depend on:
- Rate of administration (IV bolus, IV drip)
- Blood half-life
- Distribution
    - Rapid exchange between plasma and extracellular space
    - Exclusion from intracellular space
    - Agents do not cross intact blood-brain barrier
- Excretion
    - Glomerular filtration with no resorption in the tubules
    - Hepatic excretion (vicarious excretion) increases in renal failure

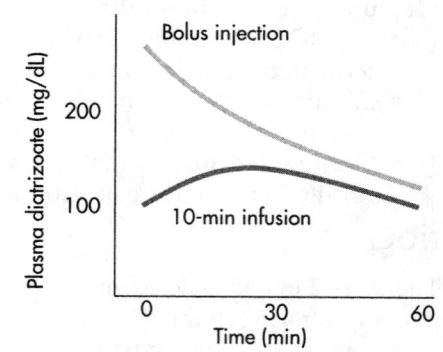

SIDE EFFECTS

OVERVIEW		
Reaction	HOCA	LOCA
Overall	5%	1%-2%
History of allergy, asthma	10%	3%-4%
Severe reaction	0.1%	0.01%
Fatal	1/40,000-170,000	1/200,000-300,000

Types of reactions
Idiosyncratic or anaphylactoid
- Urticaria
- Laryngospasm
- Bronchospasm
- Cardiovascular collapse

Nonidiosyncratic
- Vasovagal response
- Pain
- Renal failure
- Cardiac arrhythmias
- Seizures
- Nausea/vomiting

Risk factors
High-risk patients should either (1) be premedicated with steroids, (2) receive nonionic agents, or (3) be evaluated by MR/US without contrast agents. Major risk factors are:
- Allergies, asthma, atopy, 10%
- Cardiac disease, 20%
- Previous reaction to contrast agents, 25%

Other risk factors
- Pheochromocytoma
- Sickle cell disease
- Hyperproteinemic states (e.g., multiple myeloma)
- Other (e.g., myasthenia gravis, homocystinuria)

All patients now receive LOCA for contrast CT examinations

Premedication

In patients with prior anaphylactoid reactions, premedication and use of LOCA is the safest approach. There is no universally accepted premedication regimen.
- Benadryl: 50 mg PO on call
- Cimetidine: 300 mg PO q6 hours × 3; 1st dose night before
- Prednisone: 50 mg PO q6 hours × 3; 1st dose night before

Contrast-induced nephropathy

The overall incidence of contrast-induced renal failure is 0.15%. The mechanism of injury is acute tubular necrosis. Risk factors for development include:
- Creatinine > 1.5 mg/dL
- Diabetes, especially insulin dependent
- Multiple myeloma
- Dehydration

Most contrast-induced nephropathies are brief and self-limited with resolution over 2 weeks. LOCA use may be justified in azotemic patients. Prophylactic oral administration of the antioxidant acetylcysteine (600 μg bid for 3 days starting the day before contrast-administration), together with saline hydration is an effective means of preventing contrast-induced renal damage in patients with chronic renal insufficiency.

Metformin (glucophage)

Biguanide oral antihyperglycemic agents used to treat non–insulin-dependent diabetes mellitus (NIDDM). Lactic acidosis is a rare (0-0.84 cases per 1000) complication with a 50% mortality rate that occurs mainly in patients with concomitant renal failure or hepatic failure. Recommendations regarding use of iodinated contrast in patients on metformin:

Elective study
- Discontinue metformin for 48 hrs before and after the contrast study; control blood glucose.
- Before restarting metformin, reevaluate renal function

Urgent contrast study
- Obtain a serum creatinine. If the patient has normal renal function the contrast study can be performed. Note that the patient should be (1) well hydrated, (2) receive nonionic agents, (3) not receive metformin for 48 hrs after contrast, and (4) serum creatinine should be checked before reinstituting metformin.
- If the patient has abnormal renal function, metformin has to be stopped for 48 hrs before administration of contrast.

13

Other Iodinated Agents

GASTROGRAFIN

Gastrografin (Squibb; diatrizoate meglumine and diatrizoate sodium; same as Renografin 76) is an oral contrast medium for opacification of the gastrointestinal (GI) tract. Undiluted or mildly diluted. Gastrografin can be used as substitute for barium if GI perforation is suspected. A 1:40 dilution results in a CT density of 200 HU. Preparation: ¼ ounce in 10 ounces of water; 3 cups before CT.

Complications

- Aspiration can cause chemical pneumonitis
- Diarrhea (systemic dehydration) due to the osmotic activity of the preparation; a 1:4.6 dilution of Gastrografin in water is isotonic
- Hypovolemic shock has been reported if used undiluted in pediatric patients

SINOGRAFIN

Diatrizoate meglumine and iodipamide meglumine 79%. Used for hysterosalpingography.

IOPANOIC ACID (TELEPAQUE)

Iopanoic acid is an oral cholecystographic agent. Oral cholecystographic agents are incompletely substituted benzene derivatives with an amide group at the 3 position to facilitate stable triiodo substitution at 2-, 4-, and 6-. Once in the plasma, these agents bind to albumin and attach to cytoplasmic anion-binding protein in hepatocytes and are excreted after glucuronic acid conjugation. Enterohepatic recirculation occurs. Optimal visualization of these agents occurs after 10-20 hours. Standard dose is 3 g as a starting dose for adults; if no visualization occurs after the 1st administration, the examination should be repeated the next day after a 2nd 3-g dose (double-dose examination). If bilirubin is elevated, opacification of GB isusually unsuccessful.

Complications:

- Transient hyperbilirubinemia
- Nausea, vomiting, abdominal cramps, and diarrhea in up to 40%
- Renal toxicity

Contraindications:

- Hyperuricemia
- Severe liver disease
- Planned thyroid function tests

Barium

COMPOSITION

Micronized barium ($BaSO_4$, particle size 5-10 μm) is now commonly used to prepare different barium products such as:

- "Thin barium" (e.g., EZ-Jug) for upper GI studies, small bowel follow-through, barium enema: 40% w/w $BaSO_4$ solution
- "Thick barium" (e.g., EZ-HD) for double constrast studies: 85% w/w $BaSO_4$ solution
- CT barium (e.g., Readicat): 1.2% w/w $BaSO_4$ solution, 450 mL bottles

Typical additives to barium suspensions include:
- Agents to prevent flocculation (clumping)
- Antifoam agents
- Oncotically active sugars (sorbitol)
- Sweetening, flavoring, and coloring to improve palatability
- Preservatives: potassium sorbate and sodium benzoate
- Tannic acid, an astringent that precipitates proteins and results in improved mucosal coating; do not use in inflammatory bowel disease

COMPLICATIONS

- Exacerbation of GI obstruction above a preexisting large bowel obstruction (but not small bowel obstruction)
- Intraperitoneal extravasation through esophagus or bowel perforation results in extensive fibrosis
- Aspiration can cause chemical pneumonitis
- Hypersensitivity reaction may be caused by latex tip used in barium enema

MR Contrast Agents

There are 3 classes of contrast agents based on magnetic properties:
- Diamagnetic agents (generally not used as IV contrast agents)
- Paramagnetic agents
- Superparamagnetic agents

Unlike CT contrast agents, the effect of MRI contrast agents is indirectly visualized via changes in tissue proton behavior or magnetic susceptibility.

Paramagnetic Agents

GADOLINIUM CHELATES

Gadolinium (Gd) is a paramagnetic agent that develops a magnetic moment when placed in a magnetic field. It enhances the relaxation rates of protons in its vicinity (R1 > R2). Gd-DTPA is the Gd meglumine salt of diethylenetriamine pentaacetic acid (DTPA). Each milliliter of Gd-DTPA (Magnevist, Berlex) contains 469.01 mg of Gd-DTPA dimeglumine, 0.39 mg of meglumine, 0.15 mg of DTPA and water for injection. pH = 6.5-8.0. Osmolality 1.94 osm/kg. Dosage: 0.1 mmol/kg.

Pharmacology
- Excretion
  - Glomerular fitration, 95%
  - Hepatobiliary excretion, 5%
- Half-life 90 minutes
  - $83 \pm 14\%$ excretion in 6 hours
  - $91 \pm 13\%$ excretion in 24 hours
- In renal failure there is a slower excretion of Gd-DTPA, which does not cause an increase in adverse side effects
- Exchange between plasma and extracellular fluid space similar to iodinated agents

13

Safety

The safety index (LD_{50} divided by the diagnostic dose) is approximately 10 times higher for Gd-DTPA than for diatrizoate (10 for diatrizoate vs. 100 for Gd-DTPA). Gd-related deaths are very rare but have been reported with an incidence of 1:2,500,000. The incidence of minor side effects is 1.5%, the most common ones being:

- Headache, 8%
- Injection site symptoms, 7%
- Nausea, 3%
- Allergic reactions, < 0.4%
- Seizure, 0.3 %

Biochemical abnormalities have also been reported:

- Elevated serum iron levels in 30% of patients
- Elevated bilirubin levels in 3% of patients
- Pregnancy: results of clinical studies have not been reported in pregnant women. In animal studies, however, where Gd chelates have been used at many times the human dose, teratogenic effects have been described.

GD PERFUSION AGENTS			
	Gadopentetate Dimeglumine	Gadodiamide	Gadoteridol
Trade name	Magnevist	Omniscan	Prohance
Chelator type	Linear	Linear	Macrocyclic
Molecular weight (d)	938	574	559
R1 (mM sec^{-1})	3.8 ± 0.1	3.8 ± 0.1	3.7 ± 0.1
Osmolality (mOsm/kg)	1960	789	630
Net charge	−2	0	0
Elimination half-life (hrs)	1.6 ± 0.13	1.3 ± 0.27	1.6 ± 0.08
LD_{50} (mmol/kg)	5-12	15-34	11-14

MANGAFODIPIR TRISODIUM (MN-DPDP, TESLASCAN, NYCOMED)

Weak chelate of manganese dissociates into free manganese and DPDP after IV administration. Hepatocytes take up the free manganese, which acts as an intracellular paramagnetic agent and causes marked shortening of the T1-relaxation time. The free DPDP ligand is excreted in the urine. The DPDP ligand does not contribute to the imaging properties of the agent but serves to reduce the toxicity of manganese ion. After slow intravenous infusion of mangafodipir trisodium at a dose of 5 μmol/kg, near maximal enhancement of liver parenchyma is observed from 15 minutes to 4 hours. The increased signal intensity of normal liver parenchyma, on T1-weighted (T1W) images, results in improved liver-lesion conspicuity with regard to focal hepatic lesions. Malignant and benign liver lesions of hepatocellular origin (focal nodular hyperplasia, adenoma, and well-differentiated HCC) demonstrate uptake of manganese and enhancement on delayed T1W images.

Superparamagnetic Agents

A variety of parenteral iron oxides have been developed for contrast-enhanced MRI. 2 classes of iron oxides are currently in use:

- Larger superparamagnetic iron oxides (SPIO), for example, Ferridex (Advanced Magnetics) with a high R2 relaxivity and short blood half-life (minutes)
- Ultrasmall superparamagnetic iron oxides (USPIO), for example, Ferrumoxstran (Advanced Magnetics) with a high R1 relaxivity and long blood half-life (hours)

FERRIDEX (AMI-25; ENDOREM)

This agent efficiently accumulates in liver (80% of injected dose) and spleen (6%-10% of the injected dose) within minutes after administration. Once sequestered by phagocytic cells, the agent decreases liver and spleen signal intensity T2W (liver signal intensity is maximally decreased 0.5-6 hrs after administration and returns to normal within 7 days). Malignant tumors are typically devoid of large number of phagocytic cells so that they appear as hyperintense ("bright) lesions contrasted against hypointense ("black") background of normal liver. Tumors with phagocytic elements (FNH) and hemangioma have been shown to also decrease in signal intensity.

FERRUMOXSTRAN (COMBIDEX)

This agent has a blood half-life of over 20 hours and thereafter accumulates primarily in lymph nodes, liver, and spleen (SPIO on the contrary are too rapidly cleared by liver to be able to accumulate in lymph nodes). Because the agent has a significant R1 effect, it can also be used as T1-type blood pool ("brightening") agents for imaging of tumor angiogenesis, MRA and/or hepatic lesion characterization during the equilibrium phase. Perfused lesions (e.g., hemangioma) increase in signal intensity on T1W, whereas the same lesion decreases in signal intensity on T2W.

13

Treatment of Contrast Reactions

Treating Adverse Reactions

MEDICATION			
Clinical	Medication	Dosage*	Comments
Urticaria	Diphenhydramine or hydroxyzine	25-50 mg IV/IM 25-50 mg IM	Treat if symptomatic or progressive
Facial/laryngeal edema	Diphenhydramine or hydroxyzine	25-50 mg IV/IM 25-50 mg IM	Protect the airway
	Epinephrine	0.3-0.5 mL SC 1:1000 dilution	Epinephrine may precipitate ischemia in coronary artery disease
	Epinephrine	1-3 mL slow IV 1:10,000 dilution	
Bronchospasm	β₂-Agonists	Nebulizer or MDI	Metaproterenol, albuterol
	Epinephrine	0.1-0.3 mg SC (1:1000)	
	Aminophyllline	6 mg/kg IV over 20 min	If epinephrine fails
Vasovagal	Isotonic saline	250-500 cc IV	
	Atropine	0.5-1.0 mg IV	Up to 2 mg total

*See manufacturer's packet insert for specific rates of administration.

IM, Intramuscular; IV, intravenous; SC, subcutaneous. Always monitor vital signs, and give O₂.

Emergency Drug Treatment

MEDICATION			
Clinical	Medication	Dosage	Comments
Bradycardia	Atropine	0.5–1.0 mg IV q5 min	Doses < 0.5 mg may cause paradoxical bradycardia
Ventricular tachyarrhythmia	Lidocaine	1 mg/kg bolus IV; repeat 0.5 mg/kg IV every 8-10 min	Continuous infusion at 2-4 mg/min
Supraventricular tachycardia	Verapamil	0.1 mg/kg IV slowly (maximum of 10 mg)	Contraindicated with beta blockers
	Adenosine	6 mg IV bolus	If fails, give 12 mg IV bolus
Angina	Nitroglycerin	0.3-0.4 mg SL q5 min; 10-20 mg orally	Obtain ECG and monitor BP
Hypertension	Nifedipine	10 mg SL	Lasts 2-4 hr; if refractory, consider nitroprusside
	Nitroglycerin ointment 2%	1-2 inches q4 hr	30 min to see effect
Pheochromocytoma-induced hypertension	Phentolamine	1 mg IV test dose; 5 mg IV as needed	
Hypotension (unresponsive to fluid challenge)	Dopamine	2-5 μg/kg/min (via central venous access)	Significant renal, peripheral, and mesenteric vasoconstriction occurs above 10 mg/kg/min
Seizures	Diazepam	5-10 mg IVP	Lasts 20 minutes
	Phenytoin	18 mg/kg IV at 50 mg/min	ECG monitoring

Chapter 14

Imaging Physics

Chapter Outline

X-ray Physics

Production of X-Rays

X-RAY TUBE

An x-ray tube is an energy converter receiving electrical energy and producing heat and x-rays. For a diagnostic x-ray tube operating at 100 kVp the production of heat and x-rays is:

- Heat, 99%
- X-rays, 1%
  Electron deceleration (Bremsstrahlung), 0.9%
  Characteristic radiation through ionization, 0.1%

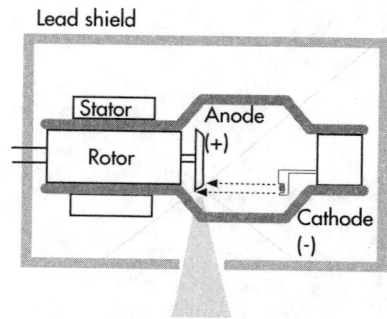

Lead shield

X-ray tubes are designed to minimize heat production and maximize x-ray output. Tubes consist of 2 main elements: a cathode (for electron production) and an anode (for conversion electron energy into x-rays). During the process of x-ray generation, x-ray beams are generated in all directions; however, the useful beam is composed only of those x-rays leaving the lead-shielded tube. All electrical components in an x-ray tube are in a vacuum. The vacuum prevents dispersion of the electrons and ionization, which could damage the filament.

Useful x-ray beam

Cathode

Cathodes produce the electrons necessary for x-ray generation. Cathodes typically consist of a tungsten filament that is heated > 2200° C. The filament is surrounded at its cathode end by a negatively charged focusing cup to direct the electrons in a small beam toward the anode.

Anode

The anode has 2 functions: to convert electron energy into x-rays and to dissipate heat. Heat dissipation is achieved by rotating the angulated target (at approximately 3600 rpm or 60 cycles/sec). The amount of x-rays produced depends on the atomic number (Z) of the anode material and the energy of electrons. Common anode materials include tungsten (W, Z = 74) or W/rhenium (Re) alloys (90%/10%). These materials are used because of their high melting point and the high yield of x-rays. Mammography units frequently use different anode materials (e.g., molybdenum [Mo]).

The focal spot is the small area on the anode in which x-rays are produced. The size of the focal spot is determined by the dimensions of the electron beam and the anode angulation. Typical angles are 12°-20°; however, smaller angles (6°) are used for neuroangiography. Tubes with smaller focal spot size are used when high image quality is essential.

X-RAY TUBE OUTPUT

Exposure delivered by an x-ray generator is controlled by selecting appropriate values for mA, kVp, and exposure time. The output of an x-ray tube increases:

- Linearly with mA
- Linearly with Z (number of protons) of the target element
- As the square of kVp

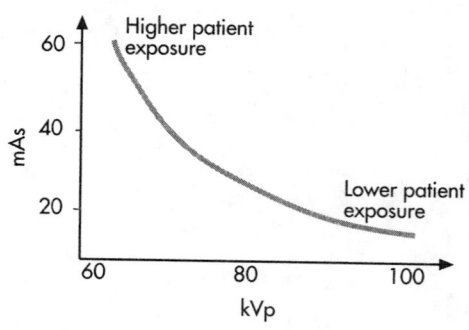

Milliampere (mA)

A milliampere (mA) is a measure of current, referring to the number of electrons flowing per second (one A corresponds to 6.25×10^{18} electrons). The higher the mA, the higher the electron flux, the higher the x-ray production. An increase in mA changes only the amount of x-rays (i.e., the intensity or exposure rate), not the maximum energy of the x-rays produced. Typical mA values range from 25 to 500 on a given x-ray unit. The use of small focal spot sizes (for high resolution) also limits the number of mAs that can be used. General rules for selecting mA:

- Use lower mA for smaller focal spots when image detail is important
- Select high mA to reduce exposure time (i.e., to limit motion blurring)
- Select high mA and reduced kVp when high image contrast is desired

Voltage

The voltage of an x-ray tube is measured in kVp (peak kilovolts). The kVp determines the maximum energy of the x-rays produced. 100 kVp means that the maximum (peak) voltage across the tube causing electron acceleration is 100,000 V. The term keV (kiloelectron volt) refers to the energy of any individual electron in the beam. When an x-ray tube is operated at 100 kVp, only a few electrons will acquire kinetic energy of 100 keV because the applied voltage usually pulsates between lower values and the maximum (peak) selected. The mean energy of an x-ray beam is approximately ⅓ of its peak energy. For 100 kVp the mean energy would be 33-40 keV. An increase in kVp translates into:

- Increased photon frequency
- Increased photon penetration
- Shortening of photon wavelength
- Increased anode heat production
- Decreased skin dose
- Decreased contrast

Film exposure is more sensitive to changes in kVp than to changes in mA or exposure time. General rules for selecting kVp:

- A 15% increase in kVp doubles exposure at the recording system (e.g., film) and has the same effect on film density as a 100% increase in mA
- An increase in kVp of 15% will decrease the contrast, so that doubling of mA is usually preferred
- mA generally needs to be at least doubled when changing from a nongrid to a grid technique (depending on field size and patient thickness)

Exposure time

Exposure times are set either by the operator (setting of a timer) or by a circuit that terminates the exposure after a selected amount of x-rays have reached the patient. General rules for selecting exposure time:

- Short exposure time minimizes blurring
- Long exposure times can be used to reduce either mA or kVp when motion is not a problem

HEAT UNIT

Heat is the factor that limits the uninterrupted use of x-ray generators. Heat units (HU) are calculated as:

$$HU = Voltage\ (kVp) \times Current\ (mA) \times Time\ (sec)$$

This formula holds true only for single-phase generators. For 3-phase generators the HU has to be multiplied by 1.35.

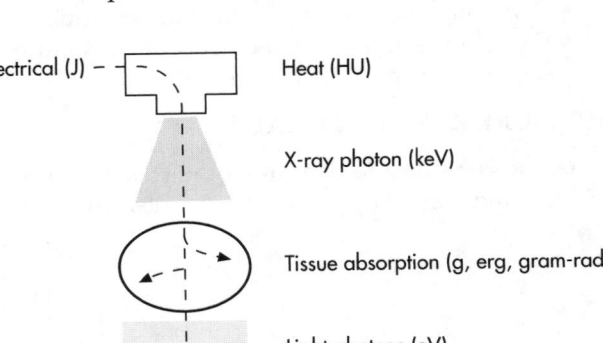

Electrical (J)

Heat (HU)

X-ray photon (keV)

Tissue absorption (g, erg, gram-rad)

Light photons (eV)

14

RATING CHARTS

The safe limit within which an x-ray tube can be operated for a single exposure can be determined by the tube rating chart. Always convert mA into mA and time before reading the charts.

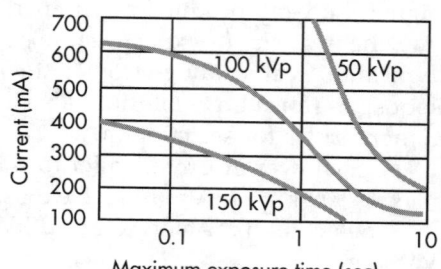

Example

What is the maximum safe kVp for a 500 mA exposure at 0.1 sec?

Answer

Approximately 100 kVp (see chart).

FOCAL SPOT (FS)

The FS is the small area on the anode in which x-rays are produced. NEMA specifications require that focal spots of < 0.3 mm have to be measured with the line pair resolution test (star pattern) and that larger focal spots can be measured with a pinhole camera. The apparent focal spot increases with:

- Increase in mA ("blooming effect")
- Increase in target angle
- Decrease in kVp

FSs SIZES	
FS (mm)	**Application**
0.1	Magnification x-ray
0.3*	Mammography
0.6	Typical small FS size
1.2	Typical large FS size
1.7 × 2.4	Maximum size of 1.2-mm FS by NEMA standards

*NEMA standards allow a 0.3 mm FS to have a tolerance of −0% and +50% (i.e., a maximum of 0.45 mm).

FOCAL SPOT AND RESOLUTION

Resolution is related to the size of the FS, the FS-object distance (FOD), and the object-detector distance (ODD):

$$\text{Resolution (lines/mm)} = \frac{1.1 \text{ FOD}}{\text{FS (mm)} \times \text{ODD}}$$

From this equation it is evident that:

- The smaller the FS, the better the resolution
- The shorter the ODD, the better the resolution
- The longer the FOD distance, the better the resolution

MEASUREMENT OF FOCAL SPOT SIZE

2 methods are used to determine the FS size: pinhole method (determines the actual FS size) and star test pattern (determines effective blur size).

Star test pattern

A star test pattern is positioned midway between FS and film. An image is then obtained in which there is a zone of blurring at some distance from the center of the object. The FS is calculated as:

$$FS = \frac{(\delta \times D \times \pi)}{(180 (M - 1))}$$

where δ = angle of one test pattern segment, D = diameter of the blur circle, and M = magnification factor.

Pinhole method

A pinhole is placed halfway between the FS and the film. The image of the FS on the exposed film will be the same size as the actual physical dimension of the FS. Pinholes are usually 0.03 mm in diameter.

MAGNIFICATION

The true magnification (M) for a point source is:

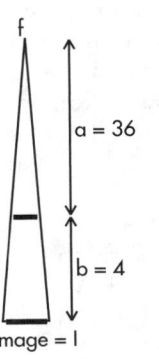
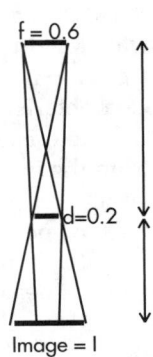

$$M = Focus - \frac{Film\ distance\ (a + b)}{}$$

In the figure on the right, the magnification would be 36 + 4/36 = 1.11 (equivalent to 11% magnification). However, because FSs are not true point sources, the real magnification of images (including penumbra) depends on the size of the FS and is given by:

$$M = m + (m - 1)\ (f/d)$$

where m = geometric magnification (a + b)/a, f = FS size, and d = object size. For this example the true magnification would thus be: M = 1.11 + (1.11 − 1) (0.6/0.2) = 1.44 (equivalent to 44% magnification).

Penumbra: zone of geometric unsharpness (edge gradient) that surrounds the umbra (complete shadow).

Unsharpness

$$Unsharpness = FS\ size \times (Magnification - 1)$$

Geometric unsharpness is highest with:
- Large FS
- Short focus object distance

Other sources of unsharpness are:
- Intensifying screen (i.e., slow single-screen films)
- Motion

RADIATION EXPOSURE AND DISTANCE

X-ray exposure to a patient increases as the square of the focus-film distance.

Example

What is the increase in exposure when the focus-film distance is changed from 50 to 75 cm?

Answer

$$Exposure_{new}/Exposure_{old} = (Distance_{new}/Distance_{old})^2 = (75/50)^2 = 2.25\text{-fold increase.}$$

14

SPECTRUM OF X-RAYS

X-rays are generated by 2 different processes:
- Bremsstrahlung: produces a continuum of photon energy radiation
- Characteristic radiation: produces defined peaks of photon energy

Bremsstrahlung

Bremsstrahlung refers to the process by which electrons, when slowed down near the nucleus of a target, give off a photon of radiation. The energy of a photon (E) is inversely proportional to its wavelength:

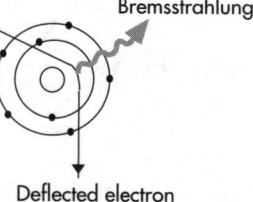

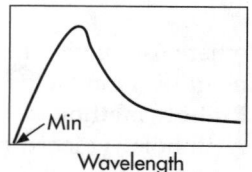

$$E \text{ (in keV)} = \frac{12.4}{\text{Wavelength (Å)}}$$

For 100 kVp the maximum energy of an electron would be 100 keV and its minimum wavelength would therefore be 12.4/100 keV = 0.124 Å. The maximum wavelength of a photon is open ended and only determined by the absorption through glass or filters.

Characteristic radiation

Characteristic radiation results when bombarding electrons eject a target electron from the inner orbits of a specific target atom. Characteristic energies from a tungsten target are:

- α_1 peak: 59.3 keV
  (L shell to K shell)
- α_2 peak: 57.9 keV
  (L shell to K shell)
- β_1 peak: 67.2 keV
  (M shell to K shell)
- β_2 peak: 69 keV
  (N shell to K shell)

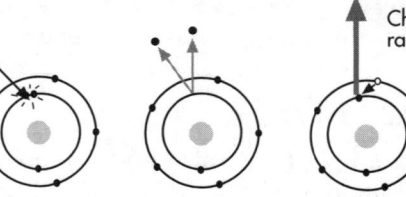

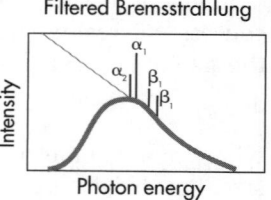

The higher the atomic number of the target atom, the greater the efficiency of x-ray production. The fraction of energy (f) released as x-rays by electrons of energy (E) in a material with atomic number (Z), is given by:

$$f = \frac{Z \times E \text{ (meV)}}{800}$$

For example, in an x-ray tube with a W target (Z = 74) and 100 keV, only 0.92% of total energy is converted into x-rays.

HEEL EFFECT

The intensity of an x-ray beam that leaves the tube is not uniform across all portions of the beam (heel effect): the intensity on the anode side is always considerably less and is close to zero for x-rays emitted along the inclined surface of the anode (cutoff). Implications of heel effect:
- Thicker parts of patient should be placed toward cathode side of tube
- Heel effect is less when large distances are used (see figure)
- Heel effect is less pronounced if smaller films are used

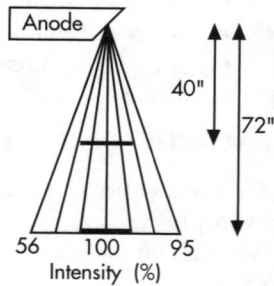

X-ray Generators

TRANSFORMER

A transformer consists of 2 wire coils wound around an iron ring. When current flows through the primary coil, a magnetic field is created within the iron ring. The magnetic field will then create a momentary current in the secondary coil. Current flows through the secondary coil only when the magnetic field is changing (i.e., when it is switched either on or off). For this reason, direct current (DC) cannot be used in the primary coil to create a steady current in the secondary coil. Rather, an alternating current (AC) has to be used in the primary coil. The voltage (V) in the 2 circuits is proportional to the number of turns (N) in the 2 coils:

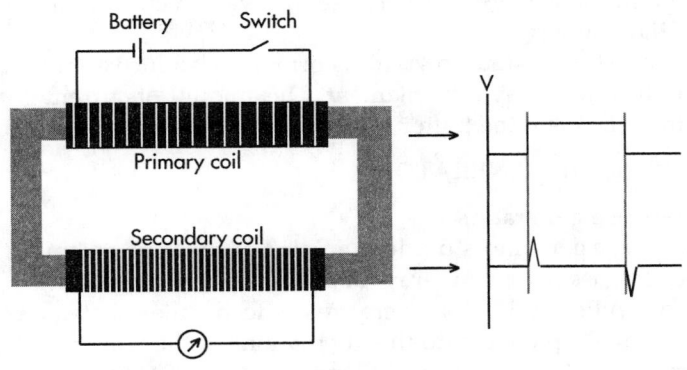

$$N_{primary}/N_{secondary} = V_{primary}/V_{secondary}$$

A transformer with more windings in the primary than in the secondary coil is called a *step-down transformer,* and a transformer with more windings in the secondary coil is called a *step-up transformer.* The product of the voltage (V) and current (I) (which is power (W): W = V × I) is always equal in both circuits:

$$V_{primary} \times I_{primary} = V_{secondary} \times I_{secondary}$$

CIRCUITS OF X-RAY GENERATORS

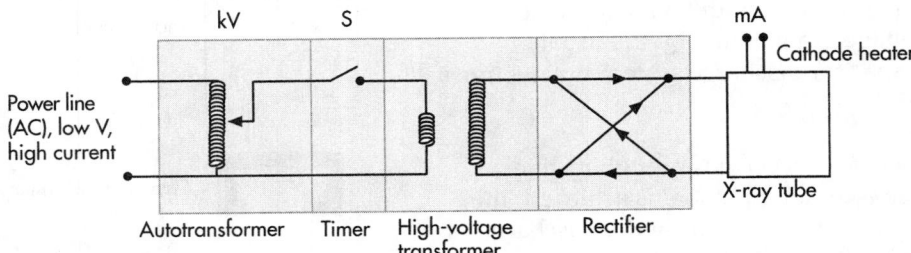

X-rays units have 2 principal circuits: a high-voltage circuit (consisting of autotransformer, timer, and high-voltage transformer) and a low-voltage filament circuit.

Autotransformer
This transformer is the kVp selector. The voltage across the primary coil can be varied by changing the number of coils in the autotransformer.

High-voltage transformer
This transformer is a step-up transformer, increasing the voltage by a factor of about 600 by having about 600 times more windings in the secondary than in the primary coil. Because the potential of the step-up transformer is up to 150,000 V, the whole transformer is immersed in oil.

Timer
Controls the exposure time.

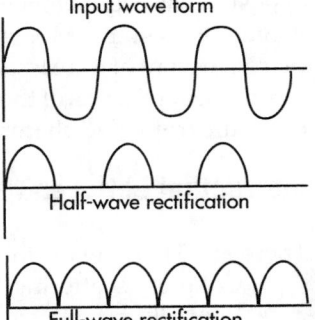

14

Rectifier

The function of the rectifier is to change AC into DC flowing in only one direction at all times. Modern rectifiers use full-wave rectification requiring 4 rectifiers.

Filament circuit

Consists of a step-down transformer to produce approximately 10 V and 3-5 A, used to heat the x-ray tube filament. The amount of current is controlled by a resistor. The more current, the hotter the filament, and the more electrons are emitted.

TYPES OF GENERATORS

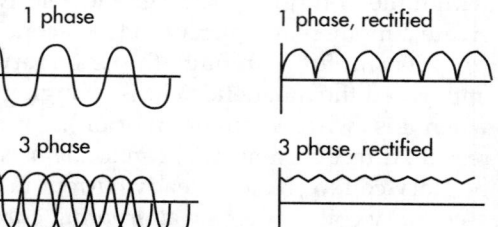

3-phase generators

3-phase generators produce an almost constant potential difference across an x-ray tube. The 3 phases lag behind each other by 120°, so there are no deep valleys between the peaks. Ripple refers to the fluctuations of the voltage across the x-ray tube (expressed as a percentage of maximum value). The theoretic ripple factor is:

- Single-phase generator: 100%
- 6-pulse, 3-phase generator: 13%
- 12-pulse, 3-phase generator: 3%

Advantages of 3-phase generators

- Higher average beam energy, less exposure for patient because unnecessary low-level radiation is reduced (higher average dose rate per time unit)
- Shorter exposure time
- Higher tube rating

Mobile generators

Most portable x-ray machines are battery powered, whereas others operate directly from a single-phase 60-Hz power outlet. The DC supply in battery-powered units is converted to AC with 60-Hz or higher kilohertz frequency. The high voltage is generated by the usual transformer-rectifier system. A capacitor discharge system is sometimes used for x-ray tube operation.

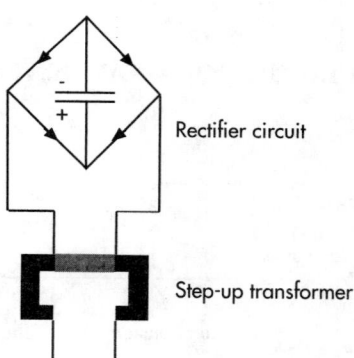

Capacitor discharge generators

The capacitor stores the electrical charge received through rectifiers from a step-up transformer. When a certain potential is achieved, the capacitor is discharged through an x-ray tube. During this discharge both the tube kV and the tube mA fall exponentially.

PHOTOTIMERS

Phototimers are used to terminate unnecessary x-ray generation after optimum exposure has been achieved. In older equipment, photomultiplier tubes were located behind the cassette. Modern x-ray equipment uses radiolucent ionization chambers placed in front of the cassette. Ionization chambers are frequently used in triplets to sample several areas of the radiographic field. A detector then averages the recorded exposure from the 3 chambers.

Interaction between X-rays and Matter

There are 5 basic ways in which an x-ray or a gamma ray interacts with matter:

- Coherent scattering
- Photoelectric effect
- Compton scattering
- Pair production
- Photodisintegration

COHERENT SCATTERING

Coherent scattering refers to radiation that undergoes a change in direction without a change in wavelength. It is the only type of interaction that does not cause ionization. Coherent scattering usually represents less than 5% of x-ray matter interaction and does not play a major role in radiology.

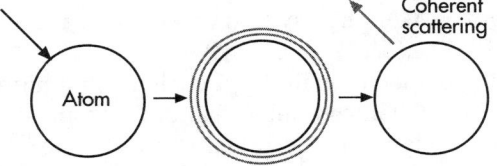

PHOTOELECTRIC EFFECT

An incident photon ejects an electron from its orbit. An electron from an outer shell then fills the gap in the K-shell, and characteristic radiation (with wavelength specific for that element) is emitted. For x-ray emission to occur the orbit must usually be in the K-shell. The end result of the photoelectric effect is:

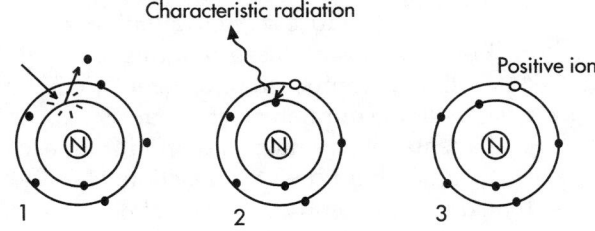

- Characteristic radiation
- A photoelectron
- A positively charged ion

The probability of the photoelectric effect occurring depends on the following:

- The incident photon must have sufficient energy to overcome the binding energy of the electron.
- A photoelectric effect is most likely to occur when the photon energy and electron binding energy are similar.
- The more tightly an electron is bound in its orbit, the more likely it is to be involved in a photoelectric reaction. Electrons are more tightly bound in elements with high atomic numbers.

ELECTRON-BINDING ENERGY		
Atomic Number	Atom	K-Shell Binding Energy (keV)
6	Carbon	0.28
8	Oxygen	0.53
20	Calcium	4
53	Iodine	33.2
82	Lead	88

The statistical probability of the photoelectric effect (PE) occurring per unit mass of a given element is proportional to atomic number (Z) and inversely proportional to the energy (E) of the x-ray:

$$PE \approx \frac{Z^3}{E^3}$$

14

Pearls

- More tightly bound electrons are more likely to interact in the photoelectric effect (K > L > M)
- Electrons in the K-shell are at a higher energy level than electrons in the L-shell
- Characteristic radiation is produced by the photoelectric effect by exactly the same process as discussed in the section on production of x-rays; the only difference is the method of ejecting the inner shell electron
- Advantages of photoelectric effect
    Does not produce scatter radiation
    Enhances natural tissue contrast by magnifying the difference between tissues composed of different elements
- Disadvantage of photoelectric effect
    Patients receive more radiation from each photoelectric reaction than from any other type of interaction
- If lead (K-shell binding energy of 88 keV) is irradiated with 1-MeV photons, the emitted photoelectrons will have a minimum energy of 912 keV

COMPTON SCATTERING

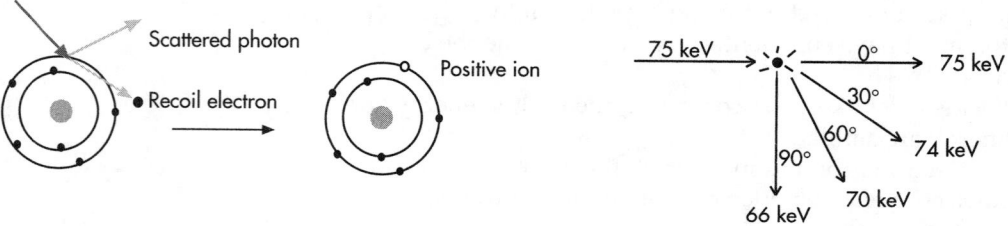

A photon is deflected by an electron so that it assumes a new direction as scattered radiation. The initial photon always retains part of its original energy. Note that the recoil electron is always directed forward, but scattered x-ray may occur in any direction. 2 factors determine the amount of energy that the photon retains:

- Its initial energy
- Angle of deflection from the original photon direction

Calculation of the change in wavelength of a scattered photon:

$$\Delta \text{ wavelength} = 0.024 \ (1 - \cos \text{ angle of deflection})$$

The maximum energy of a Compton electron in keV is given by:

$$E_{max} = E_{incident} \times \frac{2a}{(1 + 2a)}$$

$$\text{where } a = \frac{E_{incident}}{511 \text{ keV}}.$$

At very high energies (e.g., 1 MeV), most photons are scattered in a forward direction. With lower energy radiation, fewer photons scatter forward and more scatter at an angle greater than 90°. Therefore the distribution of scattered photons (e.g., 100 keV) assumes a probability curve as shown in the graph (gray shading).

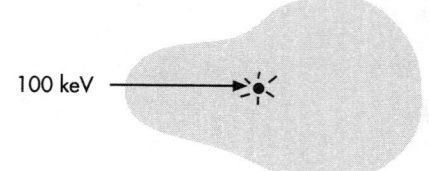

Probability of Compton scatter
- The higher the atomic number, the higher the probability of Compton scatter per atom
- The probability relative to the photoelectric effect increases with increasing energy
- Increases with electron density (electrons/cm^3)
- Increases with field size and patient thickness
- Does not depend on mA or FS size

Pearls
- Almost all the scatter in diagnostic radiology is a result of Compton scatter
- Scatter radiation from Compton reactions is a major safety hazard: a photon that is deflected 90° still retains most of its original energy in the diagnostic range

OTHER TYPES OF INTERACTIONS

Pair production
Occurs only with photons whose energy is > 1.02 MeV. The photon interacts with the electric field around the nucleus, and its energy is converted into 1 electron and 1 positron. Pair production is the dominant mode of interaction of radiation with tissue above 10 MeV.

Photodisintegration
Occurs only with photons whose energy is > 7 MeV. In photodisintegration, part of the nucleus is ejected. The ejected portion may be a neutron, proton, alpha particle, or a cluster of particles.

COMPARISON OF INTERACTION

Only 2 interactions are important to diagnostic radiology: Compton scatter and the photoelectric effect. Compton scattering is the dominant interaction except at very low energies (20-30 keV).

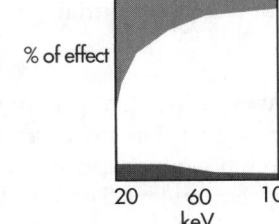 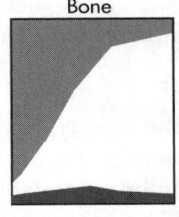 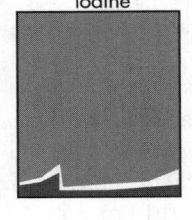 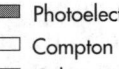

Pearls
- High keV (chest films): Compton effect predominates (determined by electron density), lower bone contrast
- Low keV (mammography): photoelectric effect predominates (determined by Z^3 and E^{-3}), high calcification contrast
- Iodine contrast material: photoelectric effect predominates for photons of energy > 33.2 keV

ATTENUATION

Attenuation refers to the reduction in intensity of an x-ray beam as it traverses matter, either by absorption or by deflection. The amount of attenuation depends on:
- Energy of the beam (high energy have increased transmission)
- Characteristics of absorber (high Z number material results in decreased transmission)
    Atomic number (the higher, the larger the percentage of photoelectric absorption)
    Density of absorber
    Electrons per gram ($6 \times 10^{23} \times$ atomic number/atomic weight). The number of electrons per gram of substance is almost the same for all materials except hydrogen (which is approximately twice that of other elements)

14

ATTENUATION COEFFICIENTS

Linear attenuation coefficient (cm⁻¹)

This coefficient represents the actual fraction of photons interacting per unit thickness of an absorber and is expressed as the fraction of attenuated photons per centimeter.

Mass attenuation coefficient

This coefficient equals the linear attenuation coefficient but is scaled per gram of tissue (cm^2/g) to reflect the attenuation of materials independent of their physical state. For example, the mass attenuation coefficient of ice, water, and vapor is the same, whereas the linear attenuation coefficient is not.

DENSITY		
Material	Effective Atomic Number (Z)	Density (g/cm³)
Water	7.41	1.0
Muscle	7.5	1.0
Fat	5.9	0.9
Air	7.6	0.00129
Calcium	20.0	1.5
Iodine	53.0	4.9
Barium	56.0	3.5

MONOCHROMATIC RADIATION

Monochromatic means that all photons have exactly the same energy (i.e., wavelength). The attenuation of monochromatic radiation is exponential:

$$N = N_o \times e^{-\mu x}$$

where N = number of transmitted photons, N_o = number of incident photons, μ = linear attenuation coefficient, and x = absorber thickness (cm). The linear absorption coefficient is the fractional rate of photon removal from a beam per centimeter of absorber (e.g., $\mu = 0.1$ cm⁻¹ means 10% absorption per centimeter). The half-value layer (HVL) refers to the absorber thickness required to reduce the intensity of the beam to 50% (n = number of HVL):

$$HVL = 0.693/\mu$$
$$\text{Fraction transmitted} = e^{-0.693\,n} \text{ where n = thickness/HVL}$$
$$\text{Fraction transmitted} = (0.5)^{thickness/HVL}$$
$$\text{Fraction absorbed} = 1 - \text{fraction transmitted}$$

The typical HVL in mm Al for film-screen mammography is approximately kVp/100. For example, if kVp is 27, then the HVL of the beam is roughly 0.27 mm Al.

Example

HVL of 140 keV beam through a given material is 0.3 cm. What is the percentage of x-rays transmitted through 1.2 cm?

Answer

Fraction transmitted = $(0.5)^{1.2/0.3} = 0.0625 = 6.25\%$

K-edge

K-edge refers to a sharp increase in the attenuation coefficient depending on the material and photon energy, which occurs at the binding energy of the K-shell electron being ejected at that specific photon energy (e.g., 29 keV for tin, 88 keV for lead). There are also increases at the binding energy for other shells (e.g., the L-shell), which occur at lower energies. The adjacent graph indicates that on a gram-for-gram basis, tin is a better absorber of x-rays than lead (between 29 and 88 keV).

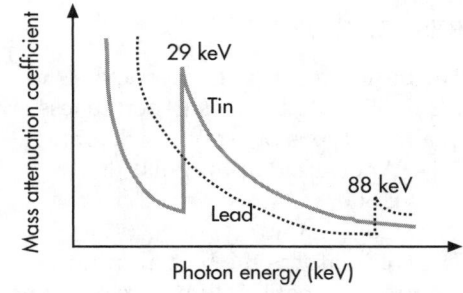

POLYCHROMATIC (TYPICAL X-RAY) RADIATION

Polychromatic radiation consists of a spectrum of photons with different energies. Unlike monochromatic radiation, attenuation of polychromatic radiation is not exponential. In polychromatic radiation a large percentage of low-energy photons is absorbed throughout the absorber, so that the mean energy of remaining photons increases.

Factors that affect scatter radiation in radiographic images are:

- Field size (most important): the larger the field size, the more scatter
- Part thickness
- Kilovoltage (not as important as the other 2 factors). At low kV (< 30 keV) there is little scatter because the photoelectric effect predominates; as radiation energy increases, the percentage of Compton scatter increases

Example

Fetus receives the hypothetical x-ray dose of 1 rem. What is the maternal skin entrance dose assuming $\mu = 0.2$ cm^{-1} and fetus is 5 cm below the skin surface?

Answer

A μ of 0.2 means that 20% of the beam is attenuated per centimeter and that 80% of the dose is transmitted. For 5 cm, the transmitted dose is $0.8 \times 0.8 \times 0.8 \times 0.8 \times 0.8 = 0.33$ rem. To obtain 1 rem to the fetus, the incident ray has to be 2.7 rem.

FILTERS

Filters are sheets of metal placed in the path of an x-ray beam near the tube to absorb low-energy radiation before it reaches the patient. The function of a filter is to protect the patient from absorption of unnecessary low-energy radiation, reducing the skin dose by as much as 80%. Use of filters typically has to be compensated for by longer exposure times. Generally one of 2 filter types is used:

- Aluminum filter: good filter for low energies. National Council of Radiation Protection (NCRP) recommendations

Below 50 keV:	0.5 mm Al
50-70 keV:	1.5 mm Al
Above 70 keV:	2.5 mm Al

- Copper filter: better filter for high energies. Typically about 0.25 mm thick and backed with 1.0 mm Al to filter out the low-energy scatter and characteristic x-rays from the copper

14

RESTRICTORS

The basic function of a restrictor is to regulate the size and shape of the x-ray beam. Well-collimated beams generate less scatter and thus improve image quality. 3 types of x-ray restrictors:

- Aperture diaphragms
- Cones
- Collimators

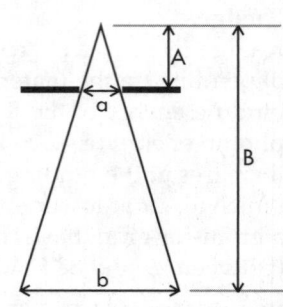

The collimator is the best all-round x-ray beam restrictor. Federal regulations require automatic collimators on all new x-ray equipment. To calculate the geometry of the aperture:

$$a/b = A/B$$

Grids

Grids consist of lead strips separated by plastic spacers. Grids are used to absorb scatter and to improve radiographic image contrast.

GRID RATIO

The grid ratio is defined as the ratio of the height of the lead strips (H) to the distance between them (D):

$$\text{Grid ratio} = H:D$$

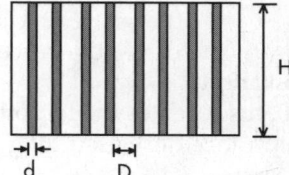

The thickness of the lead strip (d) does not affect the grid ratio, although it does affect the Bucky factor. The higher the grid ratio:

- The better the image contrast
- The higher the patient exposure
- The better the grid function (more scatter absorbed)

COMPARISON OF GRIDS		
Parameter	12:1 grid	8:1 grid
Contrast	Better	Worse
Patient exposure	Higher	Lower
Lateral decentering artifact*	More prominent	Less prominent
Scatter	Lower	Higher

*Loss of density across the image.

Rules of thumb regarding grids:

- < 90 kVp x-ray: use 8:1 grid
- > 90 kVp x-ray: use 12:1 grid
- Mammography: carbon fiber grids, 4:1 ratio, 150 lines/inch (i.e., 60 lines/cm)
- Mobile units: 6:1 ratio grid, 110 lines/inch
- Common reciprocating Bucky: 12:1 ratio grid, 80 lines/inch
- High line density for stationary grids

TYPES OF GRIDS

Linear grid
Lead strips are parallel to each other. Advantage: angle of x-ray tube can be adjusted along the length of the grid without cutoff.

Crossed grid
Made up of 2 superimposed linear grids. Cannot be used with oblique techniques (disadvantage). Only used when there is a great deal of scatter (e.g., in biplane cerebral angiography).

Focused (convergent) grid
Lead strips are angulated so that they focus in space (the convergent line). The focal distance is the distance between the grid and the convergent line or point and should be close to the focus-film distance in use.

Moving grid (Bucky grid)
If grids are moved during x-ray exposure the shadow casts produced by lead strips (grid lines) can be blurred out and the image quality can thus be improved. Although it is advantageous to use moving grids, there are certain disadvantages:

- Moving grids increase the patient's radiation dose for 2 reasons
    Lateral decentering (see below)
    Exposure is spread out over the entire surface of film
- Longer exposure times are needed (because of lateral decentering)
- Higher cost (because of film advancement mechanism)

A grid-controlled x-ray tube is a tube in which a large negative voltage can be applied to a 3rd electrode near the cathode. This negative voltage repels electrons before they reach the target and prevents x-ray production. Using this method, the x-ray beam can be rapidly switched on and off. When the grid voltage is synchronized with film advancement, this tube is suitable for rapid cinefluoroscopy (e.g., cardiac fluoroscopy).

GRID PERFORMANCE

Grid performance is usually measured by one of 3 parameters:

- Contrast improvement factor
- Bucky factor
- Primary transmission

Contrast improvement factor (K)
Measurement of a grid's ability to improve contrast. High-ratio grids with a high lead content have a high contrast improvement factor.

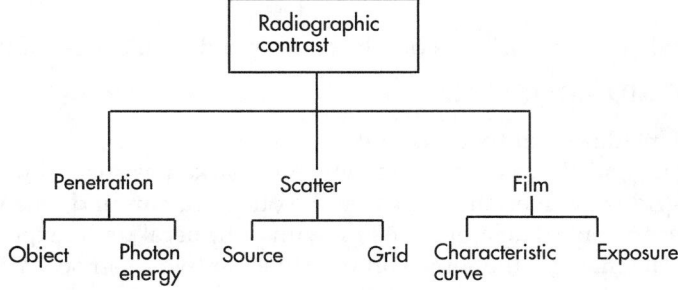

$$K = \frac{\text{Contrast with grid}}{\text{Contrast without grid}}$$

A disadvantage of this parameter is that it depends on kVp, field size, and phantom thickness, the classic 3 parameters that determine the amount of scatter. The contrast improvement factor is usually determined at 100 kVp with a large field and a phantom thickness of 20 cm.

Bucky factor (BF)
Related to the fraction of the total radiation (primary radiation and scatter) absorbed by a grid. Bucky factors (BFs) usually range from 3-7 depending on the grid ratio. The BF indicates:

14

- How much exposure factor must be increased because of use of a grid
- How much extra radiation the patient receives

The BF is calculated as follows:

$$BF = \frac{Incident\ radiation}{Transmitted\ radiation}$$

BUCKY FACTOR BY GRID RATIO		
Grid Ratio	**B at 70 kVp**	**B at 120 kVp**
No grid	1	1
5:1	3	3
8:1	3.5	4
12:1	4	5
16:1	4.5	6

Pearls

- The BF increases as the grid ratio increases
- The BF increases with the thickness of the patient
- Although a high BF is desirable (good film quality), it has the disadvantage of a higher exposure to the patient

Primary transmission

Measurement of the primary radiation (scatter excluded) transmitted through a grid. The scatter is excluded in the experimental setup by the use of a lead diaphragm and placing the phantom a long distance from the grid. The observed transmission is always lower (60%-70%) than calculated transmission (80%-90%) partly because the spacer absorbs some primary beam. The transmission (T) can be calculated by:

$$T_{calc} = (D/D + d) \times 100\%$$

where D = thickness of the spacer and d = thickness of the lead strip.

GRID ARTIFACTS

Upside-down focused grid

All grids have a tube side, which is marked as such. If the grid is inadvertently inserted the other way around, one will see a central area of exposure with peripheral underexposure. One may get the same sort of artifact in two other scenarios:

- A parallel grid is used (i.e., lead strips are not convergent)
- Focus-grid decentering (i.e., x-ray tube is too close or too far from convergent line)

Focus-grid distance decentering

The x-ray tube focus is above (far) or below (near) the convergent line. The artifact is the same as with an upside-down grid.

Normal exposure

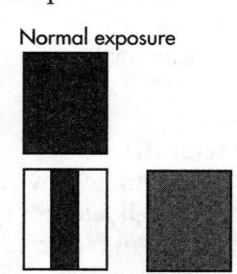

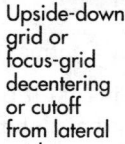

Upside-down grid or focus-grid decentering or cutoff from lateral grid

Lateral decentering, 2 inch

Lateral decentering, 3 inch

Combined lateral and focus-grid distance decentering

Lateral decentering

The more lateral the misalignment of a grid and x-ray focus, the more severe this artifact. The artifact consists of a homogeneous underexposure of the entire film. This artifact is probably the most difficult to recognize. The loss of primary radiation (in %) due to lateral decentering is given by:

$$\text{Loss} = \frac{\text{Grid ratio} \times \text{Lateral decentering (cm)}}{\text{Focal distance (cm)}} \times 100$$

When exact centering is not possible (as in portable films), low ratio grids and long focal distances should be used.

Combined lateral and focus-grid distance decentering

Probably the most commonly recognized artifact. Causes uneven exposure, resulting in a film that is light on one side and dark on the other side.

AIR GAP TECHNIQUES

Air gap techniques are an alternative method of eliminating scatter with large radiographic fields. This method is often employed for chest radiographs. Patient exposure is usually lower with this technique than with grids. The intensity of scatter is maximum at the patient's exit surface and diminishes rapidly at increasing distance from the surface. If the film is placed at a distance (gap), most scatter misses the film. Focal film distance is increased in an attempt to maintain image sharpness. As a result, x-ray exposure factors (mAs) is usually greater than with grid techniques.

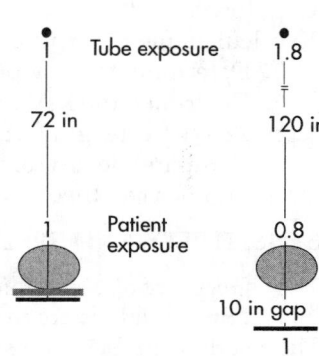

Screens

Intensifying screens are thin sheets of fluorescent material that surround radiographic film within the casette or film changer. Screens are used because light is approximately 100 times more sensitive in exposing film than is radiation. Almost all x-ray absorption in the screen is caused by the photoelectric effect (high atomic number). Implications of using screens:

- Reduces the x-ray dose to the patient
- Allows lowering of mAs, which results in shorter exposure times and fewer motion artifacts
- Main disadvantage of using screens is that they cause blurring of film

A variety of intensification screens are available. Whereas calcium tungstate ($CaWO_4$) screens were used until the 1970s, only rare earth (such as gadolinium [Ga] and lanthanium [La]) are used today because they are faster.

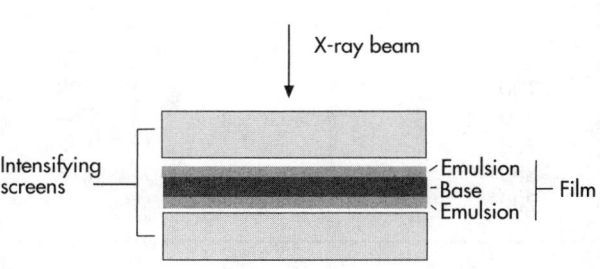

ABSORPTION EFFICIENCY

The main function of a screen is to absorb x-rays, and the best screen would be the one that absorbs all radiation leaving the patient's body (100% absorption efficiency). In reality, the absorption efficiency is only 20%-70%. Absorption efficiency depends on:

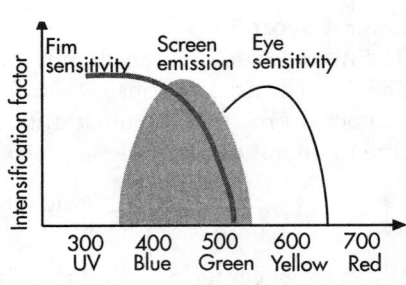

- Screen thickness: the thicker the screen the better the absorption (but also the more blur)
- Screen material: absorption efficiency is 5% for $CaWO_4$ screens, and 20%-70% for rare earth screens
- Photon energy spectrum
- Intrinsic efficiency: conversion of x-rays to light

To calculate the absorption efficiency:

1. Determine the keV of an x-ray photon (e.g., 100 keV)
2. Determine the keV of a visible light photon: keV = 12.4/wavelength (typically 3-5 eV/photon)
3. Compare the keV of x-ray and light photon: 15,000-50,000 light photons can theoretically be generated per x-ray photon

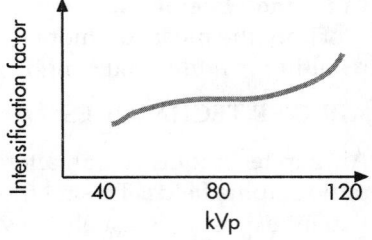

SENSITIVITY AND SPEED

The "speed" of a screen refers to the duration of exposure required to obtain a good image. Speed values are usually provided as 100, 200, 400, etc. by the manufacturer. The relationship between sensitivity (mR) and speed is given by:

Sensitivity (mR) = 128/Speed
Speed of screens ~ Absorption efficiency × Conversion efficiency
Noise of a screen ~ Conversion efficiency

FILM SPEED	
Speed	Sensitivity (mR)
12	10
25	5
50	2.56
100	1.28
200	0.64
400	0.32
800	0.16
1200	0.1

The speed of screens can be increased by:

- Increasing the thickness of the phosphor layer
- Increasing the size of the phosphor crystals (grains)
- Adding light-absorbent dyes

IMAGE BLUR

The selection of an appropriate screen is a compromise between minimizing patient exposure and maximizing image quality. Thinner screens absorb less photons and have better detail, whereas thicker screens absorb more photons but have more blur. Image screens are usually categorized into:
- Mammographic
- Detail (slow)
- Par speed
- Medium speed
- High speed

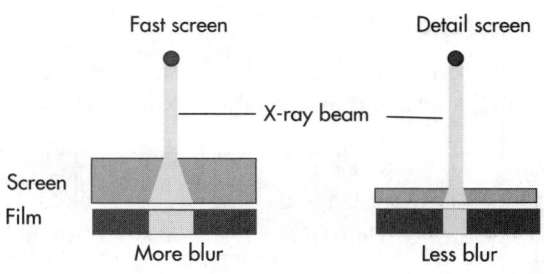

COMPARISON OF SCREEN PERFORMANCE (ASSUMING THE SAME SCREEN MATERIAL)		
	Medium Screen	**Detail Screen**
Thickness	Medium	Thin
Speed	Faster	Slower
Resolution	Lower	Higher
Patient dose	Lower	Higher
Noise	Same	Same

COMPARISON OF SCREEN PERFORMANCE (ASSUMING DIFFERENT SCREEN MATERIALS OF SAME THICKNESS)		
	Tungsten Screen	**Rare Earth Screen**
Speed	Slower	Faster
Resolution	Lower	Higher
Patient dose	Higher	Lower
Noise	Lower	Higher

RARE EARTH SCREENS

These screens contain:
- Terbium-activated gadolinium oxysulfide (Gd_2O_2S:Tb)
- Thulium-activated lanthanum oxybromide (LaOBr:Tm)

The reason for the higher efficiency of these screens is the higher absorbance of x-rays because of the lower K-edge of rare earth elements compared to W (La: 39, Gd: 50, W: 70 keV) and the higher light output per photon absorbed. At 40-70 keV the rare earth screens have a significant absorption advantage over $CaWO_4$. Emission spectrum of rare earth screens:
- Tb emits green light
- Tm emits blue light

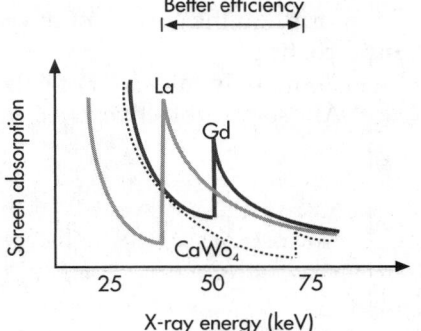

14

QUANTUM MOTTLE

Quantum mottle is due to statistical fluctuation of photons in an x-ray beam. The more photons that are utilized, the less mottle there is.

QUANTUM MOTTLE	
Source of Mottle	**Ways to Reduce Quantum Mottle (i.e., Less Noisy Image)**
X-RAY TUBE	
mA	Increase the mA (generates more photons)
kVp	Increase the kVp (generates more photons)
Dose	Increase the dose (generates more photons)
Contrast	Decrease the contrast
CT slice thickness	Increase the slice thickness
SCREEN	
Absorption efficiency	Use thicker screens (capture more photons)
Conversion efficiency	Decrease the conversion efficiency
Speed	Use slower screens
FILM SPEED	Use slower film

Film

COMPOSITION

Film base
- Glass plates were used before 1920, then cellulose (flammable), and now polyester
- May contain blue tint to produce less eye strain and less crossover for blue light

— Supercoat
— Adhesive
— Plastic base (175 μm)
— Emulsion (12 μm)

Emulsion
- Contains silver halide crystals (AgBr 90%-99%, AgI 1%-10%) in gelatin; these crystals have a cubic lattice structure; crystal size 1-2 μm
- Crystals are sensitized by adding allylthiourea to the emulsion. As a result, AgS forms on the surface of the crystal (sensitivity speck)

Supercoating
- Commonly made out of gelatin
- Antistatic protective layer

FORMATION OF LATENT IMAGE

The Gurney-Mott hypothesis explains how a latent image is created:

1. Light photon strikes Br (only 3%-10% of photon energy is used to produce photolytic Ag)
2. Free electron from Br travels until it finds a crystal impurity (i.e., the sensitivity speck)
3. Free electron is captured. Negatively charged sensitivity speck now attracts positively charged Ag ions
4. Ag ions form elemental Ag
5. Electron trapping continues with new free electrons. At least 2 Ag atoms must be present at the latent image center to allow a grain to be developed
6. Latent image formation

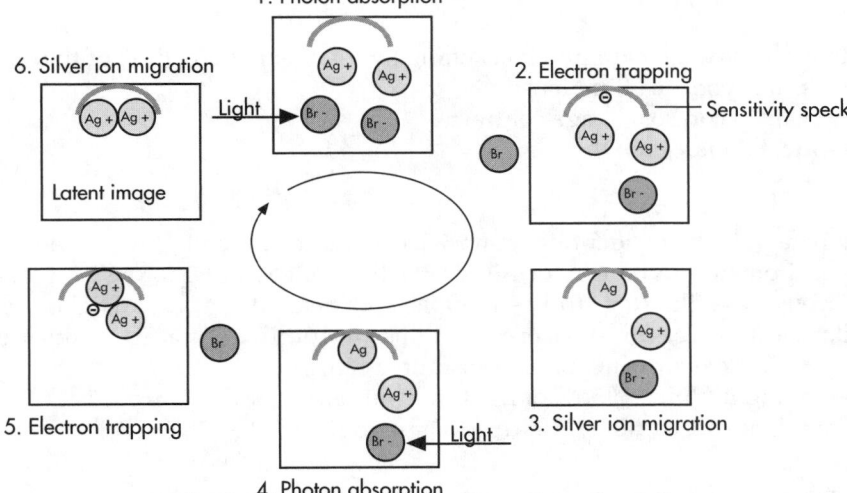

PROCESSING

Chemical processing of x-ray films amplifies the latent image by a factor of 10^6. This process is necessary since 2 Ag atoms per sensitivity speck would not be enough to be detectable by the eye. Film processing includes 3 steps:

- Development (reducing Ag), initiated at the site of a latent image speck
- Fixing: removal of nonreduced Ag in emulsion
- Washing, drying

The typical developer temperature is 93°-95° F. Operating a processor at higher temperatures may result in:

- Increased fog (this will decrease contrast)
- Increased sensitivity and speed
- Increased contrast

Developing solutions

- Reducers: hydroquinone or phenidone (reduce Ag and produce hydrogen)
- Alkali, buffers at pH 10-12
- Preservatives: sodium sulfite

Replenishment solutions have to be added to the developer to maintain its activity.

	REPLENISHER		
Error	Hydroquinone Concentration	Bromide Concentration	pH
Underreplenishment	Low	High	Low
Overreplenishment	High	Low	High
Oxidized developer	Low	Normal	High

14

Fixing solutions
- Thiosulfate to produce water-soluble silver thiosulfite complexes
- Chromium or Al to harden the gelatin

FILM DENSITY

Film density refers to film blackening by x-ray exposure. Rule of thumb:
- mA controls film density
- kVp controls image contrast

Optical density (OD)

$$OD = \log_{10} (I_{in}/I_{out})$$

where I_{in} is the incident light and I_{out} is the transmitted light (in a viewing system or densitometer). A density of 1 indicates that for each 10 photons only 1 will get through the film ($\log 10/1 = 1$). Opacity is defined as I_{in}/I_{out}. Higher density means a darker film. The densities of x-ray films are additive. Typical densities are:
- Black x-ray film: 2 (1% transmitted light)
- Light film: 0.3 (50% of light transmitted)
- Unexposed film: 0.12 (due to base fog)

PHOTOGRAPHIC DENSITY		
Opacity (I_{in}/I_{out})	Density ($\log I_{in}/I_{out}$)	Transmitted Light (%)
1	0	100
2	0.3	50
4	0.6	25
8	0.9	12.5
10	1	10
100	2	1
1,000	3	0.1
10,000	4	0.01

Note: Log 100 = 2; Log 2 = 0.3.

To change the density of x-ray film from 2 to 1, one can:
- Decrease kVp 15%
- Decrease mA by 50%
- Change from nongrid to grid technique
- Add one HVL of plastic to collimator

Example
2 films within OD of 1.5 are placed on top of each other. What is the fraction of transmitted light?

Answer
OD = 1.5 + 1.5 = 3. Antilog of 3 is 1000, therefore 0.001 of incident light is transmitted.

HD CURVE

HD (**H**urter and **D**riffield) curves provide information about contrast, speed (sensitivity), and latitude of film. The exposure is usually plotted as log on the x axis. Film density is plotted on the y axis.

Film contrast

Film contrast (best assured by HD curve) depends on:

- Film density
- Screen or direct x-ray exposure
- Film processing

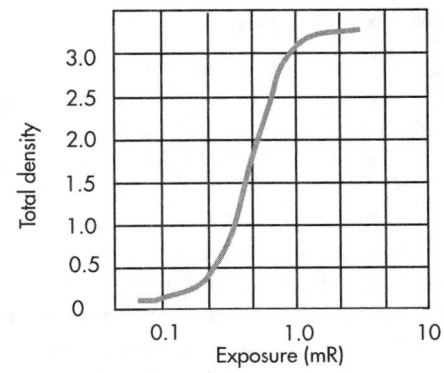

Shape of HD curve

The slope of the curve is given by:

$$\text{Slope (gamma)} = \frac{D2 - D1}{\log E2 - \log E1}$$

where D = density and E = exposure. The average gradient is measured from D1 = 0.25 to D2 = 2.0 (i.e., the D2 − D1 is always 1.75). If the average slope (gradient) is > 1 (as in all x-ray films), the film will amplify subject contrast. Usually the gradient ranges from 2-3.5.

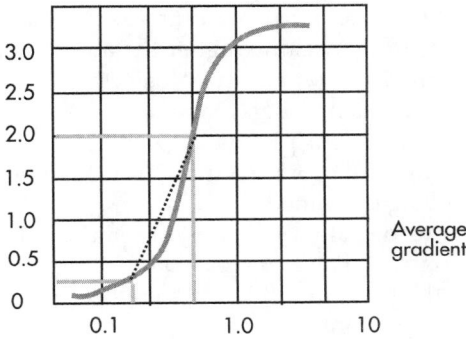

Average gradient = 1.75/0.8-0.2

Example

Calculate the average gradient if an exposure of 10 gives a density of 1 and an exposure of 100 gives a density of 2.

Answer

Gamma = 2 − 1/(log 100 − log 10) = ½ − 1 = 1

Density

Proper film exposure should always be made in the linear portion of the HD curve, not at toes or shoulders.

Speed

Film speed refers to the reciprocal value of the exposure (in roentgens) to produce a density of 1.0 above base and fog density:

$$\text{Speed} = 1/\text{roentgens}$$

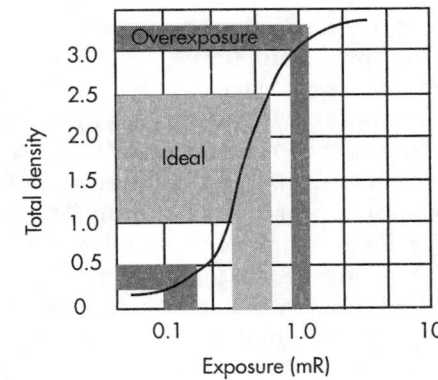

Latitude

Latitude refers to the range of log exposure that will produce density within acceptable limits. The more latitude a film has, the less critical the exposure time. Latitude varies inversely with contrast: the more latitude, the less contrast.

Darkroom safelights

- Infrared laser film: green
- Ortho film: red
- Film for $CaWO_4$ screens: yellow or red

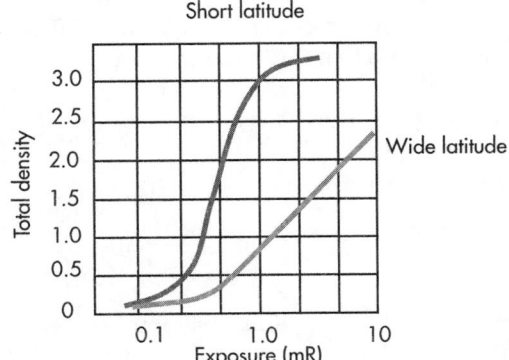

14

IMAGE QUALITY

Quality of an x-ray is primarily determined by contrast, resolution, and noise (quantum mottle). The higher the contrast-to-noise ratio, the better the image.

Contrast

Radiographic contrast depends on 3 factors:
- Subject contrast
- Film contrast (HD curve)
- Fog and scatter

Subject contrast refers to the difference in x-ray intensity transmitted through one part of the subject as compared to another. Subject contrast depends on:

- Thickness of different portions of the subject (the thicker the subject part, the higher the absorption)
- Density difference (mass per unit volume [i.e., g/cm^3]); the greater the difference, the higher the absorption
- Atomic number difference (photoelectric absorption increases with high atomic numbers)
- Radiation quality (kVp); low kVp will produce high contrast (mammography), provided the kVp is high enough to penetrate the part being examined

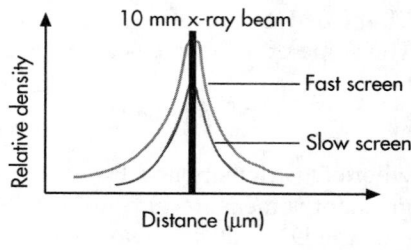

Fog and scatter (especially Compton) are undesirable because they decrease radiographic contrast. Fog is increased by:
- Use of high-speed film (highly sensitive grains)
- Improper film storage
- Contaminated or exhausted development solution
- Excessive time or temperature of development

Line spread function

Parameter of image quality. Tested with a vertical 10 μm collimated x-ray beam, which exposes a film-screen combination. The "observed" width of the image (usually the full width at half maximum [FWHM]) is greater than 10 μm and depends on the film-screen combination.

Modulation transfer function (MTF)

Parameter of image quality. The MTF can be expressed as the ratio of the diagnostic information recorded on film divided by the total information available presented as a function of spatial frequency (e.g., line-pairs per millimeter). A ratio of 1 indicates perfect utilization of information. The lower the ratio, the more information is lost in the recording process. The individual MTF factors of x-ray film, intensifying screen, and x-ray tube can be multiplied to result in the total MTF of the x-ray system.

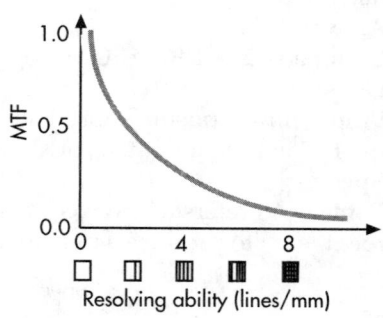

$$MTF \text{ (at a given line-pair/mm)} = \frac{\text{Contrast output}}{\text{Contrast input}} = \frac{I'_{max} - I'_{min}}{I_{max} - I_{min}}$$

where I = intensity

$$\text{Contrast output} = \frac{I'_{max} - I'_{min}}{I_{max} + I_{min}}$$

$$\text{Contrast input} = \frac{I_{max} - I_{min}}{I_{max} + I_{min}}$$

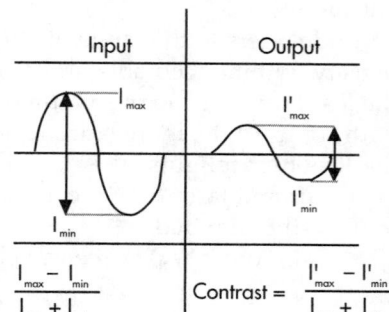

$$\text{Contrast} = \frac{I_{max} - I_{min}}{I_{max} + I_{min}} \qquad \text{Contrast} = \frac{I'_{max} - I'_{min}}{I_{max} + I_{min}}$$

Fluoroscopy

Fluoroscopes produce immediate and continuous images. Historically, flat fluorescent screens were used to intercept and visualize x-ray beams as they left the patient. Today, image intensifier tubes are used, which greatly improve image quality by amplifying x-ray beams. TV systems are now also routinely used to transfer the image from the output of the image intensifier tube to a large screen.

IMAGE INTENSIFIER

An image intensifier is an electronic vacuum tube that converts an incident x-ray image into a light image of small size and high brightness. Image intensifiers are required to amplify the x-ray signal to the light level needed for photopic (cone) vision. The individual components of an image intensifier consist of:

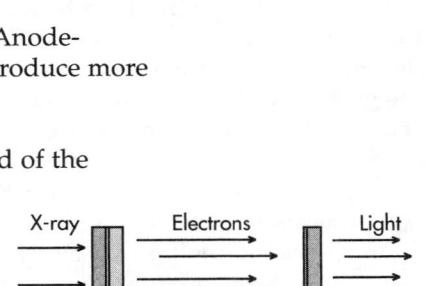

- Input phosphor: absorbs x-ray and converts it to light photons
- Photocathode: light photons strike photocathode and electrons are emitted
- Accelerating anode: electron stream is focused by lens system onto a small area (e.g., 1-inch diameter) and accelerated to anode. Anode-cathode potential is 25 kV; because electrons are accelerated they produce more light on the output phosphor (50-fold increase)
- Output phosphor: converts electron stream to light
- A video camera is usually used to record the small image at the end of the intensifier tube

Input phosphor and photocathode
- Input phosphor: thin layer of CsI
- Photocathode composed of antimony and cesium compounds
- Output phosphor composed of Ag-activated zinc-cadmium sulfide

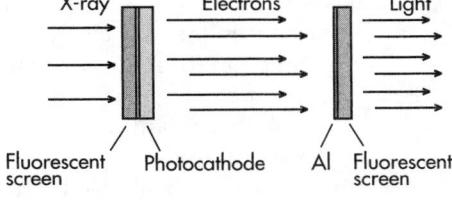

Brightness gain
The brightness gain of an image intensifier is measured by the conversion factor: candelas/m^2 at the output phosphor divided by mR/sec input exposure. Brightness gain deteriorates as the image intensifier ages (approximately 10% per year). Flux gain refers to the increase in number of output screen light photons relative to the input screen light photons.

$$\text{Brightness gain} = \text{Minification gain} \times \text{Flux gain}$$

Example
What is the brightness gain with an input screen of 6 inches, an output screen of 0.5 inch, and a 50-fold light flux gain?
Answer

$$\text{Gain} = (6/0.5)^2 \times 50 = 7200 \text{ times}$$

Minification gain

$$\text{Minification gain} = \frac{\text{Diameter input screen}^2}{\text{Diameter output screen}^2}$$

Because the output screen is usually 1 inch in diameter, the minification gain is usually the square of the image intensifier diameter (e.g., 81 for a 9-inch intensifier).

14

Example

What are the consequences when a 9-inch-diameter image intensifier is switched to intensify a 6-inch-diameter image?

Answer

First, the exposure to the patient will increase to maintain the same image brightness. Secondly, the new image will be magnified, at the ratio of 9:6.

Resolution of intensifiers

- 1-2 line-pairs/mm for old zinc-cadmium intensifiers (similar to old direct fluoroscopic screens with red light adaptation)
- 4 line-pairs/mm for modern CsI intensifiers

Distortion of intensifiers

- Refers to nonuniform electron beam focusing
- Distortion is most severe at the periphery of the intensifier
- Distortion is always more severe with large intensifiers
- Fall-off in brightness toward the periphery of the image is called vignetting

TV RECORDING SYSTEM

TV recording systems are usually employed to record the image from the 1-inch screen of the image intensifier. Although different designs of video cameras are available, only the vidicon system is widely used. The camera has the following components:

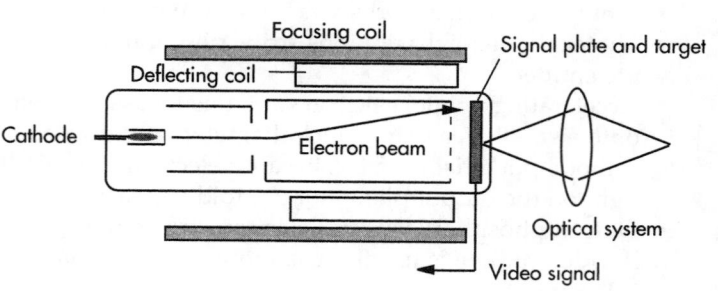

- Vacuum glass tube
- Target assembly that records the image; this assembly contains 3 structures:
    - Glass faceplate of the tube
    - Signal plate (thin film of graphite, which acts as an electrical conductor)
    - Vidicon target (antimony trisulfide suspended as globules in a mica matrix)
- Cathode electron beam to discharge the vidicon globules once they have been exposed to light. The electron beam is focused and scanned along the target by means of focusing and deflecting coils
- Anode potential: 250 V (electrons fly fast from cathode to anode); signal plate potential: 25 V (electrons flow very slowly from anode to signal plate). Deceleration of the electron beam has 2 functions:
    - Straightening the final path of the beam
    - Electrons need to strike the signal plate slowly

Video signal

- Photons strike globule and electrons are emitted
- Globule becomes positively charged
- Electron beam from the cathode neutralizes positively charged globule and a positive signal (video signal) is generated on the signal plate

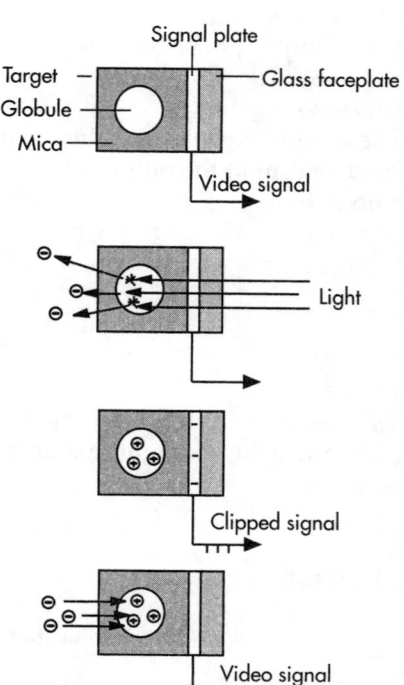

TV monitor

- Electron beam is focused onto a picture tube (fluorescent screen) by means of focusing and deflecting coils
- The anode-cathode potential is 10 kV (fast electrons emit a lot of photons when they strike the screen)
- Lag refers to the "stickiness" of an image when image detail changes rapidly; lag can be reduced with lead monoxide photoconductors (plumbicon tubes) in the videocamera
- TV resolution

  Horizontal resolution depends on bandwidth

  Vertical resolution depends on number of scan lines per millimeter

  Image resolution can be increased by increasing lines per millimeter or by decreasing FOV

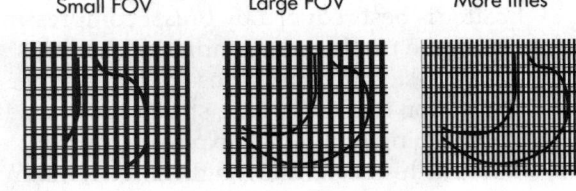

Small FOV   Large FOV   More lines

Interlaced horizontal scanning

TV monitor usually displays 30 frames/second, which is visually perceived as flicker. Instead of scanning all 525 TV lines consecutively, only the even-numbered lines are displayed in one image and the odd-numbered in the 2nd image. The frequency is thus increased to 60 fields/second (no flicker).

Kell factor

Ratio between the perceived vertical resolution and the number of horizontal scan lines. A resolution of 525 × 370 lines (185 white lines, 185 black lines) is usually maximum for a TV. The Kell factor is thus 0.7 (370/525).

Example

What is the maximum vertical resolution of a 525-line TV system with a 23-cm input?

Answer

Only about 490 lines are used to trace out image. It takes 2 lines to form a line-pair (i.e., 490/2 = 245 line-pairs). Multiply by Kell factor: 245 × 0.7 =172 line-pairs. If input screen is 23 cm, resolution is 172/230 mm or 0.74 line-pair/mm.

Mammography

TARGET FILTER COMBINATIONS

Mo is used as anode material for mammography because the characteristic x-rays with energies 17.5 and 19 keV are more desirable for maximum subject contrast. Other target/filter combinations for mammography:

OVERVIEW	
Target	**Filter**
Mo	Mo
W with Be window	Al or carbon fiber (lower glandular dose with the latter)
W	Palladium (experimental)
Rhodium	

14

TECHNICAL REQUIREMENTS OF FILM SCREEN MAMMOGRAPHY

- A small FS (~ 0.3-0.4 mm) is required for high resolution (the larger the FS, the worse the geometric unsharpness). Mammography units should also have 0.1-mm normal FS for magnification views.
- Low KVp (24-25) to obtain good soft tissue contrast
- Long distance of tube-object (65 cm) for high resolution
- Short imaging time (high mA) to reduce motion and dose
- Scatter is best reduced by breast compression and the use of a grid; a grid of 5:1 should be used when compressed breast is > 6 cm
- Compression decreases dose due to thinner tissue plane, shorter exposure, and separation of overlapping structures
- Phototiming (automatic exposure control)
- Rare earth screens and single-emulsion film help to decrease dose and crosstalk
- Processing at 95°C (normal 88°-92°C) and doubling time in the developer (from 23 to 46 seconds) can be used to increase contrast; this modified processing protocol, however, also increases noise

Tomography

Tomography is an x-ray technique in which shadows of superimposed structures are blurred out by a moving x-ray tube. Conventional tomography is now less commonly used because of the availability of cross-sectional imaging techniques such as US, CT, and MRI. There are 2 basic types of tomography: linear and nonlinear. In both techniques, the tube moves in one direction while the film cassette moves in the opposite direction, both motions centered around a fulcrum.

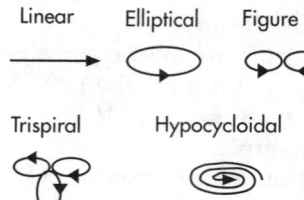

LINEAR VS. NONLINEAR TOMOGRAPHY		
Parameter	**Linear Tomography**	**Circular Tomography**
Cost	Inexpensive	Expensive
Blur margins	Indistinct	Distinct
Objects outside plane	May be visible (parasite streaks)	No parasite streaks
Phantom images	No	Yes (narrow angle tomography)
Section thickness	Not uniform	Uniform

The amount of blurring depends on the following factors:
- Amplitude of tube travel (more blur with wide-angle motion)
- Distance from focal plane (more blur at long object–focal plane distances)
- Distance from film (more blur at long object-film distances)
- Orientation of tube travel: object needs to be oriented perpendicular to motion
- Blurring is unrelated to size of the object

The amplitude of tube traveling is measured in degrees (tomographic angle)
- The wider the angle, the thinner the section
- The narrower the angle, the thicker the section

WIDE- VS. NARROW-ANGLE TOMOGRAPHY		
Parameter	Wide-Angle Tomography	Narrow-Angle Tomography
Angle	30°-50°	< 10°
Section thickness	Thin	Thick
Blurring	Maximum	Minimum
Use	Tissue with high contrast (bone)	Tissue with low contrast (lung)
Type of tomography	Linear or circular	Circular only
Phantom images	Unlikely	Yes
Exposure times	Long	Short

Disdvantages of tomography
- High patient dose with multiple cuts
- High cost of circular tomography
- Long exposure times (exposure time determined by time it takes to move the tube 3-6 seconds)
- Motion artifacts with long exposure times are more common

Stereoscopy

Stereoscopy is now rarely used. The original advantage of stereoscopy was that confusing shadows could be "untangled" when CT and MRI were not available. However, there are many disadvantages to stereoscopy:

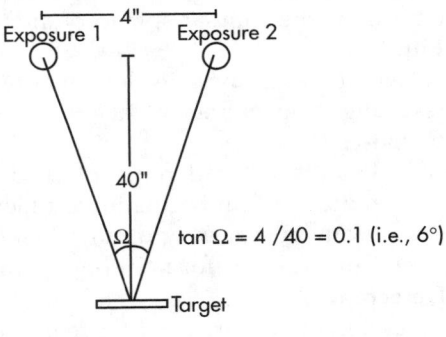

- Twice as much patient exposure
- Patient has to hold absolutely still

Stereoscopic imaging techniques require the exposure of 2 films (1 for each eye), with the x-ray tube minimally shifted between exposures. A good rule of thumb is that the shift should be 10% of the target-film distance (i.e., a 4-inch shift for a 40-inch target-film distance). The 10% shift will produce an angle of approximately 6°.

Pearls
- Best direction of tube shift is along the long axis of a grid (shift across short axis causes cutoff from lateral decentering)
- It is best to use 8:1 or lower grids
- To view films stereoscopically, film must be viewed
    From the tube side, not the other side (as is usually done on PA films)
    With the eyes converging along the direction of the tube shift
    Left film with left eye and right film with right eye

There are a number of viewing systems for stereoscopic films:
- Wheatstone stereoscope: uses mirror to match films
- Binocular prism stereoscope
- Polarized images seen through polarizing glasses
- Green (left) and red (right) images seen through green/red glasses

14

CT

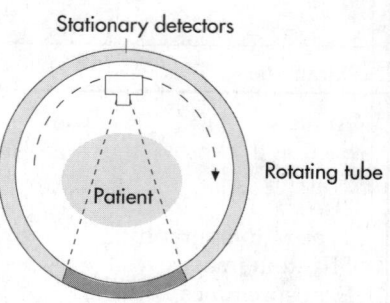

OVERVIEW

In CT a thin fan-shaped x-ray beam is projected through a slice of the body to be imaged. Penetrating radiation (or attenuation μ) is then measured by a detector. Images are reconstructed from multiple "views" obtained at different angles as the x-ray beam rotates around the patient.

CT NUMBERS

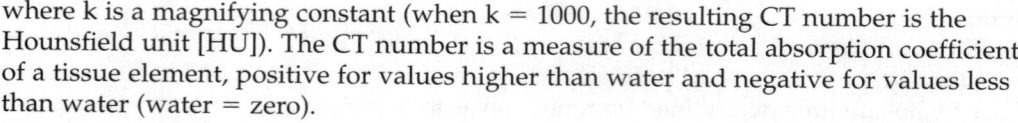

$$\text{CT number} = \frac{k\,(\mu\ \text{tissue} - \mu\ \text{water})}{\mu\ \text{water}}$$

where k is a magnifying constant (when k = 1000, the resulting CT number is the Hounsfield unit [HU]). The CT number is a measure of the total absorption coefficient of a tissue element, positive for values higher than water and negative for values less than water (water = zero).

CT COMPONENTS

X-ray tube and gantry
The x-ray tube is mounted on a gantry that allows rotation of the tube around the patient's body. The x-ray tube typically has a FS size of < 0.6 mm. Collimators determine the angular spread of the beam and the slice thickness.

Filtration
As with other x-ray units, low-energy radiation is attenuated by filtration, typically resulting in an average of 70 keV. Besides reducing radiation, filtration has 2 specific purposes:
- Results in "hardening" of the beam (increased average photon energy), which reduces beam-hardening artifacts occurring within the patient (e.g., at rib/soft tissue interfaces or around metal clips)
- Compensates for nonuniform thickness of human body

Detectors
Several materials are used for manufacturing CT detectors. Basically there are 2 types of detectors:
- Scintillation crystals attached to photomultiplier tubes: disadvantage is afterglow
- Gas-filled ionization chambers (25 atm xenon gas): no afterglow

CT SCANNER GENERATIONS

OVERVIEW OF CT SCANNERS		
Generation	Description	Comment
1st	Pencil-like x-ray beam, 1 detector Rotary (1°) motion and linear motion Time: 8-10 min/slice	Historical
2nd	Fan-shaped beam, multiple (30) detectors Rotary (30°) motion and linear motion Time: 20-120 sec/slice	Historical
3rd	Wider fan beam and more (300) detectors No linear-type movements Time: 2-10 sec/slice	Rotating detector configuration
4th	Ring of stationary detectors surrounds patient Time: < 2 sec/slice	Easy calibration, fast, 3D (helical)

IMAGE RECONSTRUCTION

Several methods are available for image reconstruction, however, filtered backprojection is used almost exclusively today.

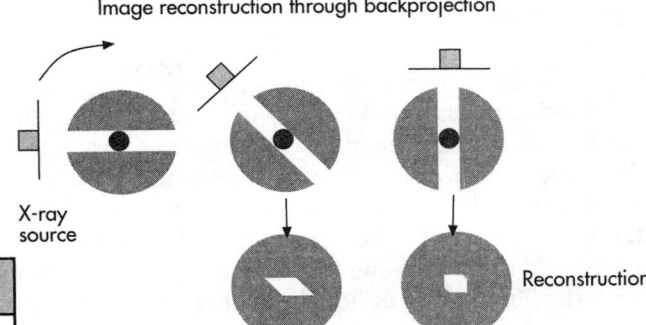

Image reconstruction through backprojection

X-ray source

Reconstruction

CT IMAGE QUALITY

Factors that affect image quality

OVERVIEW				
Parameter	Noise	Heat	Detail	Patient Dose
FS	−	+	+	−
kV	−	+	−	+
mA	+	+	−	+
Slice thickness	+	−	+	−
Matrix size	+	−	+	−
FOV	+	−	+	−
Filter algorithm	+	−	+	−

Example: to decrease the noise on a CT scanner, one could:
- Increase mA
- Increase slice thickness (however, this causes averaging of anatomical structures, and partial volume effects)
- Decrease matrix size
- Decrease FOV

Windowing

Adjustments in window levels allow one to expand any segment of the CT number scale to cover the entire gray spectrum. Contrast can therefore be easily controlled. A narrow (small) window produces high contrast (because small differences in CT numbers are viewed with large differences in gray scale). Conversely, a wide (large) window produces low contrast.

CT artifacts

- Patient movement: streak artifacts
- Aliasing: streak artifacts
- Beam hardening (cupping): reduced CT numbers in center of image
- Detector imbalance or miscalibration: ring artifacts

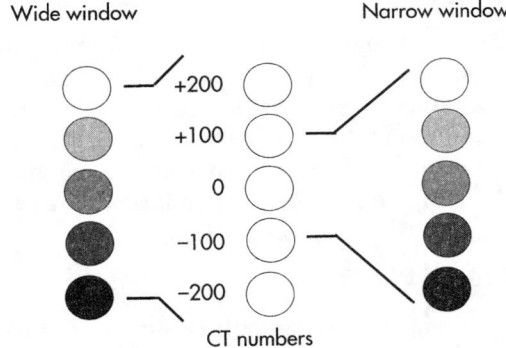

Wide window   Narrow window

+200

+100

0

−100

−200

CT numbers

14

Multislice CT

Multislice CT scanners are third-generation scanners with helical capabilities and low voltage slip rings, which acquire up to 16 (or even 32) CT slices per x-ray tube rotation. These scanners can scan large volumes with high z-axis resolution. Multirow CT scanners perform differently from single-slice scanners especially in the spiral mode. The multislice scanners use a narrow angle, cone beam of x-rays to illuminate the subject and excite the detectors. With cone beam CT, the relationship between the source and individual detector is variable, with detector elements in the periphery of the array illuminated obliquely while those in the center are not. The concept of pitch, used in helical scanners, is different when applied to multidetector scanners. The two definitions for pitch used in multidetector scanners are "$pitch_x$"(x-ray beam pitch) and "$pitch_d$" (detector pitch). $Pitch_x$ is determined solely by x-ray collimation and table speed, whereas $pitch_d$ varies, depending on the number of slices reconstructed. Manufacturers use different terminology to assign pitch values. For example, the General Electric (GE) multislice system allows the use of two modes: high-quality (HQ) and high-speed (HS) modes. In HQ mode, $pitch_d = 3$ when four images per rotation are reconstructed. In HS mode, $pitch_d = 6$ for four reconstructed images. In terms of $pitch_x$, in HQ mode it is equal to 0.75, and in HS mode it is 1.5, regardless of the number of images reconstructed. The clinical advantages of multislice scanners can be attributed to the increased speed and volume coverage. The speed can be used for trauma, thoracic, and pediatric examinations. The increased z axis resolution provides isotropic MPRs and excellent 3D reconstructions used in CT angiography and virtual endoscopy.

Digital Radiography

GENERAL

Digital radiography (computed radiography) replaces the screen/film system of conventional radiographic techniques by processing image data in digital (computer) rather than analog form. The essential parts of a digital radiography system are the image plate and the image reader. Any conventional x-ray system can be used for the x-ray generation.

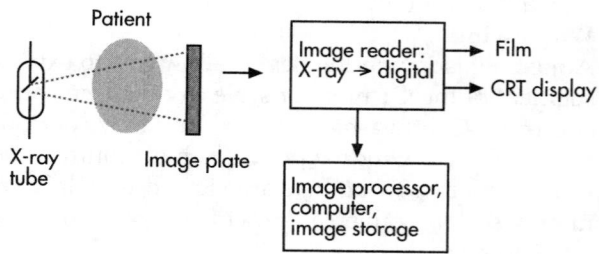

IMAGE PLATE

The image plate has features similar to those of a regular screen. However, instead of rare earth elements it contains phosphor, which can be photostimulated. The phosphor consists of europium (Eu)-containing barium (Ba) fluorohalides (Eu^{2+}:BaFX, where X is Cl, Br, I, etc.). This material changes its molecular/ionic structure by exposure to x-ray (primary stimulation), is capable of storing this information, and releases luminescence corresponding to the x-ray image when a 2nd light stimulus (reading light) is applied to the plate. Sequence of events:

1. X-ray strikes the plate
2. Eu^{2+} is ionized to Eu^{3+}
3. Electron from Eu is captured by the halide, producing a semistable F center (the x-ray is stored in this form)
4. If visible light (> 500 nm, usually applied in form of a scanning helium/neon laser) is now applied to the plate, the electron from the F center is released again
5. Eu recaptures electron and causes luminescence (emission of blue-purple light at 400 nm)
   - The particle size of the Eu:BaFX in the film is approximately 5-10 μm. The larger the grain, the greater the light-emitting efficiency. The smaller the grain, the sharper the image
   - The luminescence of Eu:BaFX decays exponentially as soon as the reading light is turned off (half-luminescence time is 0.8 μsec)
   - Fading refers to loss of the stored x-ray information in the image plate with time. As a rule of thumb, light emission will decrease about 25% within 8 hours after acquisition of the x-ray
   - The image plate is also sensitive to other forms of radiation, including gamma rays, alpha rays, beta rays, etc. Therefore the cassettes should be kept away from other sources of radiation.

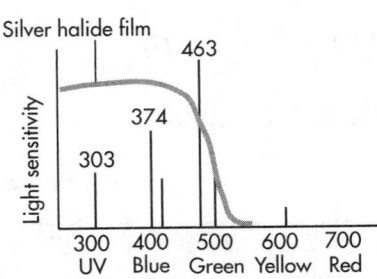

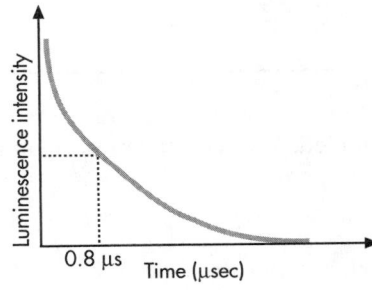

IMAGE READING

A laser scanner is used to convert the stored information of the image plate into digital signals. The photostimulated light excited by the laser spots is directed to the photomultiplier tube by high-efficiency light guides.

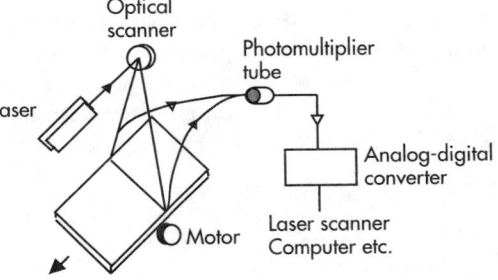

MEMORY

128 shades of gray (or colors) require 2^7 bits of information.
256 shades of gray (or colors) require 2^8 bits of information.

A 256×256 matrix image with 256 colors therefore requires $256 \times 256 \times 1$ byte of storage = 65,536 bytes. Since 1 kB ≈ 1024 bytes, approximately 64 kB are needed. Likewise, a 512×512 matrix with 64 colors would also require 64 kB.

BINARY CODE								
8	7	6	5	4	3	2	1	0
2^8	2^7	2^6	2^5	2^4	2^3	2^2	2^1	2^0
256	128	64	32	16	8	4	2	1
10000000	01000000	00100000	00010000	00001000	00000100	00000010	00000001	00000000

Example
What is 18 in binary code?
Answer
18 = 16 + 2 = 00001000 + 00000001 = 00001001

14

Nuclear Physics

Atomic Structure

Atoms consist of protons, neutrons, and electrons.

ATOMS		
	Charge (C)	**Relative Mass**
Proton	$+1.6 \times 10^{-19}$	1820
Neutron	None	1840
Electron	-1.6×10^{-19}	1

Protons and neutrons are approximately 1800 times heavier than electrons. The nucleus is small in comparison to the entire atom (approximately 10^{-5} times smaller, 10^{-13} cm in size).

$$\text{Number of electrons per gram of material} = \text{Avogadro's number} \times Z/A$$

where Z = atomic number and A = atomic mass number (described below).

Electrons are ordered in shells (K < L < M < N) and subshells (p, q, r, etc.). The binding energy (BE) of electrons in each shell is measured in eV. One eV is the energy acquired by 1 electron accelerated though a potential of 1 volt. Rules:

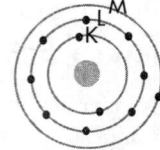

K = 2
L = 8
M = 18
N = 32

- BE decreases from inner to outer shell
- For each shell, BE increases with increasing Z
- The K-shell binding energy for elements increases roughly proportional to Z^2

BINDING ENERGY			
Element	**Z**	**K-Shell BE (keV)**	**L-Shell BE (keV)**
Hydrogen (H)	1	0.014	—
Carbon (C)	6	0.28	0.007
Oxygen (O)	8	0.53	0.024
Iron (Fe)	26	7.11	0.85
Iodine (I)	53	33.2*	5.19
Indium (In)	69	59.4	10.1
Tungsten (W)	74	69.5	12.1
Lead (Pb)	82	88	15.9

*Ideal KeV setting for contrast-enhanced studies.

FORCES

4 generic types of forces are known:
- Strong (nucleus; relative strength 1)
- Electromagnetic (relative strength 10^{-2})
- Weak (relative strength 10^{-13})
- Gravitational (relative strength 10^{-39})

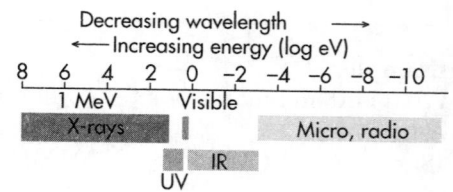

Charged particles in motion produce electromagnetic forces. Electromagnetic radiation is emitted during interaction of charged matter. The energy (E) of this radiation depends on its wavelength (λ), Planck's constant (h), and the velocity (c) of electromagnetic radiation (or light).

$$E = \frac{hc}{\lambda}$$

For the specific case where wavelength is measured in Å and E expressed in keV, the formula is simplified to:

$$E\,(\text{KeV}) = \frac{12.4}{\lambda\,(\text{Å})}$$

Energy and mass (m) are related as follows:

$$E = mc^2$$

where c = speed of light. Mass is measured in atomic mass units (amu), ½ the mass of a carbon atom. Mass energy is measured in million electron volts (MeV). At high kinetic energies (e.g., 20 MeV) electrons travel near the speed of light. The masses of subatomic structures are:

Electron	0.000549 amu	0.511 MeV
Proton	1.00727 amu	937.97 MeV ($\approx 10^9$ eV)
Neutron	1.00866 amu	939.26 MeV

Example
What is the energy required to separate a deuteron (mass = 2.01359 amu) into its components: proton and neutron ?

Answer
Mass of deuteron = 2.01359 amu; mass of proton + neutron = 2.01593 amu; difference = 0.00234 amu. This mass is equivalent to 2.18 MeV since 1 amu = 931.2 MeV.

Nuclides

An element is defined by the number of protons (Z). There may be multiple isotopes of a given element varying in the number of neutrons (N). The particles (Z + N) within the nucleus are referred to as nucleons. The atomic mass number (A) is given by:

$$A = 2 + N$$

<table>
<tr><th colspan="4">NUCLIDES</th></tr>
<tr><th></th><th>Constant</th><th colspan="2">Examples</th></tr>
<tr><td>Isotopes</td><td>Same number of protons</td><td>Z</td><td>$^{131}_{53}$I and $^{125}_{53}$I</td></tr>
<tr><td>Isobars</td><td>Same atomic mass</td><td>A</td><td>$^{131}_{53}$I and $^{131}_{54}$Xe</td></tr>
<tr><td>Isotones</td><td>Same number of neutrons</td><td>N</td><td>$^{13}_{7}$N and $^{14}_{8}$O</td></tr>
<tr><td>Isomers</td><td>Different energy state</td><td>A + Z</td><td>^{99}Tc and ^{99m}Tc</td></tr>
</table>

14

An isomer refers to the excited state of a nuclide. The isomer is distinguished from its ground state by placing an asterisk after the symbol of the nuclide. The half-life of the excited state may be fairly long and is then called *metastable,* abbreviated with an *m* (e.g., ^{99m}Tc). Unstable nuclides are called *radionuclides.* Radionuclides try to become stable by emitting radiation or particles. The stability of a nuclide is determined by 2 opposing forces:

- Strong forces (between a pair of nucleons: proton/proton, proton/neutron) are attractive and act when the distance is very small
- Electrostatic forces act only between protons and are repulsive

For a "light" stable nuclide (A < 50) the number of protons roughly equals or is slightly less than the number of neutrons. In "heavy" nuclides, the number of neutrons needs to be much higher than the number of protons to maintain stability. Nuclides with neutron excess usually decay by the beta (−) decay route. The binding energy or mass defect of a nucleus is a measure of stability. The stability of a nuclide depends on the number of protons and neutrons.

STABILITY		
Z	**N**	**Number of Stable Nuclei**
Even	Even	164
Even	Odd	56
Odd	Even	50
Odd	Odd	4

Decay

The 3 routes through which a radionuclide can decay and thus attain stability are: alpha, beta, and gamma decay.

RADIONUCLIDE DECAY			
Decay	**Z Change**	**A Change**	**Example**
ALPHA	−2	−4	^{226}Ra
BETA (ISOBARIC TRANSITION)			
Beta (−)	+1	No change	^{131}I, ^{133}Xe
Beta (+)	−1	No change	^{11}C, ^{15}O, ^{18}F, ^{68}Ga
Electron capture	−1	No change	^{123}I, ^{201}Tl, ^{111}In, ^{67}Ga
GAMMA (ISOMERIC TRANSITION)			
Gamma emission Internal conversion	No change	No change	^{99m}Tc, ^{113m}In, ^{81m}Kr

ALPHA DECAY

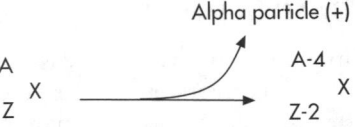

An alpha particle (2 protons and 2 neutrons: $_2^4$He) is released from the nucleus during decay. The mass of alpha particles is great and their velocity relatively low so that they do not even penetrate paper. Alpha emitters are not used for imaging. An example of alpha decay is the decay of $_{88}^{226}$Ra to $_{88}^{222}$Rn. Alpha particle decay occurs most frequently with nuclides of atomic masses > 150. The energy of the alpha particles is usually high (e.g., 4.78 MeV from ^{226}Ra).

BETA DECAY

In this type of decay, a neutron or a proton inside the nucleus is converted to a proton or a neutron, respectively. Beta decay occurs through one of the following processes:
- Beta (−): electron emission
- Beta (+): positron emission
- Electron capture

Beta (−) electron emission

A neutron is transformed into a proton and as a result, a beta particle (= electron) is released from the nucleus (not the shell) accompanied by an antineutrino (no charge). A 2 MeV beta particle has the range of 1 cm in soft tissue and is therefore not used in imaging.

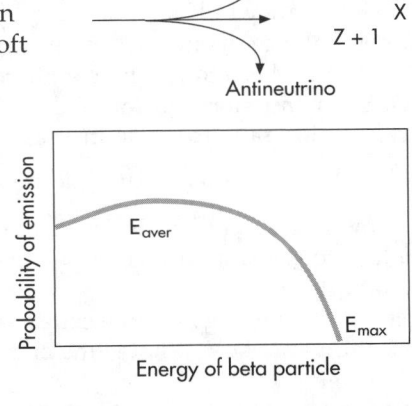

An antineutrino has no rest mass and no electrical charge. It rarely interacts with matter and therefore has little biological significance. The kinetic energy of the emitted electron is not fixed, because the total available energy in the decay is shared between the electron and the antineutrino. Therefore the spectrum of beta (−) radiation is continuous. The maximum energy (E_{max}) differs for different beta-emitters (e.g., ^{3}H decay: 0.018 MeV; ^{32}P decay: 1.71 MeV). The average electron energy (E_{aver}) is approximately ⅓ of E_{max}.

Beta (+) positron emission

A proton is converted into a neutron and the excess energy is emitted as a pair of particles, a positron (beta +) and a neutrino. Positron emission does not occur unless > 1.02 MeV (twice the mass of an electron) of energy is available to the nucleus. Positrons travel only short distances and annihilate with electrons. When this occurs, 2 photons of 511 KeV are emitted in a process known as pair production. Positron-emitting isotopes (^{11}C, ^{13}N, ^{15}O, ^{18}F, ^{82}Rb) are used in PET imaging.

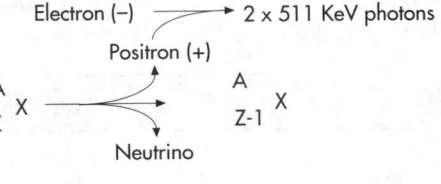

The emitted energy varies from 0 to E_{max}, known as the positron spectrum. E_{av} is approximately ⅓ of E_{max}.

Electron capture (positron → neutron)

This route of decay is an alternative to positron decay. A proton is converted into a neutron by capturing an electron from one of the shells (K-shell: K-capture). The probability of a capture from the K-shell is generally much higher than that from the L- or M-shell. During electron capture a neutrino is emitted. Electron capture may be accompanied by gamma emission and is always accompanied by characteristic radiation, both of which may be used for imaging.

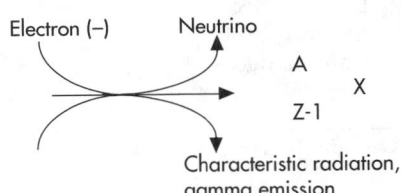

14

GAMMA DECAY

In gamma decay, energy is emitted in the form of gamma rays or as a conversion (Auger) electron without change in neutrons or protons (A and Z remain constant). The decay of an excited state to a lower energy state is known as isomeric transition (as opposed to isobaric transition in the case of beta decay) and proceeds through one of 2 processes (within the same material):

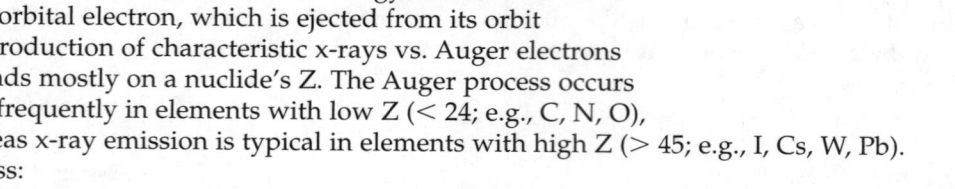

- Gamma emission of a high-energy photon
- Internal conversion: excess energy is transferred to an orbital electron, which is ejected from its orbit

The production of characteristic x-rays vs. Auger electrons depends mostly on a nuclide's Z. The Auger process occurs most frequently in elements with low Z (< 24; e.g., C, N, O), whereas x-ray emission is typical in elements with high Z (> 45; e.g., I, Cs, W, Pb). Process:

- Vacancy is created by bombardment of K-shell
- Vacancy in K-shell is filled by electron from M-shell
- Balance of energy can be emitted (x-ray) or transferred to another electron
- A 2nd electron can be emitted (Auger electron)

Gamma emission and internal conversion usually compete with each other. The conversion ratio (α) is defined as:

$$\alpha = \text{Number of electrons emitted}/\text{Number of gamma rays emitted}$$

A low ratio is always desirable to decrease the dose absorbed by the patient. ^{99m}Tc has a low conversion ratio: 0.1.

Example

The K-shell energy of an electron of W is 69.5 keV and the energy of an L-shell electron is 11 keV. What is the energy of an Auger electron?

Answer

69.5 keV − 11 keV = 58.5 keV is the energy released to fill up the empty K-shell. 58.5 keV − 11 keV = 47.5 keV is the energy of an Auger electron.

SUMMARY OF RADIATION PRODUCTION				
Decay	Beta (−) Production	Beta (+) Production	Gamma Radiation	Auger Electron
Beta (−) decay	+	−	+*	−
Beta (+) decay	−	+	511 keV	−
Electron capture	−	−	+	−
Gamma decay	−	−	+	−
Internal conversion	−	−	−	+

*Cascade effect (e.g., ^{131}I decay).

DECAY SCHEMES

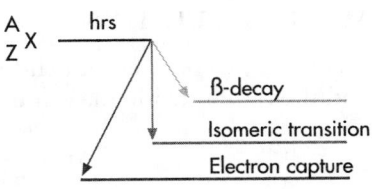

Rules:

- Nuclides are arranged in order of increasing Z from left to right
- Negative beta − decay: arrow to the right
- Positive beta + decay: arrow to the left
- Electron capture: arrow to the left
- Isomeric transitions: vertical arrow
- Energy decreases from top to bottom

Decay scheme for ^{99}Mo:

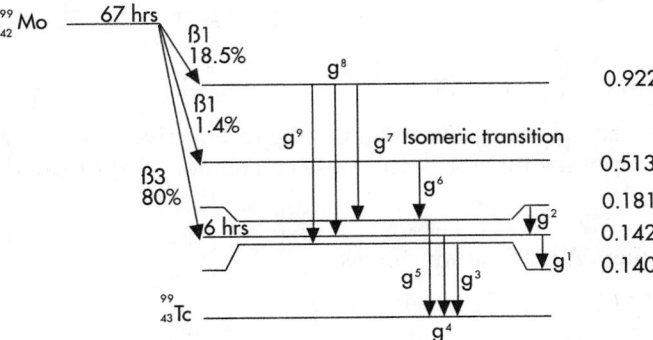

- Except for the 0.142-MeV state (half-life of 6 hours) other excited states are short-lived
- ^{99}Mo decays via beta emission to the 0.142, 0.513-, and 0.922-MeV excited state of ^{99m}Tc
- ^{99m}Tc decays from 0.142 MeV to 0.14 (99%) state (g1); from there it decays to ^{99}Tc via emission of a 0.14-MeV gamma ray or a corresponding conversion electron

RANGE OF CHARGED PARTICLES

The range (R) that particles travel in matter depends on:

- Energy: the range increases with the energy of the particle; $R = aE + b$, where a and b are constants
- Mass: lighter particles have longer ranges (e.g., electron > proton)
- Charge: particles with less charge travel farther; the signs of charge (negative, positive) do not affect the range
- Density of medium: the denser the medium, the shorter the traveling range

Radioactivity

UNITS

1 curie (Ci) = 3.7×10^{10} disintegrations per second
1 bequerel (Bq) = 1 disintegration per second
1 mCi = 37 megabequerels
1 megabequerel (MBq) = 27.03 μCi

NUMBER OF NUCLEI

The number of nuclei disintegrating per unit time (activity at a given time, A_t) is the product of the decay constant (c), unique for each nuclide, and the number of radioatoms (N_t) present:

$$A = c \times N$$

Because the constant for each nuclide is unique, 1 mCi of activity of ^{99}Tc and ^{131}I differ in the number of atoms. For example:

$$N \, (^{99m}Tc) = \frac{3.7 \times 10^7}{} = 1.15 \times 10^{12} \text{ atoms}$$

$$N \, (^{131}I) = \frac{3.7 \times 10^7}{10^{-6}} = 3.7 \times 10^{13} \text{ atoms}$$

14

MASS CALCULATION

The mass (M) of a radionuclide sample is calculated from the number of atoms (N_t) and the radionuclide mass number (A):

$$M = \frac{(N_t)}{6 \times 10^{23}} \times \text{Atomic mass number (A)}$$

For example, the M of a 1 mCi ^{99m}Tc sample is:

$$M = \frac{(1.15 \times 10^{12})}{6 \times 10^{23}} \times 99 = 1.8 \times 10^{-10} \text{ g}$$

SPECIFIC ACTIVITY

Specific activity (SA) refers to the radioactivity per gram of substance (mCi/g) and is simply the inverse of the mass calculation. SA is related to half-life ($T_{1/2}$):

$$SA \approx 1/(T_{1/2} \times A)$$

where A is the atomic mass.

HALF-LIFE

The half-life of a radionuclide refers to the time by which half of the original radioactivity (A_o) has decayed. The remaining activity (A_t) can be calculated for any time point (t) if the half-life of the isotope is known:

$$A_t = A_o e^{-(\lambda t)}$$

$$c = \frac{0.693}{T_{1/2}}$$

$$A_t = A_o (0.5)^{t/T_{1/2}}$$

Example
10 mCi of ^{99m}Tc at 8 AM ($T_{1/2}$ 6 hours). What is the remaining activity at 5 PM?
Answer
Time difference = 9 hours. $A_t = 10 \text{ mCi} (0.5)^{9/6} = 10 \times 0.35 \text{ mCi} = 3.5 \text{ mCi}$.

LOOK-UP TABLE FOR $(0.5)^x$	
x	$(0.5)^x$
0.5	0.707
1.5	0.35
2	0.25
3	0.125
4	0.0625
6	0.0156

Example
If a source decays at 1% per hour, what is the $T_{1/2}$?
Answer
$T_{1/2} = 0.693/1\% = 0.693/0.01 = 69.3$ hours.

EFFECTIVE HALF-LIFE

The disappearance of a radionuclide in the human body depends not only on its decay ($T_{phys} - T_{1/2}$) but also on biological clearance (T_{bio}). The effective half-life (T_{eff}) is given by:

$$T_{eff} = \frac{T_{phys} \times T_{bio}}{T_{phys} + T_{bio}}$$

Example

^{131}I has a physical half-life of 8 days and biological half life of 64 days. What is the effective half-life?

Answer

$T_{eff} = (8 \times 64)/(8 + 64) = 7.1$ days.

CUMULATED ACTIVITY

$$A_{cum} = A_o \times \text{Fraction of dose to organ} \times 1.44 \times T_{eff}$$

STATISTICS

3 types of calculations are frequently performed:
- Confidence and limit calculations
- Count rate calculations
- Count time calculations

Confidence calculations

For a given sample size N, the standard deviation of the sample is:

$$SD = \sqrt{N}$$

Therefore:

$$N \pm \sqrt{N} \text{ is 68\% confidence limit}$$
$$N \pm 2\sqrt{N} \text{ is 95\% confidence limit}$$
$$N \pm 3\sqrt{N} \text{ is 99\% confidence limit}$$

The fractional uncertainty for a given confidence level is:

$$\text{Uncertainty} = n\sqrt{N}/N \text{ or } n(SD/N)$$

where n is the number of SD (e.g., 1 for 68%, 2 for 95%, 3 for 99% level). The % uncertainty is the fractional uncertainty multiplied by 100. Since the desired uncertainty and confidence levels are usually known, the number of counts to achieve these is given by:

$$N = (n/\text{Uncertainty})^2$$

Example

Calculate the number of counts required to give a 1% uncertainty limit and 95% confidence level.

Answer

$N = (2/0.01)^2 = 40,000$ counts .

Count rate calculations

The count rate (R) is obtained by dividing the total number of counts (c) by the time (t):

$$R = \frac{c}{t}$$

14

A frequently asked question is to calculate the SD of the net count rate (NR) where the count rate of the sample and the background are given. The NR is simply defined as the difference between two count rates:

$$NR = R_{sample} - R_{background}$$

Example

A sample has 1600 cpm and background is 900 cpm (each counted for one minute). What is the SD of the net count rate?

$$NR = \sqrt{\frac{Sample\ (cpm)}{Time\ (min)} + \frac{Background\ (cpm)}{Time\ (min)}}$$

Answer

$NR = 1600 - 900 = 500$ cpm

$SD = \sqrt{1600 + 900} = 50$ cpm

$NR = 500 \pm 50$ cpm

Count time calculations

Counting time (t) to achieve a certain accuracy is given by (this formula can be deduced from the above formulas):

$$t\ (min) = 10{,}000/Activity\ (cpm) \times Error\ (\%)$$

Example

A sample has 3340 cpm. How long does this sample need to be counted to achieve an accuracy of 1%?

Answer

$t = 10{,}000/(3340 \times 1) \approx 3$ minutes.

Radionuclide Production

Radioactive material can be produced by 3 methods:
- Irradiation of stable nuclides in a reactor (bombardment with low-energy neutrons)
- Irradiation of stable nuclides in a cyclotron (bombardment with high-energy protons)
- Fission of heavy nuclides

REACTOR (NEUTRAL PARTICLE BOMBARDMENT)

A nuclear reactor is a source of a large number of thermal neutrons of low energy (0.025 eV). At these energies, neutrons can easily be captured by stable nuclides because there are no repulsive Coulomb forces. Note that:
- The mass number during capture increases by 1
- There is no change in element (i.e., isotopes)
- The resulting nuclide often decays through beta (−) decay
- Products are usually contaminated with other products (not carrier-free)

Examples

$^{50}_{24}Cr + ^{1}_{0}n \rightarrow ^{51}_{24}Cr$ + gamma rays

$^{98}_{42}Mo + ^{1}_{0}n \rightarrow ^{99}_{42}Mo$ + gamma rays

$^{132}_{54}Xe + ^{1}_{0}n \rightarrow ^{133}_{54}Xe$ + gamma rays

$$^{A}_{Z}X + ^{1}_{0}n \longrightarrow ^{A+1}_{Z}X + Gamma\ rays$$

CYCLOTRON (CHARGED PARTICLE BOMBARDMENT)

A cyclotron or accelerator is a source of a large number of high energy (Mev) charged particles such as protons ($_1^1P$), deuterons ($_1^2D$), $_2^3He$ or alpha particles ($_2^4He$). For each charged particle there is an energy threshold below which no interaction occurs because of Coulomb forces. The threshold is usually in the MeV range. Note that:

- There is a change of element during a cyclotron reaction
- Cyclotron-produced isotopes are neutron deficient and decay by electron capture or positron emission

Examples

$$_{30}^{68}Zn + _1^1p \rightarrow _{31}^{67}Ga + 2n$$

$$_Z^A X + _1^1 p \longrightarrow _{Z+1}^A Y + n$$

Indirect formation of radionuclides occurs through decay, for example:

$$_{52}^{122}Te + _2^4He \rightarrow _{54}^{123}Xe + 3n \rightarrow _{53}^{123}I$$
$$_{81}^{203}Tl + p \rightarrow _{82}^{201}Pb + 3n \rightarrow _{81}^{201}Tl$$

$$_Z^A X + _1^1 p \longrightarrow _{Z+1}^{A-1} Y + 2n$$

FISSION

Fission refers to the splitting of heavy nuclei into two small nuclei of roughly half the atomic number. Virtually any element with Z = 30-60 has been described as the result of fission. 1 neutron is needed to start the reaction, but 4 neutrons are released per reaction. Fission is a good source of energy (electricity) but, if uncontrolled, causes an uncontrolled chain reaction exploited in the A-bomb. ^{131}I and ^{99}Mo are produced by fission.

Example

$$_{92}^{235}U + n \rightarrow _{56}^{141}Ba + _{36}^{91}Kr + 4n$$

COMMON DIAGNOSTIC RADIONUCLIDES				
Isotope	**Energy (keV)**	**$T_{1/2}$**	**Production**	**Best Collimator**
^{99m}Tc	140	6 hrs	Generator	Low energy
^{123}I	159, 529	13.2 hrs	Accelerator, cyclotron	Low energy
^{133}Xe	80	5.2 days	Fission	Low energy
^{201}Tl	80, 135, 167	3 days	Cyclotron	Low energy
^{131}I	80, 284, 364, 637	8 days	Fission	Medium energy
^{111}In	172, 247, 392	2.8 days	Cyclotron	Medium energy
^{67}Ga	93, 185, 300, 393	3.3 days	Cyclotron	Medium energy
^{133}Ba	81, 276, 303, 356	10 yrs	Fission	—
^{137}Cs	622	30 yrs	Fission	—

Generators

A radionuclide generator ("cow") is an
assembly in which a long-lived radionuclide
decays into a daughter nuclide. The most
common generator is the ^{99}Mo/^{99m}Tc generator.

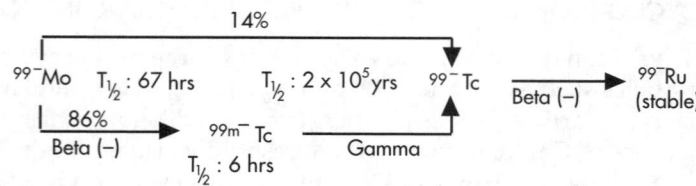

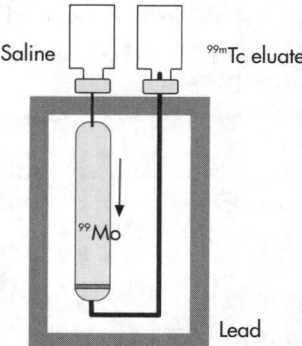

The parent nuclide, ^{99}Mo, is currently produced through fission of ^{235}U (the
historic production of ^{99}Mo was through neutron activation of ^{98}Mo). After
^{99}Mo production, it is chemically purified and then firmly absorbed onto an
anion exchange alumina (Al$_2$O$_3$) column. The loaded column is placed in a lead
container and sterilized. The daughter product, ^{99m}Tc, can be eluted from the
column with saline because it is water-soluble, whereas ^{99}Mo is not.

GENERATOR OPERATION

The adjacent graph shows the decay of ^{99}Mo (half-life of 67 hours) and the
ingrowth of ^{99m}Tc (half-life of 6 hours). Since it takes approximately 4 daughter
half-lives to reach equilibrium, this generator can be "milked" daily. If elutions
are performed more frequently, less ^{99m}Tc will be available:

- 1 half-life: 44% available
- 2 half-lives: 67% available
- 3 half-lives: 80% available
- 4 half-lives: 87% available

Equilibrium

The state of equilibrium between parent and daughter nuclides can
be classified into 2 categories:

- *Transient:* half-life of parent > half-life of daughter (e.g.,
  ^{99}Mo/^{99m}Tc generator). The activity of the daughter nuclide is
  slightly higher than the activity
  of the parent nuclide. This is true
  only if the decay from parent to
  daughter nuclide is 100% decay.
  For ^{99}Mo, however, only 86%
  decays from ^{99}Mo to ^{99m}Tc (14%
  decays directly to ^{99m}Tc). For this
  reason, the real activity of ^{99m}Tc is
  slightly lower than that of ^{99}Mo

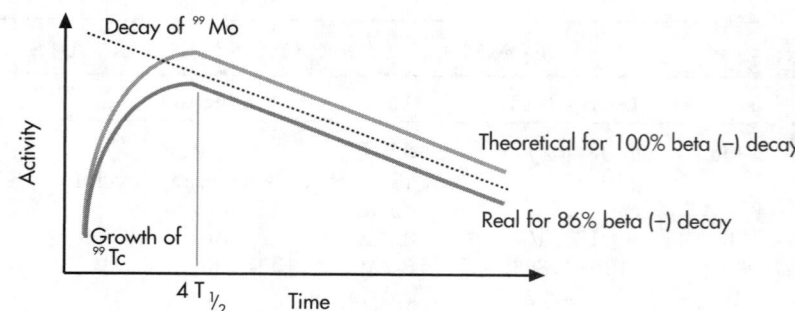

- *Secular:* half-life of parent >>
  half-life of daughter (e.g.,
  ^{113}Sn/^{113m}In, ^{226}Ra/^{222}Rn generators). The activities of parent and daughter
  nuclides become nearly equal

Efficiency of a generator

Efficiency (E) is defined as:

$$E = \frac{\text{Amount of activity eluted}}{\text{Daughter activity in column}}$$

^{99m}Tc generators have an approximate efficiency of 70%-90%.

Dosimetry

CUMULATIVE DOSE

The cumulative dose is defined as organ dose (rads) per unit of cumulative activity (μCihr) and is calculated using the S factor. This factor is a single term combining several physical and biological terms. The S factor is unique for each radionuclide and each organ. The dose (D) in a target (T) organ from a source (S) organ is given by the formula:

$$D\ (T \leftarrow S) = 1.44 \times \text{Activity in source organ} \times T_{\frac{1}{2}\,eff} \times S\ \text{factor}$$
$$D\ (T \leftarrow S) = A_{cum}\ (\mu Cihr) \times S\ \text{factor}$$

Example

What is the radiation dose to liver and testes of 2 mCi of Tc colloid (assuming 90% of activity distributes to the liver and is retained there indefinitely)? S (liver $\leftarrow$ liver) = $4.6 \times 10_{-5}$; S (testes $\leftarrow$ liver) = 6.2×10^{-8}. $T_{\frac{1}{2}eff}$ = 6 hours.

Answer

Activity in source organ (liver) = 0.9×2.0 mCi = 1.8 mCi
D (liver $\leftarrow$ liver) = $1.44 \times 1800 \times 6 \times 4.6 \times 10^{-5}$ = 0.72 rad
D (testes $\leftarrow$ liver) = $1.44 \times 1800 \times 6 \times 6.2 \times 10^{-8}$ = 0.001 rad

DOSE

$$\text{Dose} = 3.07 \times \text{Activity}\ (\mu Ci/g) \times T_{\frac{1}{2}eff}\ (h) \times \text{Energy of radiation (MeV)}$$

Detectors

TYPES OF DETECTORS

- Gas-filled detectors (ionization chambers, proportional counters, Geiger counters)
- Scintillation counters (NaI crystal counters)
- Solid state detectors (GeLi counters)

Efficiency (E) of a detector

OVERVIEW OF DETECTORS				
Detector	Efficiency	Dead Time	Energy Discrimination	Use
Ionization chambers	Very low	NA	None	Dose calibration
Proportional counters	Very low	msec	Moderate	Not used
Geiger counters	Moderate	msec	None	Radiation survey
Scintillation counters	High	μsec	Moderate	Universal detector
Solid state counters	Moderate	$< 1\ \mu$sec	Very good	Neutron activation

$$E = \frac{\text{Number of rays detected}}{\text{Number of incident rays}}$$

14

Dead time of a detector

Refers to the time interval after a count in which a detector is insensitive to radiation. There are 2 types of detectors:

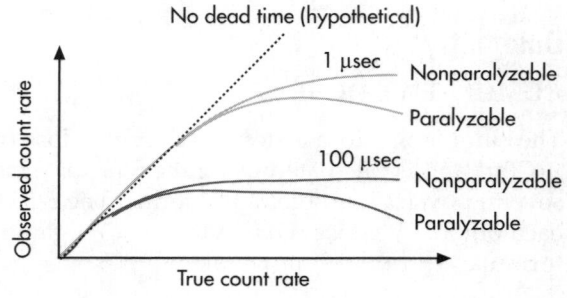

- Paralyzable detector: 2nd ray prolongs the dead time. For example, if the dead time is 100 μsec and ray arrives after 30 μsec, the detector is insensitive for 130 μsec
- Nonparalyzable detector: 2nd ray does not prolong the dead time; if dead time is 100 μsec and ray arrives after 30 μsec, the detector is still only insensitive for 100 μsec

GAS-FILLED DETECTORS

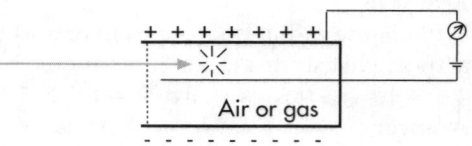

Detectors contain inert gas (argon), usually doped with ether to quench luminescence. Initially an incident beam will create an ion pair, which then produces a current. The amount of current depends on several factors:

- Voltage difference applied (most important)
- Electrodes: separation, shape, geometry
- Gas: type, pressure, temperature

5 distinct responses to increasing voltage exist in detectors:

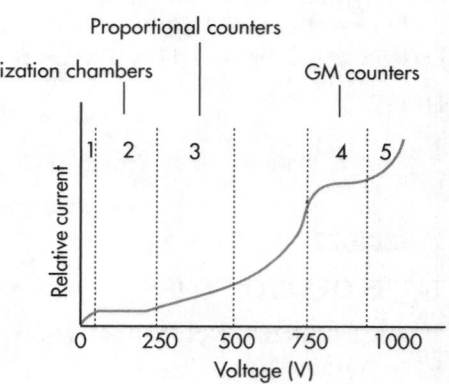

- Region 1 (< 100 V). Voltage is low enough so that ion pairs combine before they reach the electrodes.
- Region 2 (100-250 V). Voltage is sufficiently high to attract all ion pairs produced by radiation. Changes in voltage do not increase the current (ionization chambers are therefore stable and reliable). Ionization chambers (i.e., dose calibrators) work in this voltage range.
- Region 3 (250-500 V). Voltage is high enough so that secondary ion pairs are produced by collision. Current varies considerably with change in voltage. Proportional detectors operate in this voltage range (rarely used in nuclear medicine).
- Region 4 (750-900 V). Voltage is so high that the beam causes a discharge (ionization, excitations, UV light production) in the gas. This region is very sensitive to radiation and is ideal for radiation surveys (Geiger counters operate in this range). After the discharge the voltage has to be reduced to zero so that discharge can no longer be sustained. In addition, alcohols, ethers, or halogens are added to the inert gas to quench luminescence. It takes 50-200 μsec to quench the discharge (dead time of the detector). Maximum usable count rate is 50,000/minute. Ion recombination may be a problem in this region.
- Region 5 (> 900 V). Voltage is so high that radiation is not necessary to produce discharges.

PHOTOMULTIPLIER (PM) TUBES

The most common PM tubes contain sodium iodide (NaI) crystals (moderate density, effective atomic number) that are doped with small amounts of thallium, which enhance light output tenfold. NaI crystals are hygroscopic and therefore have to be sealed in aluminum. Dynodes within vacuum PM tubes amplify the primary signal (a photon) by creating secondary electrons. Typically 10^5-10^8 electrons are generated for each incident photon.

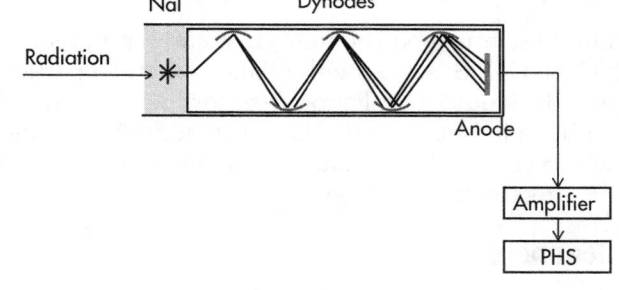

The amplifier increases the millivolt peaks of the PM tube to volt peaks. The pulse height selector (PHS) is an electronic device that allows the operator to select specific voltage pulses within a preselected range. The PHS is important for:

- Discriminating scatter from characteristic radiation
- Discriminating different peaks (and thus isotopes) in a given spectrum

The response of a PM tube to monochromatic radiation is shown in the graph:

$$\text{Energy resolution (\%)} = \frac{\text{FWHM} \times 100}{\text{Peak voltage}}$$

where FWHM = full width at half maximum. In good detector sytems, the energy resolution ranges from 10%-14% (140 keV of ^{99m}Tc). Besides the photopeak and the Compton plateau, other peaks that can be detected in PM tubes include:

- K-escape peak: lies 28 keV below the photopeak of the gamma rays (photoelectric interactions of the K-shell of I = 28 keV)
- Summation peak: refers to additional peaks corresponding to the sum of the individual gamma ray energies. Summation peaks are artifactual
- Back-scattered and lead x-ray peaks result from lead shielding

WELL COUNTERS

The total efficiency (E_{tot}) of a well counter is given as the product of geometric and intrinsic efficiency:

$$E_{tot} = E_{geom} \times E_{int}$$

where E_{int} = Number of rays detected/Number of rays incident on detector and E_{geom} = Number of rays incident on detector/Number of rays emitted by source. The accuracy of a dose calibrator should be better than ± 5%. The geometric efficiency depends on:

- The geometric arrangement of sample in the detector
- The count rate: high count rates ($> 10^6$ cpm) underestimate the true count rate because of the dead time
- Sample volume: high sample volumes (> 2 mL) lower the efficiency

Calculation of photopeak count rate

$$\text{True count rate} = \text{Number of rays emitted} \times E_{tot}$$

Example

What is the count rate for ^{99m}Tc (140 keV; 1 μCi)?

Answer

Since 1 μCi = 37,000 cps (1 mCi = 37 MBq), the count rate is $3.7 \times 10^4 \times 60$ sec/min $\times 0.84 = 1.86 \times 10^6$.

14

LIQUID SCINTILLATION DETECTORS

Liquid scintillation counters are mainly used for counting beta-emitting elements (^{3}H, ^{14}C, N, O, P, S) since their radiation (charged particles) has a short range in solids and liquids. Liquid scintillation detectors differ from well counters in that the PM tube is within a light-tight box. The substance to be counted (e.g., tissue sample) is incubated with a chemical scintillator (PPO, BBOT) whose purpose is to emit light, which is then detected by the PM tube.

Scanners

ANGER CAMERA

A typical camera consists of a 0.25-0.5-inch-thick NaI crystal (total diameter usually 11-20 inches) and multiple PM tubes.

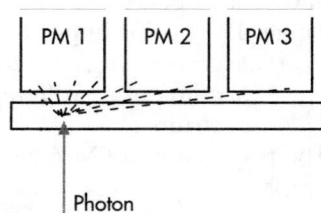

- Small FOV, portable cameras: 37 PM tubes
- Large FOV, older cameras: 55 PM tubes
- Large FOV, modern cameras: 55-91 PM tubes

Specially designed Anger circuits allow the spatial localization of incident photons. The PM tube closest to the incident light beam will receive the largest amount of signal, and the adjacent PM tube will receive less. Resolution is approximately 1 cm at 10-cm depth. The conversion efficiency to light photons is approximately 10%-15%.

Information density

Information density (ID) refers to the number of counts per unit area of crystal surface.

$$ID = \frac{\text{Counts}}{\text{Crystal area (cm}^2)}$$

$$\text{Crystal area} = \pi \times \text{Radius}^2$$

Image uniformity

- The most important source of image inhomogeneity is electronic (e.g., response to PM tubes).
- To keep inhomogeneities to a minimum, scintillation cameras must be tuned. Since the PM tube gain may drift (because of fluctuations in voltage), it is important that the uniformity of response be checked routinely.
- Desirable image inhomogeneity should be < 3% for conventional imaging and < 1% for SPECT and PET.

COLLIMATOR

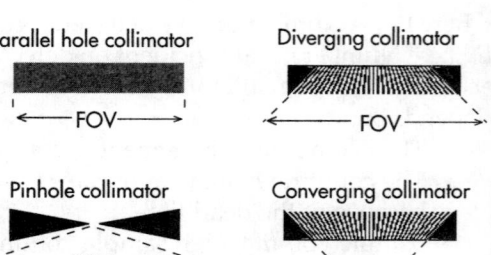

A collimator reduces the amount of scattered photons (usually 50% of all photons are scattered) and defines the geometric FOV. For imaging purposes, only primary photons that arise from the object and that travel parallel to the axis of the collimator are useful. A variety of collimators are available. Parallel collimators have the advantage of no distortion and no magnification. Converging collimators are useful for small organs (magnification views), and diverging collimators may be used for organs larger than the size of the crystal. Pinhole collimators have the best resolution; this is the reason why they are used for thyroid imaging. The resolution (R) of a collimator is given by:

$$R = \frac{d(F + L + c)}{}$$

where d is the hole diameter, F the distance of the source from the collimator, L the length, and c the thickness of the crystal. The best resolution is achieved at the face of the collimator.

Pearls

- Parallel collimators are used for most imaging tasks
- Converging and diverging collimators are no longer in use because the magnification can be done electronically

SINGLE-PHOTON EMISSION COMPUTED TOMOGRAPHY (SPECT)

SPECT uses parallel hole collimators mounted on a camera head that rotates (32, 64 stops) around the patient like a CT. Software programs allow reconstruction of slices. Problems inherent in SPECT:

- Sensitivity for each pixel is not the same
    Sensitivity of collimator is depth dependent
    Radiation originating from different tissues is attenuated at different degrees
- Difficult to collect data for a specific column
    Compton scattering
    Diverging field of collimator (therefore special collimators with longer holes are used)

POSITRON EMISSION TOMOGRAPHY (PET)

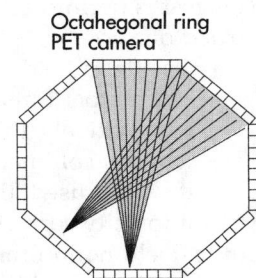

Octahegonal ring
PET camera

PET imaging utilizes the detection of annihilation coincidence. Annihilation is based on the fact that 2 photons of 511 keV are emitted in opposite directions after the annihilation of a positron with an electron. Positron emitting radionuclides are ^{11}C, ^{13}N, ^{15}O, ^{18}F, ^{68}Ga. The 2 emitted photons can be detected by a pair of detectors. A coincidence circuit records only those events that are detected within a narrow time interval (usually 5-20 ns). Photons registered in only 1 detector but not the other are rejected electronically. This mechanism defines a sensitive volume between the detectors, hence the term *electronic collimation* has been used (no physical collimators are used in PET).

Spatial resolution

The spatial resolution of PET systems (system resolution is typically 4-8 mm) depends on (1) detector resolution and (2) positron range and angular spread of photons. The range of positrons in tissues is determined by their energy and is thus characteristic of a radionuclide (e.g., 2.8 mm for ^{18}F, 3.8 mm for ^{11}C, 9 mm for ^{68}Ga). Deviation from the exact 180° emission of annihilation photons results from the fact that the positron and electron are not completely at rest when annihilation occurs.

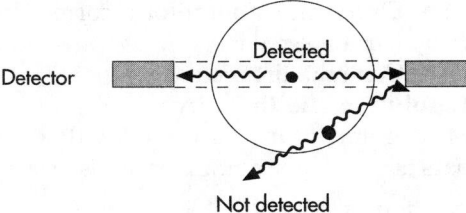

Detector

Detected

Not detected

Detector systems

511-keV annihilation photons require detectors with greater stopping power than is provided by conventional NaI crystals. Bismuth germanate (BGO) is currently the preferred detector material. BaF_2 has the advantage of a shorter decay time but the disadvantage of lower detection efficiency. Gadolinium orthosilicate (GOS) has favorable properties of both detector materials but is expensive.

14

Sensitivity

To increase sensitivity, multiple pairs of detectors are mounted on a ring or hexagonal array (multiple coincidence detection) where each detector is in coincidence with large number of detectors on the opposite side. This arrangement provides a tenfold to twentyfold increase in sensitivity when compared with SPECT.

Quality Assurance (QA)

QA FOR PLANAR IMAGING

The 3 most commonly tested quality parameters are:
- Peaking
- Field uniformity
- Spatial resolution

Peaking

Refers to tuning of the energy window so that it is centered around the photopeak of the isotope:
- Performed daily
- Assures that the PHS is correctly set on the desired photopeak
- Method
  - 1-2 mCi ^{99m}Tc
  - Set 140 keV, 20% window

Field uniformity

This test is performed daily with the automatic uniformity correction turned on and turned off.
- Use flood field image; this may be done with a point source (e.g., ^{99m}Tc without collimator) 2 m away from the camera and with the collimator removed. Alternatively, this can be achieved with a disk flood source (^{57}Co) with and without collimator.
- If ^{57}Co is used, the photopeak has still to be adjusted with ^{99m}Tc.

The uniformity correction is done on every image according to the flood field as a guide. Field nonuniformity can be due to:
- Crystal: may be damaged
- PM tube: uneven gain, old PM tubes
- Electronics: nonuniform correction, not centered on photopeak window
- Dirt on screen
- Camera: dirt on lens

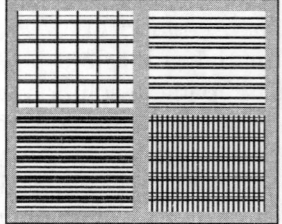

Resolution and linearity

Measurements are performed with a bar phantom. The spacing between closest bars is usually 3 mm. Linearity is assured when lines appear straight.

QA FOR SPECT

- Rotation coordinates calibration. Shift of a few pixels may produce ring artifacts.
- Image uniformity has to be better than 1% (for conventional imaging < 3%).
- Uniformity is tested at different angles of tube rotation.

QA FOR DOSE CALIBRATOR

Precision and accuracy

Measure ^{57}Co (122 keV; near Tc peak) and ^{137}Cs (662 keV; near Mo peak) phantoms daily. Fluctuation should be < 5%.

Linearity

Linearity is measured quarterly by repeated measurement of a ^{99m}Tc sample over 48 hours. The decay curve should give a straight line on semilog paper. Accuracy should be < 5%.

Radiobiology

General

Ionizing radiation consists of either electromagnetic waves, which are indirectly ionizing (x-rays and gamma rays), or particulates, which are directly ionizing (alpha and beta rays, neutrons). Because all radiations initiate damage by ionization, differences are quantitative rather than qualitative. In vivo energy deposition occurs by ionization (minimum energy necessary: 13 ev) of cellular molecules:

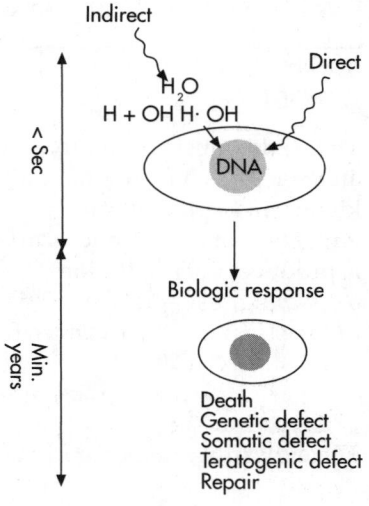

- Total energy absorbed per gram of tissue is small, but the energy transferred to isolated molecules may be relatively large; a dose of 400 rad/human is severely damaging, but if this energy were to be transferred into heat it would only heat the tissue by 10^{-3}° C
- Relatively few molecules per gram of water or tissue are ionized by 400 rad, but each ionization is very harmful to molecules
- Ionization initiates a chain of chemical reactions that may ultimately result in radiation damage

LINEAR ENERGY TRANSFER (LET)

LET is defined as the ratio of energy transferred by a charged particle (dE_{local}) to the target atoms along its path through tissue (dx). In other words, LET is a measure of the density of ionizations along a radiation beam.

$$LET\ (keV/\mu m) = dE_{local}/dx$$

Higher LET radiations (particles: alpha particles, protons, and neutrons) produce greater damage in a biological system than lower LET radiations (electrons, gamma, x-rays). For example, radiation cataracts are 10 times more likely to occur after neutron radiation than after x-ray radiation, with the same amount of absorbed dose. The relationship between relative biological effectiveness (RBE) and LET is shown in the adjacent graph.

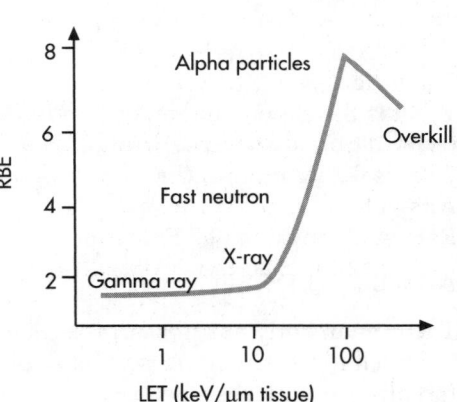

Radiation Units

Different units and quantities are used to quantify radiation.

OVERVIEW OF UNITS			
Quantity	**Conventional**	**SI Unit**	**Conversions**
Exposure	Roentgen (R)	Coulomb/kg of air (C/kg)	1 C/kg = 3876 R
			1 R = 258 μC/kg
Dose	Rad	Gray (Gy)	1 Gy = 100 rad
Dose equivalent	Rem	Sievert (Sv)	1 Sv = 100 rem
Activity	Curie (C)	Becquerel (Bq)	1 mCi = 37 MBq

EXPOSURE

This is the most common measure to determine the amount of radiation delivered to an area. The conventional unit is roentgen (R) and the SI unit is coulomb (C) per kilogram. Exposure can be directly measured by quantitating the amount of ionization of air in an ionization chamber placed in an x-ray beam. By definition, one R produces 2.08×10^9 ion pairs per cubic centimeter. Since 1 cm³ of air has a mass of 0.001293 g, 1 R = 2.58×10^{-4} C (of ionization)/kg of air. The exposure falls inversely to the square of the distance from the radiation source:

$$\text{Exposure at distance d} = \frac{\text{Dose at unit distance} \times 1}{}$$

The exposure rate of a gamma-emitting source rate is determined by:

$$\text{Exposure rate} = \frac{(\text{Activity} \times \text{Rate constant})}{\text{Distance}^2 \text{ (cm}^2)}$$

Example
What is the exposure rate for hands, 5 cm away from 20 mCi of ^{99m}Tc for 2 minutes (typical dose during preparation of a dose for bone scintigraphy)? Rate constant for ^{99m}Tc is 0.7 Rcm²/mCi/hr.

Answer
Rate = (20 mCi) × (0.7 Rcm²/mCi/hr)/(5 cm)² = 0.56 R/hr or 18.7 mR in 2 minutes.

ABSORBED DOSE

The human body absorbs approximately 90% of diagnostic radiation to which it is exposed. Absorbed dose is defined as the quantity of radiation energy absorbed per unit mass of tissue. The conventional unit is the rad and the SI unit is the Gray (Gy):

$$1 \text{ Gy} = 100 \text{ rad} = 1 \text{ J/kg} = 10,000 \text{ erg/g}$$

$$1 \text{ rad} = 100 \text{ erg/g} = 0.01 \text{ J/kg}$$

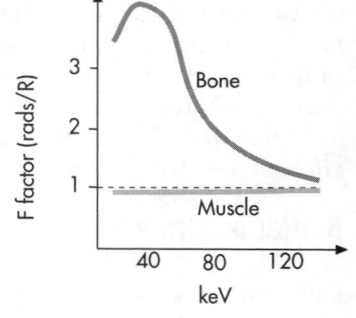

For a specific photon energy spectrum and type of tissue, the absorbed dose is proportional to the exposure. The F factor is the ratio between absorbed dose (rad) and exposure (R) and thus allows conversion. Rules of thumb for F factor:
- Depends on the energy of radiation
- Different for different materials but constant for air
    Air: 0.873 rad/R
    Bone: 3 rad/R for diagnostic x-rays (range is 2.8 to 4+)
    Soft tissue: 1 rad/R for diagnostic x-rays (range is 2.8 to 4+)
- Greater for high-Z materials and for low-energy photons

The integral dose is the total amount of energy absorbed in the body. It is determined not only by absorbed dose values but also by the total mass of tissue exposed. The conventional unit is the gram-rad (= 100 ergs of absorbed energy), and the SI unit is the joule (J):

$$1 \text{ J} = 10^7 \text{ ergs} = 100{,}000 \text{ gram-rad}$$

BIOLOGICAL IMPACT

Not all types of radiation have the same biological impact. Two quantities are associated with biological impact: dose equivalent (H) and RBE. H is the most commonly used measure to record personnel exposure. The conventional unit of H is the rem and the SI unit is the Sievert (Sv). One Sv = 100 rem.

$$\text{H (rem)} = \text{Dose (rad)} \times W_R \times \text{Dose distribution factor (DF)} \times \text{Other modifying factors}$$

where W_R is the radiation weighting factor, previously known as the quality factor (NCRP report 91, 1987). The W_R was introduced in 1991 (ICRP report 60, 1991) and updated in 1993 (ICRP report 116, 1993). W_R is defined as an average LET-dependent RBE factor to be used as a common scale in calculating biologically effective doses in humans.

RADIATION WEIGHTING FACTOR (W_R)		
LET (keV/μm) in Water	W_R	Typical Radiations
≤ 3.5	1	Beta, gamma, and x-ray
7-23	5-10	Slow neutrons
23-53	20	Fast neutrons
53-175	20	Alpha particles, heavy nuclei

The RBE of a radiation for producing a given biological effect is defined as:

$$\text{RBE} = \frac{D_{\text{x-ray}}}{D_{\text{radiation}}}$$

where $D_{\text{x-ray}}$ is the dose of standard radiation (250-kVp x-ray) needed to produce a biological effect and $D_{\text{radiation}}$ is the dose of the test radiation needed to produce the same biological effect. Because x-rays are used as a reference, the RBE of x-rays is 1.

Radiation Effect

Stages of radiochemical reactions:
- Physical damage (primary event: ionization) takes $\sim 10^{-12}$ seconds
- Physiochemical damage (production of free radicals) takes $\sim 10^{-10}$ seconds
- Chemical damage (DNA, RNA changes) takes $\sim 10^{-6}$ seconds
- Biological damage lifetime, lasts minutes to years

TARGET THEORY OF RADIATION EFFECT

The target theory assumes that the radiation effect is due to alteration of a sensitive site within a cell (e.g., DNA). According to this theory, the ionizing event must involve this site directly, and all other ionizations (those outside the sensitive site) are ineffective. The target theory was originally developed to explain observed dose-response curves (biological end-effect) purely on the basis of the physical nature of the radiation and the statistical distribution of ionizing events in the cell. This theory is now judged to be outdated because it is known that ionizing radiation produces free radicals in cells (see Indirect Theory section).

14

INDIRECT THEORY OF RADIATION EFFECT

This theory assumes that the effect of radiation on target molecules is mediated through free radicals produced by ionization; radical formation requires the presence of water. Evidence for an indirect effect of radiation comes from Dale's experiments with the enzyme carboxypeptidase. He found that the number of inactivated enzyme molecules in solution was independent of the concentration. Free radical reactions include:

Ionization reactions (primary event)
- $H_2O \rightarrow H_2O^+ + e^-$
- $H_2O + e^- \rightarrow H_2O^-$

Radical reactions (where OH· and H· are free radicals)
- $H_2O^+ \rightarrow H^+ + OH·$
- $H_2O^- \rightarrow OH^- + H·$

Factors modifying aqueous radiochemical reactions:
- LET
    High LET (i.e., particulate radiation) favors formation of molecular products (forward reactions): $H_2O \rightarrow ·H + ·OH \rightarrow H_2$ or H_2O_2
    Low LET favors OH and H radical formation and recombination of ·OH and ·H to water
- Oxygen effect
    High oxygen tension leads to formation of O_2 and HO_2 radicals, increases formation of H_2O_2, and tends to prevent back reactions
    Sensitizing effect of oxygen (radiosensitizer) in complex biological systems is probably due to reaction with organic free radicals leading to peroxydation: ($R· + O_2 \rightarrow RO·_2 \rightarrow R\text{-}OOH$
- Radioprotectors (scavengers of free radicals)
    Cysteine, cystamine, cysteamine (sulfhydryls)

REACTIONS IN MACROMOLECULES

Production of organic free radicals:
- Aqueous radicals usually produce organic radicals by abstraction of hydrogen atoms
- Free radicals may break up CH, CO, CN, CS, C=C bonds
- Fate of organic radicals
    Repair: recombination with hydrogen radical
    Reaction with another organic radical (on same or different molecule) can lead to rearrangements of molecules, degradation, polymerization, cross-linking, etc.
    Combination with oxygen results in abnormal (damaged) molecule
- Effects on DNA
    Chain breakage at sugar-phosphate bond producing single- or double-strand breaks
    Specific degradation of bases (pyrimidine or purine)
    Disruption of sugar-based bond with release of base from polynucleotide chain leading to apurinic or apyrimidinic sites in DNA

Energy transfer:
- Energy from initial ionization may be transferred by several chemical reactions to a target molecule (i.e., different intermediate organic radicals are formed).
- In a large molecule, the energy may be transferred from the point of initial damage to a sensitive site of the molecule.

CELLULAR DAMAGE

Law of Bergonie and Tribondeau: cell radiosensitivity is related to:
- Degree of cell differentiation
- Degree of mitotic activity

Differentiated cells (e.g., hepatocytes, nerve cells) are less sensitive to radiation from undifferentiated cells such as erythroblasts and myeloblasts. Order of radiosensitivity: myeloblasts, erythroblasts > lymphocytes (B > T cells) > granulocytes > intestinal crypt cells > nerve cells.

DNA repair processes in cells

Mammalian cells possess efficient molecular processes for repairing radiation induced DNA damage. The efficiency and accuracy of these processes may determine in large part the nature and the extent of the ultimate biological damage (i.e., survival vs. mutations). Repair pathways:
- Rejoining of DNA strand breaks
- Excision-resynthesis repair of damaged DNA base (unscheduled DNA synthesis)
- Repair associated with DNA replication (postreplication repair)

Cell cycle and radiosensitivity

Cells are most radiosensitive when they are in mitosis (M phase) or in RNA synthesis phase (G2 phase). Cells are relatively radioresistant in the latter part of the DNA synthesis phase (S phase).

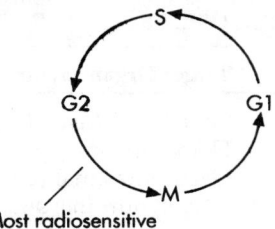

S = DNA synthesis
G2 = (gap 2) interval between DNA synthesis and mitosis
M = mitosis
G1 = (gap 1) variable time
S + G2 + M = 10-15 hours

DOSE-RESPONSE CURVES

Dose-response models have been developed to predict the risk of cancer in humans. The most relevant dose-response curves are:
- Cell culture: linear-quadratic (linear at low dose and quadratic at higher dose)
- In vivo cancer induction: National Academy of Sciences/National Research Council Committe on Biological Effects of Ionizing Radiation (BEIR) published a report in 1990 (BEIR V) indicating that the linear dose response model was best for all cancers, except for leukemia and bone cancer, for which a linear-quadratic model was suggested.

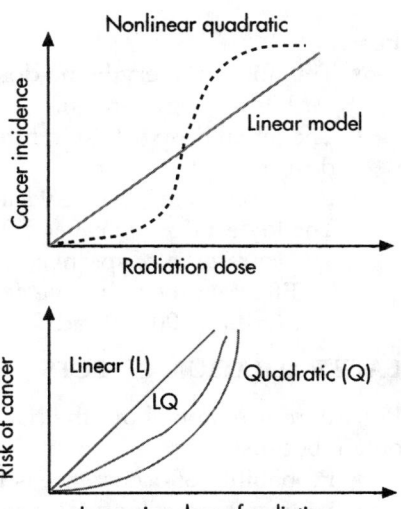

14

Risk in Humans

Biological effects of radiation are either stochastic or deterministic. A stochastic effect refers to a radiation effect in which the probability, rather than the severity, increases with dose (i.e., there is no threshold). Deterministic (nonstochastic) effects of radiation refer to effects in which the severity rather than the probability increases with dose (e.g., cataract formation in posterior portion of the lens: minimum dose for cataract formation after x-ray exposure is estimated to be 200 rad;

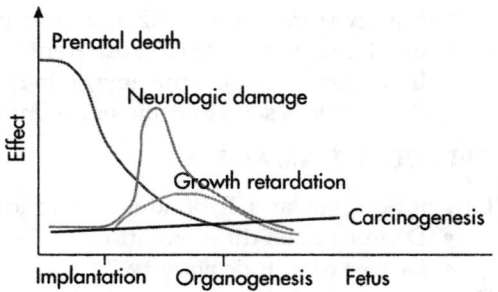

latency period is 6 months to 35 years). High dose rates (high exposure for short time) are more deleterious than low dose rates (low dose for long period of time). The effect of radiation is also less deleterious if the dose is split up into several fractions and if fractions are spaced at > 6 hours, giving time to repair sublethal damage. Children are twice as sensitive to radiation as adults. Minimum latent period (induction time) is short for leukemia (2-5 years) but much longer for most solid tumors (10-15 years).

ACUTE RADIATION EFFECTS

Acute effects occur when the dose and the dose rate are high. There are 4 stages:

	ACUTE EFFECTS OF RADIATION EXPOSURE	
Stage	Dose (rad)	Target Organ, Symptoms
1	0-200	Subclinical (usually unobservable), transient nausea
2	200-600	Hematopoietic syndrome: survival chance falls to zero at about 600 rads
3	600-1000	Gastrointestinal (GI) syndrome: death in 10-24 days
4	> 1000	CNS syndrome: shock, burning, death in hours

Pearls

- The minimum erythema dose is 200-300 rads for diagnostic x-ray (500-1000 rad for high-energy x-rays).
- The lethal dose (LD_{50}) in humans is approximately 450 rad given as a single dose.
- Epilation occurs 2-3 weeks after radiation exposure.
- The lowest dose to cause:
    Depression of sperm count: 15 rad
    Effect on reproductive capability: 25 rad
    Sterility: 300-500 rad

LATE RADIATION EFFECTS

Precise information about the risk involved with low radiation doses is difficult to obtain because:

- Probability of occurrence is low at low doses
- Latency time is long (on average 20-40 years)
- Late effects also occur from natural (ambient) radiation

The estimations on page 1007 are based on NCRP report 115 and are derived from animal experiments and Hiroshima/Nagasaki survivors.

RISK OF RADIATION-INDUCED CANCER		
Type of Cancer	Relative Risk* (% Increased/rad)	Absolute Risk† (Incidence/10^6/yr/rad)
Leukemia	2.0	1.0
Thyroid	—	1.0
Bone	0.3	0.1
Skin	< 0.3	15
Breast	1.0	0.8
Lung	0.5	1.5
Others	—	1.0

*Relative risk: percentage of increase in cancer risk over that which exists because of natural causes.
†Absolute risk: number of cancer cases per year as a result of 1 rad exposure to 1 million persons.

Rule of thumb: population exposed to 1 rad has an expected incidence of malignancies (leukemia and solid tumors included) of 2 in 10^5 per year. Increased lifetime cancer risk estimate = 0.1% per rad

Genetically significant dose (GSD)

GSD is a parameter of the gonadal radiation exposure to an entire population. In 1970, the GSD in the US was approximately 20 mrad. Diagnostic radiation contributes much more to the GSD (more people have x-rays) than therapeutic radiation. Recommended average dose limit to gonads of a population: 5 rem in 30 years.

INCREASED CANCER INCIDENCE	
Radiation Source	Increased Cancer Incidence
Radiation for tinea capitis	Thyroid, brain
Hiroshima survivors	Thyroid, leukemia, lung, breast, GI tract
Marshall Islands population	Thyroid
Radium dial painters	Tongue from licking brushes, bone
Radiation for ankylosing spondylitis	Leukemia
Repeated fluoroscopy for TB	Breast

FETUS

For diagnostic levels of radiation (0-10 rad) the following figures of malformations and cancers have been reported.

MALFORMATION		
Weeks	Gestation	Malformation
<2	Preimplant	Death
2-8	Organogenesis	1% per rad; may have smaller head size above a 5-rad threshold
8-16	CNS development	Mental retardation, likely 10-rad threshold
16-38	Growth	None at diagnostic levels

14

RISK OF CHILDHOOD CANCER*				
Time	0 rad (%)	1 rad (%)	5 rad (%)	10 rad (%)
1st trimester	0.07	0.25	0.88	1.75
2nd + 3rd trimester	0.07	0.12	0.30	0.52

*These numbers are still controversial.

Pearls

- Children are more susceptible to radiation than adults
- Most sensitive stage of radiation damage: 2nd-6th week of pregnancy
- Congenital malformations occur with > 5 rad
- 1 rem in 12th week results in 1% of birth defects with likely 5-rad threshold

DIAGNOSTIC X-RAY DOSES

RADIATION DOSE FOR TYPICAL X-RAY PROCEDURES			
Examination	Skin Dose (mrad)	Gonadal Dose (mrad)	Marrow Dose (mrad)
Chest x-ray, PA	30	0.1	10
Femur, AP	200	1	20
Abdomen, AP	300	60 (F)	25
Upper GI	500	100	70
Barium enema	1500	450 (F)	150
LS spine, lat	1500	220 (F)	100
Abdominal angiography	3700	700 (F)	300
Neuro angiography	1700	< 1	100
Mammography*	600	—	1
Abdominal CT scan	3000-4000	1500 (F)	500

F, Female.
*Glandular dose (not the skin dose) per CC view is typically 200 mrad and should be < 300 mrad (< 3 mGy) by ACR recommendations.

RISK IN MAMMOGRAPHY

- The average glandular dose from mammography is approximately 80 mR/view (no grid) and < 200 mR (with grid).
- With a typical 2-view mammography (200 mrad each view) there is a 0.1% increased cancer risk.
- The mean risk of cancer from mammography is 6-8 cancers/rad/million.

RISK IN NUCLEAR MEDICINE

RADIATION DOSE FOR ADULT SCINTIGRAPHY			
Study	Activity (mCi)	Target Organ Dose (mrad)	Whole Body Dose (mrad)
Liver scan (^{99m}Tc)	5	1400	90
Thyroid (^{123}I)	0.3	10,000	12
Bone scan	2.5	5000 (bladder)	250
Gallium scan	5	4500 (colon)	1400

RADIATION DOSE FOR PEDIATRIC SCINTIGRAPHY		
Isotope	Activity (mCi)	Whole Body Dose (mrad)
Cardiac scan (^{201}Tl)	2	800
Renal (^{99m}Tc DTPA)	10	120
Liver (^{99m}Tc)	2,5	100
Bone scan (^{99m}Tc MDP)	10	320

Radiation Protection

FILM BADGE

Anyone who might receive 10% or more of the maximum permissible dose (MPD) is required to wear a film badge. One of the badges should be worn on the front collar above the apron to be close to lens and thyroid or on the outside of the thyroid shield. A second badge should be worn under the apron or at waist level if high usage of fluoroscopy is intended or if pregnant. The window in the radiation badge is for estimation of beta radiation dose. Peak sensitivity of the emulsion in a film badge is 50 kVp.

APRON

A 0.5-mm lead apron (typical thickness) lets only 1%-3% of diagnostic x-ray radiation pass through (i.e., thirty-fold reduction of scattered radiation). When the distance to the x-ray source and collimation are taken into account, radiation exposure from diagnostic x-rays is very low beneath an apron. The recommended minimum thickness of an apron is 0.25 mm lead equivalent, often worn by technologists who are not close to the patient during fluoroscopy.

X-RAY EQUIPMENT

The workload (W) is a measure of how much an x-ray machine is used during a week and reflects the total amount of radiation generated.

W (in mA minutes) = Total exposure in mAs/week $\times$ 0.0166 (i.e., total mAs/60)

The total exposure (E) in a radiological workroom is calculated as:

$$E = (W \times 60) \times k$$

where k = average exposure in R/mAs at a distance of 1 m from the x-ray source, which depends on kVp used. Each R of primary beam exposure of a 20 $\times$ 20-cm field produces about 1 mR of scatter at a distance of 1 m from the patient. Since a typical C-arm fluoroscope exposure to a patient is approximately 3R/minute, the exposure to the radiologist (no apron) at 1 foot from the patient is approximately 27 mR/min; this translates to 270 mR for 10 minutes of fluoroscopy time or to approximately 3 times the MPD for a week.

Pearls
- Maximum permissible leakage from an x-ray tube is 100 mR in 1 hour (when the tube is operated at its highest continuous-rated current (mA) and its maximum-rated kVp).
- The average amount of radiation exposure per frame during cinefluorography is now 30 μR/frame or 27 R/min.
- High kVp, low mA has a lower skin entrance dose than low kVp, high mA.

14

RADIATION IN WORKING AREAS

A High Radiation Area must be clearly marked if the exposure rate is > 100 mR/hr.

GUIDELINES FOR EXPOSURE LIMITS

Guidelines for exposure limits are recommended by the NCRP. Government agencies such as the NRC establish the regulations and do not always agree with the NCRP. The recommended levels do not represent levels that are absolutely harmless but levels that represent an acceptable risk. For radiation workers the MPD is 5 rem/yr for whole body exposure. For the lens of the eye and the extremities, the annual limits are 15 rem and 50 rem, respectively. The MPD for nonoccupational persons is 0.1 rem/yr and 0.5 rem for "infrequent" exposure. The MPD for a fetus is 0.5 rem for the entire gestation period.

MAXIMUM PERMISSIBLE DOSES (NCRP)	
	Limit*
RADIATION WORKERS	
Whole body (prospective)	5 rem/yr
Whole body (retrospective)	10-15 rem in any 1 yr
Whole body (accumulative to age N)	N in rem
Pregnant radiation worker	0.5 rem in gestation period (< 0.05/mon)
Skin, extremities	50 rem/yr
Lens, head	15 rem/yr
Life-saving emergency	50 rem
NONRADIATION WORKERS	
Whole body	0.1 rem/yr
Whole body, infrequent exposure	0.5 rem/yr
Embryo	0.5 rem/pregnancy

*The dose limits (especially from radioactive materials) are now specified by the NCRP and the ICRP in terms of effective dose (E), which is the weighted sum of the doses to about 10 "critical" organs and not strictly for a "whole body" dose.
NOTE: Old NCRP reports (Report 91, 1987) have numbers that differ from the above, taken from NRCP report 116, 1993. ALARA principle: as low as reasonably acceptable.

Environmental Radiation

MEAN RADIATION EXPOSURE IN UNITED STATES	
Source	Annual Dose (mrem)
Radon (whole body effective)	200
Other natural radiation*	100
Medical procedures	50

*People in high radiation areas (e.g., Denver) have not been shown to have increased risk of cancer development.

RADON

Radon (Rn) is a radioactive decay product of uranium that has been implicated as a common cause of lung cancer (inhaled alpha-emitting daughter products). Rn is a gas that accumulates in nonventilated basements. It is currently estimated to be the largest contributor to radiation in the United States (200 mrem/yr compared to 100 mrem from all other sources). According to EPA standards, the proportion of lung cancers caused by radon is 10%.

RISK OF DEATH FROM ENVIRONMENTAL SOURCES

EQUIVALENT DEATH RISKS (1:10⁶)		
Amount	**Activity**	**Cause of Death**
1.2 mrem	CXR	Cancer
3 days	Live in United States	Homicide
1 day	Live in Boston	Air pollution
1	Cigarette	Cancer
0.5 L	Wine	Cirrhosis
10 spoons	Peanut butter	Liver cancer (aflatoxin)
1 gallon	Miami drinking water	Chloroform
6 min	Canoeing	Drowning
50 miles	Automobile	Accident
5 miles	Motorcycle	Accident
1 week	Visit to Denver	Cosmic rays

Ultrasound Physics

Characteristics of Sound

Unlike x-rays, sound waves are preserved waves (not electromagnetic radiation) that require a medium for transmission (sound waves cannot propagate in a vacuum). Ultrasound (US) waves propagate similarly to other sound waves: an initial US wave hits a molecule, which itself travels for a short distance (μm) and then hits another molecule. Individual molecules move only a few μm, whereas a resulting reflected wave travels for a long distance. Clinical US uses frequencies of 1-20 MHz (1 hertz = 1 cycle per second; 1 MHz = 1 million cycles per second). By timing the period elapsed between emission of the sound and reception of the echo, the distance (D) between the transducer and the echo-producing structure can be calculated:

$$D = \text{Velocity (1540 m/sec)} \times \text{Time}$$

VELOCITY OF SOUND

US velocity depends on the physical characteristics of the material the sound wave is traveling through. Most human tissues (except bone) behave like liquids and transmit sound at ~ 1540 m/sec. The denser the tissue, the faster the sound wave (more molecules to transmit the wave per unit volume). Sound velocity is determined only by compressibility and/or density of material (not viscosity). Density (g/cm³) and compressibility are inversely proportional.

14

VELOCITY OF SOUND WAVES			
Medium	Velocity (m/sec)	Acoustic Impedance (Rayls)	Absorption Coefficient (dB/MHz/cm)
Air	331	0.0004	12
Fat	1450	1.38	0.63
Soft tissue	1540	1.6	0.94*
Bone	4080	7.8	20

*Rule of thumb: ≈ 1 dB/MHz/cm.

When the velocity of the US beam increases (e.g., transition from fat to muscle), the wavelength decreases.

ATTENUATION

Sound attenuation refers to loss of sound waves from reflection, scattering, and absorption. Absorption depends mainly on:
- Frequency (therefore the absorption coefficient is expressed in dB/MHz/cm)
- Viscosity of medium
- Acoustic relaxation time of the medium

FREQUENCY

Refers to the cycles per second with which sound is generated. The higher the frequency, the "shriller" the sound.

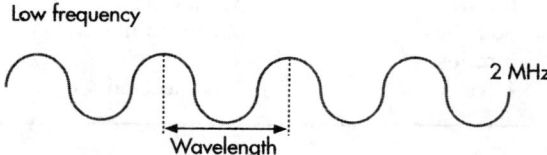

$$\text{Velocity of sound} = \text{Frequency (Hz)} \times \text{Wavelength (m)}$$

The frequency of sound is determined by the source. For example, in a piano each string has a certain frequency. In US each transducer has its own frequency (e.g., 2, 3, 5, 7.5 MHz). The only way to change US frequencies is to change the transducer.

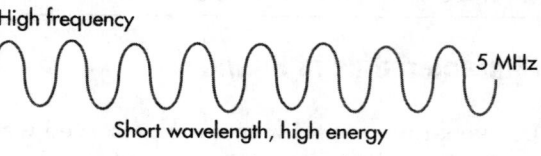

As sound waves pass from one medium to another, their frequency remains constant but their wavelength changes to accommodate the new velocity in the 2nd medium.

WAVELENGTH

The distance sound travels during one vibration is known as the wavelength. The wavelength (in meters) is measured from the top of one wave to the next.

ACOUSTIC IMPEDANCE (Z)

Acoustic impedance of a tissue is the product of its density and the velocity of sound in that tissue. Since the velocity of sound in tissue is fairly constant over a wide range of frequencies, a tissue's acoustic impedance is proportional to tissue density:

$$Z \text{ (Rayls)} = \text{Density (g/cm}^3) \times \text{Velocity (cm/sec)}$$

INTENSITY

Refers to "loudness" of US beam. Loudness is determined by length of oscillation of the particles conducting the waves: the greater the amplitude of oscillation, the more intense the sound. Absolute intensity is measured in watts (W)/cm^2.

DECIBELS

Relative sound intensity is measured in decibels (dB). Positive dB indicates a gain in power; negative dB indicates a loss in power. One dB is 0.1 ("deci") of one Bell. The definition of dB is:

$$dB = 10 \log (\text{Intensity}_{out}/\text{Intensity}_{in})$$

dB	DECIBEL	
	Original Intensity	Attenuated Intensity
0	1	1
−10	10	0.1
−20	100	0.01
−30	1000	0.001

Example
If a US beam has an original intensity of 10 W/cm^2 and the returning echo is 0.001 W/cm^2, what is the relative intensity?
Answer
Log 0.001/10 = log 0.0001 = −4B = −40 dB.
Example
A 5-MHz beam passes through 6 cm of soft tissue (1 dB/MHz/cm). How much is the original intensity decreased?
Answer
(1 dB/cm/MHz) × (5 MHz) × (6 cm) = 30 dB. 30 dB = log I_{out}/I_{in} and therefore 3 B = log I_{out}/I_{in}. The original intensity is therefore reduced by a factor of 1000.
Pearls
- The wavelength of clinical US waves is 1.5–0.08 mm
- High-frequency transducers have better resolution
- High-frequency transducers have lower penetration power

Characteristics of US Beam

Waves traveling in the same direction form a wavefront. The distance at which waves become synchronous depends on their wavelength and marks the so-called point X'. The beam zone proximal to that point is called the Fresnel zone (beam is coherent). The beam zone beyond X' is called the Fraunhofer zone (beam is divergent).

14

Angle of divergence (dispersion)

$$\text{Sin } \alpha = 1.22 \times \frac{\text{Wavelength}}{\text{Transducer diameter}}$$

Therefore lateral resolution is decreased with a small-diameter transducer.

Fresnel zone

The length of the Fresnel zone is determined by:

$$\text{Length of Fresnel zone (cm)} = \frac{\text{Transducer radius}^2 \text{ (cm}^2\text{)}}{\text{Wavelength (cm)}}$$

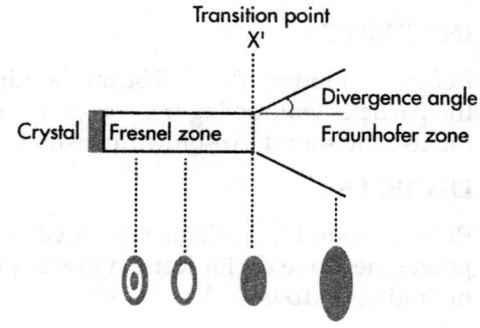

The Fresnel zone increases with:
- Increasing diameter of the transducer
- Increasing frequency

REFLECTION

The percentage of beam reflected at a tissue surface depends on:
- Acoustic impedance of tissue
- Angle of incidence into tissue

Reflection (R) can be calculated as:

$$R = [(Z2 - Z1)/(Z2 + Z1)]^2 \times 100$$

where R is percent of reflected beam, Z1 is acoustic impedance of medium 1, and Z2 is acoustic impedance of medium 2.

Pearls
- Percentage of reflection at tissue/tissue interfaces:
    Air/lung: 99.9%
    Water/kidney: 0.64%
    Skull/brain: 44%
    Muscle/bone: 80%
- Transmission (%) + reflection (%) = 100%
- The higher the angle of incidence the lower the amount of reflection

REFRACTION

The angle of refraction at media interfaces can be calculated by:

$$\frac{\sin \partial i}{\sin \partial t} = \frac{V1}{V2}$$

where ∂i is the incident, ∂t is the transmitted angle, and V1 and V2 are the velocities of sound in the 2 media. In other words, the angle of reflection depends only on the sound velocities in the 2 media. As sound propagates through the parenchyma of an organ that contains microscopic fluctuations in acoustic impedance, small quantities of US are scattered in all directions, an effect that is responsible for the pixely gray-scale appearance of an organ.

ABSORPTION

Absorption refers to the energy of an US beam that is converted into heat. Absorption is a result of friction between particles in the medium. The relationship between frequency and absorption is linear: doubling the frequency doubles the absorption.

Components

TRANSDUCER

The components of a transducer include:
- Piezoelectric crystal
- Backing block
- Quarter wave matching layer

Piezoelectric crystal

The crystal consists of many dipoles arranged in a parallel geometric pattern (approximately 0.5 mm thick). Plating electrodes on either side of the crystal produce an electric field, which changes the orientation of the crystals. When an alternating voltage (rapid change in polarity; e.g., 3 MHz) is applied, the crystals vibrate like a cymbal. Piezoelectric crystals are manufactured by heating a ceramic (such as lead-zirconium-titanate [PZT]) in a strong electric field. As the temperature of the crystal increases, the dipoles are free to move and align themselves in the magnetic field generated by the applied electricity. The crystal is then cooled in the magnetic field so that the dipoles stay aligned in their new parallel orientation. The temperature at which this polarization is lost is called the Curie temperature. Crystals lose their piezoelectric properties above the Curie temperature.

PIEZOELECTRIC MATERIALS		
Materials	Curie Temperature (°C)	Q Factor
Quartz	573	> 25,000
Barium titanate	100	
Lead zirconium titanate (PZT)-4	328	> 500
PZT-5	365	75

Resonance frequency

The resonance frequency of a piezoelectric crystal is determined by the thickness of the crystal. Like a pipe in a church organ—the larger the pipe, the lower the pitch of sound—the thinner the crystal, the higher its frequency.

Crystal thickness = ½ the wavelength of US

Transducer Q factor

The Q factor reflects:
- Purity of sound
- Length of time that the sound persists (ring-down time = time for complete stop of vibration)

High-Q crystals are good transmitters, low-Q crystals are good receivers (receiver to a broad spectrum of reflected frequencies).

Backing block

The backing block is special material at the back of the transducer that quenches the vibration and shortens the sonic pulse. Backing blocks are made of a combination of tungsten, rubber powder, and epoxy.

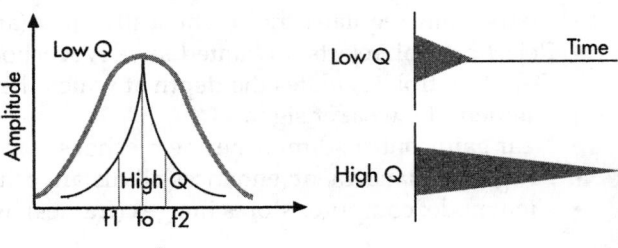

14

Quarter wave matching layer

Layer of material located in front of the transducer used to transmit the sonic energy more efficiently to the patient. The thickness of this layer must be equal to ¼ (hence "quarter wave") the wavelength. Layers consist of aluminum in epoxy resin.

US EQUIPMENT TYPES

A (amplitude) mode

Probe has a single transducer that pulses and displays echo depth and amplitude as a line on an oscilloscope screen. No longer used in medical imaging.

TM (time motion) mode

Spikes from the A mode are converted into dots and displayed on a moving strip. The amplitude of returning pulse is not displayed. Occasionally used in echocardiography to image valve motions.

B (binary) mode

Transducer attached to mechanical arm is moved across surface. A series of received echoes form the tomographic image. Gray scale assigns shades of gray to the different amplitudes of returning echos. No longer used in medical imaging.

Real-time mode

2 types of real-time scanners are commonly used today:

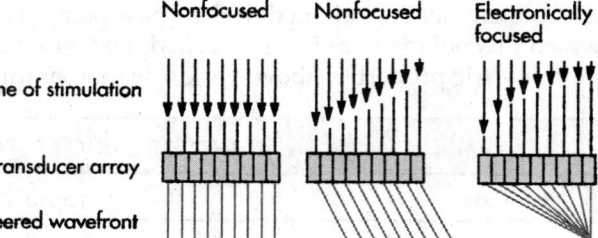

- Mechanical sector scanners: a single transducer oscillates to cover the field; alternatively, 3-4 transducers are mounted on a ball that turns in one direction
- Electronic array scanners that contain 64-200 transducers per probe
  - A steered wavefront can be created by sequential simulation of many individual transducers
  - A beam can be focused by plastic lenses and by the timing of the pulses to the transducers
  - Fresnel zone can be electronically adjusted by determining how many individual transducers are excited at once; decreasing the radius of the transducer decreases the Fresnel zone

Real-time US generates images at ~ 15 frames/sec

- A frame is composed of many vertical lines (~ 110-220 lines/frame)
- Each line corresponds to a transducer in the probe
- Relationship between spatial and temporal resolution: high spatial resolution is obtained by increasing number of lines; high temporal resolution is achieved by increasing number of frames per second

CONTROLS

Time-gain compensator (TGC) is an important control function that allows adjustment of attenuated echoes from deep structures.

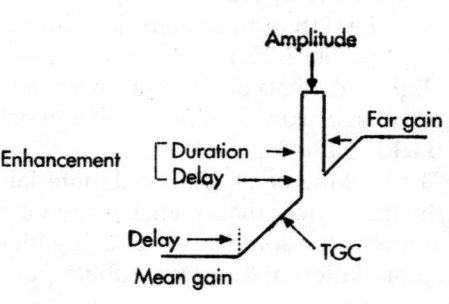

- Coarse gain: regulates the height of all echoes (amplifier)
- Reject control: rejects unwanted low-level echoes
- Delay control: regulates the depth at which the TGC begins to augment the weaker signals
- Near gain control: diminishes near echoes
- Far gain enhancement: enhances all distant echoes
- Cine mode: computer stores images (frames), which can then be displayed later

RESOLUTION

US allows measurement of distances indirectly by determining time between US waves and then converting them to distance, assuming that velocity in tissues is 1540 m/sec.

Axial resolution

Axial or depth resolution refers to the ability to separate two objects lying in tandem along the course of the beam. Two objects will be recognized as separate if the spatial pulse length (i.e., the length of each US pulse) is less than twice the distance between the objects. Therefore axial resolution can be defined as ½ the spatial pulse length.

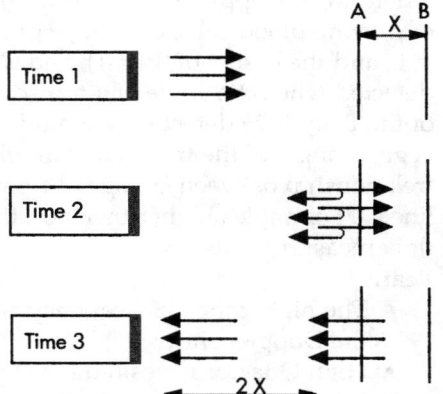

- The higher the frequency, the better the axial resolution
- Axial resolution is generally better than lateral resolution
- Axial resolution is the same at all depths
- Axial resolution is independent of the transducer diameter

Lateral resolution

To resolve two parallel objects next to each other, the US beam has to be narrower than the space separating the two objects. Narrow transducers have a short Fresnel zone, which causes poor resolution of deep structures. Lateral resolution depends on:

- Number of scan lines (the number of scan lines decreases if the frame rate increases)
- Width of US beam: the wider the beam the less lateral resolution

SCAN TIME

Scan time refers to the time required for a US pulse to be emitted and received by the transducer/receiver. The next pulse cannot be fired before the 1st one has been received. An image is made up of several scan lines, usually 110-220. The frame rate refers to the number of scan lines that can be obtained per second.

$$\text{Time of a scan line} = 2 \times \frac{\text{Imaging depth}}{1540\ \text{m} \times \text{sec}^{-1}}$$

$$\text{Time of a frame} = \text{T of a scan line} \times \text{Number of scan lines}$$
$$\text{Frame rate} = \text{Number of scan lines/sec}$$

Doppler US

The Doppler effect refers to a frequency change that occurs in a moving wave. In a stationary wave, wavelengths are equal in all directions. In a moving wave source, however, wavelengths increase and decrease depending on the direction of movement. The Doppler shift refers to the frequency of the initial signal, which is subtracted from that of the returning echo. According to the following equation, blood flow can thus be measured:

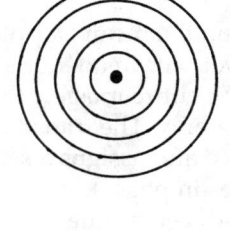
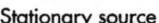
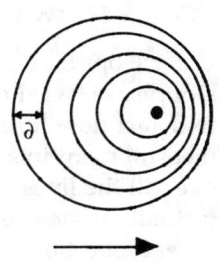

Stationary source   Moving source

$$\Delta f = 2\, f_{o}\, v \cos \varnothing / C$$

14

where Δf = Doppler shift, f_o = original frequency transmitted in MHz, v = velocity of moving blood cells, ø = angle of transducer to the moving blood cells (cosine of 90° = 0, and the cosine of 0° = 1), and C = speed of sound in soft tissues. Flow cannot be detected when the angle of a transducer is at 90° relative to the blood vessel. The optimal angle to detect flow would be close to zero degrees relative to moving blood. A good angle of the transducer in relation to the vessel for imaging is 1°-60° (relationship between change of frequency and change in velocity of the blood cells is linear). For angles higher than 60°, the relationship is exponential, causing errors in flow measurements.

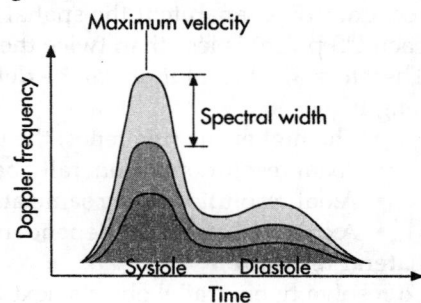

Pearls
- The higher the US frequency and the lower the angle, the larger the Doppler shift
- High Q factor is desired for Doppler US
- Long pulse length is required to increase the Q factor

Spectral broadening
Spectral broadening refers to widening of the spectral width, a parameter of flow disturbance. The larger the spectral broadening, the more flow disturbance.

CONTINUOUS WAVE DOPPLER

Continuous wave Doppler uses two separate transmitting and receiving transducers within the same transducer, both operating continuously (hence "continuous wave"). The frequency of the initial signal is subtracted from that of returning echoes. The difference is referred to as the Doppler shift and usually falls within the audible frequency range. Continuous wave Doppler is thus used mainly to measure stenosis of vessels.

PULSED DOPPLER

Pulsed Doppler allows measurement of the depth at which a returning signal has originated. This is achieved by emitting a pulse of a sound rather than a continuous sound (hence "pulsed Doppler"). Only echoes received at a precise time (and therefore from a specific depth) are thus sampled. Pulsed Doppler is a more sensitive means to determine flow than color Doppler. The duplex Doppler combines pulsed Doppler and B mode real-time imaging for obtaining real-time images. There are separate transducers within a probe, both of which usually operate at different frequencies (carotids: 7 MHz for the imaging, 5 MHz for the Doppler; abdomen: 5 MHz for the imaging, 3 MHz for the Doppler).

COLOR FLOW DOPPLER

Color Doppler US is based on the mean Doppler frequency shift, whereas pulsed Doppler is based on peak Doppler frequency shift. Color Doppler imaging allows one to detect flow throughout the entire image, whereas pulsed Doppler allows measurement in a small area only. The transducer measures the change of frequency over all the lines in the image and assigns a set color to specific frequency ranges (actually it measures changes in phase):
- Blood flowing to transducer = blue
- Blood flowing away from transducer = red
- Velocity determinations (e.g., color assignments) are angle dependent

Color Doppler imaging has several shortcomings, including a tendency for noise, angle dependence, and aliasing. Power Doppler US has been developed to overcome these shortcomings. Power Doppler US is a color Doppler US method in which the color map displays the integrated power of the Doppler signal rather than the mean Doppler frequency shift.

Pearls

- As multiple samples are required to measure velocity in the large field of view, the frame is usually reduced; this explains why the temporal resolution of color Doppler is not as good as pulsed Doppler.
- Since the sampling rate is slow, there is an increased potential for aliasing when compared to pulsed Doppler. To cut back on this, one can limit color sampling to a defined region.
- Aliasing and turbulent flow on color US is usually encoded by different color.

Artifacts

REVERBERATION ARTIFACT

Returning echoes are partially reflected at an internal boundary. This produces misregistration and assigns structures to places they do not exist (e.g., a bright line is seen in the bladder).

MIRROR IMAGE ARTIFACT (SPECULAR REFLECTION)

Because of reflection of US waves at acoustic mirrors (e.g., diaphragm), lesions can be projected into locations in which they are not really present. Typical example is that of a liver lesion near the diaphragm that can be projected into the lung because the liver-lung boundary acts as an acoustic mirror.

RING-DOWN ARTIFACT

Occurs when the US beam strikes a structure that is capable of ringing (e.g., metal, cholesterol crystals in GB wall).

SHADOWING AND ENHANCEMENT

Shadowing refers to absent through-transmission through a lesion (e.g., containing calcium). Enhancement: refers to better through-transmission (e.g., through a fluid-filled structure such as a cyst).

NONSPECULAR REFLECTIONS

Nonspecular reflections occur at objects that are smaller than the wavelength of the US beam. These reflections generally give a weak signal since only a small portion of the beam is reflected back toward the transducer. Particulate US contrast agents exploit this principle.

ALIASING

Aliasing refers to an artifact that may be introduced when converting analog to digital signal. If the digital sampling is not done frequently enough (too few scan lines), the digital signal may not contain enough information to reproduce the analog signal. In general, one should use twice as many scan lines as expected for resolving described objects without aliasing. Diagram:

14

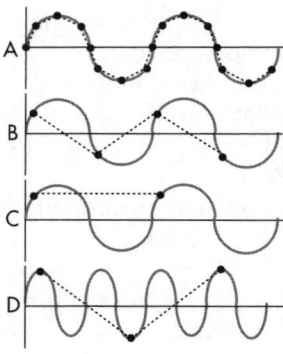

- A: digital sampling frequency (black dots) is much greater than analog frequency (sine wave) → no information is lost
- B: digital sampling taken at twice the frequency of the analog signal. This is the minimal sampling rate to preserve all the information, called the Nyquist frequency. To resolve a structure of dimension d, the Nyquist frequency (f_N) must be

$$f_N = 2/d$$

- C: all analog information is lost
- D: The digital signal has a lower frequency than the analog one. Thus information not present in the original (analog) signal is produced in the digital signal. This is aliasing.

OTHER ARTIFACTS

- Duplication artifact
- Off-axis artifact
- Section thickness artifact
- Refraction artifact

MRI Physics

General

When materials are placed in a magnetic field they can absorb and then reemit electromagnetic radiation of a specific frequency (usually in the form of radio signals). The signal intensity of a given pixel is determined by:

- Proton (i.e., hydrogen) density (N[H])
- Longitudinal relaxation rate (R_1)
- Transverse relaxation rate (R_2)
- Flow
- Other parameters
  Diffusion
  Magnetization
    exchange rate
  Magnetic
    susceptibility

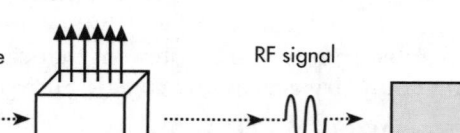

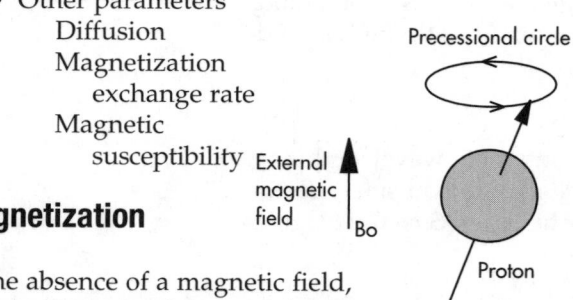

Magnetization

In the absence of a magnetic field, nuclei are randomly oriented and produce no net magnetic effect. When tissue is placed in a magnetic field, some nuclei align with the field, and their combined effect is usually referred to as a magnetization vector (referred to as M_0 when in resting state or as M_z when deflected by radiofrequency).

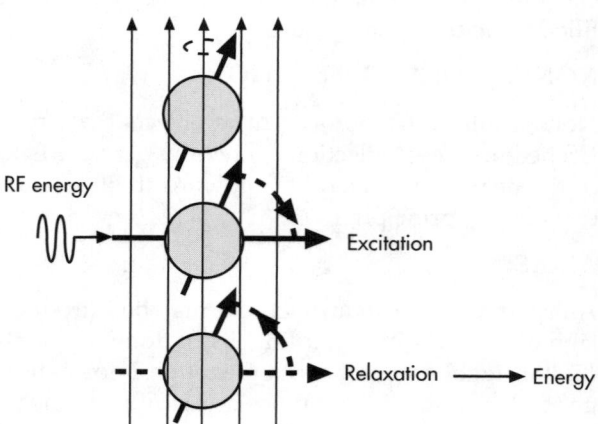

There are 2 basic directions of tissue magnetization:
- Longitudinal (spin-lattice relaxation) (T1)
- Transverse (spin-spin relaxation) (T2)

Spin-lattice relaxation is a process responsible for the dissipation of energy from radiofrequency-excited protons into their molecular environment or "lattice." T1 relaxation time is a measure of the time required for M_z to return to 63% of its equilibrium magnetization (M_0).

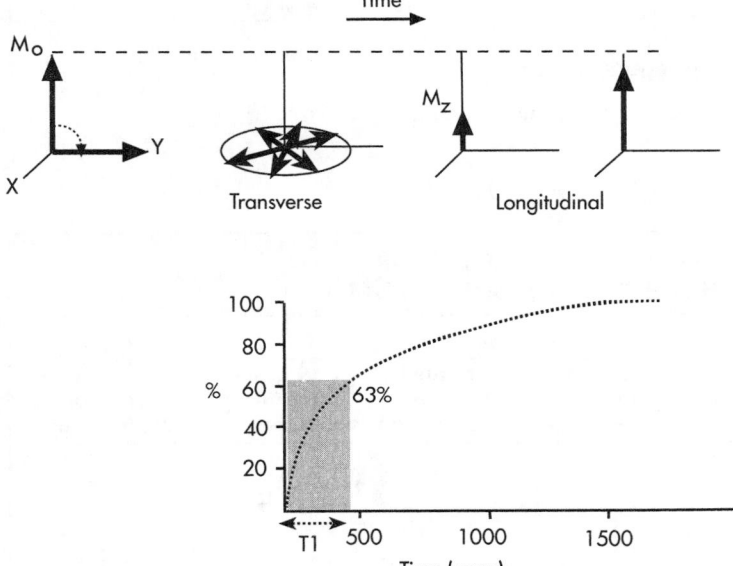

Spin-spin relaxation is a process that progressively reduces order after an excitation pulse. Individual components of magnetization lose their alignment and rotate at various rates in the transverse plane. T2 relaxation time is a measure of the time required for 63% of the initial magnetization to dissipate. T2 is usually much shorter than T1.

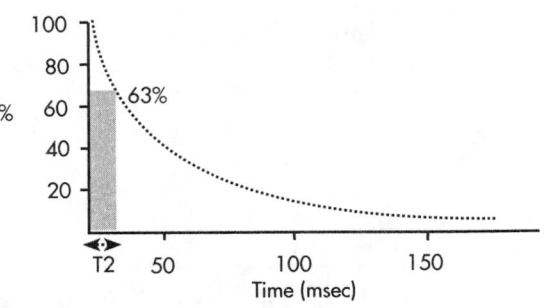

APPROXIMATE T1 AND T2 VALUES FOR HUMAN TISSUES			
Tissue	T1 at 1.5 T (msec)	T1 at 0.5 T (msec)	T2 (msec)
Skeletal muscle	870	600	47
Liver	490	323	43
Kidney	650	449	58
Spleen	780	554	62
Fat	260	215	84
Gray matter	920	656	101
White matter	790	539	92
Cerebrospinal fluid	> 4,000	> 4,000	> 2,000
Lung	830	600	79

14

Spin-Echo Imaging

Sequence composed of a series of selective 90° and 180° pulses that generate a spin echo at a specified echo time (TE) after the initial 90° pulse. The sequence is repeated at a specified repetition interval (TR). Transverse magnetization is measured in the presence of a read-out gradient (Gx) during which many samples are taken.

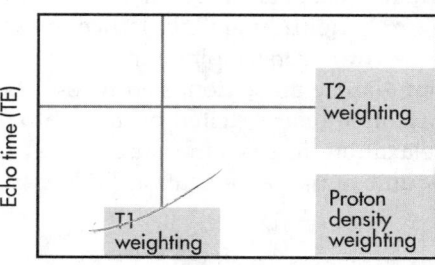

$$Sl_{se} = kN_{(H)}e^{-TE/T2}[1-2e^{-(TR-TE)/2/T1}+e^{-TR/T1}]$$

The time (T) required for the acquisition of a pulse sequence is:

$$T = TR \times \text{number of phase encoding steps } (N_{phase}) \times \text{number of signal averages (NSA)}$$

Signal-to-Noise Ratio (SNR)

			Spatial Resolution			
Goal	Imaging Parameters	SNR Change*	Section-Encoding Direction	Frequency-Encoding Direction	Phase-Encoding Direction	Time of Acquisition
Higher SNR	NSA × 2	× 1.41	—	—	—	× 2
Higher SNR	BW/2	× 1.41	—	—	—	—
Higher resolution	FOV_{phase}/2	× 0.25	—	× 2	× 2	—
Higher resolution	N_{freq} × 2	× 0.71	—	× 2	—	—
Higher resolution	N_{phase} × 2	× 0.71	—	—	× 2	× 2

EFFECTS OF IMAGING PARAMETERS ON SNR, SPATIAL RESOLUTION, AND ACQUISITION TIME

BW, Bandwith in frequency-encoding direction; *FOV_{freq}*, field of view in frequency-encoding direction; *FOV_{phase}*, field of view in phase-encoding direction; *N_{freq}*, number of pixels across FOV_{freq} (without interpolation); *N_{phase}*, number of phase-encoding steps; *NSA*, number of signals averaged; *SL*, section thickness.
*0.71 = $1/\sqrt{2}$, 1.41 = $\sqrt{2}$.

Imaging Parameters

EFFECT OF IMAGING PARAMETERS ON SNR AND WEIGHTING

Parameter	Parameter Increased	Parameter Decreased
Slice thickness	Increases SNR	Decreases SNR
	Increases image detail	Decreases image detail
TR	Increases SNR	Decreases SNR
	Longer imaging time	Shorter imaging time
	More sections	Fewer sections
	Less T1W	More T1W
TE	Decreases SNR	Increases SNR
	More T2W	Less T2W
NSA	Increases SNR	Decreases SNR
	Longer imaging time	Shorter imaging time
Matrix size	Decreases SNR	Increases SNR
	Longer imaging time	Shorter imaging time
	Better resolution	Worse resolution

Statistics

Testing

MEASUREMENTS

MEASUREMENT SCALES			
Type	Example	Appropriate Statistics	Information Content
Nominal	Sex, blood type	Counts, rates, proportions, relative risk, chi-square	Low
Ordinal	Degree of pain	In addition to the above: median, rank correlation	Intermediate
Continuous	Weight, length	In addition to the above: mean, standard deviation, t-test, analysis of variance	High

STATISTICAL TESTING

STATISTICAL METHODS TO TEST HYPOTHESES					
Type of Data	2 Groups, Different Individuals	≥ 3 Groups, Different Individuals	Single Treatment, Same Individual	Multiple Treatments, Same Individual	Association Between 2 Variables
Continuous (normally distributed population)	Unpaired t-test	Analysis of variance	Paired t-test	Repeated measures analysis of variance	Linear regression and Pearson product-moment correlation
Nominal	Chi-square analysis or contingency table	Chi-square analysis or contingency table	McNemar's test	Cochran Q	Contingency coefficent
Ordinal	Mann-Whitney rank-sum test	Kruskal-Wallis statistic	Wilcoxon signed rank test	Friedman statistic	Spearman rank correlation

Accuracy, Precision

The accuracy of a variable is the degree to which it represents what it is supposed to represent. Precision is the degree to which a variable can be repeated. The 2 measures are thus different and not necessarily linked.

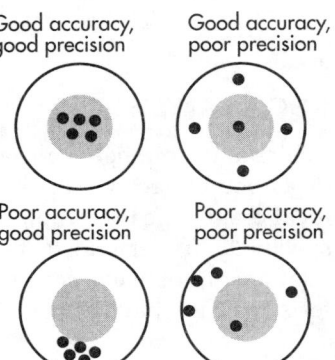

Good accuracy, good precision
Good accuracy, poor precision
Poor accuracy, good precision
Poor accuracy, poor precision

PRECISION AND ACCURACY		
	Accuracy	**Precision**
Definition	The degree to which a variable actually represents what it is supposed to represent	The degree to which a variable has nearly the same value when measured several times
Best way to assess	Comparison with a reference standard	Comparison among repeated measures
Threatened by	Systematic error (bias)	Random error (variance)

SENSITIVITY

Number of patients with disease that have been correctly detected (true positive [TP]) divided by all patients with disease (TP + FN where FN = false negative):

$$\text{Sensitivity} = \frac{TP}{TP + FN}$$

Test result

		Positive	Negative	
Truth	Positive	TP	FN error type 2	Sensitivity
	Negative	FP error type 1	TN	Specificity

PPV   NPV

SPECIFICITY

Number of patients with no disease that have not been detected (true negative [TN]) divided by all patients without disease (TN + FP where FP = false positive):

$$\text{Specificity:} \frac{TN}{TN + FP}$$

PREDICTIVE VALUES

The value of a diagnostic test depends not only on its sensitivity and specificity but also on the prevalence of the disease in the population being tested.

Positive predictive value (PPV)

This is the probability that a person with a positive test result actually has the disease.

$$PPV = \frac{TP}{TP + FP}$$

Negative predictive value (NPV)

This is the probability that a person with a negative test result does not have the disease.

$$NPV = \frac{TN}{TN + FN}$$

ROC ANALYSIS

The relationship between sensitivity and specificity is usually described by receiver operating characteristics (ROC) curves. An ideal diagnostic test would have 100% sensitivity and 100% specificity. If a diagnostic test has no predictive value, the relationship between sensitivity and specificity is linear. Diagnostic tests typically have a curve shape in between.

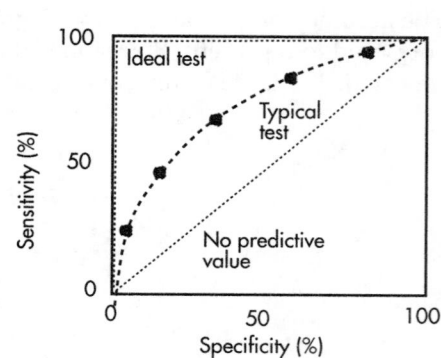

SUGGESTED READINGS

Chandra R: *Introductory physics of nuclear medicine*, Philadelphia, 1992, Lippincott Williams & Wilkins.

Curry TS, Dowdey J, Murry RC: *Christensen's introduction to the physics of diagnostic radiology*, Philadelphia, 1990, Lippincott Williams & Wilkins.

Edelman RR, Hesselink JR, Zlatkin MB: *Clinical magnetic resonance imaging*, Philadelphia, 1996, WB Saunders.

Sorenson JA et al: *Physics in nuclear medicine*, Philadelphia, 1986, WB Saunders.

Sprawls P: *Physical principles of medical imaging*, Rockville, Md, 1993, Aspen Publishers.

14

Index